Injuries and Health Problems in Football

Editor-in-Chief
João Espregueira-Mendes

Editors
C. Niek van Dijk • Philippe Neyret
Moises Cohen • Stefano Della Villa
Helder Pereira • J. Miguel Oliveira

Injuries and Health Problems in Football

What Everyone Should Know

Springer

Editor-in-Chief
João Espregueira-Mendes
Clínica do Dragão, Espregueira-Mendes
Sports Centre - FIFA Medical Centre of
Excellence
Porto
Portugal

Dom Henrique Research Centre
Porto
Portugal

3B's Research Group–Biomaterials,
Biodegradables and Biomimetics,
University of Minho, Headquarters of the
European Institute of Excellence on
Tissue Engineering and Regenerative
Medicine, AvePark, Parque de Ciência
e Tecnologia, Zona Industrial da Gandra
Barco, Guimarães
Portugal

ICVS/3B's–PT Government Associate
Laboratory
Braga/Guimarães
Portugal

Orthopaedics Department of Minho
University
Minho
Portugal

Editors
C. Niek van Dijk
Department of Orthopaedic Surgery
Academic Medical Centre
Amsterdam Zuidoost
Noord-Holland
The Netherlands

Philippe Neyret
Hopital de la Croix-Rousse
University of Lyon 1 Hopital de la
Croix-Rousse
Lyon
France

Moises Cohen
Department of Orthopedics & Traumatology
Federal University of São Paulo
Vila Clementino - São Paulo
Brazil

Stefano Della Villa
Isokinetic Medical Group
FIFA Medical Centre of Excellence
Bologna
Italy

Helder Pereira
3B's Research Group–Biomaterials,
Biodegradables and Biomimetics,
University of Minho, Headquarters of the
European Institute of Excellence on Tissue
Engineering and Regenerative Medicine,
AvePark, Parque de Ciência e Tecnologia,
Zona Industrial da Gandra
Barco, Guimarães
Portugal

ICVS/3B's–PT Government Associate
Laboratory
Braga/Guimarães
Portugal

J. Miguel Oliveira
3B's Research Group–Biomaterials,
Biodegradables and Biomimetics,
University of Minho, Headquarters of the
European Institute of Excellence on Tissue
Engineering and Regenerative Medicine,
AvePark, Parque de Ciência e Tecnologia,
Zona Industrial da Gandra
Barco, Guimarães
Portugal

ICVS/3B's–PT Government Associate
Laboratory
Braga/Guimarães
Portugal

ISBN 978-3-662-53923-1 ISBN 978-3-662-53924-8 (eBook)
DOI 10.1007/978-3-662-53924-8

Library of Congress Control Number: 2017938163

Printed on acid-free paper

This Springer imprint is published by Springer Nature
The registered company is Springer-Verlag GmbH Germany
The registered company address is: Heidelberger Platz 3, 14197 Berlin, Germany

Foreword

Not so long ago, the medical world was not interested in the world of sport, although there were some exceptions, like the well-known Galenus, who was also, besides his other duties, the doctor of the Roman gladiators.

Sport medicine, related to football, was limited to one single question: "Can he play next Sunday?"

Indeed, the relation between medicine and sport only concerned the treatment of lesions.

Times changed: progressively, sports medicine received more attention, essentially due to the worldwide development of sport itself, becoming one of the most important social surroundings for young people.

This resulted in general principles, valuable for the global world of sport.

There was, however, no differentiation: the medical approach concerned, without specification, all sports disciplines.

Later, times changed again: the specificity of each sport discipline resulted in sports-medical challenges, completely different from one discipline to another.

Even in the same discipline, differences became evident and led to important medical repercussions.

One of the most important specific approaches concerned football medicine: indeed, football, today, is played in every country of the world, and brings together, under the worldwide umbrella of FIFA, some 300 million football players.

This gives us, football doctors, an important place in the contemporary society. It also gives us, however, an important responsibility.

That is why I enthusiastically support the edition of this ISAKOS – book about injuries and health problems in football.

This book is, naturally, essentially focused on locomotoric problems, but it also concerns other aspects of football medicine, essentially cardiologic, nutritional and respiratory aspects.

It follows the different steps in the medical guidance of football medicine, from prevention to diagnosis, conservative and surgical therapy, rehabilitation and, finally, "return to play".

This is not the end of the story. Like so many other aspects in our human society, the medicine of football will be influenced, and directed tomorrow, by the "BINC" revolution: **B**iophysiology, **B**iotechnology, **I**nformatics and artificial **I**ntelligence, **N**anotechnology and **C**ognitive sciences.

The techniques of diagnosis and therapy will change. What must remain is our constant care for the health and the physical condition of the young football players.

Football doctors must never forget
that football is a game before being a product,
that football is a sport before being a market,
that football is a spectacle before being a business.

Baron Dr Michel D'Hooghe
Chairman of the Medical Commission of FIFA and UEFA

Preface

Medical education is a noble mission, where basic sciences together with medical skills, innovations, and applied technology compete to improve the quality of life and performance of sports practitioners.

Football is the world's number one sport, played by 300 million men and women, including referees and officials. It is interesting that 69.6% of registered female and 54.7% of registered male players are young, which shows that FIFA and its member associations are on track toward enhancing the popularity of this sport further in the future.

This new publication on football medicine is dedicated to all those who love football and presents insights into the most frequent problems in the sport and some of the hot topics in a friendly, clear, and practical way. In **injuries and health problems in football – what everyone should know**, we sought to provide an update on the state of the art. To achieve this goal, we gathered valuable contributions from some of renowned experts in the field, selected from FIFA, UEFA, ISAKOS, and ESSKA.

We used our experience to put together a team that could contribute to the leverage of education in this field, providing knowledge of high-performance skills, offering guidance on the current rules for best practice, and ensuring high standards in football medicine with regard to prevention, diagnosis, conservative and surgical treatment, complications, time and criteria for return to sports, and prognosis. We are now entering the era of biologics, tissue engineering, and a molecular understanding of healing, and starting to leave the gray area of experimental therapies behind in favor of evidence-based treatments.

In the subsequent pages of this book, the reader will become acquainted with a generous amount of cognitive knowledge, conveying a comprehensive resource for understanding the most frequent problems in football medicine. Talented and passionate authors in sports medicine bring science to you. We hope you will join us on this priceless mission.

"I hear and I forget. I see and I remember. I do and I understand" Confucius, 551–479 BC.

Thank you so much to all the contributors. It is an honor, a privilege, and a great pleasure to share with you this exciting challenge.

João Espregueira-Mendes

Contents

Part I

The Athlete in the Field

1 The Relevance of Medicine in Football

José Ferraz, José Pereira, Jacques Menetrey, and Paulo Lobo

The management of the athlete's health requires a close cooperation between coaches and medical staff. A large part of professional football trainers, who run the big teams, are in agreement and demand the presence of medical experts in their teams.

After so many deaths in sport, but mainly in football, technical offices were set up to discuss standard procedures and measures to prevent sudden death in sport, but little has been published to date on the subject. The medical advice and recommendations for deciding whether or not an athlete should continue its sport activity, at its most basic level, comprise physical exams, electrocardiograms, and other tests.

There are very frequent muscle injuries after certain types of physical efforts, without being able to say that there is a physical therapy with demonstrated validity. The best treatment will always rely in prevention. Adequate progression in training will enable to achieve specific exercises (e.g. the eccentric exercises) that might bring long standing benefits. However, any type of therapy still lack scientific high-level evidence.

Medication might play a role, including anti-inflammatory drugs for pain management. However, its use is not fully clarified or established. The drugs need to be prescribed in a suitable dose for the beneficial effects to be maximized, and the adverse and toxic effects minimized. It should be prescribed individually and in a correct dose to ensure the best risk/benefit ratio for this to have rapid and positive effects; the presence of health experts is necessary, with the technical team.

It is regrettable, from the legal point of view, that there is still no worldwide obligation for athlete's clinical assessment prior to regular competition. Medical screening for all athletes is mandatory.

J. Ferraz (✉)
Revista Treino Científico,
Rua Humberto Cruz, 412, 2º esqº,
4450-694 Leça Da Palmeira, Porto, Portugal
e-mail: jose.ferraz60@netcabo.pt

J. Pereira
Associação Nacional Treinadores de Futebol e Futsal (National Association of Football Coaches),
Associação Nacional dos Treinadores de Futebol
Largo dos Arcos da Ribeira, nº 114,
4050-062 Porto, Portugal
e-mail: josepereira@antf.pt

J. Menetrey
Centre de médecine du sport et de l'exercice,
Hirslanden Clinique La Colline, University Hospital of Geneva, Geneva, Switzerland

Faculty of Medicine, University of Geneva,
Geneva, Switzerland
e-mail: Jacques.Menetrey@hcuge.ch

P. Lobo
Orthopedic and Medical Specialized Hospital – FIFA Medical Centre of Excellence, Brasília, Brasil
e-mail: paulolobojr@gmail.com

J. Espregueira-Mendes et al. (eds.), *Injuries and Health Problems in Football*,
DOI 10.1007/978-3-662-53924-8_1

The importance of the integrated work of the technical committee with the medical department should be done every day. Emotional self-control, the importance of the psychological side, the physiotherapist, the sociologist, the traumatologist, etc. are areas of activity that require from the experts attention and follow-up, next to the technical team and the nearest possible to the athlete. The main objective is to assure the fastest return of the athlete to sports activity after an injury. Physiotherapeutic guidance covers the preparation and athlete's training, prevention and treatment of injuries, and early return to activity. The professional ceased to operate only in the rehabilitation, leaving the office and acting directly on the edge of the field, in order to detect possible muscle imbalances present and biomechanical performance, with full-time professional. Attention is focused on the integration with the professional coaching staff, making everyone work towards the same objective, which is to make the athlete always prepared and ready to perform their work at the highest level possible.

In summary, we must consider that the integration of the doctor in the team must be on a daily basis.

Epidemiology: The Most Frequent Lesions

2

Henrique Jones, Pedro Cantista, and Matteo Denti

Contents

H. Jones (✉)
Montijo Orthopaedic and Sports Medicine Clinic, Montijo, Portugal
e-mail: ortojones@gmail.com

P. Cantista
Hospital de Santo António, ICBAS – Universidade do Porto, Porto, Portugal
e-mail: pedro.cantista@gmail.com

M. Denti
Galeazzi Orthopaedic Institute IRCCS, Milan, Italy
e-mail: matteo@denti.ch.it

2.1 Introduction

Injury was defined as any physical damage that occurred during football activities (scheduled matches or training sessions) and resulted in the player being unable to participate fully in future training sessions or matches.

A player was considered injured until the team doctor allowed full participation in team training and match play. Reinjury was defined as an injury in the same location and of the same type as the player had suffered previously.

2.2 Football Injury Epidemiological Studies

Epidemiological studies on football injuries have been implemented in Europe since the end of the 1970s, particularly in the northern countries, namely, on amateur or semi-professional footballers. Typical injuries for footballers were described and the possibility of reducing their incidence [1]. In the last three decades, professionalism in football has increased, and injury surveys have been performed at all levels of football: amateur, semi-professional, professional and elite. Moreover, they have also been performed at youth level and in women's football and implemented in many countries. Simultaneously prevention programmes were implemented to avoid injuries regarding

J. Espregueira-Mendes et al. (eds.), *Injuries and Health Problems in Football*,
DOI 10.1007/978-3-662-53924-8_2

muscles, tendons and ligament severe injuries. Mostly in women, the ACL injury incidence was drastically decrease with programmes like the Santa Monica PEP or FIFA 11+. In men, the incidence of groin pain or muscle injuries has also decreased with such programmes, and the exponential increase in children sports participation allows us to think in future specific children prevention programmes.

2.3 The Football Associations Contribution

Injuries are common in football, and FIFA, UEFA and national football organizations are all concerned about the safety of players.

In 2001, UEFA initiated a research project with the aim of increasing sports safety.

One of the initial goals of the research programme was to monitor the increasing load on professional football players and the correlation between this increasing load and injuries, i.e. to study the possible effects of "overmatching". The results from the first years of the study suggest that although normally the professional clubs have effective strategies to avoid overloading their players, the intense match schedule for many top players towards the end of the season might have some negative effects on these players' performance and health, namely, in the final season of the European and World Cups.

2.4 The Injury Incidence in National Teams in European Competitions

In Euro 2004 in Portugal, 45 injuries occurred (39 in matches and 6 during training); in Euro 2008 in Austria and Switzerland, 56 injuries occurred (46 in matches and 10 during training); and in Euro 2012 in Poland and Ukraine, 28 injuries occurred (19 in matches and 9 during training) (Fig. 2.1). Probably the differences in climate, stadium and training camp conditions, adequate rest and fatigue control, coaches methodology, fair play, referee intervention and effective prevention and more adequate treatments could justify this injury incidence and differences between different realities.

During Euro 2004, the thigh was the most common injury location (22%) followed by the ankle (17%), lower leg (14%) and hip/groin (14%).

Sprains (ligament injury) were the most dominant type of injury at Euro 2008 (n = 16, 29%), and nine of these injuries comprised the ankle joint and seven the knee joint. The 15 muscle strain injuries mainly occurred in the thigh (n = 6), calf (n = 4) and groin (n = 2).

In terms of risk injury Euro 2004 had a rate of 9.0/1000h of exposure; during Euro 2008, the total risk of injury was 10.0/1000 h of exposure and during Euro 2012, the total risk of injury was 6.0/1000 h of exposure (4.2/1000 h in the Portuguese team).

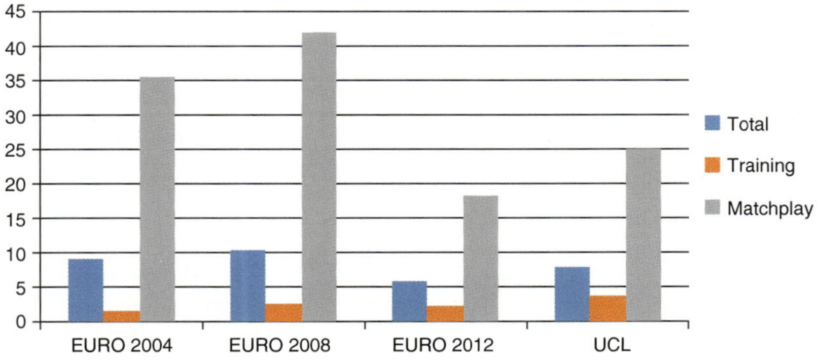

Fig. 2.1 Incidence of injuries during training sessions and matches

In Euro 2012, the injury incidence was about 16 times higher during match play (41.8 injuries/1000 match hours) than during training (2.6 injuries/1000 training hours).

2.5 Clubs Competitions: The UEFA Champions League Injury Study

The UEFA Champions League represents the highest expression of club level football in the world. Since 2001, UEFA has implemented an injury survey among Champions League clubs [2], with the aim of reducing injuries, which, at this level, have a high sporting and economic impact. Prof Jan Ekstrand, one of the pioneers of football injury epidemiology, leads the group study for this project. The UEFA Champions League (UCL) injury study involves the most important clubs in European football from several countries and with different levels of competition success. Each day, injury data together with information on the football activity exposure of each player are collected by the medical staff of these clubs and sent to the group study. Feedback on the club's injury profile is sent periodically by the study group to the club in order to improve specific prevention programmes. Until now, the results of this survey have been extensively published in the scientific literature [2, 3] and have helped to identify the most common injuries at that level of football as well as their specificity and fundamental characteristics, namely, the total injury risk in top-level club football in Europe (8.0/1000 h).

According to the UCL injury study, a professional football team can expect about 50 injuries that cause time loss from play each season, which equates to two injuries per player per season [3]. The impact of injuries on team performance can therefore be considerable as on average; 12% of the squad is unavailable due to injury at any point during the season. Most injuries occur during a match where there is a five times higher risk of injury compared with training. Data from the UEFA Champions League show that the risk of injury remained constant in the last decade (Fig. 2.1).

During a match, data show that injury incidence increases during the last part of each half (Fig. 2.2).

There is also evidence that overuse injuries have a higher incidence during the preseason (Fig. 2.3), while there are different trends of seasonality linked to different regions and their specific environmental conditions. In modern football, where a considerable amount of money is invested, this has a notable economic impact with some teams reportedly losing millions of euros due to injury [4]. These data suggest the importance of the medical staff, whose role in many clubs and federations is still undervalued.

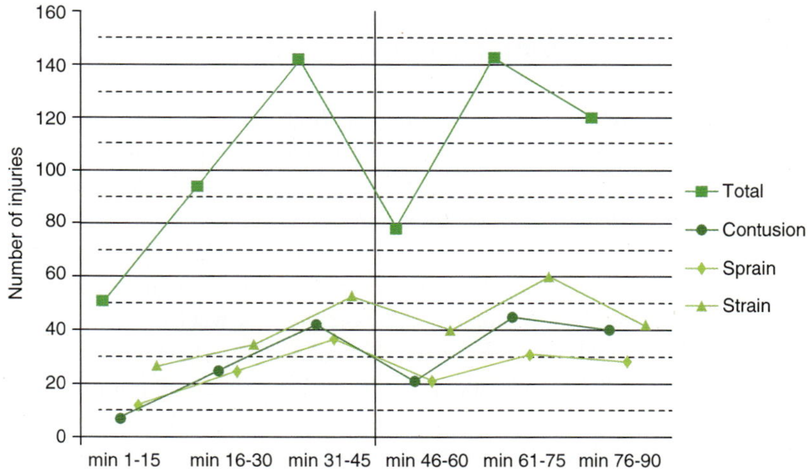

Fig. 2.2 Injury incidence during matches (courtesy of Waldén M et al. [2])

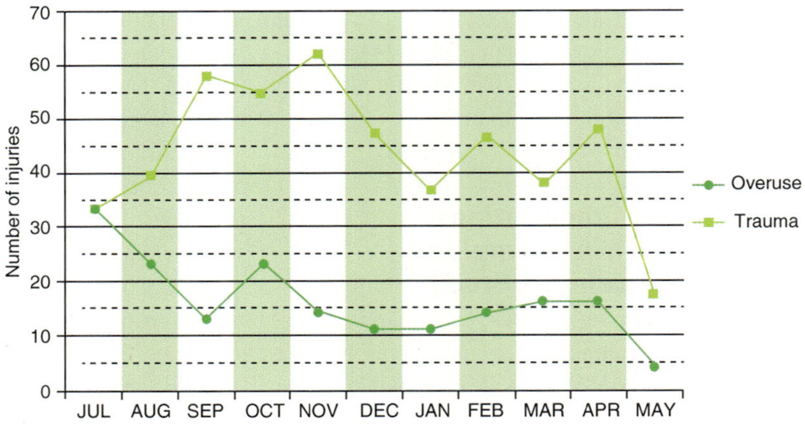

Fig. 2.3 Distribution of injuries during season (courtesy of Waldén M et al. [2])

In injury study by Ekstrand et al.[2], some conclusions were evident:

1. Low risk of injuries in training
2. The injury risk at matches is higher
3. No difference in injury risk between group phase and final phase
4. Higher injury risk for younger players
5. Higher risk of severe injuries
6. Injury patterns – less head and knee injuries/ less severe injuries
7. Most injuries occurred at the end of each half
8. Many players left the tournament still injured
9. Few reinjuries
10. Higher injury risk to forwards

2.6 The Most Common Injuries

The most common injury in football is thigh strain, typically affecting the hamstrings muscle group. Thigh strain represents about 17% of all injuries, and a typical 25-player squad can expect 10 thigh strains each season, with seven hamstrings and three quadriceps strains [5]. Figure 2.4 shows the football gestuality and potential location of injury (thigh 23%, knee 20%, ankle 14%, groin/hip 12%, lower leg 11%, back 6% and foot 5%).

In general, muscle injuries represent almost one third of all time-loss injuries in men's professional football, and 92% of all injuries affect the four big muscle groups in the lower limbs. Again, if we consider a team of 25 players at elite level, we can expect about 15 muscle injuries each season, with approximately 2 weeks missed for each injury (Fig. 2.5). Muscle injuries tend to occur more frequently towards the end of each half.

The knee is the second most common location of injury in football players (Fig. 2.4). Despite their relatively low incidence (< 1% of all injuries), anterior cruciate ligament (ACL) lesions are the most attention-drawing pathology in football medicine [6].

The hip and groin are another common injury location. It seems that the real magnitude of injuries in this location has been initially misevaluated due to the relatively difficult diagnosis and injury definitions, which do not always allow a clear identification and classification of such injuries. According to Werner et al. [7], a team will have seven groin injuries each year. In addition to this considerable incidence, which has been shown to be consistent over consecutive seasons, prevention programmes have been included in training sessions, but groin and hip injuries have a significant severity: more than half of them imply a lay-off time of more than 4 weeks.

The ankle is the most common injury location in sports traumatology. In football, around 90% of ankle injuries are sprains. The first football epidemiological studies were performed in the early 1980s and reported that the ankle is the

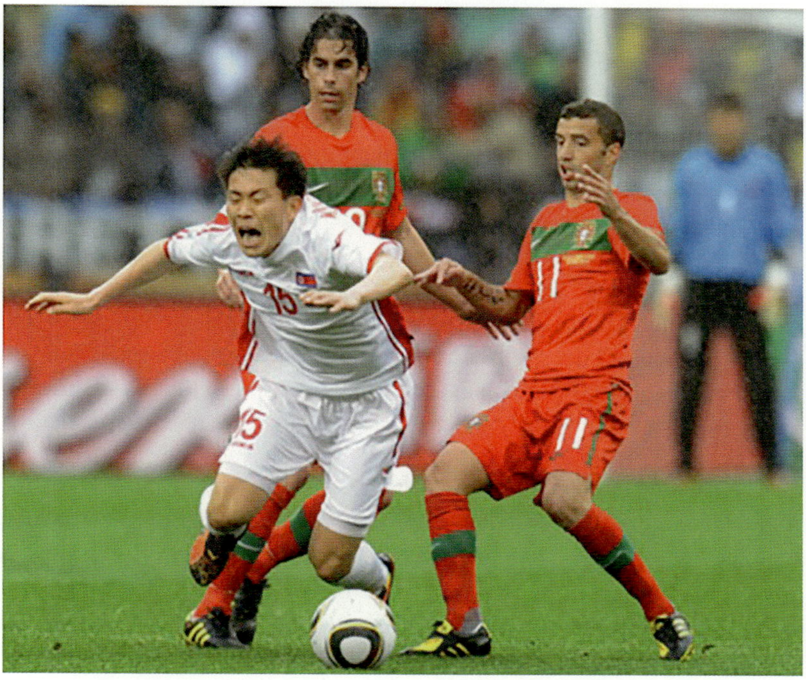

Fig. 2.4 Football gestuality and potential injuries

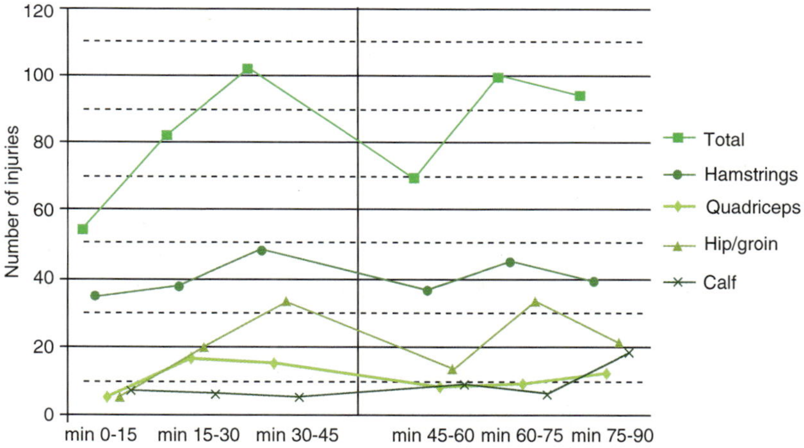

Fig. 2.5 Location and percentage of total injuries (courtesy of Waldén M et al. [2])

most common location of injury (around 30% of total injuries). More recent reports show a decrease of about 50% of ankle injuries. This can be the result of prevention strategies (e.g. neuromuscular training, bracing, taping, individualized shoes), which have proved to be effective in reducing the incidence of ankle sprains [8]. The sanctions to aggressive behaviour also contributed to decrease the ankle injury incidence [9]. A correlation has been found between major injuries (causing absence >4 weeks) and performance. There is a considerable variation in the number of matches played per season in European professional leagues. Top-level players are obliged to play many matches, especially during the final period of the season. A correlation was found between many matches at the end of a season and an increased injury risk and/or underperformance during subsequent world tournaments [10].

2.7 Are Women Injuries Different from Men?

Women's football has gained more and more importance in the last few years. The number of participants is rapidly increasing together with the discipline's professionalism. Male players have an increased risk of training and match injury compared with female players, but the risk of sustaining a moderate to severe injury (>1 week absence) does not differ between men and women. Injury patterns are largely similar, but females suffer relatively more knee injuries, and men suffer more groin injuries.

Female players have a two to three times higher risk of ACL injury compared with their male counterparts. Females also tend to sustain their ACL injury at a younger age and have a higher risk of injury, especially during match play, whereas no relevant gender-related difference seems to exist during training. These data have provided the basis for an extensive programme of prevention for ACL injury in female footballers.

2.8 Are Children and Adolescents at Risk?

The knee is the most frequent site of musculoskeletal injury in the paediatric athlete. The higher participation rate of children (in earlier ages) and adolescents in competitive sports has led to a dramatically increase in knee injuries over the past decade. Concerns in children sports participation (Fig. 2.6) are expressed in most of football academies where young boys' (7 years old) training sessions and competitions represent more than 15 h a week including gym sessions. This means a high impact and frequency load training, as well as, abnormal chondral load with frequent severe injuries presenting abnormal

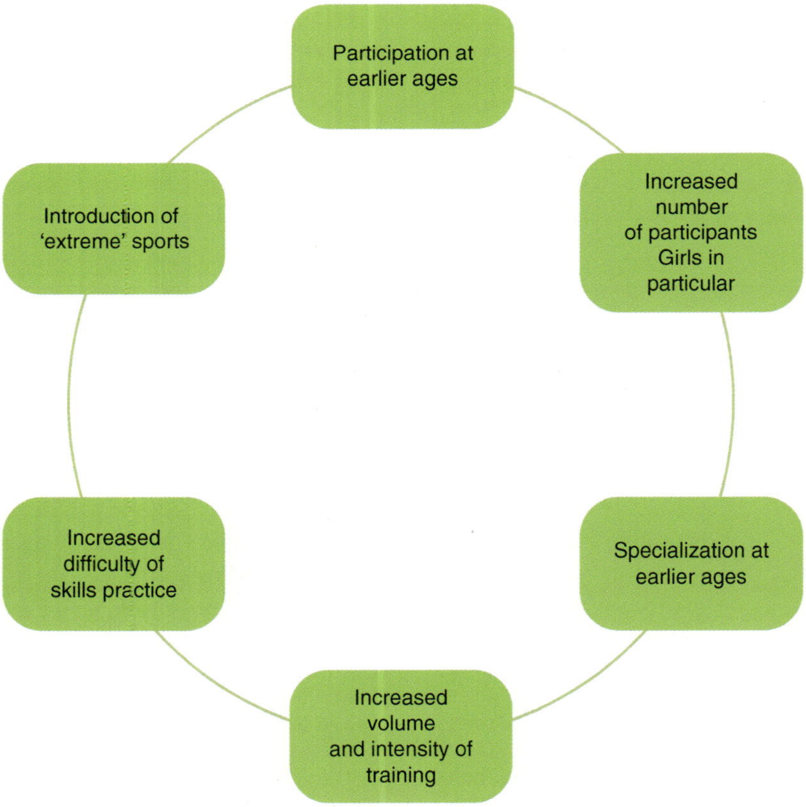

Fig. 2.6 Trends in children and youth's sports

patterns involving structures like the ACL, bone apophyses and cartilage. At the moment, we need to better identify children at risk for ACL and other injuries and add injury prevention programmes to workouts.

Conclusion

The injury risk decreased in male professional football during recent years. At elite level, the risk of ankle sprain has been decreased, and thigh muscle strain is the most common injury. A period with a congested match calendar can lead to fatigue increasing the risk of injury and to poor performance during the following period.

References

1. Eirale C, Tol JL, Farooq A, Smiley F, Chalabi H. Low injury rate strongly correlates with team success in Qatari professional football. Br J Sports Med. 2013; 47:807–8.
2. Waldén M, Hägglund M, Ekstrand J. UEFA Champions League study: a prospective study of injuries in professional football during the 2001–2002 season. Br J Sports Med. 2005;39:542–6.
3. Ekstrand J, Hägglund M, Waldén M. Injury incidence and injury patterns in professional football: the UEFA injury study. Br J Sports Med. 2011;45:553–8.
4. Eirale C, Farooq A, Smiley FA, Tol JL, Chalabi H. Epidemiology of football injuries in Asia: a prospective study in Qatar. J Sci Med Sport. 2013; 16:113–7.
5. Ekstrand J, Hägglund M, Waldén M. Epidemiology of muscle injuries in professional football (soccer). Am J Sports Med. 2011;39:1226–32.
6. Ekstrand J. A 94% return to elite level football after ACL surgery: a proof of possibilities with optimal caretaking or a sign of knee abuse? Knee Surg Sports Traumatol Arthrosc. 2011;19:1–2.
7. Werner J, Hägglund M, Waldén M, Ekstrand J. UEFA injury study: a prospective study of hip and groin injuries in professional football over seven consecutive seasons. Br J Sports Med. 2009;43:1036–40.
8. Fuller CW, Ekstrand J, Junge A, Andersen TE, Bahr R, Dvorak J, et al. Consensus statement on injury definitions and data collection procedures in studies of football (soccer) injuries. Scand J Med Sci Sports. 2006;16:83–92.
9. Hawkins RD, Hulse MA, Wilkinson C, Hodson A, Gibson M. The association football medical research programme: an audit of injuries in professional football. Br J Sports Med. 2001;35:43–7.
10. Ekstrand J. Epidemiology of football injuries. Sci Sports. 2008;23:73–7.

Teamwork in Football/Bringing Science to the Pitch

3

José Neto

Contents

3.1 Introduction

To be invited to draw up a critical reflection on the subject *teamwork in football/bringing science to the pitch*, I could eventually evolve my reflection in the context of the prevalence and incidence of sports injuries, in a historical and

J. Neto
Instituto Universitário da Maia, Maia, Portugal
e-mail: zeneto7@gmail.com

J. Espregueira-Mendes et al. (eds.), *Injuries and Health Problems in Football*,
DOI 10.1007/978-3-662-53924-8_3

evolutionary approach of the most common injuries, explaining with examples the most significant predisposing factors for your appearance.

In this context, I could refer to the contraindications for the practice of sports and physical activity, age and gender, weather conditions, time zones, planning on coaching, preparation for the activity, and finally at the level of the sports facilities and the material used.

However, bearing in mind that under psychological and mental, in terms of evaluation and presentation of strategies for the recovery of injured athletes, becoming a field of greater impact in the context of the great theme, I will seek to develop, albeit very concisely, what I think of greater relevance to the effect required.

3.2 Part I

3.2.1 Psychological Factors Associated with the Prevention and Recovery of Sports Injuries

Several reasons lead us to consider the injuries as negative events in life of practitioners and may result in loss of verve, monetary awards, physical condition and fitness sports, etc. and also changes in the personal family life (irritability, depressive states, concerns and doubts about the future).

It has been noted that psychological variables such as motivation, stress, attention, aggressiveness, self-confidence, persistence, or the mood may influence the possibility of athletes' injuries and contribute to the processes of recovery of injuries and prevention of further relapses. The psychosocial stress is a key variable in this process, essentially before and when the injury takes place; in fact, studies conducted by Davis, Hardy, Richman, and Rosenfeld [4] and Petrie [18] proved that stress appears to increase considerably the probability of causing injury.

3.2.2 Stress and Sports Injuries

Anderson and Williams [1] made a risk assessment of injuries suggesting intervention strategies for their reduction, particularly in high-risk and more vulnerable athletes, from the psychological point of view.

We identify three important factors (personality, history of stress factors, and confrontational resources) that prevent sports situations that are potentially *stress*-generating. In which concerns the personality, there is a set of variables such as psychological tendency, locus of control, competitive anxiety, motivation for achievement, and demand of sensations. According to our conclusions, all these potentially stress-generating situations can cause psychological and attentional changes, increased muscle tension, limitation and reduction of the visual field, and increased distractibility, thus creating "great" conditions for the competition of sports injuries.

3.2.3 Model of Vulnerability to Sports Injuries

Buceta [6] suggested a model of psychological vulnerability to sports injuries, which the main assumption is the interaction between potentially stressful situations and individual and personal variables. Thus, the higher the frequency, the duration and/or the intensity of potentially stressful situations, the greater the probability of appearance of stress conducive to greater vulnerability to injury.

Adapted from Buceta [6], we identify various *potentially stressful situations*:

- Failure of general type (e.g., family conflicts, loss of loved ones, financial problems, etc.)
- Successes related to the sports activity (e.g., exchange of statute or contractual issues paper, exchange of team or coach, etc.)
- Lifestyle
- Training requirements
- Requirements of the competition

Table 3.1 Effect on stressful situations according to personal variables (Adapted from Buceta 1996) [6]

Previous history of injuries	(>)
Anxiety state, related to the activity and athletic competition	(>)
"Stiffness" (righteousness, commitment, and control)	(<)
Confrontational styles	(>) (<)
Confrontation skills domain	(<)
Social support	(>) (<)
High motivation to sporting goals	(>) (<)
High self-confidence	(<)
High self-esteem	(<)
Tendency for optimism	(<)
System of beliefs and attitudes	(>)

- Other situations related to the sports activity (e.g., the opinion of the media, the relationship with directors, etc.)
- More specifically, background stimuli associated with sports injuries earlier

In a context of competitive sport, we can assume the following *effects* (Table 3.1) (Adapted from Buceta 1996 [6]):

3.2.4 Psychological Injury Recovery and Prevention

One of the most important issues facing the person who has responsibility to retrieve an injured person consists in the evaluation of their behavioral reactions to injury.

Brewer [5] mentioned various situational and personal variables, related to the psychological and emotional reactions to injury. With regard to *situational variables, the severity of the injury and the time required for recovery appear to be the most stress-generating factors*. On the contrary, when there is a strong social support and there is evolution in recovery, stress levels seem to drop significantly. As regards personal variables, Brewer [5] referred the success had on previous injury recovery; the type of practice and sporting competition; the patient's age, with more negative emotional phenomena in young and older athletes; and extremely negative ways of thinking and pessimistic also generating higher levels of stress, calling into question the emotional stability of the athlete.

Main signs of *psychological adjustment* in the face of injury:

(a) *Loss of identity* – An injury that requires an athlete to abandon definitely practice or sporting competition generates naturally a loss in personal identity of the athlete. The fact that a major loss in itself "was lost" negatively affects seriously the athlete's self-concept and self-esteem
(b) *Fear and anxiety* – Injured athletes may also experience high levels of fear and anxiety, experiencing particularly high levels of concern about their ability to fully recover from injury, about the possibility of turning the injured, and about the possibility of being able to be away from the team and replaced by other colleagues. The fact that they cannot train or compete allows them to have much time to worry about these aspects
(c) *Lack of confidence* – The lack of trust and training time will likely lead to declines or significant decreases in income after the injury. Many athletes have a huge difficulty in lowering their expectations and personal requirements after an injury and, on the contrary, continue to have expectation levels identical to those that had before injuries

Psychological reactions associated with sports injuries (Table 3.2) (adapted from Petitpas and Danish 1995; Source: Cruz and Dias 1996 [8]):

The fact that athletes experience negative emotional reactions can contribute to a good or a bad injury recovery. Buceta [6] indicates several steps of the stress associated with the post-injury period: at the time of hospitalization, in recovery, in resumption of training functions, the fact that

Table 3.2 Signs of a potentially problematic adjustment to sports injuries (Adapted from Petitpas and Danish 1995; Source: Cruz and Dias 1996) [8]

Feeling of irritation, anger, and confusion
Obsessive thoughts about the day he can return to compete
Negation (e.g., "the injury is nothing...")
Return repeatedly to competition too quickly, and they suffer injuries
Pride over the top ("wife") about the benefits and achievements
Insistence on physical complaints without importance
Blame for the weak earnings of team
Isolation and/or removal of other significant people
Rapid changes in moods
Claims, regardless what is done, the recovery will not be possible

the athlete competes injured, and in cases where athletes have to stop leaving his practice compete.

Ievleva and Orlick [15], through interviews, showed that athletes who resorted to the practice of positive thinking, and the mental visualization of the state of its development, recovered more effectively and faster.

Weinberg and Gould [23] drawed attention to some practical techniques of psychological intervention in recovery, mainly:

- The relationship with the athlete should be based on the seriousness and optimism. The training methodology to perform must be known to the injured athlete
- Using psychological skills such as visualization and relaxation should be conveniently prepared
- The injured athlete should be prepared to overcome any unforeseen factors
- A dynamic of constant emotional support and help for people who share more directly to the athlete's life

According Buceta [6] psychological intervention must have four post-injury central objectives:

(a) Improve well-being and psychological functioning of athletes
(b) Contribute and promote the effectiveness of rehabilitation
(c) Help athletes in return to sports practice and competition
(d) Prevent relapses or new lesions

Given the important role of psychological processes in injury recovery, we can conceptualize the psychological intervention, in this kind of cases, according to four main points suggested by Cruz and Dias [8]:

(a) Analyze the behaviors of athletes before the injury, as well as their resources to deal with the same
(b) Train athletes in some psychological strategies that help them in reducing control of stress associated with injuries
(c) Teach all those who deal with the injured athlete about the behaviors that may have to assist the recovery process
(d) Cooperate with all components of the medical team, in a way that it can be a permanent and clear communication with the athlete about the evolution of the recovery

It is in this sense that Buceta [6] points out the goals of the work of the sports psychologist:

(a) The contribution to the development and personal growth of the athletes
(b) Performance optimization
(c) The prevention and recovery of injuries
(d) The general well-being of the athletes

3.2.5 Effectiveness of Psychological Intervention in the Prevention of Sports Injuries

A study of Ievleva and Orlick [15], which analyzes the strategies and psychological factors associated with a rapid recovery from injury, evaluated the following factors:

(a) *Attitude to injury* – We all know that the way they face the injury has a positive or negative influence to their recovery
(b) *Stress control* – High levels of stress may predispose to illness and injury and can also hinder

a rapid recovery. It depends on the individual's way of dealing with the stress, as well as the circumstances in which the subject lives

(c) *Social support* – Those who have high levels of social support experienced less stress when faced with unforeseen events

(d) *Formulating objectives* – It is the first step to start any task, including a rapid recovery from injury

(e) *Internal positive speech* – Internal positive speech as we all know contributes to personal well-being. Athletes cannot change the fact that they were injured, but they can control their thoughts about the injury and his recovery

(f) *Mental visualization* – Images of a complete rehabilitation, as well as a positive recovery process, have beneficial results [19]

(g) *Beliefs* – All of the above strategies have the greatest chance of success if the athlete believes and feels what is to be done

3.3 Part II

3.3.1 Psychological Assessment and Diagnosis of Sports Injuries

The injury often occurs and can suddenly stop the realization of the objectives of the athlete's income [14]. All injuries can drag something psychological: physical, social, and psychological factors that are dependent on the role that sport represents in the life of an athlete. Due to the large investment in terms of time, energy, and money, an athlete experiences a greater loss and a greater threat to self-esteem.

In this sense, authors such as Buceta [6] and Heil [14] emphasize the need and importance to assess and/or diagnose various aspects and psychological factors associated with sports injuries.

3.3.2 The Preceding Factors of the Lesion

The personal attitudes and behaviors, as well as events in the recent past and remote, are reflected in the athlete and in his ability to face and deal with the weight of an injury. Thus it becomes important to assess factors such as medical and psychological history and the experience of significant changes in sport and personal life.

Another significant factors are major team competitions, the effects of the player who is furthest from the working group, and other risk factors such as drug use or eating disorders, as well as relapses of injury or prolonged hospitalizations for multiple surgeries.

For Taylor [22], the well-known phenomenon of "somatization" can be seen as a process of deficient information to the athlete where overvalued many times are the somatic sensations. In its extreme form, the somatization disorder is characterized by a long history of pain and various somatic complaints, by the frequent use of medicines, and by a penchant for medical consultations, with vaguely defined phenomenon origin.

3.3.3 Life with Stress and Change

Athletes with a lower capacity or psychological skills to fight against psychosocial adversities are at greater risk of injury [20]. Therefore, it is essential to pay greater attention to the athlete who gets injured in a negative phase, because the solution may not be compatible with the requirement to solve other problems in his life [6].

3.3.4 Stress and Change in Sports

All athletes have to be trainer for winning and losing, but a change/challenge still being positive can also be stressful [6, 14].

The psychologist/methodologist-retriever training/physical therapist and others can obtain important information by contacting the coaches. A change of "status" on the team, a growing improvement, or the sudden decline of income can be detected easily. In addition, a higher competitive level requires greater physical and mental requirements.

3.3.5 Approximation of the Major Competitions

Some studies, in sporting contexts, refer that as we approach the games of greater significance and importance, it also increases the risk of injury, and such risk may be related to overloads of training prior to the competitions and associated with psychological stress that competition in itself causes [6].

3.3.6 The Psychological State of the Player Sidelined

It should also identify the case of athletes "marginalized" and tend to "hide" injuries, with fear or fear of losing the opportunity of being summoned to a game.

3.3.7 Training Overload

The workout overload occurs when training exceeds the psychological ability of the athlete to give response to effort. It is mainly manifested in emotional and psychological instability, increasing susceptibility to infectious diseases and sleep disorders.

3.3.8 The Risk Factors of Illness of Sportsmen

Some athletes are identified within a population at higher risk for substance abuse, and food, and drug use leading to a mental and psychological change. Substances which may generate additional anxiety in competition include nicotine, caffeine, tranquilizers, alcohol, and cocaine among other compounds.

3.3.9 The Emotional Stress

According to Heil [14], when greater psychological trauma is associated with an injury, greater is the likelihood of psychological problems during rehabilitation. The psychological impact can be evidenced by certain symptoms, such as fear, anxiety, pessimism, catastrophic thoughts at the time of occurrence of injury, depersonalization, among others.

3.3.10 The Location of the Lesion

The injury of the body parts particularly "admired" by the athlete has a greater impact and psychological effect (negative) compared to injuries in other parts of the body.

3.3.11 Pain

Pain is an immediate response to injury and reflects not only the seriousness of the "damage" but also the anxiety and hopes to face the future impact. The feeling of pain, as well as the stress Heil [14] and Buceta [6], is conditioned by the state of mind of the athlete.

3.3.12 Time of Occurrence of Injuries

Even minor injuries, whether they happen in a focal point of an athlete's career, could have tremendous consequences. For example, the end-of-season injuries can create a feeling of lack of achievement, dragging the athlete to serious psychological problem.

3.3.13 Cases and Unforeseen Situations

A professional competition can lead to much more disturbing reactions, before a serious injury, compared with those who are least prepared and which are more inexperienced in the activity.

3.3.14 Subsequent to the Injury Factors

Rehabilitation effectiveness, complications in the treatment, pain, use of medicines, psychological state, social support, personal conflicts, and reactions of the fans and the press are key factors and potentially decisive for own progress in rehabilitation and full recovery from injury [6].

3.3.15 Auto-Scapegoating of the Athlete

The athlete experiences increased feeling of guilt on injury problems. So, if this assumes responsibility for the occurrence of the injury or the plays as a result of a fault or mistake guys, often arise the feel of guilt in the athlete.

3.3.16 Social and Emotional Support

The positive role of the social, emotional, and psychological support in the recovery of sports injuries is widely recognized and evidenced by the literature in the field of sport psychology [8, 9]. The social support transmits confidence, helping to better address the problems and psychological difficulties associated with the injury.

3.3.17 "Secondary" Benefits

Although the injury is a negative event, it can also get "secondary" benefits and some positive consequences, for example, increased attention, sympathy, or social support by others or the break free from the responsibilities of everyday life or escape to stressful situations.

3.3.18 Psychological Assessment of the Injury (or Post Injury)

Heil [14] and Buceta [6] refer to the most pertinent issues in the process of psychological evaluation of the lesion:

1. *Identity*: What is exactly the lesion? Does the lesion produce too much or little pain?
2. *Pain*: What area of the body is injured? Is there some medication being administered?
3. *Activity*: Does the injury interfere with the activity of the sport? Must interrupt the activity? For how long? Implies limitations? Which?
4. *Hospitalization*: Needed? For how long? Are you going to have surgery? Which?
5. *Aids*: What impact, for the injured, does the measures adopted have? Need help or not to move, dress, etc.? How to fill in the time? Will have difficulty in sleeping?
6. *Recovery*: What is the prognosis? How long for the reappearance? May yield as before? Should you restrict the future activity? Will likely be a decrease of capacity?

3.4 Part III

3.4.1 Strategies for Monitoring Physical and Psychological Recovery of Injured Athletes

Some investigations are able to demonstrate the emotional responses of athletes to injury [24]. Some injured athletes show a variety of negative emotional reactions such as mood disturbances, tension, and anger [12, 20]. In the study of Smith et al. [20], it was evidenced that the severity of the injury was the biggest determinant of emotional response and that athletes with minor injuries had less mood disturbance.

As suggested by the work of Gordon et al. [11], some injured athletes have behavioral reactions similar to states of grief, as identified by Kübler-Ross [16] in his work with the terminally ill. Psychological recovery strategies should be used as soon as the injury is diagnosed.

3.4.2 Mental and Psychological Training in the Treatment of Injuries

Buceta [6] addressed and suggested some mental training techniques in the treatment of sports injuries. These psychological techniques usually include the following combinations:

(a) *Relaxation training*, to develop body awareness, enhance relaxation resting muscle, and increase muscle efficiency
(b) *Imagination and mental visualization*, consisting in the use of imagination to rehearse repeatedly sports situations
(c) *Internal discourse*, where the athlete uses assertive statements to increase the self-confidence or refocus his/her attention. The internal discourse can also be used to modify or stop negative thoughts detrimental to performance
(d) *Biofeedback training* using the psychophysiological measures to provide fast and accurate *feedback* to subtle changes in muscle tension or in other activities mediated by the autonomic nervous system (e.g., heart rate and brain activity, among others)
(e) *Hypnotic techniques*, based on focus of attention so that the athlete uses suggestions to be confident and to deal with the *stress* associated with the injury

3.4.3 Recovery Training Field

We seek to attain the foundation ideas of the various *factors* that can determine the integration in the normal group. According to the type of injury and its evolution in recovery, we can also associate the field training in the gym and swimming pool.

(a) *Aerobic endurance* – establishment of the organic balance by increasing the aerobic capacity of the muscle fiber, establishing the bases of other functional capabilities, until a gradual adaptation of the increasing loads of practice
(b) *Anaerobic resistance* – ability to make efforts with oxygen deficit, revealing this work at a more advanced stage of training. This approach is characterized by efforts over a period of time to intense short duration or intense and long-lasting, calling the combined forms of continuous training, interval or circuit
(c) *Strength* – muscular strength is a fundamental physical ability to carry out the sports gesture, assuming that is why the musculoskeletal system has a preponderant role in improving performance [21]
(d) *Speed* – is strongly conditioned by the genetic endowment of the sportsman, but it is known that this ability can be greatly improved with a qualification of specific training, in particular, as regards race, playing technique, range coordination, and synchronization of movements that an athlete in recovery can so subsequently optimize
(e) *Flexibility* – primarily intended for the execution of large muscle movements and jointd. It should be always the intended movement synchronized with the optimization of the technique

Furthermore, the use of some psychological techniques, which are associated with the task execution, results in a *new vision of sports training*:

(a) *Communication skills* – being the methodologist of the workout directly responsible for the operationalization of recovery, he/she should undertake clear information about the processes that are being worked on and use some strategies as enthusiasm in dialogue and strong messages of support, seriousness, optimism and keep an optimistic state in athlete, stimulating compensations in recovery
(b) *Relaxation techniques* – relaxation techniques whose fundamental objectives in its use can take to improve the field of *stress* and anxiety control, increase the concentration, facilitate quick mobilization and great energy through stimulation of the field to use attention, and improve self-control
(c) *Formulation of objectives* – defining and accomplishing positive and specific objectives (challenging, but realistic) as well as avoiding the idea of unrealistic goals
(d) *Imagination and mental visualization* – is a valid instrument for the acquisition of a great

state of sports performance and may also be used to simulate and anticipate predictable emotional states in the face of pressure to appear even "impossible" for maximum performance

3.4.4 Influence of Sports Injury Changes in Mood and Precompetitive Anxiety in Football Players

According Olmedilla et al. [17], players before the injury demonstrate higher levels of stress and self-confidence and after suffering an injury demonstrate higher levels of depression, anxiety, and cognitive and somatic anxiety. The relationship between injury and the psychological aspects of sport is closely related [3].

The scientific literature indicates that the risk, causation, and etiology of sports injury include the interaction between intrinsic (biological characteristics and psychological aspects) and extrinsic (physical and sociocultural characteristics) aspects and its influence on sport behavior [25]. In this sense, some authors stress the importance of cognitive processes, both emotional and behavioral occurring in the rehabilitation of injuries [13].

There are difficulties in assessing the precompetitive anxiety, manifested immediately before starting the competition and the state of mind of professional or semiprofessional athletes. For anxiety, in most cases, there have been studies of anxiety trait and descriptive models [4].

3.4.5 Injured Athletes' Perceptions About Social Support

Clement and Shannon [7] refer in their study that the social support moderates the harmful effects of stress, which in turn affects indirectly the health of injured athletes and their well-being. Previous research suggests that the lack of influence of social support on the psychological reactions of athletes benefits accession to rehab.

Social support can be defined as an exchange of resources between two individuals with the intention of increasing the welfare of the recipient. The social support operates through two mechanisms, the chance and the direct effect, that influence the injured athletes in rehabilitation experiences. Social support, according to the hypothesis of time, moderates the harmful effects of stress and indirectly affects the health of injured athletes and their well-being.

3.4.6 Relationship Between the Perception of Pain and Fatigue with Mood

García and Más [10] refer a case study of a young man who starts sport after 6 months of recovery for having suffered different injuries during the period of 1 year. The POMS was used and by rating scales subjective were measured variables pain, fatigue and satisfaction, the resulting higher threshold of pain at the beginning of the competition and in this same scenario, low fatigue and satisfaction ratings.

New studies show that the Profile of Mood States (POMS) provides information on the psychological evaluation of the athlete, that some authors claim "there is a certain preference for the use of this questionnaire, especially the smaller versions, evaluating mood during the period of training" [2].

Conclusion

As conclusive, I can mention, that in each of the chapters mentioned, we could develop a way, by chance, more explicit and circumstantial for the general theme proposed.

Then, with the sense of gathering more syncretism when I was asked, "I left" the way some notes in technical and pedagogical order, which could and should be larger object.

As a final note, I would not fail to point out that a project of rehabilitation or recovery of an injured athlete, it is fundamental the involvement of different professionals from the most diverse areas of intervention, in turns by a single goal, passing a reassuring aura who meets expectations high.

From my experience as methodologist, in this function, in addition to the elements that contain the medical and technical team, in the recovery of injured players, family and friends always become a source of endless support and construction, day by day, a properly and sustained design of principles, honor, duty, and guarantees, for the revival of a "god" dropped.

References

1. Anderson MB, Williams JM. A model of stress and athletic injury prediction and prevention. J Sport Exerc Psychol. 1988/1993;10:294–306.
2. Andrade E, Arce C, Seoane G. Aportaciones del POMS a la medida del estado de ánimo de los deportistas: estado de la cuestión. Revista de Psicología del Deporte. 2000;9(1–2):7–20.
3. Ardern CL, Taylor NF, Feller JA, Whitehead TS, Webster KE. Psychological responses matter in returning to preinjury level of sport after anterior cruciate ligament reconstruction surgery. Am J Sports Med. 2013;41(7):1549–58.
4. Aslan SH, Aslan RO, Alparslan ZN. Anxiety levels of the football players participating in the U-21 national team infrastructure selection. Turk J Sports Med. 2000;35(2):51–8.
5. Brewer B. Review and critique of models of psychological adjustment to athletic injury. J Appl Sport Psychol. 1994;6:87–100.
6. Buceta JM. Psicologia y Lesiones Deportivas: Prevencion y Recuperacion. Madrid: Dykinson; 1996.
7. Clement D, Shannon VR. Injured athletes' perceptions about social support. J Sport Rehabil. 2011;20(4):457.
8. Cruz JF, Dias MA. Factores psicológicos associados às lesões desportivas. In: Cruz J, editor. Manual de Psicologia do Desporto. Braga: SHO; 1996.
9. Duda JL, Smart AE, Tappe MK. Predictors of adherence in the rehabilitation of athletic injuries. J Sport Exerc Psychol. 1989;11:367–81.
10. García RL, Más AG. Fercepción de dolor y fatiga en relación con el estado de ánimo. Cuadernos de Psicología del Deporte. 2011;11(2):93–106.
11. Gordon S, Milios D, Grove JR. Psychological aspects of the recovery process from the injury: the perspective of sports physiotherapists. Aust J Sci Med Sport. 1991;3:17–29.
12. Grove, Stewart, Gordon, Smith, Scott, O'Fallon and Young (1990). Emotional reactions of athletics to knee rehabilitaion. Paper presented at the Annual Meeting of the Australian Sports Medicine Federation. Alice Springs.
13. Hackfort D, Kleinert J. Research on sport injury development: former and future approaches from an action theory perspective. Int J Sport Psychol. 2007;5:324–39.
14. Heil J. Psychology of sport injury. Champaign: Human Kinetics; 1993.
15. Ievleva L, Orlick T. Mental links to enhanced healing: an exploratory study. Sport Psychol. 1991;5:25–40.
16. Kübler-Ross E. On death and dying. New York: MacMillan; 1969.
17. Olmedilla A, Ortega E, Gómez J. Influence of sports injury changes in mood and precompetitive anxiety in soccer players. Cuadernos de Psicología del Deporte. 2014;14(1):55–61.
18. Petrie TA. Coping skills, competitive trait auxiety, and playing status: moderating effects on the life stress – injuries relationship. J Sport Exerc Psychol. 1993;15:261–74.
19. Simonton OC, Matthews-Simonton S, Creighton JL. Getting well again. New York: Bantam Books; 1978.
20. Smith AM et al. The psychological effects of sports injuries: coping. Sports Med. 1990;9:352–69.
21. Soares J. O treino do futebolista. Porto: Editora; 2005.
22. Taylor J. Predicting athletic performance with self-confidence and somatic and cognitive anxiety as a function of motor and physiological requirements in sports. J Psychol. 1987;55:139–53.
23. Weinberg R, Gould D. Foundations of sport and exercise psychology. Champaign: Human Kinetics; 1995.
24. Wiese-Bjornstal DM, Smith AM. Counseling a strategies for enhanced recovery of injured athletes within a team approach. In: Pargman D, editor. Psychological buses of sport injuries. Morgantown: WV Fitness Information Technology; 1993. p. 149–82.
25. Wiese-Bjornstal DM. Sport injury and college athlete health across the lifespan. J Intercollegiate Sport. 2009;2:64–80.

The Field Case

4

Rodolfo Moura

Contents

R. Moura
Rodolfo Moura's Center, Porto, Portugal
e-mail: rodolfomoura@sapo.pt

J. Espregueira-Mendes et al. (eds.), *Injuries and Health Problems in Football*,
DOI 10.1007/978-3-662-53924-8_4

4.1 Introduction

Whenever I got into the field with my field case, it meant that an athlete had, somehow, suffered an injury and, consequently, it was a reason to stop the game. I have no doubt that all the attentions were drawn to the place where I and my case were with the mission to assist the injured athlete. Many times have I opened the field case to withdraw the most suitable product and applied it in a safe and fast way to assure that the athlete returned to the game in his perfect physical and mental condition.

The field case has been an essential item in my work as a sport health professional. My long experience in the sports health area, particularly in football, the most popular sport in Portugal, enables me to reflect about several and different issues on this matter. Reading and studying several authors such as Arliani et al. [1], Costa [2], Moreno [3], and Pinto [4] that have written about sports and health allowed me to go further in the topic.

This research work is on:

- What is the origin of the field case?
- What is it used for?
- How has it evolved?
- What is its content?
- What are the main principles for its use?

Along with these questions, many others may be equally relevant. However, they will be object of future reflections.

4.2 The Origin of the Field Case

The field case is as old as football itself, and its origin goes back to the United Kingdom, the birthplace of football. Right from the beginning, this sport has always required the need to assist injured footballers during the game (including first aid help). Water and bandages have probably been the first products used in the field.

As professional sports have become more and more demanding, other products have been used and included in the field case. Nowadays the field case is very different from the one used 20 years ago.

4.3 The Use of the Field Case

Sports, particularly football, have been characterized by an increase in the effort and competitiveness. Pinto [4] (Page 23) when trying to define the effort in football refers that "the rhythm, the motor density, the body contact and the game complexity are higher and higher, as well as occasional", which increases the risk of injures that can affect the athlete's well-being and health. This very same author states that "modern football requires a strong and fast player able to overcome obstacles and handle charges (…) as well as keep high effort levels even though being physically exhausted." (Page 32). In this context where effort is taken to the limit, the field assistance is vital to the athlete (Fig. 4.1).

The field case has countless times been a quick response to different traumatic situations. This quick response justifies its use in all occasions.

4.4 Field Case Evolution

The field case has followed the scientific and technological progress over the last years. In fact, we can say that there have been major changes in it, especially when it comes to human resources (more competent professionals in the sports area) and more knowledge when it comes to material resources (new treatment techniques and new products). There has been a major investment in the academic education as well as in the professionalism of all the agents that work in sports health area. Modern football has led to the creation of a group of health professionals with a degree in sports that ensure a high-quality medical assistance to the athlete. These professionals use modern techniques and have new approaches which

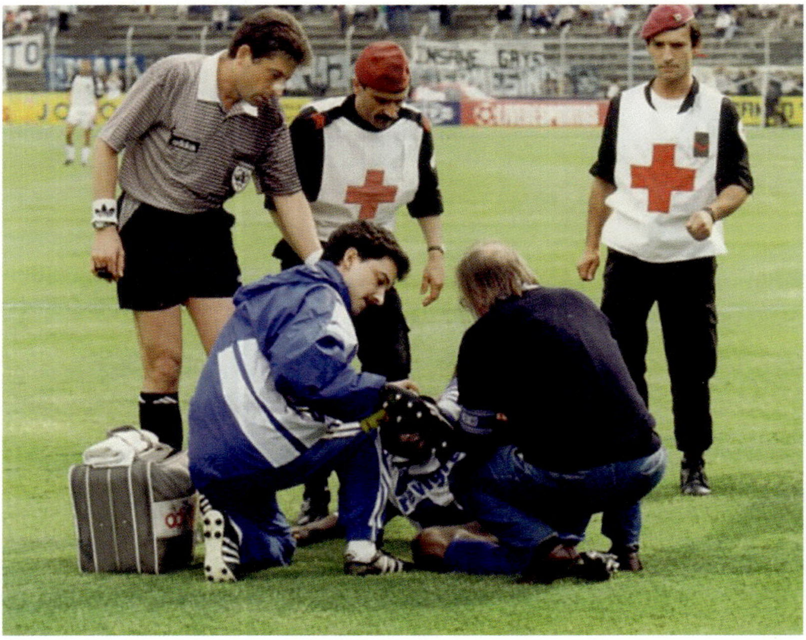

Fig. 4.1 Field case being used during a football game

solve in a very fast and effective way the athletes' injuries and traumas. New treatment techniques along with new products are the result of medical innovation and new technologies. Thus, the field case has included a wide range of products that respond effectively to the needs of modern football. Further ahead, a list of the products that are usually part of a field case will be presented.

4.5 Principles of Its Use: Cautions, Treatment, and Preservation

Footballers work very close to their limits and therefore are extremely predisposed to injuries. Studies and statistical data on field injuries allow us to know how frequently injuries happen. According to Arliani et al. [1], football injuries are estimated in about 10–15 cases to 1000 hours of physical exercise. Most of the injuries affect the lower limbs (70–80%), and most of them are related to knee and ankle joints and thigh brawniness. The same author points out that most of these injuries happen during games and that data help to conclude that an athlete will suffer an injury related to football at least one time a year.

There is a high probability for an athlete to suffer an injury during competition. However, the preventive behavior of the health professionals has deeply contributed to diminish the number of injury occurrences. This way, the athlete's body and balance is always taken into serious consideration. This complex concept – body and balance – is all about achieving the top when it comes to health and well-being [3] (Fig. 4.2).

These perceptions have always led to a wide range of actions that help to avoid or diminish the risks of top-level sport practice, such as football. Being able to properly evaluate an injury is of extreme importance to make the right decisions. In some cases, the best thing to do is to withdraw the player from the game as the injury may get worse. All in all, the response to a serious injury must be quick and efficient so that the situation evolves for the best. The ready use of the first aid kit and the use of specific recovery techniques assure a positive recovery of the athlete's physical condition. This way, it is necessary that the field case includes products and equipment ready to be used in the field.

4.6 The Field Case: Features and Content

The field case must be light, easy to carry, and functional. The products must be stored in a way that facilitates the quick and efficient use of them. The action of properly placing the products is essential. The field case should be ordered

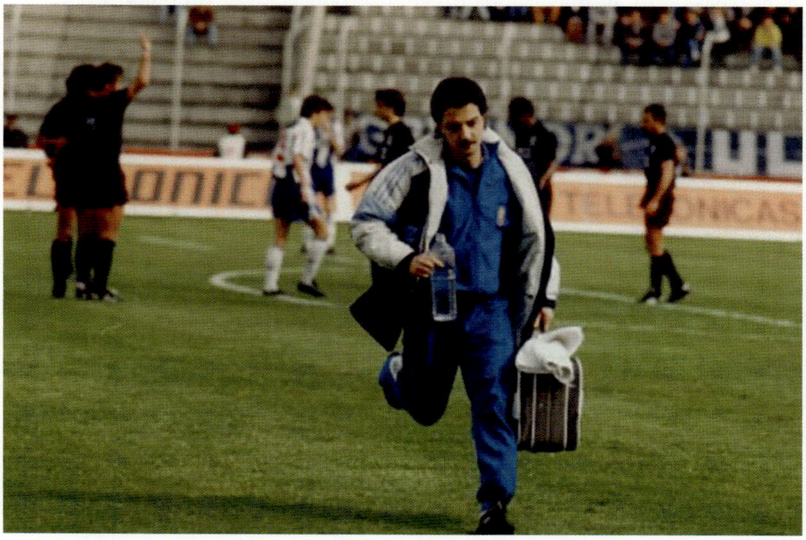

Fig. 4.2 Leaving the football field after a quick use of the field case

Table 4.1 List of products

Iodine solution	Stitch adhesive strips
Hydrogen peroxide	Disposable gloves
Ethyl alcohol	Spray patch
Saline solution	Hambu
Ether solution	Mayo tube
Spongostan	Portable defibrillator
Sterile gauze	Splints (boot and glove type)
Cotton	Scissors
Normal and hypoallergenic patch	Tweezers
Cold spray ethyl	Scalpel
Gel ice power	Elastic wraps
Elastic bandages	Anti-inflammatory drugs
Binding bandages	Painkillers
Adhesive elastic bandage	Antacids
Adhesive nonelastic tapes	Hydrotricine
Neuromuscular patches	Vaseline
Mousse pretape	Antihistamine (cream or gel)
Liquid spray pretape	Cool box
Syringes and needles	Instant ice
Soludacortina	
Tourniquet	
Staples and device	

according to the health professional that is going to use it. The products that make part of it should be of different types in order to give the right response to the different injuries that may occur in a game situation (Table 4.1).

This list of products is presented on an indicative basis, and it may include other products according to the health professional that uses it.

4.7 Guidelines for the Use of the Field Case

Taking decisions in an emergency situation is of huge responsibility since there is a serious risk of affecting the physical, psychological, and emotional condition of the athlete. The health professional that uses the field case must have the adequate education and professional training in order to do his work properly.

My experience allows me to present a wide range of guidelines that all health professionals should take into consideration. The items presented below are just guidelines for the best use of the field case.

The health professional must:

(i). Always act according to the decisions of the Medical Department
(ii). Know about basic life support
(iii). Give first aid efficiently
(iv). Know how to use the products and devices that make part of the field case in a quick and efficient way
(v). Not stress (must stay calm and undisturbed)
(vi). Have the field case ready to use
(vii). Have an ethic attitude when approaching the athlete
(viii). Act to prevent the spread of transmissible diseases
(ix). Be aware that his action plays an important pedagogical role

The presented guidelines point out the fact that these precautions go further than the sport medical area and appeal to the health professional's ecological attitude.

In fact, many agree that football is a violent sport, and we should not ignore this reality. Football is "probably the most spectacular, popular and worldwide sport but also one of the most violent" [2].

Taking this reality into consideration, any field action should contribute to the peace process of sports and appeal to the protection of social positive attitudes. Thus, in an emergency situation, the health professional should reveal his solidary humanism.

Conclusion

The field case is as old as football, and its use has been gaining importance as time goes by. Its content and use have been approved by the scientific community that points out the importance of preserving the athletes' health conditions.

The field case must be handled by professionals with the right education training and that follow the guidelines that assure the best use of it.

References

1. Arliani GG et al. Classificações em Ortopedia e Traumatologia. 1st ed. Manole: São Paulo; 2011.
2. Costa AS. Saúde, violência e desporto. In Desporto, Saúde Bem Estar – Atas das jornadas científicas. Universidade do Porto. Jorge Bento e António Marques ed. 1991, p. 61–74.
3. Moreno A. Desporto, saúde e bem estar. In Desporto, Saúde, Bem Estar – Atas das jornadas científicas. Universidade do Porto. Jorge Bento e António Marques ed. 1991, p. 33–40.
4. Pinto J. A caracterização do esforço no futebol e algumas das suas implicações no treino. In As Ciências do Desporto e a Prática Desportiva – Atas do II Congresso da Educação física dos Países de Língua Portuguesa. Universidade do Porto. Jorge Bento e António Marques ed. 1991, p. 23–34.

5 How to Examine an Athlete on the Field: What You Should Not Miss

Frederico Varandas, Nuno Oliveira, João Pedro Araújo, Paulo Beckert, and Paco Biosca

Contents

5.1 Introduction

Team physicians are part of the game of football. They have the difficult task of having to quickly evaluate the injured athlete, determining the lesion severity and assessing return-to-play strategies.

The environment in which decisions are taken, in the middle of the rush of the game, with the added pressure of the public, referees, and sometimes coaches, makes this a difficult job.

The vast majority of injuries in football are small contusions and bruises that pose no harm to the athlete and allow a safe return to play. On the other hand, the increasing speed and athleticism of the modern game contributes to a vast list of severe injuries that one should be prepared to deal with occasionally.

On this chapter we will focus on the immediate evaluation on the field, approaching medical emergencies and the most frequent musculoskeletal injuries. We will rely on practical examples in order to answer some of the readers' questions.

F. Varandas (✉) • N. Oliveira
Medical Department, Sporting Clube Portugal, Lisbon, Portugal

Comcorpus Clinic – Sports Rehabilitation Center, Lisbon, Portugal
e-mail: frederico_varandas@hotmail.com; npoliveira@sporting.pt

J.P. Araújo
Medical Department, Al Jazira Sports Club, Abu Dhabi, UAE

Clínica do Dragão, Espregueira-Mendes Sports Centre - FIFA Medical Centre of Excellence, Porto, Portugal
e-mail: joaopedroaraujo@gmail.com

P. Beckert
Medical Department, Portuguese National Football Team, Oeiras, Portugal

Clínica CUF Alvalade, Lisbon, Portugal
e-mail: paulobeckert@hotmail.com

P. Biosca
Medical Department, Chelsea Football Club, London, UK
e-mail: Paco.biosca@ChelseaFC.com

J. Espregueira-Mendes et al. (eds.), *Injuries and Health Problems in Football*, DOI 10.1007/978-3-662-53924-8_5

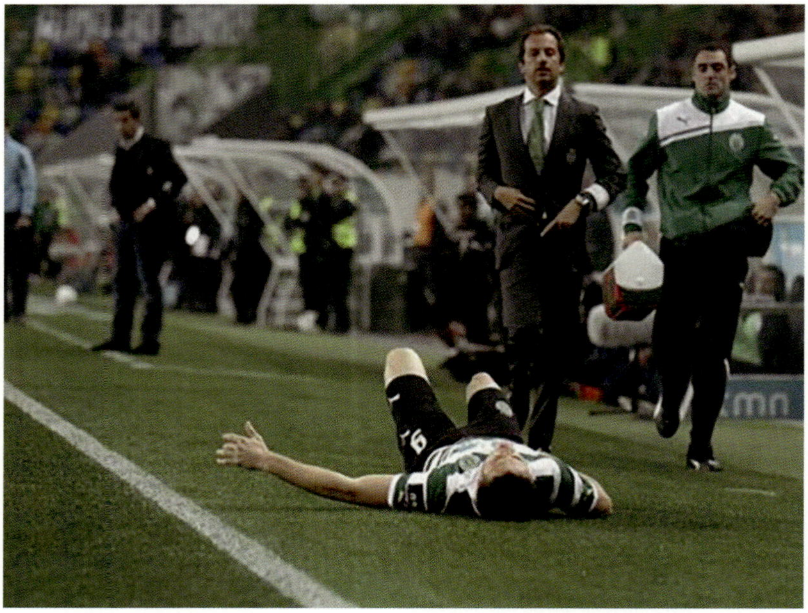

5.2 Emergencies

5.2.1 Head Injuries

In the world of sports, football is unique because of the purposeful use of the unprotected head for controlling and advancing the ball. This skill obviously places the player at risk of head injury.

Head injury can be a result of contact of the head with another head (or other body parts), ground, goalpost, other unknown objects, or even the ball. Such impacts can lead to contusions, fractures, eye injuries, concussions, or even, in rare cases, death.

Correct heading of the ball can rarely be accountable as a cause of acute injury; however, the long-term effects of this repetitive trauma are yet to be determined.

Case 1 A striker is running toward the goal. As he is challenged by the goalkeeper, he incidentally hits his head. The goalkeeper remains lying on the floor, apparently unconscious.

It is thought that the goalkeeper is the position most at risk for head injury and concussions in particular.

Players who exhibit signs or have symptoms of possible head injury must immediately be removed from play and medically evaluated. Unconscious players should be assumed to have a cervical spine injury, and quick attention should be made to address their airway, breathing, and circulatory status, while maintaining spinal immobilization.

Unconscious and unresponsive players should immediately have their cervical spine stabilized.

Immobilization of the cervical spine often complicates airway management in an injured athlete because the cervical spine is ideally splinted in a neutral position. This is most often accomplished by positioning someone at the head of the supine athlete to hold the head in a neutral (in-line) position. Unfortunately, this necessary procedure allows for less access to the airway, with less physical space for the physician to maintain or control the airway at the head of the athlete [1].

Players that have suffered a loss of consciousness should be referred to the emergency department (ED) for further evaluation and head CT scan.

Case 2 As they try to reach for the ball after a goal kick, the central defender from one team

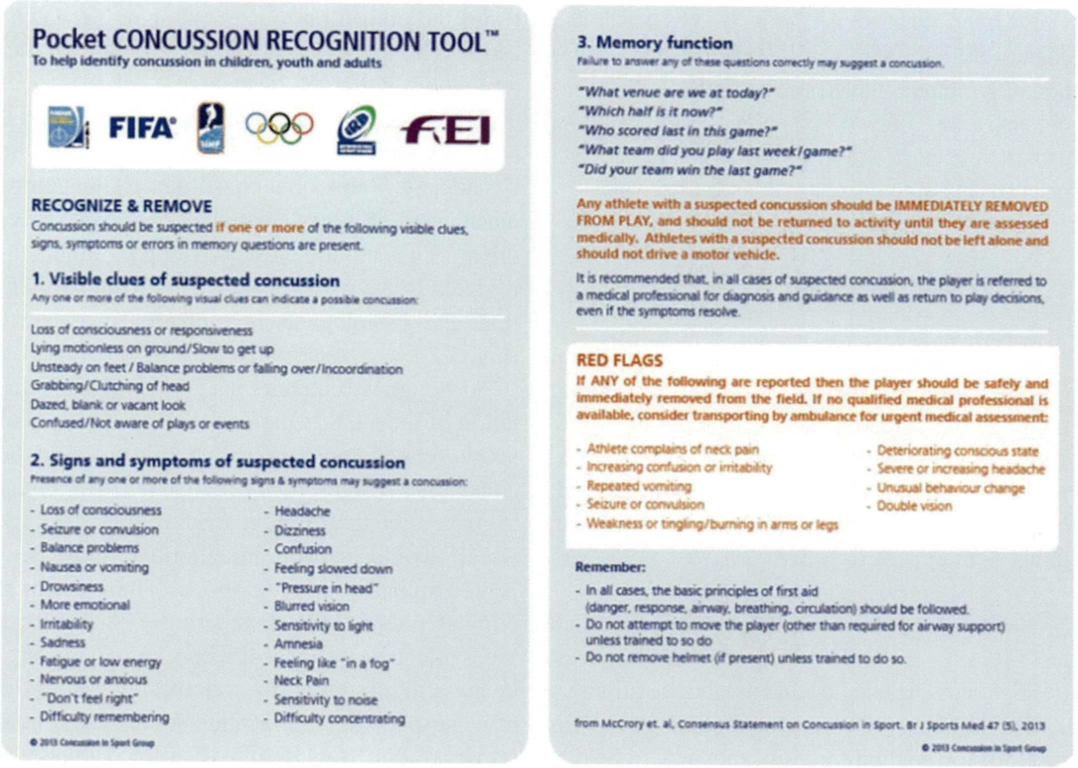

Pocket CONCUSSION RECOGNITION TOOL™
To help identify concussion in children, youth and adults

FIFA FEI

RECOGNIZE & REMOVE
Concussion should be suspected if one or more of the following visible clues, signs, symptoms or errors in memory questions are present.

1. Visible clues of suspected concussion
Any one or more of the following visual clues can indicate a possible concussion:

Loss of consciousness or responsiveness
Lying motionless on ground/Slow to get up
Unsteady on feet / Balance problems or falling over/Incoordination
Grabbing/Clutching of head
Dazed, blank or vacant look
Confused/Not aware of plays or events

2. Signs and symptoms of suspected concussion
Presence of any one or more of the following signs & symptoms may suggest a concussion:

- Loss of consciousness
- Seizure or convulsion
- Balance problems
- Nausea or vomiting
- Drowsiness
- More emotional
- Irritability
- Sadness
- Fatigue or low energy
- Nervous or anxious
- "Don't feel right"
- Difficulty remembering
- Headache
- Dizziness
- Confusion
- Feeling slowed down
- "Pressure in head"
- Blurred vision
- Sensitivity to light
- Amnesia
- Feeling like "in a fog"
- Neck Pain
- Sensitivity to noise
- Difficulty concentrating

© 2013 Concussion in Sport Group

3. Memory function
Failure to answer any of these questions correctly may suggest a concussion.

"What venue are we at today?"
"Which half is it now?"
"Who scored last in this game?"
"What team did you play last week/game?"
"Did your team win the last game?"

Any athlete with a suspected concussion should be IMMEDIATELY REMOVED FROM PLAY, and should not be returned to activity until they are assessed medically. Athletes with a suspected concussion should not be left alone and should not drive a motor vehicle.

It is recommended that, in all cases of suspected concussion, the player is referred to a medical professional for diagnosis and guidance as well as return to play decisions, even if the symptoms resolve.

RED FLAGS
If ANY of the following are reported then the player should be safely and immediately removed from the field. If no qualified medical professional is available, consider transporting by ambulance for urgent medical assessment:

- Athlete complains of neck pain
- Increasing confusion or irritability
- Repeated vomiting
- Seizure or convulsion
- Weakness or tingling/burning in arms or legs
- Deteriorating conscious state
- Severe or increasing headache
- Unusual behaviour change
- Double vision

Remember:
- In all cases, the basic principles of first aid (danger, response, airway, breathing, circulation) should be followed.
- Do not attempt to move the player (other than required for airway support) unless trained to so do
- Do not remove helmet (if present) unless trained to do so.

from McCrory et. al, Consensus Statement on Concussion in Sport. Br J Sports Med 47 (5), 2013

© 2013 Concussion in Sport Group

Fig. 5.1 FIFA's pocket concussion recognition tool

struck his opponent on the head. They both remain sitting on the floor as the two medical teams arrive. The central defender has a vacant look into the sky.

Football is a sport not traditionally identified as high risk for concussions, yet several studies have shown that concussion rates in football are comparable to, and often exceed those of, other contact sports [2].

In conscious patients, a quick survey of the ABCs should be followed by evaluation of spinal tenderness and a neurologic assessment of the upper and lower extremities. Unstable patients should be transported immediately to a medical facility for additional imaging and management.

Symptoms may include headaches, nausea, dizziness, photophobia, fatigue, and difficulty with concentration and memory. Outward signs include loss of consciousness, confusion, amnesia, loss of balance and coordination, and personality changes.

Loss of consciousness (LOC) is not required for a diagnosis of concussion. Only approximately 10% of sports-related concussions include LOC.

There are several pocket guides to help the physician to quickly diagnose a concussion on the field; we normally use the one from the FIFA medical group (Fig. 5.1).

Thorough physical and neurological examination, followed by a quick questionnaire as exampled above, normally provides the diagnosis.

Concussion is a complex pathophysiological process affecting the brain, induced by traumatic biomechanical forces. Direct or indirect transmitted forces due to rotational and/or acceleration-deceleration forces to the brain cause changes at the cellular environment.

All concussed players should be removed from the contest and should not return to play that day. A graded return-to-play guideline should be applied to each athlete, allowing progression based on the individual.

Each individual should be rested physically and cognitively until symptoms resolve. Upon resolution of symptoms, athletes can progress to light aerobic exercise, followed by sport-specific exercise, then non-contact drills, followed by full-contact practice, and eventual return to unrestricted play.

5.2.2 Cervical Spine

Case 3 During a goal kick, a striker and a central defender jump for the ball. On their descending moment, the defender quits and flexes his upper body, leaving the striker falling unchallenged with his head first. At the medical team's arrival, he complains of cervical pain and some tingling in his right upper extremity.

Neck injuries are much less common than head injuries in football. Most are mild injuries (mild sprains, abrasions, and small lacerations).

The mobility of the cervical spine allows for much of the applied forces of the neck to be dissipated through lateral bending, flexion, and extension.

These forces are effectively absorbed through the paravertebral muscles and intervertebral disks. When these mechanisms fail, serious injury occurs.

Most serious neck injuries resulting in fracture or dislocation of the cervical spine usually occur as a result of a fall.

When approaching an athlete complaining with neck pain, the priority is to stabilize cervical spine to prevent further injury.

The next step is to establish the mechanism of injury if it was not witnessed. The following questions will then have to be answered:

- Is the athlete alert and orientated?
- Is there any midline pain?
- Is there any midline effusion, bony tenderness, and step-off on palpation?
- Are there any neurological signs of central injury or paresthesias in the extremities?
- Is he able to actively rotate his head 45° to each side without pain?

The sequence of the questions is fundamental. A negative answer to any of the questions establishes the obligation to cervical spine immobilization and to proceed to the ED for further evaluation (X-ray, CT scan, etc.).

The example above, frequent in recreational and professional football according to the Canadian C-Spine rule, constitutes a "dangerous mechanism of injury" that one could compare to diving. This and the presence of upper limb neurological signs would make C-spine immobilization and radiological investigation mandatory (Fig. 5.2).

Although we consider it a good tool, the limitation of the CCR is the fact that the majority of sports-related mechanisms of injury could be considered dangerous mechanisms (force equal to or greater than falling from a height >3 ft), which would require imaging for most suspected spinal injuries in sports. Thus, personal clinical judgment and experience still play a vital role in assessing sideline spinal injuries, keeping in mind that if a serious spinal injury is ever suspected, appropriate stabilization and transportation for definitive care should be implemented [3].

5.3 Upper Extremity

5.3.1 Shoulder

Case 4 During an under-19 game, two players try to reach the same ball; as they try to gain control of the ball, they run shoulder to shoulder, and one of them succumbs to the pressure and falls, landing on his right shoulder. The referee immediately calls for medical assistance.

In the last years, shoulder injuries have represented an increasing health problem in football players. The modern football has been characterized by high-speed game, "dangerous" tactical solutions such as pressing and marking, and augmented number of legal and illegal physical contacts.

It is always helpful for the medical staff to watch the mechanism of injury. When dealing with shoulder injuries, this assumes a capital importance in order to rapidly perform a diagnosis.

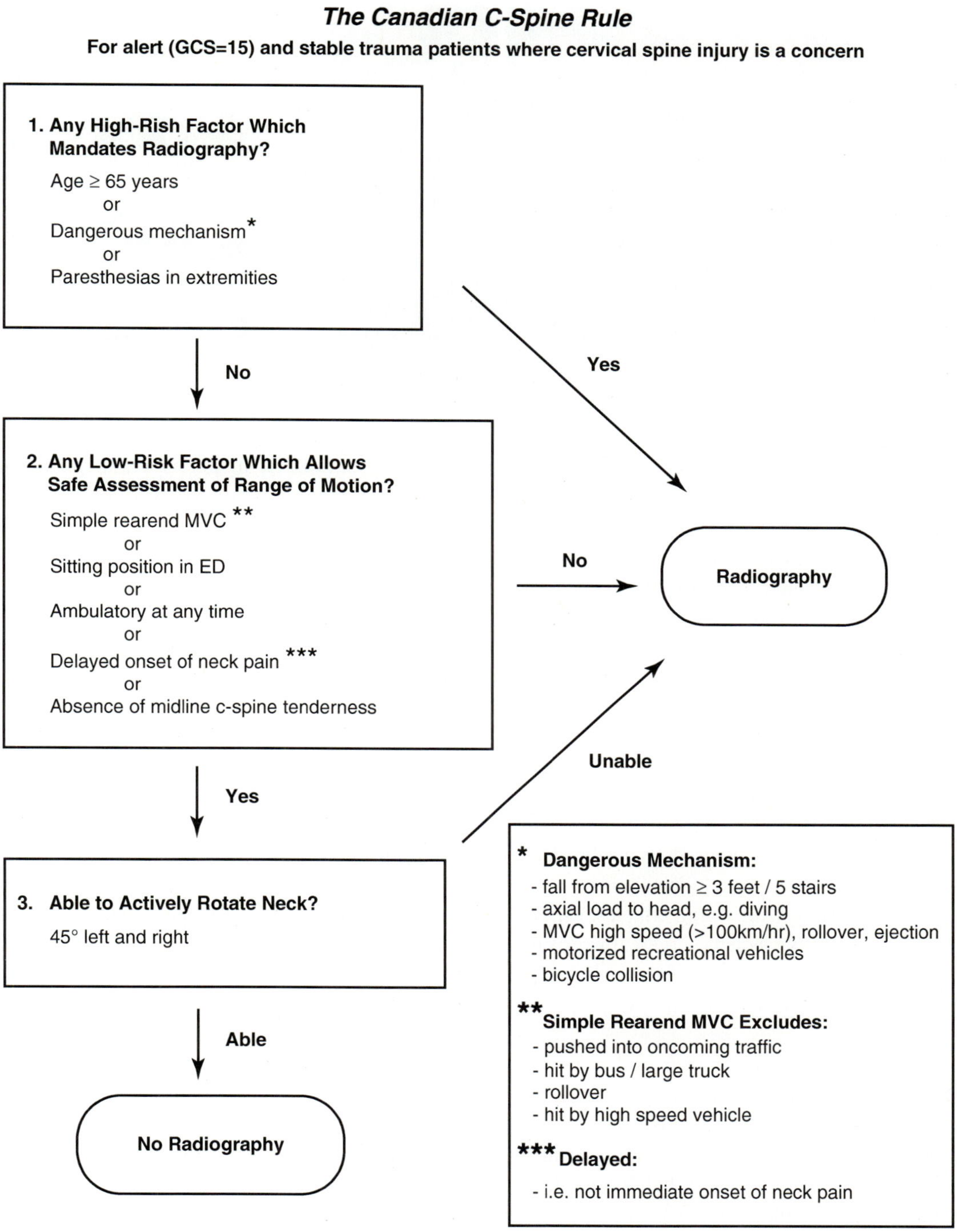

Fig. 5.2 Canadian C-spine rule

The first question to answer is: What was the position of the arm at the time of trauma? Was it in abduction or in adduction?

One should then proceed to do a careful inspection and palpation of the shoulder girdle on the field.

5.3.1.1 Shoulder

Dislocation normally occurs after a trauma where the arm is in abduction and external rotation. The athlete may have a history of shoulder instability, but most often in football, we deal with a traumatic isolated episode.

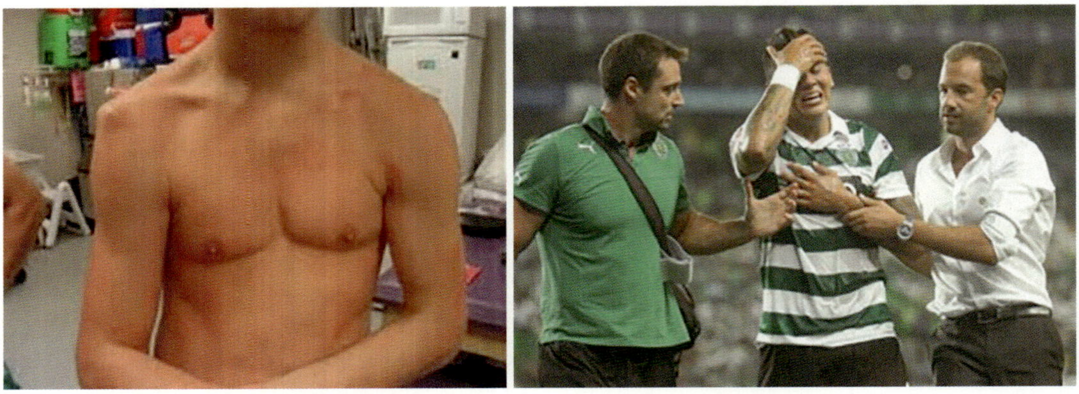

Removing of the shirt will facilitate clinical examination. Inspection reveals the loss of the round shape of the shoulder, and as 90% of the luxations are anteroinferior, palpation of the humeral head on the armpit is possible.

Shoulder dislocations are very stressful events both for the athlete and for the medical team. Players are in pain, anxious, and most often unwilling to move their arm. We discourage any attempt to make the reduction of the articulation on the field by inexperienced personnel. Neurovascular status should be checked. Presence of numbness on the arm, forearm, or hand is a sign of neurological damage. Asymmetry of the radial pulse should also be checked. These athletes should be immobilized on an arm sling and proceed to the hospital for X-ray evaluation and then reduction [4].

When dealing with young athletes, especially under-12, team physicians should always suspect of a proximal humeral fracture through the epiphysis when confronted with major deformity of the shoulder.

5.3.1.2 Acromioclavicular

Acromioclavicular (AC) joint separations are common injuries of the shoulder girdle; in football they account for nearly half of all shoulder injuries among athletes involved in contact sports.

Typically, the mechanism of this injury is a direct force against the lateral aspect of the adducted shoulder or a fall on an outstretched hand (FOOH), the magnitude of which affects injury severity.

The acromioclavicular joint is a diarthrodial articulation with an interposed fibrocartilaginous meniscal disk that links the hyaline cartilage articular surfaces of the acromial process and the clavicle. The joint is horizontally and vertically stabilized in anterior and posterior translation by a combination of dynamic muscular and static ligamentous structures, which allow a normal anatomic range of motion. Because of the transverse orientation of the articulation, direct downward forces may result in shear stresses that cause disruption of these stabilizing structures and create displacement beyond the normal limits. This is evidenced by abnormal positioning of the clavicle relative to the acromion, usually in the superior direction [5].

Rockwood classified AC joint dislocations in six grades as seen on the table below (Fig. 5.3):

When approaching an athlete with shoulder trauma, the medical staff should mentally reconstitute the mechanism of injury. Acromioclavicular injuries in football are usually low energy (I–III).

Clinical signs vary from:

- Pain/tenderness on AC joint with no deformity (Grade I)
- Pain on AC joint and lateral clavicle becomes a little more prominent (Grade II)
- In type III sprains, the force applied to the shoulder completely disrupts the acromioclavicular and coracoclavicular ligaments, leading to complete separation of the clavicle and obvious changes in appearance. The lateral clavicle is very prominent

Grade I injuries do not compromise AC joint stability and are compatible with completion of

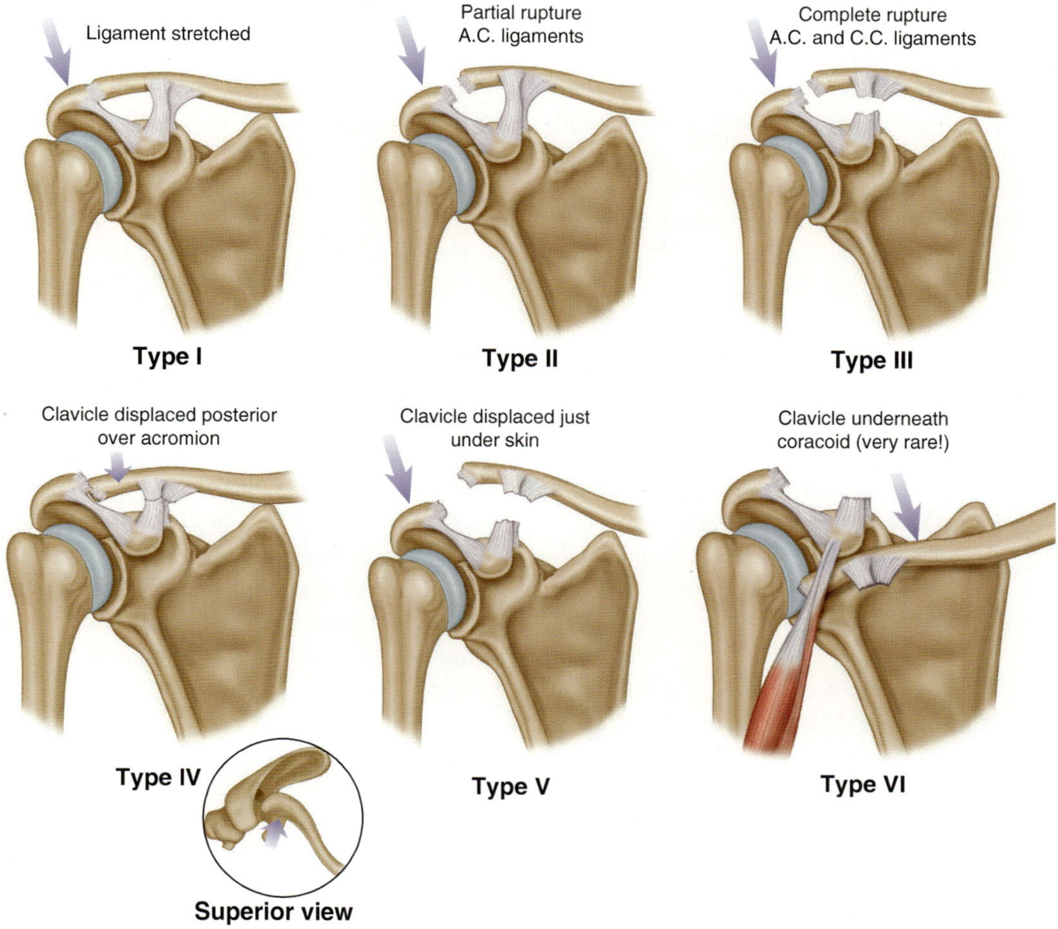

Fig. 5.3 Rockwood classification of AC joint dislocations

the game especially on the professional setting, depending on the athlete's pain tolerance.

Grade II and III injuries are painful; ligamentous rupture dictates that the athlete abandons the field and shoulder put to rest on an arm sling until further investigation.

5.3.1.3 Clavicle

Case 5 A 9-year-old player incidentally steps on an opponent; he falls on his left shoulder. As the coach and referee approach, he is sitting, yelling in pain. His shoulder has no gross deformity, but there is a small bruising and pain when the middle third of his clavicle is palpated.

Clavicle fractures can occur after a direct impact on the shoulder or FOOH mechanism.

Athletes will pinpoint the site of injury. Inspection will most often show some degree of deformity, bruising, and occasionally skin suffering as the clavicle lays subcutaneously [6].

When there is a suspicion of clavicle fracture, the athlete should be withdrawn from the field and immobilized on an arm sling, and further X-ray investigation should be provided.

Pediatric population is especially vulnerable to this type of injury.

5.3.2 Elbow

Elbow injuries are less common in football than in other contact sports. The vast majority are small soft tissue contusions that allow for safe return to play. However, elbow dislocations and fractures can occur.

When evaluating a painful elbow, the following aspects should be taken into consideration:

- Is there any major deformity?
- Does the athlete have full range of motion?
- Is strength symmetrical?
- Can he perform football-specific activity?

If an elbow dislocation (90% of which are posterior or posterolateral displacement of the forearm relative to the humerus) or fracture is suspected, the athlete should be immobilized in a 90 degree, well-padded posterior splint and evacuated to ED for further investigation.

5.3.3 Wrist and Hand

Case 6 During the preparation of a corner kick, the index finger of the central defender gets stuck on the shirt of his opponent. As they fight for positioning, he feels a "pop." He approaches the bench with an obvious deformity on the proximal interphalangeal joint.

Wrist and hand injuries can be assessed in a similar manner to elbow injuries – the previously listed questions will need to be answered.

When evaluating a wrist injury, attention should be placed on bony tenderness, especially snuffbox tenderness, crepitus, local swelling, and obvious deformity, as well as functional status.

Hand and finger injuries account for 9% of all sports injuries because they are the most active portion of the upper extremity and the least protected. Again, athletes with suspected fractures should be withheld from play until appropriate X-rays can be obtained. Interphalangeal (IP) joint dislocations, collateral ligament sprains of IP joints, and mallet fingers typically can be reduced on the sideline and protected by buddy taping if the athlete wants to return to play. In cases of jersey fingers, ulnar collateral ligament sprains, and metacarpophalangeal dislocations, return is not advised.

5.4 Lower Extremity

Injuries of the lower extremities have a greater incidence in football. The fact that the ball is driven by the feet makes understandably more likely that traumatic incidents affecting the knee, leg, ankle, and foot occur.

Fortunately, the vast majority of these injuries are abrasions and contusions that do not endanger players. However, physicians should be prepared to deal with complex patterns of lesion especially concerning the knee and ankle joints.

When evaluating lower extremity injuries, the most important question is: can the athlete bear weight? An athlete unable to bear weight obviously increases the likelihood of long bone fracture. However, the ability to fully or partially bear weight does not exclude all fractures and definitely does not clear the athlete to restart competition.

5.4.1 Hip

Traumatic injuries of the femoroacetabular joint and labrum are relatively infrequent in contact sports, including football. Extra-articular injuries to the hip region are reported more frequently, such as bone and soft tissue contusions to the iliac crest and fossa, and sprains and strains of the soft tissues of the hip and pelvic girdle [7].

Again, team physicians should have a systematic approach and evaluate:

- Can the athlete bear weight?
- Does he have full range of motion?
- Is strength symmetrical?
- Can he perform football-specific tasks?

When evaluating muscle injuries around the hip, one should ask how the beginning of pain was. In case of rupture, athletes will mention a sudden "stinging" and the region involved will be easily pointed. Isometric contraction and especially resisted contraction will elicit pain.

Muscle strains can happen in any of the muscles crossing the hip joint with a higher incidence on the hip flexors. Forceful contraction against resistance is the most common mechanism of injury as well as sprinting.

In pediatric populations, one should be alert to growth plate avulsion fractures. Although avulsion fractures of the anterior superior iliac spine are rare, it can be seen in adolescents, as a result of sudden vigorous contraction or repetitive contraction of the sartorius and tensor fasciae latae muscles. This injury is typically accompanied by a "pop" at the time of injury, can be quite painful, and can be very difficult to put weight on the leg.

5.4.2 Knee

The on-the-field assessment of an acute knee injury should be as brief but as thorough as possible and include history taking and initial physical exam. The goal is to rule out a fracture, dislocation, or neurovascular injury.

5.4.2.1 Mechanism

Regarding the mechanism of injury, the following questions should be answered. Was there contact with another player? What was the position of the leg/foot? What sensations were felt?

In contact injuries it is important to determine where the site of the blow was. Most often ligamentous injuries will occur on the opposite site to the blow (e.g., external impact, valgus stress, medial collateral injury).

A description of the athlete's injury-related sensations, such as tearing or an audible pop, can also facilitate the diagnosis. For example, a pop typically indicates an anterior cruciate ligament (ACL) tear, while a tearing sensation often accompanies a medial collateral ligament (MCL) tear.

5.4.2.2 Initial Evaluation

Immediate on the field examination includes inspection of the skin and major deformity.

Contact injuries such as fractures or dislocations are not subtle; deformity, hemarthrosis, and even abnormal distal pulses can be observed.

It is especially important to check neurovascular status of the limb if a tibiofemoral dislocation is suspected.

Fortunately, these injuries are rare, and priority will be to gently align (with axial traction) and stabilize the lower extremity in order to safely proceed to hospital facility where further investigation will be done.

Patellar dislocations can be reduced on the field by medial traction and knee extension.

Inspection of the skin is important as the site of the blow will be evident. Immediate effusion may indicate hemarthrosis and intra-articular injury such as LCA rupture, meniscal fracture, or osteochondral lesion.

In more subtle cases where initial inspection is normal and the team physician is asked to clear the athlete for competition, one should perform a systematic examination of the knee on the sideline:

- Range of motion: Full extension (comparison with the opposite site) and full flexion. Pain or blocking could be present in meniscal tears or osteochondral injuries
- Stability tests (tibiofemoral joint): Varus/valgus stress tests, Lachman test and anterior/posterior drawer tests, and dial test
- Patellofemoral joint: Palpation of the extensor mechanism looking for pain or any step-off. Pain on the medial patellofemoral ligament/internal retinaculum confirmed by a positive patellar apprehension test could indicate patellofemoral instability

Normally, on the sideline the athlete can indicate the area of pain and guide the medical staff in order to shorten the examination. For the injured athlete to return to play, he must have full range of motion of the knee, nonsignificant swelling, weight-bearing ability, and the ability to play his specific position [8].

It is especially important on the cases where the athlete is cleared to finish the game, to perform a full post-match examination, in proper facilities after cooling down.

5.4.3 Ankle and Foot

Ankle and foot injuries have a high incidence in football. While the most common injury is the ankle sprain, complex injuries like fractures, ligament tears, and cartilage damage can occur. Such injuries have a high impact on the player's career.

The majority of injuries are caused by tackles involving lateral or medial forces that created a corresponding eversion or inversion rotation of the foot or ankle.

Case 7 A striker suffers a tackle during his progression with the ball. He sustains a direct blow on his medial malleolus causing the inversion of his left ankle (Fig. 5.4). When approaching the athlete, he complains of pain around the ankle and especially on the external aspect of his foot.

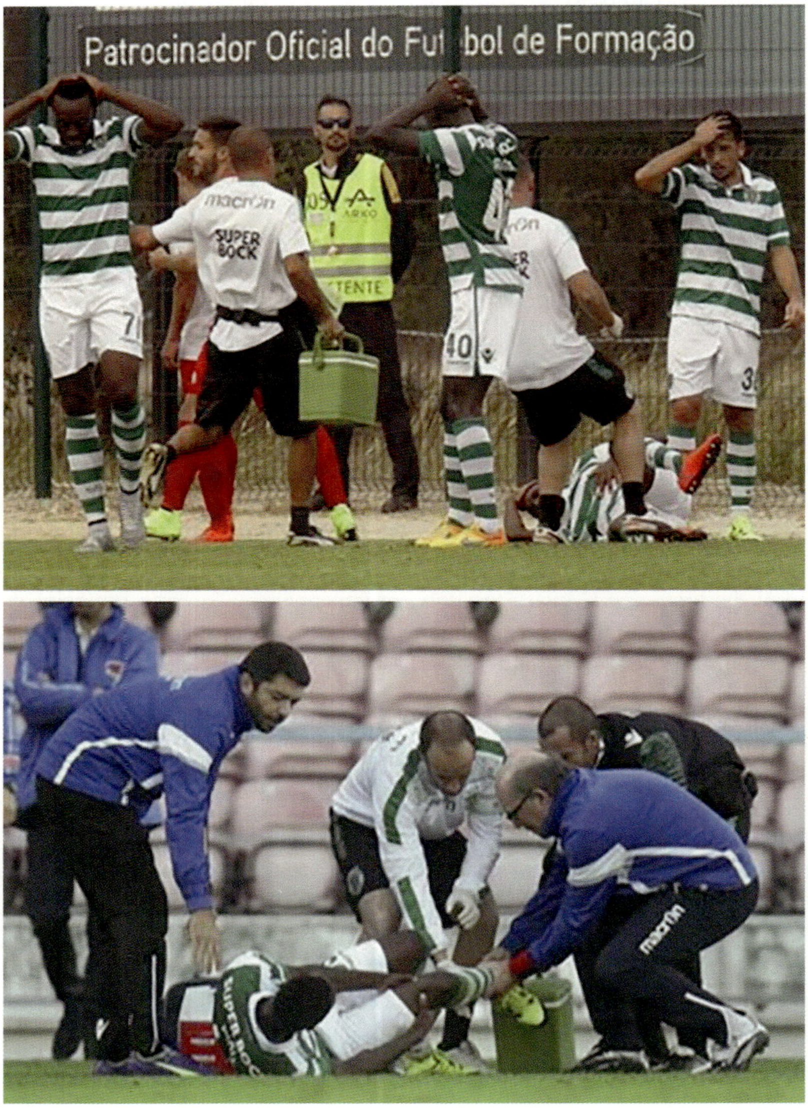

Fig. 5.4 Field injury

As with other lower limb injuries, the initial focus should be to distinguish between potentially dangerous injuries and the ones that can allow a safe (sometimes protected) return to play.

Ankle fractures and fracture/dislocations are rare in football but can occur. In these situations, the priority is to obtain a correct alignment of the ankle in order to reduce pain, avoid neurovascular compromise, and allow splinting of the extremity for a safe transfer to hospital facilities.

Open fractures should be suspected when a laceration is seen overlying the deformity. Care should be taken to clean the wound and cover it with moist sterile dressings. These injuries require emergent care, including intravenous antibiotics, irrigation, and debridement in the operating room.

Fortunately, the vast majority of ankle injuries are more subtle. As mentioned above, soft tissue injuries including external ankle sprains have a high incidence in football.

When approaching the athlete, the focus should be in finding the answer to these questions:

- Mechanism of injury
- Site of pain
- Bony or soft tissue tenderness
- Swelling
- Ability to bear weight

Given the strong correlation between the mechanism of injury and diagnosis, identifying the joint position at the time of injury is a useful first step in the clinical evaluation.

The Ottawa ankle rules can guide physicians on a systematic approach and avoid unnecessary X-ray (Fig. 5.5).

When performing physical examination of football athletes after what they consider "another ankle sprain," attention should be given to the base of the fifth metatarsal. Varus alignment of the knee and ankle, common in footballers, with increased loads on the external aspect of the feet

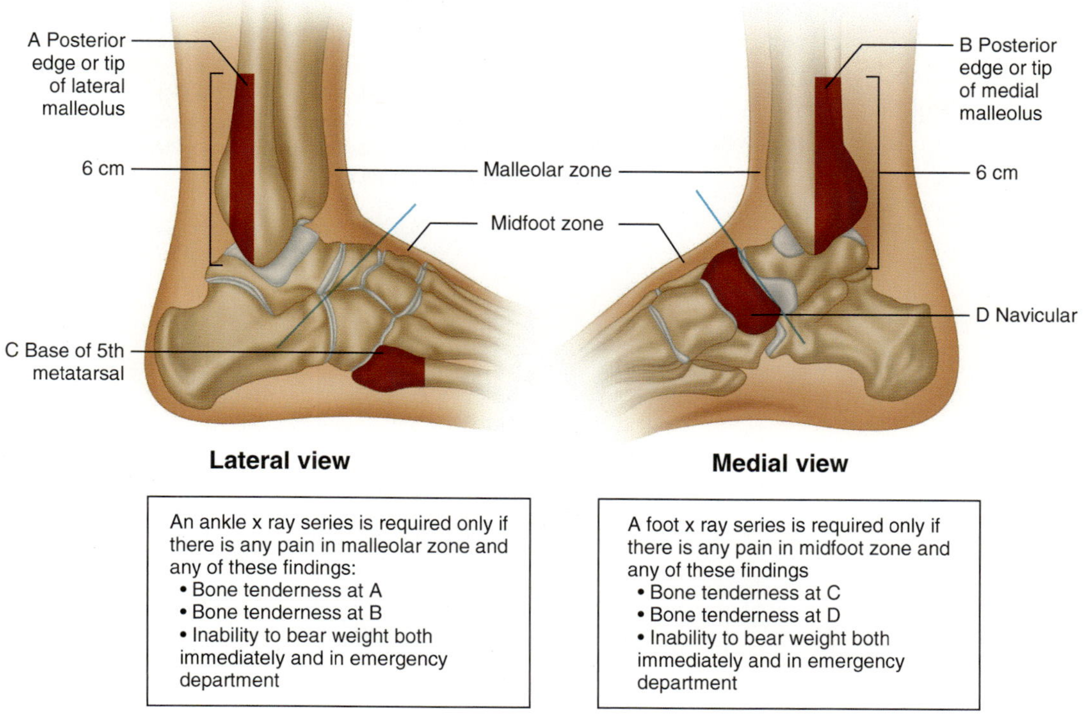

Fig. 5.5 Ottawa ankle rules

predisposes them to "stress" fractures of the fifth metatarsal. Such fractures can become clinically evident after a minor ankle sprain.

Special attention should be given to syndesmotic ankle sprains or "high" ankle sprains. Pain/tenderness over the anterior syndesmotic ligament, pain in dorsiflexion, inability to bear weight, and a positive "squeeze test" should raise suspicion of an injury to the syndesmosis. The fact that there is often not much edema on the external side of the ankle may confuse the medical staff.

Lisfranc injuries also can occur in football and are often misdiagnosed. An axial load on a plantar flexed foot can be the mechanism of injury. Pain will be disproportionate when comparing with the physical findings. Weight bearing, single toe raises, and mobilization of the middle foot will elicit pain. These players should be withdrawn from the game.

Conclusion

The sideline management of football injuries is a difficult and complex task for team physicians. Priority is to quickly triage potentially life- or limb-threatening situations. Prompt assessment of neurovascular and functional status by the sideline provider is required. Decisions have to be made in a short time frame with no imaging available.

One should rely on evidenced-based guiding tools to help in decision-making on such a difficult environment.

The safety of the player, especially in the youth teams, should always be in the mind of the medical staff.

References

1. Delaney JS, Al-Kashmiri A, Baylis PJ, Troutman T, Aljufaili M, Correa JA. The assessment of airway maneuvers and interventions in university Canadian football, ice hockey, and soccer players. J Athl Train. 2011;46(2):117–25.
2. Levy ML, Kasasbeh AS, Baird LC, Amene C, Skeen J, Marshall L. Concussions in soccer: a current understanding. World Neurosurg. 2012;78(5):535–44.
3. Al-Kashmiri A, Delaney JS. Head and neck injuries in football (soccer). Trauma. 2006;8:189–95.
4. Longo UG, Loppini M, Berton A, Martinelli N, Maffulli N, Denaro V. Shoulder injuries in soccer players. Clin Cases Miner Bone Metab. 2012;9(3):138–41.
5. Warth RJ, Martetschläger F, Gaskill TR, Millett PJ. Acromioclavicular joint separations. Curr Rev Muscoskelet Med. 2013;6(1):71–8.
6. Schupp CM. Sideline evaluation and treatment of bone and joint injury. Curr Sports Med Rep. 2009;8(3):119–24.
7. Callahan W, Chang CJ. Sideline evaluation and management of acute hip trauma in a collegiate athlete. Curr Sports Med Rep. 2008;7(5):281–3.
8. LaPrade RF, Wentorf F. Acute knee injuries on-the-field and sideline evaluation. Phys Sports Med. 1999;27(10):55–61.

Principles of Rehabilitation

6

João Pedro Araújo, Isabel Lopes,
Filipe Guimarães, and Vítor Moreira

Contents

J.P. Araújo (✉)
Clínica do Dragão, Espregueira – Mendes Sports Centre – FIFA Medical Centre of Excellence, Porto, Portugal

Medical Department, Al Jazira Football Club, Dubai, UAE
e-mail: joaopedroaraujo@gmail.com

I. Lopes
Clínica do Dragão, Espregueira – Mendes Sports Centre – FIFA Medical Centre of Excellence, Porto Portugal
e-mail: isabelcameiralopes@gmail.com

F. Guimarães • V. Moreira
Sporting Clube de Braga, Football SAD, BRAGA Portugal
e-mail: filipeguimaraes@hotmail.com; vitorvarandasmoreira@gmail.com

After the injury occurrence and the start of rehabilitation period, several factors need to be addressed for a correct diagnosis, prognosis, and progression throughout this period. The progression should be carried in a way to assure simultaneous quickest return of the player to training and competition while minimizing the risk of recurrence or future associated injuries. To attend to the two latter conditions, the player should fulfill a number of specific criterions, set after the establishment of an accurate diagnosis and a full comprehensive rehabilitation program. While professional sport very often presents competition timings and very often economic interests (for both entities and players) that may increase the demand of a quick return to training and competition, the factor time should never be taken in isolation for decision-making processes.

6.1 Diagnosis

Establishing a correct diagnosis is a key aspect for a right planning of a rehabilitation plan. Diagnostic sequence and tests have been addressed in other chapters of this book, according to each type of injury. However, for the purposes of a correct establishment of the rehabilitation plan, there are four main issues that are crucial for a correct diagnosis:

J. Espregueira-Mendes et al. (eds.), *Injuries and Health Problems in Football*,
DOI 10.1007/978-3-662-53924-8_6

Mechanism of injury – valuable information to the diagnosis and further rehabilitation is obtained solely for understanding how the injury happened, not only because different mechanisms will typically affect different anatomic locations [1] with different healing characteristics and rehabilitation needs but also because a proper reeducation of the injury gesture should be achieved before a return to training. This could be, e.g., a progression in running speeds and distances while sprinting in the case of hamstring injuries sustained under this mechanism, or a progressive shooting plan after a rectus femoris muscle strain, also if this was the gesture responsible for the injury.

Previous injury – history of previous injuries in the same location as the injury currently under examination or it is also a valuable addiction when collecting information from the player. This fact is especially related with (re)injury risk as it is from general consensus that a previous injury increases the risk for (re) injury [2].

Location – the importance of the injury location is specifically related with the healing properties of the injured tissue due to vascularization issues or factors such as load absorption which may predispose more the structure to failure if compared with locations with less demands regarding the latter.

Grade – the aim of grading is to reflect the extension of the injury, after a location is identified. Although there is ongoing discussion around the currently grading systems for certain types of injuries [3, 4, 5], a higher or lower grade of an injury is generally related with its prognosis.

6.2 Healing Stages and Loading Throughout Rehabilitation

For a correct implementation of a rehabilitation plan, it is essential to understand the course of healing after injury, either if this refers to a minor joint injury such as a grade I sprain or a postsurgery process. Loading through exercise is an essential component of a rehabilitation plan, once it will be through loading the right stimulus for human tissue proliferation and collagen synthesis, components of all types of musculoskeletal structures [6, 7, 8, 9]. It will also be through the form of strength training and other types of exercises (e.g., neuromuscular control, balance, mobilization) that improvements in the tolerance thresholds of load absorption by the injured structured will be achieved, allowing progressions during the rehabilitation. However, this loading input through exercise needs to be adapted or even suspended according to the injury nature and the stage of the healing process, in order to not compromise the latter; otherwise, it may result in a delayed or insufficient rehabilitation.

Therefore, one have to attend that if in a muscle injury addressed conservatively, the acute stage and protective phase after injury may require no more than a few days, with loading through full weight bearing and strength exercises starting after 3 to 5 days post injury, modified according to the athlete's tolerance, the same will not be applied after, e.g., a fracture, in which immobilization and protection are normally required for longer periods.

6.3 Progression Criterion

The importance of establishing markers for progression during sports injury rehabilitation will have the double purpose of helping to implement a plan of treatment to achieve the goals of each stage while also promoting a safe progression and therefore decreasing the risk of setbacks or reinjury.

We can define "Progression criteria in rehabilitation as a combination of subjective and objective markers that the athlete must fulfill before progressing in the treatment program, considering the biological healing process, injury risk factors, and injury mechanism." These markers are established considering several clinical and functional parameters, and although there are some minor variations between musculoskeletal structures (e.g., the presence of visual effusion should be addressed when assessing a joint such as the knee and the ankle, while a muscle does not present an identical typical sign), most of them are similar across different injury locations.

Acute stages following characterized by inflammatory signs such as pain, swelling, and redness along with functional limitations such as loss of range of motion and strength or intolerance to weight bearing in case of lower limb injuries are normally present in a first moment and should be controlled before progressing to the following stage. Decreases in these acute signs and strength and range of motion improvements, tolerance to weight bearing, or decreases in pain during daily life activities (e.g., for lower limb injuries) are normally signs that indicate that the affected area is ready for a progression. Higher markers of functionality such as maximum strength capability, full range of motion, and ability to full weight bearing while performing neuromuscular control and balance tasks are additional indicators to allow progression until a final stage where specific football-related tasks are introduced during monitored outfield work.

For a better understanding of the practicality of these markers, we suggest an example of progression for a grade 2 muscle injury during the course of rehabilitation. Fig. 6.1 shows how to link the different stages during the progression of the rehabilitation and the markers that should be reached before introducing load increments to the injured muscle.

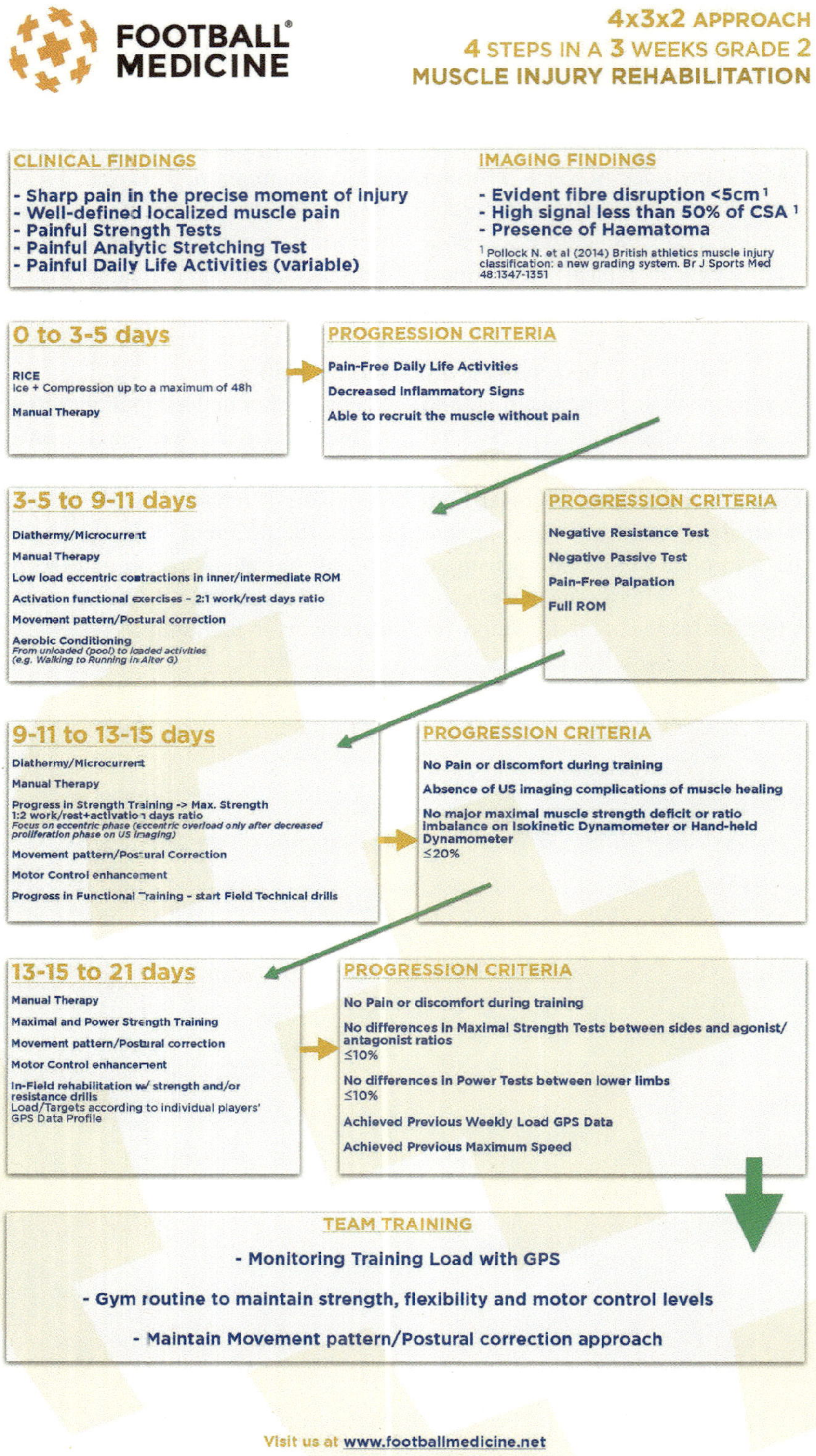

Fig. 6.1 Grade 2 muscle injury rehabilitation and progression criterion (adapted from www.footballmedicine.net and used under permission of Football Medicine®)

References

1. Askling C, Saartok T, Thorstensson A. Type of acute hamstring strain affects flexibility, strength, and time to return to pre-injury level. Br J Sports Med. 2006;40(1):40–4.
2. Hägglund M, Waldén M, Ekstrand J. Risk factors for lower extremity muscle injury in professional soccer: The UEFA Injury Study. Am J Sports Med. 2013;41(2):327–35.
3. Tol JL, Hamilton B, Best TM. Palpating muscles, massaging the evidence? An editorial relating to 'Terminology and classification of muscle injuries in sport: The Munich consensus statement'. Br J Sports Med. 2013;47(6):340–1.
4. Pollock N, James SL, Lee JC, Chakraverty R. British athletics muscle injury classification: A new grading system. Br J Sports Med. 2014;48(18):1347–51.
5. Mueller-Wohlfahrt HW, Haensel L, Mithoefer K, Ekstrand J, English B, McNally S, et al. Terminology and classification of muscle injuries in sport: The Munich consensus statement. Br J Sports Med. 2013;47(6):342–50.
6. Järvinen TA, Järvinen TL, Kääriäinen M, Äärimaa V, Vaittinen S, Kalimo H, et al. Muscle injuries: Optimising recovery. Best Pract Res Clin Rheumatol. 2007;21(2):317–31.
7. LaStayo PC, Woolf JM, Lewek MD, Snyder-Mackler L, Reich T, Lindstedt SL. Eccentric muscle contractions: their contribution to injury, prevention, rehabilitation, and sport. J Orthop Sports Phys Ther. 2003;33(10):557–71.
8. Simanski CJ, Maegele MG, Lefering R, Lehnen DM, Kawel N, Riess P, et al. Functional treatment and early weightbearing after an ankle fracture: A prospective study. J Orthop Trauma. 2006;20(2):108–14.
9. Vasarhelyi A, Baumert T, Fritsch C, Hopfenmüller W, Gradl G, Mittlmeier T. Partial weight bearing after surgery for fractures of the lower extremity–is it achievable? Gait Posture. 2006;23(1):99–105.

Part II

Anatomy, Biomechanics and Imaging

Basics on Knee (dys)Function

7

Rogério Pereira, Ricardo Vidal, Ana Leal, and Maria Amélia Ferreira

Content

R. Pereira (✉)
Clínica do Dragão, Espregueira-Mendes Sports Centre – FIFA Medical Centre of Excellence, Porto, Portugal

Faculty of Health Sciences, University of Fernando Pessoa, Porto, Portugal

Faculty of Sports, University of Porto, Porto, Portugal

Dom Henrique Research Centre, Porto, Portugal
e-mail: rp@espregueira.com

R. Vidal
Clínica do Dragão, Espregueira-Mendes Sports Centre – FIFA Medical Centre of Excellence, Porto, Portugal
e-mail: rvidal@espregueira.com

A. Leal
Clínica do Dragão, Espregueira-Mendes Sports Centre – FIFA Medical Centre of Excellence, Porto, Portugal

Dom Henrique Research Centre, Porto, Portugal

CMEMS Center for MicroElectroMechanical Systems, Mechanical Engineering Department, University of Minho, Guimarães, Portugal
e-mail: anaisabeleal@gmail.com

7.1 Introduction

The athlete's body is in constant adaptation, i.e., the mechanotransduction phenomenon in *stricto sensu* and all the genotype-environment interactions in *lato sensu* occur in a continuum, delivering structural and functional effects which have their implications for recovering, maintenance, and development of the human organism. Part of these effects can be somewhat predictable, and therefore we can establish goals such as motor and physical improvements. This is possible through specific exercise prescription that can offer recovering, enhancing, and/or preventive physical and functional alterations. This has particular importance in the lower limb injuries since epidemiological studies clearly report the high incidence and severity in this body segment [1, 2]. Among etiological factors, several are non-modifiable such as height, race, genetic and hereditary factors, gender, bone morphology, and others [3, 4]. In which concerns modifiable factors, it is crucial to know the etiology and risk factors related with the different injuries. It is indispensable to comprehend the regional sports biomechanics, the interdependence with the other body segments, and the cross implications within

M.A. Ferreira
Faculty of Medicine, University of Porto, Porto, Portugal
e-mail: mameliaferreira@gmail.com

J. Espregueira-Mendes et al. (eds.), *Injuries and Health Problems in Football*,
DOI 10.1007/978-3-662-53924-8_7

skeleton, passive stabilizers, nervous system, muscular actions, and, clearly, normal functioning of all the other organic systems. Nonetheless, within the particular scope of human motion, the subsequent discussion aims a succinct and integrative overview on global lower limb function. Thus, lower limb kinematics, passive and active stabilizers, and kinetics determinants are implied for targeted, safe, and effective performance. Even so, all this acting together and properly is not, by its own, a warranty of safeness and high performance for footballers. It has been reported the factors such as kinesiophobia, being more likely after a severe injury such as an anterior cruciate ligament tear, may impair significantly the ability to return and perform at the previous level [5–7].

7.2 Motor Control is a Challenge

Dynamic and static stability, normal patterns of motion, and limb symmetry, when suitable for motor goals, require integrity and correct alignment of lower limbs and different structures to function adequately and synergically. In fact, when high-intensity and multiplanar dynamic actions are in play, there is an impressive need to a complex interplay between different segments based on an almost perfect formula for force distribution over joints, time, and space, leading to safe and goal-oriented motor skills.

7.3 Lower Limb Dysfunction: Theoretical Rationale

Beyond the classification, degrees of freedom, movement patterns, and normal range of motion of the major joints (Tables 7.1, 7.2, and 7.3) [8] – without underestimating the relevance of foot joints for biomechanical behavior of the all superjacent joints – we intend to draw attention to abnormal conditions that can result or lead to lower limb dysfunction and predispose to injury and/or performance impairment or reinjury. In which concerns laxity, understood as described by Musahl et al. [9] as the passive articular response to an externally applied force or torque, and particularly taking as example posteroanterior knee laxity resulting from anterior cruciate ligament rupture [10–12], it correlates with higher peak of ACL strain in situations of anterior tibial translations and cadaveric simulated landing [13]. Thus, this arthrokinematic permissiveness (which can be greater if we add other ligaments with potential insufficiency or major menisci tear) along with perturbations driven by motor tasks [14] and specially by dynamic high-risk activities may cause an insta-

Table 7.1 Type, degrees of freedom, movement patterns, and range of motion of the hip joint

Joint	Plane	Movement	Range of motion
Hip (ball-and-socket synovial joint)	Sagittal	Flexion Extension Hyperextension	120 120 20
	Frontal	Adduction Abduction	25 40
	Transverse	Internal rotation External rotation	45 45

Table 7.2 Type, degrees of freedom, movement patterns, and range of motion of the knee joint

Joint	Plane	Movement	Range of motion
Knee (synovial hinge joint)	Sagittal	Flexion Extension Hyperextension	135 135 0
	Frontal	None	None
	Transverse	Rotation (full extension) Rotation (70° flexion)	0 45

Table 7.3 Type, degrees of freedom, movement patterns, and range of motion of the ankle joint

Joint	Plane	Movement	Range of motion
Ankle (synovial hinge joint)	Sagittal	Plantar flexion Dorsiflexion	45 20
Rearfoot and midfoot joints	Multiplanar	Inversion Eversion	35 15

bility with large and unpredictable displacements [15]. Moreover, it is of utmost importance to lunch several hypotheses and acknowledge evidences on the risk that a lack of motor control, stability [16, 17], and biomechanical asymmetries [18] may arise. Therefore, all the previous alterations consubstantiate a dysfunction that may result in severe injuries which implies great health and economic and societal losses. Going back to the basics of normal function of the lower limb and recalling some evidence on potentially modifiable risk factors for reinjury [17], it is imperative to understand that frontal, sagittal, and transversal planes embrace a multitude of biomechanical behaviors, in relation with the degrees of freedom of each joint, structural and functional integrity of passive stabilizers, and, particularly, performance delivered for active stabilizers that can become outstanding motor skills or turn into biomechanical risk factors. An osteokinematic abnormal range of adduction and internal rotation of the femur may be a matter of kinetics, motor control, or both, i.e., a lack of strength can exist or an inadequate recruitment of the hip abductors and external rotators or even both scenarios may concur. Nevertheless, if we have a footballer with increased dynamic valgus (Fig. 7.1) [19] and this rises the odds of a ACL rupture, there is a need to deliver the most efficient strategies for motor learning enhancement, such as those based on external focus of attention which increase the effectiveness in learning safe movement techniques [20, 21]. The importance of what was previously said may be stressed out bringing for discussion the scarce 40 msec in which an ACL rupture may occour seen as a consequence of an altered/discoordinated pattern of motion at landing, i.e., no time for muscle preventive actions at in the time window meaning that we need to improve through motor learning landing safe techniques to reduce incidence of sports injuries [19, 22, 23]. This chapter should help the reader to recall the importance and the need to focus on deviations from normal function, taking as example some evidence and critical thinking concerning the knee but with theoretically transfer for the other joints.

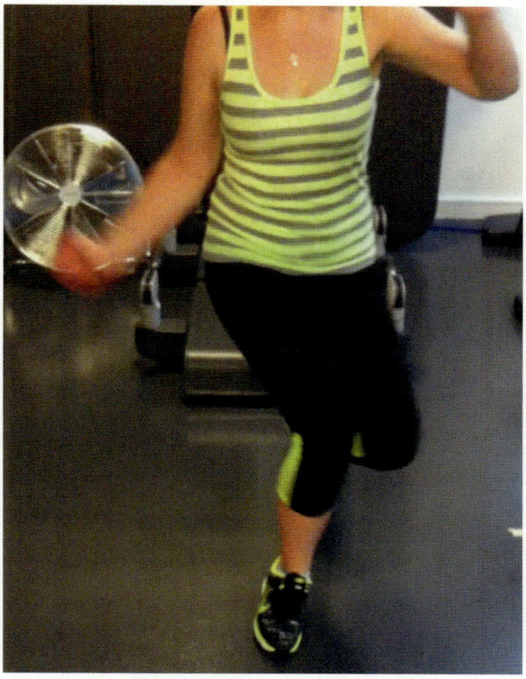

Fig. 7.1 Dynamic valgus at landing

References

1. Ekstrand J, Hägglund M, Waldén M. Injury incidence and injury patterns in professional football: the UEFA injury study. Br J Sports Med. 2009;bjsports60582.
2. Waldén M, Hägglund M, Ekstrand J. Time-trends and circumstances surrounding ankle injuries in men's professional football: an 11-year follow-up of the UEFA Champions League injury study. Br J Sports Med. 2013;47:748–53.
3. Andrade R, Vasta S, Sevivas N, Pereira R, Leal A, Papalia R, et al. Notch morphology is a risk factor for ACL injury: a systematic review and meta-analysis. J ISAKOS. 2016;1:70–81.
4. Alentorn-Geli E, Mendiguchía J, Samuelsson K, Musahl V, Karlsson J, Cugat R, et al. Prevention of anterior cruciate ligament injuries in sports—Part I: systematic review of risk factors in male athletes. Knee Surg Sports Traumatol Arthrosc. 2014;22:3–15.
5. Flanigan DC, Everhart JS, Pedroza A, Smith T, Kaeding CC. Fear of reinjury (kinesiophobia) and persistent knee symptoms are common factors for lack of return to sport after anterior cruciate ligament reconstruction. Arthroscopy J Arthrosc Relat. 2013;29:1322–9.
6. Ardern CL, Webster KE, Taylor NF, Feller JA. Return to the preinjury level of competitive sport after anterior cruciate ligament reconstruction surgery two-thirds of patients have not returned by 12 months after surgery. Am J Sports Med. 2011;39:538–43.

7. Ardern CL, Webster KE, Taylor NF, Feller JA. Return to sport following anterior cruciate ligament reconstruction surgery: a systematic review and meta-analysis of the state of play. Br J Sports Med. 2011;bjsports76364.
8. Brukner P. Brukner & Khan's clinical sports medicine. North Ryde: McGraw-Hill; 2012.
9. Musahl V, Hoshino Y, Becker R, Karlsson J. Rotatory knee laxity and the pivot shift. Knee Surg Sports Traumatol Arthrosc. 2012;20:601–2.
10. Espregueira-Mendes J, Pereira H, Sevivas N, Passos C, Vasconcelos JC, Monteiro A, et al. Assessment of rotatory laxity in anterior cruciate ligament-deficient knees using magnetic resonance imaging with Porto-knee testing device. Knee Surg Sports Traumatol Arthrosc. 2012;20:671–8.
11. Ohashi B, Ward J, Araujo P, Kfuri M, Pereira H, Espregueira-Mendes J, et al. Partial Anterior Cruciate Ligament Ruptures: knee laxity measurements and pivot shift. Sports injuries: prevention, diagnosis, treatment and rehabilitation; 2015. p. 1245–58.
12. Espregueira-Mendes J, Andrade R, Leal A, Pereira H, Skaf A, Rodrigues-Gomes S, et al. Global rotation has high sensitivity in ACL lesions within stress MRI. Knee Surg Sports Traumatol Arthrosc. 2016; doi:10.1007/s00167-016-4281-0.
13. Kiapour AM, Wordeman SC, Paterno MV, Quatman CE, Levine JW, Goel VK, et al. Diagnostic value of knee arthrometry in the prediction of anterior cruciate ligament strain during landing. Am J Sports Med. 2014;42:312–9.
14. Tashman S, Collon D, Anderson K, Kolowich P, Anderst W. Abnormal rotational knee motion during running after anterior cruciate ligament reconstruction. Am J Sports Med. 2004;32:975–83.
15. Nishizawa Y, Tashman S. In vivo biomechanics: laxity versus dynamic stability. In: Mushal V, Karlsson J, Kuroda R, Zaffagnini S, editors. Rotatory knee instability. Springer; 2017. p. 37–48.
16. Hewett TE, Myer GD, Ford KR, Paterno MV, Quatman CE. Mechanisms, prediction & prevention of ACL injuries: Cut risk with 3 sharpened & validated tools. J Orthop Res. 2016;34:1843–55.
17. Paterno MV, Schmitt LC, Ford KR, Rauh MJ, Myer GD, Huang B, et al. Biomechanical measures during landing and postural stability predict second anterior cruciate ligament injury after anterior cruciate ligament reconstruction and return to sport. Am J Sports Med. 2010;38:1968–78.
18. Paterno MV, Ford KR, Myer GD, Heyl R, Hewett TE. Limb asymmetries in landing and jumping 2 years following anterior cruciate ligament reconstruction. Clin J Sport Med. 2007;17:258–62.
19. Hewett TE, Myer GD, Ford KR, Heidt RS, Colosimo AJ, McLean SG, et al. Biomechanical measures of neuromuscular control and valgus loading of the knee predict anterior cruciate ligament injury risk in female athletes a prospective study. Am J Sports Med. 2005;33:492–501.
20. Gokeler A, Benjaminse A, Hewett TE, Paterno MV, Ford KR, Otten E, et al. Feedback techniques to target functional deficits following anterior cruciate ligament reconstruction: implications for motor control and reduction of second injury risk. Sports Med. 2013;43:1065–74.
21. Benjaminse A, Gokeler A, Dowling AV, Faigenbaum A, Ford KR, Hewett TE, et al. Optimization of the anterior cruciate ligament injury prevention paradigm: novel feedback techniques to enhance motor learning and reduce injury risk. J Orthop Sports Phys Ther. 2015;45:170–82.
22. Dallinga J, Benjaminse A, Gokeler A, Cortes N, Otten E, Lemmink K. Innovative video feedback on jump landing improves landing technique in males. Int J Sports Med. 2016; doi:10.1055/s-0042-106298.
23. Waldén M, Krosshaug T, Bjørneboe J, Andersen TE, Faul O, Hägglund M. Three distinct mechanisms predominate in non-contact anterior cruciate ligament injuries in male professional football players: a systematic video analysis of 39 cases. Br J Sports Med. 2015; bjsports-2014-094 57349: 1452–60.

Biomechanics of Lower Limb Injuries

8

Manuel Vieira da Silva and Bruno Pereira

Contents

M.V. da Silva (✉)
Orthopaedic Department Hospital de Braga, Braga, Portugal

ICVS/3B's Laboratório Associado, PT Government Associate Laboratory, Braga, Portugal
e-mail: vieira.silva@hospitaldebraga.pt

B. Pereira
Orthopaedic Department Hospital de Braga, Braga, Portugal

Clínica do Dragão, Espregueira-Mendes Sports Centre - FIFA Medical Centre of Excellence, Porto, Portugal

Universitat de Barcelona, Barcelona, Spain

School of Health Sciences (ECS), University of Minho, Braga, Portugal
e-mail: pereira.bac@gmail.com

8.1 What Is it?

Biomechanics is a discipline among the sciences derived from the natural sciences, which deals with physical analysis of biological systems, therefore, the physical analysis of the human body movements. When dimensioned biomechanics in the context of related sciences, whose aim's to study the movement, we must remember that this scientific context rests on two fundamental facts: (a) the biomechanics has clearly defined its subject matter, thus defining its basic structure of knowledge, and (b) the results of investigations are obtained through the use of scientific methods [20, 22, 35].

As opposed to a rigid body, the biological structure of the human body allows the production of strength through muscle contraction, which turns the body into an autonomous and independent system. In this way, science is define that describes, analyses and models biological systems as the biomechanics and then a highly interdisciplinary science of relations given the nature of the phenomenon investigated. Thus, the biomechanics of movement seeks to explain how the waveforms of the bodies of living things happen in nature from kinematic indicators and dynamic. Through sport biomechanics and their areas of expertise applied, we can analyse the causes and parameters related to sports movement. So, it is considered the movement as the central object of study and

J. Espregueira-Mendes et al. (eds.), *Injuries and Health Problems in Football*,
DOI 10.1007/978-3-662-53924-8_8

analysing causes and effects generated for the optimization of income [20, 25, 44].

In the field of sports movement analysis area, overloading the normal behaviour of the joint and the effects of motor mechanisms in the learning process are examples of topics that relate to the diagnosis of sports technique. Therefore, we refer also to biomechanics of sport, dedicated to the study of the human body and the sporting movement relative laws and physical-mechanical principles including anatomical and physiological knowledge of the human body. In the broadest sense of its application, it is still the task of biomechanics of sport, characterization and optimization of motion techniques through scientific knowledge which delimit the operating area of science that has the sports movement [22, 39].

The biomechanics can be divided into internal and external, given the large difference in their approach and application. The internal biomechanics is concerned with the internal forces transmitted by the internal biological structures of the body, such as muscle strength and strength in the tendons, ligaments, bone and articular cartilage, among others. The determination of the internal forces of the muscles and joints still represents a methodological problem not fully resolved in biomechanics but surely if it constitutes fundamental basis for better understanding of criteria for motion control. The external biomechanics constitutes the parameters for quantitative and/or qualitative determination referring to the place change and position of the human body in sports movements, with the aid of descriptive measures kinematic and/or dynamic therefore those which refer to the observable characteristics outside the structure movement [20, 29].

8.2 Football Injuries

The risk of injury is present in all sporting activity. However, prospective and retrospective research studies have described the risk of injury in football as considerable and high compared to other sports. Certain risk factors can make football more dangerous than some high-risk industrial occupations, such as agriculture and construction [4, 24].

Suffering an injury can have physical, psychological and financial consequences for the player. For example, a loss of playing time can cause a reduction in revenue from supporters wanting to see the best players. Teams may also fail to do as well in competitions, which can directly influence the prize monies won and further discourage supporters from watching their team. Furthermore, if the player continues to train and/or compete with an injury, their performance could be impaired, which could lower the chance of being successful. Also, if these injuries are repeatedly sustained, they can have long-term effects on the participant's mental and physical well-being. In the most extreme case, multiple minor injuries can lead to a more serious injury and ultimately result in the player having to retire early.

Treatment of injury is also a huge financial burden on the health service. Sports and exercise contribute significantly to this high cost of treatment. Serious injury can also affect their long-term health of both professional and amateur football players as they may be unable to participate in an active lifestyle, if the injury becomes untreatable. Therefore, the pain and discomfort, along with the frustrations that come from the rehabilitation of injury, and the high financial cost provide clear reasons for research into the understanding and prevention of injury risk in football [32, 35, 37].

Van Michelin, Hlobil and Kemper presented a four-step paradigm by which the prevention of injury could be addressed [44]:

Step 1: To establish the extent of the sports injury problem
Step 2: To establish the specific aetiology (risk factors) and mechanisms of injuries
Step 3: To introduce preventative measures
Step 4: To assess the effectiveness of the preventative interventions by repeating step 1

Steps 1 and 2 of this framework are used in this literature review to discuss the existing research that relates to the occurrence and severity of certain football injuries. It is also used to highlight the biomechanical characteristics of football players while experiencing the various risk factors. In addition, the framework is used to identify research that is needed to further knowledge behind the characteristics of football players when these injuries potentially occur and the interventions presently prescribed to reduce similar injuries in other sports [44].

8.2.1 Problem in Football Injury

Football is one of the most popular sports worldwide and requires the player to have considerable stamina while superimposing sprinting, jumping, tackling, rapid changes of direction and kicking. This contact sport has a significant risk for acute and overuse injuries.

The term football injury encompasses all injuries that occur during participation which vary in terms of their anatomical location and severity. Therefore, the overall injury value does not provide enough detail into which injuries are the most common and as such isn't particularly useful, when trying to lower the occurrence of injury. Instead, it is more valuable to identify the specific, most problematic injuries which are the largest contributor towards the high rate of injury found in football. As such, it may be possible to apply suitable interventions to lower the risk of these specific injuries [35, 36].

Due to the bipedal nature of football, many injuries occur to the lower extremity. Across this region, the ankle and knee joints are most commonly injured, with muscle and tendon strains and ligament sprains being consistently reported. However, although these sites are most common, the risk of injury to these regions can vary throughout the year [30, 32].

In sports such as football that start in summer and early autumn, the risk of injury can increase during this time. Woods et al. observed the presence of an early season *bias* towards certain injuries, which is not typically reported in summer football competition or indoor sports such as basketball. These injuries are generally less severe than those experienced at other times, with a significantly greater percentage of slight and minor injuries being observed. However, it has been shown that the experience of an initial injury will put the participant at a considerably greater risk of reinjury at a later date. Indeed, one third of football players who experience a minor injury in the first instance, sustaining a more serious injury at the same location. Likewise, in response to the first injury, participants may change their movement patterns. This can put other previously less used structures at an increased load and unexpected stress, accentuating the risk of a new injury to result. Therefore, much of the high injury rate observed in football may be reduced by establishing the causes of the most common injuries during the preseason period [53].

8.3 Biomechanics of Football Injury

Sports medicine professionals use biomechanical principles to understand injury mechanisms, select appropriate injury prevention and rehabilitation protocols and monitor recovery. The qualitative analysis of exercise technique can help sports medicine professionals ensure that the client's technique achieves the desired training effect. Qualitative analysis of therapeutic exercise also requires an interdisciplinary approach, especially integrating clinical training and experience with biomechanics. Other issues sports medicine professionals must take into account beyond biomechanical principles are pain, fear, motivation and competitive psychology [29, 38].

Biomechanical studies on injuries in football are increasing, and the need to optimize the recovery and avoidance of injuries has largely focused on the two most frequently injured joints, the knee and ankle, but the most common injuries in football are the muscle and tendon injury.

8.3.1 Biomechanics of Pelvis, Hip and Groin Injury

The biomechanical studies that evaluate the pelvis movement in football were poor. The pelvis contains the centre of gravity of the body and acts as the fulcrum for all athletic movement in football.

Anatomically and functionally, this area is extremely complex with several mobile and fixed articulations associated with powerful muscle groups, aponeuroses and ligaments that make it difficult to calculate accurately forces and associated moments [54].

The hip joint is the main area of the pelvis that has been formally evaluated biomechanically with in vivo prosthesis monitoring. The hip effectively acts as a multiaxial ball-and-socket joint upon which the upper body is balanced during stance and gait. Stability of this joint is critical to allow motion while supporting the forces encountered during activity. Nearly all motion between the femoral head and acetabulum is rotational, with no detectable translation because of the congruency of the articulating surfaces. The high degree of articular congruency is provided by the bony architecture of the joint and the acetabular labrum, articular cartilage, joint capsule and surrounding musculature [1, 6, 16, 38, 43, 47].

The joint reactive forces calculated through the hip joint are five times the body weight while jogging and over eight times the body weight during athletic activity or stumbling. These forces are further increased in single stance, which commonly occurs in football with kicking, jumping or cutting-in.

The labrum is a complex structure consisting of a fibrocartilaginous rim composed of circumferential collagen fibres spanning the entirety of the acetabulum and becoming contiguous with the transverse acetabular ligament. The complete physiologic function of the labrum is not entirely defined, but it appears to serve multiple purposes including a limitation of extreme range of motion and deepening the acetabulum to enhance the stability of the hip joint. The labrum contributes approximately 22% of the articulating surface of the hip and increases the volume of the acetabulum by 33%. In athletic motion, the labrum undergoes shearing forces while limiting femoral head motion, which can result in acute labral tears or chronic degeneration. Indeed, in retired football players, there is a high incidence of premature hip osteoarthritis, and there is now an increasing recognition of osteochondral and labral injuries occurring during active playing careers [6].

In football, considerable reactive forces also act through the anterior pelvis, in particular the symphysis pubis, inguinofemoral aponeuroses and parasymphyseal muscles. The symphysis pubis and rami function as an effective strut modulating reactive forces between the lower limbs and axial skeleton. Biomechanical studies have attempted to reproduce running and single stance forces in fresh cadaver pelvis and measured forces of the order of 300 N across the symphysis with normal relative pubic body movement of up to 2 mm in the vertical plane. The pelvis is normally tilted anteriorly in relation to the hip and lower limb, and this relationship must be maintained through all the complex athletic movements that occur in football. This core stability is thought to be crucial for normal and repetitive athletic activity of the pelvis, which in turn acts as the stabilizer for effective athletic function of the lower limb kinetic chain. Studies have shown that preseason weakness of the hip abductors and external rotators predisposes to lower limb injury and decreased adductor function predisposes to further ipsilateral adductor injury [1, 16].

In football players, a prospective study of the elite teams in UEFA during seven seasons found a total of 628 hip/groin injuries accounting for 12–16% of all injuries per season. Acute groin injuries in football include myotendinous strain of adductor longus or abdominal muscles, but have a good response to rehabilitation. Chronic injury and pain in this region may be career ending as it can be extremely difficult to diagnose and treat effectively. The increased incidence of chronic injury in sports that require constant cutting-in may relate to chronic shearing forces being further exacerbated, if the player develops one dominant leg and is commonly in single stance. Groin injury has been described more frequently in football players and is a significant problem estimated to constitute 10% of acute and 18% of chronic football-related injuries [12, 16, 17, 54].

8.3.2 Biomechanics of Knee Injury

Knee injuries are prevalent among a variety of competitive sports, especially those that involve sprinting, jumping and landing both with and without passing a ball, cutting-in and direct impact. The incidence of knee injuries during competition is 15–19% of all injuries. Of these, 35–37% are strains, 20–21% sprains and 16–24% contusions. However, knee injuries account for 58% of all major injuries. Two of the most common sports-related knee injuries are patellofemoral pain syndrome (PFPS) and anterior cruciate ligament (ACL) injuries [14, 31].

The three main factors that contribute to an increased risk of knee injury in football are the age of the player, a previous injury and the ligamentous status of the knee. Females sustain more injuries during training than males, whereas males sustain more injuries during competition, and particularly during competition in contact situations, with the tackled player being the more susceptible to injury. The playing environment has a role, with a higher number of injuries in indoor football, of which the majority are non-contact. It is not surprising that foul play was identified as a risk for a major knee injury, with 20% of illegal activity-related knee injuries requiring surgery [15, 43].

The high incidence of major knee injuries in female players is of great concern. The majority are non-contact injuries that occur with a change in direction. Many aetiological factors have been considered and include anatomical and structural differences between men and women, muscle strength and neuromuscular activation patterns as well as hormonal influences on knee stability. Although there has been little reported gender-related difference in injury patterns elsewhere in the body, there seems to be a significant increase in the incidence of non-contact internal derangement of the knee in female football players relative to male counterparts [2].

The different biomechanics of muscle and joint recruitment in running and especially landing after jumping have been studied in female football players and matched male controls. When an athlete lands on one leg after jumping, considerable translational force is produced across the knee joint. This is increased in sports where the athlete wants to push off immediately in another direction, requiring forceful thigh muscular contraction resulting in further femur rotation and ligament stress. Muscular recruitment can significantly modify the degree of knee flexion and stress directed across the joint, with the hamstrings in particular acting to decrease tibial anterior translation. Concomitant injury or fatigue of these muscles can precipitate a serious knee injury on landing as more force is transmitted through the knee ligaments alone.

8.3.2.1 ACL Injury

ACL injuries have the highest morbidity of knee injuries for football players and result in the most time lost. The incidence of ACL injury ranges from 0.06 to 3.7 per 1000 h of active football play, with females being two to eight times more likely to sustain non-contact ACL injury than males. ACL injuries occur as a result of a combination of a deceleration and twisting on a planted foot with an extended or near fully extended knee. The result is a varus or valgus strain combined with internal or external rotation of the tibia on a fixed foot, combined with an anterior translation force. The player usually describes a “popping” feeling with a sensation of giving way. The presence of a knee haemarthrosis is positive for an ACL injury in 70% of cases [13, 15, 43].

The active patient with an ACL-deficient knee is at risk for repeated episodes of instability, meniscal and articular cartilage injury, early joint degeneration and a decline in joint function. There is a large variation in the management and rehabilitation approach by surgeons on different continents. Few football players are able to remain competitive with an ACL-deficient knee despite strengthening and bracing, and surgical reconstruction should be recommended for all players wishing to continue the sport. Surgery is usually delayed to start 'pre-rehabilitation' until the swelling has subsided and near to normal range of motion has been achieved [4, 24].

Successful return to a pre-injury level of football is possible, although the success rates may vary from 50% to 90%. Players participating at a higher level of competition tend to have a more successful outcome. Recent studies specific to football have shown that a high percentage of players studied gave up football because of poor knee function or fear of a new injury regardless of the treatment. The role of neuromuscular control, proprioception and landing error assessment has now been successfully employed in the reduction of ACL injuries through the institution of preventive programmes [19, 51].

8.3.2.2 Patellofemoral Pain Syndrome (PFPS)

Several factors have been implicated in the aetiology of PFPS. The aetiology remains uncertain, which identified three major predisposing factors: bone abnormalities, malalignment of the lower limb, and muscle-tendon imbalances and periarticular soft tissues.

(a) Bone Abnormalities

With the knee in full extension, the patella is in a higher position on the femoral trochlea. As the knee flexion is initiated, the distal portion of the rod comes into contact with the lateral femoral condyle, between 10° and 20° bending. Then the patella describes an S curve during their contact with the femoral trochlea, linking up with the femur in the distal-proximal direction as the bending increases from 30° to 90°. The 120° contact between the patella and femur is small, remaining only the most proximal facet in contact with the femur. The configurations of the femoral condyles, with greater prominence of lateral V shape, and the patella are two key factors in maintaining the patella centred in the trochlea. Different degrees of dysplasia of the femoral trochlea can compromise the effectiveness of static stabilizer contributing to greater instability femoropatellar joint. The asymmetry of patella aspects also contributes to a decrease in congruence. The normal ratio of the lateral to medial facet is 3:2; this lateral facet is longer and more oblique corresponding to higher and wider lateral femoral condyle [49, 50, 51]

(b) Bad Lower Limb Alignment

The misalignment of the lower limbs has been considered a determining factor in the development of PFPS. Significant deviations in the secondary alignment patellar femoral anteversion, valgus knee, external tibial torsion and excessive subtalar pronation can contribute to the onset of femoropatellar pain by increasing the contact pressure between the patella and the facet trochlear lateral. The study of cadaveric knees showed that the femoral anteversion leads to an increase in contact between the patella and the lateral surface of the trochlear pressure that can theoretically trigger patellar symptomatology. The Q angle measurement is used in clinical practice as an indicator of a possible misalignment of the lower limb. Many authors consider that a Q angle greater than 15–20° is a risk factor for the development of PFPS to condition a lateral deviation of the alignment rod; however, only few patients with PFPS feature a Q angle higher than normal, and many people with increased Q angles show no complaints. We conclude, therefore, that the Q angle is just one of multiple etiologic factors that determine the appearance of PFPS [49, 52]

(c) Imbalances in Muscle-Tendon and Periarticular Soft Tissue

The balance established between the medial and lateral heads of the quadriceps is one of the most important anatomical factors in the dynamic stabilization of the patella. Lateral dynamic forces are produced by the vastus lateralis, biceps femoris, gluteus and tensor fascia lata, through its inclusion in the iliotibial band and lateral retinaculum. The vastus is responsible for producing a force vector with medial direction and the vastus medialis muscle (VM) considered the leading medial stabilizer of the patella. In situations of weakness or late activation of the VM, the lateral forces acting on the bearing exceed the medial, which results in an increase in its lateral mobility. Anomalies of periarticular soft tissues may also affect biomechanics of femoropatellar joint. Retractions of the quadriceps, hamstrings, iliotibial band and peripatellar retinacula, contribute to an increase in the contact pressure between the lateral patella and femoral trochlea and lateral displacement of the patella [49, 52]

8.3.3 Biomechanics of Ankle Injury

The ankle is one of the most common acutely injured areas in football players with a reported incidence of 17% of all injuries, most of them occur during activity between the ages of 15 and 35 years. The ankle is exposed to stresses during sprinting, sudden changes of direction and tackling and the actual kicking mechanism [3, 8, 48].

8.3.3.1 Lateral Complex Injury

In the neutral position, the bony anatomy of the ankle joint is responsible for the stability. Bone stability is increased by the compressive loads on the body loading position. Stormont demonstrated that, under load, the joint surface provides rotational stability of 30% and 100% stability inversion. In no load conditions, stabilization is promoted by the ligamentous structures. With increased plantar flexion, bone containment is decreased, and the soft tissues are more prone to injury. The main side stabilizing soft tissue ankle ligaments is the lateral ligament complex: the anterior talofibular ligament (ATFL), the calcaneofibular ligament (CFL) and the posterior talofibular ligament (PTFL) [5, 7, 10, 11].

The ATFL really is nothing more than a thickening of the tibiofibular cover that comes from the leading edge and the tip of the lateral malleolus and earlier runs to insert into the talar neck. Its width is 6 mm to 10 mm, 20 mm length and 2 mm thickness. It runs almost parallel to the neutral axis of the foot. When the foot is in plantar flexion, however, the ligament runs parallel to the leg axis. Due to most sprains occur when the foot is in plantar flexion, this ligament is the most frequently involved in twisting inversion [7, 11, 18, 50].

The CFL originates at the tip of the lateral malleolus and runs with a slight posterior tilt to the side portion of calcaneus. The ligament is extra-articular and is positioned below the peroneal tendons. It has 20 mm to 25 mm long with a diameter of 6 mm to 8 mm. Since this ligament runs more perpendicular to the axis of the foot in a neutral position, isolated breaks are less common with the typical lesions in plantar flexion. It is most commonly ruptured during moderately severe kinks when rupturing the ATFL, and the lesion progresses around the outer side of the ankle, also breaking the CFL. Isolated lesions may occur but are rare and occur when the ligament is under maximum stress on the foot in dorsiflexion [7, 11, 18, 50].

The PTFL emerges from the posteromedial portion of the lateral malleolus and runs posterior medially to the posterior process of the talus. It has an average diameter of 6 mm. The ligament is under maximum stress when the foot is in dorsiflexion. Isolated lesions of PTFL are extremely rare. Many injuries occur as a result of a very serious ankle sprain, when both ATFL and CFL were previously severed at break of PTFL while the lesion progresses around the lateral side of the ankle.

The ATFL and PTFL contain the anterior and posterior displacement, respectively, of the talus relative to the tibia and fibula. The CFL limits calcaneal inversion in relation to fíbula.

8.3.3.2 Deltoid Injury

The deltoid ligament, fan-shaped, is composed of a vertical surface layer and an innermost layer, smaller and horizontal. The surface part consists of the above tibionavicular ligament, the ligament in tibiocalcaneal means (originating from 1 or 2 cm above the tip of the medial malleolus and inserted into the sustentaculum tali of the calcaneus) and subsequently linking tibiotalar surface. The deepest horizontal layer of the deltoid ligament is the strongest ligament posterior and anterior tibiotalar. The deepest layer is most important for ankle stability than the superficial layer. During the mobility of the ankle, however, all parts of the deltoid ligament function as a single unit, giving static support for the ankle in abduction, eversion and pronation of the foot. The tibionavicular ligaments and medial tibiocalcaneal ligament give stability to both the subtalar joints and hock, while the deep tibiotalar ligaments are solely responsible for the medial stability of the hock joint [33, 34].

Isolated lesions of the deltoid ligament are very rare. In a number of acute injuries of 281 ankles studied by Brostrom, only 3% of these were located on the medial side. Almost all of the medial side injuries were partial ruptures of the ligament. Complete ruptures of the deltoid ligament most often occur in combination with ankle fractures. In reviewing Harper, of the 42 patients with complete deltoid ligament ruptures, all were associated with other injuries. The three major characteristics of the deltoid ligament injury mechanisms are due to pronation-abduction, external rotation and pronation-supination-external rotation of the foot. The first component describes the position of one foot, and the second indicates the relative mobility of the foot when the supported leg rotates. Then in injury-prone abduction, the foot is supported in pronation when the body falls to the lateral side of the foot, exerting great force abduction ankle and deltoid ligament. Since the forces required to damage the strong deltoid ligament are great, the injury usually continues for syndesmosis and the action of the lateral malleolus on the side of the talus [18].

8.3.3.3 Syndesmosis Injury

The tibiofibular syndesmosis is a structure that maintains the relationship between the distal tibia and fibula. The syndesmosis consists of four components: anterior inferior tibiofibular ligament (AITFL), posterior-inferior tibiofibular ligament (PITFL), transverse ligament and interosseous membrane. The anterior and posterior tibiofibular ligaments are attached superiorly and medially to the tibia and inferiorly and laterally to the fibula. The most distal aspect of the lower tibiofibular ligament and posterior tibiofibular ligament is called transverse.

There is a small groove on the distal tibia where the fibula rotates on its vertical axis during plantar flexion and dorsal ankle. The AITFL and PITFL are responsible for holding the fibula in the groove. The interosseous membrane melts in the anterior and posterior tibiofibular ligaments in approximately from 1 cm to 2.5 cm on the talus dome. This place remains the top connecting adjacent rough surfaces of the tibia and fibula. The AITFL controls the external rotation and posterior displacement of the fibula with respect to the tibia, but all three tibiofibular ligaments prevent excessive lateral displacement of the fibula. The lateral displacement of the fibula will cause increased ankle shroud [18, 42, 45].

Diastasis syndesmosis occurs with partial or complete rupture of the syndesmosis complex. Isolated complete syndesmosis injuries are rare, and there is relatively little information in the literature on the ankle diastasis in the absence of fracture.

Partial ruptures of the lower tibiofibular ligaments, however, are not common. As the above isolated breaks, they occur most commonly in a violent external rotation of the foot while the ankle is in dorsiflexion. Isolated partial syndesmosis injuries occur with some frequency; it is much more common for the associated injury with a fracture and/or deltoid ligament injury. The frequency of the syndesmosis disruption is directly related to the type and level of associated fibular fractures. This is predicted by Lauge-Hansen in his injury mechanism for the classification of ankle fractures. In this classification scheme, ligament injuries or fractures occur when the lesion pattern continues around the circular mode ankle. The most characteristic syndesmosis injury mechanism is from the pronation-external rotation of the foot. Then in the pronation-external rotation injury the foot is placed prone with the rotations of the body and causes the relative external rotation of the foot. It has a lot of strength, first in the deltoid ligament, then the anterior inferior tibiofibular ligament in the shaft above the syndesmosis and finally the posterior-inferior tibiofibular ligament. Since the forces required to completely break the strong deltoid ligament are so great, the injury usually continues through the syndesmosis like a strong lever arm of the lateral malleolus on the side of the talus [21, 27, 43].

8.3.4 Biomechanics of Muscle and Tendon Injury

Muscle and tendon injuries occur at areas of transition (anatomical or functional) because these sites represent potential weaknesses in the functional unit involving the muscle, tendon and bone.

8.3.4.1 Muscle Injury

Muscular strains of the lower limb are among the most common injuries in sport. They make up one third of all referrals to sports physicians, and their frequency and disabling effect is well documented. Hamstring injuries in particular are the most common type of muscular strain to effect the lower limb in the elite athlete.

Muscle injury to the thigh is the single most common injury subtype in top-level football and accounts for 23% of all injuries. The risk of sustaining a thigh muscle injury is 1.6/1000 h of exposure, which means that a team with 25 players in the squad can expect (as a mean) ten such injuries each season [23, 27, 40].

Although nonsurgical treatment results in a good prognosis for most athletes with muscle injuries, the consequences of treatment failure may be dramatic, postponing the return to physical activity for weeks or even months. Knowledge of certain basic principles of the regeneration and repair mechanisms of skeletal muscles may help to avoid imminent hazards and accelerate the return to sport.

Muscle fibres generally originate in a bone or in dense connective tissue and insert in another bone through a tendon insertion. There are muscles that cross one or more joints to generate movement. Muscles with a tonic or postural function are generally wide, planar and located at a single joint with a low contraction velocity and a capacity to generate and maintain large contractile force. They are generally located in deeper compartments. Muscles involving two joints have greater contraction velocity and greater capacity to change length, but less capacity to withstand tension. They are generally located in superficial compartments. With regard to shape, fusiform muscles allow greater range of motion, while pennate muscles have greater contractile strength. Fibre length is an important determinant of the quantity of contraction possible in a muscle. Since myofibrils generally present oblique distribution within a muscle belly, they are generally shorter than the total length of the muscle [4, 24, 43].

Muscle injuries can be caused by bruising, spraining or laceration. More than 90% of all sports-related injuries are bruises or sprains. On the other hand, muscle lacerations are the least frequent injuries resulting from sports. The tensile force exerted on a muscle may lead to excessive stretching of the muscle fibres, and consequently a tear closes to the muscle-tendon junction. Muscle sprains are typically observed in the superficial muscles that work by traversing two joints, such as the rectus femoris, semitendinosus and gastrocnemius muscles [4].

Acute injuries commonly occur at the distal myotendinous junction of rectus femoris, proximal or distal myotendinous junction of biceps femoris and the myotendinous junction of the gastrocnemius-soleus. Other potential areas of injury include the muscular-aponeurosis junction or midsubstance tear. Although avulsion of the iliac spine epiphysis is not an uncommon injury from tackling and kicking in adolescents, avulsion or a proximal injury of rectus femoris in skeletally mature players is rare. This type of injury may occur in goalkeepers, presumably involving the transition zone at the interface of the straight and reflected tendons of rectus femoris. In the goal kicks, these players strike the dead ball from their goal area into the opposition half. To generate this power, the kicking leg is hyperextended at the hip and flexed at the knee, resulting in severe eccentric tensing of both proximal tendon components anterior to the hip joint and the potential for proximal rectus injury [43].

8.3.4.2 Tendon Injury

Athletes may have acute injuries that come from breaking them being partial or total, often related to trauma or may have chronic injuries, which are caused by overload. The function of the tendon is divided into two categories, one is the transmission of tensile strength, and the other is the storage and release of elastic energy during locomotion. The action of the tendons in the storage and release of energy is found mainly in sports with stretching and shortening cycles.

To store and release high-energy loads without damage to the tendon tissue, tendons require greater energy absorption capacity. If this capacity is insufficient, the demands on the energy absorption and release can quickly exceed the capacity of the tendon, so the more intense, the more problems activity can be developed in the tendons [15,17, 23].

In sports such as running and jumping, the tendon muscle unit acts as elastic spring, with the risk of further injury, due to increased overhead. So it is essential to increase the capacity of tendon energy absorption as prevention and treatment of tendon injuries [23].

The method of the tendon increase capacity is by eccentric exercise, and the other is reducing the rigidity of the tendon by increasing the elasticity. These two modes are interconnected as to make quality eccentric exercise; the tendon must be elastic.

The causes of tendon injuries, according to *Guillet*, are the wrong use of technical movements, lack of training, physical fatigue and, in particular, the association workforce. Among all the problems caused by overuse and related to physical activity, tendonitis is the most common [43].

Tendinopathy in the Achilles tendon is a common overuse injury but can also be caused by muscle hard or weak calves or any condition that causes the tendon to become less flexible and more rigid, such as reactive arthritis or normal ageing.

Achilles tendon is a band of tissue that connects the heel bone to the calf muscle and can support forces of 3000 N to 5000 N during athletic movement.

The lesions involve irritation, stretch or tear of the tendon that connects the calf muscle to the back of the heel. The break in this structure results from jump manoeuvre or cutting, common in football and in other sports. Tendon rupture can require surgery or just plaster cast for up to 10 weeks [26].

A partial disruption of tendon can only cause pain and limited range of motion but when giving a total disruption may present significant deformity, so that the tendon may present spherical shape or a muscle peat. In such cases, it applies the Thompson test, which is done by squeezing the calf muscle to see if bending occurs in the foot; if not, the total breakup is proven [26].

During muscular activity, the tendon must move or slide on other structures around whenever the muscle contracts. If a particular motion is performed repeatedly, the tendon becomes irritated and inflamed. This inflammation is manifested by pain during movement, swelling and possibly some heating usually sputtering.

Immediately should be use immobilization and application of ice pack. It is necessary to perform compression and local protection with bandage. The use of functional bandage has the aim of promoting joint positioning without causing restriction in the same, only limiting unwanted movement or symptom reported by the patient, maintaining joint mobility. This allows proper mechanical operation and avoids overload tendon structures, capsular ligament and muscle [26].

References

1. Al-Dirini RM, Thewlis D, Paul G. A comprehensive literature review of the pelvis and the lower extremity FE human models under quasi-static conditions. Work. 2012;41(Suppl 1):4218–29. doi:10.3233/WOR-2012-1039-4218.
2. Alentorn-Geli E, Myer GD, Silvers HJ, Samitier G, Romero D, Lázaro-Haro C, Cugat R. Prevention of non-contact anterior cruciate ligament injuries in soccer players. Part 1: mechanisms of injury and underlying risk factors. Knee Surg Sports Traumatol Arthrosc. 2009;17(7):705–29. doi:10.1007/s00167-009-0813-1.

3. Babbs CF. Biomechanics of heading a soccer ball: implications for player safety. Sci World J. 2001 8;1:281–322.
4. Bahr R, Krosshaug T. Understanding injury mechanisms: a key component of preventing injuries in sport. Br J Sports Med. 2005;39(6):324–9. doi:10.1136/bjsm.2005.018341.
5. Beumer A, van Hemert WL, Swierstra BA, Jasper LE, Belkoff SM. A biomechanical evaluation of the tibiofibular and tibiotalar ligaments of the ankle. Foot Ankle Int. 2003;24(5):426–9.
6. Bowman Jr KF, Fox J, Sekiya JK. A clinically relevant review of hip biomechanics. Arthroscopy. 2010;26(8): 1118–29. doi:10.1016/j.arthro.2010.01.027.
7. Butler AM, Walsh WR. Mechanical response of ankle ligaments at low loads. Foot Ankle Int. 2004;25(1): 8–12.
8. Deschamps K, Roosen P, Nobels F, Deleu PA, Birch I, Desloovere K, Bruyninckx H, Matricali G, Staes F. Review of clinical approaches and diagnostic quantities used in pedobarographic measurements. J Sports Med Phys Fitness. 2015;55(3):191–204.
9. DiStefano LJ, Padua DA, DiStefano MJ, Marshall SW. Influence of age, sex, technique, and exercise program on movement patterns after an anterior cruciate ligament injury prevention program in youth soccer players. Am J Sports Med. 2009;37(3): 495–505.
10. Doherty C, Bleakley C, Hertel J, Caulfield B, Ryan J, Delahunt E. Dynamic balance deficits 6 months following first-time acute lateral ankle sprain: a laboratory analysis. J Orthop Sports Phys Ther. 2015;45(8):626–33.
11. Dowling GJ, Murley GS, Munteanu SE, Smith MM, Neal BS, Griffiths IB, Barton CJ, Collins NJ. Dynamic foot function as a risk factor for lower limb overuse injury: a systematic review. J Foot Ankle Res. 2014;7(1):53. doi:10.1186/s13047-014-0053-6.
12. Ekstrand J, Hägglund M, Waldén M. Epidemiology of muscle injuries in professional football (soccer). Am J Sports Med. 2011;39(6):1226–32.
13. Ekstrand J, Timpka T, Hägglund M. Risk of injury in elite football played on artificial turf versus natural grass: a prospective two-cohort study. Br J Sports Med. 2006;40(12):975–80.
14. Flandry F, Hommel G. Normal anatomy and biomechanics of the knee. Sports Med Arthrosc. 2011;19(2): 82–92.
15. Fuller CW, Ekstrand J, Junge A, Andersen TE, Bahr R, Dvorak J, Hägglund M, McCrory P, Meeuwisse WH. Consensus statement on injury definitions and data collection procedures in studies of football (soccer) injuries. Clin J Sport Med. 2006;16(2):97–106.
16. Goldman EF, Jones DE. Interventions for preventing hamstring injuries. Cochrane Database Syst Rev. 2010;1:CD006782.
17. Hägglund M, Waldén M, Ekstrand J. Risk factors for lower extremity muscle injury in professional soccer: the UEFA Injury Study. Am J Sports Med. 2013;41(2): 327–35.
18. Haraguchi N, Armiger RS, Myerson MS, Campbell JT, Chao EY. Prediction of three-dimensional contact stress and ligament tension in the ankle during stance determined from computational modeling. Foot Ankle Int. 2009;30(2):177–85.
19. Hewett TE, Ford KR, Hoogenboom BJ, Myer GD. Understanding and preventing ACL injuries: current biomechanical and epidemiologic considerations – update 2010. N Am J Sports Phys Ther. 2010;5(4):234–51.
20. Karandikar N, Vargas OO. Kinetic chains: a review of the concept and its clinical applications. PM R. 2011;3(8):739–45.
21. Kaumeyer G, Malone TR. Ankle injuries: anatomical and biomechanical considerations necessary for the development of an injury prevention program. J Orthop Sports Phys Ther. 1980;1(3):171–7.
22. Knudson D. Fundamentals of biomechanics. 2nd ed. New York: Springer; 2007.
23. Kristensen LB, Andersen TB, Sørensen H. Optimizing segmental movement in the jumping header in soccer. Sports Biomech. 2004;3(2):195–208.
24. Kucera KL, Marshall SW, Kirkendall DT, Marchak PM, Garrett Jr WE. Injury history as a risk factor for incident injury in youth soccer. Br J Sports Med. 2005;39(7):462.
25. Lees A, Nolan L. The biomechanics of soccer: a review. J Sports Sci. 1998;16(3):211–34.
26. Maffulli N, Sharma P, Luscombe KL. Achilles tendinopathy: aetiology and management. J R Soc Med. 2004;97(10):472–6.
27. Napier C, Cochrane CK, Taunton JE, Hunt MA. Gait modifications to change lower extremity gait biomechanics in runners: a systematic review. Br J Sports Med. 2015;49(21):1382–8.
28. Neely FG. Biomechanical risk factors for exercise-related lower limb injuries. Sports Med. 1998;26(6): 395–413.
29. Nigg BM. Biomechanics, load analysis and sports injuries in the lower extremities. Sports Med. 1985;2(5):367–79.
30. Nigg BM, Wakeling JM. Impact forces and muscle tuning: a new paradigm. Exerc Sport Sci Rev. 2001;29(1):37–41.
31. Ortiz A, Micheo W. Biomechanical evaluation of the athlete's knee: from basic science to clinical application. PM R. 2011;3(4):365–71.
32. Parkkari J, Kujala UM, Kannus P. Is it possible to prevent sports injuries? Review of controlled clinical trials and recommendations for future work. Sports Med. 2001;31(14):985–95.
33. Pavei G, Cazzola D, La Torre A, Minetti AE. The biomechanics of race walking: literature overview and new insights. Eur J Sport Sci. 2014;14(7): 661–70.
34. Pelletier-Galarneau M, Martineau P, Gaudreault M, Pham X. Review of running injuries of the foot and ankle: clinical presentation and SPECT-CT imaging patterns. Am J Nucl Med Mol Imaging. 2015;5(4): 305–16.

35. Rahnama N, Reilly T, Lees A. Injury risk associated with playing actions during competitive soccer. Br J Sports Med. 2002;36(5):354–9.
36. Reilly T, Williams M. Science and soccer. 2nd ed. London: Routledge 2003.
37. Reilly T, Williams AM, Nevill A, Franks A. A multidisciplinary approach to talent identification in soccer. J Sports Sci. 2000;18(9):695–702.
38. Robinson P, White LM. The biomechanics and imaging of soccer injuries. Semin Musculoskelet Radiol. 2005;9(4):397–420.
39. Sasaki S, Koga H, Krosshaug T, Kaneko S, Fukubayashi T. Biomechanical analysis of defensive cutting actions during game situations: six cases in collegiate soccer competitions. J Hum Kinet. 2015;46:9–18.
40. Serbest K, Çilli M, Eldoğan O. Biomechanical effects of daily physical activities on the lower limb. Acta Orthop Traumatol Turc. 2015;49(1):85–90.
41. Shan G, Zhang X. From 2D leg kinematics to 3D full-body biomechanics-the past, present and future of scientific analysis of maximal instep kick in soccer. Sports Med Arthrosc Rehabil Ther Technol. 2011;3(1):23.
42. Simonsen EB. Contributions to the understanding of gait control. Dan Med J. 2014;61(4):B4823.
43. Toda H, Nagano A, Luo Z. Age and gender differences in the control of vertical ground reaction force by the hip, knee and ankle joints. J Phys Ther Sci. 2015;27(6):1833–8.
44. van Mechelen W, Hlobil H, Kemper HC. Incidence, severity, aetiology and prevention of sports injuries: a review of concepts. Sports Med. 1992;14(2):82–99.
45. Waldén M, Hägglund M, Ekstrand J. Time-trends and circumstances surrounding ankle injuries in men's professional football: an 11-year follow-up of the UEFA Champions League injury study. Br J Sports Med. 2013;47(12):748–53.
46. Waldén M, Hägglund M, Ekstrand J. The epidemiology of groin injury in senior football: a systematic review of prospective studies. Br J Sports Med. 2015;49(12):792–7.
47. Waldén M, Hägglund M, Ekstrand J. UEFA Champions League study: a prospective study of injuries in professional football during the 2001–2002 season. Br J Sports Med. 2005;39(8):542–6.
48. Wannop JW, Luo G, Stefanyshyn DJ. Footwear traction and lower extremity noncontact injury. Med Sci Sports Exerc. 2013;45(11):2137–43.
49. Weiss K, Whatman C. Biomechanics associated with patellofemoral pain and ACL injuries in sports. Sports Med. 2015;45(9):1325–37.
50. Willems T, Witvrouw E, Verstuyft J, Vaes P, De Clercq D. Proprioception and muscle strength in subjects with a history of ankle sprains and chronic instability. J Athl Train. 2002;37(4):487–93.
51. Wojtys EM, Brower AM. Anterior cruciate ligament injuries in the prepubescent and adolescent athlete: clinical and research considerations. J Athl Train. 2010;45(5):509–12. doi:10.4085/1062-6050-45.5.509.
52. Wong P, Hong Y. Soccer injury in the lower extremities. Br J Sports Med. 2005;39(8):473–82.
53. Woods C, Hawkins R, Hulse M, Hodson A. The Football Association Medical Research Programme: an audit of injuries in professional football: an analysis of ankle sprains. Br J Sports Med. 2003;37(3):233–8.
54. Zoric I. Anatomy, physiology and biomechanics of hamstrings injury in football and effective strength and flexibility exercises for its prevention. J Hum Sport Exerc. 2012;7:208–17.

Imaging in Football Lesions

9

Sérgio Rodrigues-Gomes,
José Carlos Vasconcelos, Pedro Portugal,
Rui Aguiar, Abdalla Skaf, and Nuno Sousa

Contents

9.1 Radiologic Perspective

Sports medicine is one of the most rapidly growing subspecialties in orthopedics. It has been estimated that 25% of patients seen by primary care physicians complain of musculoskeletal problems, many of which are sports or activity related [1]. Sports injuries often generate nonspecific symptoms and clinical findings, demanding further imaging investigations for accurate diagnosis and optimal treatment planning.

Over the last 10 years, imaging techniques have become increasingly important as a diagnostic tool for sports injuries without replacing the traditional methods of management [2, 3].

The discipline of musculoskeletal radiology has evolved into a major imaging subspecialty in recent years since the first use of X-rays to diagnose fractures. Musculoskeletal radiology expertise has experienced enormous developments in diagnostic sensitivity and specificity and in image-guided treatment options, in addition to technologic advances far beyond X-rays. Advances in cross-sectional imaging such as CT and MR imaging and educational and research endeavors have contributed further to the growth of musculoskeletal radiology as a distinct subspecialty.

S. Rodrigues-Gomes (✉)
Clinica do Dragão, Espregueira-Mendes Sports Centre - FIFA Medical Centre of Excellence, Porto, Portugal

Dom Henrique Research Centre, Porto, Portugal

Smic Group, Portugal
e-mail: sergiorodgomes@gmail.com

J.C. Vasconcelos • P. Portugal • R. Aguiar
Smic Group, Santarém, Portugal
e-mail: vaspor@sapo.pt; drpedroportugal@gmail.com; ruiaguiar@gmail.com

A. Skaf
Hospital do Coração, São Paulo, Brazil

Musculoskeletal Department, Clínica Alta Excelência Diagnóstica, São Paulo, Brazil
e-mail: abskaf@gmail.com

N. Sousa
Life and Health Sciences Research Institute (ICVS), School of Medicine, University of Minho, Braga, Portugal

ICVS/3B's - PT Government Associate Laboratory, Braga/Guimarães, Portugal

J. Espregueira-Mendes et al. (eds.), *Injuries and Health Problems in Football*,
DOI 10.1007/978-3-662-53924-8_9

Diagnostic imaging plays an increasingly important role in the detection, management, and follow-up of sports disorders.

The use of a wide range of imaging modalities such as routine radiography and ultrasound, as well as advanced imaging modalities such magnetic resonance imaging (MRI) and computed tomography (CT), allows an accurate diagnosis of a broad range of osseous, articular, and soft tissue abnormalities.

However, over-imaging can cause problems in high-level athletes, who have easy access to imaging modalities.

The choice of the imaging modality depends on multiple factors inherent to the radiologist, athlete, and type of lesion, and the optimal imaging process may not exist and should be individually tailored.

While diagnostic imaging allows for accurate characterization of a lesion and local anatomy, it must be emphasized that clinical correlation is mandatory to avoid diagnostic discrepancies and promote optimal athlete management. Good communication between the radiologist and the sports physician is essential.

The sports medicine radiologist can provide confirmation of specific injury, monitoring of the healing process and the return to play, screening and evaluation before competition/signing, and technical assistance in invasive procedures.

The radiology department of sports medicine should provide different imaging techniques (X-ray, ultrasound, CT, MRI), radiologists with experience in sports medicine imaging, and availability 24 h/7 days with rapid response.

In an ideal setting, the radiologic exams should be available at the training center of the athlete. In recent years, there has been a crescent recognition of the importance of the imaging department within the medical departments of clubs, national and international federations, and Olympic committees. Top European clubs and Olympic Games have been establishing partnerships with imaging medical systems companies to provide radiologic equipment within their own medical and training centers and the Olympic village. It's predictable the integration of radiologists in the medical department staff of top clubs, federations, and Olympic delegations.

9.2 Role of Imaging

The athlete's population differs from the normal population. In sports medicine, especially elite sports medicine, there is always the dichotomy between lesion severity and the pressure of time to resume to play.

Radiological imaging is often required to obtain accurate diagnosis in sports injuries. Even if symptoms and clinical findings in sports injuries are specific, sports medicine physicians often request additional and costly imaging more easily, as they often need a more rapid and accurate diagnosis for lesion severity grading and to optimize treatment planning [4]. Imaging techniques are also readily used to monitor ongoing pathology and to facilitate return-to-play decisions [5].

Imaging can play an important role allowing a fast and accurate diagnosis, helping in evidence-based decision for conservative versus surgical treatment, and also by demonstrating to the athlete the presence of the lesion and reinforcing his adherence to treatment. Imaging can also guide treatment interventions.

9.3 Overview of Imaging Modalities

This chapter aims to review the role of imaging techniques available to the diagnosis and grading of injuries inherent to football practice, enlightening their specific advantages and limitations and delineating possible imaging strategies and pathways to evaluate most frequent problems and injuries in football, with additional practical guidelines that may be useful in daily clinical practice.

9.4 Conventional Radiology (CR)

Plain radiography is the initial screening examination for osseous disorders due to its ability to visualize osseous structures with high spatial resolution, low cost, and widespread availability [6].

The characterization of the cortical bone is excellent, but the trabecular bone is underdiagnosed. Bone lesions producing cortical disruption, namely, fractures, are relatively easily visualized. Bone loss limited to the trabecular bone from osteoporosis is more difficult to characterize.

The presence of metal is not a limiting factor for CR, allowing assessment of the postoperative bone lesions safely and without artifacts.

CR has important limitations in the evaluation of soft tissue lesions due to poor contrast resolution. It may play a role in the evaluation of the presence of calcifications within the lesion, for example, in myositis ossificans lesions.

Indications for radiography include trauma, pain, instability, impingement, infection, preoperative or postoperative evaluation and/or follow-up, and evaluation of soft tissues in an extremity (e.g., suspected foreign body) (ACR–SPR–SSR Practice Parameter for the Performance of Radiography of the Extremities [7]).

The minimum recommended views in routine circumstances most often include two orthogonal perpendicular projections. Views may be modified for any given clinical situation. Additional views (e.g., oblique views, stress views) may be warranted as part of the initial examination, or after review of the initial images, to clarify suspected pathology. In the evaluation of the shaft of a long bone, the X-ray should include both proximal and distal joints.

While standard radiographs are a static form of imaging, stress radiography is employed to dynamic evaluation, allowing assessment of alignment and stability. These stressed views may demonstrate misalignment or signs of instability not visualized in neutral position.

CR plays an important role in assessing bone position following the treatment of a fracture or dislocation, in monitoring the progress of fracture healing with callus formation and in the diagnosis of fracture complications or complications arising from treatment. Two or more views are usually required to accurately assess bone position after any treatment procedure.

There are numerous normal anatomical variants which may mimic fractures. Correlation of X-ray findings with clinical features is often useful to eliminate significant injury. Some fracture mimics have characteristic features.

Conventional arthrography (X-ray joint evaluation after injection of intra-articular contrast medium) has evolved during the last century from crude techniques with postprocedural radiographic imaging to modern CT and MR arthrographic techniques. Arthrography saw its widest use in the 1960s and 1970s, but indications for its use in many joints decreased significantly after the introduction of cross-sectional imaging modalities such as CT and MR imaging. Arthrography nowadays is only performed as part of CT or magnetic ressonance arthrography (MRA) [8].

CR uses ionizing radiation. Medical ionizing radiation has great benefits and should not be feared, especially in urgent situations. Radiological dose and risk depends on good methodology and quality control, taking into account the possible risk from radiation exposure and the diagnostic image quality necessary to achieve the clinical objective ("as low as reasonably achievable").

The prescribing physician must justify the examination and determine relevant clinical information before referring the patient to a radiologist. Indications and decisions should reflect the possibility of using nonionizing radiation examinations, such as MRI or ultrasonography. Repetition of examinations should be avoided at other institutions.

9.5 Ultrasound (US)

US technology is rapidly advancing and being refined, and is aimed at both increasing image quality and opening new fields of applications.

Acute skeletal muscle injury is one of the major causative factors for loss of playing time in all athletes and is the most common injury in professional football. A recent study on male professional footballers showed that injuries to muscle represent more than 30% of all injuries and are responsible for approximately one quarter of total injury absence. Over 90% of muscle injuries affect the four major muscle groups of the lower extremity: hamstrings, adductors, quadriceps, and gastrocnemius. Injury to the hamstring muscle group is reported to be the most common injury subtype [9].

Over the last 15 years, musculoskeletal ultrasonography has become an important imaging modality used in sports medicine, being considered the sports medicine stethoscope. This technique has become an indispensable tool in the clinical management of sports injuries and degenerative and traumatic lesions of the articulations and periarticular soft tissues. With the rapid development and sophistication of this modality, essential information for a better understanding of the pathophysiologic assessment of many disorders has been established, allowing crucial decisions regarding treatment planning and monitoring the effects of therapy.

Major advantages for the diagnostic accuracy of US in sports medicine practice are the ready availability, portability, affordability, speed, real-time and dynamic imaging, high spatial resolution, and absence of ionizing radiation. The possibility of using Doppler imaging is another advantage.

US main disadvantages are the inadequate characterization of bone and deep structures, operator dependency, and the short field of view. Despite the former, ultrasound is sensitive to rule out cortical fractures of superficially located bones and is more accurate to detect rib fractures compared to radiographs [10].

US is able to recognize the internal muscle architecture. Intramuscular vessels coursing within the hyperechoic septa are visible on color and power Doppler imaging. The outer muscle fascia (epimysium) appears as a well-delineated echogenic envelope circumscribing the hypoechoic muscle. Large hyperechoic septa (aponeuroses) directed within the muscle belly can be seen arising from it. In complex muscles, an individual hyperechoic fascial sheath surrounds each muscle belly thus helping the examiner to recognize the different heads. The interstice between juxtaposed fasciae of two adjacent muscles appears as a hypoechoic band and corresponds to loose connective tissue that allows some sliding of the muscles during contraction [11].

Dynamic US scanning performed during muscle contraction can show changes in size and relationship of fascicles and fibro-adipose septa.

High-frequency (7–18 MHz) linear-array probes are used to perform musculoskeletal US examinations. Broadband transducers use a spectrum of frequency distribution (i.e., 12–5 MHz) instead of a single fundamental frequency (i.e., 10 MHz): the high-frequency components tend to increase the intensity maximum in the focal zone but cause a prompt decrease in intensity with depth, whereas the low-frequency components extend the penetration depth [12]. Other systems use the total transducer bandwidth for the transmitted pulse and then adjust the receiver bandwidth to lower frequencies as deeper depths are sampled. These systems give increased flexibility to the US examination, enabling the same transducer to change the image acquisition parameters during scanning based on the desired clinical information. In musculoskeletal imaging, this is particularly important when the study focuses on both superficial (i.e., subcutaneous tissue planes) and deep (i.e., muscle tissue layers) tissues in the same study and body area to be explored.

A variety of linear-array transducers, including large (>40 mm), medium-sized (<40 mm) and small-FOV (hockey-stick-shaped) probes, are currently available in the frequency range used for musculoskeletal examinations. Selection of the adequate transducer primarily depends on the frequency. Hockey-stick probes are the best choice for imaging small superficial structures at sites in which the skin surface does not allow adequate contact with larger probes (i.e., soft tissues adjacent to bony prominences) or while performing dynamic maneuvers, but they are characterized by a restricted field of view. Compared with small transducers, high-frequency large-diameter transducers tend to have a large near-field beam width leading to a poor lateral resolution at shallow depths. Because they maintain beam shape to greater depths with less divergence of the US beam, they have the best potential for imaging deep-seated structures [11].

Recent technologic innovations in US have resulted in improved diagnostic performance for the evaluation of the musculoskeletal system, including wideband Doppler imaging, spatial compound imaging, extended field-of-view imaging, steering-based gray-scale imaging, elastography, and 3D imaging [11].

The ability of high-frequency color and power Doppler to detect low flow states in superficial structures and to correlate hyperemic changes with structural abnormalities has allowed for the noninvasive study of blood flow and vascularity within anatomic structures and lesions, opening new perspectives in the evaluation of a variety of musculoskeletal disorders.

The most studied example is the detection of intra-tendon neovascularization in tendinopathy, considered of diagnostic and prognostic value, related to clinical outcome, and the exclusive target of some therapeutic interventions [13–16], but with discrepant results, and recent studies have been questioning the value of neovascularization in tendinopathy [17–19].

Spatial compound imaging indicates an acquisition mode in which the information is obtained from several angles of insonation and is combined to obtain a single image [20, 21].

The advantages of compound mode are many, including reduction of image artifacts (e.g., speckle, clutter, noise, angle-generated artifacts), sharper delineation of tissue interfaces and better discrimination of lesions over the background, as well as improvement in detail resolution and image contrast. In the musculoskeletal system, compound imaging leads to an improved delineation of structures composed of specular echoes, such as tendons and muscles [21].

The extended field-of-view technique contributes to an improved presentation of the US information for the referring physician [22–25], displaying the full extent of an abnormality and showing its relationship with adjacent structures on a single image.

Three-dimensional acquisition can be achieved with US using either 2D conventional transducers equipped with a small electromagnetic positional sensor or dedicated "3D volume transducers," which are larger than standard probes and more difficult to handle but have the advantage of providing more exact assessment of each scanning plane.

Ultrasound elastography (EUS) is a method to assess the mechanical properties of tissue, by applying stress and detecting tissue displacement using ultrasound. There are several EUS techniques used in clinical practice; strain (compression) EUS is the most common technique that allows real-time visualization of the elastographic map on the screen. There is increasing evidence that EUS can be used to measure the mechanical properties of musculoskeletal tissue in clinical practice, with the future potential for early diagnosis to both guide and monitor therapy [11].

Due to the excellent spatial resolution and definition of muscle structure, US has become an indispensable tool for evaluation of muscle pathology, not only for the diagnosis of the lesion, allowing an accurate characterization most of the times, especially in superficial muscles, but also for the follow-up of lesions during healing process, with detection of healing complications such as fibrosis, hematomas/seromas, hernias, or myositis ossificans.

The ideal time for the US examination of fresh traumatic muscle lesions is between 2 and 48 h after trauma. Before 2 h, the hematoma is still in formation. After 48 h, the hematoma can be spread outside of the muscle [26]. However, with some muscles it can stay for much longer. It is recommended that for lesions in the hamstrings, the US examination be done as soon as possible after the 2 h delay. For rectus femoris and gastrocnemius lesions, the examination can be postponed for as long as 2 or 3 days, or even longer sometimes [27].

Dynamic US study may be very helpful to the correct diagnosis, e.g., to search for muscle hernia (during muscle contraction) or to evaluate the snapping hip syndrome (during hip flexion and lateral rotation). To avoid artifacts or pitfalls, comparison with the contralateral side may be necessary.

US has intrinsic limitations in the assessment of the bone. In some applications, however, it can be useful to assess selected bone disorders, especially if performed as a complement to standard radiographs [28]. With US, the interface between the soft tissue and cortical bone is highly echogenic because of an inherent high acoustic impedance mismatch [29]. The bone cortex appears as a regular continuous bright hyperechoic line with strong posterior acoustic shadowing and some reverberation artifact.

US can detect cortical outgrowths (exostoses, anatomic variants), defects (fracture, osseous tunnels, impact lesions), and erosions. Some authors have suggested that the process of fracture healing can be followed with color Doppler imaging and spectral analysis [30].

Bone abnormalities seen at US can easily be correlated with clinical findings and can suggest the requirement for additional radiographic views or other imaging studies if further evaluation is warranted.

The indications for joint US are rapidly expanding due to the refinement of high-resolution transducers and to the fact that both radiologists and clinicians are increasingly aware of the potential of US [31].

US allows visualization and characterization of superficial ligaments, intra-articular fat pads, and intra-articular fluid. Some ligaments located in the central portion of joints (i.e., the interosseous tarsal sinus ligaments and the cruciate ligaments of the knee) cannot be visualized with US because of the overlying osseous structures.

In most joints, small amounts of normal intra-articular fluid can be detected in the articular cavity by means of high-resolution US.

Many joints contain fibrocartilaginous structures, including the meniscus in the knee, the labrum in the hip and the shoulder, the triangular fibrocartilage in the wrist, and the volar and plantar plates in the hand and foot. Because of their deep location and close contact with the bone, these structures can be evaluated with US only in part and not reliably. However, some conditions involving the superficial part of these structures, such as an extruded meniscus, a meniscocapsular detachment with fluid intervening between the capsule and the fibrocartilage or a meniscal ossicle can be inferred on US.

In contrast to the results of fibrocartilage evaluation, US has proved to be an effective modality for diagnosing parameniscal and paralabral cysts [32–34].

Ligament tears can be demonstrated with US at different sites, including the ankle and foot [35, 36], the wrist and hand [31, 37–39], the knee [40–42], and the elbow [43]. The US features of a torn ligament vary depending on whether the lesion is acute or has healed. In acute phases, a partially torn ligament appears swollen and hypoechoic but continuous; an anechoic band over the superficial aspect of the ligament may be observed representing reactive soft tissue edema [35]. In complex ligaments, US can distinguish the abnormal hypoechoic portion of the ligament from the unaffected one retaining a normal appearance. In acute complete ruptures, a hypoechoic cleft reflecting the hematoma can be detected through the ligament substance, and the free ends of the severed ligament may appear retracted and wavy. In doubtful cases, the ability to assess the ligament dynamically is a definite advantage of US: under stress, a normal ligament tightens preventing excessive widening of the joint space; if the ligament is torn, a paradoxical movement is obtained reflecting joint instability [44, 45]. In chronic partial tears, the ligament always appears thicker than normal on US images. Calcifications within the ligament substance in old tears and irregularities of the bony insertions in avulsion injuries may be observed [45]. A typical example is the Pellegrini-Stieda syndrome (calcification of the proximal end of the medial collateral ligament of the knee).

One of the major limitations of US in evaluating osteoarthritis is the incomplete evaluation of the cartilage surface, which is, for the most part, masked by the ends of opposing bones. This is true for both tight and large joints. In the knee, for instance, articular cartilages that are vulnerable to tears and ulcerations are mainly located at the posteroinferior aspect of the femoral condyle and on the lateral facet of the patella: both surfaces are barely evaluated with US. Similarly, geodes (subchondral cysts) are not visible at US because they are completely surrounded by the bone. On the other hand, osteophytes can be readily appreciated as beak-like bone projections covered by hypoechoic cartilage adjacent to the joint line. They increase the surface area of the articular cartilage, thus lessening the stress and loading forces that are experienced by the joint and, at the same time, increasing its stability: typical locations of osteophytes are the posterior humeral head, the internal femorotibial, and the anterior tibiotalar joints [46].

Finally, US can be useful in assessing para-articular soft tissue abnormalities that can be responsible for pain in osteoarthritis and may help to guide intra-articular drug injection.

Detection and localization of postoperative infection and complications may be a challenging task and underdiagnosed with US.

9.6 Multidetector Spiral CT (MDCT) Scan

CT is a frequently and an increasingly used imaging modality with multiple musculoskeletal applications. Technological improvements and innovations have refined and broadened the utility of CT for clinical imaging.

CT has distinct advantages and inherent limitations in the assessment of bones, joints, and soft tissues, both need to be considered when choosing CT for a specific imaging task.

CT technology has evolved since the first scanner was introduced in 1972. The past four decades have witnessed major improvements. These include development of spiral CT, rapid acquisition and processing of raw data, and improvements in spatial resolution. These have resulted in the ability to generate isotropic volume data sets and multiplanar reformations (MPRs). There have been multiple generations of CT scanners, but most of the current clinical scanners use a third-generation geometry in which the X-ray tube or tubes and detector arrays are opposed and mounted to a rotating gantry. Advances in tube, detector and software design continue to refine and redefine clinical applications.

Multislice CT has brought about major advances in bone and joint imaging. A volumetric image set with isotropic properties can be obtained in a single acquisition with a 0.5-mm slice width. Multislice CT allows extended anatomic coverage with thin slices; large patients and patients with metal hardware in their bodies now can be scanned without sacrificing diagnostic quality. To take full advantage of these capabilities, production of multiplanar reformatted images has become an integral part of the examination. Different three-dimensional rendering techniques can be applied to reduce the large image sets into clear pictures for the referring physician and the patient.

Most musculoskeletal applications demand high spatial resolution. The progressive increase in the number of detector elements in each row and decrease of detector width have improved spatial resolution. A typical 64 multidetector computed tomography (MDCT) scan can achieve a spatial resolution of 0.33–0.47 mm.

Reconstruction algorithms can be applied to image data in order to enhance detail or contrast resolution depending on the purpose of the study. High spatial resolution filters can enhance image detail and sharpness to better evaluation of bone trabecular structure. Lower space resolution filters can generate a smoother image, better for evaluation of soft tissues and low contrast structures.

Isotropic data sets also improved the quality of three-dimensional (3D) rendering techniques, like volume rendering, shaded surface display, and maximum intensity projection (MIP). The generated 3D overview provides good visualization of structure spatial relationship, helpful in presurgical planning.

Recent advances in technology and software development also allowed improvements in some disadvantages of CT. The most observable changes are the availability of radiation dose reduction and metal artifact reduction.

The optimal CT protocol for musculoskeletal imaging contemplates several parameters with the objective of achieving the best diagnostic image quality for the specific clinical scenario.

Major musculoskeletal clinical applications of CT are trauma; nontraumatic osseous, soft tissue, and periarticular lesions; and imaging around metal hardware.

Possibly the most obvious ideal application for spiral CT is in the evaluation of musculoskeletal trauma. Once a volumetric data set is generated, the images can be used for multiplanar and three-dimensional reconstruction. The value of rapid acquisition is particularly apparent in trauma patients when the trauma involves areas where patients may have difficulty remaining still such as the shoulder, sternoclavicular joint, elbow, or wrist.

More common CT applications in musculoskeletal trauma include the pelvis and acetabulum, the knee including the tibial plateau, the ankle joint, the wrist, and the spine. Transaxial CT supplemented by multiplanar reconstruction and 3D imaging could have a major impact on both diagnosis and patient management. The use of MPR and 3D imaging can alter the patient management versus the use of transaxial CT alone. These changes in management are predominantly two types: tentative surgery scheduled due to a situation worse than anticipated and acute surgery deferred in favor later definitive arthrodesis or arthroplasty, again usually when the images revealed a clinical picture worse than anticipated.

In acetabular and pelvic trauma, spiral CT data sets coupled with a real-time 3D volume-rendering program allow visualization of the entire pelvis through any plane or perspective [47]. By scanning and creating 3D maps of the entire pelvis, we can easily detect any associated sacral or sacroiliac injuries.

CT is especially useful in lower extremity trauma involving either the knee joint or the ankle. In the patient with a tibial plateau fracture, spiral CT with sagittal and coronal reformatting of data is an important study in defining whether or not a patient needs surgical intervention. The use of these displays coupled with 3D images is ideal for defining plateau depression and quantifying it. In cases of proximal tibiofibular dislocation, the 3D images are especially valuable. Severe ankle trauma also illustrates the role of multiplanar and 3D imaging in finalizing assessment and surgical planning [48]. Pilon fractures, with severe impaction and destruction of the articular plafond, may be triaged into those patients needing immediate surgery and those who will be treated later with arthroplasty. Injuries to the talus, calcaneus, or tarsal bones are well imaged with spiral CT protocols.

Spiral CT with direct coronal reconstructions is an excellent approach to the traumatized wrist [49], allowing successful evaluation of occult or complex fractures.

Trauma to the spine can be routinely visualized successfully with a combination of transaxial CT, MPR images, and 3D studies.

One limitation of CT in acute trauma is the poor depiction of bone marrow edema and soft tissue injuries compared with magnetic resonance imaging (MRI), which is more accurate for detecting non-displaced fractures, bone contusions, ligament and tendon tears, and other soft tissue lesions.

In addition to acute trauma, CT can be used in the setting of chronic trauma. Fractures require serial follow-up to assess healing and to look for potential complications. Although radiographs alone are sufficient in most cases, certain situations may warrant additional cross-sectional evaluation. CT is used commonly to assess fracture complications like malunion, nonunion, hardware failure, and infection. CT allows more precise determination of the relative volume of osseous to fibrous union and cortical bone bridging. The cortical bone destruction of infection is easier to visualize at CT than MRI, particularly in cases with adjacent metal hardware.

CT can provide advantages over radiography for characterization of nontraumatic osseous, soft tissue, and periarticular lesions. CT can improve the detection of focal lesions if they are small or located in anatomic complex regions, like the pelvis, and characterization of the lesion, like the matrix mineralization or presence of cortical shell, nidus, or sequestrum.

The evaluation of soft tissue or muscle infection and/or tumor is another clinical application for spiral CT. With the use of iodinated contrast material, the scan can evaluate an area of suspected musculoskeletal abnormality during peak levels of contrast enhancement. It has been previously documented that contrast enhancement allows for better detection of intramuscular pathology whether it is inflammatory or neoplastic [50, 51]. CT is also useful in distinguishing vascular masses from hematoma, abscess, or tumor.

Artifacts from metal hardware traditionally have been a major limitation to diagnostic imaging, including CT.

Recently metal artifacts have become less problematic in CT imaging by using optimal scanning technique in conjunction with advances in scanner hardware and software. These artifacts can be reduced by adapting the acquisition protocol and scanning technique to the clinical question and type of the hardware.

CT arthrography (CTA) consists of intra-articular injection of iodinated contrast solution performed under fluoroscopic observation [52]. The volume of contrast medium injected depends on which joint is studied: shoulder, 10–15 ml; wrist, 5 ml; hip, 10 ml; knee, 20 ml; and ankle, 6–12 ml. After injection of contrast material, patients are asked to perform full-range mobilization of the joint. Anteroposterior, lateral, and oblique views are routinely obtained to image the entire articular cavity. Subsequently, multidetector CT is performed.

CTA can be an acceptable alternative to MRI and MRA for evaluation of internal derangements of joints in several situations; in some cases it can be the study of choice. Technical advances in CT have improved the usefulness of CTA.

The main advantages of CTA over MR and MRA include faster acquisition speed, higher spatial resolution, and fewer artifacts near metal hardware. MR has some contraindications, like cardiac pacemakers, and CTA can replace MR in these cases.

The advantage of CTA for the assessment of the cartilage is the excellent conspicuity of focal morphologic cartilage lesions that result from the high spatial resolution and the high attenuation difference between the cartilage substance and the joint contrast filling the lesion [53]. A limitation of CTA imaging of the cartilage is its complete insensitivity to alterations of the deep layers of the cartilage.

The faster acquisition speed may constitute an important strength of CTA in patients with claustrophobia, pain, and other constraints that would limit MR scan.

Metal artifacts are less problematic in CT than MRI, and CTA is a useful technique in many postoperative scenarios.

Other limitations of CTA include its invasiveness, possible allergic reaction, use of ionizing radiation, and poor soft tissue contrast resolution.

Radiation dose from CT has received considerable attention from the imaging community and from the public. Adapting protocols to the particular patient body region and clinical scenario is critical to optimization of the radiation dose. Efforts to lower the dose begin by determining the appropriateness of CT as an imaging technique for the specific clinical problem; alternative nonionizing or low-dose imaging techniques must be considered.

Radiologist and technologist should anticipate cases where dose is wasted and should be eliminated, excessive and can be reduced, or inadequate and should be increased.

It is therefore important to understand the clinical questions to be answered prior to performing the spiral CT examination. There are a variety of current CT techniques available for imaging musculoskeletal problem, and radiologists must decide judiciously to when and where they should be applied.

9.7 Magnetic Resonance Imaging (MRI)

Since its introduction in the 1970s, magnetic resonance imaging (MRI) has revolutionized the diagnosis and treatment of musculoskeletal disorders. Excellent soft tissue contrast, spatial resolution, and multiplanar imaging are among the major advantages of MRI. The majority of applications for musculoskeletal MRI fall into one of three major categories of disease: (i) derangement within and about joints, (ii) infectious processes, and (iii) tumors and tumorlike conditions. MRI for sports medicine includes high spatial resolution multiplanar depiction of anatomy and abnormalities in almost every joint in the body, as a result of its ability to assess a wide variety of anatomy and pathology ranging from ligament injuries to articular cartilage lesions [54–56]. The field of musculoskeletal radiology is constantly advancing as MRI applications in the musculoskeletal field continue to grow enormously. Remarkable advances have taken place in both hardware and software technology that allow for improved visualization of anatomy and pathology.

Specialized non-contrast sequences enable the direct quantitative assessment of articular cartilage and other joint structures, thereby providing indirect assessment of tissue health and biochemistry. T2 mapping displays local water content and collagen fibril orientation, and the method of T1 rho mapping displays the local proteoglycan content of the tissue. Ultrashort echo imaging improves the contrast of joint structures with high tissue isotropy or low water content, such as ligament, tendon, and meniscus.

Traditionally, most MRI of the musculoskeletal system is done at intermediate field strengths of 1.5 T or lower. However, imaging at 3.0 T has become increasingly more common for clinical evaluation, while other higher field systems are being evaluated in the research field. Despite initially being used for neurological imaging, availability of specialized coils and numerous studies have confirmed the benefits and abilities of higher field systems in musculoskeletal imaging [57–59]. The most valuable benefit includes an improved signal to noise (SNR) which can result in increased image resolution and decreased exam time. However, with the increase to a 3.0 T or higher field strength comes numerous issues that must be considered in order to optimize its intrinsically superior imaging capabilities.

The gain in SNR that is afforded by 3 T MR imaging systems has tremendous clinical applications in the musculoskeletal system. The potential for demonstrating and enhancing the visibility of normal osseous, tendinous, cartilaginous, and ligamentous structures is exciting. Radiologists have enjoyed great success in assessing joint disease with current MRI field strengths; however, many intrinsic joint structures remain difficult to evaluate, which leads to a golden opportunity for 3 T MRI. The articular cartilage of the knee, the glenoid labrum of the shoulder, the intrinsic ligaments and TFC of the wrist, the collateral ligaments of the elbow, the labrum and articular cartilage of the hip, and the collateral ligaments of the ankle have been evaluated suboptimally on 1.5 T systems using routine non-arthrographic MRI. Because of the enhanced SNR, the higher spatial resolution, and the greater CNR of intrinsic joint structures at higher field strengths, 3 T MRI has the potential to improve diagnostic abilities in the musculoskeletal system vastly, which translates into better patient care and management. As coil technology advances and as the use of parallel imaging becomes more available in the extremities, it's expected to see even more dramatic improvements in image quality.

The quality of MRI depends on the lack of motion, signal and resolution, and tissue contrast.

Although appropriate selection of imaging planes will depend on the location and desired coverage of the anatomical region to be examined and the pathology to be expected, a complete MR examination requires that images be obtained in the axial, coronal, and sagittal planes. Oblique planes may also be useful, e.g., in the shoulder (paracoronal and parasagittal images). A typical musculoskeletal examination includes three to six sequences obtained in various anatomic planes.

The number of pulse sequences and combinations is almost infinitive. Conventional spin echo (SE) include T1-weighted (T1 W), T2-weighted (T2 W), and proton density weighted (PDW). Fast spin echo (FSE) allows for much more rapid acquisition than the conventional spin echo method. Decreased overall acquisition time lessens the potential for patient motion. FSE sequences are commonly used in musculoskeletal imaging. This technique has some drawbacks; the signal intensity of fat remains intensely bright on FSE-T2 W images and consequently can obscure pathology in subcutaneous fat and bone marrow. FSE can result in blurring tissue margins, making some pathology difficult to detect, like meniscal tears.

Short tau inversion recovery (STIR) is a fat saturation technique that results in markedly decreased signal of fat and strikingly increased signal from fluid and edema. As a result, STIR sequences are a very sensitive tool to detection of soft tissue and bone marrow pathology. FSE-STIR sequences are widely used in musculoskeletal protocols.

Gradient echo (GRE) sequences were originally developed to generate T2 images more rapid than SE sequences. Ligaments, cartilage, and fibrocartilaginous structures like knee menisci and glenoid labrum are well shown in GRE sequences. GRE imaging can be performed using a two-dimensional technique or a three-dimensional (3D) volumetric technique.

One feature of GRE sequences is a heightened sensitivity to susceptibility artifacts. This refers to artifactual signal loss at the interface between tissues of widely different magnetic properties. This can be advantageous to detect subtle areas of hemorrhage, loose bodies, and soft tissue gas. Susceptibility effects can be problematic when imaging patients with metallic hardware.

Fat signal suppression can be achieved with two main techniques: frequency-selective (chemical) fat saturation and STIR imaging.

The frequency-selective technique can be used with T1 W imaging, like in MR arthrography and after intravenous injection gadolinium contrast material, and FSE-T2 W imaging to highlight areas of soft tissue and bone marrow pathology. A major problem with frequency-selective technique is the potential for inhomogeneous suppression of fat signal.

STIR technique tends to produce more homogeneous suppression of fat signal but cannot be used with IV or intra-articular injection of gadolinium because its signal would be saturated along with fat in STIR sequences.

Most useful sequences to evaluate the bone are STIR, FSE-T2, and T1 and GRE T2*, articular cartilage are STIR or fat-saturated FSE-T2 and 3D–T1 W gradient echo with fat saturation, fibrocartilage are SE PD and GRE T2* and T1, tendons and ligaments are STIR or FSE-T2 with or without fat saturation and GRE T2* and T1, muscle are T1 and STIR, and synovium is T1 W fat-saturated images after IV administration of Gd-DTPA.

Because each anatomic site contains multiple different structures being imaged, it is necessary to use protocols that adequately characterize these structures. Pulse sequences and imaging planes must be carefully selected to optimal characterization in the shortest time achievable in order to clarify the clinical indication for the imaging study.

MRI allows characterization of multiple clinical scenarios at different body regions by adapting MRI protocols and is an excellent diagnostic tool for evaluation of the bone marrow, tendons and muscles, peripheral nerves, arthritis and cartilage, osseous trauma, musculoskeletal infections, tumors, and internal derangements of the different joints.

Recently, diffusion tensor imaging (DTI) has been used to study muscle architecture and structure. In the future, DTI may become a useful tool for monitoring subtle changes in skeletal muscle, which may be a consequence of age, atrophy, or disease [60]. Furthermore, important information about muscle biomechanics, muscle energetics, and joint function may be obtained with unique MRI contrast such as T2-mapping, spectroscopy, blood-oxygenation-level-dependent (BOLD) imaging, and molecular imaging.

The contrast medium injected for MRA separates the articular capsule from other structures and, due to considerable T1 shortening, outlines intra-articular structures on T1-weighted images. Direct MRA has been successfully used in many joints of the body for a variety of conditions. MRA is a technique which is mainly used in the shoulder, wrist, ankle, knee, and hip joint. Compared with standard MRI, MRA improves the detection of intra-articular bodies and osteochondral lesions in any of the peripheral joints. Moreover, direct MRA improves the assessment of internal joint derangements, such as the detection of labral and ligamentous abnormalities in the shoulder and hip. In the wrist, MRA improves confidence in the diagnosis of interosseous ligament tears and tears of the triangular fibrocartilage complex (TFCC).

In the direct arthrography technique, the contrast medium is a 2 mmol/l solution of Gd-DTPA in 0.9% NaCl. Eventually add 1–5 ml 1% lidocaine. Fluoroscopy is used to bring the needle tip into a correct intra-articular position. To assure the correct position, 1–2 ml of 60% nonionic contrast medium is injected. The amount of the MR contrast medium injected depends on the selected joint. MRI (with FS SE T1-WI) is initiated within 30 min after injection to minimize the absorption of contrast solution and the loss of capsular distension. In the indirect arthrography technique, there is intravenous administration of 10–20 ml 0.1 mmol Gd-DTPA/kg body weight. Synovial excretion of contrast medium occurs in minutes after injection to shorten the relaxation time of the synovial fluid and is heightened by rigorous exercise (joint movements) for about 10 min. MR imaging (with FS SE T1-WI) is initiated within 30 min after injection, when maximal enhancement is reached blanc line.

Gadolinium contrast agents, however, have not been approved for intra-articular injection by the Food and Drug Administration (FDA). Intra-articular administration of gadolinium contrast agents, therefore, represents an unapproved use of an approved drug. Intra-articular administration of gadolinium contrast agents is currently considered safe, and FDA approval is not required for use on an individual patient. Future contrast agents for MRA may incorporate paramagnetic contrast agents entrapped in liposomes to prevent diffusion into articular cartilage.

A major disadvantage of the direct technique is its invasiveness. The indirect technique has the advantage of not requiring direct access to the joint but lacks the advantages of joint distension.

MRI has become the dominant imaging modality in the assessment of sports-related injury, because sports medicine and high-quality imaging are inextricably linked. There are, however, many findings on MRI that may not represent clinically significant disorders. Therefore, optimization of image acquisition and interpretation requires correlation with clinical findings.

9.8 General Principles and Indications

There is no doubt that radiography is the first-line imaging modality for assessment of bone disorders: it allows a panoramic, low-cost, and reproducible evaluation of the bone. Conventional radiography should always be the first diagnostic modality performed to depict associated skeletal or joint abnormalities. More accurate analysis can be obtained by means of CT, especially if complex anatomic areas must be examined. CT can be used for better evaluation of fracture, for assessment of fracture healing process and complications, or for biometric views. While CT allows an optimal assessment of the bone cortex, MRI is the technique of choice to evaluate the bone marrow. US has intrinsic limitations in the assessment of the bone. In some applications, however, it can be useful to assess selected bone disorders, especially if performed as a complement to standard radiographs [28].

As a general rule, MRI and US are most accurate for grading soft tissue injuries, while bone injury can be assessed with conventional radiography and MRI. Bone scintigraphy has a high sensitivity but low specificity and lacks spatial resolution and has been largely superseded by MRI, providing excellent sensitivity and specificity, as it can also identify alternative sources of pain [61].

For the diagnosis of muscle and tendon lesions, US is considered the best imaging modality (*sports medicine stethoscope*), both in the initial phase for recognition of a lesion and also for the assessment of the various changes it undergoes until complete healing has been achieved. Complementary characterization and detection of associated abnormalities and complications can be obtained by MRI.

For internal derangements of joints, MRI is the preferred technique because of its noninvasive character and soft tissue contrast, allowing detailed characterization of the different intra- and periarticular structures.

Concomitant knee multiaxial laxity quantification and ligaments structure and functional assessment is useful for clinical management in the ACL-ruptured individual. Thus, the availability of laximeters, which are safe and compatible with MRI environment (e.g. Porto Knee Testing Device), may embody an opportunity for further understanding of specific patterns of tissue damage and knee arthrokinematics changes [62, 63].

If plain radiographs and/or US are negative or reveal unequivocal findings and clinical symptoms are suspicious for musculoskeletal lesion, MRI must be performed.

Due to the recent developments in CT technology, multidetector CTA has become a valuable alternative to MRI for the assessment of internal derangement of joints and has proved to be an accurate technique to detect articular cartilage lesions. A major drawback of spiral CTA, however, is its invasive character and use of ionizing radiation.

MRA is considered the reference standard of arthrographic techniques for joint imaging. The choice between multidetector CTA and MRI for assessment of internal joint derangement depends on the clinical situation. Multidetector CTA constitutes a valid alternative when MRA is contraindicated or the acquisition time is a major concern. CTA may be preferred if osseous lesions can be present and constitute a decisional element in the surgical strategy.

Familiarity with mechanisms of injury, position of the player, and the need for rapid diagnosis and reporting will help radiologists with imaging of football players. Although plain radiographs are typically the first imaging modality used, magnetic resonance imaging has become the cornerstone on which diagnoses and treatment decisions are based. As football athletes become stronger, faster, and more skilled, the ability to accurately assess their injuries becomes even more important, and understanding the challenges that these patients present becomes critical.

Medical imaging has attained a preeminent role in the treatment of these athletes. Although history and physical examinations remain the primary means of diagnosis, and plain radiographs are often the first line of imaging for these players, MRI has become the definitive imaging examination, particularly as the level of player becomes more elite. MR imaging is relied on by players, coaches, and team physicians because of its ability to confirm suspected diagnoses, add additional unknown information, and provide a roadmap for surgical or conservative treatment planning. When dealing with professional football players, time is always a pressure, and rapid diagnosis of an injury can be critical. This is where imaging, and, namely, advanced imaging, can play an important role for both the sports physician and the athlete, by helping in making an accurate diagnosis as well as guiding therapy and monitoring response to treatment and return to play.

References

1. Johnson R. Sports medicine in primary care. Philadelphia: Saunders; 2000.
2. Geertsma T, Maas M. Beeldvormende diagnostiek in de sportgeneeskunde. Geneesk Sport. 2002;35:12–6.
3. De March A, Robba T, Ferrarese E, et al. Imaging in musculoskeletal injuries: state of the art. Radiol Med. 2005;110:15–131.
4. Cook JL, Purdam CR. Is tendon pathology a continuum? A pathology model to explain the clinical presentation of load-induced tendinopathy. Br J Sports Med. 2009;43(6):409–16.
5. Mcurdie I. Imaging in sports and exercise medicine " a sports physician's outlook and needs". Br J Radiol. 2012;85(1016):1198–200.
6. Pathria MN. Physical injury: spine. In: Resnick D, Niwayama G, editors. Diagnosis of bone and joint disorders. 3rd ed. Philadelphia: WB Saunders; 1995. p. 2825–98.
7. ACR–SPR–SSR practice parameter for the performance of radiography of the extremities 2014
8. Peterson JJ et al. History of arthrography. Radiol Clin. 2009;47(3):373–86.
9. Ekstrand J et al. Injury incidence and injury patterns in professional football: the UEFA injury study. Br J Sports Med. 2011;11:553–8.
10. Evans CS, Harris NS. Ultrasound and ski resort clinics: mapping out the potential benefits. Wilderness Environ Med. 2012;23(3):239–47.
11. Bianchi S, Martinoli C. Ultrasound of the musculoskeletal system. Berlin Heidelberg: Springer-Verlag; 2007.

12. Whittingham TA. Broadband transducers. Eur Radiol. 1999b;9:298–303.
13. Alfredson H, Ohberg L, Forsgren S. Is vasculo-neural ingrowth the cause of pain in chronic Achilles tendinosis? An investigation using ultrasonography and colour Doppler, immunohistochemistry, and diagnostic injections. Knee. Surg Sports Traumatol Arthrosc. 2003;11(5):334–8.
14. Alfredson H, Ohberg L. Sclerosing injections to areas of neo-vascularisation reduce pain in chronic Achilles tendinopathy: a double-blind randomised controlled trial. Knee Surg Sports Traumatol Arthrosc. 2005;13(4):338–44.
15. Reiter M, Ulreich N, Dirisamer A, Tscholakoff D, Bucek RA. Colour and power Doppler sonography in symptomatic Achilles tendon disease. Int J Sports Med. 2004;25(4):301–5.
16. Zanetti M, Metzdorf A, Kundert HP, Zollinger H, Vienne P, Seifert B, Hodler J. Achilles tendons: clinical relevance of neovascularization diagnosed with power Doppler US. Radiology. 2003;227(2):556–60.
17. Tol J, de Jonge S, Weir A, de Vos RJ, Verhaar J. Relationship between neovascularization and clinical severity in Achilles tendinopathy: a prospective analysis of 556 paired measurements. Knee Surg Sports Traumatol Arthrosc. 2012;20(suppl 1):S63.
18. de Vos RJ, Weir A, Cobben LP, Tol JL. The value of power Doppler ultrasonography in Achilles tendinopathy: a prospective study. Am J Sports Med. 2007;35(10):1696–701.
19. van Sterkenburg MN, de Jonge MC, Sierevelt IN, van Dijk CN. Less promising results with sclerosing ethoxysclerol injections for midportion achilles tendinopathy: a retrospective study. Am J Sports Med. 2010;38(11):2226–32.
20. Entrekin RR, Porter BA, Sillesen HH, et al. Real-time spatial compound imaging: application to breast, vascular and musculoskeletal ultrasound. Semin Ultrasound CT MR. 2001;22:50–64.
21. Lin CD, Nazarian LN, O'Kane PL, et al. Advantages of real-time spatial compound sonography of the musculoskeletal system versus conventional sonography. AJR Am J Roentgenol. 2002;171:1629–31.
22. Weng L, Tirumalai AP, Lowery CM, et al. US extended field-of-view imaging technology. Radiology. 1997;203:877–80.
23. Barberie JE, Wong ADW, Cooperberg PL, et al. Extended field-of-view sonography in musculoskeletal disorders. AJR Am J Roentgenol. 1998;171:751–7.
24. Lin EC, Middleton WD, Teefey SA. Extended field of view sonography in musculoskeletal imaging. J Ultrasound Med. 1999;18:147–52.
25. Sauerbrei EE. Extended field-of-view sonography: utility in clinical practice. J Ultrasound Med. 1999;18:335–41.
26. Peetrons P, Allaer D, Jaenmart L. Cysts of the semilunar cartilages of the knee: a new approach by ultrasound imaging. Study of six cases and review of the literature. J Ultrasound Med. 1990;9:333–7.
27. Brandser EA, El-Khoury GY, Kathol MH, et al. Hamstring injuries: radiographic, conventional tomographic, CT and MR imaging characteristics. Radiology. 1995;197:257–62.
28. Cho KH, Lee YH, Lee SM, et al. Sonography of bone and bone-related diseases of the extremities. J Clin Ultrasound. 2004;32:511–21.
29. Erickson SJ. High-resolution imaging of the musculoskeletal system. Radiology. 1997;205:593–618.
30. Caruso G, Lagalla R, Derchi L, et al. Monitoring of fracture calluses with color Doppler sonography. J Clin Ultrasound. 2000;28:20–7.
31. Boutry N, Lapegue F, Masi L, et al. Ultrasonographic evaluation of normal extrinsic and intrinsic carpal ligaments: preliminary experience. Skelet Radiol. 2005;34:513–21.
32. Peetrons P. Ultrasound of muscles. Eur Radiol. 2002; 12:35–43.
33. Rutten MJ, Collins JM, van Kampen A, et al. Meniscal cysts: detection with high-resolution sonography. AJR Am J Roentgenol. 1998;171:491–6.
34. Seymour R, Lloyd DC. Sonographic appearances of meniscal cysts. J Clin Ultrasound. 1998;26:15–20.
35. Peetrons P, Creteur V, Bacq C. Sonography of ankle ligaments. J Clin Ultrasound. 2004;32:491–9.
36. Campbell DG, Menz A, Isaacs J. Dynamic ankle ultrasonography. A new imaging technique for acute ankle ligament injuries. Am J Sports Med. 1994;22:855–8.
37. Jones MH, England SJ, Muwanga CL, et al. The use of ultrasound in the diagnosis of injuries of the ulnar collateral ligament of the thumb. J Hand Surg (Br). 2000;25:29–32.
38. Noszian IM, Dinkhauser LM, Orthner E, et al. Ulnar collateral ligament: differentiation of displaced and nondisplaced tears with US. Radiology. 1995;194:61–3.
39. Finlay K, Lee R, Friedman L. Ultrasound of intrinsic wrist ligament and triangular fibrocartilage injuries. Skelet Radiol. 2004;33:85–90.
40. Ptasznik R, Feller J, Bartlett J, et al. The value of sonography in the diagnosis of traumatic rupture of the anterior cruciate ligament of the knee. AJR Am J Roentgenol. 1995;164:1461–3.
41. Miller TT. Sonography of injury of the posterior cruciate ligament of the knee. Skelet Radiol. 2002;31: 149–54.
42. O'Reilly MA, O'Reilly PM, Bell J. Sonographic appearances of medial retinacular complex injury in transient patellar dislocation. Clin Radiol. 2003;58:636–41.
43. Nazarian LN, McShane JM, Ciccotti MG, et al. Dynamic US of the anterior band of the ulnar collateral ligament of the elbow in asymptomatic major league baseball pitchers. Radiology. 2003;227:149–54.
44. De Smet AA, Winter TC, Best TM, et al. Dynamic sonography with valgus stress to assess elbow ulnar collateral ligament injury in baseball pitchers. Skelet Radiol. 2002;31:671–6.
45. Brasseur JL, Morvan G, Godoc B. Dynamic ultrasonography. J Radiol. 2005;86:1904–10.

46. Gupta KB, Duryea J, Weissman BN. Radiographic evaluation of osteoarthritis. Radiol Clin N Am. 2004;42:11–41.
47. Scott Jr WW, Fishman EK, Magid D. Acetabular fractures: optimal imaging. Radiology. 1987;165:537.
48. Magid D, Michelson JD, Ney DR, Fishman EK. Adult ankle fractures: Comparison of plain films and interactive two- and three-dimensional CT scans. AJR. 1990;154:1017–23.
49. Kuszyk BS. Fishman EK. Direct coronal CT of the wrist: helical acquisition with simplified patient positioning. AJR Am J Roentgenol. 1996;166(2):419–20.
50. Magid D, Fishman EK. Musculoskeletal infections in patients with AIDS: CT findings. AJR. 1992;158:603–7.
51. Ayala A, Murray JA, Erling MA. Osteoid osteoma: intraoperative tetracycline-fluorescence demonstration of the nidus. J Bone Joint Surg Am. 1988;68:747–51.
52. Newberg AH, Munn CS, Robbins AH. Complications of arthrography. Radiology. 1985;155:605–6.
53. Vande Berg BC, Lecouvet FE, Poilvache P, et al. Spiral CT arthrography of the knee: technique and value in the assessment of internal derangement of the knee. Eur Radiol. 2002;12:1800–10.
54. Ahn JM, El-Khoury GY. Role of magnetic resonance imaging in musculoskeletal trauma. Top Magn Reson Imaging. 2007;18:155–68.
55. Gold GE, Hargreaves BA, Beaulieu CF. Protocols in sports magnetic resonance imaging. Top Magn Reson Imaging. 2003;14:3–23.
56. Mosher TJ. Musculoskeletal imaging at 3 T: current techniques and future applications. Magn Reson Imaging Clin N Am. 2006;14:63–76.
57. Craig JG, Go L, Blechinger J, et al. Three-tesla imaging of the knee: initial experience. Skelet Radiol. 2005;34:453–61.
58. Gold GE, Han E, Stainsby J, Wright G, Brittain J, Beaulieu C. Musculoskeletal MRI at 3. 0 T: relaxation times and image contrast. AJR Am J Roentgenol. 2004;183:343–51.
59. Uematsu H, Takahashi M, Dougherty L, Hatabu H. High field body MR imaging: preliminary experiences. Clin Imaging. 2004;28:159–62.
60. Galban CJ, Maderwald S, Uffmann K, et al. Diffusive sensitivity to muscle architecture: a magnetic resonance diffusion tensor imaging study of the human calf. Eur J Appl Physiol. 2004;93(3):253–62.
61. Anderson MW, Greenspan A. Stress fractures. Radiology. 1996;199:1–12.
62. Espregueira-Mendes J, Pereira H, Sevivas N, Passos C, Vasconcelos JC, Monteiro A, et al. Assessment of rotatory laxity in anterior cruciate ligament-deficient knees using magnetic resonance imaging with Porto-knee testing device. Knee Surg Sports Traumatol Arthrosc. 2012;20:671–8.
63. Espregueira-Mendes J, Andrade R, Leal A, Pereira H, Skaf A, Rodrigues-Gomes S, et al. Global rotation has high sensitivity in ACL lesions within stress MRI. Knee Surg Sports Traumatol Arthrosc. 2016:1–11.

Part III

Ankle and Foot Injuries

Injury of Ankle Ligaments

10

Renato Andrade, Hélder Pereira, João Paulo Vilas-Boas, João Espregueira-Mendes, and C. Niek van Dijk

Contents

R. Andrade (✉)
Clínica do Dragão, Espregueira-Mendes Sports Centre, FIFA Medical Centre of Excellence, Porto, Portugal

Dom Henrique Research Centre, Porto, Portugal

Faculty of Sports, University of Porto, Porto, Portugal
e-mail: randrade@espregueira.com

H. Pereira
3B's Research Group – Biomaterials, Biodegradables and Biomimetics, University of Minho, Headquarters of the European Institute of Excellence on Tissue Engineering and Regenerative Medicine, AvePark, S. Cláudio de Barco, 4806-909 Taipas, Guimarães, Portugal

ICVS/3B's – PT Government Associated Laboratory, Braga, Portugal

Orthopedic Department, Centro Hospitalar Póvoa de Varzim Vila do Conde, Póvoa de Varzim, Portugal

Ripoll y de Prado Sports Clinic—FIFA Medical Centre of Excellence, Murcia-Madrid, Spain

J.P. Vilas-Boas
Faculty of Sports, CIFI2D, and Porto Biomechanics Laboratory (LABIOMEP), University of Porto, Porto, Portugal

J. Espregueira-Mendes
Clínica do Dragão, Espregueira-Mendes Sports Centre, FIFA Medical Centre of Excellence, Porto, Portugal

Dom Henrique Research Centre, Porto, Portugal

3B's Research Group – Biomaterials, Biodegradables and Biomimetics, University of Minho, Headquarters of the European Institute of Excellence on Tissue Engineering and Regenerative Medicine, AvePark, S. Cláudio de Barco, 4806-909 Taipas, Guimarães, Portugal

ICVS/3B's – PT Government Associated Laboratory, Braga, Portugal

Orthopedic Department, Minho University, Braga, Portugal

C. Niek van Dijk
Amsterdam Medical Centre, Amsterdam, The Netherlands

J. Espregueira-Mendes et al. (eds.), *Injuries and Health Problems in Football*,
DOI 10.1007/978-3-662-53924-8_10

10.1 Introduction

Ankle sprains are the most common athletic injury in modern sports and represent one of the most frequent causes of time lost from sports participation [1, 2]. An estimated incidence rate of 2.1 and 2.15 per 1000 person-years in the general population was reported regarding the emergency departments within the Netherlands [3] and the United States [4], respectively. When focusing in the athletic population, the incidence rate increases, accounting up to 21% of all injuries [1, 5] and 14–21% within football specifically [1, 6–8]. Along this line, the UEFA Champions League injury study recorded a total of 1080 ankle injuries during a period of 11 years, representing a reported total of 13% of all injuries [9]. The presence of chronic ankle instability (defined as history of recurrent sprains and a sensation of "giving way") was assessed in 512 college/high school athletes (total of 17 sports, 118 football players). The authors reported 65.8% of the athletes indicated previous ankle injuries and 23.4% of the athletes developed chronic ankle instability (half of them bilaterally). Focusing on football, it was found that 79.7% of players suffered from previous lateral ankle sprains and 23.7% had chronic ankle instability [10]. In addition, Jain et al. [11] recorded the injury incidence of anEnglish Premier League football team over a 4-season period and reported 14 ATLF injuries (31%), six tibiofibular syndesmosis injuries, (13%) and one deltoid ligament injury (2%).

The majority of ankle sprains comprise younger individuals, as they represent the most physically active population. The most common injury mechanism is a high-velocity excessive inversion of the rear foot or combined adduction of the plantar flexed foot [12, 13], that is, sometimes exacerbated by external rotation of the lower leg [14]. Specifically in football, the mechanism of ankle injury is mainly triggered by (1) player-to-player contact with impact by an opponent on the medial aspect of the leg just before or at foot strike, resulting in a laterally directed force causing the player to land with the ankle in a vulnerable, inverted position, or (2) forced plantar flexion where the injured player hit the opponent's foot when attempting to shoot or clear the ball [15].

These injuries, if not treated properly, can lead to chronic ankle instability and long-term associated morbidity [16–18]. Moreover, it is possible that bony, cartilage, and tendon injuries may occur concomitantly [19], which must be addressed along with the ankle ligament surgery. In addition, the recurrence rate of acute ankle lateral ligament injury has been reported to be up to 70%, and 20–74% develop chronic ankle instability [12, 20–24]. These patients often experience an early onset of ankle posttraumatic osteoarthritis [12].

At the elite level of football, the absence of a key player may result in the game defeat and associated economic costs for the club. Moreover, the high loads imposed in the ankle joint of these players represent an unfavorable prognostic factor for developing further damage and extend the clinical symptomatology [25], augmenting the challenge of treating these patients [19].

10.2 Lateral Ankle Instability

The majority of the ankle sprains occurs in the lateral ankle ligament complex [9] and may occur in an isolated or multiligamentous fashion [19]. The lateral ankle ligament's complex is composed of three ligaments: the anterior talofibular ligament (ATFL), the calcaneofibular ligament (CFL), and the posterior talofibular ligament (PTFL) (Fig. 10.1). The ATFL has been reported to be the weakest and the first to be injured upon an ankle sprain, which ruptures in 66% of the ankle sprains as an isolated injury, and in 20% of the cases, it occurs in combination with a CFL rupture [26]. Isolated capsular lesion or partial rupture of the ATFL is only present in 1% of all the supination injuries [27, 28]. In addition, the subtalar ligaments are also injured in combination when a lateral ankle sprain occurs, with an estimated incidence of 75–80% of individuals with chronic ankle instability [20, 29].

10.2.1 Predisposing Risk Factors

Over the last few decades, several predisposing intrinsic and extrinsic risk factors for acute lateral ankle sprains have been investigated (Table 10.1). The most commonly cited intrinsic risk factors for lateral ankle sprain are previous injury [30–36], poor neuromuscular postural control [31, 37–40], and decreased ankle joint range of movement [41, 42]. Conversely, gender [32, 43], age [30, 33, 43], biometry (height, weight) [30, 31, 33, 36, 44], strength (ankle and hip) [39, 41], and anatomical alignment [33, 44–49] still show conflicting evidence on the scientific literature. Regarding the extrinsic risk factors, improper lace-up of ankle brace [50, 51], third and fourth generation of artificial turf [52, 53], absence of or incorrect warm-up [54], player position [33, 34, 55], time into the game/season (which may be associated with accumulated fatigue) [34], and lack of use of external support have been suggested [36, 56] (Table 10.1).

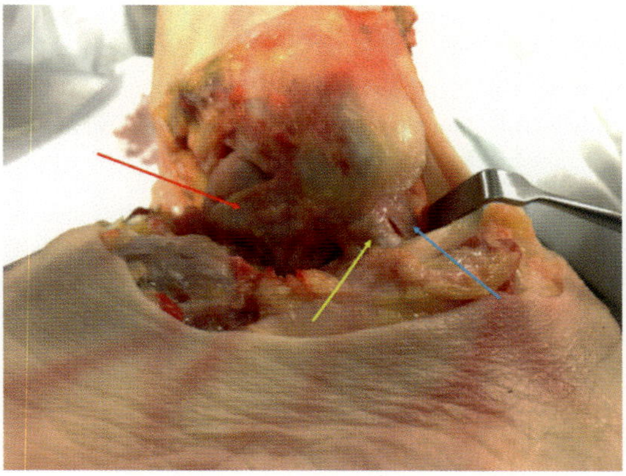

Fig. 10.1 The lateral ligaments of the ankle comprise of the anterior talofibular ligament (ATFL – *red arrow*), the calcaneofibular ligament (CFL – *yellow arrow*), and the posterior talofibular ligament (PTFL – *blue arrow*)

10.2.2 Classification

Ankle sprain has been defined as a morphologic pathological condition of the ankle ligamentous complex, ranging from an overstretching to complete rupture of the ligament [19]. Thus, after an acute ankle supination trauma, it is essential to differentiate a simple sprain from a ligament rupture [57]. In this sense, several grading systems for lateral ankle ligament injuries have been developed, based on the anatomical injury, clinical symptoms, trauma mechanism, stability, and the severity of the injury [19]. In addition, grading of the injury may allow the clinician to better

Table 10.1 Predisposing intrinsic and extrinsic risk factors for lateral ankle sprains

Intrinsic risk factors			Extrinsic risk factors		
Variable	Negative effect	No effect	Variable	Negative effect	No effect
Previous injury	[30–36]	–	Improper lace-up of ankle brace	[50, 51]	–
Gender	[43]	[32]	third/fourth generation of artificial turf	[52, 53]	–
Age	[43]	[30, 33]	Absence of or incorrect warm-up	[54]	–
Biometry (height, weight)	[36, 44]	[30, 31, 33]	Player position	[34, 55]	[33]
Poor NM postural control	[31, 37–40]	[33, 43]	Time into the game/season	[34]	–
ROM (ankle)	[41, 42]	[31]	Lack of use of external support	[36, 56]	–
Strength	–	[39, 41]			
Anatomical alignment[a]	[44, 45]	[33, 45–49]			

[a]*Anatomical alignment*: tibial varum, foot type, arch type, forefoot position, rearfoot position, toe deformity, Q angle, and tibiofemoral angle
Legend: NM, neuromuscular, ROM, range of movement

Table 10.2 Classification system adapted from Konradsen et al. [59]

Grade	Severity	Grading criteria (compared to the uninjured side)			
		Anatomical damage	Swelling, tenderness, and pain	Laxity	Function
I	Mild	Stretching of the ligament without macroscopic rupture	Minor swelling and tenderness	Normal	Minimal
II	Moderate	Partial macroscopic rupture of the ligaments	Moderate swelling, tenderness, and pain	Mild to moderate	Some loss of motion and moderate functional disability
III	Severe	Complete rupture of the ligaments and the joint capsule	Severe swelling and pain	Increased	Major loss of function and reduction of motion

Table 10.3 Classification of acute lateral ankle sprains in athletes, adapted from Malliaropoulos et al. [60]

Grade	Grading criteria (compared to the uninjured side)		
	Decreased ROM	Edema	Stress radiography
I	Up to 5°	Lower 0.5 cm	Normal
II	5–10°	0.5–2.0 cm	Normal
IIIA	Greater than 10°	Greater than 2.0 cm	Normal
IIIB			Laxity greater than 3 mm

Legend: ROM – range of movement

Table 10.4 Functional classification of ankle sprains

Grade	Grading criteria
I	The ankle feels stable and the patient is able to walk with minimal pain
II	The ankle sometimes feels stable, and tender damaged areas and walking are clearly painful
III	The ankle is unstable and the patient may feel some "wobbly" of the ankle joint. Walking is usually not possible due to "giving away" symptomatology and intense pain

judge the prognosis and design the rehabilitation program [19, 58].

Konradsen and colleagues [59] proposed, in 1991, a severity classification system grouped into three grades according to the injury severity: mild (grade 1), moderate (grade 2), and severe (grade 3). This classification is easily reproducible and should be applied 5 days after the injury (Table 10.2) [59].

However, when dealing with elite athletes, providing a precise prognosis as soon as possible plays a crucial role, as time to return to competition is a determinant factor. Thus, Malliaropoulos and colleagues [60] proposed a simple grading system for the severity of acute lateral ankle sprains in athletes based in accurate objective criteria (Table 10.3).

In addition, a functional classification of ankle sprains, based on the patient's ambulatory ability, may also be made (Table 10.4).

When considering the ankle joint stability, two types of instability may be considered [14, 61]:

- *Mechanical ankle instability*: clinical and radiographic evidence of pathological laxity (excessive talar movement) after ankle ligamentous injury
- *Functional ankle instability*: occurrence of the recurrent ankle instability and the sensation of joint instability due to the contributions of proprioceptive and neuromuscular deficits, without radiographic and clinical evidence of tibiotalar laxity

Chronic ankle instability implicates the occurrence of repetitive bouts of episodes of lateral ankle instability, resulting in numerous ankle sprains, associated with biomechanical instability [14].

Dynamic ankle joint stiffness, defined as passive and active resistance of the joint structures (muscles and other soft tissues which cross the ankle joint), generating a net joint moment response [62], should also be considered when assessing ankle stability. It has been suggested that there may be an optimal volume of stiffness that allows the player's performance with lower risk of injury, taking into account the type of activity or task, gender, and the degree of muscle activation [63–65]. In this sense, increased stiffness may be associated to bony injuries, as decreased stiffness might be correlated with soft tissue injuries. Nevertheless, increased stiffness has been advocated to yield clinically relevant benefits toward performance, diagnosis, and injury prevention programs [63, 65, 66].

10.2.3 Diagnosis

Lateral ankle sprain is known to be the most frequent traumatic sports-related ankle injury. The correct diagnosis and accurate subgrouping of the patients are essential for the treatment success. In this sense, it is important to exclude all differential diagnosis including fracture, high ankle sprain, cuboid syndrome, medial ankle sprain, and osteochondral lesion [58]. In addition, neural, muscular, and vascular structures should also be assessed [67].

Usually, a comprehensive medical history taking and an accurate physical examination are enough to the diagnosis of an acute lateral ankle sprain [67]. Performing the physical examination in an acute setting is not recommended, once the results may be unreliable and once the results may be biased or limited due to ankle mechanical pain [57]. It has been reported that delayed physical diagnostic examination (within 4–5 days post-injury) provides better diagnostic accuracy, with high sensitivity and specificity values (96% and 84%, respectively) [68]. Hence, physical examination should be performed as soon as the athlete's swelling and pain have decreased, and it has been confirmed that the etiology of the swelling is edema or hematoma [57]. The physical examination must include inspection of the ankle complex, palpation of the ATFL (Fig. 10.2), the talar inversion tilt test, and

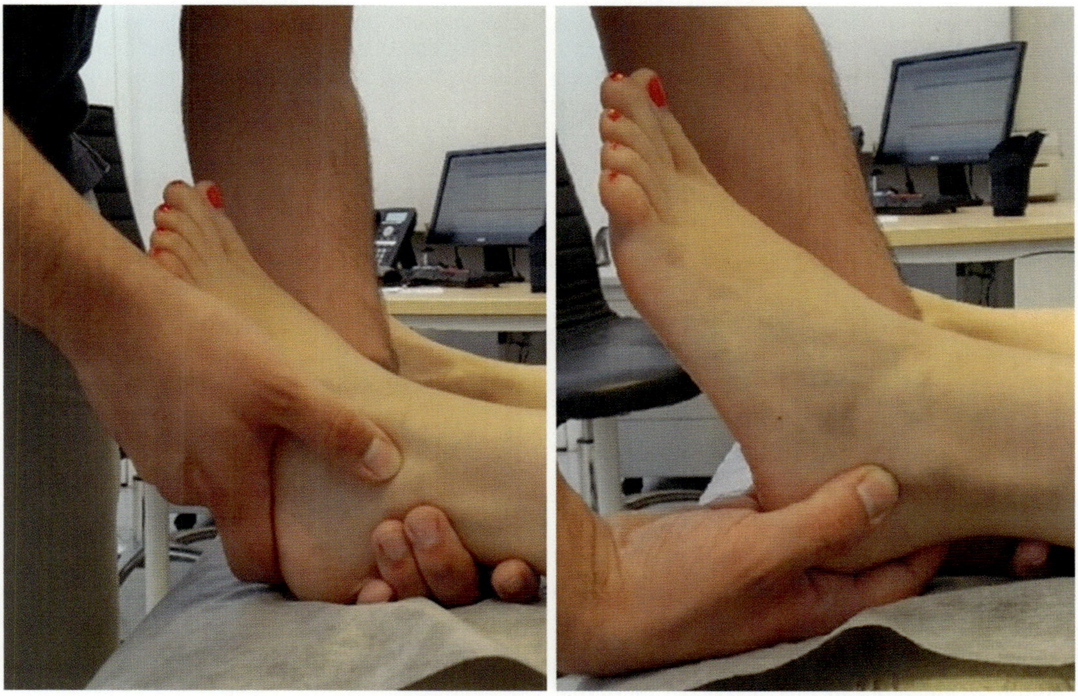

Fig. 10.2 Evaluation of tender spots–anterior talofibular ligament (on the *left*) and calcaneofibular ligament (on the *right*)

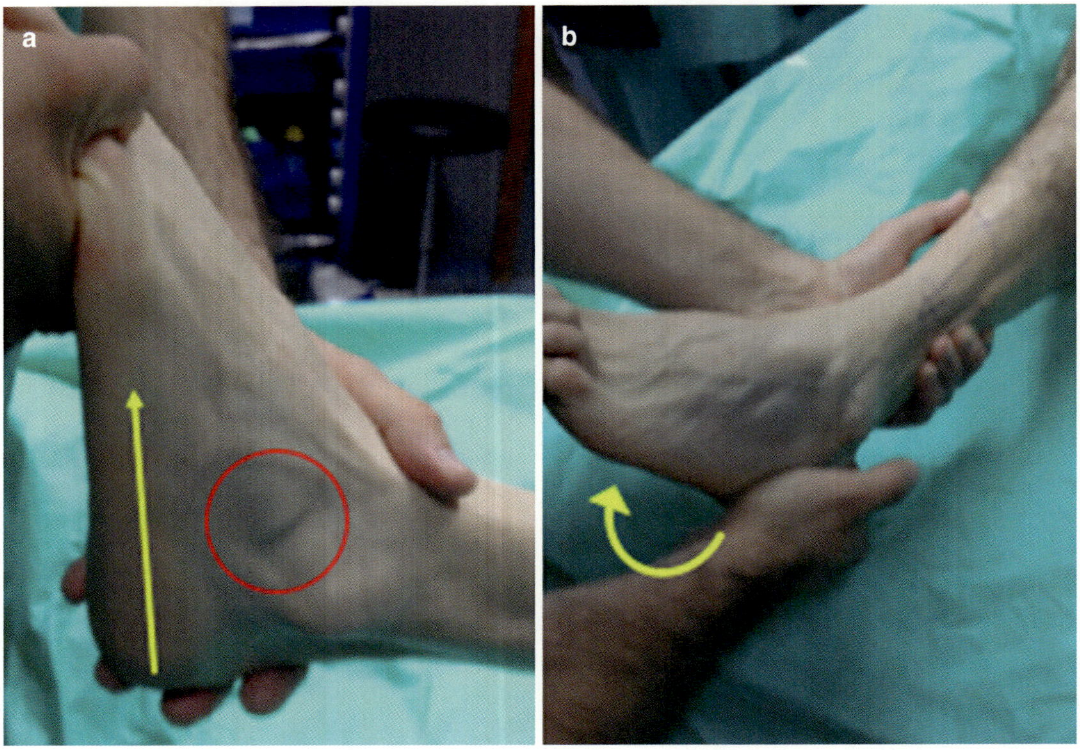

Fig. 10.3 (**a**) Anterior drawer test for involvement of anterior talofibular ligament injury. The test determines the amount of talus anterior displacement over the tibiofibular mortise. It is used to assess mainly the ATFL. A force is applied in the anterior direction from the calcaneus (*yellow arrow*), and the amount of talar displacement is observed anteriorly to the tip of the fibula (*red circle*) (**b**). Talar inversion tilt test: The foot and ankle are maintained in the neutral position. The examiner stabilizes the distal lower leg while cupping the calcaneus with the opposite hand. The talus is then rolled inward to inversion. This test checks the integrity of the lateral ligaments, specifically the calcaneofibular, anterior talofibular, and posterior talofibular ligaments (in order of involvement)

the anterior drawer test (Fig. 10.3), and a few considerations may be made regarding the lateral ankle ligaments rupture [57, 69]:

- Pain during palpation combined with hematoma discoloration (90% chance of rupture)
- Pain during palpation combined with a positive anterior drawer test and hematoma discoloration (sensitivity of 100% and specificity of 77%)

When assessing athletes with suspicion of ankle lateral ligamentous injury, in addition to the considerations above, the clinician should also assess the ankle and subtalar joint range of motion, ligamentous mechanical laxity, muscular strength, and functional performance (such as single-limb balance, star excursion balance test, and hop tests) [58, 60, 67]. In addition, several outcome instruments [70–75] may be used to further qualify the lateral ankle joint status (Table 10.5).

Table 10.5 Outcome measure scales for rating ankle stability, functionality, and activity limitation

Purpose	Scale
Stability	Cumberland Ankle Instability Tool [70]
	Chronic Ankle Instability Scale [71]
Functionality	Foot and Ankle Ability Measure (FAAM) [72, 73]
	Foot and Ankle Outcome Score (FAOS) [74]
Activity limitation	Sports Ankle Rating System [75]

Diagnostic physical examination is known to be dependent of the clinician's sensitivity and experience [76]. Hence, several mechanical testing devices have emerged as a potential instrument to objectively measure the ankle ligamentous laxity [77–83].

After a lateral ankle sprain, if there are recurrent episodes of giving away and/or "feelings of instability," the clinician should suspect of the development to chronic ankle instability [13, 14]. In this sense, the chronic ankle instability may be subgrouped into biomechanical (mechanical and functional) instability, or even the presence of both types of ankle instability [84]. By subgrouping the patients into different categories, the clinician may tailor the rehabilitation protocol in accordance to the specific deficits associated with the type of instability and personalize it in order to address each player's needs and expectations.

10.2.4 Imaging Evaluation

When dealing with athletes with an acute lateral ankle trauma, radiography is of upmost importance to exclude the presence of any ankle fracture [19]. In this sense, the Ottawa and Bernese ankle rules may be used as criteria to exclude ankle fractures; however, the Ottawa ankle rules seem to be more reliable [85, 86].

Stress radiography has no role in the routine diagnosis of acute lateral ankle ligament injuries [19]. In addition, during the acute setting, performing stress radiography evaluation may appear difficult due to pain, edema, and muscle spasms [87]. This diagnostic tool is able to measure the soft tissue structures' passive stiffness and identify the presence of increased laxity within the talocrural and subtalar joints (Fig. 10.4) [88, 89]. Hence, it provides the possibility to further characterize the ankle instability and better direct the treatment.

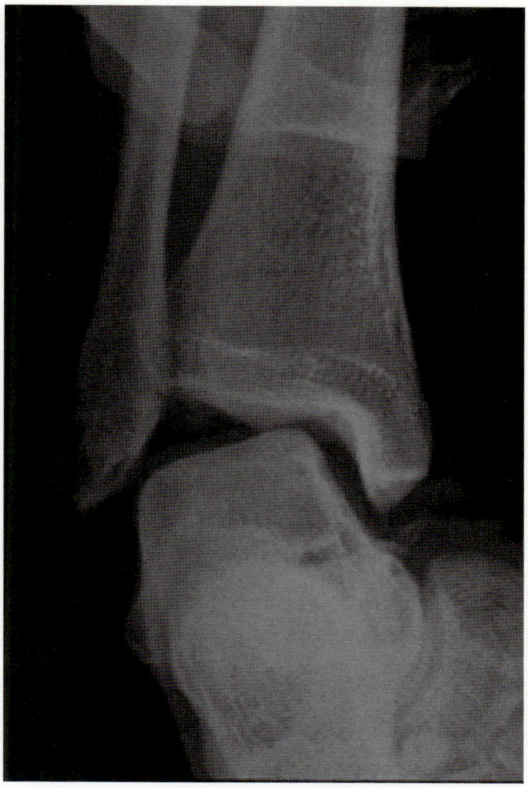

Fig. 10.4 Stress radiography evaluation of the right foot

Magnetic resonance imaging (MRI) may be useful to assess the integrity and morphology of the lateral ankle ligamentous complex and its peripheral tissues (Fig. 10.5) [67]. In addition, it has a valuable role in the differential diagnosis of osteochondral lesions, tendon disorders, and occult fractures [90, 91]. It has been suggested that performing the imaging studies with resort to superficial coils and with the ankle at 20 degrees of flexion improves the ligament visualization [19]. Nevertheless, osteochondral lesions may be better identified using computed tomography (CT) [19]. Moreover, CT scans may be useful to assess the articular surface, abnormal osseous anatomy, and avulsion fractures [92].

The ultrasound is able to provide a detailed and accurate depiction of the normal ankle's anatomic structures and ligament integrity [93]. In which concerns ankle ligament ruptures, it has high sensitivity (92%) and moderate specificity (64%), with positive and negative predictive values of 85 and 77%, respectively [76, 94]. Although stress ultrasonography may cause some discomfort and requires some level of expertise, it may augment the accuracy of the diagnosis [19, 95].

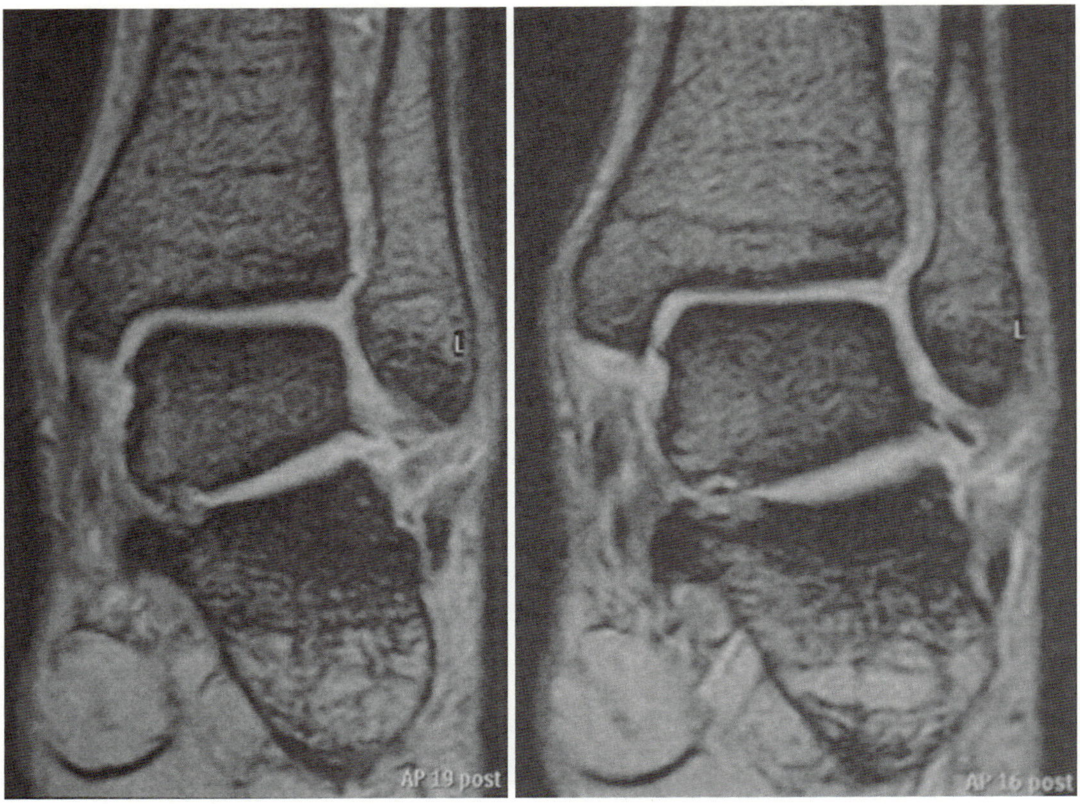

Fig. 10.5 Magnetic resonance imaging of the left foot. It has visible signal changes in the lateral ligament complex (mainly in the CFL)

10.2.5 Surgical Versus Conservative Management

It has been discussed over the past decades which treatment approach provides better outcomes after an acute lateral ankle ligament injuries. In this sense, Kekhoffs et al. [96] performed, in 2007, a Cochrane systematic review of randomized control trials (20 randomized control trials and 2562 patients included) assessing the surgical versus conservative treatment for acute injuries of the lateral ligament complex of the ankle in adults. The authors found no statistical significant superiority in which concerns the two treatment approaches. More recently, two randomized control trials also compared the surgical treatment against functional treatment, showing, likewise, no clear superiority of one approach over the other [97, 98]. Thus, the decision between surgical and conservative treatment must be on an individual basis, taking into account the relative benefits and risks of each treatment approach [96], as also, other relevant sports-related features, such as athlete's individual and team expectations, time into the season and/or career, expected ankle load, medical history, time since the trauma/injury, and concomitant injuries [99].

Several plausible advantages in favor of primary repair of acute lateral ankle ligaments' rupture may be enunciated, such as enhanced ligament healing, reduced layoff days from training/competition, inferior rate of recurrence episodes, and lower risk of developing chronic ankle instability [98, 100]. In addition, surgical repair provides better objective stability to the ankle joint (positive talar tilt on stress radiographs or positive anterior drawer sign) [19], which plays a crucial role in the elite athlete.

When considering elite athletes, expert consensus (level V) [19, 69] suggests the surgical treatment as a primary approach once it provides a better chance in maintaining the ankle joint stability. In addition, it has also been recommended that the surgical repair of acute lateral ankle ligaments injury should be performed by an experienced surgeon, once it will likely improve the outcomes [19, 101, 102].

10.2.6 Surgical Management

Since its first report in 1932 by Nilsonne [103], ankle ligament surgery has been gaining its place in the orthopedic and traumatology community (specially within the sports medicine scope), and dozens of new techniques have been developed [104].

In relation to ankle ligament surgery, two main approaches appear: anatomic and nonanatomic reconstruction. The nonanatomic reconstruction using local tendons has been proposed; however, it can lead to functional and mechanical instability, restricted ankle range of movement, subtalar and tibiotalar stiffness, higher rate of reoperations, development of chronic pain, degenerative joint disease changes, and impaired sports performance [105–110]. The anatomic reconstruction (Fig. 10.6) usually provides good long-term outcomes in which concerns stability, decreased symptomatology, and functional ability [111–114]. In this sense, the Broström procedure, along with its modifications, has been accepted and has the gold standard procedure to surgically treat lateral ankle ligament injuries [57, 115]. In addition, anatomic reconstruction with tenodesis augmentation with autograft or allograft tissue (usually from the hamstrings) has been proposed, with good results [116–119]. In fact, it has been demonstrated that anatomic reconstruction of the ATLF with semitendinosus allografts provides similar strength and stiffness as the native ligament at time zero in a fresh-frozen cadaveric model. This approach is clearly useful in clinical situations where a Broström repair is unlikely to be successful or has previously failed [120]. Additionally, it may be considered a suture-tape augmentation of ATFL [121, 122], once it is at least as strong and stiff as the native one at time zero in a cadaveric model [121]. Moreover, other modified techniques have emerged to address the specific needs of high-demanding athletes [123, 124].

More recently, arthroscopic techniques for repair of the lateral ankle ligaments (Fig. 10.7) have been gaining increasing interest as they provide an improved diagnosis of the lesion diagnosis, also reduce the surgical aggression, and shorten the rehabilitation process [57, 125, 126]. In this sense, and along with the development of novel anchor and fixation devices, several arthroscopic techniques have been developed to repair the lateral ankle ligaments [125, 127–140]. However, there is still limited evidence to support the arthroscopic repair since most available studies are either technical notes or case series (level IV and V) [141]. Nevertheless, biomechanical cadaveric studies comparing open vs arthroscopic approach for lateral ankle instability found that the minimal invasive approach provided an effective ankle stabilization, and,

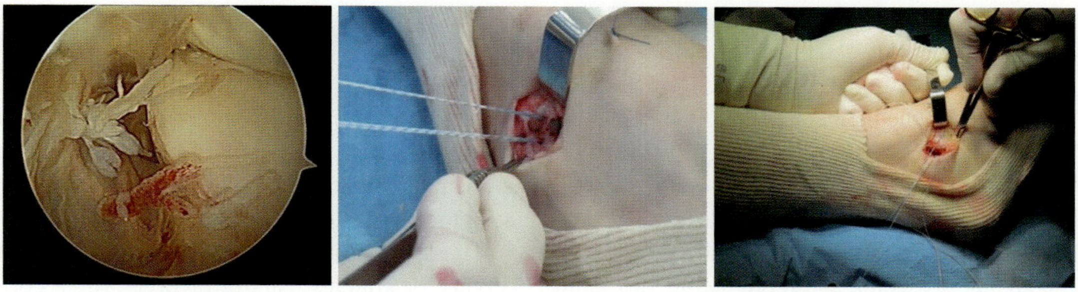

Fig. 10.6 Anatomic reconstruction. Arthroscopic evaluation confirms a poor ATFL remnant (on the *left*). Mini-open approach is then used for ATFL and CFL repair

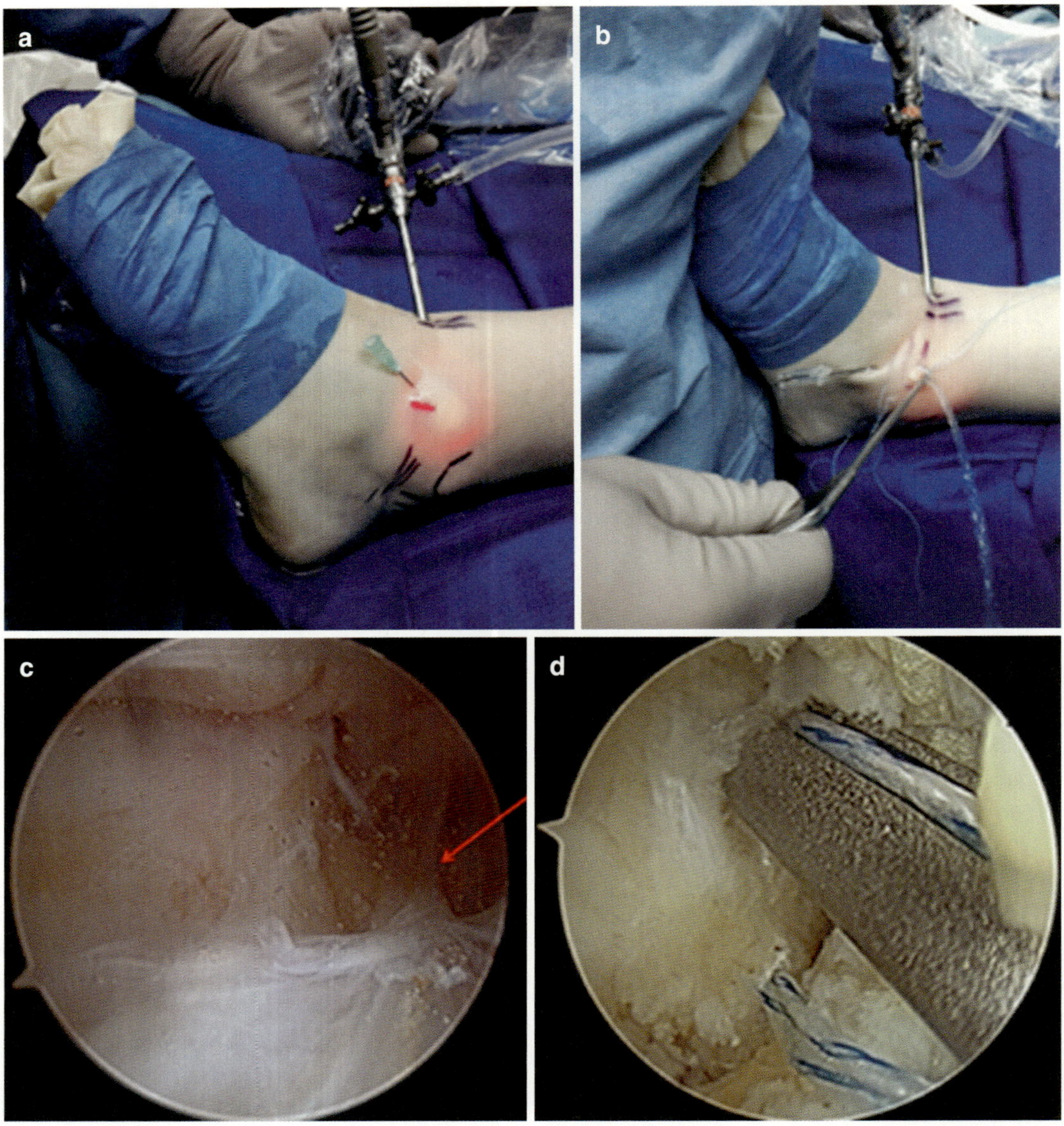

Fig. 10.7 Arthroscopic Broström repair: (**a**) and (**b**) after introducing the arthroscope in the media portal, the lateral gutter is inspected, and the lateral portal is created by transillumination, and instruments can be introduced. (**c**) The ATFL remnant is inspected (*red arrow*). (**d**) Two anchors are placed for final ligament's repair

therefore, a minimally invasive, arthroscopic approach may be deliberated for the treatment of lateral ankle instability [142, 143]. In addition, ESSKA-AFAS Ankle Instability Group consensus opinion suggests that the arthroscopic anatomical reconstruction of the lateral ankle ligaments is feasible and reproducible procedure if performed by an experienced surgeon used to the arthroscopic techniques [144].

When dealing with athletes, a direct anatomic repair of the ruptured ligaments by an expert ankle/sports surgeon in order to provide the best surgical approach without compromising or delaying return to competition is suggested [145].

The rehabilitation following ankle ligament surgery in athletes usually involves some controversy due to the conflict between the athlete safety concerns and the return to play as soon as possible. In the postsurgical phase (10–14 days), the athlete's ankle is immobilized. After wound inspection, it is allowed for the patient to walk in full weight-bearing while using a walker boot. However, walking without any protection should not be allowed until the sixth week. In the early rehabilitation phase (6–10 weeks), the athlete is allowed to walk with any support, and the rehabilitation goals include increased muscular strength and lower limb range of motion, restored full ankle/foot active range of motion, and improved gait symmetry. To progress to the late rehabilitation phase (8–12 weeks), the athlete should be able to walk with turns without pain, good static balance, and at least 90% of muscular strength compared to the contralateral side. At this phase, the muscular strengthening is performed unilaterally, and rehabilitation goals are based in the balance and functional performance improvement. As soon as the athlete demonstrates good ankle functional performance (functional tests at least 90% compared to the contralateral side), the athlete progresses to the sports-specific training phase, which is usually between the 12th week and the 14th month. In this last phase, the athlete returns to running and agility exercises, as sport-specific drills are added to the rehabilitation [146].

10.2.7 Conservative Management

Conservative management of lateral ankle ligament injuries is based on the early functional rehabilitation focusing on the controlling of clinical symptomatology and restoration of the neuromuscular deficits (such as proprioceptive deficits and peroneal muscle latency [147, 148]). In this sense, the early rehabilitation should include the PRICE protocol (protection, rest, ice, compression, and elevation), early range of movement exercises, progressive weight-bearing and peroneal strengthening, and proprioceptive training [87, 149–151].

In the healing phase, the PRICE protocol helps to control the clinical symptomatology (specially pain and swelling). The cryotherapy should be performed intermittently and may be applied through immersion or direct approach [152, 153]. The application of ice with nonsteroidal anti-inflammatory medication may enhance a faster healing [150].

Progressive early weight-bearing with support has shown to have significant clinical and functional benefits and cost-effectiveness in the treatment of acute lateral ankle sprains [154–156]. During the healing phase, the use of crutches or other walking supports may prevent the occurrence of reinjury and reduce the pain during walking, providing improved conditions to the athlete and the rehabilitation exercises [67].

Short-term plaster immobilization or similar rigid supports (± 10 days) in the acute healing phase may provide a hasten decrease on pain and swelling [69, 157]. Nevertheless, a 4–6-week functional treatment is preferable [69, 158, 159]. Several external ankle supports have shown to be helpful in the treatment of acute lateral ankle sprains [160, 161]. Within this scope, lace-up ankle orthosis has shown better results than semi-rigid ankle support, elastic bandage, and tape [161] and should be recommended [69].

Therapeutic exercises should be added to the treatment plan and should be tailored to increase ankle range of motion, strengthen the peripheral muscles, and restore the neuromuscular deficits [162–168]. Trunk and hip strengthening exercises may also be included in order to address potential hip strength deficits and consequently reduce the risk of reinjury [39, 58]. In addition, the incorporation of early manual therapy, such as articular mobilization, soft tissue massage, and lymphatic drainage, may be helpful in decreasing the joint stiffness and swelling, as well as increase the ankle range of movement [163, 169–171]. Correcting ankle joint malpositions in pre-landing to post-landing stages will improve muscle recruitment and co-contraction, enhancing the ankle dynamic postural control in patients with chronic ankle instability [172].

In which concerns the use of physical agents, the scientific literature provides conflicting evidence regarding electrotherapy [173–175], low-level laser therapy [176, 177], and therapeutic ultrasound [178] and therefore are not recommended for acute lateral ankle sprains. Pulsating shortwave diathermy seems to be beneficial in decreasing edema and associated gait deviations [179].

Sports-specific training is important and should be included in the more advanced phase of ankle ligament injuries' rehabilitation [67]. This sports-specific training should focus to the reestablishment of mobility, strength, and coordination while performing the sport-specific exercises [58, 146].

10.2.8 Prevention

One of the bases to design a prevention program is a comprehensive and accurate screening of the athlete's biomechanical performance. This initial screening will allow the physiotherapist to identify the athletes at risk of sustaining an ankle ligament injury and measure potential neuromuscular, proprioceptive, and ligamentous laxity deficits. As soon as the modifiable risk factors are identified, the physiotherapist should focus on correcting those impairments to prevent future injury/reinjury. Even after a successful return to the competition, the athlete should continue with his prevention exercises in order to prevent further damage, recurrence of the injury, or new injuries (secondary prevention). In this sense, the follow-up screening is crucial to measure the effects of the preventive strategies and keep tailoring the prevention program to address each athlete's individual deficits.

Several preventive strategies have been suggested in the scientific literature. The use of brace to prevent an inversion injury is recommended, and different systematic reviews have shown to be an effective strategy [160, 180, 181]. Although exercise therapy shows conflicting evidence in the literature [39, 163, 180, 182–187], the implementation of balance and coordination training within the preventive programs is recommended [69].

These prevention programs are proven to be cost-effective and able to reduce the associated cost of €69 and €332 for non-injured and injured athletes, with an overall €35.9 million reduction per year in the Netherlands [183]. Thus, promoting adherence and compliance strategies to these prevention programs is of upmost importance.

10.3 Tibiofibular Syndesmotic Injuries

Tibiofibular syndesmotic injuries are also known as high ankle sprains. Compared to the lateral ankle ligament injuries, tibiofibular syndesmotic injuries are rare once they require higher loads to fail [87]. Several injury mechanisms have been described; however, the most common involves hyperdorsiflexion and external rotation of the ankle [188], which can also injure the deltoid ligament [189]. In football, the injury mechanism usually involves (1) quick internal twist of the externally rotated foot with lateral impact on the leg or (2) external lateral trauma to the lower leg (proximal to the heel), forcing the footballer ankle to external rotation [190].

The ESSKA-AFAS consensus panel has provided a definition to isolate syndesmotic injuries as "injury of one or more ligaments of the tibiofibular syndesmosis with or without the association of the injury of the deltoid ligament" [191]. Moreover, they classified these injuries based on the time from injury, as it affects the management:

- *Acute*: less than 6 weeks
- *Subacute*: between 6 weeks and 6 months
- *Chronic*: more than 6 months

In addition, a distinction between total and partial rupture of the syndesmotic ligament is crucial [192]. Medical history may assist in determining the extent of the injury [57]. Physical examination involves palpation of the membrane interossea, and manual test includes cotton test, dorsiflexion-compression test, external rotation stress test, fibular translation, palpation test, and squeeze test [191]. If the pain and swelling extend proximally through the interosseus membrane, an unstable ankle mortise should be suspected, since they have direct correlation [192]. Nevertheless, in the acute setting, the diagnosis may be difficult since 40% of the patients may also present pain on the anterior distal talofibular ligament with no rupture of the syndesmotic ligaments [193]. The MRI provides high sensitivity (95%) and specificity (90%) figures [190, 194] and may be reliably used in the diagnosis and prognosis of syndesmotic ligament injuries in football players [193]. Stress ultrasonography may be considered as it provides a cheaper and faster examination [195].

The ESSKA-AFAS consensus panel [196] recommends that acute isolated syndesmotic ruptures with rupture of the anterior-inferior talofibular ligament, with or without interosseus ligament, and with an intact deltoid ligament should be treated conservatively: non-weight-bearing with initially rest, cryotherapy, and walker boot (3 weeks). Following these for 3 weeks, proprioceptive training, strengthening, and mobility exercises should be included into the conservative treatment [196, 197]. Acute syndesmotic injuries with deltoid ligament rupture (unstable) should be treated surgically [196]: screw fixation, dynamic fixation with a suture button, or direct repair of the anterior inferior talofibular ligament with or without suture anchors/button [196, 197].

10.4 Deltoid Ligament Injuries

Isolated deltoid ligament injuries are uncommon and mostly associated with lateral malleolar and fibular fractures [198]. The primary mechanism of injury mainly involves eversion or external rotation of the ankle, which in athletes usually occurs during an off-balanced, pronated foot landing [199]. This injury is often associated with anteromedial pain instead of recurrent medial ankle instability [57]. Hintermann et al. [200] classified these injuries into three grades based on the location and severity of injury (Table 10.6).

Table 10.6 Hintermann classification of medial ankle injuries [200]

	Grading criteria	
Grade	Localization	Ligaments involved
I	Proximal tear or avulsion	Tibionavicular or tibiospring
II	Intermediate tear	
III	Distal tear or avulsion	Tibionavicular and spring

Radiography should include anteroposterior, mortise, and lateral views, providing moderate sensitivity (57%) and specificity (60%) [201]. On the other hand, MRI provides high sensitivity and specificity figures to superficial and deep deltoid ligament layers [202], with clinical use at the acute setting [198]. In addition, ultrasonography has high diagnostic accuracy, with 100% sensitivity and specificity reported [201]. CT scans may be used in cases with associated fracture or avulsion or when bony morphology is unclear on radiographs or MRI [198].

Isolated superficial deltoid ligament injury may be treated with short-term immobilization and rehabilitation program similar to the one discussed for lateral ankle ligament injuries [198, 203]. Acute and chronic deltoid ligament injury and deltoid ligament insufficiency may be treated surgically through direct repair or reconstruction, once it might provide an early stabilization and anatomical reduction of the talus and, therefore, facilitate the early rehabilitation [198, 203].

10.5 Return to Training and Competition

In the majority of the players that have suffered an ankle sprain, the initial inflammatory symptomatology may be resolved through conservative management in a short period of time [152, 160, 162]. Nevertheless, these athletes often present disabling symptomatology and decreased performance due to loss of strength and power and functional deficits (poor balance and neuromuscular control), which may persist even after returning to practice [37, 204–207]. In this sense, Konradsen et al. [23] followed 648 patients with lateral ankle sprains for a period of 7 years. They found that 32% of the patients still presented clinical symptomatology (pain and/or swelling) and/or recurrent sprains. Around 70% of these patients also reported functional impairments at the 7-year follow-up. In addition, Perron et al. [208] reported persistence of eversion and plantar flexion concentric strength deficits in 32 male military units at 6 months post-injury.

After an acute lateral ankle sprain, there is a high likelihood of a rapid return to training and competition [209–211], which can be enhanced with accelerated rehabilitation protocols [211], nevertheless with a twofold increased risk of reinjury within the following year [212, 213]. In addition, it has been reported that, even after successful return to play, residual deficits may persist leading to a higher risk of injury recurrence [214]. These include pain (30%), instability (20%), crepitus (18%), weakness (17%), stiffness (15%), and swelling (14%) [6].

It was reported that successful return to training and competition after acute lateral ligament repair (grade III injuries) was 63 days (49–110) and 77 days (56–127), respectively. However, when associated injuries were present, the return was delayed to 86 days (63–152) and 105 days (82–178). Still, all patients return to their pre-injury athletic level [102]. In another study, with a short- to medium-term follow-up after a modified Broström repair with immediate postoperative weight-bearing, a 94% return to sports at the pre-injury levels was reported, and the remaining athletes abandoned sports due to associated injuries [215]. In a case series with a 9-year follow-up of 42 athletes after isolated ATFL ligament Broström repair, 58% of the athletes return to practice at the pre-injury levels as other 16% lowered their athletic levels, but were still performing less demanding sports [114].

In which concerns tibiofibular syndesmotic injuries, Calder et al. [216] found that patients with anterior inferior tibiofibular ligament and deltoid ligament tenderness and presented positive squeeze and external rotation tests had unstable syndesmosis at arthroscopy. They reported a mean time to return to sports of 45 days (23–63) for patients treated conservatively (grade IIa injuries) compared with 65 days (27–104) for those with treated with surgical fixation (grade IIb injuries). Patients that had injured both the anterior inferior tibiofibular ligament and deltoid ligament took longer to return to sports, as well as the ones that required concomitant chondral surgical procedure. The authors suggested that the cornerstone for a successful treatment relies on preserving the anatomic restoration of the syndesmosis throughout the duration of treatment until full healing is achieved.

Athletes with lateral ligament surgical repair should expect a successful return to competition, within 2–3 months postsurgery. Regarding tibiofibular syndesmotic injuries, it should be expected that the return to competition is within 1–2 months and 1–3 months for patients treated conservatively or with surgical fixation, respectively.

10.6 Final Remarks and Future Directions

Ankle ligament injury management underwent important developments in the last few decades. Nowadays, trend of arthroscopic anatomic reconstruction/repair provides the closest replication of the ligament's native anatomy, showing promising results. Diagnostic procedures have also experienced several advancements, providing good figures of diagnostic accuracy. Both conservative and surgical managements have proved to be effective, with preference of the surgical treatment for athletes due to the increased ligament stability provided. Neuromuscular and functional prevention programs are cost-effective and might help to prevent the injury recurrence. Acute syndesmotic injuries with deltoid ligament rupture (unstable) should be treated through surgical approach. Deltoid ligament injury/insufficiency may be treated through direct repair or reconstruction. After an acute injury, a rapid return to competition may be expected, however often associated with long-term residual deficits. Future research should be focused in:

- Refined arthroscopic repair techniques
- Improved arthroscopic ATLF fixation
- Developed biomechanical dynamic testing protocols
- Developed effective secondary prevention programs
- Improved adherence and compliance with prevention programs
- Defined objective criteria to allow returning to training/competition

References

1. Fong DT-P, Hong Y, Chan L-K, Yung PS-H, Chan K-M. A systematic review on ankle injury and ankle sprain in sports. Sports Med. 2007;37:73–94.
2. Kerkhoffs GM, Kennedy JG, Calder JD, Karlsson J. There is no simple lateral ankle sprain. Knee Surg Sports Traumatol Arthrosc. 2016;24:941–3.
3. Kemler E, Port I, Valkenberg H, Hoes A, Backx F. Ankle injuries in the Netherlands: trends over 10–25 years. Scand J Med Sci Sports. 2015;25:331–7.
4. Waterman BR, Owens BD, Davey S, Zacchilli MA, Belmont PJ. The epidemiology of ankle sprains in the United States. J Bone Joint Surg Am. 2010;92:2279–84.
5. Hootman JM, Dick R, Agel J. Epidemiology of collegiate injuries for 15 sports: summary and recommendations for injury prevention initiatives. J Athl Train. 2007;42:311.
6. Yeung M, Chan K-M, So C, Yuan W. An epidemiological survey on ankle sprain. Br J Sports Med. 1994;28:112–6.
7. Hawkins RD, Fuller CW. A prospective epidemiological study of injuries in four English professional football clubs. Br J Sports Med. 1999;33:196–203.
8. Hägglund M, Waldén M, Ekstrand J. Injuries among male and female elite football players. Scand J Med Sci Sports. 2009;19:819–27.
9. Waldén M, Hägglund M, Ekstrand J. Time-trends and circumstances surrounding ankle injuries in men's professional football: an 11-year follow-up of the UEFA Champions League injury study. Br J Sports Med. 2013;47:748–53.
10. Tanen L, Docherty CL, Van Der Pol B, Simon J, Schrader J. Prevalence of chronic ankle instability in high school and division I athletes. Foot Ankle Spec. 2014;7:37–44.
11. Jain N, Murray D, Kemp S, Calder J. Frequency and trends in foot and ankle injuries within an English Premier League Football Club using a new impact factor of injury to identify a focus for injury prevention. Foot Ankle Surg. 2014;20:237–40.
12. Gribble PA, Bleakley CM, Caulfield BM, Docherty CL, Fourchet F, Fong DT-P, et al. Evidence review for the 2016 International Ankle Consortium consensus statement on the prevalence, impact and long-term consequences of lateral ankle sprains. Br J Sports Med. 2016;bjsports-2016-096189.
13. Gribble PA, Delahunt E, Bleakley C, Caulfield B, Docherty C, Fourchet F, et al. Selection criteria for patients with chronic ankle instability in controlled research: a position statement of the International Ankle Consortium. Br J Sports Med. 2013;bjsports-2013-093175.
14. Hertel J. Functional anatomy, pathomechanics, and pathophysiology of lateral ankle instability. J Athl Train. 2002;37:364.
15. Andersen TE, Floerenes TW, Arnason A, Bahr R. Video analysis of the mechanisms for ankle injuries in football. Am J Sports Med. 2004;32:69S–79S.
16. Bonnel F, Toullec E, Mabit C, Tourné Y. Chronic ankle instability: biomechanics and pathomechanics of ligaments injury and associated lesions. Orthop Traumatol Surg Res. 2010;96:424–32.
17. Choi WJ, Lee JW, Han SH, Kim BS, Lee SK. Chronic lateral ankle instability the effect of intra-articular lesions on clinical outcome. Am J Sports Med. 2008;36:2167–72.
18. Ferkel RD, Chams RN. Chronic lateral instability: arthroscopic findings and long-term results. Foot Ankle Int. 2007;28:24–31.
19. van den Bekerom MP, Kerkhoffs GM, McCollum GA, Calder JD, van Dijk CN. Management of acute lateral ankle ligament injury in the athlete. Knee Surg Sports Traumatol Arthrosc. 2013;21:1390–5.
20. Hertel J, Denegar CR, Monroe MM, Stokes WL. Talocrural and subtalar joint instability after lateral ankle sprain. Med Sci Sports Exerc. 1999;31:1501–8.
21. Beynnon BD, Webb G, Huber BM, Pappas CN, Renström P, Haugh L. Radiographic measurement of anterior talar translation in the ankle: determination of the most reliable method. Clin Biomech (Bristol, Avon). 2005;20:301–6.
22. Fong DT, Chan Y-Y, Mok K-M, Yung PS, Chan K-M. Understanding acute ankle ligamentous sprain injury in sports. BMC Sports Sci Med Rehabil. 2009;1:1.
23. Konradsen L, Bech L, Ehrenbjerg M, Nickelsen T. Seven years follow-up after ankle inversion trauma. Scand J Med Sci Sports. 2002;12:129–35.
24. Anandacoomarasamy A, Barnsley L. Long term outcomes of inversion ankle injuries. Br J Sports Med. 2005;39:e14–e.
25. Linde F, Hvass I, Jürgensen U, Madsen F. Early mobilizing treatment in lateral ankle sprains. Course and risk factors for chronic painful or function-limiting ankle. Scand J Rehabil Med. 1985;18:17–21.
26. Broström L. Sprained ankles. I. Anatomic lesions in recent sprains. Acta Chir Scand. 1964;128:483–95.
27. Broström L. Sprained ankles: a pathologic, arthrographic and clinical investigation. PhD thesis. 1966.
28. Prins JG. Diagnosis and treatment of injury to the lateral ligament of the ankle. A comparative clinical study. Acta Chir Scand Suppl. 1978;486:3.
29. Meyer J-M, Garcia J, Hoffmeyer P, Fritschy D. The subtalar sprain: a roentgenographic study. Clin Orthop Relat Res. 1988;226:169–73.
30. Arnason A, Sigurdsson SB, Gudmundsson A, Holme I, Engebretsen L, Bahr R. Risk factors for injuries in football. Am J Sports Med. 2004;32:5S–16S.
31. Md N, Franca L, Haupenthal A, Nunes G. Intrinsic predictive factors for ankle sprain in active university students: a prospective study. Scand J Med Sci Sports. 2013;23:541–7.
32. Emery C, Meeuwisse W. The effectiveness of a neuromuscular prevention strategy to reduce injuries in youth soccer: a cluster-randomised controlled trial. Br J Sports Med. 2010;44:555–62.

33. Engebretsen AH, Myklebust G, Holme I, Engebretsen L, Bahr R. Intrinsic risk factors for acute ankle injuries among male soccer players: a prospective cohort study. Scand J Med Sci Sports. 2010;20:403–10.
34. Kofotolis ND, Kellis E, Vlachopoulos SP. Ankle sprain injuries and risk factors in amateur soccer players during a 2-year period. Am J Sports Med. 2007;35:458–66.
35. Steffen K, Myklebust G, Andersen TE, Holme I, Bahr R. Self-reported injury history and lower limb function as risk factors for injuries in female youth soccer. Am J Sports Med. 2008;36:700–8.
36. Tyler TF, McHugh MP, Mirabella MR, Mullaney MJ, Nicholas SJ. Risk factors for noncontact ankle sprains in high school football players the role of previous ankle sprains and body mass index. Am J Sports Med. 2006;34:471–5.
37. McKeon PO, Hertel J. Systematic review of postural control and lateral ankle instability, part I: can deficits be detected with instrumented testing? J Athl Train. 2008;43:293–304.
38. Munn J, Sullivan SJ, Schneiders AG. Evidence of sensorimotor deficits in functional ankle instability: a systematic review with meta-analysis. J Sci Med Sport. 2010;13:2–12.
39. McHugh MP, Tyler TF, Tetro DT, Mullaney MJ, Nicholas SJ. Risk factors for noncontact ankle sprains in high school athletes the role of hip strength and balance ability. Am J Sports Med. 2006;34:464–70.
40. Trojian TH, McKeag DB. Single leg balance test to identify risk of ankle sprains. Br J Sports Med. 2006;40:610–3.
41. de Noronha M, Refshauge KM, Herbert RD, Kilbreath SL. Do voluntary strength, proprioception, range of motion, or postural sway predict occurrence of lateral ankle sprain? Br J Sports Med. 2006;40:824–8.
42. Pope R, Herbert R, Kirwan J. Effects of ankle dorsiflexion range and pre-exercise calf muscle stretching on injury risk in army recruits. Aust J Physiother. 1998;44:165–72.
43. Waterman BR, Belmont PJ, Cameron KL, DeBerardino TM, Owens BD. Epidemiology of ankle sprain at the United States Military Academy. Am J Sports Med. 2010;38:797–803.
44. Milgrom C, Shlamkovitch N, Finestone A, Eldad A, Laor A, Danon YL, et al. Risk factors for lateral ankle sprain: a prospective study among military recruits. Foot Ankle Int. 1991;12:26–30.
45. Beynnon BD, Renström PA, Alosa DM, Baumhauer JF, Vacek PM. Ankle ligament injury risk factors: a prospective study of college athletes. J Orthop Res. 2001;19:213–20.
46. Baumhauer JF, Alosa DM, Renström PA, Trevino S, Beynnon B. A prospective study of ankle injury risk factors. Am J Sports Med. 1995;23:564–70.
47. McGuine TA, Keene JS. The effect of a balance training program on the risk of ankle sprains in high school athletes. Am J Sports Med. 2006;34:1103–11.
48. Pefanis N, Papaharalampous X, Tsiganos G, Papadakou E, Baltopoulos P. The effect of Q angle on ankle sprain occurrence. Foot Ankle Spec. 2009;2:22–6.
49. Pefanis N, Karagounis P, Tsiganos G, Armenis E, Baltopoulos P. Tibiofemoral angle and its relation to ankle sprain occurrence. Foot Ankle Spec. 2009.
50. McGuine TA, Brooks A, Hetzel S. The effect of lace-up ankle braces on injury rates in high school basketball players. Am J Sports Med. 2011;39:1840–8.
51. McGuine TA, Hetzel S, Wilson J, Brooks A. The effect of lace-up ankle braces on injury rates in high school football players. Am J Sports Med. 2012;40:49–57.
52. Williams S, Hume PA, Kara S. A review of football injuries on third and fourth generation artificial turfs compared with natural turf. Sports Med. 2011;41:903–23.
53. Ekstrand J, Timpka T, Hägglund M. Risk of injury in elite football played on artificial turf versus natural grass: a prospective two-cohort study. Br J Sports Med. 2006;40:975–80.
54. LaBella CR, Huxford MR, Grissom J, Kim K-Y, Peng J, Christoffel KK. Effect of neuromuscular warm-up on injuries in female soccer and basketball athletes in urban public high schools: cluster randomized controlled trial. Arch Pediatr Adolesc Med. 2011;165:1033–40.
55. Anderson KM. Movement control and cortical activation in functional ankle instability. ProQuest; 2008.
56. Surve I, Schwellnus MP, Noakes T, Lombard C. A fivefold reduction in the incidence of recurrent ankle sprains in soccer players using the Sport-Stirrup orthosis. Am J Sports Med. 1994;22:601–6.
57. van Dijk CN. Ankle arthroscopy: techniques developed by the Amsterdam Foot and Ankle School. Heidelberg: Springer Science & Business; 2014.
58. McGovern RP, Martin RL. Managing ankle ligament sprains and tears: current opinion. Open Access J Sports Med. 2016;7:33.
59. Konradsen L, Hølmer P, Søndergaard L. Early mobilizing treatment for grade III ankle ligament injuries. Foot Ankle Int. 1991;12:69–73.
60. Malliaropoulos N, Papacostas E, Papalada A, Maffulli N. Acute lateral ankle sprains in track and field athletes: an expanded classification. Foot Ankle Clin. 2006;11:497–507.
61. Hertel J. Functional instability following lateral ankle sprain. Sports Med. 2000;29:361–71.
62. Davis RB, DeLuca PA. Gait characterization via dynamic joint stiffness. Gait Posture. 1996;4:224–31.
63. Butler RJ, Crowell HP, Davis IM. Lower extremity stiffness: implications for performance and injury. Clin Biomech (Bristol, Avon). 2003;18:511–7.
64. Farley CT, Morgenroth DC. Leg stiffness primarily depends on ankle stiffness during human hopping. J Biomech. 1999;32:267–73.
65. Gabriel RC, Abrantes J, Granata K, Bulas-Cruz J, Melo-Pinto P, Filipe V. Dynamic joint stiffness of the ankle during walking: gender-related differences. Phys Ther Sport. 2008;9:16–24.

66. Jalaleddini S, Sobhani TE, Kearney R. A subspace approach to the structural decomposition and identification of ankle joint dynamic stiffness. IEEE Trans Biomed Eng. 2016; doi:10.1109/TBME.2016.2604293.
67. Martin RL, Davenport TE, Paulseth S, Wukich DK, Godges JJ, Altman RD, et al. Ankle stability and movement coordination impairments: ankle ligament sprains. J Orthop Sports Phys Ther. 2013;43:A1–A40.
68. Van Dijk C, Lim L, Bossuyt P, Marti R. Physical examination is sufficient for the diagnosis of sprained ankles. Bone Joint J. 1996;78:958–62.
69. Kerkhoffs GM, van den Bekerom M, Elders LA, van Beek PA, Hullegie WA, Bloemers GM, et al. Diagnosis, treatment and prevention of ankle sprains: an evidence-based clinical guideline. Br J Sports Med. 2012;46:854–60.
70. Hiller CE, Refshauge KM, Bundy AC, Herbert RD, Kilbreath SL. The Cumberland ankle instability tool: a report of validity and reliability testing. Arch Phys Med Rehabil. 2006;87:1235–41.
71. Eechaute C, Vaes P, Duquet W. The chronic ankle instability scale: clinimetric properties of a multidimensional, patient-assessed instrument. Phys Ther Sport. 2008;9:57–66.
72. Martin RL, Irrgang JJ. A survey of self-reported outcome instruments for the foot and ankle. J Orthop Sports Phys Ther. 2007;37:72–84.
73. Martin RL, Irrgang JJ, Burdett RG, Conti SF, Van Swearingen JM. Evidence of validity for the Foot and Ankle Ability Measure (FAAM). Foot Ankle Int. 2005;26:968–83.
74. Roos EM, Brandsson S, Karlsson J. Validation of the foot and ankle outcome score for ankle ligament reconstruction. Foot Ankle Int. 2001;22:788–94.
75. Williams GN, Molloy JM, DeBerardino TM, Arciero RA, Taylor DC. Evaluation of the sports ankle rating system in young, athletic individuals with acute lateral ankle sprains. Foot Ankle Int. 2003;24:274–82.
76. van Dijk CN. On diagnostic strategies in patients with severe ankle sprain. PhD thesis. Rodopi; 1994.
77. De Vries J, Kerkhoffs G, Blankevoort L, Van Dijk C. Clinical evaluation of a dynamic test for lateral ankle ligament laxity. Knee Surg Sports Traumatol Arthrosc. 2010;18:628–33.
78. Hubbard TJ, Kaminski TW, Griend R, Kovaleski JE. Quantitative assessment of mechanical laxity in the functionally unstable ankle. Med Sci Sports Exerc. 2004;36:760–6.
79. Hubbard TJ. Ligament laxity following inversion injury with and without chronic ankle instability. Foot Ankle Int. 2008;29:305–11.
80. Kerkhoffs G, Blankevoort L, Schreurs A, Jaspers J, Van Dijk C. An instrumented, dynamic test for anterior laxity of the ankle joint complex. J Biomech. 2002;35:1665–70.
81. Kerkhoffs G, Blankevoort L, Van Dijk C. A measurement device for anterior laxity of the ankle joint complex. Clin Biomech (Bristol, Avon). 2005;20:218–22.
82. Kovaleski JE, Heitman RJ, Gurchiek LR, Hollis JM, Liu W, Pearsall IV AW. Joint stability characteristics of the ankle complex after lateral ligamentous injury, part I: a laboratory comparison using arthrometric measurement. J Athl Train. 2014;49:192–7.
83. Kovaleski JE, Heitman RJ, Gurchiek LR, Hollis J, Liu W, Pearsall IV AW. Joint stability characteristics of the ankle complex in female athletes with histories of lateral ankle sprain, part II: clinical experience using arthrometric measurement. J Athl Train. 2014;49:198.
84. Hiller CE, Kilbreath SL, Refshauge KM. Chronic ankle instability: evolution of the model. J Athl Train. 2011;46:133–41.
85. Beceren GN, Yolcu S, Tomruk O, Atay T, Baykal YB. Ottawa versus Bernese: which is better? Eur J Trauma Emerg Surg. 2013;39:147–50.
86. Derksen RJ, Knijnenberg LM, Fransen G, Breederveld RS, Heymans MW, Schipper IB. Diagnostic performance of the Bernese versus Ottawa ankle rules: results of a randomised controlled trial. Injury. 2015;46:1645–9.
87. van Dijk CN, Vuurberg G. Ankle ligament lesions. In: Volpi, editor. Football traumatology: new trends. 2nd ed. Cham: Springer; 2015. p. 333–42.
88. Leardini A, O'Connor JJ, Catani F, Giannini S. The role of the passive structures in the mobility and stability of the human ankle joint: a literature review. Foot Ankle Int. 2000;21:602–15.
89. Bahr R, Pena F, Shine J, Lew WD, Lindquist C, Tyrdal S, et al. Mechanics of the anterior drawer and talar tilt tests: a cadaveric study of lateral ligament injuries of the ankle. Acta Orthop Scand. 1997;68:435–41.
90. Breitenseher MJ, Trattnig S, Kukla C, Gaebler C, Kaider A, Baldt MM, et al. MRI versus lateral stress radiography in acute lateral ankle ligament injuries. J Comput Tomogr. 1997;21:280–5.
91. Campbell SE, Warner M. MR imaging of ankle inversion injuries. Magn Reson Imaging Clin N Am. 2008;16:1–18.
92. van Dijk CN, Mol BWJ, Lim LS, Marti RK, Bossuyt PM. Diagnosis of ligament rupture of the ankle joint: physical examination, arthrography, stress radiography and sonography compared in 160 patients after inversion trauma. Acta Orthop Scand. 1996;67:566–70.
93. Sconfienza LM, Orlandi D, Lacelli F, Serafini G, Silvestri E. Dynamic high-resolution US of ankle and midfoot ligaments: normal anatomic structure and imaging technique. Radiographics. 2015;35:164–78.
94. Lee KT, Park YU, Jegal H, Park JW, Choi JP, Kim JS. New method of diagnosis for chronic ankle instability: comparison of manual anterior drawer test, stress radiography and stress ultrasound. Knee Surg Sports Traumatol Arthrosc. 2014;22:1701–7.
95. Croy T, Saliba S, Saliba E, Anderson MW, Hertel J. Talofibular interval changes after acute ankle

sprain: a stress ultrasonography study of ankle laxity. J Sport Rehabil. 2013;22:257–63.
96. Kerkhoffs GM, Handoll HH, de Bie R, Rowe BH, Struijs PA. Surgical versus conservative treatment for acute injuries of the lateral ligament complex of the ankle in adults. Cochrane Database Syst Rev. 2007;2:CD000380.
97. Pihlajamäki H, Hietaniemi K, Paavola M, Visuri T, Mattila VM. Surgical versus functional treatment for acute ruptures of the lateral ligament complex of the ankle in young men. J Bone Joint Surg Am. 2010;92:2367–74.
98. Takao M, Miyamoto W, Matsui K, Sasahara J, Matsushita T. Functional treatment after surgical repair for acute lateral ligament disruption of the ankle in athletes. Am J Sports Med. 2012;40:447–51.
99. Kerkhoffs GM, Tol JL. A twist on the athlete's ankle twist: some ankles are more equal than others. Br J Sports Med. 2012;46:835–6.
100. Chaudhry H, Simunovic N, Petrisor B. Cochrane in CORR®: surgical versus conservative treatment for acute injuries of the lateral ligament complex of the ankle in adults (review). Clin Orthop Relat Res. 2015;473:17–22.
101. van Dijk C, editor. The athletes' ankle: lateral ligament injury. Consensus Meeting ESSKA-AFAS. Warsaw; 2011.
102. White WJ, McCollum GA, Calder JD. Return to sport following acute lateral ligament repair of the ankle in professional athletes. Knee Surg Sports Traumatol Arthrosc. 2016;24:1124–9.
103. Nilsonne H. Making a new ligament in ankle sprain. J Bone Joint Surg Am. 1932;14:380–1.
104. Di Matteo B, Tarabella V, Filardo G, Tomba P, Viganò A, Marcacci M, et al. A historical perspective on ankle ligaments reconstructive surgery. Knee Surg Sports Traumatol Arthrosc. 2016;24:971–7.
105. Baumhauer JF, O'brien T. Surgical considerations in the treatment of ankle instability. J Athl Train. 2002;37:458.
106. Becker HP, Ebner S, Ebner D, Benesch S, Frössler H, Hayes A, et al. 12-year outcome after modified Watson-Jones tenodesis for ankle instability. Clin Orthop Relat Res. 1999;358:194–204.
107. Caprio A, Oliva F, Treia F, Maffulli N. Reconstruction of the lateral ankle ligaments with allograft in patients with chronic ankle instability. Foot Ankle Clin. 2006;11:597–605.
108. Maffulli N, Ferran NA. Management of acute and chronic ankle instability. J Am Acad Orthop Surg. 2008;16:608–15.
109. Krips R, Brandsson S, Swensson C, Van Dijk C, Karlsson J. Anatomical reconstruction and Evans tenodesis of the lateral ligaments of the ankle. Bone Joint J. 2002;84:232–6.
110. Krips R, van Dijk CN, Halasi T, Lehtonen H, Corradini C, Moyen B, et al. Long-term outcome of anatomical reconstruction versus tenodesis for the treatment of chronic anterolateral instability of the ankle joint: a multicenter study. Foot Ankle Int. 2001;22:415–21.
111. Lassus J, Tulikoura I, Konttinen Y, Santavirta S. Anatomical reconstruction of ruptured lateral ligaments of upper ankle joint. Ann Chir Gynaecol. 2000;90:213–7.
112. Bell SJ, Mologne TS, Sitler DF, Cox JS. Twenty-six-year results after Broström procedure for chronic lateral ankle instability. Am J Sports Med. 2006;34:975–8.
113. Karlsson J, Eriksson BI, Bergsten T, Rudholm O, Swärd L. Comparison of two anatomic reconstructions for chronic lateral instability of the ankle joint. Am J Sports Med. 1997;25:48–53.
114. Maffulli N, Del Buono A, Maffulli GD, Oliva F, Testa V, Capasso G, et al. Isolated anterior talofibular ligament Broström repair for chronic lateral ankle instability 9-year follow-up. Am J Sports Med. 2013;41:858–64.
115. de Vries JS, Krips R, Sierevelt IN, Blankevoort L, van Dijk C. Interventions for treating chronic ankle instability. Cochrane Database Syst Rev. 2011;8:CD004124.
116. Coughlin MJ, Matt V, Schenck RC. Augmented lateral ankle reconstruction using a free gracilis graft. Orthopedics. 2002;25:31–5.
117. Coughlin MJ, Schenck RC, Grebing BR, Treme G. Comprehensive reconstruction of the lateral ankle for chronic instability using a free gracilis graft. Foot Ankle Int. 2004;25:231–41.
118. Dierckman BD, Ferkel RD. Anatomic reconstruction with a semitendinosus allograft for chronic lateral ankle instability. Am J Sports Med. 2015;43:1941–50.
119. Giza E, Whitlow SR, Williams BT, Acevedo JI, Mangone PG, Haytmanek CT, et al. Biomechanical analysis of an arthroscopic Brostrom ankle ligament repair and a Suture anchor-augmented repair. Foot Ankle Int. 2015;36:836–41.
120. Clanton TO, Viens NA, Campbell KJ, LaPrade RF, Wijdicks CA. Anterior talofibular ligament ruptures, part 2 biomechanical comparison of anterior talofibular ligament reconstruction using semitendinosus allografts with the intact ligament. Am J Sports Med. 2013:0363546513509963.
121. Viens NA, Wijdicks CA, Campbell KJ, LaPrade RF, Clanton TO. Anterior talofibular ligament ruptures, part 1 biomechanical comparison of augmented Broström repair techniques with the intact anterior talofibular ligament. Am J Sports Med. 2013:0363546513510141.
122. Cho BK, Park KJ, Kim SW, Lee HJ, Choi SM. Minimal invasive suture-tape augmentation for chronic ankle instability. Foot Ankle Int. 2015;36:1330–8.
123. Cho BK, Kim YM, Shon HC, Park KJ, Cha JK, Ha YW. A ligament reattachment technique for high-demand athletes with chronic ankle instability. J Foot Ankle Surg. 2015;54:7–12.
124. Kennedy JG, Smyth NA, Fansa AM, Murawski CD. Anatomic lateral ligament reconstruction in the

ankle a hybrid technique in the athletic population. Am J Sports Med. 2012;40:2309–17.

125. Pereira H, Vuurberg G, Gomes N, Oliveira JM, Ripoll PL, Reis RL, et al. Arthroscopic repair of ankle instability with all-soft knotless anchors. Arthroscopy Tech. 2016;5:e99–107.
126. Thès A, Klouche S, Ferrand M, Hardy P, Bauer T. Assessment of the feasibility of arthroscopic visualization of the lateral ligament of the ankle: a cadaveric study. Knee Surg Sports Traumatol Arthrosc. 2016;24:985–90.
127. Corte-Real N, Moreira RM. Arthroscopic repair of chronic lateral ankle instability. Foot Ankle Int. 2009;30:213–7.
128. Vega J, Golanó P, Pellegrino A, Rabat E, Peña F. All-inside arthroscopic lateral collateral ligament repair for ankle instability with a knotless suture anchor technique. Foot Ankle Int. 2013;34:1701–9.
129. Takao M, Matsui K, Stone JW, Glazebrook MA, Kennedy JG, Guillo S, et al. Arthroscopic anterior talofibular ligament repair for lateral instability of the ankle. Knee Surg Sports Traumatol Arthrosc. 2016;24:1003–6.
130. Guillo S, Cordier G, Sonnery-Cottet B, Bauer T. Anatomical reconstruction of the anterior talofibular and calcaneofibular ligaments with an all-arthroscopic surgical technique. Orthop Traumatol Surg Res. 2014;100:S413–S7.
131. Lui TH. Modified arthroscopic Brostrom procedure. Foot Ankle Surg. 2015;21:216–9.
132. Guillo S, Archbold P, Perera A, Bauer T, Sonnery-Cottet B. Arthroscopic anatomic reconstruction of the lateral ligaments of the ankle with gracilis autograft. Arthroscopy tech. 2014;3:e593–e8.
133. Matsui K, Takao M, Miyamoto W, Innami K, Matsushita T. Arthroscopic Broström repair with Gould augmentation via an accessory anterolateral port for lateral instability of the ankle. Arch Orthop Trauma Surg. 2014;134:1461–7.
134. Cottom JM, Rigby RB. The "all inside" arthroscopic Broström procedure: a prospective study of 40 consecutive patients. J Foot Ankle Surg. 2013;52:568–74.
135. Acevedo JI, Mangone PG. Arthroscopic lateral ankle ligament reconstruction. Tech Foot Ankle surg. 2011;10:111–6.
136. Kim ES, Lee KT, Park JS, Lee YK. Arthroscopic anterior talofibular ligament repair for chronic ankle instability with a suture anchor technique. Orthopedics. 2011;34:273.
137. Nery C, Raduan F, Del Buono A, Asaumi ID, Cohen M, Maffulli N. Arthroscopic-assisted Broström-Gould for chronic ankle instability a long-term follow-up. Am J Sports Med. 2011;39:2381–8.
138. Labib SA, Slone HS. Ankle arthroscopy for lateral ankle instability. Tech Foot Ankle Surg. 2015;14:25–7.
139. Matsui K, Takao M, Miyamoto W, Matsushita T. Early recovery after arthroscopic repair compared to open repair of the anterior talofibular ligament for lateral instability of the ankle. Arch Orthop Trauma Surg. 2016;136:93–100.
140. Prissel MA, Roukis TS. All-inside, anatomical lateral ankle stabilization for revision and complex primary lateral ankle stabilization a technique guide. Foot Ankle Spec. 2014:1938640014548418.
141. Matsui K, Burgesson B, Takao M, Stone J, Guillo S, Glazebrook M. Minimally invasive surgical treatment for chronic ankle instability: a systematic review. Knee Surg Sports Traumatol Arthrosc. 2016;24:1040–8.
142. Drakos MC, Behrens SB, Paller D, Murphy C, DiGiovanni CW. Biomechanical comparison of an open vs arthroscopic approach for lateral ankle instability. Foot Ankle Int. 2014;35:809–15.
143. Giza E, Shin EC, Wong SE, Acevedo JI, Mangone PG, Olson K, et al. Arthroscopic suture anchor repair of the lateral ligament ankle complex a cadaveric study. Am J Sports Med. 2013;41:2567–72.
144. Guillo S, Takao M, Calder J, Karlson J, Michels F, Bauer T. Arthroscopic anatomical reconstruction of the lateral ankle ligaments. Knee Surg Sports Traumatol Arthrosc. 2016;24:998–1002.
145. Kerkhoffs GM, Van Dijk CN. Acute lateral ankle ligament ruptures in the athlete: the role of surgery. Foot Ankle Clin. 2013;18:215–8.
146. Pearce CJ, Tourné Y, Zellers J, Terrier R, Toschi P, Silbernagel KG. Rehabilitation after anatomical ankle ligament repair or reconstruction. Knee Surg Sports Traumatol Arthrosc. 2016;24:1130–9.
147. Hopkins JT, Brown TN, Christensen L, Palmieri-Smith RM. Deficits in peroneal latency and electromechanical delay in patients with functional ankle instability. J Orthop Res. 2009;27:1541.
148. Willems T, Witvrouw E, Verstuyft J, Vaes P, De Clercq D. Proprioception and muscle strength in subjects with a history of ankle sprains and chronic instability. J Athl Train. 2002;37:487.
149. DiGiovanni CW, Brodsky A. Current concepts: lateral ankle instability. Foot Ankle Int. 2006;27:854–66.
150. Inklaar H, Van Beek P. Guideline for diagnosis and treatment of acute inversion trauma of the ankle in athletes. Ned Tijdschr Geneeskd. 2010;155:A3324-A.
151. Karlsson J, Rudholm O, Bergsten T, Faxen E, Styf J. Early range of motion training after ligament reconstruction of the ankle joint. Knee Surg Sports Traumatol Arthrosc. 1995;3:173–7.
152. Bleakley CM, McDonough SM, MacAuley DC. Cryotherapy for acute ankle sprains: a randomised controlled study of two different icing protocols. Br J Sports Med. 2006;40:700–5.
153. Bleakley C, McDonough S, MacAuley D. The use of ice in the treatment of acute soft-tissue injury a systematic review of randomized controlled trials. Am J Sports Med. 2004;32:251–61.
154. Kerkhoffs GM, Rowe BH, Assendelft WJ, Kelly KD, Struijs PA, van Dijk CN. Immobilisation for acute ankle sprain. Arch Orthop Trauma Surg. 2001;121:462–71.

155. Cooke MW, Marsh JL, Clark M, Nakash R, Jarvis RM. Treatment of severe ankle sprain: a pragmatic randomised controlled trial comparing the clinical effectiveness and cost-effectiveness of three types of mechanical ankle support with tubular bandage. The CAST trial. Health Technol Assess. 2009;13:144.
156. Kemler E, van de Port I, Backx F, van Dijk CN. A systematic review on the treatment of acute ankle sprain: brace versus other functional treatment types. Sports Med. 2011;41:185–97.
157. Lamb SE, Marsh J, Hutton J, Nakash R, Cooke M, Trial CAS. Mechanical supports for acute, severe ankle sprain: a pragmatic, multicentre, randomised controlled trial. Lancet. 2009;373:575–81.
158. Kerkhoffs GM, Rowe BH, Assendelft WJ, Kelly KD, Struijs PA, Van Dijk C. Immobilisation and functional treatment for acute lateral ankle ligament injuries in adults. Cochrane Database Syst Rev. 2002;3:CD003762.
159. Jones MH, Amendola AS. Acute treatment of inversion ankle sprains: immobilization versus functional treatment. Clin Orthop Relat Res. 2007;455:169–72.
160. Petersen W, Rembitzki IV, Koppenburg AG, Ellermann A, Liebau C, Brüggemann GP, et al. Treatment of acute ankle ligament injuries: a systematic review. Arch Orthop Trauma Surg. 2013;133:1129–41.
161. Kerkhoffs GM, Struijs PA, Marti RK, Assendelft WJ, Blankevoort L, Van Dijk C. Different functional treatment strategies for acute lateral ankle ligament injuries in adults. Cochrane Database Syst Rev. 2002;3:CD002938.
162. Bleakley CM, McDonough SM, MacAuley DC. Some conservative strategies are effective when added to controlled mobilisation with external support after acute ankle sprain: a systematic review. Aust J Physiother. 2008;54:7–20.
163. van der Wees PJ, Lenssen AF, Hendriks EJ, Stomp DJ, Dekker J, de Bie RA. Effectiveness of exercise therapy and manual mobilisation in acute ankle sprain and functional instability: a systematic review. Aust J Physiother. 2006;52:27–37.
164. van Os AG, Bierma-Zeinstra SM, Verhagen AP, de Bie RA, Luijsterburg PA, Koes BW. Comparison of conventional treatment and supervised rehabilitation for treatment of acute lateral ankle sprains: a systematic review of the literature. J Orthop Sports Phys Ther. 2005;35:95–105.
165. Bleakley CM, O'Connor SR, Tully MA, Rocke LG, MacAuley DC, Bradbury I, et al. Effect of accelerated rehabilitation on function after ankle sprain: randomised controlled trial. BMJ. 2010;340:c1964.
166. Hale SA, Hertel J, Olmsted-Kramer LC. The effect of a 4-week comprehensive rehabilitation program on postural control and lower extremity function in individuals with chronic ankle instability. J Orthop Sports Phys Ther. 2007;37:303–11.
167. van Rijn RM, van Heest JA, van der Wees P, Koes BW, Bierma-Zeinstra SM. Some benefit from physiotherapy intervention in the subgroup of patients with severe ankle sprain as determined by the ankle function score: a randomised trial. Aust J Physiother. 2009;55:107–13.
168. Hall EA, Docherty CL, Simon J, Kingma JJ, Klossner JC. Strength-training protocols to improve deficits in participants with chronic ankle instability: a randomized controlled trial. J Athl Train. 2015;50:36–44.
169. Eisenhart AW, Gaeta TJ, Yens DP. Osteopathic manipulative treatment in the emergency department for patients with acute ankle injuries. J Am Osteopath Assoc. 2003;103:417–21.
170. Collins N, Teys P, Vicenzino B. The initial effects of a Mulligan's mobilization with movement technique on dorsiflexion and pain in subacute ankle sprains. Man Ther. 2004;9:77–82.
171. Brantingham JW, Globe G, Pollard H, Hicks M, Korporaal C, Hoskins W. Manipulative therapy for lower extremity conditions: expansion of literature review. J Manipulative Physiol Ther. 2009;32:53–71.
172. Lin C-F, Chen C-Y, Lin C-W. Dynamic ankle control in athletes with ankle instability during sports maneuvers. Am J Sports Med. 2011;39:2007–15.
173. Mendel FC, Dolan MG, Fish DR, Marzo J, Wilding GE. Effect of high-voltage pulsed current on recovery after grades I and II lateral ankle sprains. J Sport Rehabil. 2010;19:399.
174. Wilson D. Treatment of soft-tissue injuries by pulsed electrical energy. Brit Med J. 1972;2:269–70.
175. Man IO, Morrissey MC, Cywinski JK. Effect of neuromuscular electrical stimulation on ankle swelling in the early period after ankle sprain. Phys Ther. 2007;87:53–65.
176. Stergioulas A. Low-level laser treatment can reduce edema in second degree ankle sprains. J Clin Laser Med Surg. 2004;22:125–8.
177. de Bie RA, de Vet HC, Lenssen TF, van den Wildenberg FA, Kootstra G, Knipschild PG. Low-level laser therapy in ankle sprains: a randomized clinical trial. Arch Phys Med Rehabil. 1998;79:1415–20.
178. van den Bekerom MP, van der Windt DA, ter Riet G, van der Heijden GJ, Bouter LM. Therapeutic ultrasound for acute ankle sprains. Cochrane Database Syst Rev. 2011;6:CD001250.
179. PasHa M, Visuri T, Sundholm A. Pulsating shortwave diathermy: value in treatment of recent ankle and foot sprains. Arch Phys Med Rehabil. 1978;59
180. Verhagen EA, van Mechelen W, de Vente W. The effect of preventive measures on the incidence of ankle sprains. Clin J Sport Med. 2000;10:291–6.
181. Handoll HH, Rowe BH, Quinn KM, de Bie R. Interventions for preventing ankle ligament injuries. Cochrane Database Syst Rev. 2011;5:CD000018.
182. Hupperets MD, Verhagen EA, Van Mechelen W. Effect of unsupervised home based proprioceptive training on recurrences of ankle sprain: randomised controlled trial. Brit Med J. 2009;339:b2684.
183. Hupperets MD, Verhagen EA, Heymans MW, Bosmans JE, van Tulder MW, Van Mechelen

W. Potential savings of a program to prevent ankle sprain recurrence economic evaluation of a randomized controlled trial. Am J Sports Med. 2010;38:2194–200.
184. Cumps E, Verhagen E, Meeusen R. Efficacy of a sports specific balance training programme on the incidence of ankle sprains in basketball. J Sports Sci Med. 2007;6:212–9.
185. McGuine TA, Greene JJ, Best T, Leverson G. Balance as a predictor of ankle injuries in high school basketball players. Clin J Sport Med. 2000;10:239–44.
186. Emery CA, Cassidy JD, Klassen TP, Rosychuk RJ, Rowe BH. Effectiveness of a home-based balance-training program in reducing sports-related injuries among healthy adolescents: a cluster randomized controlled trial. Can Med Assoc J. 2005;172: 749–54.
187. Verhagen E, Van der Beek A, Twisk J, Bouter L, Bahr R, Van Mechelen W. The effect of a proprioceptive balance board training program for the prevention of ankle sprains a prospective controlled trial. Am J Sports Med. 2004;32:1385–93.
188. Mulligan EP. Evaluation and management of ankle syndesmosis injuries. Phys Ther Sport. 2011;12:57–69.
189. Dubin JC, Comeau D, McClelland RI, Dubin RA, Ferrel E. Lateral and syndesmotic ankle sprain injuries: a narrative literature review. J Chiropr Med. 2011;10:204–19.
190. Williams GN, Allen EJ. Rehabilitation of syndesmotic (high) ankle sprains. Sport Health. 2010;2:460–70.
191. van Dijk CN, Longo UG, Loppini M, Florio P, Maltese L, Ciuffreda M, et al. Classification and diagnosis of acute isolated syndesmotic injuries: ESSKA-AFAS consensus and guidelines. Knee Surg Sports Traumatol Arthrosc. 2016;24:1200–16.
192. van Dijk C, Vuurberg G, Amendola A, Lee J. Anterior ankle arthroscopy: state of the art. J ISAKOS. 2016;1:105–15.
193. Howard DR, Rubin DA, Hillen TJ, Nissman DB, Lomax J, Williams T, et al. Magnetic resonance imaging as a predictor of return to play following syndesmosis (high) ankle sprains in professional football players. Sport Health. 2012;4:535–43.
194. Brown KW, Morrison WB, Schweitzer ME, Parellada JA, Nothnagel H. MRI findings associated with distal tibiofibular syndesmosis injury. AJR Am J Roentgenol. 2004;182:131–6.
195. Mei-Dan O, Kots E, Barchilon V, Massarwe S, Nyska M, Mann G. A dynamic ultrasound examination for the diagnosis of ankle syndesmotic injury in professional athletes a preliminary study. Am J Sports Med. 2009;37:1009–16.
196. van Dijk CN, Longo UG, Loppini M, Florio P, Maltese L, Ciuffreda M, et al. Conservative and surgical management of acute isolated syndesmotic injuries: ESSKA-AFAS consensus and guidelines. Knee Surg Sports Traumatol Arthrosc. 2016;24:1217–27.
197. Jones CB, Gilde A, Sietsema DL. Treatment of syndesmotic injuries of the ankle. JBJS Rev. 2015;3:e1.
198. McCollum GA, van den Bekerom MP, Kerkhoffs GM, Calder JD, van Dijk CN. Syndesmosis and deltoid ligament injuries in the athlete. Knee Surg Sports Traumatol Arthrosc. 2013;21:1328–37.
199. O'Loughlin PF, Murawski CD, Egan C, Kennedy JG. Ankle instability in sports. Phys Sportsmed. 2009;37:93–103.
200. Hintermann B. Medial ankle instability. Foot Ankle Clin. 2003;8:723–38.
201. Henari S, Banks LN, Radiovanovic I, Queally J, Morris S. Ultrasonography as a diagnostic tool in assessing deltoid ligament injury in supination external rotation fractures of the ankle. Orthopedics. 2011;34:e639–e43.
202. Koval KJ, Egol KA, Cheung Y, Goodwin DW, Spratt KF. Does a positive ankle stress test indicate the need for operative treatment after lateral malleolus fracture? A preliminary report. J Orthop Trauma. 2007;21:449–55.
203. Savage-Elliott I, Murawski CD, Smyth NA, Golanó P, Kennedy JG. The deltoid ligament: an in-depth review of anatomy, function, and treatment strategies. Knee Surg Sports Traumatol Arthrosc. 2013;21:1316–27.
204. Van Rijn RM, Van Os AG, Bernsen RM, Luijsterburg PA, Koes BW, Bierma-Zeinstra SM. What is the clinical course of acute ankle sprains? A systematic literature review. Am J Sports Med. 2008;121:324–31.
205. Hertel J. Sensorimotor deficits with ankle sprains and chronic ankle instability. Clin Sports Med. 2008;27:353–70.
206. Wikstrom EA, Naik S, Lodha N, Cauraugh JH. Bilateral balance impairments after lateral ankle trauma: a systematic review and meta-analysis. Gait Posture. 2010;31:407–14.
207. Holme E, Magnusson S, Becher K, Bieler T, Aagaard P, Kjaer M. The effect of supervised rehabilitation on strength, postural sway, position sense and re-injury risk after acute ankle ligament sprain. Scand J Med Sci Sports. 1999;9:104–9.
208. Perron M, Moffet H, Nadeau S, Hebert LJ, Belzile S. Persistence of long term isokinetic strength deficits in subjects with lateral ankle sprain as measured with a protocol including maximal preloading. Clin Biomech (Bristol, Avon). 2014;29:1151–7.
209. Gerber JP, Williams GN, Scoville CR, Arciero RA, Taylor DC. Persistent disability associated with ankle sprains: a prospective examination of an athletic population. Foot Ankle Int. 1998;19:653–60.
210. McKeon JMM, Bush HM, Reed A, Whittington A, Uhl TL, McKeon PO. Return-to-play probabilities following new versus recurrent ankle sprains in high school athletes. J Sci Med Sport. 2014;17:23–8.
211. Miyamoto W, Takao M, Yamada K, Matsushita T. Accelerated versus traditional rehabilitation after

anterior talofibular ligament reconstruction for chronic lateral instability of the ankle in athletes. Am J Sports Med. 2014;42:1441–7.
212. Verhagen E, Van Tulder M, van der Beek AJ, Bouter L, Van Mechelen W. An economic evaluation of a proprioceptive balance board training programme for the prevention of ankle sprains in volleyball. Br J Sports Med. 2005;39:111–5.
213. Beynnon BD, Murphy DF, Alosa DM. Predictive factors for lateral ankle sprains: a literature review. J Athl Train. 2002;37:376.
214. Steib S, Hentschke C. Fatigue-induced alterations of static and dynamic postural control in athletes with a history of ankle sprain. J Athl Train. 2013;48:203.
215. Petrera M, Dwyer T, Theodoropoulos JS, Ogilvie-Harris DJ. Short-to medium-term outcomes after a modified Broström repair for lateral ankle instability with immediate postoperative weightbearing. Am J Sports Med. 2014:0363546514530668.
216. Calder JD, Bamford R, Petrie A, McCollum GA. Stable versus unstable grade II high ankle sprains: a prospective study predicting the need for surgical stabilization and time to return to sports. Arthroscopy. 2016;32:634–42.

Osteochondral Ankle Injuries

11

Ricardo Telles Freitas, Hélder Pereira, John Kennedy, and C. Niek Van Dijk

Contents

11.1 Introduction

An osteochondral ankle defect (OCD) is a lesion of the talar cartilage and subchondral bone mostly caused by a single or multiple traumatic events, leading to partial or complete detachment of the fragment (Figs. 11.1 and 11.2) [1].

The defects cause deep ankle pain associated with weight bearing. Impaired function, limited range of motion, stiffness, catching, locking, and swelling may be present [2]. These symptoms place the ability to walk, work, and perform sports at risk.

R.T. Freitas (✉)
CUF Descobertas Hospital, Lisbon, Portugal

H. Pereira
3B's Research Group–Biomaterials, Biodegradables and Biomimetics, University of Minho, Headquarters of the European Institute of Excellence on Tissue Engineering and Regenerative Medicine, AvePark, Parque de Ciência e Tecnologia, Zona Industrial da Gandra, 4805-017 Barco, Guimarães, Portugal

Ripoll y De Prado Sports Clinic – FIFA Medical Centre of Excellence, Murcia-Madrid, Spain

Orthopedic Department, Centro Hospitalar Póvoa de Varzim – Vila do Conde, Póvoa de Varzim, Portugal

J. Kennedy
Hospital for Special Surgery, New York, NY, USA

C.N. Van Dijk
Department of Orthopaedic Surgery, Academic Medical Center Amsterdam, Meibergdreef 9, 1105 AZ Amsterdam, The Netherlands

J. Espregueira-Mendes et al. (eds.), *Injuries and Health Problems in Football*, DOI 10.1007/978-3-662-53924-8_11

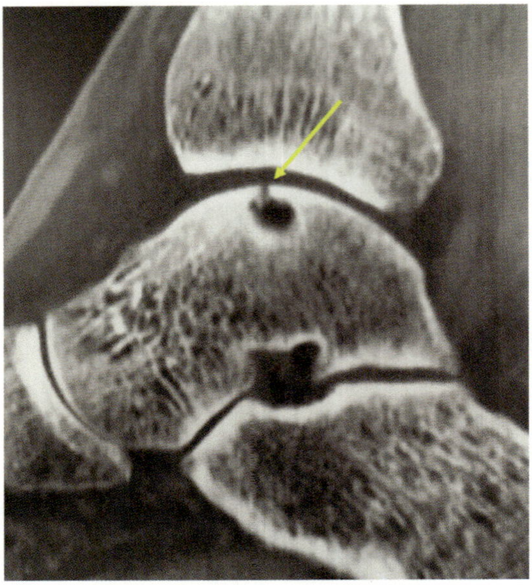

Fig. 11.1 CT image of talus osteochondral defect with bone cyst formation (*yellow arrow*). A cartilage defect in a congruent joint enables joint fluid to penetrate the subchondral bone leading to osteolysis. Bony defects are better evaluated in CT opposing to MRI

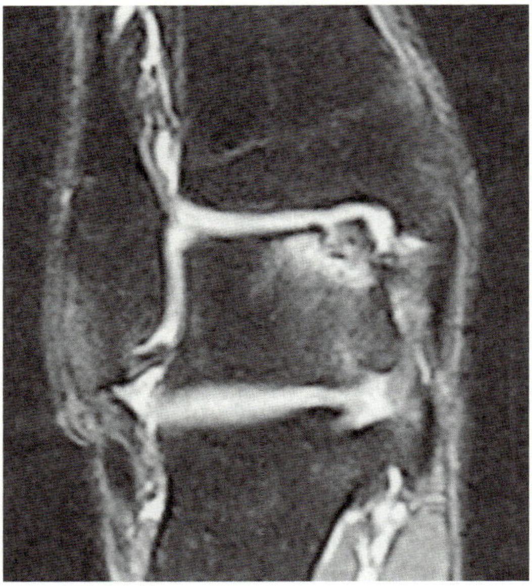

Fig. 11.2 MRI T2 image of medial talus osteochondral defect (*yellow arrow*). Edema is sometimes related to "active" (more symptomatic) lesions

Symptomatic osteochondral ankle defects often require surgical treatment [3].

11.2 Etiology

A traumatic insult is widely accepted as the most important etiologic factor of an OD of the talus [1].

The injury was classified by Berndt and Harty in 1959 [4].

Ankle sprains cause intra-articular pressure impact and have a prominent role in the development of traumatic OCD. For lateral talar defects, trauma has been described in 93–98% and for medial defects in 61–70% [1].

The trauma causing the lesion can be a single event or a series of less intense (micro) traumas, which may remain unrecognized in some cases.

As not all patients report a history of ankle injury, a subdivision can be made in the etiology of nontraumatic and traumatic defects [2]. Ischemia, subsequent necrosis, and possibly genetics are etiologic factors in nontraumatic OCD [2].

11.3 Epidemiology

Symptomatic OCDs of the talus usually appear in the second or third decade of life. Men are affected more often than women.

Approximately 1 in 10,000 people per day suffers an ankle injury [2]. Talar OCDs occur in 15–25% of these injuries. These data suggest that OCDs are common but not always cause symptoms [5].

11.4 Clinical Presentation

In the acute situation, an OCD of the talus often remains unrecognized since the swelling and pain from the lateral ligament lesion prevail.

When the symptoms of the ligament injury have resolved after some weeks, symptoms of persistent swelling, limited range of motion, and pain on weight bearing may continue. If symptoms have not resolved within 4–6 weeks, an osteochondral defect should be suspected. Locking and catching are symptoms of a displaced fragment [2].

Chronic lesions typically present as persistent or intermittent deep ankle pain during or after activity. Most patients demonstrate a normal range of motion with the absence of recognizable tenderness on palpation and absence of swelling. However, reactive swelling or stiffness may be present [6].

11.5 Cause of Pain in Osteochondral Ankle Lesions

Several factors can play a role in the cause of pain in ODs.

A rise in intra-articular pressure can be a cause of pain in degenerative joint disease [7]. However, it is unlikely that in a localized osteochondral talar defect, a raise in intra-articular pressure plays a role [8]. These patients typically do not demonstrate relevant joint effusion.

Nerve endings can be found in the synovium and joint capsule. Patients with an OD of the ankle, however, generally do not show much synovitis. The synovium of the anterior ankle joint can be palpated since it lies directly under the skin. These patients usually can differentiate this secondary synovial pain from the deep ankle pain caused by the OD. The disabling deep ankle pain on weight bearing cannot be reproduced during physical examination.

The most probable cause of this pain is the nerve endings in the subchondral bone that have been firstly detected in the early 1990s [5, 9] [3].

Pain probably develops as a rise in fluid pressure, and a decrease in pH excitates nerve fibers present in bone [4].

11.6 Natural History

The lesions can either heal and remain asymptomatic or progress to deep ankle pain on weight bearing and formation of subchondral bone cysts [10].

The natural history of osteochondral lesions of the talus whether treated or not is benign [3]. Reports of ankle arthrodesis following ODs of the talus are rare [5].

11.7 Joint Congruency Versus Cartilage Thickness

The cartilage of the talar dome is thin in comparison with the cartilage of other articulating surfaces. The average cartilage thickness of the talar dome is 1.11 (±0.28 mm) in women and 1.35 (±0.22 mm) in men [5].

Braune and Fischer proposed that articular cartilage is thicker in regions of low congruence. Simon et al. related joint congruence to cartilage thickness [11].

Shepherd and Seedhom hypothesized that congruent joint surfaces, such as those in the ankle and elbow, are covered only by thin articular cartilage because the compressive loads are spread over a wide area, decreasing local joint stresses and eliminating the necessity for large cartilaginous deformations. Incongruent joints are covered by thicker cartilage which more easily deforms, thereby increasing the load-bearing area and decreasing the stress per unit area [12].

11.8 Cartilage, Subchondral Bone, and Loading

Ramsey and Hamilton found that a 1-mm lateral talar shift, as occurs after an ankle fracture malunion, reduces the contact area by 42% and a 2-mm lateral shift reduces the contact area by 58% [13]. A 1-mm shift generally is considered acceptable, while a 2-mm shift should be surgically corrected because of the high risk of degenerative changes [13].

Apparently, the talar cartilage can adapt to an increase in contact stress as great as 42%.

Christensen et al. evaluated the effect of talar OCDs graduated in size. Significant changes in contact stresses were demonstrated only for larger lesions (diameter, ≥15 mm) [14].

It has been postulated by van Dijk that the increase in load caused by a small OCD probably is not large enough to cause damage to the remaining cartilage in a normally aligned ankle [5]. However, any varus or valgus malalignment increases the likelihood of cartilage damage by high contact stresses [14].

11.9 Types of Osteochondral Defects in the Ankle and Subchondral Cyst Formation

The consecutive stages of local ODs may help us to understand the development of the defects. Superficial lesions consist of sheared off flakes with an intact subchondral bone plate. In a more severe defect, the subchondral bone is damaged, as with microfractures and bone bruises [9]. The reticular type bone bruise is not continuous with the adjacent articular surface. In general, this type heals normally, and the healing occurs from the periphery to the center.

Subchondral cyst formation (Fig. 11.1) has been hypothesized to be caused by the damaged cartilage functioning as a valve [10, 15]. This valve mechanism would allow intrusion of fluid from the joint space into the subchondral bone, but not in the opposite direction [5].

On the weight-bearing phase of gait, there is full contact between major parts of the talar and tibial cartilage, with most contact over the talar shoulders. During this phase, pressures in opposing talar and tibial cartilage are theoretically identical, which may result in the forcing of fluid in the direction of the least resistance, i.e., the damaged subchondral bone. Backflow is prevented by the direct contact of opposing cartilage. During unloading of the joint, joint space fluid may reenter the articular cartilage. On the next weight-bearing cycle, this fluid again is intruded in the subchondral bone. This repetitive mechanism represents a vicious circle, causing the intermittent shift of synovial fluid under high pressure into the damaged subchondral talar bone. Development of a subchondral cyst is then just a matter of time.

11.10 Imaging

Radiographs (weight-bearing anteroposterior mortise and lateral views) are the preferred initial investigation for a suspected OCD. The sensitivity and specificity of the combination of medical history, physical examination, and radiography are 59% and 91% [16].

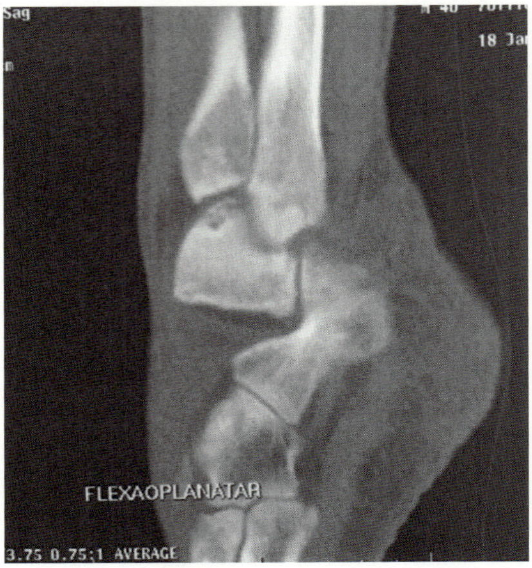

Fig. 11.3 Plantar-flexed CT sagittal view for preoperative planning (*yellow arrow* represents possible approach by surgical instruments)

An anteroposterior heel rise view with the ankle in a plantar-flexed position may reveal a posteriorly located defect.

The radiographs may show an area of detached bone or radiolucency. Initially, the damage may be too small to be visualized on routine radiography. By repeating the imaging in a later stage, the abnormality sometimes becomes apparent.

The sensitivity and specificity of CT to detect an OCD are 81% and 99%, respectively; those of MRI are 96% and 96% [16].

In diagnosing a talar OCD, CT is as accurate as MRI ($p = 0.33$). CT is useful in determining the size, location, shape, and degree of displacement of osteochondral fragments and is therefore valuable in preoperative planning [16].

Moreover, CT (particularly plantar-flexed sagittal view) can be helpful when deciding if the lesion is reachable by arthroscopic approach (Fig. 11.3) or requires open surgery (combined with osteotomy or ligament's release).

MRI offers the advantage of visualizing bone bruises, articular cartilage damage, and other soft tissue insults, but signal patterns in the talus may overestimate the severity of the bone injury [16].

Two types of bone bruises can be found on MRI. The reticular type bone bruise is not continuous with the adjacent articular surface [5]. In general, this type heals normally, and the healing occurs from the periphery to the center. The geographic type bone bruise is continuous with the adjacent articular surface [5]. It is this type that is often associated with ODs of the talus. Spontaneous healing is impaired or absent [5].

11.11 Surgical Treatment Strategies

The surgical treatment strategies to OCD of the ankle can be divided in three groups.

Debridement and bone marrow stimulation (microfracturing, drilling, abrasion arthroplasty, retrograde drilling), with or without loose body removal (Figs. 11.4 and 11.5) [3].

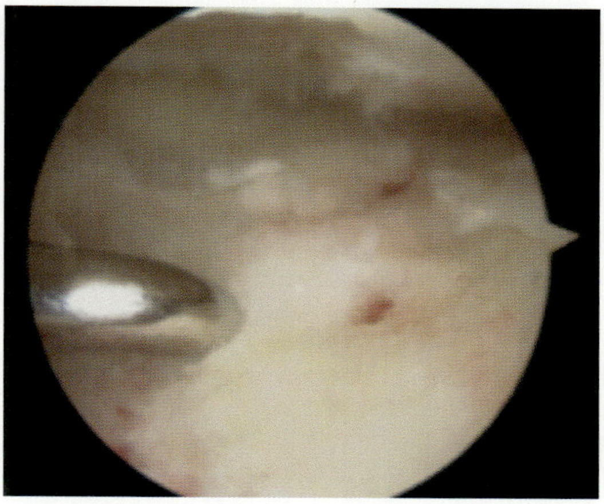

Fig. 11.4 Debridement and microfractures for talar osteochondral defect

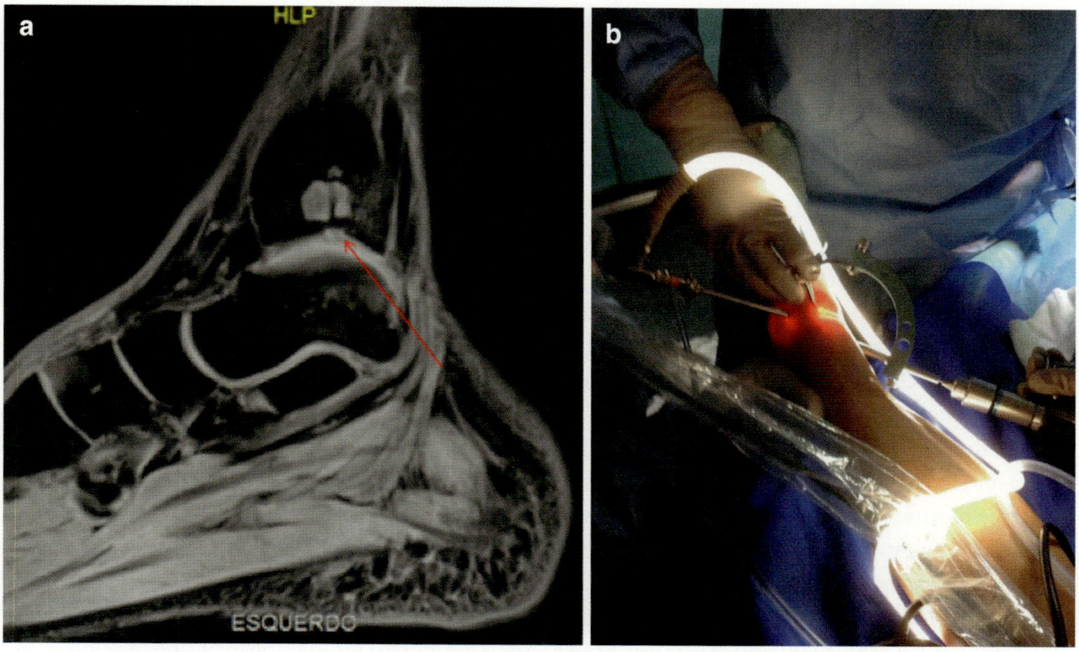

Fig. 11.5 MRI image of tibial osteochondral defect (**a**). Retrograde drilling using specific aiming device (**b**)

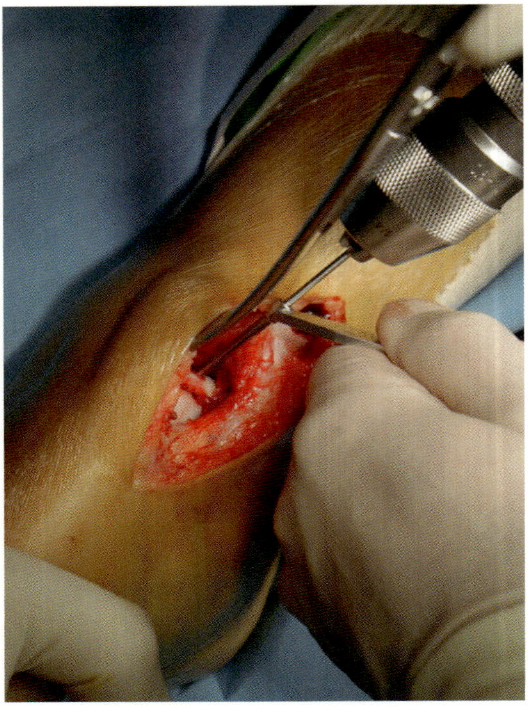

Fig. 11.6 Fixation of a loose osteochondral fragment after lifting, debridement and drilling, filling with bone autograph, and ultimately screw fixation

Fixing a lesion to the talar dome (fragment fixation, cancellous bone grafting) (Fig. 11.6) [7].

Development or replacement of hyaline or hyaline-like cartilage (osteochondral autograft transfer [OATS], autologous chondrocyte implantation [ACI]) [6, 17].

Tissue engineering is promising to have a growing role in the present and also for the future (growth factors, cytokines, stem cells, hydrogels) especially in ankle lesions [8, 18–24].

Based on the current best available evidence, at present, treatment by means of debridement and bone marrow stimulation is the most effective treatment strategy for symptomatic osteochondral lesions of the talus with an average success rate of 85% (41–93%). Large lesions (>15 mm) and secondary cases may be treated by OATS (success rate 76%) or ACI (success rate 87%) [9].

The surgical approach is determined by the size and location of the lesion as well as the type of surgical treatment.

The preferred approach of most lesions is by means of anterior arthroscopy [25].

Alternative approaches are posterior arthroscopy by means of a two-portal hindfoot approach and open arthrotomy with or without a medial malleolar osteotomy [16].

Arthroscopy offers less postoperative morbidity, faster and functional rehabilitation, and earlier resumption of sports [6].

11.12 Debridement and Bone Marrow Stimulation (BMS)

Advantages of this technique are the possibility of arthroscopy, the relatively easy procedure, and early rehabilitation. A disadvantage is the formation of fibrous cartilage rather than hyaline cartilage. Although often successful, this may be insufficient for large defects [26].

In this surgical procedure, all unstable cartilage is removed including the underlying necrotic bone. Any cysts underlying the defect are opened and curetted. Several connections with the subchondral bone are created by drilling or microfracturing. The objective is to partially destroy the calcified zone that is often present and to create openings into the subchondral bone. The formation of local new blood vessels is stimulated, marrow cells are introduced in the defect, and fibrocartilaginous tissue is formed [10].

11.13 Pre-op Planning: Lesion Size, Location, and Accessibility

Most of the lesions can be treated by anterior arthroscopy in the anterior working area by full plantar flexion of the ankle. As a rule, lesions located in the anterior half or in the anterior part of the posterior half of the talus in patients with unlimited plantar flexion can be reached and treated this way.

Computed tomography of the ankle in full plantar flexion is a reliable method for preoperative planning of arthroscopic access to osteochondral defects of the talus [9]. If the anterior border of the defect is located anteriorly to the anterior distal tibial rim on the plantarflexion scan – the OCD will be accessible through anterior arthroscopy. Access in posterior lesions depends on various parameters, such as ankle range of motion, joint laxity, and the presence of osteophytes, as well as surgical methods. Removal of osteophytes and joint opening in case of ligament laxity will ease the access.

11.14 Surgical Technique

After performing the appropriate debridement of the lesion, the subchondral bone can be perforated using a 2-mm drill, a microfracture awl, or a 1.4-mm Kirschner wire (K-wire).

A K-wire has the advantage of flexibility, whereas a drill may break more easily if the position of the ankle is changed during drilling.

A microfracture awl offers the possibility to work "around the corner" and results in microfractures of the trabeculae rather than destruction of the bone.

Any created small bony particles should be carefully removed.

Sufficient bleeding can be checked by loosening of the tourniquet.

11.15 Rehabilitation

Active plantar flexion and dorsiflexion are encouraged from the first day.

Partial weight bearing is allowed as tolerated. We allow progress to full weight bearing within 4 weeks in patients with central or posterior lesions of up to 1 cm. Larger lesions and anterior lesions require partial weight bearing up to 6 weeks.

Running on even ground is permitted after 12 weeks.

Full return to sporting activities is usually possible 4–6 months after surgery.

Conclusion

Most osteochondral talar defects are caused by trauma.

They may heal and remain asymptomatic or progress to subchondral cysts with deep ankle pain on weight bearing.

The pain in osteochondral defects is most probably caused by an intermittent local rise in intraosseous fluid pressure which occurs on every step and which thus sensitizes the highly innervated subchondral bone.

Based on the current best available evidence, at present, treatment by means of debridement and bone marrow stimulation is the most effective treatment strategy for symptomatic osteochondral lesions of the talus.

References

1. Schachter AK, Chen AL, Reddy PD, Tejwani NC. Osteochondral lesions of the talus. J Am Acad Orthop Surg. 2005;13(3):152–8.
2. O'Loughlin PF, Heyworth BE, Kennedy JG. Current concepts in the diagnosis and treatment of osteochondral lesions of the ankle. Am J Sports Med. 2010;38(2):392–404.
3. Zengerink M, Struijs PA, Tol JL, van Dijk CN. Treatment of osteochondral lesions of the talus: a systematic review. Knee Surg Sports Traumatol Arthrosc. 2010;18(2):238–46.
4. Berndt AL, Harty M. Transchondral fractures (osteochondritis dissecans) of the talus. J Bone Joint Surg Am. 1959;41-A:988–1020.
5. van Dijk CN, Reilingh ML, Zengerink M, van Bergen CJ. Osteochondral defects in the ankle: why painful? Knee Surg Sports Traumatol Arthrosc. 2010;18(5):570–80.
6. Ferreira C, Vuurberg G, Oliveira JM, Espregueira-Mendes J, Pereira H, Reis RL, et al. Good clinical outcome after osteochondral autologous transplantation surgery for osteochondral lesions of the talus but at the cost of a high rate of complications: a systematic review. J ISAKOS. 2016;1(4):184–91.
7. Bruns J, Rosenbach B. Pressure distribution at the ankle joint. Clin Biomech. 1990;5:153–61.
8. Lloyd J, Elsayed S, Hariharan K, Tanaka H. Revisiting the concept of talar shift in ankle fractures. Foot Ankle Int. 2006;27(10):793–6.
9. Gomoll AH, Madry H, Knutsen G, van Dijk N, Seil R, Brittberg M, et al. The subchondral bone in articular cartilage repair: current problems in the surgical management. Knee Surg Sports Traumatol Arthrosc. 2010;18(4):434–47.
10. Durr HD, Martin H, Pellengahr C, Schlemmer M, Maier M, Jansson V. The cause of subchondral bone cysts in osteoarthrosis: a finite element analysis. Acta Orthop Scand. 2004;75(5):554–8.
11. Braune W, Fischer O. Die Bewegungen des Kniegelenks nach einer neuen Methode am lebenden Menschen gemessen. Leipzig: Hirzel S; 1891. p. 75–150.

12. Shepherd DE, Seedhom BB. Thickness of human articular cartilage in joints of the lower limb. Ann Rheum Dis. 1999;58(1):27–34.
13. Ramsey PL, Hamilton W. Changes in tibiotalar area of contact caused by lateral talar shift. J Bone Joint Surg Am. 1976;58(3):356–7.
14. Christensen JC, Driscoll HL, Tencer AF. 1994 William J. Stickel Gold award. Contact characteristics of the ankle joint. Part 2. The effects of talar dome cartilage defects. J Am Podiatr Med Assoc. 1994;84(11):537–47.
15. Buckwalter JA, Mankin HJ. Articular cartilage: degeneration and osteoarthritis, repair, regeneration, and transplantation. Instr Course Lect. 1998;47:487–504.
16. Van Dijk CN. Osteochondral lesions. In: Van Dijk CN, editor. Ankle arthroscopy – techniques developed by the Amsterdam foot and ankle school. Berlin, Heidelberg: Springer; 2014. p. 149–86.
17. Kennedy JG, Murawski CD. The treatment of osteochondral lesions of the talus with autologous osteochondral transplantation and bone marrow aspirate concentrate: surgical technique. Cartilage. 2011;2(4):327–36.
18. Kim IL, Mauck RL, Burdick JA. Hydrogel design for cartilage tissue engineering: a case study with hyaluronic acid. Biomaterials. 2011;32(34):8771–82.
19. Kreuz PC, Muller S, Freymann U, Erggelet C, Niemeyer P, Kaps C, et al. Repair of focal cartilage defects with scaffold-assisted autologous chondrocyte grafts: clinical and biomechanical results 48 months after transplantation. Am J Sports Med. 2011;39(8):1697–705.
20. Martel-Pelletier J, Wildi LM, Pelletier JP. Future therapeutics for osteoarthritis. Bone. 2012;51(2):297–311.
21. Qi Y, Feng G, Yan W. Mesenchymal stem cell-based treatment for cartilage defects in osteoarthritis. Mol Biol Rep. 2012;39(5):5683–9.
22. Rush SM. Trinity Evolution: mesenchymal stem cell allografting in foot and ankle surgery. Foot Ankle Spec. 2010;3(3):140–3.
23. Vinatier C, Mrugala D, Jorgensen C, Guicheux J, Noel D. Cartilage engineering: a crucial combination of cells, biomaterials and biofactors. Trends Biotechnol. 2009;27(5):307–14.
24. Weil Jr L. Biologics in foot and ankle surgery. Foot Ankle Spec. 2011;4(4):249–52.
25. van Dijk CN, van Bergen CJ. Advancements in ankle arthroscopy. J Am Acad Orthop Surg. 2008;16(11):635–46.
26. Doral MN, Bilge O, Batmaz G, Donmez G, Turhan E, Demirel M, et al. Treatment of osteochondral lesions of the talus with microfracture technique and postoperative hyaluronan injection. Knee Surg Sports Traumatol Arthrosc. 2012;20(7):1398–403.

Ankle and Foot Fractures and Dislocations

12

Marta Massada, Gino Kerkoffs, and Paulo Amado

Contents

M. Massada (✉)
Hospital de Santa Maria – Porto, Porto, Portugal
e-mail: martamassada@gmail.com

G. Kerkoffs
Department of Orthopedic Surgery, Academic Medical Center, University of Amsterdam, Amsterdam, Netherlands

Academic Center for Evidence based Sports medicine (ACES), Amsterdam, Netherlands

Amsterdam Collaboration for Health and Safety in Sports (ACHSS), AMC/VUmc IOC Research Center, Amsterdam, Netherlands

Team NL, NOC-NSF, Arnhem, Netherlands
e-mail: g.m.kerkhoffs@amc.nl

P. Amado
Paulo Amado – Hospital Lusíadas – Porto, Porto, Portugal
e-mail: paulo.amado@pauloamado.pt

J. Espregueira-Mendes et al. (eds.), *Injuries and Health Problems in Football*,
DOI 10.1007/978-3-662-53924-8_12

Football is one of the most popular sports in the world not only with regard to increasing match attendances and TV audiences but also to the number of people around the globe who actually plays the game. According to impressive findings of the Big Count, a Fédération Internationale de Football Association (FIFA) survey of its member associations, 265 million male and female players and a further five million referees, coaches, and other officials or a grand total of 270 million people, or 4% of the world's population, are involved in football [1].

Football is a high-demand team sport involving constantly changing complex movement patterns. Walking, running, sprinting, sudden changes in direction, jumping, and body contact require a high grade of coordination and body control. Several studies have investigated the incidence and nature of injuries during football play [2–4]. This incidence, due to the specificity of football movement patterns, is higher in the lower extremity [4, 5] with foot and ankle accounting for most of it [2, 3, 6, 7]. From the results of previous studies, it can be estimated that the incidence of foot and ankle injuries in elite football competition is between three and nine injuries per 1000 player-hours of competition [8]. Ankle injuries as part of overall injury rates for each sport as reported by Fong et al. [6] are shown in Fig. 12.1. Detailed video analysis of the mechanism of acute foot and ankle injuries in football shows that the two main situations where they occur are during player-to-player contact or during extreme joint ranges of motion. The player-to-player contact often occurred just above the ankle joint, and before or at foot strike, which pushes the foot into high-speed inversion or eversion. When, during a shot or long pass, the high-velocity movement of plantar flexion at the ankle is followed by a contact with an opponent's foot, hyperflexion is created that stresses the tissues at the front and back of the ankle and results in injury [9].

Energy transfer to the lower leg by a direct-impact trauma, such as a miskick or slide tackle, can result in a fracture [10]. The incidence of fractures in football has been reported to range from 2 to 20% of all reported injuries, one-third of which are located in the lower extremities. Of all lower-leg fractures, ankle fractures are the most common (36%), followed by fractures of the foot (33%) and the tibia (22%) [11].

To our knowledge, there is no data on the exact classification and morphology of ankle fractures in football. Overall, supination and

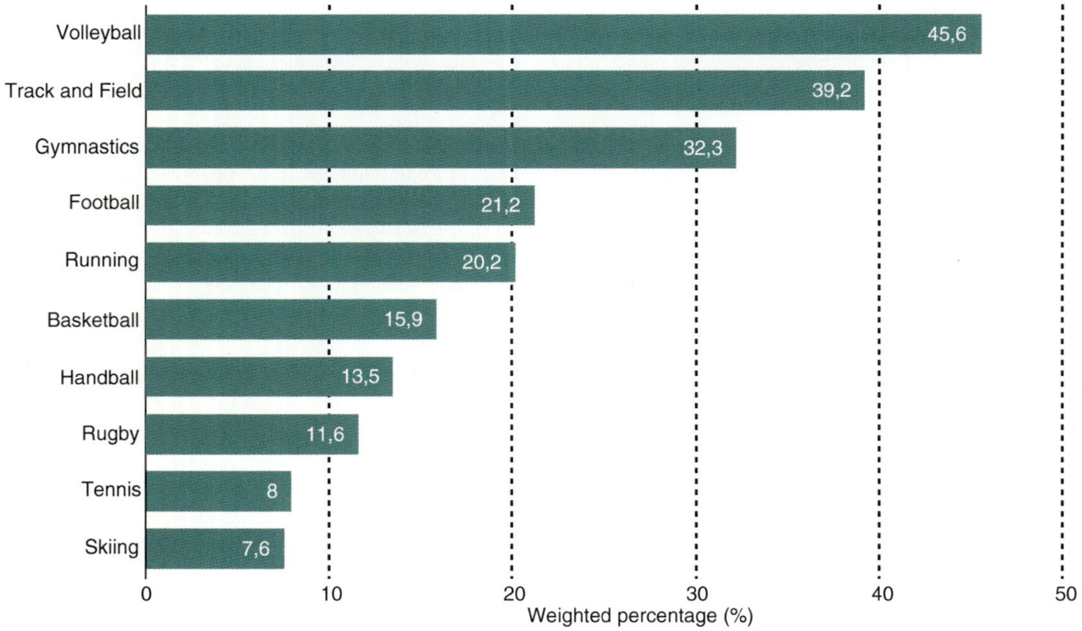

Fig. 12.1 Weighted percentage of ankle injury in different sports (Adapted from "A systematic review on ankle injury and ankle sprain in sports" by Fong et al. [6])

external rotation (according to Lauge-Hansen Classification) are the most common mechanism of ankle fractures in sports. Another pattern of fractures in football is the metatarsal fractures and Lisfranc fractures/lesions. In football players, stress fractures of the fifth metatarsal account for up to 78% of all stress fractures [12].

The high injury rate among football players constitutes a considerable problem for the player, the team, the club, and, given the popularity of this phenomenon, the society at large. Health consequences may be seen not just in the short term but also in medium/long term with the risk of early consequences, like ankle osteoarthritis which has a high prevalence among retired players (6%) [8].

12.1 Ankle Fractures

We already know that the ankle is the most affected segment in football. Overall, almost all ankle injuries are due to trauma, and about two-thirds involve a collision or tackle with an opponent [4]. As referred previously, of the reported football injuries, 2–20% are fractures, one-third of which are located in the lower extremities [11]. In a prospective study of ankle injuries in the UK youth football population, there were only three fractures reported in a total of 56 ankle injuries (5.4%) [2]. During the 2010 FIFA World Cup, only one ankle fracture was diagnosed (n=229) [3].

Ankle fractures result from higher energy trauma and can require more extensive treatment and may result in a greater loss of time from sports and work than mild strains and sprains. Fractures with or without ligament trauma can result in long-term disability and preclude return to sports [13].

12.1.1 Anatomy

The ankle joint is the junction of three bony structures: the distal ends of the tibia and fibula, forming a mortise-like cavity that receives the trochlea of the talus. Stability of the joint is due to the congruity of the osseous structures and associated ligaments. The tibia and fibula are bound by the ligamentous structures of the syndesmosis (interosseous membrane; anterior, posterior, and transverse tibiofibular ligaments) [14]. Powerful collateral ligaments stabilize the joint against stress: the medial malleolus is supported by the broad fan of the deltoid ligament and the plantar calcaneonavicular ligament (spring ligament); the lateral aspect of the joint is reinforced by the lateral complex which consists the anterior fibulotalar ligament (AFTL), fibulocalcaneal ligament (FCL), and posterior fibulotalar ligament (PFTL). The ankle joint is not a pure hinge. It moves as a rotatory hinge around the helical axis of the joint due to the asymmetric shape of the talus. To function properly, exact congruence is crucial. Ankle fractures are regarded as articular fractures even if there is no joint involvement. Nonanatomical reductions and restraints in the ankle joint may have major adverse effects as premature degeneration of the joint, as they alter the biomechanics of the joint and cause pathological compressive stress [15, 16]. Hence, competent anatomical reconstruction and reduction, often involving surgery, are required in order to prevent long-term sequels.

12.1.2 Classification

The two most widely used classification systems for ankle fractures are the Danis-Weber and AO-Müller and Lauge-Hansen systems [17–19]. According to Danis-Weber and AO-Müller, a fracture is classified based on the level of the fibular fracture in relation to the syndesmotic ligaments. The Lauge-Hansen classification [17] describes the trauma mechanism of fractures based on the position of the foot at the time of injury and the direction of the deforming force. There are five types of Lauge-Hansen fracture each with progressive stages of injury: supination adduction, supination external rotation, pronation external rotation, pronation abduction, and pronation dorsiflexion. This classification was initially proposed to guide the closed reduction of ankle fractures by reversing the injury mechanism. Although it can be useful in describing the pathomechanics of ankle injuries and inferring their stability [20], we find it too complicated for routine use. We favor the Danis-Weber classification in which a lateral malleolar fracture below the syndesmosis is designated a type A injury; a fracture at the level of the syndesmosis, a type B injury; and a fracture above the syndesmosis, a type C injury. The Maisonneuve fracture is a special case, as it involves a proximal fracture of the fibula, typically below the fibular head that is usually caused by an indirect pronation mechanism. In this type of fracture, a tear of the entire interosseous membrane of the lower leg, the syndesmosis, and the deltoid ligament destabilizes the ankle joint.

12.1.3 Physical Examination

Evidence of an ankle fracture includes swelling, hematoma formation, and tenderness to pressure over the medial and/or lateral malleolus or over the proximal head of the fibula (proximal fibular fracture, the so-called Maisonneuve fracture). It can be hard, though, to differentiate a fracture from a more common ligamentous injury, especially during on-the-field evaluation. Visible malposition of the joint should be immediately reduced with manual axial traction, followed by joint immobilization in a splint or an appropriate alternative. Careful neurovascular status and associated soft tissue damage should always be assessed.

12.1.4 Radiographic Examination

Plain radiographs are needed in practically all cases of a fracture or a sprain with ligamentous instability suspicion. Ottawa ankle rules, first introduced by Stiell et al. in 1992, serve as guidelines in terms of ruling out serious ankle and midfoot fractures [21]. Although useful to reduce costs and increase time effectiveness (e.g., decrease wait times) in the emergency department, they do not correspond to the diagnostic standard in Europe. We believe that the costs and low radiation dose do not overweigh the risk of missing a fracture, particularly in the athlete.

Standard x-ray imaging of the ankle joint should be performed in the anteroposterior and lateral views. The mortise view is not a true anteroposterior view – it is obtained with the leg internally rotated 15–20° to optimize visualization of the ankle joint without being overlapped by the fibula. Depending on the associated injuries that may be suspected, additional views or a lateral image of the foot (to rule out fifth metatarsal base fractures) may be indicated. Computed tomography (CT) can also be helpful for the evaluation of articular fractures. On the other side, magnetic resonance imaging (MRI) is not indicated on the acute setting, but it can be valuable later on for the assessment of associated cartilaginous or ligamentous injuries.

12.1.5 Treatment

In the general population, treatment of ankle fractures involves open reduction and internal fixation (ORIF) or nonoperative treatment. The ideal treatment of ankle fractures in the athlete remains relatively undetermined as the options are affected by concerns such as time to full return to sporting activity, amount of time of immobilization required, and ability to rehabilitate while recovering and healing. We believe that surgical treatment offers the potential for a more rapid and healthy recovery than nonsurgical management, allowing for early rehabilitation and preventing the deleterious effect of joint immobilization (muscle inactivity, osteopenia, joint stiffness, etc.). Nevertheless, any stable fracture with non-displaced or only slightly displaced fragments can be treated conservatively. The key factor to long-term success of treatment, regardless of the chosen method, is anatomical reduction [13]. In our practice, surgical reduction with rigid internal fixation is recommended to athletes with ankle fractures with bone displacement greater than or equal to 3 mm or if the athlete is especially concerned about a rapid return

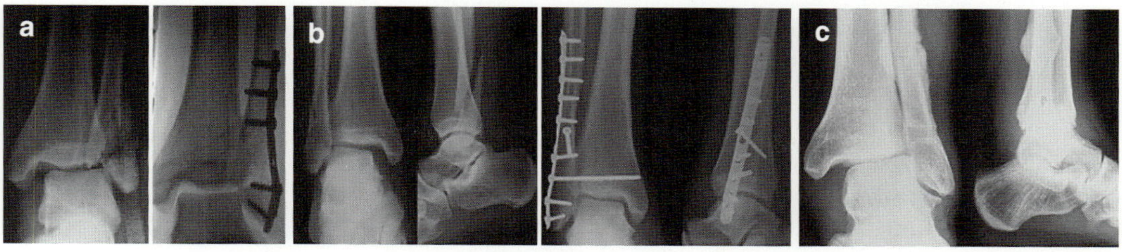

Fig. 12.2 Ankle fractures (**a**) a Danis-Weber B type fracture and its treatment, (**b**) a Danis-Weber C type fracture and its treatment, (**c**) post-Danis-Weber C fracture complication with talus lateral shift

to activity. Usually, after the surgical reduction to an anatomic position, Danis-Weber type A and B injuries are fixated with a plate and cortical lag screws with or without interfragmentary screws. For Danis-Weber type C fractures, the fibula is reduced and fixated in a manner identical to that of the type A and B fractures. If the syndesmosis is unstable to external rotation following fixation of the Danis-Weber C fibula, then we insert one or two syndesmosis screws or knotless suture fixation systems. Bimalleolar fractures require appropriate reduction and fixation of the fibula as described, as well as reduction and fixation of the medial malleolus with lag screws. Bimalleolar equivalent injuries are treated according to the protocol of type B fractures, with additional repair of the deltoid ligament with large absorbable suture, if the mortise remains unstable after fibular fixation. Early postoperative functional treatment and physiotherapy are advised to improve joint function and proprioception (especially in athletes with combined ligamentous injuries). Full return to sports is likely 12–16 weeks after the injury.

In a Cochrane Review, which included three randomized and one quasi-randomized trial with 292 patients, the complications of nonoperative treatment included malunion, nonunion, pain, loss of function, muscle atrophy, cartilage degeneration, stiff/swollen joint, deep vein thrombosis (DVT), and pulmonary embolism (PE) [22]. Postoperative wound infections are the most commonly reported complication. Other complications reported include insufficient primary osteosynthesis, soft tissue necrosis, DVT, delayed union, nonunion, secondary displacement, refracture, stiffness, muscular atrophy, tendinous insufficiency, sensory deficit, tarsal tunnel syndrome, and complex regional pain syndrome type 1 [23] (Fig. 12.2).

12.2 Pilon Fractures

Pilon fractures, also called tibial plafond fractures, are defined as fractures of the tibial metaphysis. The term pilon (hammer) was introduced by a French radiologist called Destot in 1911 to describe a compression injury which also produces severe soft tissue damage [24]. The common pathway for all pilon fractures is some form of axial compression. The rest will be a product of varying degrees of torsion, shearing and bending, depending on the position of the foot at the moment of impact. Albeit most fractures are caused by a high-energy axial force, low-energy injuries can also occur, resulting in fewer fracture fragments, mainly assuming a spiral configuration with minimal displacement and soft tissue insult. Pilon fractures are relatively uncommon, making up approximately 7% of all tibial fractures and 1% of all fractures of the lower limb in the general population [25].

12.2.1 Anatomy

The distal portion of the tibia is known as the plafond, which, along with the medial and lateral malleoli, forms the mortise to articulate with the talar dome. The plafond is concave in the anteroposterior plane and convex in the lateral plane.

It is wider in the anterior plane to provide stability, especially while weight bearing (vide Ankle Fractures).

12.2.2 Classification

The two most commonly used classification systems are based on fracture patterns as seen on the radiograph: the Ruedi and Allgower [26] and the AO/OTA group classifications [27].

Ruedi and Allgower proposed the first of these classification systems in 1969. It is the classification system we use more often. Fractures are separated according to the degree of articular displacement as below:

Type 1: Simple cleavage-type fracture with little or no articular displacement

Type 2: Mild to moderate displacement of articular surface but minimal or no comminution of the articular surface or adjacent metaphysis

Type 3: Comminution of the articular surface and metaphysis with significant impaction of the metaphysis

It is also crucial to assess and grade the amount of soft tissue damage, according to the Tscherne classification [28].

12.2.3 Physical Examination

The most common signs and symptoms are pain, swelling, deformity, and crepitus about the ankle, along with the inability to bear weight. Neurovascular examination should include pulses and capillary refill and assessment of sensation and ability to move the toes. An assessment for compartment syndrome should also be performed, as often there is significant soft tissue injury with a tibial plafond fracture.

12.2.4 Radiographic Examination

In the first instance, multi-view radiographs including the foot, ankle (AP, mortise, and lateral views), and full-length leg views should be obtained. CT scans are particularly important and are necessary in most cases.

12.2.5 Treatment

The main goals of treatment are the reestablishment of articular congruity, stable fixation with anatomic reduction, prevention of soft tissue complications, and rapid return to function. This requires operative intervention in most cases. Acute ankle external fixation followed by delayed reconstruction of the tibial plafond with plating or limited internal fixation combined with external fixation is the primary treatment option in cases of extensive soft tissue injury. Long leg cast may be an acceptable treatment in patients with isolated, non-displaced fractures. Acute ORIF should be limited to low-energy fracture patterns with minimal soft tissue injury or swelling. Early motion is usually delayed 7–10 days following treatment for soft tissue considerations. Generally, in intra-articular fractures, weight bearing is restricted in the first 8 weeks. Intensive physiotherapy exercise regimes play an integral role in rehabilitation. Although satisfactory long-term outcomes are usually expected in the general population, tibial plafond fractures can be disastrous to the professional athlete.

12.3 Calcaneal Fractures

Calcaneal fractures represent about 2% of all fractures in the general population, and 65–70% of those fractures involve the articular surface of the subtalar or calcaneocuboid joint [29]. Calcaneal fractures are scarcely seen in football mainly because they are the result of high-energy trauma by an axial load on the patients' heels (most often by a fall from a height or motorcycle accidents) [30].

12.3.1 Anatomy

The *calcaneus* is the largest bone in the *hindfoot*. It articulates with the *talus* superiorly and the *cuboid* anteriorly and shares a joint space with the talonavicular joint, appropriately called the talocalcaneonavicular joint. The calcaneus transfers most of the body weight from the lower limb to the ground and acts as a lever for the force generated by the calf muscles.

12.3.2 Classification

As reported by Sanders, the classification of Essex-Lopresti divides intra-articular fractures into two types: tongue type (tuberosity fragment attached to the articular fragment) or joint depression (when it is not). Sanders further classified fractures according to the number and location of posterior facet articular fragments on CT [30].

12.3.3 Physical Examination

Patients usually present after a fall from a height with complaints of severe heel pain and a variable degree of swelling. The integrity of the soft tissues should be assessed. Patients can also develop compartment syndrome in the "calcaneal compartment," which, if left untreated, can lead to claw toe deformities.

12.3.4 Radiographic Examination

Patients should be assessed initially with plain radiographs, including lateral and axial Harris views of the hindfoot. An oblique view can be helpful for visualizing the calcaneocuboid joint. If these radiographs reveal an intra-articular component to the fracture, a computed tomographic scan should be made.

12.3.5 Treatment

The treatment of displaced intra-articular calcaneal fractures can be divided into three categories: nonoperative, open reduction and internal fixation, and primary arthrodesis. Extra-articular fractures can be treated nonoperatively with immobilization and non-weight bearing, unless the fragments are substantially displaced or impede soft tissue function, as is the case of the calcaneal tuberosity fracture still attached to the Achilles insertion. Intra-articular fractures should be treated operatively. The primary goals of surgery are to restore bony geometry (i.e., height and width) and joint congruity.

12.4 Lisfranc Injuries and Midfoot Fractures

Lisfranc fracture dislocations were first described by Jacques Lisfranc, a French surgeon, reported on midfoot injuries when cavalrymen would fall from their horses with a foot remaining plantar flexed in the stirrup [31]. Although very serious, this kind of injury is uncommon in football. It occurs as a result of trauma to the tarsometatarsal articulations of the midfoot, from forced plantar flexion or abduction of the forefoot [31, 32]. Another causative circumstance can occur with an axial force driven downward through the calcaneus, while the foot is plantar flexed.

12.4.1 Anatomy

The forefoot is comprised of five metatarsal bones and the phalanges of each toe. The midfoot consists of five bones: three cuneiforms (medial, middle, and lateral), the cuboid, and navicular. The Lisfranc joint consists of the articulations between the metatarsals and the three cuneiforms and cuboid. Its osseous architecture and soft tissue connections are critical to the stability of the foot. Soft tissue support of the tarsometatarsal (TMT) articulation consists primarily of capsular and ligamentous structures. The Lisfranc ligament is the most important and runs from the plantar medial cuneiform to the base of the second metatarsal. Injury to this ligament can destabilize the entire forefoot as well as the Lisfranc articulation [32].

12.4.2 Classification

In 1909, Quenu and Kuss first described injuries to the TMT joint based on the direction of displacement at the metatarsotarsal joint [33]. Myerson et al. classified these injuries into different types to aid in clinical decision-making [34]:

Type A – total incongruity of the TMT joint

Type B1 – partial incongruity affecting the first ray in relative isolation (i.e., partial medial incongruity)

Type B2 – partial incongruity in which the displacement affects one or more of the lateral four metatarsals (i.e., partial lateral incongruity)

Types C1 and C2 – a divergent pattern, with partial or total displacement

12.4.3 Physical Examination

Athletes with Lisfranc or other midfoot fractures will complain of midfoot pain of immediate onset and present a subsequent inability to weight bear and midfoot swelling. Classic findings of Lisfranc fracture include forefoot and midfoot edema and plantar arch ecchymosis.

12.4.4 Radiographic Examination

Computed tomography (CT) may supplement standard radiographic examination if there is need for further description and surgical planning. The images will typically reveal diastasis between the hallux and the second toe on an anteroposterior (AP) foot radiograph – a "positive gap sign" [32] – and/or multiple fractures along the TMT joints along with suggestions of ligamentous instability.

12.4.5 Treatment

Unstable Lisfranc injuries should be treated surgically with either transarticular fixation to restore anatomical alignment and stabilize the tarsometatarsal joints or arthrodesis, depending on ligamentous or bony injury and comminution. Postoperatively, patients are frequently placed in a short leg cast for up to 4 weeks. Physical therapy to regain balance, strength, and ROM is recommended. Customarily, athletes needing surgical fixation of a Lisfranc fracture-dislocation should expect to be sidelined for at least 12–16 weeks [31] (Fig. 12.3).

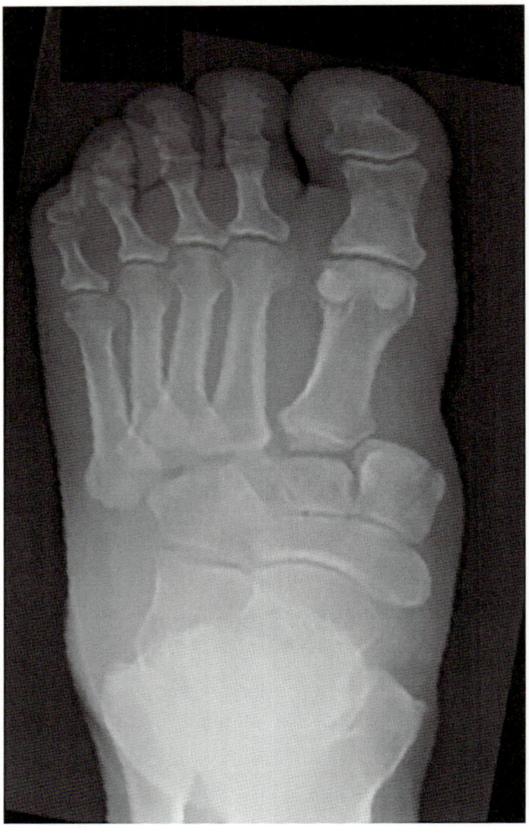

Fig. 12.3 Lisfranc fracture-dislocation

12.5 Metatarsal and Phalanges Fractures

Literature is not consensual in the diagnosis, classification, pathomechanics, and treatment of proximal fifth metatarsal fractures. This controversy goes back to 1902, when Sir Robert Jones published his well-known study *Fracture of the Base of the Fifth Metatarsal Bone by Indirect Violence*, inspired by the injury himself suffered while dancing [35]. This has been perpetuated by the universal application of the Jones fracture designation to all fifth metatarsal base fractures.

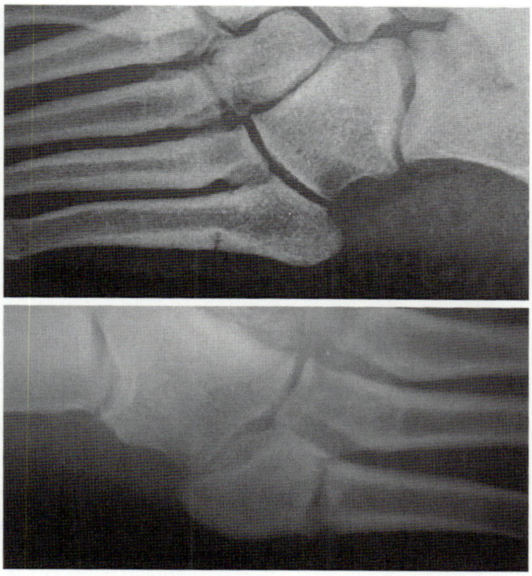

Fig. 12.4 Diaphysis fracture (zone III) of fifth metatarsal

The uniqueness of this type of fractures resides on the anatomical variations in the osseous structure of the fifth metatarsal, which enables its division in three different zones. The tuberosity avulsion fracture (zone I) is therefore distinct of the true Jones fracture (zone II, at the junction of the metaphysis and diaphysis) and of pure diaphysis fracture (zone III) (Fig. 12.4). Blood supply plays a crucial role in the healing ability of these fractures [36, 37]. Perfusion comes from metaphyseal arteries at the base. At the metaphysis-diaphysis junction, there is an area at high risk for avascularity and poor healing. Zone I fracture often results from traction forces imposed by the peroneus brevis and/or the lateral band of the plantar aponeurosis with foot inversion. This type of fractures usually heals without complications in a cast walker (4–6 weeks). Jones fractures and true diaphysis fractures (distal to the fourth and fifth metatarsal base articulation – frequently stress fractures) have been reported to have higher rates of nonunion when treated nonoperatively. Nonunion rates as high as 50% have been reported [38]. Kavanaugh et al. have suggested that almost 66% of the zone III fractures showed delayed union [39]. The authors advocate early surgical treatment in high-demand athletes and in zone III fractures with evidence of delayed union or nonhealing stress fractures in sedentary. Surgical fixation usually involves placing an intramedullary screw with or without bone graft in order to achieve compression of the fracture site and annulment of the loads acting on it. Dameron, in 1975, was the first to suggest that proximal fifth metatarsal fracture should be treated accordingly to the activity level of the patient [40]. We also believe that nonoperative treatment in the high-demand footballer could lead to higher refracture rates, delayed union, and long recovery periods. Furthermore, conservative treatment requires weeks of immobilization and non-weight bearing, which have deleterious effects in the athlete-like articulation stiffness, loss of muscle capacity, and osteopenia. Intramedular fixation of proximal fifth metatarsal fractures is our method of choice in the athlete. It is simple and minimally invasive, associated with low complication rates, and allows an early return to sports. In a previous study, we have followed 11 footballers with intramedullary fixation of proximal fifth metatarsal fractures. The average time to return to sports was 7.5 weeks (2–12), and the athletes score an average of 95 points in the midfoot AOFAS scale [41]. All of the athletes returned to previous level of activity, and no complications have been reported to date. The possibility of an almost immediate rehabilitation without the use of orthotics or casts augmented by the action of weight bearing on the affected limb has, in our opinion, benefits by allowing an early recovery of range of motion, increase of blood supply, and osteoblastic activity.

12.6 Stress Fractures of the Foot and Ankle

The first fatigue (stress) fractures were described in soldiers in 1855 by Breihaupt, a Prussian army doctor [42]. The so-called march fractures were reported after soldiers complained of painful swollen feet after long marches. Since then there have been numerous descriptions of fatigue fractures, and nowadays stress fractures are common overuse injuries in athletes.

12.6.1 Epidemiology

The most common locations for stress fractures are the metatarsals, tibia, fibula, tarsal navicular, and pars articularis. These sites of occurrence are activity related, and some anatomical sites are specific of certain sports [43]. Although less common, upper-extremity stress fractures can occur in overhead athletes. The most common stress fractures affecting footballers are fifth metatarsal fractures maybe due to the many bending moments applied to this bone during rapid changes in direction and speed [12].

12.6.2 Pathophysiology

Wolff's law states that mechanical loadings imposed to the living bone are followed by adaptation that will influence the structure of its tissue. Therefore, the repetitive cyclic loads that football imposes on the bone may lead to an imbalance between bone resorption and formation. This may be due to an excessive increase in the intensity (or duration) of the physical activity or to intrinsic factors as hormonal changes, dietary content, endocrine input, or altered osseous mineral density, common in the female athlete. Although the exact mechanical phenomenon responsible for initiating stress fractures still remains unclear, the bone response can be represented in agreement with the principles of mechanic enginery. Material properties can be described according to the response to the application of external load. Stress is defined as the force applied to the material, and the response of the material to cyclic stress is fatigue, which can result in failure of the material.

12.6.3 Clinical Evaluation

Stress fracture injuries usually present insidiously. The pain customarily occurs at the end of physical activity with a focal point of tenderness. Athletes often refer pain that only comes with activity evolving to persistent pain during activity and finally pain at rest. Physical examination consistently shows tenderness over the involved area, and swelling may or not be present.

At present, a classification system is still lacking. The more convenient grading, prognosis, and treatment system in the literature to classify stress fractures is high or low risk [44]. High-risk fractures typically require surgical repair, while low-risk stress fractures often respond to conservative treatment. Determination of low- and high-risk stress fractures should not only include anamnesis and physical evaluation but also imaging. Notwithstanding, plain radiographs often show any signs of a stress fracture, as bone reaction is time dependent. The identification is dependent of periosteal changes or gross cortical bone failure that usually takes 3–4 weeks to appear [37, 45–47]. Thus, stress fractures that are not detectable on plain radiographs should be confirmed by scintigraphy, CT scan, or even MRI.

12.6.4 Forefoot Stress Fractures

As mentioned, the most common stress fractures in football are on the fifth metatarsal (Fig. 12.5) [12]. Due to the anatomical specificity of fifth metatarsal blood supply, these fractures have high nonunion or delayed union rates (vide Metatarsal and Phalanges Fractures). Additionally, there are mechanical aspects in football that can predispose athletes to this type of fracture. Typically, there is a gradual onset of pain on the outer side of the foot but only when the pain interferes with playing does the athlete seeks treatment. Radiographs may show callus formation, medullary sclerosis, or even obliteration of the medullary canal. We believe that immediate operative treatment – internal fixation with a compression screw with or without bone grafting – should be considered in all performance athletes with fifth metatarsal stress fractures.

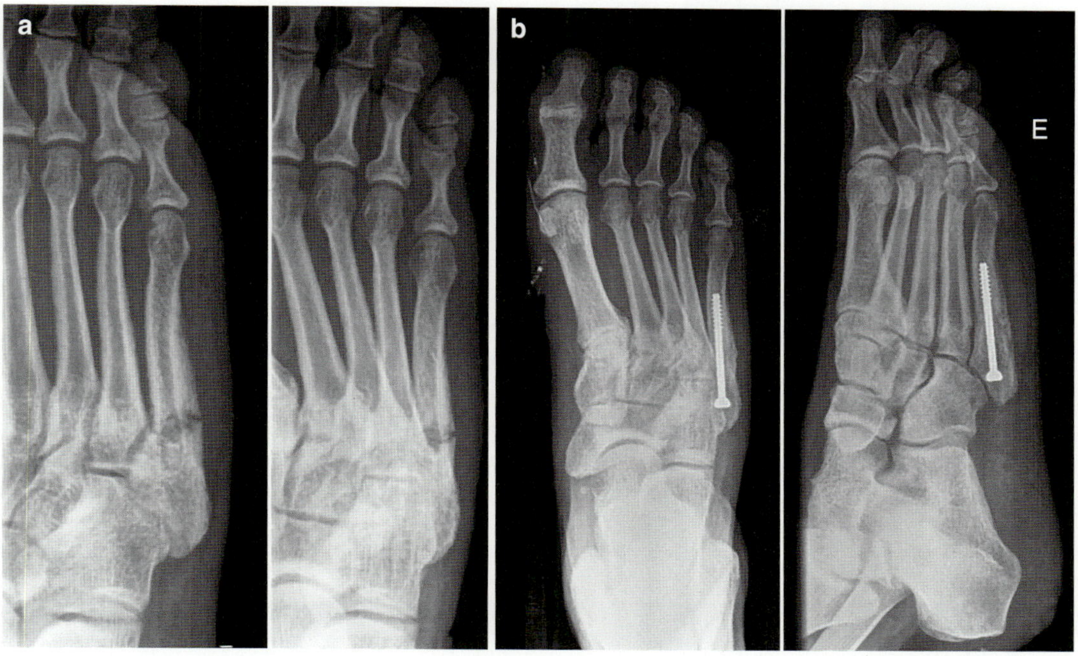

Fig. 12.5 Fifth metatarsal stress fractures treated with intramedular compression screw

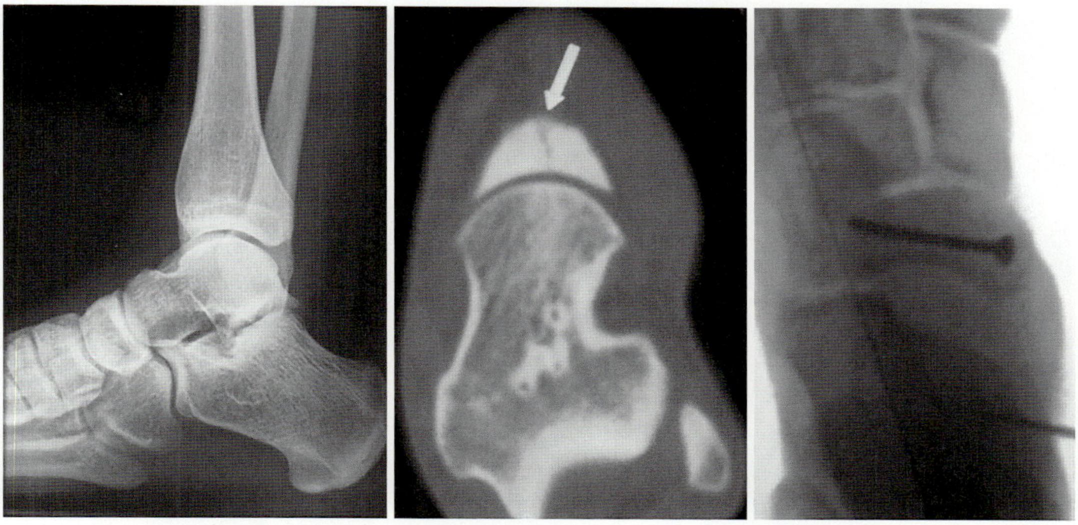

Fig. 12.6 Stress fracture of the tarsal navicular

12.6.5 Midfoot Stress Fractures

Stress fractures have been described in virtually all midfoot bones, especially in the tarsal navicular [43, 46, 48–50] (Fig. 12.6), even though they are not common in this segment nor in football. Athletes usually complain of ill-defined pain or cramping of the foot and, in the case of tarsal navicular fractures, tenderness with compression of the bone or over the medial longitudinal arch. The pain has frequently been present for a long time. Again, the diagnosis may be difficult due to the negativity of plain radiographs, a characteristic of stress fractures. Complementary exams, like a bone scan or MRI, can help. When they occur, displaced fractures should be treated with internal fixation, as should delayed unions or nonunions. Partial or complete undisplaced fractures may be treated with immobilization and non-weight bearing and athletic activity elimination. This can take several months until healing is complete.

12.6.6 Hindfoot Stress Fractures

Calcaneal stress fractures are the most common stress fractures in this region. Nevertheless, talar fractures have also been reported (Fig. 12.7). Fractures in this region, being infrequent in football, require a high index of clinical suspicion. The clinical signs and radiological findings, as in other sites, are usually subtle, making it problematic to establish an early diagnosis. If the diagnosis is uncertain, a bone scan or MRI can help differentiate stress fractures from Achilles tendinosis, painful *os trigonum*, retrocalcaneal bursitis, or plantar fasciitis. A favorable response has been reported with activity modification/limitation and the use of soft heel pads, although the authors have some reservations (vide Treatment). Becoming familiar with this rare stress fracture may prevent delayed diagnosis and long-lasting damage, both of which are important factors in competitive athletes.

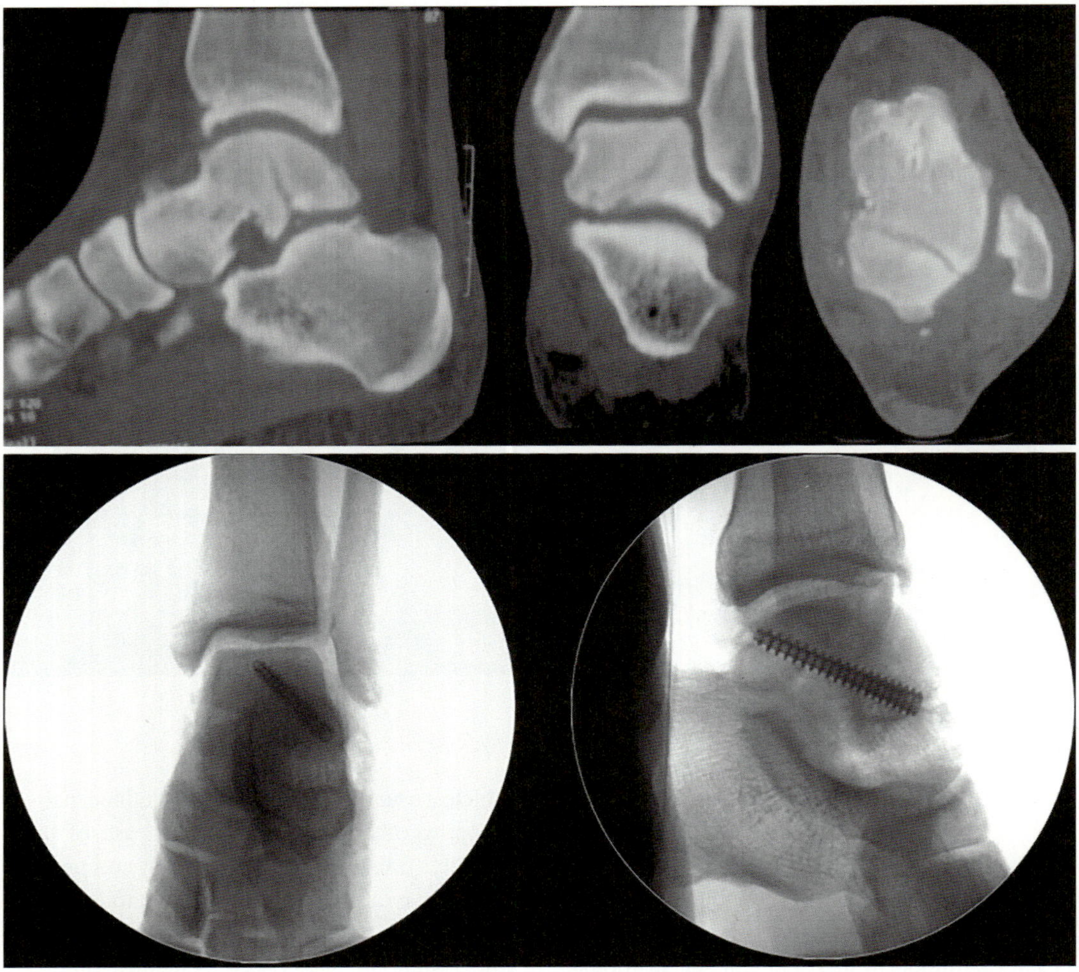

Fig. 12.7 Talar stress fracture

12.6.7 Ankle Stress Fractures

These are most commonly seen proximal to the medial malleolus or the lateral malleolus [45, 51]. They usually cause pain directly over the bone or, if in the lateral malleolus, a few centimeters proximal to the tip of the fibula. Radiographs are often negative, and a bone scan is required to confirm the diagnosis.

12.6.8 Treatment

As Ekstrand and Torstveit refers that it, stress fracture in the footballer is a rare injury but with a long absence from sports. Athletes who sustain a stress fracture may be hindered from sports for up to 6 months [12]. As a consequence, treatment of stress fractures depends on whether they behave as a high- or a low-risk injury. Authors maintain their opinion that in the high-demand athlete, to whom repetitive and intense loads are imposed, surgical fixation is a recommendation. For ankle and foot low-risk stress fractures, a rest period of 2–6 weeks of limited weight bearing progressing to full weight bearing may be necessary. This is followed by a phase of low-impact activities, such as biking, swimming, or pool running. All predisposing factors, as sudden increases in training loads and nutritional, hormonal, or medical abnormalities, need to be assessed, particularly in female athletes.

12.7 Pediatric Foot and Ankle Fractures

Approximately one-third of pediatric fractures occur during sport or recreational activity. Football is associated with an activity-specific fracture rate of 0.44 (95% confidence interval, 0.35–0.52) per 10,000 h of exposure [52]. Fractures around the ankle account for approximately 5% of pediatric fractures and carry about a 30% risk of later growth disturbances [53]. Metatarsal fractures are commonly seen in emergency departments. In children, 61% of all fractures of the foot are located in the metatarsal bones [54]. The most common pediatric metatarsal fracture seen in football is the fracture of the fifth metatarsal. Due to the unique anatomy of the immature skeleton and the risk of partial or complete growth arrest, extra care must be taken in assessing and treating patients with injuries of this type.

12.7.1 Anatomy

The physis, or growth plate, consists of chondrocytes surrounded by an extracellular matrix; it is closely connected to the epiphysis, which provides its blood supply. The chondrocytes are organized in columns along the longitudinal axis of the bones directed toward the metaphysis where endochondral ossification occurs.

12.7.2 Classification

The Salter-Harris classification system is simple and reproducible, and it remains the most widely used system for children's ankle fractures [55]. The fracture is classified in one of five different types according to its relationship to the physis

12.7.3 Physical Examination

Swelling, ecchymosis, and skin tenting are assessed, and the ankle must be visualized circumferentially to exclude a possible open fracture. Tenderness to palpation over the physis can aid in the clinical diagnosis. If there is gross deformity, urgent reduction is required. The vascular, motor, and sensory examination should be performed prior to and following any reduction maneuver.

12.7.4 Radiographic Examination

Anteroposterior and lateral views are required to fully evaluate the ankle and foot. Additional views, like the mortise radiograph, may be necessary particularly in fractures without obvious deformity. There is no indication for routine stress views as they are unlikely to change the treatment, are uncomfortable, and cause increased radiation exposure. CT is recommended for preoperative planning and postreduction assessment for intra-articular pediatric ankle fractures.

12.7.5 Treatment

The goals of treatment are to achieve and maintain a satisfactory reduction and to avoid physeal arrest. The decision to treat pediatric ankle fractures is based on the fracture type, displacement, and the ability to restore and maintain the alignment of the physis and the congruity of the ankle joint. If a satisfactory closed reduction can be achieved and maintained, pediatric fractures can be effectively managed with cast immobilization and close radiographic follow-up evaluation. However, if closed reduction is unsuccessful, open reduction with or without skeletal fixation is warranted. Before a closed reduction is attempted, the child must be comfortable and relaxed. This may need either intravenous sedation or general anesthesia to facilitate the reduction and reduce the risk of further physeal injury. Physeal ankle injuries in younger children with considerable growth remaining should be followed closely for at least 1 year after injury as growth arrest may result in substantial angular deformity and limb-length discrepancies with the eventual development of osteoarthritis, gait disturbance, and spinal disorders. Besides those that result from physeal damage, the potential complications associated with pediatric ankle fractures include those seen with adult fractures (such as posttraumatic arthritis, stiffness, and reflex sympathetic dystrophy) (Fig. 12.8).

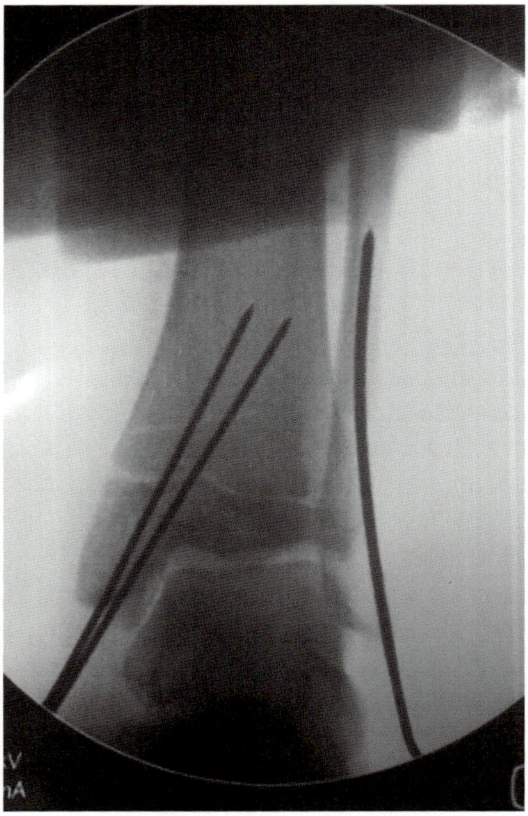

Fig. 12.8 Pediatric ankle fracture elastic fixation

References

1. Fédération Internationale de Football Association. 270 million people active in football. 2012. http://www.fifa.com/media/news/y=2007/m=5/news=fifa-big-count-2006-270-million-people-active-football-529882.html.
2. Cloke DJ, Ansell P, Avery P, Deehan D. Ankle injuries in football academies: a three-centre prospective study. Br J Sports Med. 2011;45:702–8.
3. Dvorak J, Junge A, Derman W, Schwellnus M. Injuries and illnesses of football players during the 2010 FIFA World Cup. Br J Sports Med. 2011;45:626–30.
4. Brito J, Malina RM, Seabra A, Massada JL, Soares JM, Krustrup P, Rebelo A. Injuries in Portuguese youth soccer players during training and match play. J Athl Train. 2012;47:191–7.
5. Wong P, Hong Y. Soccer injury in the lower extremities. Br J Sports Med. 2005;39:473–82.
6. Fong DT, Hong Y, Chan LK, Yung PS, Chan KM. A systematic review on ankle injury and ankle sprain in sports. Sports Med. 2007;37:73–94.
7. Jain N, Murray D, Kemp S, Calder J. Frequency and trends in foot and ankle injuries within an English Premier League Football club using a new impact factor of injury to identify a focus for injury prevention. Foot Ankle Surg. 2014;20:237–40.
8. Giza E, Fuller C, Junge A, Dvorak J. Mechanisms of foot and ankle injuries in soccer. Am J Sports Med. 2003;31:550–4.

9. Andersen TE, Floerenes TW, Arnason A, Bahr R. Video analysis of the mechanisms for ankle injuries in football. Am J Sports Med. 2004;32:69S–79S.
10. Boden BP, Lohnes JH, Nunley JA, Garrett Jr WE. Tibia and fibula fractures in soccer players. Knee Surg Sports Traumatol Arthrosc. 1999;7:262–6.
11. Vanlommel L, Vanlommel J, Bollars P, Quisquater L, Van Crombrugge K, Corten K, Bellemans J. Incidence and risk factors of lower leg fractures in Belgian soccer players. Injury. 2013;44:1847–50.
12. Ekstrand J, Torstveit MK. Stress fractures in elite male football players. Scand J Med Sci Sports. 2012;22:341–6.
13. Porter DA, May BD, Berney T. Functional outcome after operative treatment for ankle fractures in young athletes: a retrospective case series. Foot Ankle Int. 2008;29:887–94.
14. Hermans JJ, Beumer A, de Jong TA, Kleinrensink GJ. Anatomy of the distal tibiofibular syndesmosis in adults: a pictorial essay with a multimodality approach. J Anat. 2010;217:633–45.
15. Goost H, Wimmer MD, Barg A, Kabir K, Valderrabano V, Burger C. Fractures of the ankle joint: investigation and treatment options. Dtsch Arztebl Int. 2014;111:377–88.
16. Massada JL. Ankle overuse injuries in soccer players. Morphological adaptation of the talus in the anterior impingement. J Sports Med Phys Fitness. 1991;31:447–51.
17. Lauge-Hansen N. Fractures of the ankle. II. Combined experimental-surgical and experimental-roentgenologic investigations. Arch Surg. 1950;60:957–85.
18. Müller ME, Nazarian S, Koch P, Schatzker J. The comprehensive classification of fractures of long bones. Berlin: Springer-Verlag; 1990.
19. Weber BG. Die Verletzungen des oberen Sprunggelenkes. Zweite, überarbeitete und ergänzte Auflage. Vienna: Hans Huber Bern Stuttgart; 1972.
20. Michelson JD, Magid D, McHale K. Clinical utility of a stability-based ankle fracture classification system. J Orthop Trauma. 2007;21:307–15.
21. Stiell IG, Greenberg GH, McKnight RD, Nair RC, McDowell I, Worthington JR. A study to develop clinical decision rules for the use of radiography in acute ankle injuries. Ann Emerg Med. 1992;21:384–90.
22. Donken CC, Al-Khateeb H, Verhofstad MH, van Laarhoven CJ. Surgical versus conservative interventions for treating ankle fractures in adults. Cochrane Database Syst Rev. 2012;8:CD008470.
23. SooHoo NF, Krenek L, Eagan MJ, Gurbani B, Ko CY, Zingmond DS. Complication rates following open reduction and internal fixation of ankle fractures. J Bone Joint Surg Am. 2009;91:1042–9.
24. Bourne RB. Pilon fractures of the distal tibia. Clin Orthop Relat Res. 1989;240:42–6.
25. Bourne RB, Rorabeck CH, MacNab J. Intra-articular fractures of the distal tibia: the pilon fracture. J Trauma. 1983;23:591–6.
26. Ruedi TP, Allgower M. Fractures of the lower end of the tibia into the ankle joint. Injury. 1969;1:92–9.
27. Anon. Orthopaedic trauma association committee for coding and classification: fracture and dislocation compendium. J Orthop Trauma. 1996;10:57–8.
28. Oestern HJ, Tscherne H. Pathophysiology and classification of soft tissue injuries associated with fractures. Fractures with soft tissue injuries. Berlin: Springer-Verlag; 1984.
29. Talarico LM, Vito GR, Zyryanov SY. Management of displaced intra-articular calcaneal fractures by using external ring fixation, minimally invasive open reduction, and early weight bearing. J Foot Ankle Surg. 2004;43:43–50.
30. Sanders RW. Displaced intra-articular fractures of the calcaneus. J Bone Joint Surg Am. 2000;82: 225–50.
31. Haddix B, Ellis K, Saylor-Pavkovich E. Lisfranc fractures-dislocation in a female soccer athlete. Int J Sports Phys Ther. 2012;7:219–25.
32. Gotha HE, Lareau CR, Fellars TA. Diagnosis and management of lisfranc injuries and metatarsal fractures. R I Med J. 2013;96:33–6.
33. Quénu, E., Küss, G. Étude sur les luxations du métatarse (luxations métatarso-tarsiennes). Rev Chir. 1909;39:281–336 (720–91, 1093–134 [in French]).
34. Myerson MS, Fisher RT, Burgess AR, Kenzora JE. Fracture dislocations of the tarsometatarsal joints: end results correlated with pathology and treatment. Foot Ankle. 1986;6:225–42.
35. Jones R. I. Fracture of the base of the fifth metatarsal bone by indirect violence. Ann Surg. 1902;35: 697–700.
36. Dameron Jr TB. Fractures of the proximal fifth metatarsal: selecting the best treatment option. J Am Acad Orthop Surg. 1995;3:110–4.
37. Eisele SA, Sammarco GJ. Fatigue fractures of the foot and ankle in the athlete. J Bone Joint Surg Am. 1993;75:290–8.
38. Ortiguera CJ, Fischer DA. A review of the current treatment for fracture of the proximal fifth metatarsal first described by Jones. Orthop Tech Rev. 2000;2:1–2.
39. Kavanaugh JH, Brower TD, Mann RV. The Jones fracture revisited. J Bone Joint Surg Am. 1978;60: 776–82.
40. Dameron Jr TB. Fractures and anatomical variations of the proximal portion of the fifth metatarsal. J Bone Joint Surg Am. 1975;57:788–92.
41. Massada MM, Pereira MA, de Sousa RJ, Costa PG, Massada JL. Intramedullary screw fixation of proximal fifth metatarsal fractures in athletes. Acta Ortop Bras. 2012;20:262–5.
42. Fitch KD. Stress fractures of the lower limbs in runners. Aust Fam Physician. 1984;13:511–5.
43. Brukner P, Bradshaw C, Khan KM, White S, Crossley K. Stress fractures: a review of 180 cases. Clin J Sport Med. 1996;6:85–9.
44. Kahanov L, Eberman LE, Games KE, Wasik M. Diagnosis, treatment, and rehabilitation of stress fractures in the lower extremity in runners. Open Access J Sports Med. 2015;6:87–95.

45. Shelbourne KD, Fisher DA, Rettig AC, McCarroll JR. Stress fractures of the medial malleolus. Am J Sports Med. 1988;16:60–3.
46. Carreira DS, Sandilands SM. Radiographic factors and effect of fifth metatarsal Jones and diaphyseal stress fractures on participation in the NFL. Foot Ankle Int. 2013;34:518–22.
47. Kor A, Saltzman AT, Wempe PD. Medial malleolar stress fractures. Literature review, diagnosis, and treatment. J Am Podiatr Med Assoc. 2003;93:292–7.
48. Fowler JRGJ, Boden BP, Pavlov H, Torg JS. The non-surgical and surgical treatment of tarsal navicular stress fractures. Sports Med. 2011;41:613–9.
49. Lee S, Anderson RB. Stress fractures of the tarsal navicular. Foot Ankle Clin. 2004;9:85–104.
50. Luthje P, Nurmi I. Fracture-dislocation of the tarsal navicular in a soccer player. Scand J Med Sci Sports. 2002;12:236–40.
51. Gross CE, Nunley JA. Medial-sided stress fractures: medial malleolus and navicular stress fractures. Oper Tech Sports Med. 2014;22:296–304.
52. Randsborg PH, Gulbrandsen P, Benth JS, Sivertsen EA, Hammer OL, Fuglesang HF, Arøen A. Fractures in children: epidemiology and activity-specific fracture rates. J Bone Joint Surg Am. 2013;95:1–7.
53. Lohman M, Kivisaari A, Kallio P, Puntila J, Vehmas T, Kivisaari L. Acute paediatric ankle trauma: MRI versus plain radiography. Skeletal Radiol. 2001;30:504–11.
54. Singer G, Cichocki M, Schalamon J, Eberl R, Höllwarth ME. A study of metatarsal fractures in children. J Bone Joint Surg Am. 2008;90:772–6.
55. Salter RB, Harris R. Injuries involving the epiphyseal plate. J Bone Joint Surg Am. 1963;45:587–622.

13 Football Ankle Fractures and Return to Sport: A Review on the Arthroscopic Approach

Pieter d'Hooghe, Hélder Pereira, and Stefano Zaffagnini

Contents

P. d'Hooghe (✉)
ASPETAR Orthopaedic and Sports Medicine Hospital, Department of Orthopaedic Surgery, Aspire Zone, Doha, Qatar
e-mail: pieter.dhooghe@aspetar.com

H. Pereira
3B's Research Group–Biomaterials, Biodegradables and Biomimetics, University of Minho, Headquarters of the European Institute of Excellence on Tissue Engineering and Regenerative Medicine, AvePark, Parque de Ciência e Tecnologia, Zona Industrial da Gandra, 4805-017 Barco, Guimarães, Portugal

ICVS/3B's – PT Government Associate Laboratory, Minho University, Braga/Guimarães, Portugal

Orthopedic Department, Centro Hospitalar Póvoa de Varzim – Vila do Conde, Póvoa de Varzim, Portugal

Ripoll y De Prado Sports Clinic – FIFA Medical Centre of Excellence, Murcia/Madrid, Spain

S. Zaffagnini
Rizzoli Orthopedic Institute, Bologna, Italy

J. Espregueira-Mendes et al. (eds.), *Injuries and Health Problems in Football*,
DOI 10.1007/978-3-662-53924-8_13

Disclosure None

13.1 Introduction

There are more than 300 million registered football players worldwide, and the ankle is one of the most commonly reported injured joints – ankle injuries constitute 12–23% of all injuries recorded during FIFA competitions [1]. One in five of all injuries to footballers of all skill and age groups is to the ankle – this prevalence increases to 35% in low-level amateur players, children, and adolescents [1].

Arthroscopic surgery for chronic pathology post ankle fracture has been shown to have significant benefits, but evidence on its use in the acute setting is limited. In the management of acute ankle fractures in the athlete, arthroscopy becomes increasingly important – not only in optimizing diagnosis but also in offering expanded treatment options [2]. Proposed arthroscopic advantages in ankle fracture treatment include:

- Minimally invasive nature
- Ability to directly visualize joint articulation
- Evaluation of ligamentous injuries

This aids in the diagnosis and treatment of concomitant pathology that may not be obvious through open surgery alone. Arthroscopy may also help in minimizing the risk for postoperative delay in rehabilitation and return to competition [3].

There are several potential benefits to the use of arthroscopy in elite athlete ankle fracture management:

1. In up to 60% of ankle fractures, a combined cartilage lesion is also noted
2. Syndesmotic stability – and the presence of intra-articular pathology – can best be assessed by arthroscopy
3. Complex intra-articular ankle fractures need accurate tibial plafond reduction – which can best be achieved through arthroscopy
4. The minimally invasive character of arthroscopy can be beneficial for the elite athlete by allowing for a more rapid rehabilitation

The aim of this article is to offer a comprehensive review of the current medical literature on the indications and treatment options for arthroscopic ankle procedures in football players.

13.2 Materials

The generally accepted pathological indications for ankle arthroscopy are:

- Ankle osteosynthesis
- Ligament ruptures
- Impingement syndromes
- Cartilage lesions

We performed a Medline search using the keywords "ankle fracture, arthroscopy, and football." We found and reviewed 55 articles, describing either the procedure or the results of arthroscopic-assisted reduction and internal fixation (ARIF) of various ankle fractures. Only 6 of these 55 papers had a combined focus on elite sports (e.g., football) [3–8]. Ligamentous injuries will not be covered specifically, since they are considered not in the scope of this review chapter on football-related ankle fractures and the role of arthroscopy.

The indications for ARIF (arthroscopic-assisted reduction and internal fixation) in elite sports ankle fracture management are:

- Malleolar fracture
- Intra-articular fracture
- (Osteo)chondral injury
- Syndesmotic injury
- Talar body/neck fracture
- Talar process fractures

13.3 ARIF

The obvious benefits of ARIF in the management of ankle fractures are:

- Accurate reduction of damage to the soft tissue envelope and blood supply to the damaged area
- Reduced incidence of infection
- Improved visualization and accurate restoration of the articular surface

Concerns exist in terms of increased surgical time and surgeon-dependent ability to successfully use the technique – being mindful of any associated soft tissue swelling. Imade et al. describe an acute anterior compartment syndrome following ankle arthroscopy after a Maisonneuve fracture in a football player [9].

Fibrous tissue formation after an ankle fracture can cause impairment in function through impingement. This is due to remnants of torn ligaments and capsular tissue – including those from the syndesmotic, ATFL, and medial deltoid ligaments – causing inflammation and laying down of scar tissue [10]. This pathology is known to respond well to arthroscopic resection [11]. Acute arthroscopic evaluation and debridement may be beneficial, but current evidence to support this is limited [3, 4]. Hepple has described potentially significant benefits of

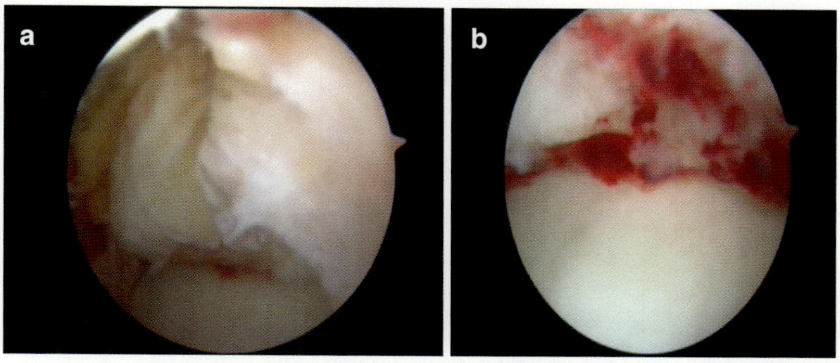

Fig. 13.1 (**a**) Intraoperative image of an arthroscopic-assisted distal tibial fracture (extending into the talocrural joint) assessment. (**b**) Intraoperative image of an arthroscopic-assisted intra-articular distal tibial fracture. Note the fracture hematoma

ankle arthroscopy in fractures with a combined need for ligamentous repair. Others, however, suggest the negative effects of fluid extravasation into soft tissues as a reason not to combine an arthroscopic procedure with a one-stage ligamentous repair [4]. There is currently no evidence to guide surgeons encountering these combined lesions acutely, and more research is required in this area. Techniques for arthroscopic lateral ligament repair in chronic cases show promising results, but further work is required for their effect to be extrapolated to acute and elite sports cases [12, 13].

ARIF has been described for fractures of the talar body, talar neck, or talar process and the distal tibia, malleolar, and transitional fractures [14–17]. Hindfoot process fracture excision/fixation – when symptomatic – is also possible through arthroscopic-assisted techniques [18]. A classic two-portal anterior/posterior arthroscopic technique is most often used prior to a combined open fracture reduction and fixation (Fig. 13.1a, b). The literature, however, on the value of arthroscopy in the management of these specific fractures in football is limited [3–5].

13.4 Indications for Combined Ankle Arthroscopy in Acute Football Ankle Fractures

13.4.1 Malleolar Fractures

Malleolar fractures are generally evaluated by physical examination and radiographs – they are then classified according to either the AO or Weber classification systems. In cases of dislocation, immediate reduction is mandatory to prevent skin necrosis and possible nerve damage. Correct treatment is chosen on the basis of:

- Mechanism of injury
- Correct classification
- Associated soft tissue damage

Weber A fractures are usually treated conservatively, while Weber B and C fractures frequently require surgery. Specific attention should be given to the intraoperative evaluation of syndesmotic joint stability – up to 66% of Weber B and C ankle fractures have some degree of syndesmotic ligamentous injury [4, 19–25]. The most frequent complications are wound hematoma and wound necrosis. Postoperative infection rate is around 2%. Stufkens et al. analyzed the long-term outcomes of these fractures and concluded that over 10% of patients develop ankle arthrosis [19]. The evidence for optimal treatment strategies is low – especially in elite sports such as football. Arthroscopy – prior to open surgery – is shown to be effective in discovering hitherto undetected osteochondral defects in the ankle and enabling the surgeon to check the anatomical reduction [2, 4, 20, 25–29]. Up to 60–75% of ankle fractures (that require surgical fixation) have demonstrated evidence of articular cartilage damage – previously undiagnosed prior to surgery [19]. Such injuries are mostly cartilaginous in nature and therefore not radiographically

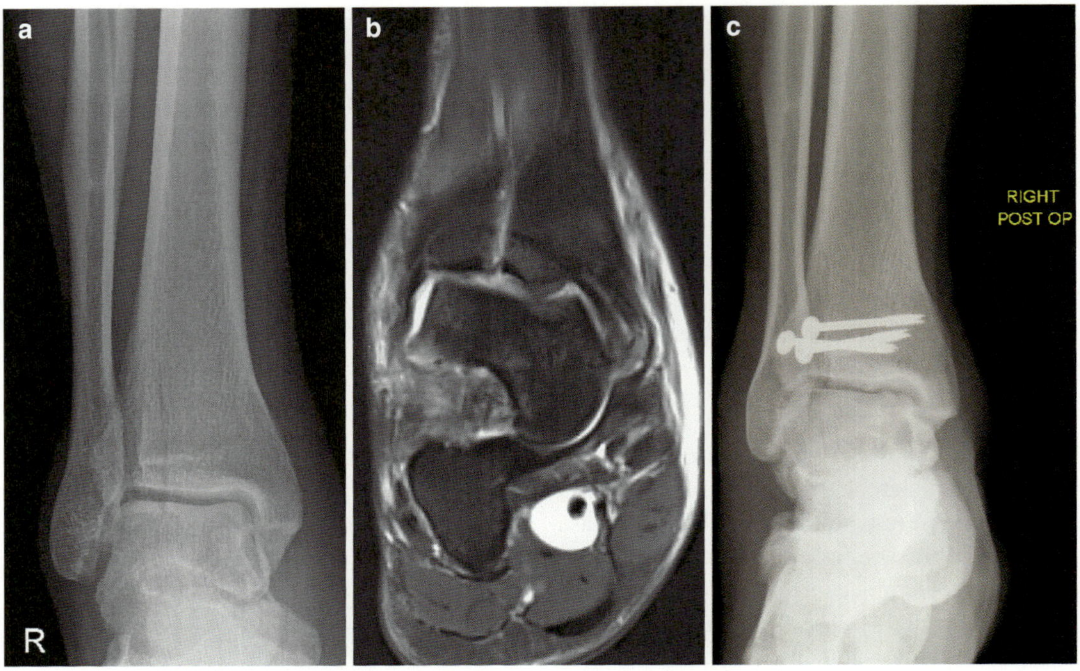

Fig. 13.2 (**a**) Anteroposterior (AP) X-ray of an elite football player with a centro-lateral distal tibial stress fracture with intra-articular excursion. (**b**) Coronal T2 MRI image of the centro-lateral distal tibial stress fracture with intra-articular excursion. (**c**) After arthroscopic-assisted percutaneous reduction and fixation with control over the anatomical reduction and articular cartilage status

visible (Fig. 13.2a–c). These lesions usually occur at locations not accessible through traditional fracture surgery incisions. Therefore, simultaneous arthroscopic assessment and management of these lesions is required to improve the rate and quality of recovery after fracture surgery.

Since radiographs are commonly used as the preferred diagnostic tool in acute ankle fractures, the very low sensitivity of plain radiography leads to many undiagnosed osteochondral lesions [4, 19, 20, 30–32].

In the only prospective randomized trial comparing arthroscopic-assisted with traditional non-assisted lateral malleolar fracture fixation, Takao et al. showed a very high rate of secondary pathology. This was mostly chondral damage and syndesmotic injury [20]. At average follow-up of 40 months, there was a small but significantly greater AOFAS outcome score in the arthroscopically assisted group compared with the traditional group [20].

13.4.2 Intra-articular Fractures

Intra-articular fractures like triplane and Tillaux fractures clearly benefit from an arthroscopic-assisted approach because fracture site clearance and accurate intra-articular realignment check can be performed. The same applies to simple malleolar or distal tibial stress fractures that have an intra-articular fracture line. Complete cartilage assessment can also be performed without the need for large exposures. Any step-off into the joint line, comminution, or depressed fragment can be recognized and realigned

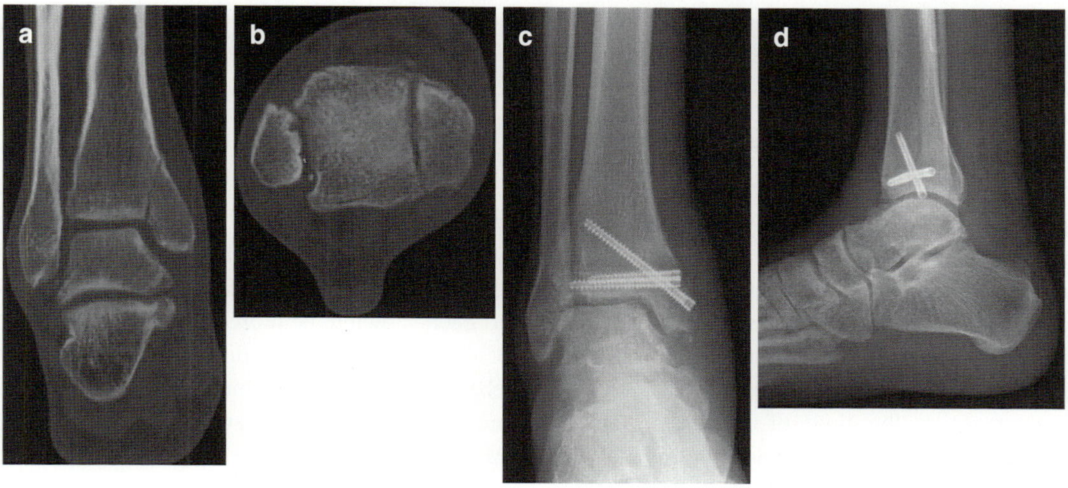

Fig. 13.3 (**a**) Coronal CT image of a medial malleolar stress fracture in the ankle of an elite football player. Note the talar varus deformity alignment. (**b**) Axial CT image of a medial malleolar stress fracture in the ankle of an elite football player. Note the anterior small fragment. (**c**) Postoperative AP X-ray after arthroscopic-assisted percutaneous fracture reduction and fixation. (**d**) Postoperative lateral X-ray after arthroscopic-assisted percutaneous fracture reduction and fixation

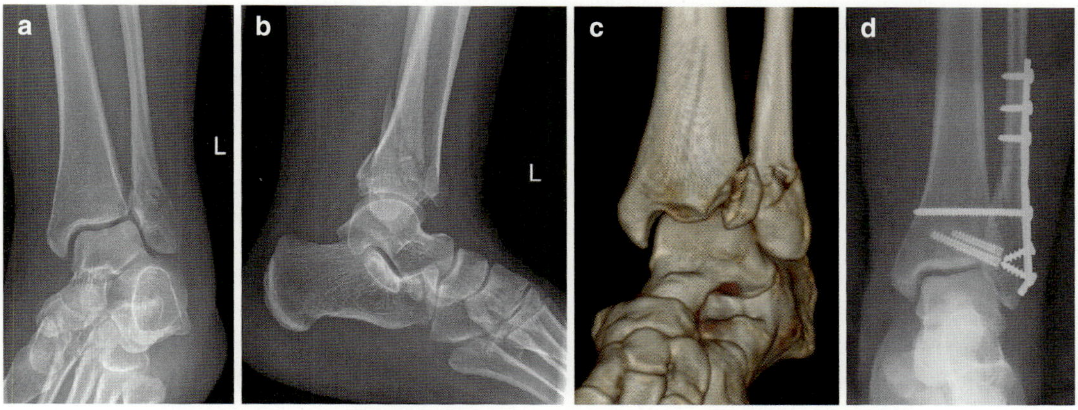

Fig. 13.4 (**a**) AP X-ray of a Weber B distal fibular fracture in a professional football player. (**b**) Lateral X-ray reveals the combined bony anterior syndesmotic fracture. (**c**) Coronal 3D CT image of the intra-articular ankle fracture. (**d**) AP X-ray image after arthroscopic-assisted fracture reduction and fixation

(Fig. 13.3a–d). Percutaneous temporary K-wires are frequently used to manipulate and aid in fracture reduction before definitive osteosynthesis is performed [33, 34] (Fig. 13.4a–d). However, the technique can be demanding, and no studies comparing conventional open techniques are available [4, 28].

13.4.3 Osteochondral Lesions

A substantial proportion of osteochondral injuries after ankle fracture will not cause long-term symptomatic problems. There remains a lack of studies over the need for combined arthroscopy as a standardized tool in fracture fixation treatment. A prospective randomized trial by Takao et al. showed no difference in outcome between patients undergoing arthroscopy and management of articular damage at the time of fixation and those that did not [20]. Ono et al. – in a larger prospective randomized trial of 72 patients – showed a statistically improved AOFAS score (91.0 vs 87.6) in patients that had arthroscopically assisted fixation [29]. Articular damage following ankle fracture may be an independent predictor for the development of post-traumatic arthritis. Hence, arthroscopic assessment at the time of fracture would be advantageous in predicting long-term outcome. Documentation of defect size, condition, and location (medial, central, lateral) can assist in adequate treatment decision-making. This is particularly true for defects over the medial malleolus that have been shown to have the poorest long-term outcomes [3, 20, 21, 31]. Frequently, acute osteochondral defects that are detected in combination with ankle fractures are amenable to arthroscopic treatment. Arthroscopy can help in decision-making and immediate treatment with regard to fragment fixation to anatomic fit or removal. Based upon the talar dome/tibial plafond defect size, bone marrow stimulation techniques (drilling, abrasion, or microfracture) can be used in the same procedure stage to treat osteochondral ankle lesions [35–39]. Cartilage regeneration procedures (autologous chondrocyte implantation [ACI], matrix-induced autologous chondrocyte implantation [MACI]) are becoming more popular in the treatment of football players with a chronic osteochondral defect of the talus [40, 41]. Arthroscopy can be beneficial in these cases – a cartilage biopsy can also be taken at the time of procedure for cell culture for cartilage implantation (ACI). The same treatment strategy is useful for the less frequent tibial plafond osteochondral lesions [33].

13.4.4 Syndesmosis

Injury to the syndesmosis after an ankle fracture is seen in 47–66% of patients and can result in chronic ankle problems [22]. Intraoperative stress views are more reliable – when compared to plain radiographs – at detecting definitive instability [23]. Nevertheless, borderline instability or partial injury to the syndesmotic complex without instability is difficult to detect. Magnetic ressonance imaging (MRI) has been shown to provide accurate information when documenting a syndesmotic injury, but has a significant false positive rate, whereas arthroscopic assessment has been shown to be more sensitive and specific [3, 4, 23, 24, 42]. In addition, arthroscopy can debride the extra-syndesmotic fibers of the ruptured ligaments that may otherwise produce chronic pain and impingement [10, 11, 43]. Good to excellent results have been reported in a few studies where arthroscopic assessment (with fixation) and/or debridement were used to manage such injuries [20, 21, 30, 32]. Arthroscopic evaluation may also detect sagittal and rotational ankle instability, which may not always be visualized on intraoperative stress radiography [3, 44]. Finally, damage to the medial area of the talocrural joint is an indirect finding commonly associated with syndesmotic injury.

13.4.5 Talar Body and Neck Fractures

Fractures of the talar neck and body (Fig. 13.5a–e) are rare injuries that can cause significant morbidity and complications. For the football player, these injuries can have a deleterious effect on their long-term functional outcome. Treatment efforts are aimed at the quality of fracture reduction and the preservation of talar blood supply. Arthroscopic-assisted surgery has been shown to be of value in both these aspects, but the technique is demanding and prolongs operative time and increases soft tissue swelling. Case reports, and small case series, provide some evidence to recommend this technique [19, 45–47]. The underlying principle in managing a talar fracture is to achieve anatomical reduction and stable fixation with minimal disturbance to the soft tissue – for the abovementioned reasons [45, 46]. Skin necrosis, infection, malunion, and post-traumatic arthritis are well-recognized complications of talar fractures, and management should be designed to minimize

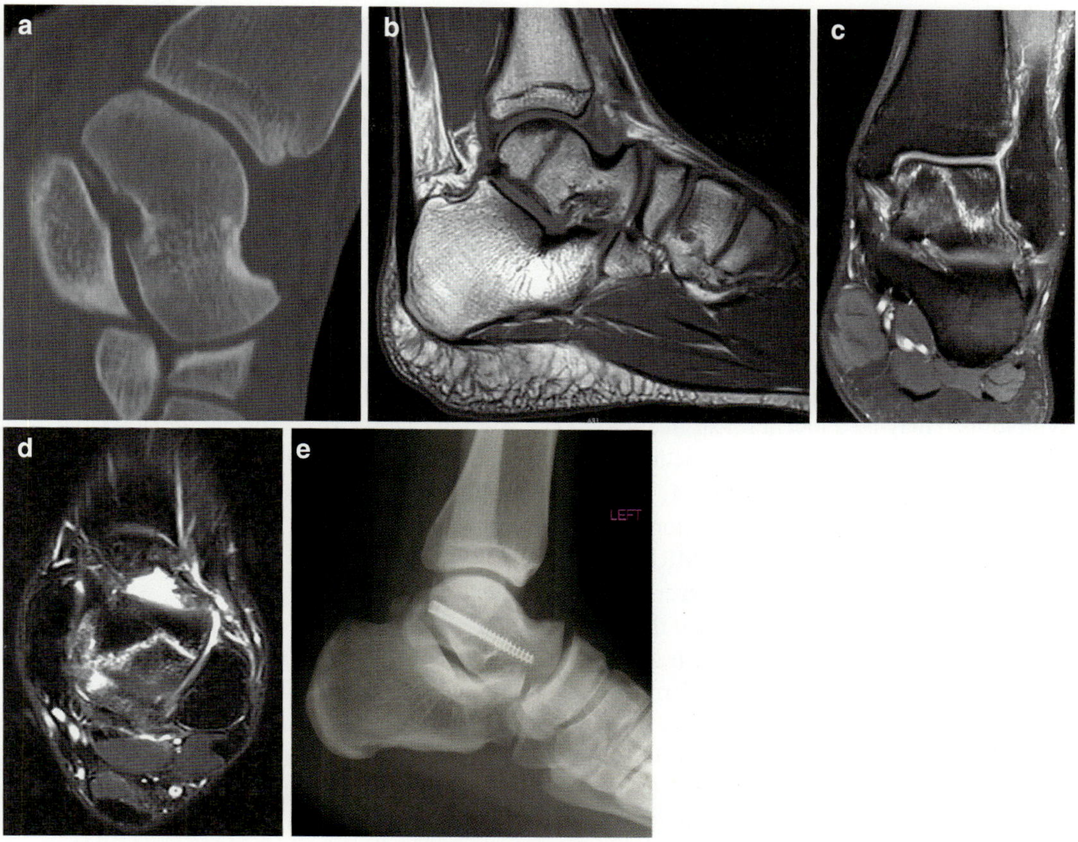

Fig. 13.5 (**a**) Sagittal CT image of a professional football player with sudden ankle pain after a preseason training camp. (**b**) Sagittal T1 MRI image of a talar body stress fracture. Note the Hawkins sign. (**c**) Coronal T2 MRI image of the progressive diastasis of the talar body stress fracture during conservative treatment. (**d**) Axial T2 MRI image of the progressive diastasis of the talar body stress fracture during conservative treatment. (**e**) Lateral X-ray of the arthroscopic-assisted talar body fracture compression screw fixation

these. Subairy et al. have shown that arthroscopic-assisted surgical stabilization of these fractures is advantageous and reduces the time to union [46].

Stress fractures are the most common overuse bony injuries in football (Fig. 13.5), but stress fractures of the talar body are extremely rare and have only rarely been reported [5, 14, 48]. More common – but still rare – are stress fractures of the talar neck or lateral talar process [5, 15, 16]. Due to their minor displacement, most stress fractures of the talar body are treated nonsurgically [5, 14, 17]. Stress fractures in football are the result of excessive, repetitive cyclic loads traumatizing bones with normal form and structure [49]. Predisposing factors may be both intrinsic and extrinsic and include malalignment, lack of flexibility, increase in training, training of excessive volume and intensity, hard or soft activity surfaces, inappropriate shoes, and inadequate coaching [5, 14]. Additional factors to be considered include age, ethnicity, gender, fitness, skill level, and menstrual history [5, 50]. Mechanical factors that may lead to a stress fatigue fracture remain unclear but may result from repeated loading or from repetitive prolonged muscular action on bone not yet conditioned to such heavy and novel action.

In football players, significant pathogenetic movements predisposing to talar stress fracture can be identified in repetitive, restricted axial loading while sprinting, kicking a ball, or landing after heading. The load that has to be absorbed during these actions, the extremes in plantar-/dorsiflexion of the foot (kicking the ball), and other traumatic actions should be considered important pathogenetic factors in repetitive strain injuries. Moreover, when playing toward the end of a match, coordination is less precise as athletes are often fatigued [5, 50]. The diagnosis of stress fracture is based on clinical suspicion, a detailed history, and a physical examination, followed by appropriate imaging investigations. The role of conventional radiography is important, although initial findings are often minimal or absent (Fig. 13.5a). The earliest sign – often delayed until after the onset of symptoms – may be a lucent linear image (more often a sclerotic band, periosteal reaction, or callus formation) seen on X-ray [5, 14, 17]. MRI has a high sensitivity for the detection of stress fractures (Fig. 13.5b). In addition, MRI signs are evident several weeks before radiographic signs. Conservative treatment is preferred if there is no, or only minor, displacement at the fracture site. There is only limited scientific information on healing times for stress fractures of the talar body but overall, stress fractures are known for their prolonged healing period [5, 51]. Generally, treatment of stress fractures is immobilization for 4–8 weeks [14, 48, 50, 51]. Avascular necrosis remains a relatively high risk – given the suboptimal talar vascular status – even after an adequate immobilization period [51, 52]. Hawkins classified (nonstress) fractures of the talus in an attempt to predict the risk of avascular necrosis [53]. Hawkins type 1 fracture has a good prognosis as the risk of avascular necrosis is less than 15% [54]. If significant diastasis/displacement (Hawkins type 2) occurs, the risk of avascular necrosis rises to 50%, and surgical repositioning and fixation is indicated [54] (Fig. 13.5c–e).

If adequate measures – with rapid intervention to reposition the displaced fracture – are taken, it is possible to achieve a positive outcome without ongoing problems [5] (Fig. 13.5e). D'Hooghe et al. described the management of progressive talar body stress fractures in professional football players through posterior arthroscopy-assisted compression screw fixation with excellent healing results [5] (Fig. 13.5a–e). No other articles were found that combine arthroscopy with talar stress fracture fixation management.

13.4.6 Talar Process Fractures

13.4.6.1 Lateral Tubercle Fractures and Os Trigonum Complex

Posterior impingement in the ankle refers to a mechanical conflict on the posterior side of the ankle. In football, it accounts for about 4 % of all ankle injuries and can present either acutely or chronically [3].

Posterior ankle impingement syndrome is a clinical pain syndrome reflecting the most common cause of posterior ankle pain. It can be provoked by a forced hyperplantar flexion movement of the ankle [18, 20, 55, 56]. In the event of bony posterior impingement of the ankle, plantar flexion induces a conflict between the posterior malleolus of the distal tibia onto the posterosuperior calcaneal bone. A hypertrophic posterior talar process or an os trigonum is present in almost 7% of the football population [3]. Not every apparent posterior bone – caused by acute or repetitive overload (micro)trauma – induces posterior ankle pain and is not necessarily associated with the posterior ankle impingement syndrome.

Acute forced hyperplantar flexion movement of the ankle can induce bony conflict in the posterior ankle joint; thus, it is frequently seen in football. The mechanism of injury is a repetitive forced plantar flexion or an acute blocked kicking action. Compression of the os trigonum between the distal tibia and calcaneal bone can also cause this lesion, thus potentially leading to displacement of an os trigonum or fracture of the processus posterior tali or distal tibia (Fig. 13.6).

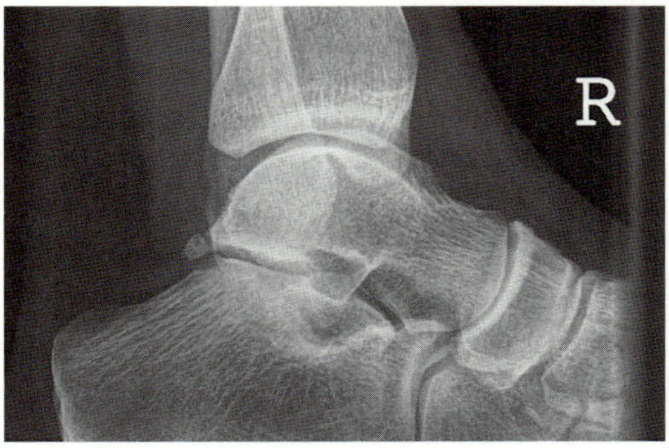

Fig. 13.6 Lateral X-ray of an os trigonum in a professional football player's ankle

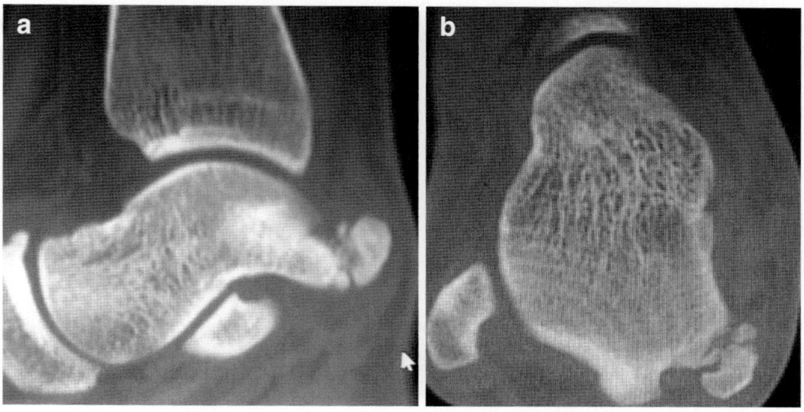

Fig. 13.7 (**a**) Sagittal CT image of a Cedell fracture in a professional football player's ankle. (**b**) Axial CT image of a Cedell fracture in a professional football player's ankle

Over the last three decades, posterior arthroscopy of the ankle joint has become a standardized procedure, with numerous indications for treating posterior (intra-articular) ankle pathology. Lack of direct access and the nature and deep location of its hindfoot structures are reasons why posterior ankle problems still pose a diagnostic and therapeutic challenge today.

The two-portal endoscopic technique by van Dijk et al. – introduced in 2000 – gives excellent access to the posterior ankle compartment and also to the surrounding extra-articular posterior ankle structures [55].

This technique has modified classic arthroscopic tools and skills and has introduced a broad spectrum of new indications in posterior ankle pathology [55–57].

The most influential indication to perform posterior ankle arthroscopy remains the treatment of os trigonum. This is an attractive alternative to open surgery for experienced arthroscopic surgeons.

Improved functional outcomes after surgery, lower morbidity and more rapid rehabilitation time, are all reasons why football players can clearly benefit from this technique [54–57].

13.4.6.2 Medial Tubercle Fractures

Fractures of the medial tubercle are rare in football [3]. They can be due to:

- Avulsion of the posterior talotibial ligament (posterior aspect of the deltoid ligament)
- Dorsiflexion and eversion (Cedell fracture)
- Direct compression of the process as above
- Impingement of the sustentaculum tali in supination

In contrast to lateral tubercle injuries, pain and swelling is usually present between the Achilles tendon and the medial malleolus. There may, however, be limited pain on walking or movement of the ankle. It is difficult to visualize fractures of the medial tubercle on plain AP and lateral radiographs, and it has been suggested that the addition of two oblique views at 45° and 70° of external rotation may significantly aid detection prior to resorting to a CT or MRI [3] (Fig. 13.7a, b). These fractures can be approached through the posterior arthroscopic technique – their extent can be visualized and the necessary treatment can be performed all in a one-stage procedure.

13.4.6.3 Entire Posterior Process Fractures

These injuries are usually fractures of the lateral or posterior process and comprise some of the most commonly missed fractures in acute ankle injuries.

Routine AP and lateral radiographs do not often show acute fractures and may be incorrectly interpreted. CT scan remains the mainstay of diagnosis, but there also needs to be a high index of suspicion by the assessing physician [3, 4].

Lateral process fractures in football often present with signs and symptoms of simple ankle sprain. Undiagnosed and untreated fractures often lead to persistent lateral ankle pain and late

Table 13.1 Hawkins classification of lateral talar process fractures [59]

Lateral talar process fractures	
Type 1	Simple fracture extending from talofibular to talocalcaneal joint
Type 2	Comminuted fracture
Type 3	Small chip fracture not involving talofibular joint

subtalar joint arthritis. Outcomes are suboptimal when diagnosis and treatment is delayed for more than 2 weeks [4, 58]. The classification of these fractures is shown in Table 13.1.

Type 1 fractures benefit from stable fixation usually via an open surgical technique. Type 3 fractures respond well to conservative treatment. Type 2 fractures, however, appear to respond best to early removal of the fracture fragments as opposed to delayed surgery. Removal of these fracture fragments by arthroscopy would reduce the surrounding soft tissue dissection and potentially accelerate return to normal activity. However, at present, there is no study available that supports this theory. Further studies are therefore necessary in this area.

Posterior process fractures usually occur as a result of forced plantar flexion injuries and are even less common than lateral process fractures. Most of these injuries are initially treated with conservative management, but a small number of cases with significant comminution (such as in elite football cases) may be appropriately treated by early arthroscopic debridement [4].

13.5 Rehabilitation

Rehabilitation is a central aspect of management of ankle fractures in football athletes. The aim of arthroscopy in ankle fracture treatment is – in the first instance – to improve functional outcome and reduce morbidity and rehabilitation time. Therefore, it is commonly used as a valuable tool in football-related ankle traumatology. Initial elevation after injury or operation, as well as early range of motion exercises as soon as safely possible, is encouraged in the early postoperative phase [3].

13.6 General Outcomes and Time to Return to Competition

Outcomes from the general population cannot be directly extrapolated to football players, who usually receive better and more intense rehabilitation. Their safe and prompt return to a highly demanding level of activity is paramount. Evidence on outcomes on the rarer fractures around the ankle (i.e., process and talar fractures) in football is scarce and has been discussed earlier. Some evidence on the more common malleolar type fractures has been documented and allows for some conclusions to be made [3]. It has to be noted that a number of studies reporting time-loss ankle injuries from training and competition provide limited information. These studies often group ankle injuries together, with the severity of injury often being defined by the time to return to sport (rather than the type of injury) [3].

Surgical treatment may allow a more rapid recovery, with earlier weight-bearing and functional rehabilitation providing a speedier return to normal daily living and work. However, a recent systematic review by Donken et al. looked at surgical versus conservative intervention for treating ankle fractures in adults. He concluded that there is insufficient evidence to determine which type of treatment provided better long-term outcomes [60]. The review only identified four controlled trials (292 adults with displaced ankle fractures) from the general population. Also, there were significant variations and limitations in the types of patients, the surgical and rehabilitation protocols applied, the outcomes reported, and the duration of follow-up. Another study by Colvin et al. looked at the functional ability of 243 patients who underwent operative fixation of unstable ankle fractures to return to "vigorous activity" and sport [6]. Younger, healthier male patients were more likely to return to sport. At 1-year follow-up – although 88% of recreational athletes were able to return to sport – only 11.6% of competitive athletes were able to do so. Specifically, those with bimalleolar fractures were more likely to return to sport, compared with those with uni-malleolar fractures.

However, the study looked only retrospectively at self-reported outcomes from a general trauma population [6]. Nevertheless, it has been suggested that surgical management (by open reduction and internal fixation of unstable ankle fractures) in football players may provide a number of advantages. Firstly, it would avoid the issues of secondary fracture displacement which delay recovery. Secondly, it would ensure anatomic fracture reduction and articular surface restoration. Finally, it allows for early range of movement exercises and early weight-bearing (within 1–2 weeks of fixation) and a more rapid recovery and return to sport [7].

Studies specifically looking at ankle fractures in football players are limited [3, 7, 8, 61], but appear to demonstrate that a successful return to high-level competition can be expected. A study by Dunley et al. on three professional American football players showed that all three returned to their pre-injury level [8]. Similar findings were reported in a study by Walsh et al. on the surgical treatment of ankle fractures in three American football and one football player [61]. Another study by Oztekin et al. looked at the time-loss from play in ankle injuries of Turkish professional football players. In this study, all patients that were surgically treated for their ankle fracture were able to return to their previous level of play [62]. A layoff of 150 days in this study was reported for two football players (one with a Maisonneuve fracture and one with a lateral malleolar fracture with deltoid rupture), while a patient that was treated for a lateral malleolus pseudoarthrosis took 200 days.

Another study by Porter documented the management, rehabilitation, and outcomes in 27 athletes with ankle fractures that underwent ORIF (including repair of any injured ligaments). The indication for surgery was either displacement of ≥3 mm or if the athlete was "especially enthusiastic" for an early return to sports [7]. The most common sport injuries were in American football (ten athletes) and baseball (three athletes), but two athletes involved in football were also included. At an average follow-up of 2.4 years (12 months to 3.7 years), all athletes reported an average 96.4% functional rating compared to their pre-injury level, with 12 athletes rating their ankle as 100%. Early rehabilitation and ambulation was encouraged, which included the use of an ankle Cryo/Cuff™, with athletes encouraged to weight-bear in a walking boot within a week postoperatively. The ability of athletes to be weaned off their rehabilitative devices and the time required to reach activity goals are shown in Table 13.2 [7]. Those athletes with isolated Weber A and B lateral malleolar fractures were able to return to sport within the shortest time. In this study, return to full activity was seen as early as 4 weeks. Two out of the six athletes did not rate their ankle 100% in either flexibility or decreased stability

Table 13.2 Time (in weeks) athletes required the use of rehabilitative devices and time when athletes were able to resume activities in 27 athletes with ankle fractures that underwent ORIF [3, 7]

Time (in weeks) athletes required the use of rehabilitative devices and time when athletes were able to resume activities							
Classification	N	Crutches	Boot	Brace	Daily living	Practice	Competition
Lateral malleolus fracture	6	1.3 ± 0.5	3.0 ± 0.9	4.3 ± 3.8	1.2 ± 0.8	5.0 ± 0.9	6.8 ± 2.4
Medial malleolus fracture	2	2.0 ± 1.4	2.0 ± 1.4	7.0 ± 1.4	2.0 ± 0.0	12.0 ± 5.7	17.0 ± 9.9
Bimalleolar fracture	10	3.7 ± 1.6	3.7 ± 2.0	4.2. ± 2.2	1.0 ± 0.5	10.9 ±4.0	12.7 ± 4.0
Syndesmosis disruption injury	4	3.3 ± 1.0	2.3 ± 1.3	6.8 ± 6.1	0.8 ± 0.5	13.5 ± 2.5	15.8 ± 1.7
Salter-Harris type fracture	4	2.0 ± 0.8	3.5 ± 1.7	9.0 ± 1.2	1.0 ±0.0	6.3 ±1.3	8.5 ± 1.0
Pilon fracture	1	4.0	2.0	2.0	1.0	8.0	16.0

issues. Two athletes in this study, with isolated medial malleolar fractures, required deltoid ligament repair at the same time. These athletes took longer to return to competition, with one patient taking 24 weeks to return to motocross racing. Athletes with bimalleolar fractures required 12.7 ± 4.0 weeks to return to competition, while athletes with syndesmotic and pilon fractures took slightly longer. The authors did not document the recovery of patients with stable and undisplaced ankle fractures that underwent nonoperative treatment. There is a lack of evidence with regard to outcomes and return to competition in athletes with such injuries, but we feel that early rehabilitation and ambulation would be possible in such cases, and a similar return to sport should be expected [3]. No study was found that documents arthroscopic-assisted ankle fracture fixation and its value in return to elite football resumption, compared to a control group (without arthroscopy). Further work is required to objectively describe the potentially added value of arthroscopy in this return-to-sport perspective.

Conclusion

The incidence of ankle fractures is small, making up less than 3% of all ankle injuries in the modern professional football game. Optimal management for the higher-level football player has to address the demand for early and safe return to a high level of activity. The evidence for current best practice in football-related ankle fractures remains limited, and there is a lack of good studies. A thorough history, examination, and adequate imaging are essential to correctly diagnose injuries and decide upon the optimal treatment plan. Early rehabilitation allows for an early return to sport within 2–4 months. Surgical reduction (when indicated) and provision of stability by fixation optimizes both outcomes and return to competition in football ankle fractures. Arthroscopy may be helpful in diagnosing (and treating) intra-articular pathology (because up to 60% of ankle fractures may have a cartilage injury). It may also have a role in the assessment of syndesmosis stability and can assist in the accurate reduction of displaced (tibial plafond, malleolar, and talar) fractures. This minimally invasive surgery allows for a more rapid rehabilitation, with less complications, than conventional techniques in football athletes.

References

1. FIFA F-MARC Football Medicine Manual 2nd Edition. Chapter 3: Ankle injuries. 2009. pp. 154–60.
2. Bonasia DE et al. The role of arthroscopy in the management of fractures about the ankle. J Am Acad Orthop Surg. 2011;19(4):226–35.
3. d'Hooghe P, Kerkhoffs G. The ankle in football. Chapter 15 on ankle fractures. 2014. pp. 159–86.
4. Hepple S, Guha A. The role of ankle arthroscopy in acute ankle injuries of the athlete. Foot Ankle Clin. 2013;18(2):185–94.
5. d'Hooghe P, Wiegerinck JI, Tol JL, Landreau P. A 22-year-old professional soccer player with atraumatic ankle pain. Br J Sports Med. 28Aug 2013. doi:10.1136/bjsports-2013-092579
6. Colvin AC et al. Return to sports following operatively treated ankle fractures. Foot Ankle Int. 2009;30(4):292–6.
7. Porter DA et al. Functional outcome after operative treatment for ankle fractures in young athletes: a retrospective case series. Foot Ankle Int. 2008;29(9):887–94.
8. Donley BG et al. Pronation-external rotation ankle fractures in 3 professional football players. Am J Orthop (Belle Mead NJ). 2005;34(11):547–50.
9. Imade S et al. Leg anterior compartment syndrome following ankle arthroscopy after Maisonneuve fracture. Arthroscopy. 2009;25(2):215–8.
10. Utsugi K, Sakai H, Hiraoka H, Yashiki M, Mogi H. Intra-articular fibrous tissue formation following ankle fracture: the significance of arthroscopic debridement of fibrous tissue. Arthroscopy. 2007;23(1):89–93.
11. Mitev K, Mladenovski S, Kaftandziev I. Posttraumatic soft tissue impingement of the ankle: arthroscopic findings and surgical outcomes. Prilozi. 2014;35(1):237–42.
12. Lui TH. Arthroscopy and endoscopy of the foot and ankle: indications for new techniques. Arthroscopy. 2007;23(8):889–902. Epub 7 May 2007. Review.
13. Corte-Real NM, Moreira RM. Arthroscopic repair of chronic lateral ankle instability. Foot Ankle Int. 2009;30(3):213–7.
14. Rossi F, Dragoni S. Talar body fatigue stress fractures: three cases observed in elite female gymnasts. Skeletal Radiol. 2005;34(7):389–94.
15. Black KP, Ehlert KJ. A stress fracture of the lateral process of the talus in a runner. A case report. J Bone Joint Surg Am. 1994;76(3):441–3.

16. Motto SG. Stress fracture of the lateral process of the talus – a case report. Br J Sports Med. 1993;27(4): 275–6.
17. Kaeding CC, Yu JR, Wright R, Amendola A, Spindler KP. Management and return to play of stress fractures. Clin J Sport Med. 2005;15(6):442–4.
18. Glazebrook MA, Ganapathy V, Bridge MA, Stone JW, Allard JP. Evidence-based indications for ankle arthroscopy. Arthroscopy. 2009;25(12): 1478–90.
19. Stufkens SA et al. Long-term outcome after 1822 operatively treated ankle fractures: a systematic review of the literature. Injury. 2011;42(2):119–27.
20. Takao M, Uchio Y, Naito K, Fukazawa I, Kakimaru T, Ochi M. Diagnosis and treatment of combined intra-articular disorders in acute distal fibular fractures. J Trauma. 2004;57(6):1303–7.
21. Loren GJ, Ferkel RD. Arthroscopic assessment of occult intra-articular injury in acute ankle fractures. Arthroscopy. 2002;18(4):412–21. Foot Ankle Int 2009 Jun;30(6):524–9.
22. Gardner MJ, Demetrakopoulos D, Briggs SM, Helfet DL, Lorich DG. Malreduction of the tibiofibular syndesmosis in ankle fractures. Foot Ankle Int. 2006;27(10):788–92.
23. Lui TH et al. Comparison of radiologic and arthroscopic diagnoses of distal tibiofibular syndesmosis disruption in acute ankle fracture. Arthroscopy. 2005;21(11):1370.
24. Oae K, Takao M, Naito K, et al. Injury of the tibiofibular syndesmosis: value of MR imaging for diagnosis. Radiology. 2003;227(1):155–61.
25. Swart EF, Vosseller JT. Arthroscopic assessment of medial malleolar reduction. Arch Orthop Trauma Surg. 2014;134(9):1287–92. doi: 10.1007/s00402-014-2031-7
26. Turhan E, Doral MN, Demirel M, Atay AO, Bozkurt M, Bilge O, Huri G, Atesok K, Kaya D. Arthroscopy-assisted reduction versus open reduction in the fixation of medial malleolar fractures. Eur J Orthop Surg Traumatol. 2013;23(8):953–9.
27. Hou ZQ, Jegan K, Peter T. The applications of arthroscopy on malleolus fractures. Chin J Traumatol. 2005;8(6):379–82.
28. Goost H, Wimmer MD, Barg A, Kabir K, Valderrabano V, Burger C. Fractures of the ankle joint: investigation and treatment options. Dtsch Arztebl Int. 2014; 111(21):377–88.
29. Ono A, Nishikawa S, Nagao A, et al. Arthroscopically assisted treatment of ankle fractures: arthroscopic findings and surgical outcomes. Arthroscopy. 2004;20(6):627–31.
30. Atesok K, Dorl MN, Whipple T, Mann G, Mei-Dan O, Atay OA, Beer Y, Lowe J, Soudry M, Schemitsch EH. Arthroscopy-assisted fracture fixation. Knee Surg Sports Traumatol Arthrosc. 2011;19(2):320–9.
31. Leontaritis N, Hinojosa L, Panchbhavi VK. Arthroscopically detected intra-articular lesions associated with acute ankle fractures. J Bone Joint Surg Am. 2009;91(2):333–9.
32. Thordarson DB et al. The role of ankle arthroscopy on the surgical management of ankle fractures. Foot Ankle Int. 2001;22(2):123–5.
33. Hammond AW, Crist BD. Arthroscopic management of C3 tibial plafond fractures: a technical guide. J Foot Ankle Surg. 2012;51(3):382–6.
34. Poyanli O, Esenkaya I, Ozkut AT, Akcal MA, Akan K, Unay K. Minimally invasive reduction technique in split depression type tibial pilon fractures. J Foot Ankle Surg. 2012;51(2):254–7.
35. Cuttica DJ, Smith WB, Hyer CF, Philbin TM, Berlet GC. Osteochondral lesions of the talus: predictors of clinical outcome. Foot Ankle Int. 2011;32(11): 1045–51.
36. Choi WJ, Park KK, Kim BS, Lee JW. Osteochondral lesion of the talus: is there a critical defect size for poor outcome? Am J Sports Med. 2009;37(10): 1974–80.
37. Aurich M, Bedi HS, Smith PJ, Rolauffs B, Mückley T, Clayton J, Blackney M. Arthroscopic treatment of osteochondral lesions of the ankle with matrix-associated chondrocyte implantation: early clinical and magnetic resonance imaging results Am J Sports Med 2011;39(2):311–9.
38. Elias I, Raikin SM, Schweitzer ME, Besser MP, Morrison WB, Zoga AC. Osteochondral lesions of the distal tibial plafond: localization and morphologic characteristics with an anatomical grid. Foot Ankle Int. 2009;30(6):524–9.
39. Mologne TS, Ferkel RD. Arthroscopic treatment of osteochondral lesions of the distal tibia. Foot Ankle Int. 2007;28(8):865–72.
40. Giannini S, Buda R, Ruffilli A, Cavallo M, Pagliazzi G, Bulzamini MC, Desando G, Luciani D, Vannini F. Arthroscopic autologous chondrocyte implantation in the ankle joint. Knee Surg Sports Traumatol Arthrosc. 2014;22(6):1311–9.
41. Giannini S, Buda R, Vannini F, Di Caprio F, Grigolo B. Arthroscopic autologous chondrocyte implantation in osteochondral lesions of the talus: surgical technique and results. Am J Sports Med. 2008;36(5): 873–80.
42. Vogl TJ, Hochmuth K, Diebold T, et al. Magnetic resonance imaging in the diagnosis of acute injured distal tibiofibular syndesmosis. Invest Radiol. 1997;32(7):401–9.
43. Sri-Ram K, Robinson AH. Arthroscopic assessment of the syndesmosis following ankle fracture. Injury. 2005;36(5):675–8.
44. Takao M et al. Arthroscopic diagnosis of tibiofibular syndesmosis disruption. Arthroscopy. 2001;17(8): 836–43.
45. Saltzman CL, Marsh JL, Tearse DS. Treatment of displaced talus fractures: an arthroscopically assisted approach. Foot Ankle Int. 1994;15(11):630–3.
46. Subairy A, Subramanian K, Geary NP. Arthroscopically assisted internal fixation of a talus body fracture. Injury. 2004;35(1):86–9. Erratum in: Injury. 2004 Jan;35(1):104.

47. Sitte W, Lampert C, Baumann P. Osteosynthesis of talar body shear fractures assisted by hindfoot and subtalar arthroscopy: technique tip. Foot Ankle Int. 2012;33(1):74–8.
48. Motto SG. Stress fracture of the talar body. Clin J Sport Med. 1996;6(4):278–9.
49. Hontas MJ, Haddad RJ, Schlesinger LC. Conditions of the talus in the runner. Am J Sports Med. 1986;14(6):486–90.
50. Fitzgerald RH, Kaufer H, Malkani AL, Potter, Mosby, McCance K. Orthopaedics. Elsevier; 2008.
51. Mulfinger GL, Trueta J. The blood supply of the talus. J Bone Joint Surg Br. 1970;52(1):160–7.
52. Travlos J, Learmonth ID. Bilateral avascular necrosis of the talus following strenuous physical activity. J Bone Joint Surg Br. 1991;73(5):863–4.
53. Hawkins LG. Fractures of the neck of the talus. J Bone Joint Surg Am. 1970;52(5):991–1002.
54. Metzger MJ, Levin JS, Clancy JT. Talar neck fractures and rates of avascular necrosis. J Foot Ankle Surg. 1999;38(2):154–62.
55. van Dijk CN, Scholten PE, Krips R. A 2-portal endoscopic approach for diagnosis and treatment of posterior ankle pathology. Arthroscopy. 2000;16:871–6.
56. van Dijk CN, de Leeuw PA, Scholten PE. Hindfoot endoscopy for posterior ankle impingment: surgical technique. J Bone Joint Surg Am. 2009;91(Suppl 2):287–98.
57. van Dijk CN. Hindfoot endoscopy. Foot Ankle Clin. 2006;11:391–414.
58. Perera A, Baker JF, Lui DF, Stephens MM. The management and outcome of lateral process fracture of the talus. Foot Ankle Surg. 2010;16(1):15–20.
59. Hawkins LG. Fracture of the lateral process of the talus. J Bone Joint Surg. 1965;47A(6):1170–5.
60. Donken CC et al. Surgical versus conservative interventions for treating ankle fractures in adults. Cochrane Database Syst Rev. 2012;8:CD008470.
61. Walsh WM, Hughston JC. Unstable ankle fractures in athletes. Am J Sports Med. 1976;4(4):173–83.
62. Oztekin HH et al. Foot and ankle injuries and time lost from play in professional soccer players. Foot (Edinb). 2009;19(1):22–8.

Part IV

Knee Injuries

Meniscal Lesions: From Basic Science to Clinical Management in Footballers

14

Ibrahim Fatih Cengiz, Hélder Pereira, Joana Silva-Correia, Pedro L. Ripoll, João Espregueira-Mendes, Rodrigo Kaz, J. Miguel Oliveira, and Rui Luís Reis

Contents

I.F. Cengiz • J. Silva-Correia • R.L. Reis
3B's Research Group–Biomaterials, Biodegradables and Biomimetics, University of Minho, Headquarters of the European Institute of Excellence on Tissue Engineering and Regenerative Medicine, AvePark, Parque de Ciência e Tecnologia, Zona Industrial da Gandra, 4805-017 Barco, Guimarães, Portugal

ICVS/3B's–PT Government Associate Laboratory, Braga/Guimarães, Portugal

H. Pereira
3B's Research Group–Biomaterials, Biodegradables and Biomimetics, University of Minho, Headquarters of the European Institute of Excellence on Tissue Engineering and Regenerative Medicine, AvePark, Parque de Ciência e Tecnologia, Zona Industrial da Gandra, 4805-017 Barco, Guimarães, Portugal

ICVS/3B's–PT Government Associate Laboratory, Braga/Guimarães, Portugal

Orthopedic Department Centro Hospitalar Póvoa de Varzim, Vila do Conde, Portugal

Ripoll y De Prado Sports Clinic – FIFA Medical Centre of Excellence, Murcia-Madrid, Spain

P.L. Ripoll
Ripoll y De Prado Sports Clinic – FIFA Medical Centre of Excellence, Murcia-Madrid, Spain

J. Espregueira-Mendes
3B's Research Group–Biomaterials, Biodegradables and Biomimetics, University of Minho, Headquarters of the European Institute of Excellence on Tissue Engineering and Regenerative Medicine, AvePark, Parque de Ciência e Tecnologia, Zona Industrial da Gandra, 4805-017 Barco, Guimarães, Portugal

ICVS/3B's–PT Government Associate Laboratory, Braga/Guimarães, Portugal

Clínica do Dragão, Espregueira-Mendes Sports Centre – FIFA Medical Centre of Excellence, Porto, Portugal

Dom Henrique Research Centre, Porto, Portugal

Orthopaedics Department of Minho University, Minho, Portugal

R. Kaz
Orthopaedic Knee and Sports Traumatolology, Americas Medical City, Rio de Janeiro (RJ), Brazil

Brazilian Athletics Confederation (Confederacao Brasileira de Atletismo), Rio de Janeiro, Brazil

Botafogo Futebol e Regatas, Rio de Janeiro, Brazil

Pontificia Universidade Catolica do Rio de Janeiro (PUC -RJ), Rio de Janeiro, Brazil

J. Espregueira-Mendes et al. (eds.), *Injuries and Health Problems in Football*,
DOI 10.1007/978-3-662-53924-8_14

J.M. Oliveira (✉)
3B's Research Group–Biomaterials, Biodegradables and Biomimetics, University of Minho, Headquarters of the European Institute of Excellence on Tissue Engineering and Regenerative Medicine,
AvePark, Parque de Ciência e Tecnologia, Zona Industrial da Gandra, 4805-017 Barco, Guimarães, Portugal

ICVS/3B's–PT Government Associate Laboratory, Braga/Guimarães, Portugal

Ripoll y De Prado Sports Clinic – FIFA Medical Centre of Excellence, Murcia-Madrid, Spain

Clínica do Dragão, Espregueira-Mendes Sports Centre – FIFA Medical Centre of Excellence, Porto, Portugal
e-mail: miguel.oliveira@dep.uminho.pt

14.1 Introduction

Prof. René Verdonk recently wrote that "Nothing has changed so much in recent years of orthopedics as the treatment algorithm of meniscus lesions" [1]. Together with Prof. Philippe Beaufils, both started a movement dedicated to saving the meniscus in order to preserve the future [2]. In the 1970s, the meniscus has even been considered as a useless structure [3] that whenever related to complaints should be completely removed in order to prevent future injuries. Today, the current trend defends the preservation of meniscus tissue whenever possible by means of repair or even replacement [1]. Nevertheless, meniscectomy is still one of the most frequent orthopedic procedures [4] despite the latest results favor meniscal repair over partial meniscectomy concerning either clinical outcome and/or risk for subsequent osteoarthritis [5].

Moreover, patient's expectations are decisive in the course of action to follow, especially when dealing with high-level athletes. A doctor who deals with this subject must be able to provide the best available knowledge concerning assessment, indications, outcome, and time to return to activity and both short- and long-term risks. The patient should be informed and afterward brought to participate in the final decision. Concerning professional athletes, they often require involving family, agents, managers, and others prior to final decision.

The menisci are heterogeneous structures with segmental variations according to its biology and function [6, 7]. The menisci are two wedge-shaped semilunar disks of fibrocartilage which have crucial roles in knee kinematics [8]. They are largely constituted of collagen fibers (mostly type I collagen) interposed between cells and an extracellular matrix (ECM) of proteoglycans and glycoproteins [7]. They are known to play a role in joint nutrition and stabilization [3], load transfer, joint congruency, proprioception, lubrication, and impact absorption [8–10].

The biological characterization of the menisci has substantially advanced in the last few years. Different cells have been described [11], while segmental variations have also been documented regarding the type of cells and density [12], ultrastructure, extracellular matrix, and biomechanical properties [6]. The lateral meniscus carries most of the load transfer on lateral compartment while in the medial compartment the load transmission is more distributed between the exposed cartilage surfaces and respective meniscus [13]. In vitro trials indicated that 50–70% of the load transmission occurs through the corresponding menisci in the lateral and medial compartment [14]. While the lateral meniscus has higher mobility, the medial meniscus also plays a role as secondary stabilizer contributing to oppose the anterior tibial displacement [8]. In the meniscus of adults, peripheral vessels penetrate no more than 10–25% of the width of the lateral meniscus and 10–30% width of the medial meniscus [15]. The meniscofemoral ligaments help to stabilize the posterior horn of the lateral meniscus to the femoral condyle [16]. The coronary ligaments connect in a somewhat "slack" way the peripheral meniscal rim to the tibia. The lateral meniscus has no attachment to the lateral collateral ligament (LCL) despite the close anatomical correlation.

The basic science research around the meniscus is of the highest relevance once it is known that it is the basis to understand the mechanism of healing and influences the indications and outcome of repair [17]. Moreover, biology and biomechanics represent the fundamentals for the development of future therapies, including tissue engineering and regenerative medicine [18].

14.2 Physiopathology of Meniscal Injuries (Traumatic Versus Degenerative)

One critical distinction when dealing with meniscus injuries/tears is recognizing its traumatic or degenerative nature though it is not always easy to perform [19]. A traumatic meniscus tear is usually related to an acute knee injury capable of producing enough energy to tear the meniscus. Usually, longitudinal, bucket-handle tears (Fig. 14.1) and radial tears (Fig. 14.2) are included in this category [20]. Flap tears can also be considered as traumatic (Fig. 14.3).

On the other hand, degenerative meniscus lesions (Fig. 14.4) have an importantly different nature. A degenerative meniscus might present characteristics such as cavitations, softened meniscal tissue, fibrillation, multiple tear patterns, or other degenerative changes [21]. Horizontal tears are most often degenerative, even in younger populations [22–24]. Considering posterior root tears, the medial meniscus ones are more frequently considered as degenerative, while the lateral ones are more frequently considered traumatic, often related to acute anterior cruciate ligament (ACL) rupture [25, 26]. This seems to influence prognosis and outcome.

Patient's age is known to play a role on the etiological and pathophysiological factors of meniscal lesions, despite these can occur in all age groups [4, 19, 27]. The tissue characteristics including water content, cells, extracellular matrix, collagen, and adhesion glycoproteins vary according to age, injury pattern, and pathological conditions [28]. During normal knee kinematics, the menisci "suffer" from compressive, radial tensile, and shear stresses [29–31]. These have consequences in meniscus injuries and on secondarily on further knee joint consequences of these injuries [32]. High-energy and sports-related trauma can be implicated in meniscus tears [33] which might also occur combined with fractures around the knee [33].

Clinical presentation of acute tears usually includes sudden onset of pain and/or swelling of the knee joint. Mechanical symptoms such as clicking, catching, or locking of the knee joint might be caused by unstable tears [34]. Young and active persons, specifically when involved in level 1 contact sports that comprise frequent pivoting (e.g., football, rugby, or American football), are more prone to meniscus tears [34]. However, apparently innocuous activities such as walking or squatting have also been connected to injuries of the menisci [35].

One of the most frequent traumatic mechanisms has been described as a twisting movement at the knee while the leg is bent which is common during football regardless of the competitive level. Torsional loading or axial loading (a high compressive force between femur and tibia) might also cause meniscus injuries [36]. Valgus impact with external rotation of the tibia can also cause a well-known triad of injuries involving meniscal damage combined with medial collateral and ACL tears [37, 38]. Another

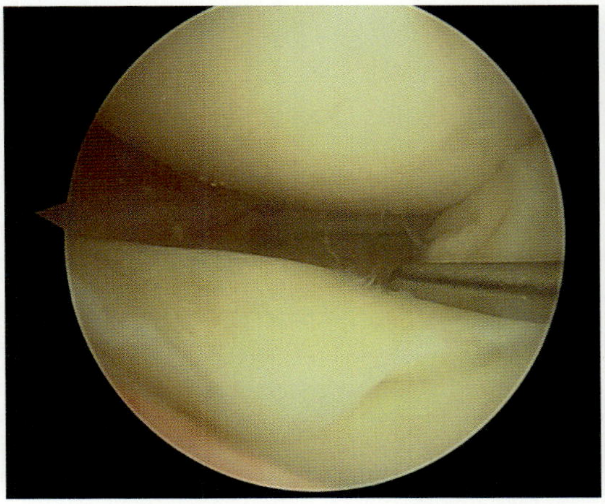

Fig. 14.1 Arthroscopic view of a bucket-handle tear inspected by a hook probe

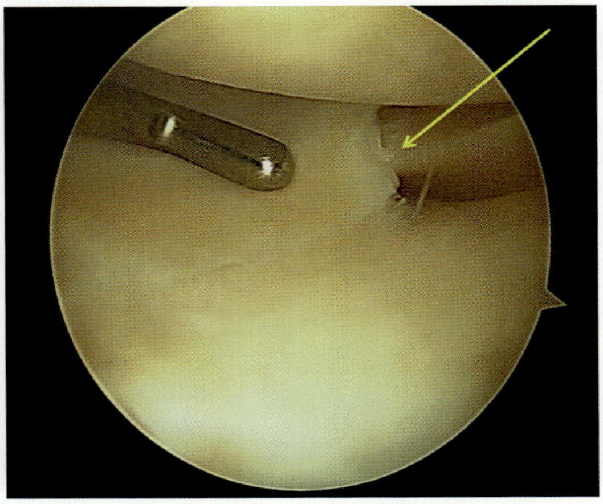

Fig. 14.2 Radial tear of medial meniscus (*yellow arrow*)

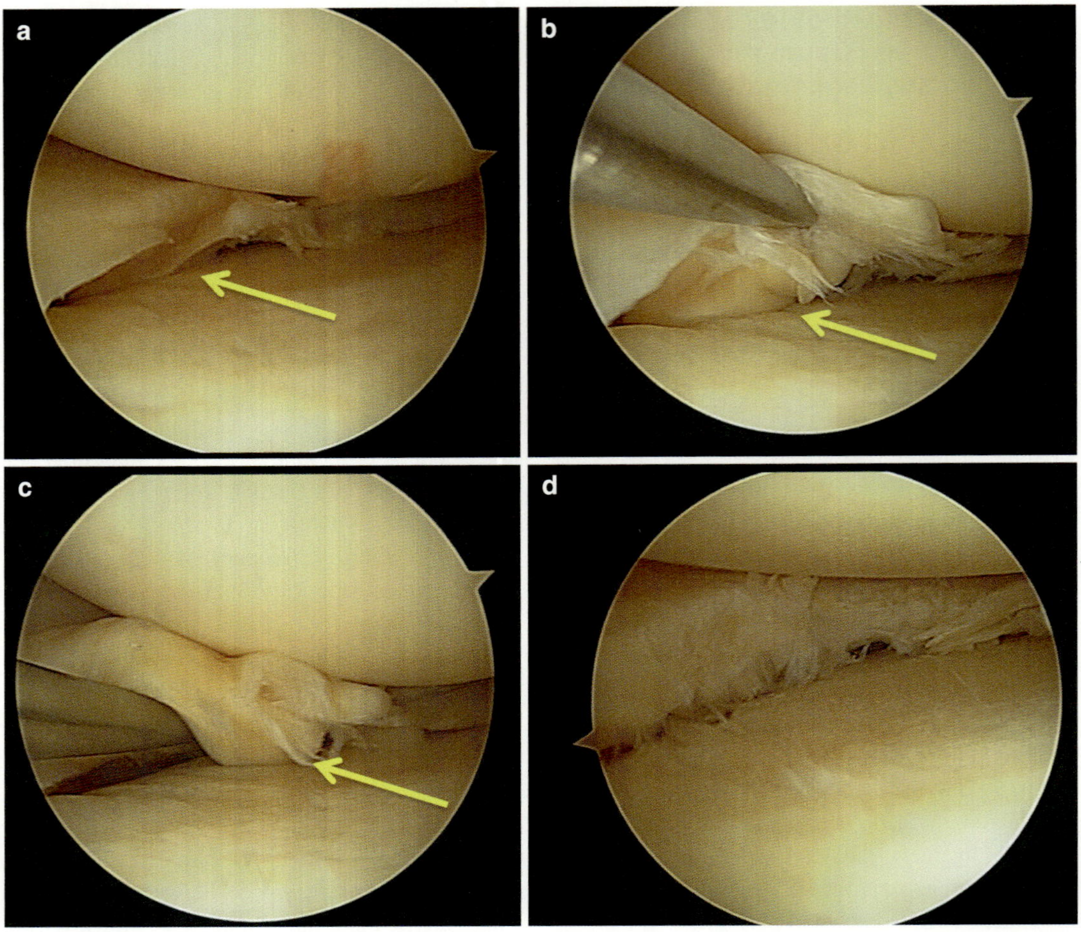

Fig. 14.3 Flap tear (*yellow arrow*) of medial meniscus dislocated to meniscotibial compartment (**a**), the meniscal flap is retrieved with the hook probe (**b** and **c**), partial meniscectomy is performed (**d**)

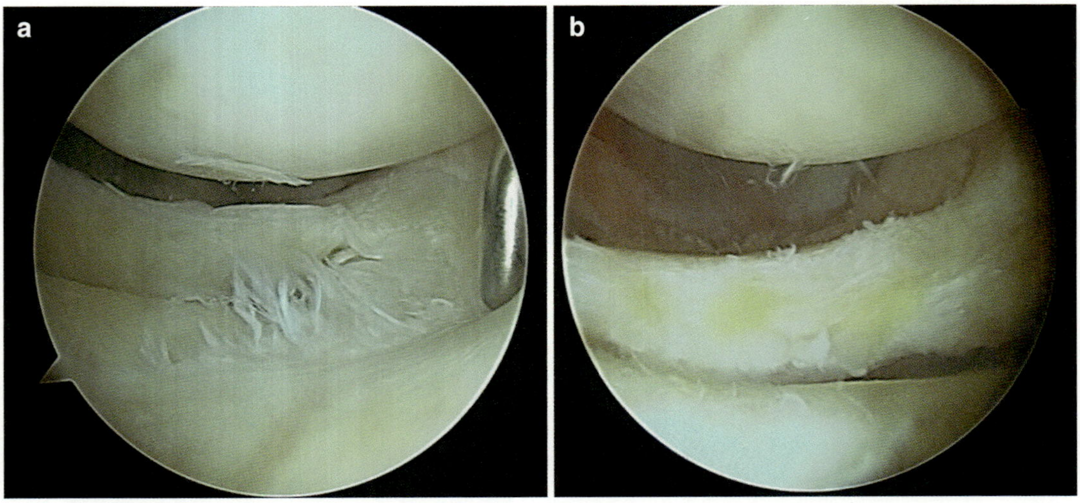

Fig. 14.4 Arthroscopic view of a complex degenerative tear (**a**) treated by partial meniscectomy and radiofrequency (**b**)

movement typically described by patients with meniscus tears is a sudden transition from knee's hyperflexion to full extension, (the meniscus gets entrapped between the femur and the tibia) [36].

Meniscal injuries are a common incidental finding on magnetic resonance imaging (MRI) in symptomatic and asymptomatic knees [39]. Most tears are found in older patients that usually result from long-term degenerative changes. Among patients with clinical and radiographic findings of osteoarthritis, the reported prevalence of meniscal lesions is comprised between 68% and 90% [40, 41]. High-level sports, given its high demand, with repetition of microtrauma, might play a role in the early degeneration of the menisci, as well as the knee joint in general [42]. In both situations, a decreased vascularization might be expected to lead to tissue degeneration [19, 43]. The assessment of the global status of the knee joint is mandatory once it is questionable if the isolated treatment of meniscal tears is effective in the reduction of symptoms caused by global joint osteoarthritis [19]. Sometimes, depending on several aspects, this is the case even in active professional football players (e.g., previous injuries, long-lasting careers, inadequate pitch or shoe wear, age).

14.3 Classification of Meniscal Injuries

Careful assessment of history and clinical examination is mandatory. There are many different clinical tests described for diagnosing a meniscal lesion (e.g., McMurray's test, joint line tenderness, Apley's grinding test) [44]. These have only low to moderate diagnostic accuracy which increases substantially when several tests are combined with adequate clinical history [44]. Standing X-ray protocol evaluations (including frontal plane, lateral, skyline patella, and "schuss" view) are useful and advised as soon as possible in order to assess alignment and global joint evaluation. MRI has high accuracy regarding the preoperative evaluation of meniscus lesions (Fig. 14.5) [45–47]. A radiologist trained in musculoskeletal radiological assessment is advised once this is associated with an increase in accuracy [48, 49].

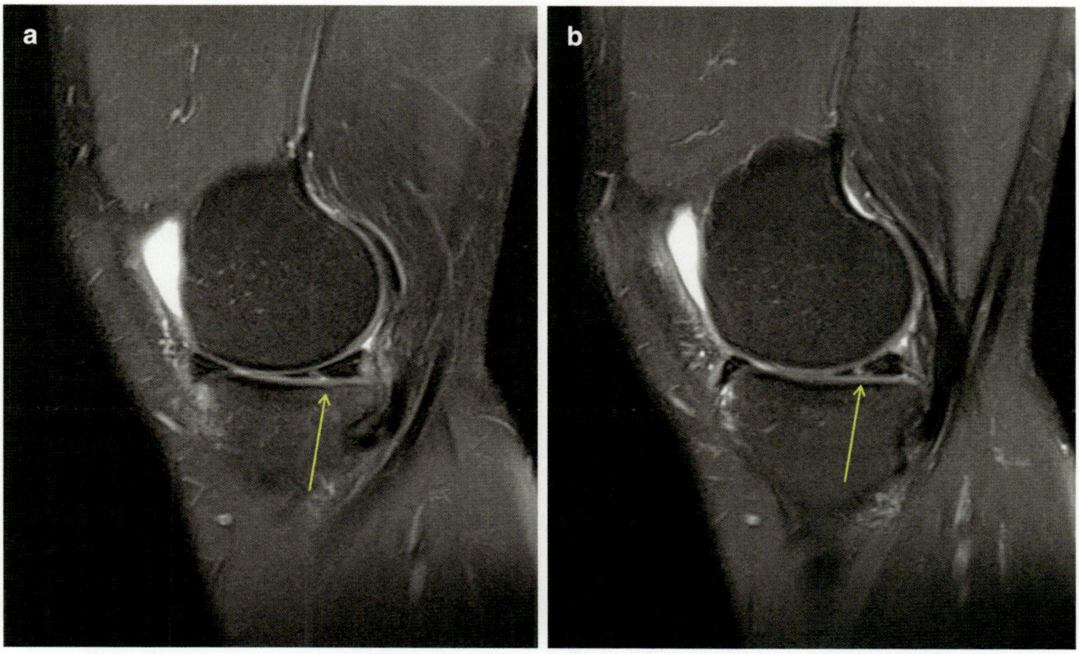

Fig. 14.5 Two consecutive MRI images (**a** and **b**) of a longitudinal medial meniscus tear (*yellow arrow*)

Meniscus lesions have different patterns, which are linked to different prognosis, clinical evolution, and implications [43]. Posterior capsular avulsions are considered out of the scope of this text. A correct diagnosis and classification and understanding the specificity of different meniscus tears are critical to determine the best choice for treatment. Several classification methods of meniscal lesions have been proposed over the years aiming to guide treatment as well as prognosis and assessment of outcome [21].

Vascularity is known to play a central role in meniscus healing; thus it has been taken into account in the most frequently used classifications. Cooper et al. [50] described a classification system in which the meniscus is divided into circumferential zones. Zone 0 corresponds to the meniscal-synovial junction, zone 1 corresponds to the outer third of the meniscus, zone 2 includes the middle third, and zone 3 is the central third of the meniscus [50].

The ISAKOS classification of meniscal tears aims to be an improvement on the classification systems by combining the best currently available clinical and basic science knowledge. It provides sufficient interobserver reliability for decisive factors, which assist surgeons in the choice of the most adequate management, as well as collecting data from clinical trials designed to evaluate the outcomes [21].

Various tear patterns and configurations have been described [51, 52]. These include radial tears, flap or parrot-beak tears, longitudinal tears, bucket-handle tears, horizontal cleavage tears, complex degenerative tears, and more recently a hot topic on meniscal root tears (Fig. 14.6). A complex tear is usually described as a combination of two or more type of tears which might occur in multiple planes [19]. It must be also considered that, in some circumstances, a degenerative meniscus injury, previously asymptomatic, might change and become symptomatic after an acute traumatic event [19].

14.4 Treatment of Meniscus Injuries: Meniscectomy, Repair, and Replacement

14.4.1 Meniscectomy

Meniscectomy is still one of the most frequent cases in orthopedic surgery [4]. However, recent results favor meniscal repair over partial menis-

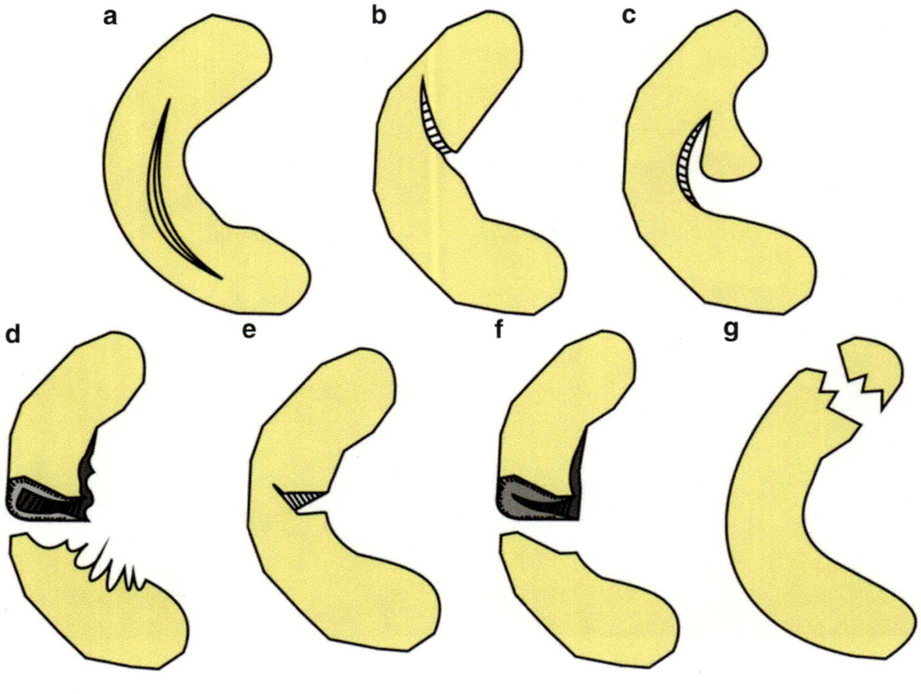

Fig. 14.6 Types of meniscal tears: longitudinal/bucket-handle tear (**a**), oblique tear (**b**), parrot-beak or flap tear (**c**), complex degenerative tear (**d**), radial tear (**e**), horizontal cleavage tear (**f**), root tear (**g**)

cectomy concerning either clinical outcome and/or risk for subsequent osteoarthritis [5]. Considering the amount of tissue that is removed, it is usually referred as partial, subtotal, or total meniscectomy. However, the "boundaries" for each of these categories are not very well established [32]. Partial meniscectomy has been linked to higher risk of radiographic changes toward osteoarthritis compared to repair on a recent systematic review (level I–IV studies) [5]. Considering traumatic meniscal tears, worse long-term results have been attributed to partial meniscectomy when compared to repair either in return to sports as well as risk for osteoarthritis [53].

The preservation of peripheral rim and the largest possible amount of meniscus tissue has positive implications for load transmission and contact area [54–56]. Joint instability (e.g., ACL repair) should be properly addressed once the risk of undergoing subsequent meniscectomies was decreased in patients undergoing a concomitant ACL reconstruction meniscus repair [57]. So there is a difference considering prognosis and outcome when dealing with meniscal tears by meniscectomy on a stable versus unstable knee [32]. Worse results are expected when performing isolated meniscectomies on unstable knees [32]. It has been defended that the indications for surgical repair can be widened for the medial meniscus given the increased risk of secondary meniscectomy (if "left alone"), even for small stable lesions [58]. On the opposite, for the lateral meniscus with small stable lesions, "let the meniscus alone" can be sometimes a good option given the low risk of subsequent meniscectomy [46]. An overall *odds ratio* of 3.50 for medial meniscal tears has been described when ACL surgery is performed more than 12 months after the ACL injury when compared to less than 12 months after ACL injury [59]. On the other hand, concerning lateral meniscus tears and the period of time comprised between ACL injury and reconstruction surgery, there was minimal to no evidence that this represents a risk factor [59]. These conclusions are in line with the documented distinctive roles of medial and lateral menisci within the knee joint.

For traumatic lateral meniscus tears approached during ACL reconstruction procedures [60], it seems plausible to provide the general recommendation to leave small tears (<1 cm) alone, repair large tears in the vascular zone, and excise only unstable, irreparable tears in the avascular zone [61]. Moreover, the risk for rapid chondrolysis after lateral meniscectomy is considerably higher when compared to medial meniscectomy [62, 63]. This is an important possible complication that patients must be informed about prior to surgery. In general, a worse outcome should be expected following a lateral meniscectomy when compared to medial [32].

It has also been demonstrated that the volume of subsequent meniscectomy after a failed meniscus repair is not more than that of the meniscectomy that would have been performed initially without repairing [64]. Despite this, partial meniscectomy has been connected to satisfactory results and faster return to activity and rehabilitation program when compared to meniscus repair [53, 65]. This creates controversy between surgeons, athletes, managers, and agents. In brief, meniscectomy remains as a possibility. However, higher risk of complications, possible lower rate of return to the same level (mainly in the lateral compartment) and a higher risk of secondary osteoarthritis must be discussed with the athlete. Nowadays, even in high-level athletes, there is an increasing strength toward the general recommendation to preserve the meniscus.

14.4.2 Meniscus Repair

Meniscus repair techniques include all-inside [66, 67], inside-out [68, 69], or outside-in [70, 71] approaches, alone or in combination. "All-inside" refers to the fact that suture/repair devices are kept inside the joint at all times during repair. Bioabsorbable meniscal repair devices, including arrows (Fig. 14.7), screws [72], darts, and staples, have been described for all-inside use. However, most of these devices were composed of the rigid poly-L-lactic-acid (PLLA) that has been linked to some concerns related to degradability. Despite some good results described in the literature [73, 74], these devices were related to higher failure rates [75, 76] and a higher number of complications including synovitis, inflammatory reaction, cyst formation, device failure/migration, and chondral damage [76]. Given the considerable prevalence of complications, these rigid (third-generation) devices have progressively lost popularity, particularly in high-level athletes.

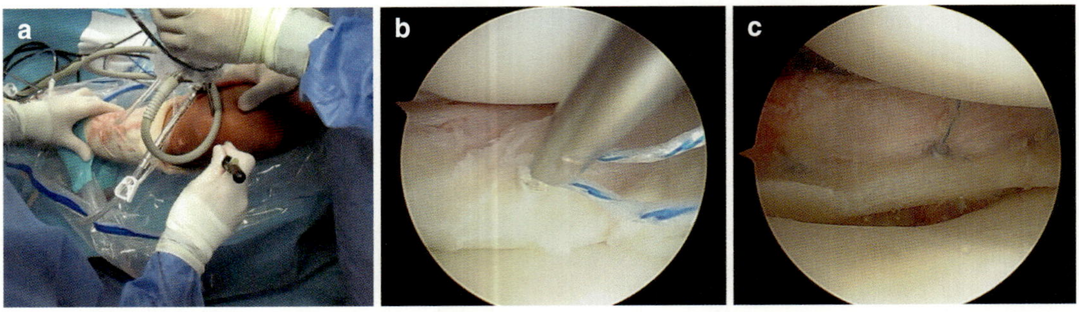

Fig. 14.7 Arthroscopic suture of the lateral meniscus using an all-inside device (**a**). The scope is introduced through the medial portal, and the suture device is managed through the lateral portal single-handed (**a**). Arthroscopic view of the device trespassing the meniscus through the capsule where a peek anchor holds the suture (**b**). The same device is similarly passed a second time in a different point of the meniscus. The suture is finally tensioned, and the final result enables a stable repair of the meniscus (**c**)

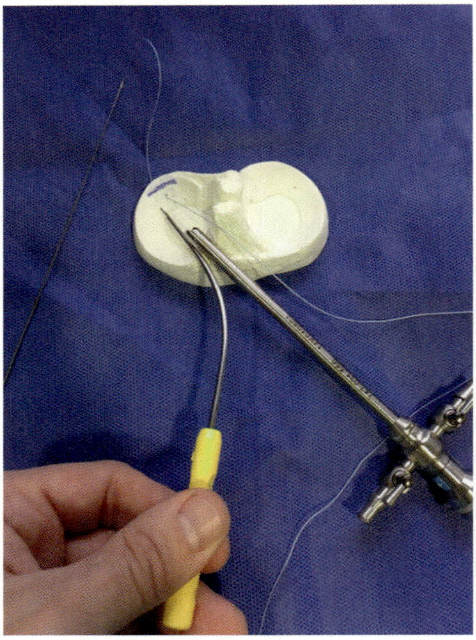

Fig. 14.8 Model representing inside-out technique of meniscal suture with curved cannulas to assess more precise approach to the injury and diminish neurovascular risk

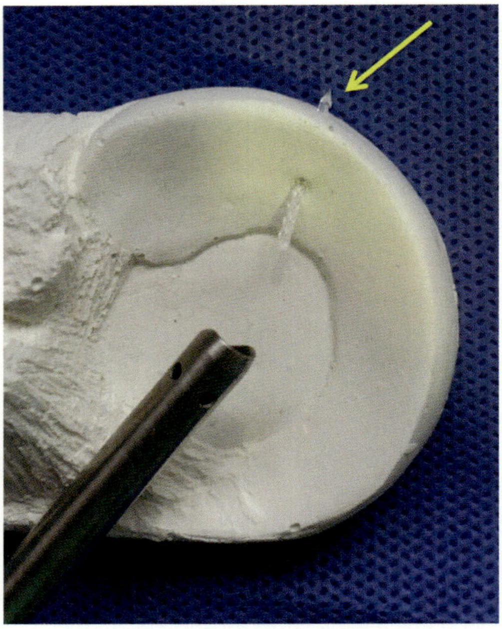

Fig. 14.9 Polylactic acid arrow for meniscal repair (*yellow arrow*). Acknowledge the risks for subsequent conflict and/or rigid loose bodies resulting from possible erratic degradation of the implant inside and/or outside the joint

The most frequently used all-inside sutures are currently considered as the fourth generation of all-inside sutures. These are usually composed of suture combined with small anchors (serving as blocks) and a prettied slipknot [66]. They have low profile and permit variable compression and retensioning of the suture. A depth-limiting sleeve on the inserter is commonly used to avoid excessive penetrations of the needle, which has an inherent risk of iatrogenic complications (neurovascular structures) [77].

Inside-out (Fig. 14.8) means that the sutures come from the inner joint where they are passed through the meniscus toward the outside (capsule) where knots are tied (or equivalent). In outside-in (Fig. 14.9), the devices for passing the sutures are introduced percutaneously into the joint catching the meniscus tissue, and afterward they are also fixed over the capsule beneath the subcutaneous tissue (Fig. 14.10). Regardless of the used technique, vertical or

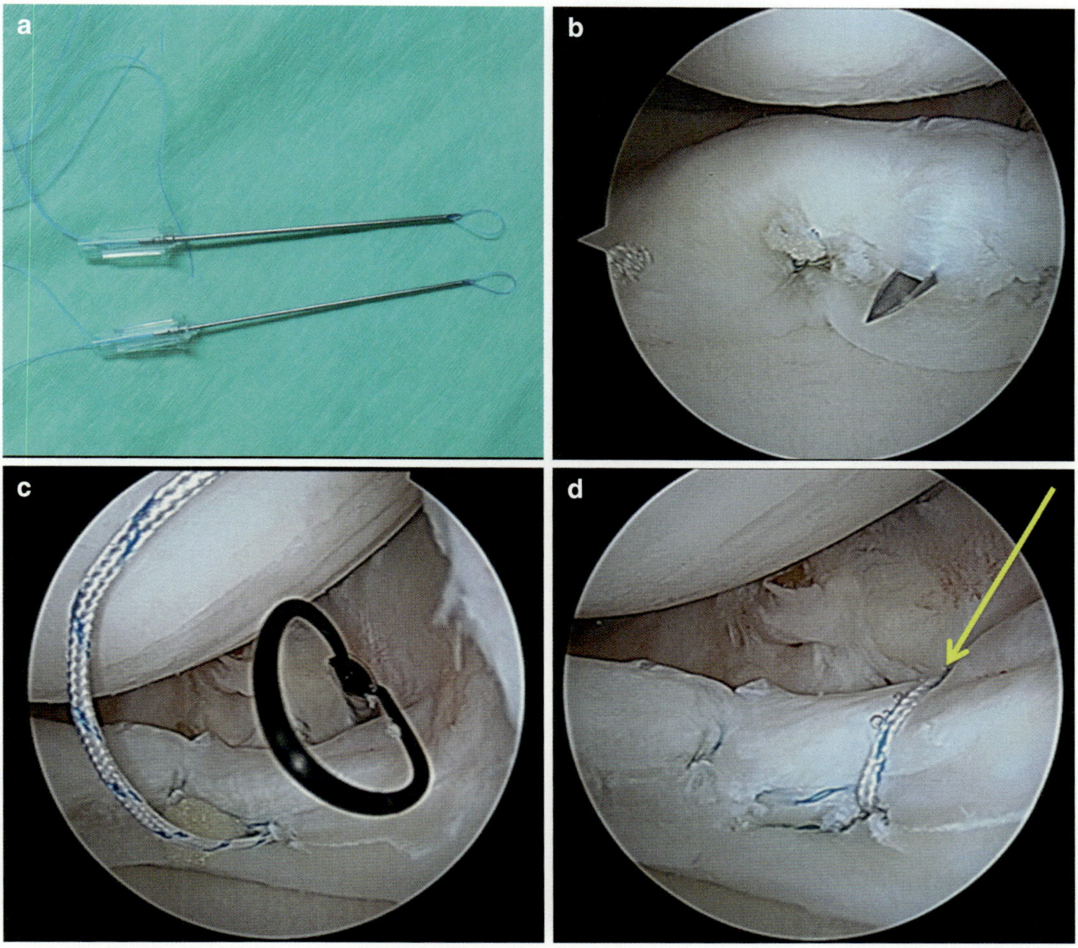

Fig. 14.10 Outside-in meniscus repair technique. Two needles used as suture passers with nylon loops (**a**) one needle trespasses the meniscus, and the first suture is passed through the meniscus (**b**) a second needle brings the suture through the capsule for the outside (**c**) and sutures are tensioned and tied percutaneously resulting in a vertical suture (*yellow arrow*) (**d**)

horizontal mattress sutures can be considered. Vertical sutures are perpendicular to the circumferential fibers of the meniscus and have been stated to have higher pullout resistance [78]. Horizontal sutures are parallel to the same fibers.

In order to increase possibilities for healing, sutures combined with grasping, trephination, or augmentation with fibrin clot have been proposed [36]. As previously mentioned, meniscal sutures are not exclusive of acute traumatic tears, once some selected degenerative injuries (including some horizontal cleavage tears) might be effectively repaired [79]. Some degenerative meniscal root tears have also been successfully repaired thus preserving meniscal functions [80].

Currently, the type of tears that can be possibly suitable for suture include horizontal injuries (degenerative nature even in younger patients) [22], vertical or longitudinal tears, bucket-handle, and some radial tears (vascular zone) which are considered in the traumatic group [20]. All these can be considered as possibly repairable depending on the classification, zone, and surgeon's experience. Flap tears (frequently traumatic) are frequently considered irreparable. This type of lesion can also be detected in complex degenerative (irreparable) lesions. Multiple factors must be considered when considering to repair a meniscus lesion [51]. These include age, activity level, tear pattern, chronicity of the tears, combined injuries (ACL injury), and healing potential/vascularization. Meniscus repair in older

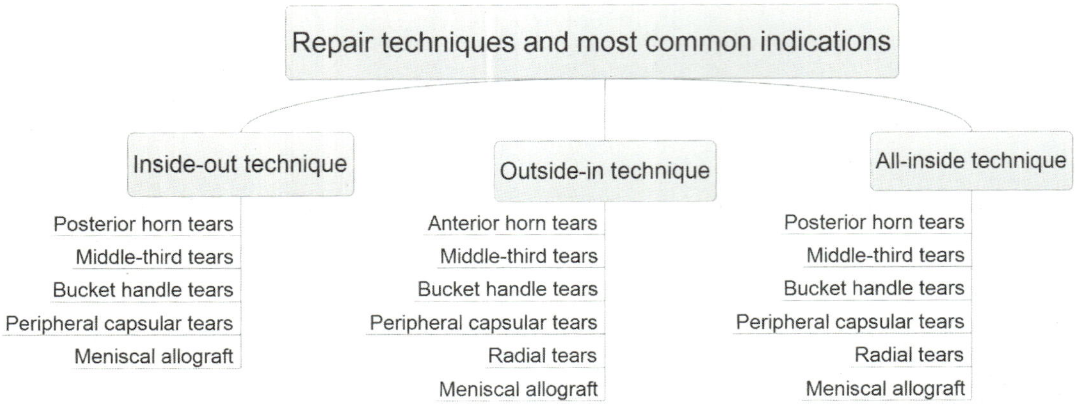

Fig. 14.11 Techniques for meniscus repair and most common indications

people provides worst outcome comparing to youngsters [81].

Several "biologic" techniques have been tried and kept under intense development aiming to enhance healing and repair of meniscus lesions even in the so-called avascular zones [18, 82]. These include fibrin clot [69, 83], fibrin glue [84], meniscal rasping, growth factors [85], and cell-based therapies [86]. Even more experimental in vivo strategies have been described. As an example, a bioabsorbable conduit has been tried to augment the healing of avascular meniscal tears by increasing vascularization (dog model) [87]. Additional tactics have been using several biomaterials such as porous polyurethane [88], porcine small intestinal submucosa [89], fascia sheaths [90], collagen scaffolds, and growth factors [82]. Tissue engineering and regenerative medicine strategies will most probably provide new answers to overcome current clinical limitations. However, this ambitious target has not yet been entirely achieved and requires ongoing research [82].

Suture/repair techniques have recently improved a lot based on increased biological and anatomical knowledge accompanied with advances in surgical techniques and medical devices [91]. So several techniques are available and can be selected according to the injury pattern, surgeon's experience, and available resources (Fig. 14.11).

14.4.2.1 Indications for Meniscal Repair

Through recent times, there has been a progressive increase in indications for potentially repairable meniscus lesions including some tears previously considered as irreparable (Fig. 14.12).

Longitudinal and Bucket-Handle Tears A vertical or longitudinal tear occurs in the same orientation as the circumferential fibers of the meniscus. If such tear reaches enough length with potential for dislocation/instability, it is referred as a bucket-handle tear which might cause locking of the knee joint. These tears, mainly those at the peripheral vascular zones, have always been considered as the most straightforward indication for repair either by horizontal or vertical sutures or combinations of both [5, 92, 93]. Stable tears are easier and have better chances for successful repair [94, 95]. In the presence of a bucket-handle dislocated/unstable tear, the first action will be to reduce bluntly the meniscus to its native site prior to repair [94].

Radial Tears These are usually related to trauma but have been also described in the degenerative meniscus. According to its peripheral extent, radial tears can be complete or incomplete. They are oriented extending from the inner edge of the meniscus toward its periphery, where there might be some healing capacity. Radial tears are generally considered as unstable [96]. They were classically considered as irreparable because once the circumferential hoop fibers are disrupted and the majority of the tear is often avascular. However, a complete radial tear has major biomechanical consequences. Hence, repair of complete radial

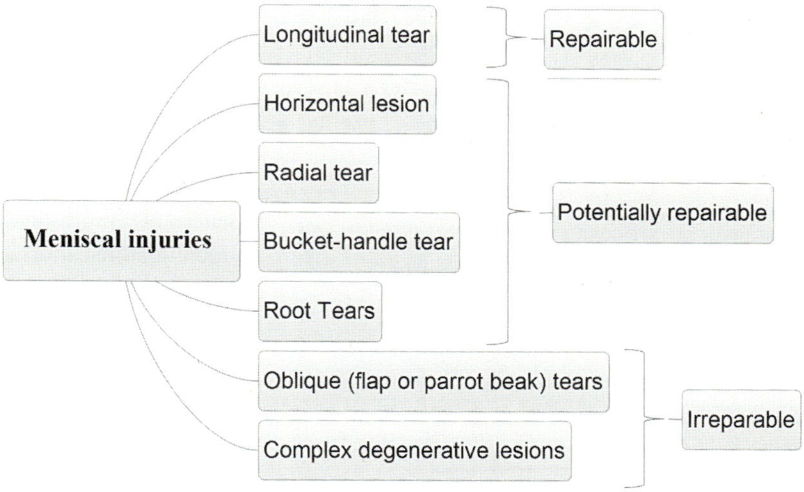

Fig. 14.12 Meniscus injury types and general potential to repair

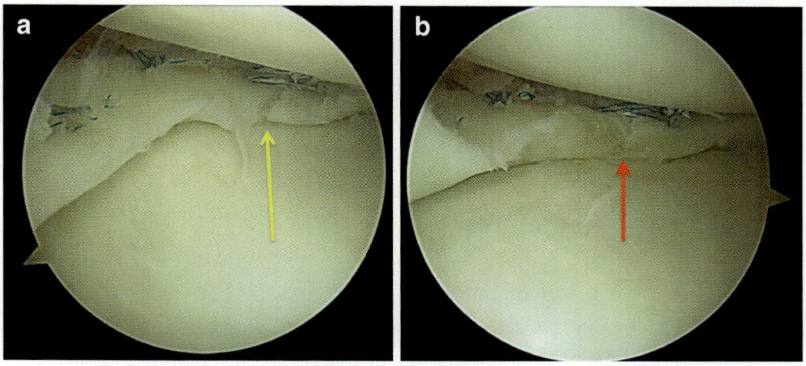

Fig. 14.13 Complex meniscus injury including a radial tear before tensioning the sutures (**a** *yellow arrow*) and after tensioning the sutures (**b** *red arrow*)

meniscal tears is critical to restore the mechanical resistance necessary to maintain hoop tension in the meniscus (Fig. 14.13). Repair of radial tears is currently considered a challenge and represents a difficult decision for the surgeon [91]. Sutures enhanced by fibrin clot have been described as providing positive results for the treatment of radial tears [79, 97].

Horizontal Cleavage Tears Symptomatic horizontal meniscal tears in young patients are a particular condition that they are often present as isolated severe meniscus injuries. Classically, the meniscus will be divided into a superior and an inferior surface. A complete resection of such tear would subsequently result in an extensive (total/subtotal) meniscectomy. Arthroscopic repair of such lesions is sometimes possible and has provided fair outcome [79]. A recent systematic review (level IV) concluded that horizontal cleavage tears show a comparable success rate to repairs of other types of meniscal tears [98]. However, the postoperative protocol is usually significantly longer opposing to meniscectomy, and this is a relevant factor in active high-level athletes. Open meniscal repair of complex horizontal tears, even those extending into the avascular zone, has proven to be effective at midterm follow-up in young and active patients with a low rate of failure [99, 100].

Meniscal Root Tears (MRTs) This type of meniscal tears is receiving increasing attention [101]. Most regularly, MRTs are degenerative in nature (medial compartment) and must be differentiated from the traumatic root tears (more often in lateral compartment and combined with ACL tear). They can be repaired by tibial fixation [80] when the tissue remnant is adequate for repair. The repair of root tears (Fig. 14.14) has been

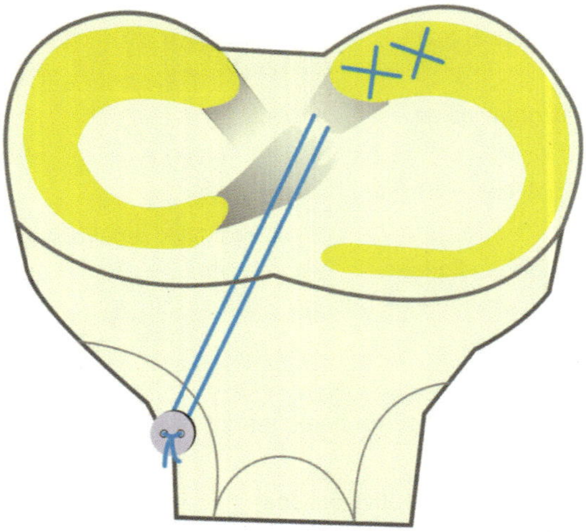

Fig. 14.14 Schematic representation of transtibial reinsertion of posterior root tear of the medial meniscus

done by trans-osseous tunnels [26] and all-inside techniques (more frequently on anterior horns) [102].

14.4.3 Meniscus Replacement

Meniscus allograft transplantation (MAT) has proven to be an effective and reproducible technique when dealing with consequences of severe meniscal loss [103, 104]. On the other hand, partial meniscus replacement by means of scaffolds (mainly acellular) has been used with promising short-term clinical outcome for chronic partial meniscus defects [82, 105–107]. The indications for both techniques are different, while, in summary, scaffold implantation requires that the meniscal roots and peripheral rim remain preserved (which is not a requirement for MAT). There is even one case report describing return to play on a professional footballer after partial lateral meniscus replacement [108]. However, we cannot find current evidence in the literature to promote such techniques in active athletes and expect consistent return to sports at the same level. Such technique, however, represents the best option in some young patients with post-meniscectomized knees as bridging procedures for more aggressive therapies (e.g., osteotomies or arthroplasties). This is quite common in footballers in the final stage of their active competitive careers.

14.5 Results and Return to Sports

Generally fair results are to be expected even allowing athletes to return to pre-injury levels of sports after partial meniscectomy particularly on the short term [109]. However, results seem to deteriorate with time concerning the lateral compartment. Chatain et al. [110] found a higher rate of lowering sports level after lateral meniscectomy [110]. Jaureguito et al. [111] reported in their series that the time of maximal improvement after arthroscopic partial lateral meniscectomy occurred at a mean of 5 months after surgery and lasted about 2 years [111]. Higher reoperation rates (about twice as much) have been reported after lateral meniscectomy comparing to medial (further arthroscopies, osteotomies, or arthroplasties) [32, 110]. Meniscectomy also has been considered to lower the outcome of ACL repair [112, 113]. Considering these, there is a growing trend toward meniscus repair and preservation.

In general, the healing rates after meniscal repair according to literature are complete healing in 60% of the cases, partial healing in 25% of the cases, and failure in 15% of the cases [56]. Moreover, partially or incompletely healed menisci are often asymptomatic [64, 99]. The failure rate after arthroscopic meniscal repair ranges from 5% to 43.5%. However, in general, a failure rate around 15% is accepted by most authors [64].

Another point is that the attempt of meniscal repair, even if it fails, does not seem to worsen the outcome of a subsequent meniscectomy [64]. According to the best available knowledge, it can be stated that arthroscopic meniscal repair provides long-term protective effects, even if the initial healing sometimes is incomplete [56]. Degenerative meniscal tears have lower possibilities for healing and subsequently for repair. Even so, it has been presented that repair horizontal of degenerative cleavage tears can achieve favorable results with a low rate of secondary meniscectomy [99]. Concerning radiographic changes, a significant difference has been observed: 78% of meniscal repairs had no radiographic degenerative changes comparing to 64% of partial meniscectomies [5]. Another study has also demonstrated that meniscal repair for isolated traumatic meniscal tears enabled better outcome in long-term follow-up concerning prevention of osteoarthritis and sports activity recovery compared with partial meniscectomy [53]. In this study, the rate of return to sports activity was 96.2% after repair compared with 50% after meniscectomy [53].

There is no consensus in the literature concerning a possible difference in failure rate for medial meniscus repair comparing to lateral [5, 114]. Despite several reports that meniscal repair combined with ACL reconstruction provides a better outcome, this fact was not confirmed in a study at more than 5 years follow-up [114]. Moreover, the initial meniscal healing rate after meniscal repair in a recent study did not significantly influence clinical or imaging outcomes, and only 12.9% of patients underwent subsequent meniscectomy [56].

In summary, the risk for subsequent meniscectomy after the meniscal repair is low (8.9%) [57]. Meniscus repair is globally a safe and effective procedure [57]. Furthermore, the volume of an eventual subsequent meniscectomy after failed meniscal repair is not significantly increased when compared to the volume of tissue removal if meniscectomy had been the option in primary surgery [64]. It should be noted that, when dealing with traumatic lateral meniscus tears during ACL reconstruction procedures [60], it seems plausible to provide the general recommendation to leave small (<1 cm) tears alone, repair large tears in vascular zone, and excise unstable tears in avascular zone (level I study) [61]. The red-white (zone 2) (rim width 3–5 mm) of menisci has been considered the "gray" area for healing; however, in selected cases, repair in zone 2 is possible and might provide good outcome [92].

In the case of meniscectomy is required, the preservation of peripheral rim and the largest possible amount of meniscus tissue has positive implications for load transmission and contact area [54–56]. In general, the most recent meta-analysis concludes and reinforces that meniscal repairs have better long-term patient-reported outcomes and better activity levels than meniscectomy. Furthermore, meniscal repair had a lower failure rate than meniscectomy [115]. As previously referred, replacement strategies by either meniscus allograft transplantation or partial replacement by scaffolds have not been settled as reproductive and consistent techniques for active footballers [82, 103, 116].

14.6 Complications

Arthroscopic or open meniscal surgery (meniscectomy, repair, or replacement) has some risks of complications which are common to any surgical procedure. After the previous, this section will dedicate attention to complications considered as specific of meniscal repair. Surgical repair of the posterior horn of either medial or lateral menisci is associated with some risk of iatrogenic damage to local neurovascular structures [117]. Concerning the posterior horn of lateral meniscus, special attention is dedicated to the popliteal artery and common peroneal nerve [117]. On the other hand, during repair of the posterior horn of medial meniscus, the saphenous nerve (mainly its infrapatellar branch) is at some risk. Popliteal artery injury (fistulas, pseudoaneurysm, or even laceration) has been reported despite being exceptionally rare [69, 118, 119]. Neuropraxia of the saphenous nerve (and its infrapatellar branch) is the most common neural injury with some authors reporting 22% of transient saphenous neuropraxia (mainly in inside-out techniques) [120]. During medial meniscus repair, few reports have described possible entrapment of the saphenous vein, medial collateral ligament, sartorius, gracilis, and semimembranosus tendons [121, 122].

The use of rigid meniscal repair devices (e.g., polylactic acid or derivatives) has been associated with possible loose fragments/bodies in or outside the joint [123]. Sometimes this might be related to the structure and erratic degradation rates of such polymers [123]. Device-specific complications include synovitis, inflammatory reaction, cyst formation, device failure/migration, and chondral damage [76]. Regarding the most commonly used all-inside devices, particu-

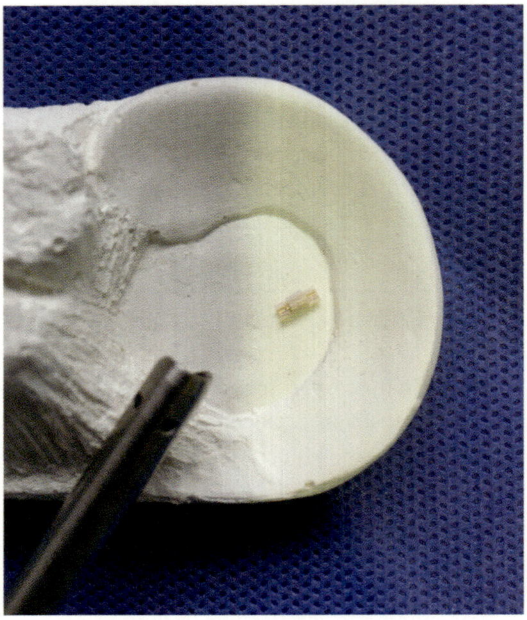

Fig. 14.15 Model demonstrating hard PEEK component of an all-inside device that can migrate intra-articularly

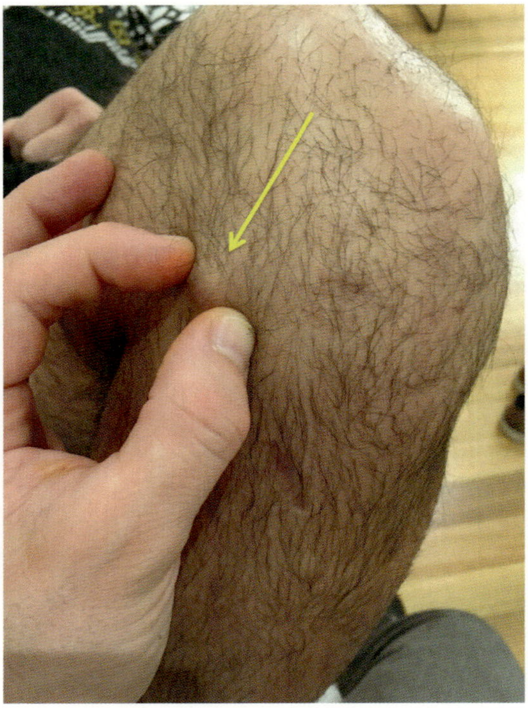

Fig. 14.16 Outside view of a late granuloma around knot sutures 4 months after outside-in medial meniscus repair (the knee is in complete flexion)

larly during the beginning of the learning curve period, complications may arise such as loosening of the implant inside the joint (Fig. 14.15), intra-articular deployment of the device, and suture failure or cutting while tensioning or bending of the device itself during its use [77]. Cartilage of meniscal damage might derive from the former [77]. It is also possible to observe some superficial granulomas around sutures and/or rigid implants of all-inside suture devices (Fig. 14.16).

Conclusion

The high-level athlete has specific demands concerning return to activity (timing and level of same return to play). Despite the fact that arthroscopic meniscectomy has provided, and still provides, satisfactory results on the treatment of irreparable meniscal lesions, there is a growing trend toward meniscal preservation. Meniscal repair has proven to be effective, reproducible, and reliable if adequate indications and techniques are elected. Some injuries previously considered as irreparable are currently found to be potentially reparable (e.g., horizontal cleavage tears, radial tears, root tears). Preoperative planning is mandatory in order to achieve more efficient classification and subsequent prognosis and treatment strategies. Currently, surgeons dedicated to the knee joint must be trained and prepared for several repair options of meniscus injuries.

References

1. Verdonk R. The meniscus: past, present and future. Knee Surg Sports Traumatol Arthrosc. 2011;19:145–6.
2. Beaufils P, Verdonk R. The meniscus. Berlin/Heidelberg: Springer-Verlag; 2010.
3. Smillie IS. Injuries of the knee joint. 4th ed. Edinburgh: Churcill Livingstone; 1972.

4. Salata MJ, Gibbs AE, Sekiya JK. A systematic review of clinical outcomes in patients undergoing meniscectomy. Am J Sports Med. 2010;38: 1907–16.
5. Paxton ES, Stock MV, Brophy RH. Meniscal repair versus partial meniscectomy: a systematic review comparing reoperation rates and clinical outcomes. Arthroscopy. 2011;27:1275–88.
6. Pereira H, Caridade SG, Frias AM, Silva-Correia J, Pereira DR, Cengiz IF, Mano JF, Oliveira JM, Espregueira-Mendes J, Reis RL. Biomechanical and cellular segmental characterization of human meniscus: building the basis for Tissue Engineering therapies. Osteoarthritis Cartilage. 2014;22: 1271–81.
7. Pereira H, Silva-Correia J, Oliveira JM, Reis RL, Espregueira-Mendes J. The meniscus: basic science. In: Verdonk R, Espregueira-Mendes J, Monllau JC, editors. Meniscal transplantation. Heidelberg/New York/Dordrecht/London: Springer; 2013. p. 7–14.
8. McDermott ID, Masouros SD, Amis AA. Biomechanics of the menisci of the knee. Current Orthopaedics. 2008;22:193–201.
9. McDermott ID, Amis AA. The consequences of meniscectomy. J Bone Joint Surg Br. 2006;88: 1549–56.
10. McDevitt CA, Webber RJ. The ultrastructure and biochemistry of meniscal cartilage. Clin Orthop Relat Res. 1990;252:8–18.
11. Verdonk PC, Forsyth RG, Wang J, Almqvist KF, Verdonk R, Veys EM, Verbruggen G. Characterisation of human knee meniscus cell phenotype. Osteoarthritis Cartilage. 2005;13:548–60.
12. Cengiz IF, Pereira H, Pego JM, Sousa N, Espregueira-Mendes J, Oliveira JM, Reis RL. Segmental and regional quantification of 3D cellular density of human meniscus from osteoarthritic knee. J Tissue Eng Regen Med. 2015; Epub ahed of print. doi: 10.1002/term.2082
13. Walker PS, Hajek JV. The load-bearing area in the knee joint. J Biomech. 1972;5:581–9.
14. Bourne RB, Finlay JB, Papadopoulos P, Andreae P. The effect of medial meniscectomy on strain distribution in the proximal part of the tibia. J Bone Joint Surg Am. 1984;66:1431–7.
15. Arnoczky SP, Warren RF. Microvasculature of the human meniscus. Am J Sports Med. 1982;10:90–5.
16. Gupte CM, Bull AM, Thomas RD, Amis AA. The meniscofemoral ligaments: secondary restraints to the posterior drawer. Analysis of anteroposterior and rotary laxity in the intact and posterior-cruciate-deficient knee. J Bone Joint Surg Br. 2003;85: 765–73.
17. Smigielski R, Becker R, Zdanowicz U, Ciszek B. Medial meniscus anatomy-from basic science to treatment. Knee Surg Sports Traumatol Arthrosc. 2015;23:8–14.
18. Pereira H, Silva-Correia J, Oliveira JM, Reis RL, Espregueira-Mendes J. Future trends in the treatment of meniscus lesions: from repair to regeneration. In: Verdonk R, Espregueira-Mendes J, Monllau JC, editors. Meniscal transplantation. Heidelberg/New York/Dordrecht/London: Springer; 2013. p. 103–14.
19. Beaufils P, Englund M, Järvinen TLN, Pereira H, Pujol N. How to share guidelines in daily practice on meniscus repair, degenerate meniscal lesion, and meniscectomy. In: Zaffagnini S, Becker R, GMMJ K, Espregueira-Mendes J, van Dijk CN, editors. ESSKA instructional course lecture book Amsterdam. Berlin: Springer; 2014. p. 97–112.
20. Poehling GG, Ruch DS, Chabon SJ. The landscape of meniscal injuries. Clin Sports Med. 1990;9: 539–49.
21. Anderson AF, Irrgang JJ, Dunn W, Beaufils P, Cohen M, Cole BJ, Coolican M, Ferretti M, Glenn Jr RE, Johnson R, Neyret P, Ochi M, Panarella L, Siebold R, Spindler KP, Ait Si Selmi T, Verdonk P, Verdonk R, Yasuda K, Kowalchuk DA. Interobserver reliability of the International Society of Arthroscopy, Knee Surgery and Orthopaedic Sports Medicine (ISAKOS) classification of meniscal tears. Am J Sports Med. 2011;39:926–32.
22. Smillie IS. The current pattern of the pathology of meniscus tears. Proc R Soc Med. 1968;61:44–5.
23. Christoforakis J, Pradhan R, Sanchez-Ballester J, Hunt N, Strachan RK. Is there an association between articular cartilage changes and degenerative meniscus tears? Arthroscopy. 2005;21:1366–9.
24. Yim JH, Seon JK, Song EK, Choi JI, Kim MC, Lee KB, Seo HY. A comparative study of meniscectomy and nonoperative treatment for degenerative horizontal tears of the medial meniscus. Am J Sports Med. 2013;41:1565–70.
25. LaPrade CM, Foad A, Smith SD, Turnbull TL, Dornan GJ, Engebretsen L, Wijdicks CA, LaPrade RF. Biomechanical consequences of a nonanatomic posterior medial meniscal root repair. Am J Sports Med. 2015;43:912–20.
26. Koenig JH, Ranawat AS, Umans HR, Difelice GS. Meniscal root tears: diagnosis and treatment. Arthroscopy. 2009;25:1025–32.
27. Noble J, Hamblen DL. The pathology of the degenerate meniscus lesion. J Bone Joint Surg Br. 1975;57:180–6.
28. Sweigart MA, Athanasiou KA. Toward tissue engineering of the knee meniscus. Tissue Eng. 2001;7:111–29.
29. Nishimuta JF, Levenston ME. Response of cartilage and meniscus tissue explants to in vitro compressive overload. Osteoarthritis Cartilage. 2012;20:422–9.
30. Abraham AC, Edwards CR, Odegard GM, Donahue TL. Regional and fiber orientation dependent shear

properties and anisotropy of bovine meniscus. J Mech Behav Biomed Mater. 2011;4:2024–30.
31. Guo H, Maher SA, Spilker RL. Biphasic finite element contact analysis of the knee joint using an augmented Lagrangian method. Med Eng Phys. 2013;35:1313–20.
32. Fayard JM, Pereira H, Servien E, Lustig S, Neyret P. Meniscectomy global results-complications. Berlin/Heidelberg: The Meniscus Springer-Verlag; 2010. doi:10.1007/978-3-642-02450-4.
33. Ruiz-Iban MA, Diaz-Heredia J, Elias-Martin E, Moros-Marco S, Cebreiro Martinez Del Val I. Repair of meniscal tears associated with tibial plateau fractures: a review of 15 cases. Am J Sports Med. 2012;40:2289–95.
34. Poulsen MR, Johnson DL. Meniscal injuries in the young, athletically active patient. Phys Sportsmed. 2011;39:123–30.
35. Baker P, Coggon D, Reading I, Barrett D, McLaren M, Cooper C. Sports injury, occupational physical activity, joint laxity, and meniscal damage. J Rheumatol. 2002;29:557–63.
36. Frizziero A, Ferrari R, Giannotti E, Ferroni C, Poli P, Masiero S. The meniscus tear. State of the art of rehabilitation protocols related to surgical procedures. Muscles Ligaments Tendons J. 2012;2:295–301.
37. Dacombe PJ. Shelbourne's update of the O'Donoghue knee triad in a 17-year-old male Rugby player. BMJ Case Reports. 2013;10.1136/bcr.01.2012.5593
38. Shelbourne KD, Nitz PA. The O'Donoghue triad revisited. Combined knee injuries involving anterior cruciate and medial collateral ligament tears. Am J Sports Med. 1991;19:474–7.
39. Englund M, Guermazi A, Gale D, Hunter DJ, Aliabadi P, Clancy M, Felson DT. Incidental meniscal findings on knee MRI in middle-aged and elderly persons. N Engl J Med. 2008;359:1108–15.
40. Englund M, Niu J, Guermazi A, Roemer FW, Hunter DJ, Lynch JA, Lewis CE, Torner J, Nevitt MC, Zhang YQ, Felson DT. Effect of meniscal damage on the development of frequent knee pain, aching, or stiffness. Arthritis Rheum. 2007;56:4048–54.
41. Kornaat PR, Bloem JL, Ceulemans RY, Riyazi N, Rosendaal FR, Nelissen RG, Carter WO, Hellio Le Graverand MP, Kloppenburg M. Osteoarthritis of the knee: association between clinical features and MR imaging findings. Radiology. 2006;239:811–7.
42. Howell R, Kumar NS, Patel N, Tom J. Degenerative meniscus: pathogenesis, diagnosis, and treatment options. World J Orthod. 2014;5:597–602.
43. Makris EA, Hadidi P, Athanasiou KA. The knee meniscus: structure-function, pathophysiology, current repair techniques, and prospects for regeneration. Biomaterials. 2011;32:7411–31.
44. Smith BE, Thacker D, Crewesmith A, Hall M. Special tests for assessing meniscal tears within the knee: a systematic review and meta-analysis. Evid Based Med. 2015;20:88–97.
45. Van Dyck P, Vanhoenacker FM, Lambrecht V, Wouters K, Gielen JL, Dossche L, Parizel PM. Prospective comparison of 1.5 and 3.0-T MRI for evaluating the knee menisci and ACL. J Bone Joint Surg Am. 2013;95:916–24.
46. Beaufils P, Hulet C, Dhenain M, Nizard R, Nourissat G, Pujol N. Clinical practice guidelines for the management of meniscal lesions and isolated lesions of the anterior cruciate ligament of the knee in adults. Orthop Traumatol Surg Res. 2009;95:437–42.
47. Nam TS, Kim MK, Ahn JH. Efficacy of magnetic resonance imaging evaluation for meniscal tear in acute anterior cruciate ligament injuries. Arthroscopy. 2014;30:475–82.
48. Ben-Galim P, Steinberg EL, Amir H, Ash N, Dekel S, Arbel R. Accuracy of magnetic resonance imaging of the knee and unjustified surgery. Clin Orthop Relat Res. 2006;447:100–4.
49. Rossbach BP, Pietschmann MF, Gulecyuz MF, Niethammer TR, Ficklscherer A, Wild S, Jansson V, Muller PE. Indications requiring preoperative magnetic resonance imaging before knee arthroscopy. Arch Med Sci. 2014;10:1147–52.
50. Cooper DE, Arnoczky SP, Warren RF. Meniscal repair. Clin Sports Med. 1991;10:529–48.
51. Bernstein J. In brief: meniscal tears. Clin Orthop Relat Res. 2010;468:1190–2.
52. Ciccotti MG, Shields CLJ, El Attrache NS. Meniscectomy. In: Fu FH, Harner CD, Vince KG, editors. Knee surgery, vol. 1. Philadelphia: Williams & Wilkins; 1994. p. 591–613.
53. Stein T, Mehling AP, Welsch F, von Eisenhart-Rothe R, Jager A. Long-term outcome after arthroscopic meniscal repair versus arthroscopic partial meniscectomy for traumatic meniscal tears. Am J Sports Med. 2010;38:1542–8.
54. Anderson L, Watts M, Shapter O, Logan M, Risebury M, Duffy D, Myers P. Repair of radial tears and posterior horn detachments of the lateral meniscus: minimum 2-year follow-up. Arthroscopy. 2010;26:1625–32.
55. Hulet CH, Locker BG, Schiltz D, Texier A, Tallier E, Vielpeau CH. Arthroscopic medial meniscectomy on stable knees. J Bone Joint Surg Br. 2001;83:29–32.
56. Pujol N, Tardy N, Boisrenoult P, Beaufils P. Long-term outcomes of all-inside meniscal repair. Knee Surg Sports Traumatol Arthrosc. 2015;23:219–24.
57. Lyman S, Hidaka C, Valdez AS, Hetsroni I, Pan TJ, Do H, Dunn WR, Marx RG. Risk factors for meniscectomy after meniscal repair. Am J Sports Med. 2013;41:2772–8.
58. Pujol N, Beaufils P. Healing results of meniscal tears left in situ during anterior cruciate ligament reconstruction: a review of clinical studies. Knee Surg Sports Traumatol Arthrosc. 2009;17:396–401.
59. Snoeker BA, Bakker EW, Kegel CA, Lucas C. Risk factors for meniscal tears: a systematic review including meta-analysis. J Orthop Sports Phys Ther. 2013;43:352–67.
60. Shelbourne KD, Heinrich J. The long-term evaluation of lateral meniscus tears left in situ at the time of

anterior cruciate ligament reconstruction. Arthroscopy. 2004;20:346–51.
61. Cox CL, Huston LJ, Dunn WR, Reinke EK, Nwosu SK, Parker RD, Wright RW, Kaeding CC, Marx RG, Amendola A, McCarty EC, Spindler KP. Are articular cartilage lesions and meniscus tears predictive of IKDC, KOOS, and marx activity level outcomes after anterior cruciate ligament reconstruction? A 6-year multicenter cohort study. Am J Sports Med. 2014;42:1058–67.
62. Mariani PP, Garofalo R, Margheritini F. Chondrolysis after partial lateral meniscectomy in athletes. Knee Surg Sports Traumatol Arthrosc. 2008;16:574–80.
63. Sonnery-Cottet B, Archbold P, Thaunat M, Carnesecchi O, Tostes M, Chambat P. Rapid chondrolysis of the knee after partial lateral meniscectomy in professional athletes. Knee. 2014;21:504–8.
64. Pujol N, Barbier O, Boisrenoult P, Beaufils P. Amount of meniscal resection after failed meniscal repair. Am J Sports Med. 2011;39:1648–52.
65. El Ghazaly SA, Rahman AA, Yusry AH, Fathalla MM. Arthroscopic partial meniscectomy is superior to physical rehabilitation in the management of symptomatic unstable meniscal tears. Int Orthop. 2015;39:769–75.
66. Chang JH, Shen HC, Huang GS, Pan RY, Wu CF, Lee CH, Chen Q. A biomechanical comparison of all-inside meniscus repair techniques. J Surg Res. 2009;155:82–8.
67. Chang HC, Caborn DN, Nyland J, Burden R. Effect of lesion location on fixation strength of the meniscal viper repair system: an in vitro study using porcine menisci. Arthroscopy. 2006;22:394–9.
68. Henning CE. Arthroscopic repair of meniscus tears. Orthopedics. 1983;6:1130–2.
69. Henning CE, Lynch MA, Yearout KM, Vequist SW, Stallbaumer RJ, Decker KA. Arthroscopic meniscal repair using an exogenous fibrin clot. Clin Orthop Relat Res. 1990;252:64–72.
70. Warren RF. Arthroscopic meniscus repair. Arthroscopy. 1985;1:170–2.
71. Morgan CD, Casscells SW. Arthroscopic meniscus repair: a safe approach to the posterior horns. Arthroscopy. 1986;2:3–12.
72. Tsai AM, McAllister DR, Chow S, Young CR, Hame SL. Results of meniscal repair using a bioabsorbable screw. Arthroscopy. 2004;20:586–90.
73. Albrecht-Olsen P, Kristensen G, Burgaard P, Joergensen U, Toerholm C. The arrow versus horizontal suture in arthroscopic meniscus repair. A prospective randomized study with arthroscopic evaluation. Knee Surg Sports Traumatol Arthrosc. 1999;7:268–73.
74. Petsche TS, Selesnick H, Rochman A. Arthroscopic meniscus repair with bioabsorbable arrows. Arthroscopy. 2002;18:246–53.
75. Gifstad T, Grontvedt T, Drogset JO. Meniscal repair with biofix arrows: results after 4.7 years' follow-up. Am J Sports Med. 2007;35:71–4.
76. Kurzweil PR, Tifford CD, Ignacio EM. Unsatisfactory clinical results of meniscal repair using the meniscus arrow. Arthroscopy. 2005;21:905.
77. Miller MD, Kline AJ, Gonzales J, Beach WR. Pitfalls associated with FasT-Fix meniscal repair. Arthroscopy. 2002;18:939–43.
78. Seil R, Rupp S, Kohn DM. Cyclic testing of meniscal sutures. Arthroscopy. 2000;16:505–10.
79. Kamimura T, Kimura M. Meniscal repair of degenerative horizontal cleavage tears using fibrin clots: clinical and arthroscopic outcomes in 10 cases. Orthop J Sports Med. 2014;2(11):2325967114555678. doi:10.1177/2325967114555678.
80. Ahn JH, Wang JH, Yoo JC. Arthroscopic all-inside suture repair of medial meniscus lesion in anterior cruciate ligament--deficient knees: results of second-look arthroscopies in 39 cases. Arthroscopy. 2004;20:936–45.
81. Barrett GR, Field MH, Treacy SH, Ruff CG. Clinical results of meniscus repair in patients 40 years and older. Arthroscopy. 1998;14:824–9.
82. Pereira H, Frias AM, Oliveira JM, Espregueira-Mendes J, Reis RL. Tissue engineering and regenerative medicine strategies in meniscus lesions. Arthroscopy. 2011;27:1706–19.
83. Arnoczky S, Warren R, Pivak J. Meniscal repair using an exogenous fibrin clot: an experimental study in dogs. J Bone Joint Surg Am. 1998;70:1209–17.
84. Klompmaker J, Veth RP, Jansen HW, Nielsen HK, de Groot JH, Pennings AJ, Kuijer R. Meniscal repair by fibrocartilage in the dog: characterization of the repair tissue and the role of vascularity. Biomaterials. 1996;17:1685–91.
85. Griffin JW, Hadeed MM, Werner BC, Diduch DR, Carson EW, Miller MD. Platelet-rich plasma in meniscal repair: does augmentation improve surgical outcomes? Clin Orthop Relat Res. 2015;473:1665–72.
86. Peretti GM, Gill TJ, Xu JW, Randolph MA, Morse KR, Zaleske DJ. Cell-based therapy for meniscal repair: a large animal study. Am J Sports Med. 2004;32:146–58.
87. Cook JL, Fox DB. A novel bioabsorbable conduit augments healing of avascular meniscal tears in a dog model. Am J Sports Med. 2007;35:1877–87.
88. Kobayashi K, Fujimoto E, Deie M, Sumen Y, Ikuta Y, Ochi M. Regional differences in the healing potential of the meniscus-an organ culture model to eliminate the influence of microvasculature and the synovium. Knee. 2004;11:271–8.
89. Cook JL, Fox DB, Malaviya P, Tomlinson JL, Kuroki K, Cook CR, Kladakis S. Long-term outcome for large meniscal defects treated with small intestinal submucosa in a dog model. Am J Sports Med. 2006;34:32–42.
90. Kobayashi Y, Yasuda K, Kondo E, Katsura T, Tanabe Y, Kimura M, Tohyama H. Implantation of autogenous meniscal fragments wrapped with a fascia sheath enhances fibrocartilage regeneration in vivo in a large harvest site defect. Am J Sports Med. 2010;38:740–8.
91. Matsubara H, Okazaki K, Izawa T, Tashiro Y, Matsuda S, Nishimura T, Nakanishi Y, Kawamura H, Iwamoto Y. New suture method for radial tears of the meniscus: biomechanical analysis of cross-

suture and double horizontal suture techniques using cyclic load testing. Am J Sports Med. 2012;40:414–8.
92. Barber-Westin SD, Noyes FR. Clinical healing rates of meniscus repairs of tears in the central-third (red-white) zone. Arthroscopy. 2014;30:134–46.
93. Pasa L, Visna P. Suture of meniscus. Scripta Medica (Brno). 2005;78:135–50.
94. Espejo-Reina A, Serrano-Fernandez JM, Martin-Castilla B, Estades-Rubio FJ, Briggs KK, Espejo-Baena A. Outcomes after repair of chronic bucket-handle tears of medial meniscus. Arthroscopy. 2014;30:492–6.
95. Ahn JH, Kim KI, Wang JH, Kyung BS, Seo MC, Lee SH. Arthroscopic repair of bucket-handle tears of the lateral meniscus. Knee Surg Sports Traumatol Arthrosc. 2015;23:205–10.
96. Weiss CB, Lundberg M, Hamberg P, DeHaven KE, Gillquist J. Non-operative treatment of meniscal tears. J Bone Joint Surg Am. 1989;71:811–22.
97. Ra HJ, Ha JK, Jang SH, Lee DW, Kim JG. Arthroscopic inside-out repair of complete radial tears of the meniscus with a fibrin clot. Knee Surg Sports Traumatol Arthrosc. 2013;21:2126–30.
98. Kurzweil PR, Lynch NM, Coleman S, Kearney B. Repair of horizontal meniscus tears: a systematic review. Arthroscopy. 2014;30:1513–9.
99. Pujol N, Bohu Y, Boisrenoult P, Macdes A, Beaufils P. Clinical outcomes of open meniscal repair of horizontal meniscal tears in young patients. Knee Surg Sports Traumatol Arthrosc. 2013;21:1530–3.
100. Salle de Chou E, Pujol N, Rochcongar G, Cucurulo T, Potel JF, Dalmay F, Ehkirch FP, Laporte C, Le Henaff G, Seil R, Lutz C, Gunepin FX, Sonnery-Cottet B. Analysis of short and long-term results of horizontal meniscal tears in young adults. Orthop Traumatol Surg Res. 2015;101:S317–22.
101. Bhatia S, LaPrade CM, Ellman MB, LaPrade RF. Meniscal root tears: significance, diagnosis, and treatment. Am J Sports Med. 2014;42:3016–30.
102. Osti L, Del Buono A, Maffulli N. Anterior medial meniscal root tears: a novel arthroscopic all inside repair. Transl Med UniSa. 2015;12:41–6.
103. Elattar M, Dhollander A, Verdonk R, Almqvist KF, Verdonk P. Twenty-six years of meniscal allograft transplantation: is it still experimental? A meta-analysis of 44 trials. Knee Surg Sports Traumatol Arthrosc. 2011;19:147–57.
104. Chalmers PN, Karas V, Sherman SL, Cole BJ. Return to high-level sport after meniscal allograft transplantation. Arthroscopy. 2013;29:539–44.
105. Zaffagnini S, Grassi A, Marcheggiani Muccioli GM, Holsten D, Bulgheroni P, Monllau JC, Berbig R, Lagae K, Crespo R, Marcacci M. Two-year clinical results of lateral collagen meniscus implant: a multicenter study. Arthroscopy. 2015;31:1269–78.
106. Zaffagnini S, Grassi A, Marcheggiani Muccioli GM, Bonanzinga T, Nitri M, Raggi F, Ravazzolo G, Marcacci M. MRI evaluation of a collagen meniscus implant: a systematic review. Knee Surg Sports Traumatol Arthrosc. 2015;23:3228–37.
107. Bouyarmane H, Beaufils P, Pujol N, Bellemans J, Roberts S, Spalding T, Zaffagnini S, Marcacci M, Verdonk P, Womack M, Verdonk R. Polyurethane scaffold in lateral meniscus segmental defects: clinical outcomes at 24 months follow-up. Orthop Traumatol Surg Res. 2014;100:153–7.
108. Zaffagnini S, Marcheggiani Muccioli GM, Grassi A, Bonanzinga T, Filardo G, Canales Passalacqua A, Marcacci M. Arthroscopic lateral collagen meniscus implant in a professional soccer player. Knee Surg Sports Traumatol Arthrosc. 2011;19:1740–3.
109. Andersson-Molina H, Karlsson H, Rockborn P. Arthroscopic partial and total meniscectomy: a long-term follow-up study with matched controls. Arthroscopy. 2002;18:183–9.
110. Chatain F, Adeleine P, Chambat P, Neyret P. A comparative study of medial versus lateral arthroscopic partial meniscectomy on stable knees: 10-year minimum follow-up. Arthroscopy. 2003;19:842–9.
111. Jaureguito JW, Elliot JS, Lietner T, Dixon LB, Reider B. The effects of arthroscopic partial lateral meniscectomy in an otherwise normal knee: a retrospective review of functional, clinical, and radiographic results. Arthroscopy. 1995;11:29–36.
112. Kartus JT, Russell VJ, Salmon LJ, Magnusson LC, Brandsson S, Pehrsson NG, Pinczewski LA. Concomitant partial meniscectomy worsens outcome after arthroscopic anterior cruciate ligament reconstruction. Acta Orthop Scand. 2002;73:179–85.
113. Brophy RH, Gill CS, Lyman S, Barnes RP, Rodeo SA, Warren RF. Effect of anterior cruciate ligament reconstruction and meniscectomy on length of career in National Football League athletes: a case control study. Am J Sports Med. 2009;37:2102–7.
114. Logan M, Watts M, Owen J, Myers P. Meniscal repair in the elite athlete: results of 45 repairs with a minimum 5-year follow-up. Am J Sports Med. 2009;37:1131–4.
115. Xu C, Zhao J. A meta-analysis comparing meniscal repair with meniscectomy in the treatment of meniscal tears: the more meniscus, the better outcome? Knee Surg Sports Traumatol Arthrosc. 2015;23:164–70.
116. Warth RJ, Rodkey WG. Resorbable collagen scaffolds for the treatment of meniscus defects: a systematic review. Arthroscopy. 2015;31:927–41.
117. Katabi N, Pujol N, Boisrenoult P. Meniscal repair: intra- and postoperative complications. In: Beaufils P, Verdonk R, editors. The meniscus. Berlin/Heidelberg: Springer-Verlag; 2010. p. 191–8.

118. Brasseur P, Sukkarieh F. Iatrogenic pseudoaneurysm of the popliteal artery. Complication of arthroscopic meniscectomy. Apropos of a case. J Radiol. 1990;71:301–4.
119. Carlin RE, Papenhausen M, Farber MA, Ronningen E, Mauro MA, Marston WA, Keagy BA, Burnham SJ. Sural artery pseudoaneurysms after knee arthroscopy: treatment with transcatheter embolization. J Vasc Surg. 2001;33:170–3.
120. Barber FA. Meniscus repair: results of an arthroscopic technique. Arthroscopy. 1987;3:25–30.
121. Espejo-Baena A, Golano P, Meschian S, Garcia-Herrera JM, Serrano Jimenez JM. Complications in medial meniscus suture: a cadaveric study. Knee Surg Sports Traumatol Arthrosc. 2007;15:811–6.
122. Coen MJ, Caborn DN, Urban W, Nyland J, Johnson DL. An anatomic evaluation of T-Fix suture device placement for arthroscopic all-inside meniscal repair. Arthroscopy. 1999;15:275–80.
123. Farng E, Sherman O. Meniscal repair devices: a clinical and biomechanical literature review. Arthroscopy. 2004;20:273–86.

Injury of Knee Ligaments

15

Frantzeska Zampeli, Anastasios Georgoulis,
Freddie Fu, Romain Seil, Jim-Dimitris Georgoulis,
and João Espregueira-Mendes

Contents

F. Zampeli (✉) • A. Georgoulis • J.-D. Georgoulis
Orthopaedic Sports Medicine Center,
Department of Orthopaedic Surgery,
University of Ioannina, Ioannina, Greece
e-mail: fzampeli@gmail.com

F. Fu
Department of Orthopaedic Surgery,
University of Pittsburgh,
3471 Fifth Avenue, Suite 1011,
Pittsburgh, PA 15213, USA

R. Seil
Département de l'Appareil Locomoteur, Centre
Hospitalier de Luxembourg – Clinique d' Eich and
Sports Medicine Research Laboratory,
Luxembourg Institute of Health,
Strassen, UK

J. Espregueira-Mendes
Clínica do Dragão, Espregueira-Mendes Sports
Centre, FIFA Medical Centre of Excellence,
Porto, Portugal

Dom Henrique Research Centre, Porto, Portugal

3B's Research Group – Biomaterials, Biodegradables
and Biomimetics, University of Minho, Headquarters
of the European Institute of Excellence on Tissue
Engineering and Regenerative Medicine,
AvePark, S. Cláudio de Barco, 4806-909 Taipas,
Guimarães, Portugal

ICVS/3B's – PT Government Associated Laboratory,
Braga, Portugal

Orthopedic Department, Minho University,
Braga, Portugal

J. Espregueira-Mendes et al. (eds.), *Injuries and Health Problems in Football*,
DOI 10.1007/978-3-662-53924-8_15

15.1 Anterior Cruciate Ligament Injuries

15.1.1 Anatomy

The anterior cruciate ligament (ACL) is an intra-articular but extra-synovial ligament that originates from the lateral femoral condyle within the intercondylar notch. The ACL inserts on the tibial plateau, medial to the insertion of the anterior horn of the lateral meniscus [1–3].

15.1.2 Biomechanics and Function

The ACL is the primary restraint to anterior tibial translation and secondary restraint to tibial rotation and is distinguished into two functional bundles, the anteromedial (AM) and the posterolateral (PL). The terminology of the bundles is based on their tibial insertion. The AM fibers originate on the most proximal part of the femoral origin and insert on the anteromedial aspect of the tibial insertion site. The PL fibers originate on the most distal aspect of the femoral origin and insert on the posterolateral aspect of the tibial insertion site. When the knee is extended, the femoral attachment of the ACL is in a vertical position, the PL bundle is tight, and the AM bundle is moderately lax. As the knee is flexed, the femoral attachment of the ACL becomes a more horizontal orientation, causing the AM bundle to tighten and the PL bundle to loosen [2, 3].

15.1.3 Mechanism of Injury

At least two-thirds of ACL tears occur during noncontact situations such as cutting, pivoting, accelerating, decelerating, or landing from a jump [4, 5]. Isolated injuries of the ACL can occur when a twisting impact is applied at the knee joint forcing either in internal rotation and hyperextension or in external rotation and valgus. Along with ACL, concurrent lesion to MCL and the capsule may be caused when the impact at the knee occurs at the lateral side, forcing the knee into valgus and external rotation. The same injury can be caused by an impact to the medial side of the foot. Concurrent lesion of the LCL and posterolateral corner may result from an impact at the medial side of the knee (or lateral side of the foot) that forces the knee into varus and internal rotation. Finally, concurrent injury or the PCL is the end result of high-energy trauma, dislocation or subluxation of the knee, lateral or medial impact, and hyperextension or hyperflexion injuries [6–8].

15.1.4 Symptoms and Diagnosis

During the initial trauma, the patient may hear a "pop" and feel sudden knee pain, giving way symptom, and inability to continue the activity; however, sometimes the athlete may be able to walk off the field. During the next hours, usually there is excessive swelling that is attributed to hemarthrosis as can be shown by knee joint aspiration. The cause of hemarthrosis is ACL rupture in 70% of cases. Limitation of range of motion (both active and passive) may be present, while catching sensation (block) that further deteriorates any flexion or extension may occur, usually as a result of concurrent meniscal lesion.

The anterior instability that results from the ACL rupture can be assessed by the Lachman-Noulis [9] and the anterior drawer test that both estimate the anterior tibial translation (ATT) in relation to the femur in 20–30° and 90° of knee joint flexion, respectively (Fig. 15.1). For both tests the ATT is evaluated according to the end point (firm, soft) [10]. The rotational instability can be assessed with the pivot shift test that is a very specific but nonsensitive test in the non-anesthetized patient. By applying an internal rotary torque and valgus load to the knee, the examiner notices the subluxation and reduction of lateral tibial plateau during passive extension and flexion of the knee causing a glide or a clunk,

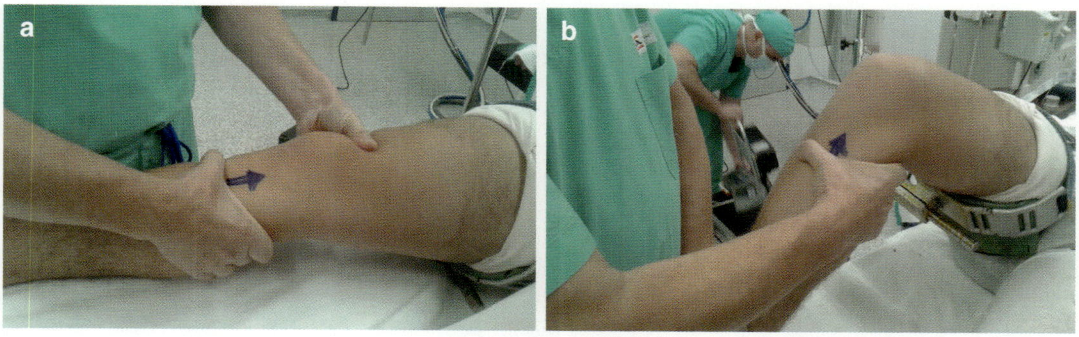

Fig. 15.1 The examination of anterior instability of the knee after ACL rupture with (**a**) the Lachman-Noulis test and (**b**) the anterior drawer test (Photo from Prof. Georgoulis ad archives)

depending on the degree of subluxation. A jump is noted at approximately 10–20° of flexion [10]. Instrumental devices such as the KT-1000 arthrometer (MEDmetric, San Diego, CA) may quantify the ATT. A side-to-side difference for ATT greater than 5 mm is indicative of ACL rupture, while that of 3–5 mm has been indicative of partial ACL rupture.

The X-ray may exclude any fracture. The MRI examination may offer several primary and secondary findings indicative of an ACL rupture.

15.1.5 Natural History and Treatment Principles

ACL rupture is functionally disabling, predisposing the knee to subsequent injuries such as tears of the menisci and cartilage degeneration thus predisposing to early onset of osteoarthritis. The level of activity of the patient and the desire to return to the prior to injury level, the recurrent giving way symptoms, and the positive pivot shift are factors that indicate operative treatment plan for patients with ACL rupture especially for athletes (professional or recreational) and athletic population. Arthroscopic ACL reconstruction aims to restore intact knee joint function, stability, and biomechanics [11]. In the long term, the restoration of abnormal knee joint biomechanics of the ACL-deficient knee may prevent the onset of early posttraumatic articular cartilage degeneration and the progression to osteoarthritis [12]. The time interval from ACL injury to reconstruction is not as important as the condition of the knee at the time of surgery. The knee should have a full range of motion with minimal effusion; the patient should have minimal pain and be mentally prepared for the reconstruction and rehabilitation after surgery.

15.1.5.1 Surgical Technique

The most commonly used grafts are the patellar tendon graft with bone blocks at both sides, the hamstrings tendon graft, and the quadriceps tendon graft. Allografts and synthetic grafts have also been used; however, these should not be considered the first choice for athletes. Several issues have been considered important, initiating a discussion on ways to improve the ACL reconstruction technique, aiming toward a more anatomic approach [13, 14]. The discussion is mainly focused either on the choice of graft or on tunnel position, which are the main considerations in an anatomic ACL reconstruction. In the first aspect, bone-patellar tendon-bone and hamstring graft (either single-bundle [SB] or double-bundle [DB] graft) are the most commonly used; they have comparable properties to the native tissue, and their effectiveness has been proven [14–16]. The second concept regarding where to place the femoral and tibial

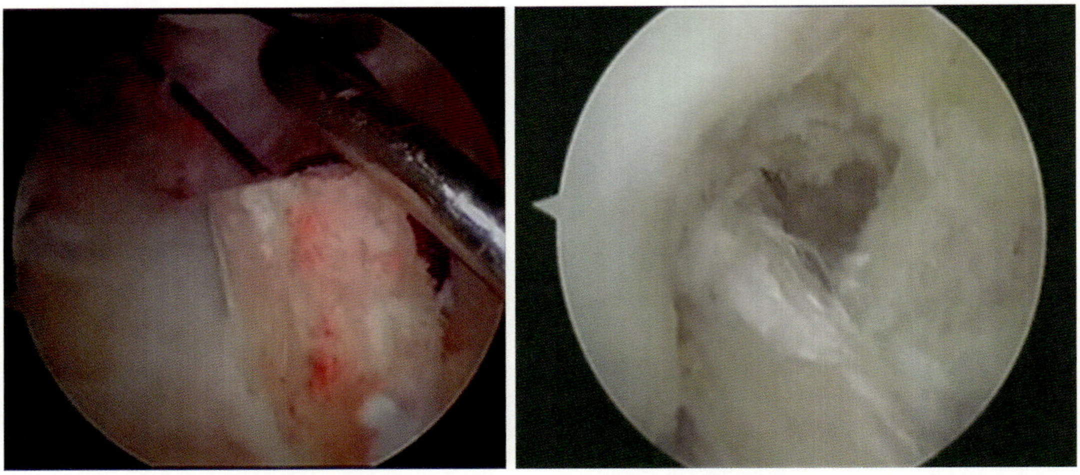

Fig. 15.2 Arthroscopic pictures demonstrating the passage of a bone-patellar tendon-bone autograft through the tibial tunnel toward the femoral tunnel (*left*) and the final graft position that imitates native anterior cruciate ligament anatomy and obliquity (*right*) (Photo from authors'study: Zampeli F, Giotis D, Bernard M, Pappas E, Georgoulis AD. Anatomic single-bundle Anterior Cruciate Ligament (ACL) reconstruction with intraoperative restoration of abnormal tibiofemoral position restores knee joint biomechanics and function to normal levels. 17th ESSKA Congress 2016, Barcelona, Spain)

tunnels has been well discussed. Most recent evidence suggests positioning of the graft at the anatomic insertions of the native ACL [17, 18]. A more detailed description of the anatomy of the ACL has been helpful in an attempt to replicate the exact anatomy and behavior of the ACL (Fig. 15.2).

15.2 Medial Collateral Ligament Injuries

MCL injury is common during contact sports, and it represents about 8% of sports injuries [19]. MCL tears present as an isolated injury or commonly in combination with injury to the ACL, posterior cruciate ligament (PCL), or both.

15.2.1 Anatomy

The MCL consists of three units, named the superficial MCL (s-MCL), the deep MCL (d-MCL) or medial capsular ligament, and the posterior oblique ligament (POL) [20]. The s-MCL is a broad ligament that attaches at the medial femoral epicondyle and inserts just below the pes anserinus, 4–5 cm distal from the joint line that is taut during flexion and lax during full extension. Just deep into the s-MCL lies the d-MCL which is a confluence of the meniscofemoral, meniscocapsular, and meniscotibial ligaments. Posterior to the MCL is the posteromedial corner (PMC), made up of a condensation of the capsule forming the POL that is tight in extension [20, 21].

15.2.2 Biomechanics

The MCL, and more specifically the s-MCL, provides 78% of the valgus restraining force of the knee. In extension, the ACL and PMC (POL, medial meniscus, and semimembranosus) also contribute to valgus stress, and the MCL provides 57% of the restraining force against valgus stress [22–24]. In general, an isolated MCL tear leads to valgus laxity in flexion, while additional injury to the secondary valgus restraints (PMC or ACL) leads to increased laxity in extension.

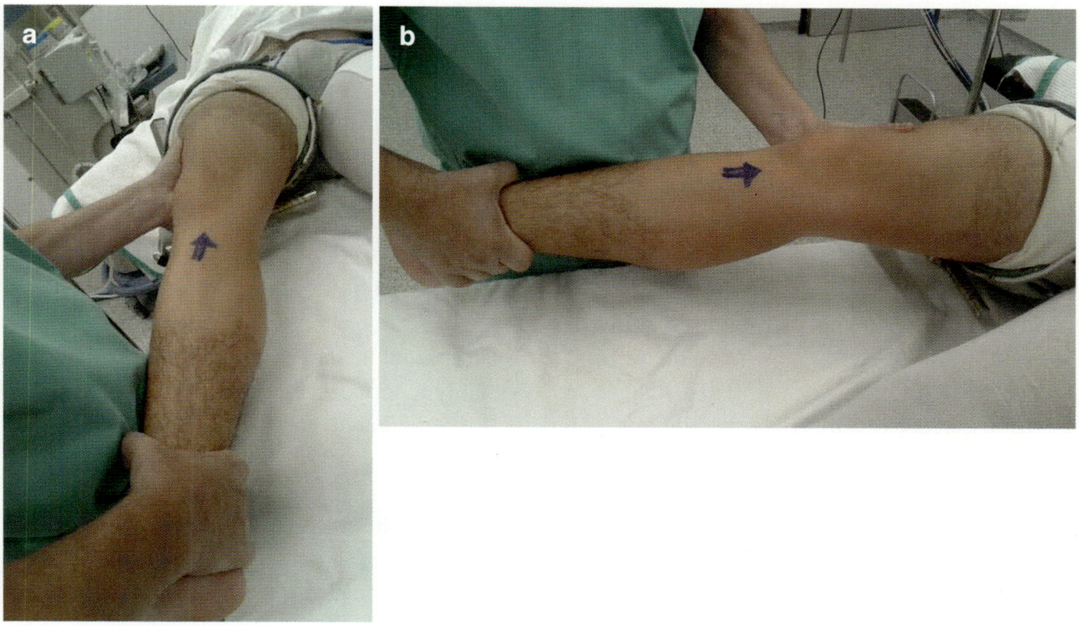

Fig. 15.3 The examination for medial collateral ligament injury. Valgus stress testing at (**a**) 0° and (**b**) 30° of knee flexion estimates the amount of laxity (Photo from Prof. Georgoulis ad archives)

15.2.3 Diagnosis

The mechanism of injury includes either contact valgus stress on the knee such as after a lateral blow to the lower thigh or upper leg or noncontact valgus stress with or without a rotational component, for example, during cutting maneuvers when an athlete plants his/her foot and then forcefully shifts directions [23]. There is pain and swelling at the site of MCL, but not knee joint swelling. If this occurs other concomitant ligamentous injuries may be suspected (ACL, PCL). The ability to walk may be impaired. Valgus stress testing at 0–30° of knee flexion estimates the amount of laxity (Fig. 15.3). At 30° of knee flexion, a grade I injury is <5 mm of medial joint opening, grade II is 5–10 mm of laxity, and grade III is >10 mm. Any laxity at 0° is indicative of associated injuries such as a cruciate tear or a posteromedial capsular injury. The location of the MCL injury refers to femoral avulsion, tibial avulsion, or midsubstance tear. Complete tibial-sided MCL tears (tears that involve both the deep and the superficial components) often do not heal. Plain radiographs may show a bony avulsion or an osteochondral fragment that could alter the treatment plan. MRI often provides significant data that assist in treatment of an MCL injury: the severity and location of the MCL tear and any associated cruciate ligament, meniscal, or capsular damage.

15.2.4 Treatment

Treatment recommendations are based on the severity, location, and chronicity of the MCL injury, as well as concomitant knee injuries.

15.2.4.1 Acute Isolated MCL Injury (<3 weeks)

Isolated grade I and II injuries are treated with nonoperative management with protected weight bearing, reestablishment of range of motion, and use of hinged bracing to avoid further valgus strain [25]. After 1–2 weeks for grade I and

2–4 weeks for grade II injuries, most patients return to sport [26–28].

For treatment of grade III (complete) isolated MCL injury, both nonoperative and operative treatments have been advocated with no subjective or objective differences between the two methods [29, 30]. Due to the lower complication rate and especially arthrofibrosis after nonoperative treatment, this is initially applied for complete tears. Most patients may require 6–12 weeks to return to sport after nonoperative treatment.

For MCL injuries with tibial-sided or bony avulsions, acute repair has been indicated [31], although it has also been proposed to follow closely the tibial-sided avulsions to assess healing and the need for operative repair. Operative repair should be considered if there is medial laxity still present after a trial of rehabilitation.

15.2.4.2 Combined MCL and Cruciate Ligament Injuries

For MCL injuries with combined ACL or PCL injuries, the optimal perspective is to evaluate each injury individually to determine the treatment plan. The general principle is a nonoperative treatment of the MCL with the delayed treatment of the ACL once the MCL is healed [32, 33]. In case of grade III MCL injuries and especially tibial avulsion injuries, operative repair should be considered if there is medial laxity still present after a trial of 4–6 weeks of rehabilitation. Once ACL surgery is initiated, examination under anesthesia will show if any valgus laxity persists, suggesting that cruciate ligament reconstruction along with MCL repair or reconstruction should be performed [34].

15.2.4.3 Chronic MCL Injuries (>6 weeks)

Chronic MCL injury that leads to chronic MCL instability may be caused either from a grade III or a tibial-sided avulsion MCL injury that failed to heal [35]. Indications for operative reconstruction include inability to participate in athletic activities. Although every effort is made to primarily repair the MCL scarring tissue does not allow to identify the torn edges, MCL reconstruction with either semitendinosus or hamstrings autograft or allograft tendon is performed [36].

15.3 Posterior Cruciate Ligament Injuries

The reported incidence of PCL injuries has been variably reported to range from 3 to 20% even up to 44% of all acute knee injuries [37–39].

15.3.1 Anatomy

The PCL originates on the posterior surface of the tibia and passes superiorly and anteromedially to insert on the lateral wall of the medial femoral condyle. It has an average width of 13 mm and length of 38 mm, and it is fan-shaped, being narrowest in the midportion and fanning out superiorly and, in a lesser extent, inferiorly. The PCL consists of a larger anterior band which is taut in flexion and relaxed in extension and a smaller posterior band which is taut in extension and relaxed in flexion.

15.3.2 Biomechanics and Function

The PCL is the strongest of the two cruciate ligaments in the knee and accounts for about 95% of the total restrain to posterior translation of the tibia in regard to the femur [40]. Secondary stabilizing functions are to restraint rotation when the knee is flexed, varus and valgus movement when the knee is extended, and restraint also overextension and hyperflexion [41, 42]. The main function of PCL (the resistance to posterior tibial translation) is also performed by other structures which are secondary stabilizers. These include the meniscofemoral ligaments and the posterolateral and posteromedial structures.

15.3.3 Mechanism of Injury

American football and football are among the most important sports activities leading to a PCL injury [43]. In football, the goalkeeper is most exposed to this type of injury [44]. The possible mechanisms of injury include:

(1) A posteriorly directed force on the upper front of flexed knee. During american football or football, a blow to the anterior surface of proximal tibia forces the tibia posteriorly and causes a PCL tear
(2) Fall on a flexed knee while the foot is in plantar flexion
(3) Knee hyperflexion while the foot is in dorsiflexion
(4) Sudden hyperextension

15.3.4 Associated Lesions

Isolated PCL injuries are not uncommon and have been estimated from 7% up to 47%, although the injury is most commonly associated with other ligamentous injuries [44–46]. The most commonly injured structure along with a PCL injury is the posterolateral corner (PLC), resulting in posterolateral rotatory instability (PLRI) [47, 48]. Associated meniscal or cartilage lesions may be found along with either an isolated PCL injury [49, 50] or when other ligament injuries exist along with the PCL rupture [46].

15.3.5 Diagnosis

Patients may present effusion, pain in the back of the knee, or pain with flexion beyond 90° or during kneeling. Instability is presented usually with combined PCL/PLC injuries rather than after an isolated PCL rupture. In general, the effusion and the pain are less than with an ACL injury. The clinical tests that indicate a PCL injury include:

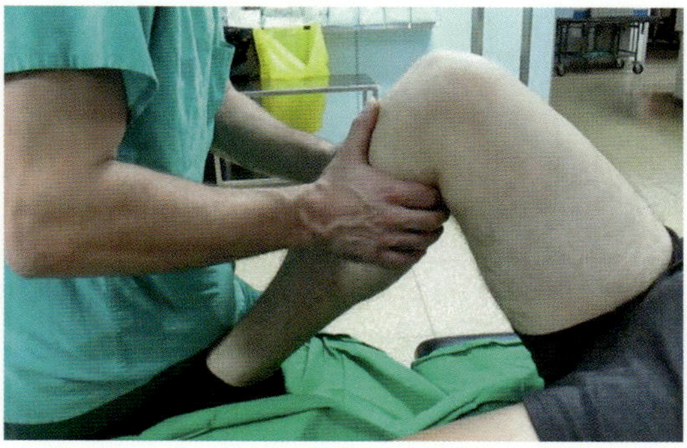

Fig. 15.4 Posterior drawer test. The biomechanical basis for this test is that the maximum posterior tibial translation occurs between 70 and 90° of knee flexion with PCL deficiency (Photo from E-writing "orthopaedics" for medical students' lessons, 2nd Department of Orthopaedics, Aristotelion University of Thessaloniki)

(a). The posterior drawer test with high sensitivity and specificity (90–99%) [51]. The biomechanical basis for this test is that the maximum posterior tibial translation occurs between 70 and 90° of knee flexion with PCL deficiency (Fig. 15.4)
(b). The step-off test is performed with the knee flexed at 90°. At this position, the medial tibial plateau normally lies approximately 1 cm anterior to the medial femoral condyle. This starting position, or step-off, is usually reduced in the PCL-deficient knee
(c). The posterior sag test
(d). The quadriceps active test

The posterior translation is graded according to the amount of posterior subluxation of the tibia. Tibial translation between 1 and 5 mm is considered a grade I injury. A grade II injury exists when posterior tibial translation is between 5 and 10 mm, and a grade III injury is seen when the tibia translates greater than 10 mm posterior to the femoral condyles.

Other clinical tests include:

(a) The Whipple-Ellis test
(b) The dynamic posterior shift test [52]

(c) The reverse pivot shift test helps identify posterolateral rotatory instability due to associated injuries of posterolateral structures
(d) The external rotation thigh-foot angle test

Instrumental devices such as the KT-1000 (MEDmetric) or rolimeter (AirCast) have been developed in order to accurately measure the posterior tibial translation [53] although these are less accurate for detecting PCL insufficiency than ACL deficiency [54].

15.3.6 Natural History

Compared to the ACL, the PCL can heal spontaneously given its abundant blood supply from the branch of the middle genicular artery and the superficial synovial layer by which is covered [38, 55–57].

15.3.7 Treatment

Nonoperative management with aggressive rehabilitation is proposed for acute grade I–II isolated PCL injuries. Conservative treatment includes a brace for 2–6 weeks and functional rehabilitation with special emphasis to quadriceps strengthening. On the other hand, surgery is recommended in patients with grade III injuries, symptomatic grade II injuries, chronic symptomatic isolated PCL lesions, and multi-ligament injuries. Arthroscopically assisted techniques are most commonly used to perform PCL reconstruction. The most commonly used grafts are patellar or quadriceps tendon autografts and Achilles tendon allografts for PCL reconstruction or hamstring tendons for PCL augmentation techniques.

For chronic posterior knee instability, some general rules for the PCL surgery are:

(1) One should not operate on a fixed posterior drawer (drawer which cannot be reduced manually) [58]
(2) The torn PCL must be only reconstructed and not repaired
(3) All the components of the instability must be corrected
(4) The reconstruction must be followed by specific rehabilitation protocols

The principal factors to be considered before surgery include graft selection, one- or two-bundle technique, drilling of a tibial tunnel, or use of a tibial inlay fixation. Also other factors are treatment of combined instabilities and necessity to perform a high tibial valgus osteotomy (HTO) [59].

15.4 Lateral Collateral Ligament Injuries and Posterior Lateral Instability

15.4.1 Anatomy and Biomechanics

The lateral collateral ligament (LCL) is the primary static restraint to varus opening of the knee [60]. The LCL inserts at femur proximal and posterior to the lateral epicondyle in a small depression between the lateral epicondyle and the supracondylar process and distally at the fibular head 8 mm posterior to the most anterior aspect of the fibular head [61, 62]. The posterior lateral corner (PLC) of the knee consists of various anatomic structures that include the iliotibial tract, LCL, popliteus tendon complex (the muscle-tendon unit and the ligamentous connections from the tendon to the proximal fibula, tibia, and meniscus), popliteofibular ligament (PFL), the biceps tendon, and the posterolateral capsule [63, 64]. The primary function of the PLC is to resist varus rotation, external tibial rotation, and posterior tibial translation [60, 65]. It should be noted that the PLC, not the PCL, is the primary restraint to posterior tibial translation near full knee extension [65].

15.4.2 Diagnosis

The LCL is most commonly injured in combination with one of the cruciate ligaments. The mechanism of injury is usually hyperextension in combination with a varus loading of the knee. Mechanisms of PLC injury include a posterolaterally directed blow to the anteromedial proximal tibia with resultant hyperextension, a noncontact hyperextension and external rotation twisting injury, direct blow to a flexed knee, or high-energy trauma [63]. PLC injuries rarely occur in isolation. They are often accompanied by other ligamentous injuries, especially PCL injury [63]. The term posterolateral rotatory instability is used to describe posterior subluxation of the lateral tibial plateau that can occur with an external rotation torque in knees with pathologic laxity of the PLC [66].

The clinical tests include the varus stress test and external rotation tests. For the former varus stress test is applied with the knee flexed at 30°. Up to 5 mm of laxity indicates LCL injury. Varus opening of 5–10 mm indicates combined LCL and popliteus injury, and more than 10 mm indicates LCL, popliteus, and ACL or PCL injury. In these cases there is also instability in the extended knee. The external rotation tests include the posterolateral drawer test, the reverse pivot shift test, the external rotation recurvatum test, and the dial or posterolateral rotation test. All allow detecting injury of the PLC complex. For the reverse pivot shift test, it should be noted that it may be positive in 35% of normal knees.

The most commonly used classification system defines injury severity based primarily on varus instability. Grade I injuries are sprains with little or no varus instability (0–5 mm opening). Grade II injuries are partial injuries with moderate laxity (6–10 mm). Grade III injuries are complete injuries with significant laxity (>10 mm). Rotational instability is then defined by the dial test, with instability defined as an increase in external tibial rotation of 10° compared with that of the contralateral knee. Since PLC injuries may have significant rotational instability with minimal varus instability, some authors proposed a grading system that combines both varus and rotational instability [1]. According to this grade I injuries have minimal instability (either varus or rotational instability of 0–5 mm or 0–5°), grade II injuries have moderate instability (6–10 mm or 6–10°), and grade III injuries have significant instability (>10 mm or >10°). It is important to note that as with all PLC classification systems, this system has not been validated.

Standard radiographs may either be normal or show avulsion or tibial plateau fractures. MRI is always indicated in order to elucidate complex PLC anatomy.

15.4.3 Treatment

In general grade III LCL injuries are treated surgically, whereas grade I and grade II injuries are treated nonoperatively. For athletes who have acute injuries of the posterolateral structures and posterolateral rotatory instability, surgical treatment within 2 weeks is widely recommended before significant capsular scarring occurs. This can be done by direct repair, with or without augmentation, or by primary reconstruction. There has been a recent trend, however, toward more nearly anatomic reconstruction, with attention paid to proper insertion site anatomy in order to restore native knee kinematics as well as possible [26]. Avulsion injuries are best treated with either rigid internal fixation or sutures, depending on the nature of the avulsion [63]. In case of combined acute injuries, an attempt should be made to address all concomitant injuries at the same setting, taking also in consideration the possible risk of arthrofibrosis [67]. In the chronic injuries of the posterolateral structures, reconstructive procedures are usually necessary. The operations that have been described include a proximal advancement of the posterolateral structures [68], biceps tenodesis [69], and reconstruction of the LCL [70, 71], PFL, or popliteotibial ligament [72, 73]. A variety of autografts or allografts have been employed for this purpose.

15.5 Knee Dislocation

Dislocation of femorotibial joint requires major trauma and may occasionally occur during sports. It is considered an orthopedic emergency because blood vessel injury may occur in 30% of these injuries. Also nerve injuries are not uncommon.

The dislocation has to be reduced immediately, and close estimation of blood supply should be done for the first days. Depending on the direction of dislocation, several ligaments of the knee may be injured. Both ACL and PCL may be torn along with LCL and posterolateral structures or MCL. Operative treatment for athletes should be performed within 2 weeks when collateral ligament and PLC structures may be repaired, while ACL and PCL may be reconstructed later. When the patient's condition does not allow early operative treatment, reconstruction may be performed later and the sequence of reconstruction should be PCL, ACL, PLC, LCL, MCL, and others (e.g., extensor mechanism, iliotibial band (ITB), biceps tendon). Most athletes face difficulty in returning to prior activity level. When possible, return to play occurs within 9–12 months.

References

1. Duthon VB, Barea C, Abrassart S, Fasel JH, Fritschy D, Menetrey J. Anatomy of the anterior cruciate ligament. Knee Surg Sports Traumatol Arthrosc. 2006;14:204–13.
2. Petersen W, Tillmann B. Anatomy and function of the anterior cruciate ligament. Orthopaede. 2002;31:710–8.
3. Girgis FG, Marshall JL, Monajem A. The cruciate ligaments of the knee joint. Anatomical, functional and experimental analysis. Clin Orthop. 1975;106:216–31.
4. Beynnon BD, Johnson RJ, Abate JA, Fleming BC, Nichols CE. Treatment of anterior cruciate ligament injuries. Part I Am J Sports Med. 2005;33:1579–602.
5. Arendt A, Dick R. Knee injury patterns among men and women in collegiate basketball and soccer. Am J Sports Med. 1995;23:694–701.
6. Boden BP, Dean GS, Feagin Jr JA, Garrett Jr WE. Mechanisms of anterior cruciate ligament injury. Orthopedics. 2000;23:573–8.
7. Cochrane JL, Lloyd DG, Buttfield A, Seward H, McGivern J. Characteristics of anterior cruciate ligament injures in Australian Football. J Sci Med Sport. 2007;10:96–104.
8. Prodromos CM, Brown C, Fu FH, Georgoulis AD, Gobbi A, Howell SM, Johnson D, Paulos LE, Shelbourne KD. The anterior cruciate ligament: reconstruction and basic science. Philadelphia: Elsevier/Saunders; 2008.
9. Soucacos PN, Papadopoulou M, Georgoulis A. The "Noulis" behind the Lachman test. Arthroscopy. 1998;14:75–6.
10. Canale ST, Beaty JH. Campbell's operative orthopaedics. 12th ed. Elsevier, Philadelphia. 2013.
11. Zantop T, Petersen W, Sekiya JK, Musahl V, Fu FH. Anterior cruciate ligament anatomy and function relating to anatomical reconstruction. Knee Surg Sports Traumatol Arthrosc. 2006;14:982–92.
12. Stergiou N, Ristanis S, Moraiti C, Georgoulis A. Tibial rotation in anterior cruciate ligament (ACL)-deficient and ACL-reconstructed knees: a theoretical proposition for the development of osteoarthritis. Sports Med. 2007;37:601–13.
13. Karlsson J, Irrgang JJ, van Eck CF, Samuelsson K, Mejia HA, Fu FH. Anatomic single- and double-bundle anterior cruciate ligament reconstruction, part 2: clinical application of surgical technique. Am J Sports Med. 2011;39:2016–26.
14. Kondo E, Yasuda K, Azuma H, Tanabe Y, Yagi T. Prospective clinical comparisons of anatomic double bundle versus single-bundle anterior cruciate ligament reconstruction procedures in 328 consecutive patients. Am J Sports Med. 2008;36:1675–87.
15. Muneta T, Koga H, Mochizuki T, Ju YJ, Hara K, Nimura A, Yaqishita K, Sekiya I. A prospective randomized study of 4-strand semitendinosus tendon anterior cruciate ligament reconstruction comparing single-bundle and double-bundle techniques. Arthroscopy. 2007;23:618–28.
16. Beynnon BD, Johnson RJ, Fleming BC, Kannus P, Kaplan M, Samani J, Renstrom P. Anterior cruciate ligament replacement: comparison of bone patellar tendon-bone grafts with two-strand hamstring grafts. A prospective, randomized study. J Bone Joint Surg Am. 2002;84:1503–13.
17. Siebold R, Ellert T, Metz S, Metz J. Tibial insertions of the anteromedial and posterolateral bundles of the anterior cruciate ligament: morphometry, arthroscopic landmarks, and orientation model for bone tunnel placement. Arthroscopy. 2008;24:154–61.
18. Siebold R, Ellert T, Metz S, Metz J. Femoral insertions of the anteromedial and posterolateral bundles of the anterior cruciate ligament: morphometry and arthroscopic orientation models for double-bundle bone tunnel placement. A cadaver study. Arthroscopy. 2008;24:585–92.
19. LaPrade RF. The medial collateral ligament complex and the posterolateral aspect of the knee. In: Arendt EA, editor. Orthopaedic knowledge update. Sports medicine 2. Rosemont: American Academy of Orthopaedic Surgeons; 1999. p. 327–40.
20. LaPrade RF, Engebretsen AH, Ly TV, Johansen S, Wentorf FA, Engebretsen L. The anatomy of the medial part of the knee. J Bone Joint Surg Am. 2007;89:2000–10.
21. Warren RF, Marshall JL. The supporting structures and layers on the medial side of the knee: an anatomical analysis. J Bone Joint Surg Am. 1979;61:56–62.
22. Warren RF, Marshall JL, Girgis F. The prime static stabilizer of the medial side of the knee. J Bone Joint Surg Am. 1974;56:665–74.

23. Indelicato PA. Isolated medial collateral ligament injuries in the knee. J Am Acad Orthop Surg. 1995;3:9–14.
24. Grood ES, Noyes FR, Butler DL, Suntay WJ. Ligamentous and capsular restraints preventing straight medial and lateral laxity in intact human cadaver knees. J Bone Joint Surg Am. 1981;63:1257–69.
25. Kannus P. Long-term results of conservatively treated medial collateral ligament injuries of the knee joint. Clin Orthop Relat Res. 1988;226:103–12.
26. Master techniques in orthopaedic surgery: sports medicine. FH Fu, LWW. Philadelphia. 2010.
27. Derscheid GL, Garrick JG. Medial collateral ligament injuries in football. Nonoperative management of grade I and grade II sprains. Am J Sports Med. 1981;9:365–8.
28. Chen L, Kim PD, Ahmad CS, Levine WN. Medial collateral ligament injuries of the knee: current treatment concepts. Curr Rev Muscoskelet Med. 2008;1:108–13.
29. Indelicato PA. Non-operative treatment of complete tears of the medial collateral ligament of the knee. J Bone Joint Surg Am. 1983;65:323–9.
30. Reider B, Sathy MR, Talkington J, Blyznak N, Kollias S. Treatment of isolated medial collateral ligament injuries in athletes with early functional rehabilitation. A five year follow-up study. Am J Sports Med. 1994;22:470–7.
31. Wilson TC, Satterfield WH, Johnson DL. Medial collateral ligament "tibial" injuries: indication for acute repair. Orthopedics. 2004;27:389–93.
32. Petersen W, Laprell H. Combined injuries of the medial collateral ligament and the anterior cruciate ligament. Early ACL reconstruction versus late ACL reconstruction. Arch Orthop Trauma Surg. 1999;119:258–62.
33. Halinen J, Lindahl J, Hirvensalo E, Santavirta S. Operative and nonoperative treatments of medial collateral ligament rupture with early anterior cruciate ligament reconstruction: a prospective randomized study. Am J Sports Med. 2006;34:1134–40.
34. Edson CJ. Conservative and postoperative rehabilitation of isolated and combined injuries of the medial collateral ligament. Sports Med Arthrosc. 2006;14:105–10.
35. Robins AJ, Newman AP, Burks RT. Postoperative return of motion in anterior cruciate ligament and medial collateral ligament injuries. The effect of medial collateral ligament rupture location. Am J Sports Med. 1993;21:20–5.
36. Yoshiya S, Kuroda R, Mizuno K, Yamamoto T, Kurosaka M. Medial collateral ligament reconstruction using autogenous hamstring tendons: technique and results in initial cases. Am J Sports Med. 2005;33:1380–5.
37. Chen CH, Chuang TY, Wang KC, Chen WJ, Shih CH. Arthroscopic posterior cruciate ligament reconstruction with hamstring tendon autograft: results with a minimum 4-year follow-up. Knee Surg Sports Traumatol Arthrosc. 2006;14:1045–54.
38. Shelbourne KD, Jennings RW, Vahey TN. Magnetic resonance imaging of posterior cruciate ligament injuries: assessment of healing. Am J Knee Surg. 1999;12:209–13.
39. Fanelli GC, Edson CJ. Posterior cruciate ligament injuries in trauma patients. II Arthroscopy. 1995;11:526–9.
40. Kannus P, Bergfeld J, Jarvinen M, Johnson RJ, Pope M, Renstrom P, Yasuda K. Injuries to the posterior cruciate ligament of the knee. Sports Med. 1991;12:110–31.
41. Kennedy NI, LaPrade RF, Goldsmith MT, Faucett SC, Rasmussen MT, Coatney GA, Engebretsen L, Wijdicks CA. Posterior cruciate ligament graft fixation angles, part 1: biomechanical evaluation for anatomic single-bundle reconstruction. Am J Sports Med. 2014;42:2338–45.
42. Malone AA, Dowd GS, Saifuddin A. Injuries of the posterior cruciate ligament and posterolateral corner of the knee. Injury. 2006;37:485–501.
43. Barrett GR, Savoie FH. Operative management of acute PCL injuries with associated pathology: long-term results. Orthopedics. 1991;14:687–92.
44. Schulz MS, Russe K, Weiler A, Eichhorn HJ, Strobel MJ. Epidemiology of posterior cruciate ligament injuries. Arch Orthop Trauma Surg. 2003;123:186–91.
45. Fanelli GC. Posterior cruciate ligament injuries in trauma patients. Arthroscopy. 1993;9:291–4.
46. Owesen C, Sandven-Thrane S, Lind M, et al. Epidemiology of surgically treated posterior cruciate ligament injuries in Scandinavia. Knee Surg Sports Traumatol Arthrosc (2015). doi:10.1007/s00167-015-3786-2.
47. Lee KH, Jung YB, Jung HJ, Jang EC, Song KS, Kim JY, Lee SH. Combined posterolateral corner reconstruction with remnant tensioning and augmentation in chronic posterior cruciate ligament injuries: minimum 2-year follow-up. Arthroscopy. 2011;27:507–15.
48. Veltri DM, Deng XH, Torzilli PA, Maynard MJ, Warren RF. The role of the popliteofibular ligament in stability of the human knee. A biomechanical study. Am J Sports Med. 1996;24:19–27.
49. Aroen A, Sivertsen EA, Owesen C, Engebretsen L, Granan LP. An isolated rupture of the posterior cruciate ligament results in reduced preoperative knee function in comparison with an anterior cruciate ligament injury. Knee Surg Sports Traumatol Arthrosc. 2013;21:1017–22.
50. Geissler WB, Whipple TL. Intraarticular abnormalities in association with posterior cruciate ligament injuries. Am J Sports Med. 1993;21:846–9.
51. Rubinstein Jr RA, Shelbourne KD, McCarroll JR, VanMeter CD, Rettig AC. The accuracy of the clinical examination in the setting of posterior cruciate ligament injuries. Am J Sports Med. 1994;22:550–7.

52. Shelbourne KD, Benedict F, McCarrol J, Rettig AC. Dynamic posterior shift test. Am J Sports Med. 1989;17:275–7.
53. Daniel DM, Stone ML, Barnett P, Sachs R. Use of the quadriceps active test to diagnose posterior cruciate – ligament disruption and measure posterior laxity of the knee. J Bone Joint Surg Am. 1988;70:386–91.
54. Huber FE, Irrgang JJ, Harner C, Lephart S. Intratester and intertester reliability of the KT-1000 arthrometer in the assessment of posterior laxity of the knee. Am J Sports Med. 1997;25:479–85.
55. Tewes DP, Fritts HM, Fields RD, Quick DC, Buss DD. Chronically injured posterior cruciate ligament: magnetic resonance imaging. Clin Orthop Relat Res. 1997;335:224–32.
56. Jung YB, Jung HJ, Song KS, Kim JY, Lee HJ, Lee JS. Remnant posterior cruciate ligament-augmenting stent procedure for injuries in the acute or subacute stage. Arthroscopy. 2010;26:223–9.
57. Bray RC, Leonard CA, Salo PT. Vascular physiology and long-term healing of partial ligament tears. J Orthop Res. 2002;20:984–9.
58. Strobel MJ, Weiler A, Schultz MS, Russe K, Eichhorn HJ. Fixed posterior subluxation in posterior cruciate ligament-deficient knees. Diagnosis and treatment of a new clinical sign. Am J Sports Med. 2002;30:32–8.
59. Christel P. Basic principles for surgical reconstruction of the PCL in chronic posterior knee instability. Knee Surg Sports Traumatol Arthrosc. 2003;11:289–96.
60. Gollehon DL, Torzilli PA, Warren RF. The role of the posterolateral and cruciate ligaments in the stability of the human knee: a biomechanical study. J Bone Joint Surg Am. 1987;69:233–42.
61. Brinkman JM, Schwering PJ, Blankevoort L, Kooloos JG, Luites J, Wymenga AB. The insertion geometry of the posterolateral corner of the knee. J Bone Joint Surg Br. 2005;87:1364–8.
62. Laprade RF, Ly TV, Wentorf FA, Engebretsen L. The posterolateral attachments of the knee. a qualitative and quantitative morphologic analysis of the fibular collateral ligament, popliteus tendon, popliteofibular ligament, and lateral gastrocnemius tendon. Am J Sports Med. 2003;31:854–60.
63. Ranawat AS, Baker III CL, Henry S, Harner CD. Posterolateral corner injury of the knee: evaluation and management. J Am Acad Orthop Surg. 2008;16:506–18.
64. Simonian PT, Sussmann PS, van Trommel M, Wickiewicz TL, Warren RF. Popliteomeniscal fasciculi and lateral meniscal stability. Am J Sports Med. 1997;25:849–53.
65. Grood ES, Stowers SF, Noyes FR. Limits of movement in the human knee: effect of sectioning the posterior cruciate ligament and posterolateral structures. J Bone Joint Surg Am. 1988;70:88–97.
66. Covey DC. Injuries of the posterolateral corner of the knee. J Bone Joint Surg Am. 2001;83:106–18.
67. Harner CD, Waltrip RL, Bennett CH, Francis KA, Cole B, Irrgang JJ. Surgical management of knee dislocations. J Bone Joint Surg Am. 2004;86:262–73.
68. Hughston JC, Jacobson KE. Chronic posterolateral rotatory instability of the knee. J Bone Joint Surg Am. 1985;67:351–9.
69. Clancy WG, Martin SD. Posterolateral instability of the knee: treatment using the Clancy biceps femoris tenodesis. Operative techniques in sports medicine. Oper Techn Sports Med. 1996;4:182–91.
70. Latimer HA, Tibone JE, ElAttrache NS, McMahon PJ. Reconstruction of the lateral collateral ligament of the knee with patellar tendon allograft. Report of a new technique in combined ligament injuries. Am J Sports Med. 1998;26:656–62.
71. Noyes FR, Barber-Westin SD. Surgical restoration to treat chronic deficiency of the posterolateral complex and cruciate ligaments of the knee joint. Am J Sports Med. 1996;24:415–26.
72. Larson RV. Anatomy and management of posterolateral corner injuries. Instructional course lecture, 67th AAOS Meeting, March, Orlando, Florida; 2000.
73. Veltri D, Warren RF. Posterolateral instability of the knee. J Bone Joint Surg Am. 1994;7:460.

Patellofemoral Pain and Instability

16

Ana Leal, Paulo Flores, Filipe Silva,
Elizabeth Arendt, Philippe Neyret,
and João Espregueira-Mendes

Contents

16.1 Anatomy, Biomechanics, and Mechanism of Injury

The patella is the largest sesamoid bone of the human body. It is enfolded by the quadriceps and patellar tendons which connect, respectively, to the quadriceps muscle and to the lower leg bone (tibia), composing the quadriceps mechanism. Along with its counterpart, the trochlear groove of the femur (also known as trochlea) constitutes together the patellofemoral joint – (Fig. 16.1) [1–4].

As an integral part of the knee, the patellofemoral joint is one of the most structurally complex articulations with high functional and

A. Leal (✉)
Clínica do Dragão, Espregueira-Mendes Sports Centre, FIFA Medical Centre of Excellence, Porto, Portugal

Dom Henrique Research Centre, Porto, Portugal

CMEMS Center for MicroElectroMechanical Systems, Mechanical Engineering Department, University of Minho, Guimarães, Portugal
e-mail: aleal@espregueira.com; aleal@dem.uminho.pt

P. Flores • F. Silva
CMEMS Center for MicroElectroMechanical Systems, Mechanical Engineering Department, University of Minho, Guimarães, Portugal
e-mail: pflores@dem.uminho.pt; fsamuel@dem.uminho.pt

E. Arendt
University of Minnesota Medical Center, Minneapolis, MN, USA
e-mail: arend001@umn.edu

P. Neyret
Centre Albert Trillat, Lyon, France
e-mail: philippe.neyret@chu-lyon.fr

J. Espregueira-Mendes
Clínica do Dragão, Espregueira-Mendes Sports Centre, FIFA Medical Centre of Excellence, Porto, Portugal

Dom Henrique Research Centre, Porto, Portugal

3B's Research Group – Biomaterials, Biodegradables and Biomimetics, University Minho, AvePark, S. Cláudio de Barco, 4806-909 Taipas, Guimarães, Portugal

ICVS/3B's – PT Government Associated Laboratory, Braga, Portugal

Orthopedic Department, Minho University, Braga, Portugal
e-mail: jem@espregueira.com

J. Espregueira-Mendes et al. (eds.), *Injuries and Health Problems in Football*,
DOI 10.1007/978-3-662-53924-8_16

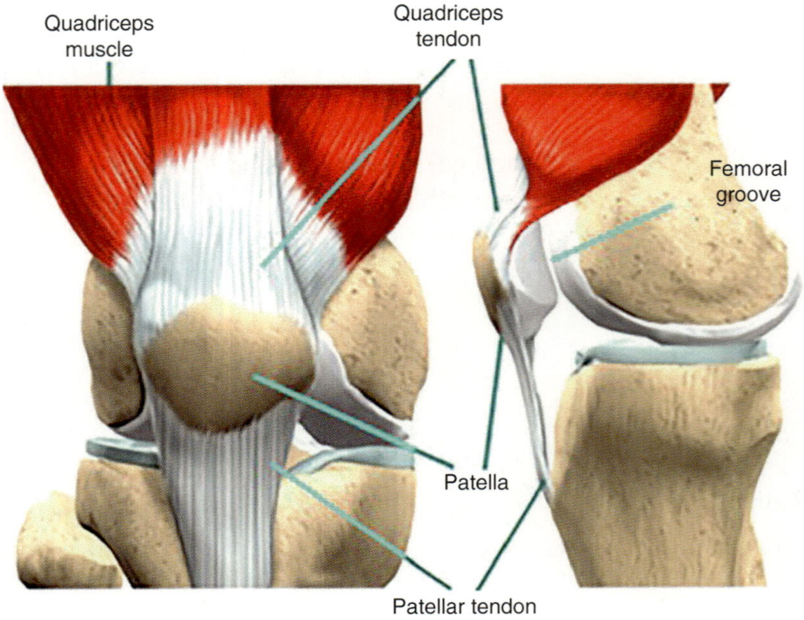

Fig. 16.1 Patellofemoral joint structure – adapted from [3]

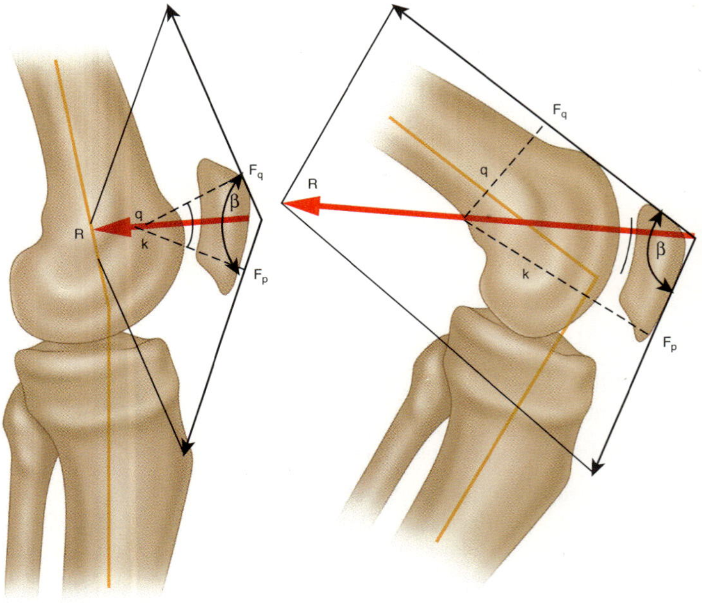

Fig. 16.2 Representation of the increasing of the patellar tendon moment arm [6]

biomechanical requirements. The biomechanical structure of this joint, along with its soft tissue complex, is able to withstand compression and tension forces (e.g., releasing the tension around the femur, by transmitting these forces to the patellar tendon), playing a major role to the flexion and extension movements of the knee. Thus, the patella acts as a biological lever arm transmitting the force of the quadriceps muscles to centralize the divergent forces. This mechanism improves the knee extension effectiveness by increasing the moment arm of the patellar tendon (Fig. 16.2). Complementarily, patella has an aesthetic

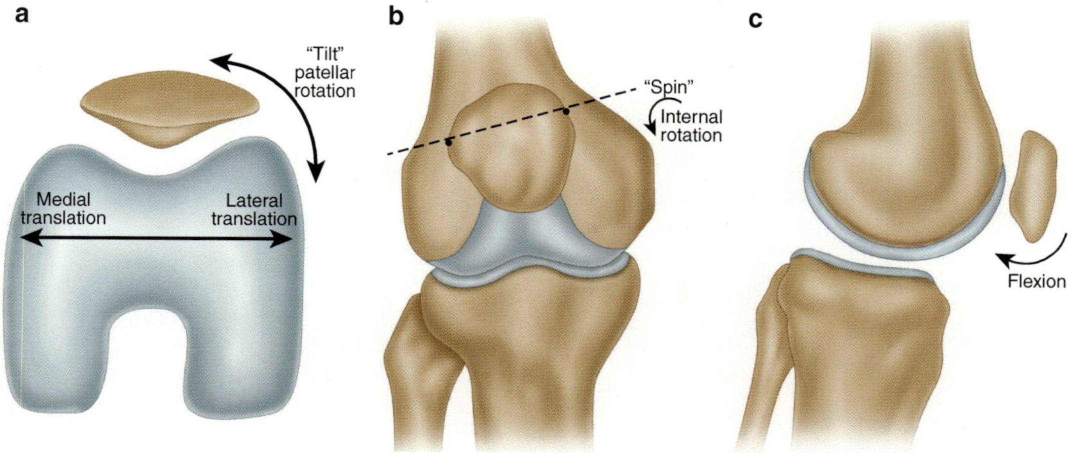

Fig. 16.3 Representation of the most relevant patellofemoral joint motion patterns: (**a**) medial-lateral translation and patellar tilt, on the axial plane; (**b**) internal and external rotation (also designated "spin"), on the coronal plane; (**c**) flexion and extension, on the sagittal plane – adapted from [7]

function for the human leg and forms a bony shield, protecting the tibiofemoral joint from direct trauma (external impacts and damage) [1, 4–6].

As a moveable osseous part, patella executes characteristic movements along the different anatomical plans of the human body (Fig. 16.3). In the axial plane, patellofemoral joint features medial-lateral translation, also called glide, and rotation, usually known as tilt. In the sagittal plane, rotation assumes the designation of flexion, and it detected a slight anterior-posterior translation. On the other hand, rotation in the coronal plane is commonly defined as spin. The fitting in the trochlear groove (at 20–30° knee flexion) is observed in this plane as well, although it is not described in the literature as a patellofemoral motion pattern. The patellofemoral joint movements depend on many factors such as the trochlear configuration, medial patellofemoral ligament (MPFL) efficiency, vastus medialis obliquus (VMO) strength, and the tibial internal rotation control (during flexion). In fact, well-developed muscles (the quadriceps and particularly the VMO) may aid the patellofemoral control and protect the joint from wear, preventing many causes of patellofemoral pain, specifically the ones related to the high athletic demands like in football [1, 5, 7].

Due to the large mobility of the patellofemoral joint (6 degrees of freedom), the contact facets of the patella are often subject to high contact loads. These contact stresses within the patellofemoral joint gradually increase with knee flexion (Fig. 16.4). For instance, a simple daily routine exercise of climbing stairs will reflect in a fourfold increase of the body weight on the patella. Along with this line, due to situations of maximum flexion (approximately 120°), where the tension increases up to sixfold the body weight, the patella is more susceptible to fracture. In this sense, the high torsional loads experienced in the football player's knee during several football maneuvers (such as pivoting or cutting) may predispose them to an early onset of patellofemoral lesions [1, 5, 6, 8].

Activities which increase the patellar compression, such as quadriceps contraction, will typically incite pain. In football, pain-inducing activities include running, kicking, landing from a jump, or falling on the knee. Out of the football field, the pain is typically experienced while kneeling, squatting, climbing stairs, or sitting with the knee flexed. Athletes may struggle with episodes of functional instability, described as collapsing or giving away of the knee, although some authors consider this

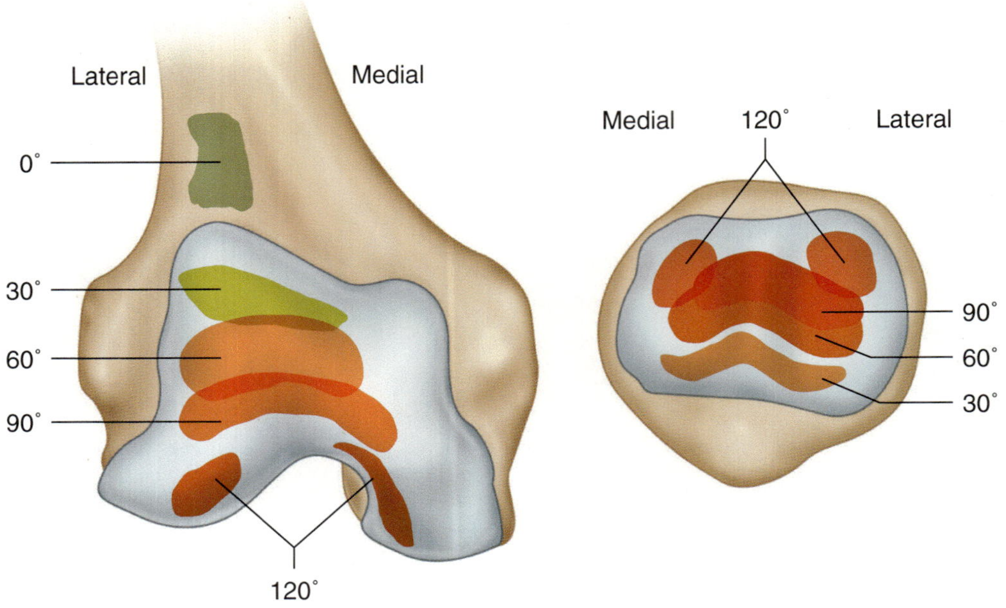

Fig. 16.4 Color gradient to represent different degrees of stress areas between the contact facets of the patellofemoral joint – adapted from [3]

dislocation of the patella as a "going out" movement of the knee. Usually, the patellofemoral symptomatology is triggered by contact forces within the knee joint. In the context of a football game, traumatic chondrosis of patellar or trochlear cartilage, or even patellar fracture, may occur due to direct trauma, as in the case of tumble on the knee. Despite the fact that the high level of training (strength or endurance, typical in elite levels) and competition may contribute to a proper neuromuscular control and muscular strength, it also can lead to a chronic overuse, often causing patellar chondrosis, as well as patellar or quadriceps tendinopathy. In this sense, other common football-related actions, such as running or kicking, may also contribute to the development of an overuse symptomatology. Scientific literature reports that higher knee abduction moments during landing are predisposing risk factors for both patellofemoral pain and anterior cruciate ligament (ACL) injuries and that these significantly greater force loading rates are verified in female football players, when compared to males [9, 10].

16.2 Etiopathogeny

Anatomical and physiological abnormalities of the patellofemoral joint may represent the cause for multiple clinical problems of the knee [1, 11]. Patellofemoral pain (also known as patellofemoral syndrome) and patellofemoral instability are the most common pathologies directly related to this joint. Four major risk factors were defined by Henri Dejour et al., in 1994, in order to characterize instability in patellofemoral problems [12]. The patellofemoral instability can be subdivided into different grades: firstly as potential instability, when it encompasses patellar subluxation; then objective instability, at least one episode of patellar dislocation has occurred; and designation of recurrent instability is applied when the patient has two or more episodes of dislocations, but there is no consensus on the terminology used worldwide [1, 4, 11, 13–20].

These pathologies often result from anatomical and biomechanical factors related to osseous and soft tissue abnormalities. In this line, four osseous abnormalities can be directly linked to the classical risk factors designated by the Lyon

School, as described in Table 16.1. Additionally, other factors related to soft tissue deficiencies can lead to instability of the patellofemoral joint, whose correlation and prevalence on patellofemoral problems have been studied: a torn MPFL, once is the most important medial stabilizer of the patella against the lateral translation; a weakened VMO that may result in significant decrease on the dynamic stabilization of the patella; an excessive femoral anteversion, which externally rotates the tibia and results in an increased quadriceps angle; an excessive tibial external rotation, which leads to a more lateralized position of the tibial tubercle, also increasing the quadriceps angle; a longer patellar tendon, increasing patellar height; as well as the patellar shape Wiberg type C – which has the facets more laterally than medially developed (medial hypoplasia), due to increased lateral stress, in association with tilt and trochlear dysplasia, affecting the articular congruency [5, 11–14, 17, 21].

Table 16.1 Lyon School classic risk factors for patellofemoral instability

Risk factor	Description
Trochlear dysplasia	Classification (Fig. 16.5) (**a**) Slight trochlear dysplasia with a concave groove – trochlear morphology preserved with a fairly shallow trochlea (**b**) Flat or convex trochlea (**c**) Asymmetry of the trochlear facets – lateral facet convex, medial facet hypoplastic (**d**) Asymmetry of the trochlea facets – vertical joint and cliff pattern
Tilt >20°	Excessive passive patellar external tilt, usually above 20° (Fig. 16.6**a**), due to quadriceps dysplasia
TT-TG ≥20 mm	Excessive distance between the tibial tubercle (TT) and the trochlear groove (TG), usually above 20 mm (Fig. 16.6**b**)
Patella *alta*	High ratio of the patellar tendon length (LT) by the patella length (LP): LT/LP > 1.2 (Fig. 16.6**c**)

16.3 Epidemiology

Regarding the epidemiological aspects, patellofemoral problems constitute one of the most common knee complaints and are more frequent among adolescents and young adults – which represent the most active population group representing a significant long-term socioeconomic burden. Usually, patellofemoral complaints are related to anterior knee pain, which make up about 20–40% of the total knee injuries, affecting up to one third of the young population. Women are known to have higher incidence and severity of the patellofemoral problems. In this sense, gender-specific, sociological, anatomical,

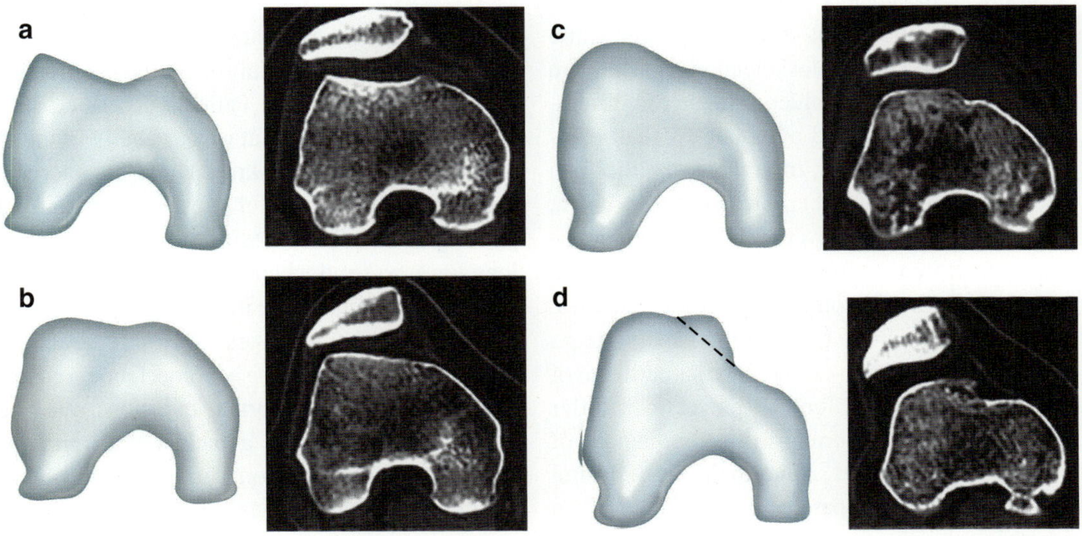

Fig. 16.5 Classification of trochlear dysplasia [16]

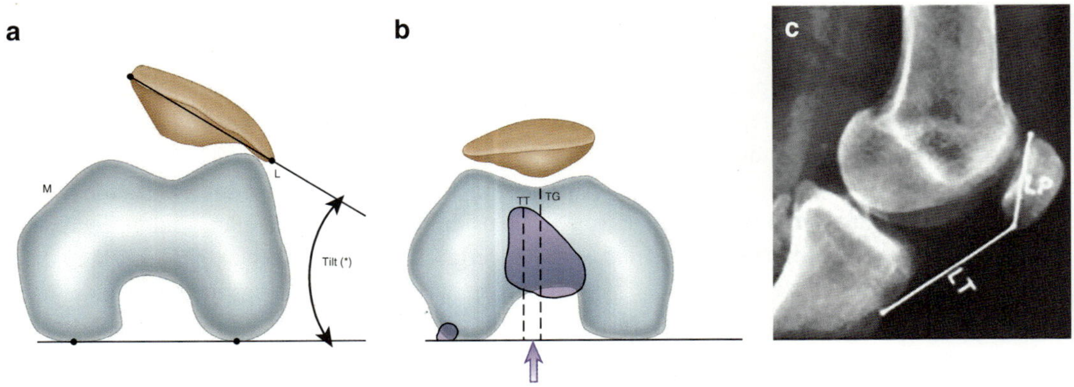

Fig. 16.6 Measurements in classic patellar instability risk factors: (**a**) patellar tilt, angle formed by lines joining the major transversal axis of the patella and the posterior femoral condyles [17]; (**b**) measurement of the true relationship of the tibial tubercle, TT, to the trochlear groove, TG, using the TT-TG distance [18]; (**c**) lateral radiograph of the knee shows the lines corresponding to patellar height ratio measurement [18]

and physiological factors might be contributing: abused high-heel wear and sitting with adducted legs, increased pelvic width and consequent excessive lateral pressure on the patella, and levels of estrogen. Both the athletic and nonathletic populations are propitious to this kind of pathology, although it is more common in the first one [3, 5, 12, 14, 19, 20].

Most recent studies state that, compared to multisport athletes, young females with early sport specialization represent a cohort with higher risk of anterior knee pain disorders, including patellofemoral pain, Osgood-Schlatter, and Sinding-Larsen-Johansson. Variations in anatomical parameters, such as patellofemoral morphology and joint stability, lower limb alignment, and musculoskeletal dysplasia, are known to have strong influence in the patellofemoral problems presented by young football players. Even at young age, these abnormalities can be so disabling that, when predisposed to them, football players may never reach the elite level – which in extreme cases, might even represent a career end. On the other hand, older athletes' injuries are often due to an overuse nature (e.g., erosion or breakdown of the articular cartilage of the patella). Besides, football players can suffer other kinds of injuries as consequence of patellofemoral-related abnormalities. Postural alterations, such as patellar malalignment, can increase the risk of traumaticorthopedic football injuries (particularly in women). This may be due to the compensatory deviations imposed to the other joints once the muscles are integrated with each other. Previous studies also identified other extrinsic (body movement, environmental conditions, shoe-surface interface, player position, and skill level) and intrinsic (joint laxity, limb alignment, notch dimensions, and ligament size) factors as possible causes to a higher rate of ACL injuries in female collegiate sports (basketball and football), compared to male [22–26].

16.4 Diagnosis

A comprehensive and accurate clinical history description plays a crucial role in the patellofemoral diagnostic process. Patients describe patellofemoral pain in different ways, usually trying to illustrate a deep anterior knee pain. Characteristic patellofemoral pain is felt, for instance, during prolonged knee flexed positions (while driving in long journeys) and when climbing or descending stairs. If the pain is more intense while exercising or afterward or if gets worse toward the evening, most probably it would be a biomechanical cause. Therefore, several important questions must be asked when evaluating a patient with anterior knee complaints: location, duration, and timing of symptoms; past clinical history; professional occupation; sports general; and specific history, among other specifications that will contribute to the analysis of previous events or complications that could be contributing to the patellofemoral complaints [13, 25].

Following the anamnesis, the physical examination of the joint is warranted. Nonetheless, there still exists inconsistencies on this topic due to lack of standardization. The exam is dependent on the clinician experience and beliefs. While assessing the patellofemoral joint, the clinician should focus the motion patterns described in Fig. 16.3, taking also into account other biomechanical and functional essential features: tight lateral retinaculum and iliotibial band, weak VMO, poor quadriceps control or endurance, abnormal hip rotation (version), excessive foot pronation, and limited flexibility of quadriceps, hamstrings, or gastrocnemius. Usually, assessment procedures may follow as described in Table 16.2. A wide range of outcome measures, scores, scales, and indexes are available in the literature to assess the patellofemoral joint. The sensitivity and specificity as well as the reliability and validity of these diagnostic and outcome assessment tools still remain unclear. In general, the majority of these tests are more use-

Table 16.2 Physical examination tests for patellofemoral joint evaluation

Test designation(s)	Test procedures	Indication(s) for diagnosis
Alignment of lower limb and extensor mechanism – Anthropometry		
Patella alignment	Observe the patient standing with the feet together, facing forward	Normal: patella face directly forward PF pain cases: patella squint or face inward, toward each other
Q angle	Measure the angle between – A line from the anterior superior iliac spine to the center of the patella – A line from the center of the tibial tubercle to the center of the patella	Normal: 15°
Foot posture	Examine the feet for evidence of overpronation or loss of medial longitudinal arch	Preexisting malalignments can be enhanced by the internal lower limb rotation, derived from foot deformity
Tubercle sulcus angle	Observe while the patient is in seated position	Normal: ≈80° males, ≈50° females
Dynamic patella tracking	Observe the patient in seated position during extension from 90° to full extension	Normal: patella moves proximally with slight lateral deviation at terminal extension PFI: greater lateral deviation
Palpation – Manual testing		
Prominence of VMO	Examine the VMO carefully, during the lower limb inspection	Asymmetry = atrophy (disease) Bilateral lack = dysplasia of the quadriceps mechanism
Patella glide	Push the patella, passively, medially, and laterally	Normal: maximum displacement is 10 mm in both directions PFI: higher risk related to hypermobility
Patella tilt	Lift the lateral facet of the patella from the femoral lateral condyle	Excessive lateral patellar syndrome is referred when pain in the lateral patellar facet and tenderness of the MPFL are observed
Apprehension test	While the patient is relaxed in supine position, with full extended knee, the clinician pushes the patella laterally as the knee is flexing over the side of the table	The patient with subluxation or recent dislocation will show apprehension and guarding
Crepitation	Palpate the patella while the patient climbs on a small step/degree	Crepitus is palpable and can be audible in cases of articular surface breakdown (patella or femoral trochlea)
Tenderness	Palpate the patellar facets, after passively subluxated medially and laterally, in full extension	MPFL and LPFL will be tense and can be palpated allowing the evaluation of tenderness

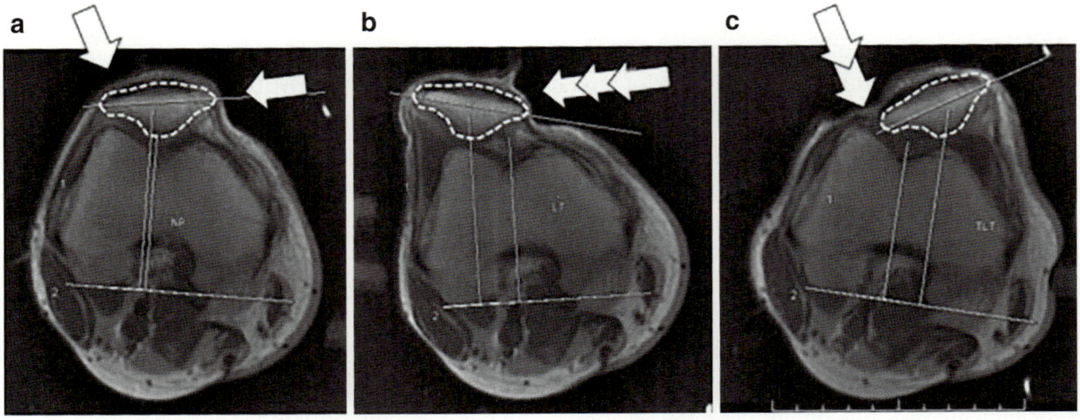

Fig. 16.7 MR images of the patellofemoral joint stress testing through instrumented assessment: (**a**) patellar neutral position without loading; (**b**) patellar lateral translation under loading; (**c**) patellar external tilt under loading, in axial view

ful for qualitative assessment, lacking objective quantitative measurement. Furthermore, poor interobserver reliability is reported, maybe due to the differences in the examination methods around the world. There is no supported accuracy and validity for the existent methods, and, until now, none is suitable for standard universal application [13, 16, 27–30].

Imaging is usually the last step in diagnosis, being performed by means of standard radiographs, computed tomography (CT) scan, and magnetic resonance imaging (MRI). The purpose of imaging is essentially to detect osteoarticular morphological changes such as degenerative arthritis or osteochondritis dissecans of the patellofemoral joint. In addition, other imaging features are important in the diagnosis: soft tissue integrity, loose bodies or other fracture fragments following an episode of patellar instability, rule out other bony pathology, and supplement the clinical assessment of patellar alignment [31–33].

There is lack of correlation between the three diagnosis phases. Consequently, many cases are still being misdiagnosed. Current evaluation tools fail in predictive and indicative value of additional health complications and therapeutic or preventive strategies, which often results in unnecessary and/or inappropriate interventions: (i) surgery instead of applying a conservative physical rehabilitation or opposing to the previous and (ii) surgical procedures not addressing critical problems (e.g., MPFL insufficiency) [3, 15–17, 19, 20].

A standardized appropriate diagnosis, applying a dynamic, anatomic, and functional assessment, with an objective, reliable, and reproducible methodology, that could better indicate the most suitable treatment to address the patient's deficits is the next step and should be expected at the clinical practice in the near future. Recently some research work has been developed in order to accomplish these goals, by means of an instrumented evaluation of the patellofemoral joint. The device should ideally allow the stress test mimicking lesions' motion patterns. The correlation of force-displacement values resulted from stress testing (Fig. 16.7) to the ones obtained by traditional methods may give us the potential to better understand the role of soft tissue restraints on the patella. Information obtained can also be correlated with subjective outcomes (scores, demographic and historical data) as well as with objective findings from classic imaging measurements. From this correlation, objective criteria for diagnosis and treatment standard algorithms can be established. Besides the scientific contribution for further research and applications on this topic, it can represent a breakthrough in clinical practice [34].

16.5 Management of the Injury and Treatment

Treatment should be progression-based and patient-tailored, respecting the patients' limitations and should address the anatomic and functional etiologic factors. Conservative treatment options available should be enough and considered as first line treatment in the patellofemoral problems. Even though, it is reported that among 60% of the rehabilitated patients experience recurrent instability. In these cases, many surgical interventions could be advocated to address the specific problem: repair or reconstruction of the medial retinaculum and MPFL, medialization of the tibial tubercle, and lateral release procedures – however remaining the lack of consensus on threshold definition and need of all factors (Lyon School classics) and need for surgical correction of all classic factors (Lyon School). Although operative management appears to result in a lower risk of patellar dislocation recurrence, it is associated with a higher risk of patellofemoral joint osteoarthritis. Nonetheless, there is insufficient evidence in this topic, and the current literature claims "powered randomized, multicentre-controlled trials conducted and reported to contemporary standards" in order to enhance the understanding on injury management [18, 20, 35–40].

Despite the high pressure imposed to the football players and everyone involved in the success of their rehabilitation, it should not push clinicians to opt for more aggressive therapeutic alternatives, in order to accelerate the return to sports. Patients with patellar instability due to significant dysplasia of the quadriceps mechanism will probably not compete at elite level, once they would be recurrently lesioned and consequently unable to play. Furthermore, players requiring a surgery may not be able to return to football even after successful surgical treatment, especially to the pre-injured level which might be due extensor mechanism dysfunction. On the other hand, patients with normal extensor mechanisms who experience patellar dislocation following specific acute trauma might be able to return to play after surgical repair. The first patellar dislocation conservative treatment and/or the postsurgical rehabilitation should be goal-based progression and can be divided into five phases that may help to plan the treatment approaches (Table 16.3); in addition, some useful tips can be pointed out. Nevertheless, it should always be borne in mind that this program is not strict and should be tailored to the individual's needs/deficits [16, 17, 39–42].

Table 16.3 Stages and tips on the rehabilitation of the patellofemoral joint

Rehabilitation stages	Rehabilitation tips
1. Resolve the symptomatology (pain, swelling, and inflammation) 2. Restore the joint normal biomechanics and flexibility 3. Recover the muscle recruitment, strength, and flexibility 4. Enhance the proprioception and neuromuscular control 5. Improve the sport-specific skills and return to sports	a. Evaluation and rehabilitation of the whole lower limb, not only the affected area b. Exercise as functionally as possible c. Prioritize control, endurance, and balance over the strength training d. Perform the exercise in a pain-free range of movement

References

1. Tecklenburg K, Dejour D, Hoser C, Fink C. Bony and cartilaginous anatomy of the patellofemoral joint. Knee Surg Sports Traumatol Arthrosc. 2006;14(3):235–40.
2. Espregueira-Mendes JDC, Pessoa P. O Joelho. Lidel: Porto; 2006.
3. Sanchis-Alfonso V. Anterior knee pain and patellar instability. Sanchis-Alfonso V, editor. London: Springer-Verlag; 2006.
4. Fulkerson JP, Hungerford DS. Biomechanics of the patellofemoral joint. Disord Patellofemoral Jt. 1990;4:24–42.
5. Panni AS, Cerciello S, Maffulli N, Di Cesare M, Servien E, Neyret P. Patellar shape can be a predisposing factor in patellar instability. Knee Surg Sports Traumatol Arthrosc. 2011;19(4):663–70.
6. Completo A, Fonseca F. Fundamentos de Biomecânica – Músculo, Esquelética e Ortopédica. Publindústria, ed. Porto; 2011.

7. Post WR, Teitge R, Amis A. Patellofemoral malalignment: Looking beyond the viewbox. Clin Sports Med. 2002;21(3):521–46.
8. Heijink A, Gomoll AH, Madry H, et al. Biomechanical considerations in the pathogenesis of osteoarthritis of the knee. Knee Surg Sports Traumatol Arthrosc. 2012;20(3):423–35.
9. Myer GD, Ford KR, Di Stasi SL, Barber Foss KD, Micheli LJ, Hewett TE. High knee abduction moments are common risk factors for patellofemoral pain (PFP) and anterior cruciate ligament (ACL) injury in girls: Is PFP itself a predictor for subsequent ACL injury? Br J Sports Med. 2014:1–7.
10. Harrisona D, Ford KR, Myer GD, Hewett TE. Sex differences in force attenuation: a clinical assessment of single-leg hop performance on a portable force plate. Br J Sports Med. 2011;45(3):198–202.
11. Ficat P, Hungerford D. Disorders of the patellofemoral joint. Baltimore: Williams & Wilkins; 1977.
12. Dejour H, Walch G, Nove-Josserand L, Guier C. Factors of patellar instability: An anatomic radiographic study. Knee Surg Sports Traumatol Arthrosc. 1994;2(1):19–26.
13. Kantaras AT, Selby J, Johnson DL. History and physical examination of the patellofemoral joint with patellar instability. Oper Tech Sports Med. 2001;9(3):129–33.
14. Merchant AC. Classification of patellofemoral disorders. Arthrosc J Arthrosc Relat Surg. 1988;4(4):235–40.
15. Dejour H, Walch G. Pathologie fémoro-patellaire. In: 6ème Journée Lyonnaise de Chirurgie du Genou. Lyon: Ameuso Editions; 1987.
16. Dejour D, Bonnin M, Servien E, Fayard JM, Al E. La Patella. In: 15éme Journées Lyonnaises de Chirurgie du Genou. Sauramps Medical: Montpellier, France; 2012.
17. Fithian DC, Neyret P, Servien E. Patellar instability: the Lyon experience. Curr Orthop Pract. 2008;19(3):328–38.
18. Arendt EA, Dejour D. Patella instability: building bridges across the ocean a historic review. Knee Surg Sports Traumatol Arthrosc. 2012;21(2):279–93.
19. Zaffagnini S, Dejour D, Arendt EA. Patellofemoral pain, instability, and arthritis: clinical presentation. Imaging and Treatment: Springer; 2010.
20. Gobbi A, Espregueira-Mendes J, Nakamura N. The patellofemoral joint: state of the art in evaluation and management. Gobbi A, Espregueira-Mendes J, Nakamura N, editors. Heidelberg: Springer; 2014.
21. Neyret P, Robinson AHN, Le Coultre B, Lapra C, Chambat P. Patellar tendon length – the factor in patellar instability? Knee. 2002;9(1):3–6.
22. Hall R, Barber Foss K, Hewett TE, Myer GD. Sport specialization's association with an increased risk of developing anterior knee pain in adolescent female athletes. J Sport Rehabil. 2015;24(1):31–5.
23. Esta R, Global P. Incidência de lesões traumato – ortopédicas no futebol de campo feminino e sua relação com alterações posturais Resultados. 2015:1–5.
24. Fulkerson JP. The etiology of patellofemoral pain in young, active patients: a prospective study. Clin Orthop Relat Res. 1983;179:129–33.
25. Reider B. Patellofemoral problems. In: Contiguglia SR, Kirkendall DT GW, ed. The U.S. soccer sports medicine book. Baltimore: Williams & Wilkins; 1996:276–294.
26. Sellars N. Book: Football medicine. BMJ Br Med J. 2004;328(7452):1384.
27. Smith TO, Clark A, Neda S, et al. The intra- and interobserver reliability of the physical examination methods used to assess patients with patellofemoral joint instability. Knee. 2012;19(4):404–10.
28. Smith TO, Davies L, Donell ST. The reliability and validity of assessing medio-lateral patellar position: a systematic review. Man Ther. 2009;14(4):355–62.
29. Fredericson M, Yoon K. Physical examination and patellofemoral pain syndrome. Am J Phys Med Rehabil. 2006;85(3):234–43.
30. Post WR. Clinical evaluation of patients with patellofemoral disorders. Arthroscopy. 1999;15(8):841–51.
31. Walch G, Dejour H. Radiology in femoro-patellar pathology. Acta Orthop Belg. 1989;55(3):371–80.
32. Sanchis-alfonso V, Montesinos-Berry E, Serrano A, Martínez-Sanjuan V. Evaluation of the patient with anterior knee pain and patellar instability. In: Anterior knee pain and patellar instability: Springer-Verlag; 2006. p. 105–23.
33. Tavernier T, Dejour D. Imagerie du genou: quel examen choisir? J Radiol. 2001;82(1):387–405.
34. Leal A, Pereira R, Pereira H, Flores P, Silva FS, Espregueira-Mendes J. Patellofemoral evaluation: do we need an objective kinematic approach? In: Gobbi A, Espregueira-mendes J, Nakamura N, editors. The patellofemoral joint: state of the art in evaluation and management. Heidelberg: Springer-Verlag; 2014.
35. Smith TO, Song F, Donell ST, Hing CB. Operative versus non-operative management of patellar dislocation. A meta-analysis. Knee Surg Sports Traumatol Arthrosc. 2011;19(6):988–98.
36. Sillanpää PJ, Mäenpää HM. First-time patellar dislocation: surgery or conservative treatment? Sports Med Arthrosc. 2012;20(3):128–35.
37. Ntagiopoulos PG, Dejour D. Current concepts on trochleoplasty procedures for the surgical treatment of trochlear dysplasia. Knee Surg Sports Traumatol Arthrosc. 2014;22(10):2531–9.
38. Nwachukwu BU, So C, Schairer WW, Green DW, Dodwell ER. Surgical versus conservative management

of acute patellar dislocation in children and adolescents: a systematic review. Knee Surg Sports Traumatol Arthrosc. 2015:1–8.
39. Respizzi S, Cavallin R. First patellar dislocation: from conservative treatment to return to sport. Joints. 2014;2(3):141–5.
40. Ménétrey J, Putman S, Gard S. Return to sport after patellar dislocation or following surgery for patellofemoral instability. Knee Surg Sports Traumatol Arthrosc. 2014;22(10):2320–6.
41. Espregueira-Mendes J, Pereira R, Monteiro A, Pereira H, Sevivas N, Varanda P. Sports and anterior cruciate lesions. Revue de Chirurgie Orthopédique et Traumatologique. 2011;97(8):S472–6
42. Wilk KE, Reinold MM. Principles of patellofemoral rehabilitation. Sports Med Arthrosc. 2001;9(4):325–36.

17 Osteochondritis Dissecans of the Knee in Football Players

Alberto Gobbi, João Espregueira-Mendes, Mustafa Karahan, Moisés Cohen, and Graeme P. Whyte

Contents

A. Gobbi (✉)
OASI Bioresearch Foundation Gobbi NPO, Milan, Italy
e-mail: gobbi@cartilagedoctor.it

J. Espregueira-Mendes
Clínica do Dragão, Espregueira-Mendes Sports Centre, FIFA Medical Centre of Excellence, Porto, Portugal

Dom Henrique Research Centre, Porto, Portugal

3B's Research Group – Biomaterials, Biodegradables and Biomimetics, University Minho, AvePark, S. Cláudio de Barco 4806-909 Taipas, Guimarães, Portugal

ICVS/3B's – PT Government Associated Laboratory, Braga, Portugal

Orthopedic Department, Minho University, Braga, Portugal

M. Karahan
Department of Orthopedics, Acibadem University, Istanbul, Turkey

M. Cohen
Traumatology and Sports Medicine Department of the Federal, University of São Paulo, São Paulo, Brazil

G.P. Whyte
Department of Orthopaedics and Rehabilitation, New York Presbyterian Hospital/Queens, New York, NY, USA

J. Espregueira-Mendes et al. (eds.), *Injuries and Health Problems in Football*,
DOI 10.1007/978-3-662-53924-8_17

17.1 Introduction

Osteochondritis dissecans (OCD) of the knee is a frequent cause of pain and functional limitation among skeletally immature and young athletes. Chronic overuse of the lower extremity in young football players can cause OCD at the knee and ankle joints; furthermore, with increased competitiveness of amateur sports, more injuries may cause OCD. Increased joint stress, such as an increased pressure at the medial femoral condyle in young patients with genu varum, might cause decreased blood flow and trigger the development of OCD.

If not recognized and appropriately treated, it can create further limitation and lead to early osteoarthritis. OCD is a disorder of one or more ossification centers, characterized by sequential degeneration or aseptic necrosis and recalcification. OCD lesions involve both bone and cartilage but appear to affect the subchondral bone primarily and secondarily affect the articular cartilage.

17.2 Etiology and Epidemiology

The etiology of OCD remains controversial; it was first described by Ambroise Paré and was named by Franz König in 1888 as a knee subchondral inflammatory process resulting in a loose fragment of cartilage from the femoral condyle; the term "dissecans" came from the Latin word *dissico* that means "to separate" [30].

Incidence of OCD has been stated to be between 0.02% and 0.03% on radiographs and 1.2% on arthroscopy [38]. Linden [31] stated the incidence of osteochondritis dissecans (OCD) in Sweden to be between 15 and 21 cases per 100,000. It occurs in patients aged 10–15 years, with a male-to-female ratio of 2:1, and occurs bilaterally in 15–30% [27].

The pathogenesis of OCD is still controversial: various theories have been proposed throughout the years but no theory is markedly superior over the other.

Theories can be divided into three major groups: genetic, vascular, and traumatic.

There has been genetic variation demonstrated in cases of OCD, and subgroups of epiphyseal dysplasia are associated with specific inheritance patterns.

OCD has been found with a variety of inherited conditions, including dwarfism, tibia vara, Legg-Calvé-Perthes disease, and Stickler syndrome [17, 32, 34, 42, 43], and there is a familial predisposition to the occurrence of OCD in other joints.

With improved techniques and decreasing costs for genetic studies, the number of genome-wide association studies (GWAS) and single-nucleotide polymorphism (SNP) studies is increasing. A mutation in the gene COL24A1, since it is known to regulate fibril diameter during fibrillogenesis, or a mutation in the signaling pathway mediated by PTH1R makes these genes a strong candidate in the onset and progression of OCD [5].

Other authors [10, 11, 23] have suggested a vascular etiology with the occurrence of a vascular event such as embolism, thrombosis, or venous stasis which can cause a secondary osteonecrosis; however, others [36] have demonstrated that the presence of an abundant vascularization does not end at the femoral epiphysis, which has refuted the vascular etiology hypothesis.

The traumatic etiology [14, 16, 18] is by far the oldest and the most well established and is based on the clinical history of previous trauma, predominantly affecting men, and the probability of reproducing similar lesions in the other parts of the body.

According to the theory of repeated microtrauma, as described by Fairbank [12] and validated by Smillie in the 1950s [41], the OCD is caused by contact of a hypertrophied tibial spine on the medial femoral condyle. This theory, despite being the most credited, does not allow an explanation of the localization of the disease in different locations of the knee. Repetitive microtrauma may be associated with vascular insufficiency, and other inherited factors are still under investigation. The exact prevalence of OCD is unknown; however, there is a male prevalence that can also be related to the number of male children practicing contact sports like football; most of the lesions are located in the posterolateral part of the medial femoral condyle.

17.3 OCD Classification

There are several types of classifications of OCD that are based upon:

1. Age of onset of the disease
2. Radiographic localization
3. Patho-anatomy
4. Arthroscopic evaluation

17.3.1 Age of Onset

Smillie [41] distinguished two forms of OCD, juvenile and adult, and suggested unique etiologies. The juvenile form OCD was supposed to be related to a disturbance of the epiphyseal development, while in the adult, a more direct traumatic causation was supposed; furthermore, the juvenile OCD lesions with an intact articular surface have better potential to heal if compared to adult OCD. However, the essential lesion is an injury of the subchondral plate resulting in destabilization of articular cartilage with loss of articular integrity.

Other authors [7] suggested a distinction based on the osseous age of the patient at the time of symptom onset: juvenile osteochondritis dissecans, which affects patients with open growth of cartilage, in a general age group between 10 and 16 years, and OCD in adults, when the cartilage physes are closed.

17.3.2 Radiographic Localization

The location of OCD can be defined topographically on standard radiographic projections of the knee [7]. On anteroposterior radiographs, the site of pathology in the coronal plane can be localized using a scale from 1–5, while on lateral radiographs, three areas are located (A, B, and C) divided between them by Blumensaat line and a midline posterior cortical from behind.

17.3.3 Anatomo-pathological Classification

Proposed by Conway and subsequently amended by Guhl [24], this classification, which was useful in the past to address the type of treatment, takes into account the anatomical characteristics of the lesion and is subdivided into five stages:

- Stage 1: Lesion evident at radiography, computed tomography (CT), or magnetic ressonance imaging (MRI), with the presence of a sclerotic line, reduced cartilage intact and only in some cases slightly soften but only in some points
- Stages 2–3: Not intact cartilage, with the presence of fissures and fragments in situ or partially detached
- Stage 4: Complete detachment but normal joint
- Stage 5: The fragment is displaced and there are phenomena of degenerative cartilage damage

17.3.4 Classification by Arthroscopy

Recently, the Board of the International Cartilage Repair Society (ICRS) defined a classification of OCD arthroscopy in four stages:

- Stage 1: Stable lesion with a continuous but softened area covered by intact articular cartilage
- Stage 2: Lesion with partial articular cartilage discontinuity but stable when probed
- Stage 3: Lesion with an unstable but not dislocated fragment "dead in situ"
- Stage 4: Empty defect with a dislocated fragment (loose body)

17.4 Clinical Evaluation

Juveniles and adolescents will complain of vague, nonspecific poorly localized anterior knee pain with variable intermittent amount of swelling, locking of the knee, grinding, or catching; pain is aggravated by activity and relieved by rest [9]. While others may be asymptomatic, a high level of suspicion should be exhibited with these types of symptoms. Symptoms are usually preceded by trauma in 40–60% of the cases [18, 31]. Others may present with Wilson's sign [49] which is performed by flexing the knee to 90° and then slowly internally rotating the leg and extending it. Patients will complain of pain at 30° of flexion and the pain is relieved by external rotation. Pain is exhibited because the tibial spine impinges on the medial femoral condyle. The test is not consistently reliable and has been shown to have an accuracy of only 70% [38, 39].

17.5 Radiographic Evaluation

The radiographic examination of a patient suspected to have OCD should always begin with plain radiographs. Standard request should be an anteroposterior, lateral, notch, and Merchant view of the knee. Notch view is specifically recommended because it demonstrates the most common areas for the occurrence of OCD and it increases the percentage of detection. Classic findings of OCD on plain film are a well-circumscribed area of subchondral bone separated by a crescent-shaped sclerotic radiolucent outline of the OCD fragment [14, 39]. In pediatric patients and adolescents, contralateral views should be requested to avoid confusion with the growth plates. Plain radiographs, however, are not ideal to assess the stability of the lesion or to examine the status of overlying cartilage; hence, additional diagnostic procedures may be necessary for us to treat these lesions.

For differentiating medial and lateral lesions and growth plate maturity, and for measuring condylar width and lesion size, plain radiographs have excellent reliability. Additionally, to evaluate lesion fragmentation, displacement, peripheral boundaries, central radiodensity, and contour, moderate to substantial reliability has been reported using plain radiographs. For evaluating the radiodensity of the lesion rim and surrounding epiphyseal bone, plain radiographs were reported to have poor to fair reliability [46].

17.5.1 CT Scan

The use of the CT scan has fallen out of favor since the advent of the MRI since the MRI gives a more detailed picture of the disease entity. CT scan is helpful in determining lesion size and loose bodies but is rarely used nowadays as part of the treatment strategy.

17.5.2 Scintigraphy

Technetium bone scans have been previously used to localize the lesion of a specific joint and follow the progression of healing in juvenile patients. Unable to provide for the status of cartilage, these have given way to the advent of the MRI. Some authors have proposed serial bone scanning of juvenile patients, however, this approach has not been widely adopted due to the time require for this study, invas venous access, and the risk of introducing a radioactive isotope.

17.5.3 Magnetic Resonance Imaging

MRI has been superior in providing valuable information as compared to other diagnostic procedures. It generally gives us the dimensions of the lesion as well as the status of cartilage and subchondral bone. The most appropriate MRI protocols for evaluating OCD lesions are fast spin echo (FSE), proton density, and T2-weighted image [39].

There is consensus on advising two sequences: FSE T2-weighted sequence and the 3D GRE T1-weighted sequence. In the FSE T2-weighted sequence, effusion, bone edema, and alteration of the cartilage surface are better evaluated, and in the 3D GRE T1-weighted sequence, alterations in cartilage thickness are better evaluated, and this sequence provides better information on the subchondral bone [26].

MRI techniques such as the delayed gadolinium-enhanced MRI of cartilage (dGEMRIC) and T2 relaxation time mapping have been available recently, providing the ability of the glycosaminoglycan content visualization, the measurement of collagen content, and the mapping of anatomical zones of cartilage. Arthrography with gadolinium has been shown to have exceptional capability in determining the status of articular cartilage using gradient echo techniques [1].

17.6 Treatment

The advent of arthroscopy has outright revolutionized the treatment of OCD. Using standard arthroscopic portals and techniques, surgeons are now visualizing lesions previously missed on standard diagnostic procedures. Open techniques have not fallen out of favor and are still utilized for lesions requiring greater exposure and visualization. Treatment options largely depend on age of the patient, lesion size, and stability. It is recommended that unstable lesions be treated surgically.

17.7 Nonoperative Treatment

Nonoperative treatment is still employed in a select group of patients with OCD. The goal of nonsurgical treatment is to promote healing of lesions in situ and prevent lesion displacement. Skeletally immature patients usually have a better prognosis. Lesions on weight-bearing surfaces and those that are greater than 1 cm^2 in size have been shown to have less successful outcomes [8, 18, 24, 29]. Symptomatic lesions in children, or skeletally immature patients, should initially be treated with conservative measures for 3 months, if there are no loose bodies upon radiographic examination [40]. The mainstay of nonsurgical treatment has been cessation of athletic activity and lifestyle modification. This is done for a period of 3–6 months with an initial 6–8 weeks of non-weight bearing and daily range of motion exercises. If at the sixth month, there are no signs of radiographic healing, then operative treatment should be considered [31, 34]. A healing rate of 50–94% has been noted with nonoperative treatment [4, 19, 31]. By contrast, adult OCD of the knee rarely responds to conservative measures [40].

Criteria described by De Smet [30] to evaluate healing after conservative treatment are based on T2-weighted MRI studies:

(i) A line of high signal intensity at least 5 mm in length between the OCD lesion and underlying bone

(ii) An area of increased homogeneous signal, at least 5 mm in diameter, beneath the lesion

(iii) A focal defect of 5 mm or more in the articular surface

(iv) A high signal line traversing the subchondral plate into the lesion

Of these signs, the high signal line behind the fragment is known to be the most predictive [40].

17.8 Operative Treatment

17.8.1 Excision of Fragments

Previously considered the most common treatments for these lesions, excision has fallen out of favor due to the dismal long-term results in juvenile and adult patients [15, 32, 45, 50]. Debridement and curretage of the lesion bed has shown to improve the results in juvenile patients [2, 16].

17.8.2 Arthroscopic Drilling

Considered as one of the first surgical treatments for OCD, either arthroscopic or open drilling is still one of the most common treatment methods for OCD. The rationale behind this procedure is that the OCD is treated as a fracture nonunion, and by penetrating the subchondral bone, it will instigate an inflammatory healing cascade, creating channels for subsequent revascularization [8]. This is a common treatment in juveniles who have failed a trial of conservative management [35, 47]. Drilling can be done in an antegrade or retrograde fashion, the former being more technically challenging in trying to center the drill and gaining the right depth over the lesion; the latter is easier to perform but violates the continuity of the articular cartilage. Anderson noted a 90% healing potential in the skeletally immature group, while the skeletally mature group had a 50% healing potential [4]. This technique is generally reserved for ICRS stage 1 lesions.

17.8.3 Open Reduction of the Fragment

Reduction and stabilization of the OCD fragment can be done with a multitude of devices such as K wires, variable pitch screws, cannulated screws, bioabsorbable pins, tack nails, and screws. This should be reserved for lesions less than 2 cm^2. Anderson et al. reported that long-term results for large lesions are poor and there is increased risk of developing early-onset arthritis [3].

Thorough evaluation of the underlying subchondral bone should be performed and assessment of stability done if the lesion is amenable to in situ fixation. Lesions with little anchoring to the base usually have abundant scar tissue, which needs to be debrided prior to reduction and fixation of the fragment. Drilling or microfracture can be employed to stimulate the healing potential prior to reduction. In cases of fragment mismatch during reduction, bone grafting can be employed. This can be taken from the proximal tibia or the intercondylar notch of the femur.

A multitude of fixation materials can be used each with its own advantages and disadvantages. Currently, there is a great deal of controversy as to which implant to choose. Pins and K wires can achieve multiple points of fixation with less risk of an iatrogenic fracture to the fragment; the disadvantage is that they provide no compression and usually loosen which eventually requires removal. The advent of biomaterials has revolutionized the way in which fragments are fixated. The concept of having to put an implant that could provide compression and be absorbed by the body was novel, but it was not without problems. Postoperative complications ranged from inflammatory reactions with effusion, to loose bodies secondary to failure of implant resorption [6, 16].

17.8.4 Osteochondral Grafting

Transplanting of either autografts or allografts to the OCD defect has the advantage of providing hyaline cartilage, providing a biomechanically stronger and more resilient tissue. Osteochondral autograft transfer (OAT) is used for lesions smaller than 2 cm^2. It is a single-step procedure which can be done arthroscopically or as a mini-open procedure. This entails harvest of cylindrical plugs from the non-weight-bearing aspect of the notch of the medial trochlear ridge, where either single or multiple plugs are harvested and transferred back to the defect. OAT can be a technically demanding procedure, and any mismatch in articular surface can cause an increase in contact pressures and shear forces. Wu et al. showed that plugs that are 1 mm prominent caused an increase in contact pressures and shear, while a 0.25-mm recess decreased pressure by 50% [51]. This is also limited by the amount of graft a donor site can give, creating a situation such as "robbing from Peter to pay Paul."

Fresh osteochondral allograft is designed to treat larger lesions (>2–3 cm^2). This could be done in either a press-fit plug technique or a shell graft technique. Advantages are the flexibility of sizing the grafts, the ability to use a single plug for a defect, and the lack of donor site morbidity. The disadvantages include reduced viability of the graft due to storing and processing, immunogenicity, transmission of diseases, and availability of the grafts (not available in many countries worldwide).

Autogenous bone has been shown to be a cost-effective and readily available matrix for large volume osteochondral defects. The autogenous nature removes the risk of complications of the allograft surgery while resulting in long-lasting biological solution for both the bone and the cartilage. Treatment for large-volume defects by this method remains salvage in nature and palliative in outcome [28].

17.8.5 First-Generation Autologous Chondrocyte Implantation (ACI)

In lesions larger than 2–3 cm^2, the transplantation of autologous chondrocytes can now be considered the technique of choice. In results reported by Peterson et al. [33], after a follow-up period of 10 years, outcomes of OCD treatment were good in 89%, with significant improvement in symptoms demonstrated in 88% of cases. They showed that autologous chondrocyte implantation (ACI) produced an integrated repair tissue with successful clinical results. In the experience of Peterson, a pioneer of ACI treatment, clinical results of treating OCD lesions, and particularly isolated lesions affecting the medial femoral condyle, have been excellent using this method.

In the first phase of his experience, Peterson performed the simple transplantation of chondrocytes in suspension. Successively he has perfected his technique for treating OCD lesions deeper than 10 mm involving significant subchondral bone loss with his "sandwich technique" in which cancellous bone is used to fill the defect and closed with a periosteal flap; the grafted chondrocytes are then suspended in between the first periosteal flap overlying the bone graft and a second flap secured superficial to this.

The recent introduction of tissue bioengineering tissues with chondrocytes seeded on the scaffold represents another possibility to fill the lesion; however, when the lesion is deep, it's necessary to reconstitute bone loss at the base of the lesion prior to application of the scaffold designed to restore the cartilage layer.

17.8.6 Second-Generation ACI

Since being introduced in 1987, the cell-based approach has gained increasing acceptance, and recent studies highlight the long-term durable nature of this form of treatment due to the production of hyaline-like cartilage that is mechanically and functionally stable and integrates into the adjacent articular surface. However, these good results have to be weighed against the number of problems that can be observed with the standard ACI methods. First-generation ACI has been associated with several limitations related to the complexity and morbidity of the surgical procedure. This technique requires a large joint exposure with a high risk of joint stiffness and arthrofibrosis. Moreover, there is a frequent occurrence of periosteal hypertrophy that often requires revision surgery. To these problems related to the surgical procedure, we must add the technical problems of the culture and transplantation procedure, such as maintenance of chondrocyte phenotype, nonhomogeneous cell distribution in the three-dimensional (3D) spaces of the defect, and cell loss using liquid suspension.

Taking into consideration all these factors, a new generation procedure for cartilage transplantation was developed. The so-called matrix-assisted ACI technique uses a new tissue engineering technology to create a cartilage-like tissue in a three-dimensional culture system with the attempt to address all the concerns related to the cell culture and the surgical technique. Essentially, the concept is based on the use of biodegradable polymers as temporary scaffolds for the in vitro growth of living cells and their subsequent transplantation onto the defect site. On the basis of published results, the matrix-assisted chondrocyte implantation guarantees results comparable to, or superior than, the traditional ACI technique and simplifies the procedure with marked advantages from a biological and surgical point of view.

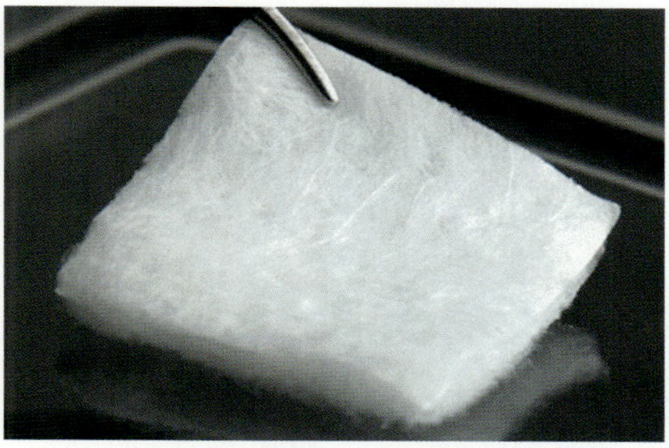

Fig. 17.1 Hyaluronic acid-based scaffold (Hyalofast, Anika Therapeutics, Padova, Italy)

Our experience with the treatment of OCD through the implant of a bioengineered tissue regards a scaffold entirely based on the benzylic ester of hyaluronic acid (Hyalofast, Anika Therapeutics, Padova, Italy). It consists of a network of 20-μm-thick fibers with interstices of variable sizes, which has been demonstrated to be an optimal physical support to allow cell-cell contacts, cluster formation, and extracellular matrix deposition (Fig. 17.1).

The cells harvested from the patient are expanded and then seeded onto the scaffold to create the tissue-engineered product Hyalograft C. Seeded on the scaffold, the cells are able to re-differentiate and to retain a chondrocyte phenotype even after a long period of in vitro expansion in monolayer culture. The efficacy of the cell-scaffold construct was also proven by in vivo implantation in an animal model. This 3D scaffold for autologous chondrocyte culture can improve the biological performance of autologous cells and overcome some of the difficulties of the ACI surgical technique. Hyalograft C constructs can be implanted by press-fitting directly into the lesion, thus avoiding suturing to surrounding cartilage and obviating the need for a periosteal flap, thereby also avoiding the possibility of periosteal hypertrophy. Moreover, the features of this device have permitted the development of an arthroscopic surgical technique, reducing patient morbidity, surgical and recovery time, and complications related to open surgery (Figs. 17.2 and 17.3).

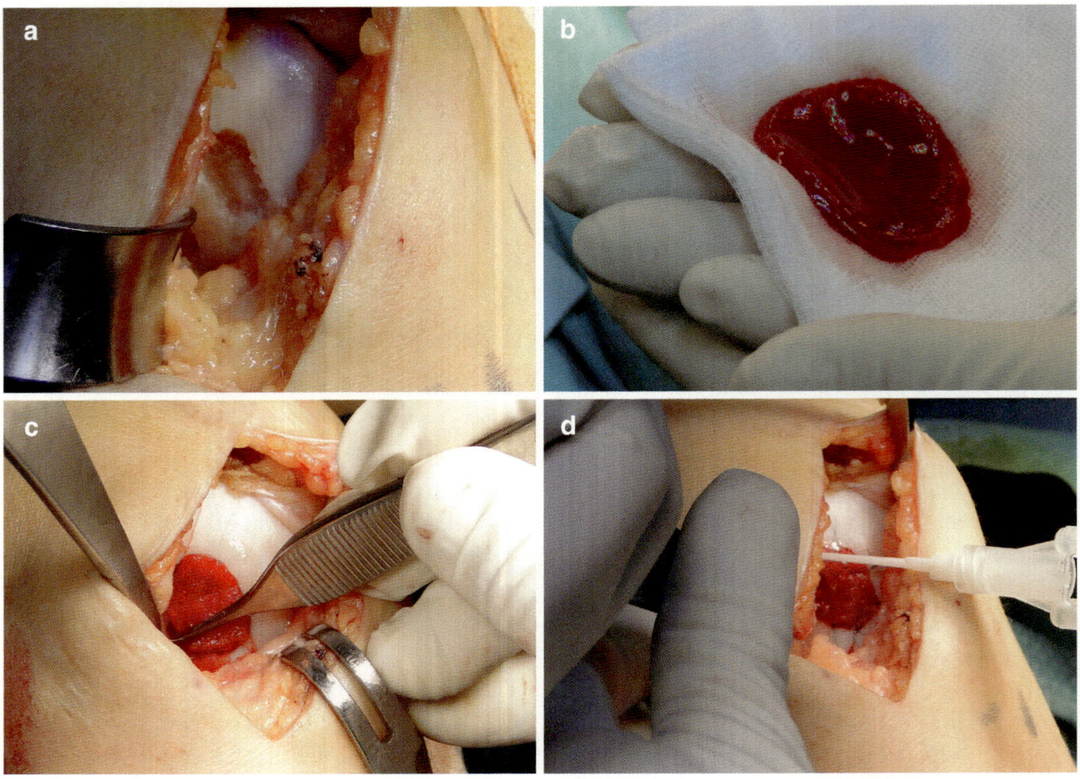

Fig. 17.2 (**a**) Grade IV chondral lesion of a knee medial femoral condyle; (**b**) clot-activated bone marrow aspirate concentrate (BMAC); (**c**) Implantation of BMAC-embedded hyaluronic acid-based scaffold (HA-BMAC) into cartilage defect, placed over clot-activated BMAC; (**d**) HA-BMAC graft secured with 6-0 PDS suture and fibrin glue

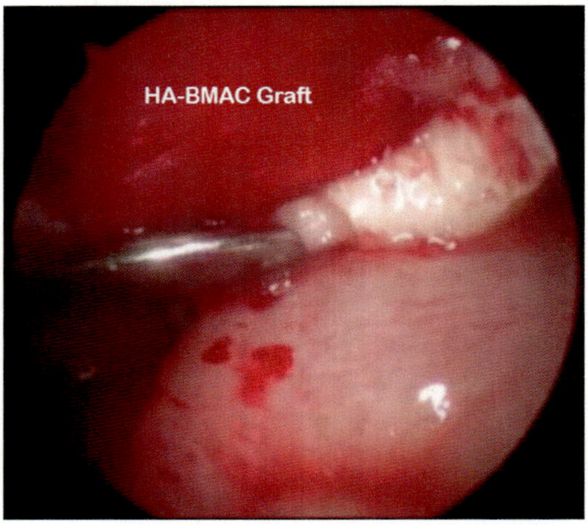

Fig. 17.3 Arthroscopic implantation of hyaluronic acid-based scaffold embedded with bone marrow aspirate concentrate (HA-BMAC) into a prepared patellar chondral defect

Since 2001, we used this tissue engineering approach for the treatment of OCD, and we implanted the bioengineered cartilage tissue in more than 50 patients. We believe that surgical goals should always try to reestablish the joint surface in the most anatomical way possible. In fact, as underlined by Linden [31] in a long-term retrospective outcome study (average follow-up of 33 years) of patients with OCD of the femoral condyle, the natural history of this osteochondral joint pathology is an earlier degeneration process [31]. Patients with adult OCD showed radiographically to develop arthritis about 10 years earlier in life than primary gonarthrosis.

The use of the autologous bioengineered tissue Hyalograft C in OCD lesions presents the problem of promoting only cartilage restoration, but not the bone regeneration. For this reason, in case of deep lesions, we utilized a two-step technique. When necessary, second-generation autologous transplantation was preceded by an autologous bone grafting, in order to restore the entire osteochondral structure and, therefore, a more anatomical articular surface. The first arthroscopic surgical step consists of the implant of a bone graft harvested from the omolateral tibia to fill the bone loss. In the same surgical procedure, healthy cartilage is harvested from the intercondylar notch for the autologous chondrocyte culture expansion. The second surgical procedure is performed 4–6 months later, after the integration of the autologous bone graft is achieved, and consists of the second-generation arthroscopic autologous chondrocyte transplantation according to the technique described by Marcacci et al.

We have reviewed the patients with a minimum follow-up of 3 years. A total of 38 OCD of the knee was treated and evaluated at a mean follow-up of 4 years. The mean age were 21.2 years (range 15–46), 84 % of patients was active and practiced sports at least at nonprofessional level, and 42% underwent previous surgery. The most common location of the lesion was the medial femoral condyle (76%) and the mean size was 2.9 cm^2 (range 1.5–4 cm^2). The mean number of Hyalograft C patches used was 2.8 (range 1–4), and in 62% of the cases, the additional bone graft step was required to restore the articular surface. The results were evaluated with the ICRS-IKDC 2000 and the Tegner scores. No complications related to the Hyalograft C implant and no serious adverse events were observed during the treatment and follow-up period.

ICRS and Tegner scores showed an overall satisfactory clinical outcome. At a mean follow-up of 4 years, the average ICRS-IKDC 2000 was increased from 41.4 to 74.9 in cases of OCD of the femoral condyle (increase 80. 4%). In cases of OCD of the patella, a lower, but still significant, improvement was observed: the mean score increased from 47 to 68. The Tegner score increased from 1.5 preoperatively to 5 at the latest follow-up with a significant improvement, even if still lower than the previous sport activity level of 6.

Second-look arthroscopy was performed in 5 cases, and according to ICRS grading criteria, 2 were considered normal, and 3 considered almost normal.

MRI examination showed a good appearance in the anatomical location of the transplant, with a concentration of glycosaminoglycans (GAG) similar to that of a normal cartilage. In few cases, persistent irregularities of the subchondral bone and incomplete filling were observed.

17.8.7 New Scaffolds

Recently, a biomimetic 3-layer scaffold, composed of type I collagen and nanostructured hydroxyapatite, was conceived with the aim of confining bone formation to the deepest portion of the construct without involving any superficial layer where the process of cartilaginous-like connective tissue formation should begin.

Preclinical studies showed good results in terms of both cartilage and bone tissue formation, and preclinical findings supported the use of the scaffold alone, suggesting that osteochondral regeneration occurred by harnessing and guiding the body's self-regenerative potential. Thus, this cell-free scaffold was introduced into clinical practice with promising preliminary results in a heterogeneous patient population [13].

The osteochondral (OC) biomimetic scaffold (Fin-Ceramica Faenza SpA, Faenza, Italy) has a porous 3-D composite trilayered structure, which mimics the whole osteochondral anatomy. The cartilage-like layer, consisting of type I collagen, has a smooth surface. The intermediate layer (tidemark-like) consists of a combination of type I collagen (60%) and hydroxyapatite (40%), whereas the lower layer consists of a mineralized blend of type I collagen (30%) and hydroxyapatite (70%) reproducing the subchondral bone layer. The final construct was obtained by physically combining the layers on top of a Mylar sheet; the product was then freeze-dried and gamma-sterilized at 25 kGy.

A recent study published by Filardo analyzed the results in 27 consecutive patients who were affected by symptomatic knee OCD of the femoral condyles grade 3 or 4 on the ICRS scale and were enrolled and treated with the implantation of this 3-layer collagen-hydroxyapatite scaffold [13].

Patients were prospectively evaluated by subjective and objective International Knee Documentation Committee (IKDC) and Tegner scores preoperatively and at 1- and 2-year follow-up. An MRI was also performed at the two follow-up times. A statistically significant improvement in all clinical scores was obtained at 1 year, and a further improvement was found the following year. At the 2-year follow-up, the IKDC subjective score had increased from 48 preoperatively to 82, the IKDC objective evaluation from 40% to 85% of normal knees, and the Tegner score from 2.4 to 4.5.

The MRI evaluations showed good defect filling and implant integration but nonhomogeneous regenerated tissue and subchondral bone changes in most patients at both follow-up times. No correlation between the MOCART (magnetic resonance observation of cartilage repair tissue) score and clinical outcome was found.

The authors concluded that this biomimetic collagen-hydroxyapatite osteochondral scaffold, which requires a minimally invasive 1-step and a cell-free surgical approach, is a valid treatment option for knee OCD and might offer a good clinical outcome at 2-year follow-up, despite some postoperative adverse events such as swelling and stiffness in some patients; furthermore, less favorable findings were obtained with MRI evaluation.

17.8.8 Mesenchymal Stem Cells (MSCs)

Recent directions in cartilage repair are moving toward the possibility of performing one-step surgery: the scaffold-based approach represents a fascinating treatment option for osteochondral lesions, providing a structural basis for defect repair and stimulating the healing processes of damaged tissues. In this scenario, cell cultivation occupies a controversial role, and the use of cell-free scaffolds showed good results and avoided cell manipulation and its regulatory obstacles; several groups are analyzing the possibility of using MSCs with chondrogenic potential and growth factors (GF), thus avoiding the first surgery for cartilage biopsy and subsequent chondrocyte cell cultivation, with a significant reduction of the cost of the total procedure. MSCs represent an appealing tool for regenerative medicine, thanks to their unique characteristics and their self-renewal characteristics, their maintenance of "stemness" thus their potential for differentiation into cells forming multiple mesodermal tissues, and finally their trophic and immune-modulatory effects. Many authors demonstrated that MSCs have a self-renewal capacity and multi-lineage differentiation potential and they can be characterized by their cultivation behavior and their differentiation potential into adipogenic, osteogenic, and chondrogenic cells; therefore, once MSCs are cultured in the appropriate microenvironment, they can differentiate to chondrocytes and form cartilage [25, 44]. In this regard, the use of bone marrow aspirate concentrate (BMAC) cells, which contain multipotent MSCs and growth factors, can represent a possible alternative for regenerating cartilage tissue.

Recently we published a prospective nonrandomized study comparing a two-step technique (Hyalofast scaffold with cultivated chondrocytes) with a single-step technique using the same Hyalofast scaffold and BMAC implantation in a single-step technique, with no need for culture, thereby avoiding the expenditure for an extra procedure to retrieve chondral biopsy, decreasing the total costs of the procedure and donor site morbidity [20].

Both groups showed significant improvement in all scores, from preoperative to final follow-up ($P = 0.001$), but there was no significant difference in improvement between the two groups.

MRI showed complete filling of the defects in 76% of patients treated with MACI, and 81% of those treated with the BMAC-embedded scaffold. Histologic analysis consistently revealed hyaline-like features of restored cartilage after both treatments. We concluded that both techniques are excellent options for the treatment of large chondral lesions of the knee, with the BMAC technique being the preferrable option due to the one-step nature of the procedure.

MSC implantation offers potential advantages, including a single surgery, and no need of cartilage biopsy and cell cultivation, thus reducing the total cost of medical care.

Another recently published study was performed on athletes operated for grade IV cartilage lesions of the knee with MSCs covered with a Hyalofast membrane (Anika Therapeutics, Padova, Italy) [21]. In these patients bone marrow was harvested from the ipsilateral iliac crest and subjected to concentration and activation with Batroxobin solution (Plateltex®act-Plateltex SRO, Bratislava, SK) in order to produce a sticky clot, which was implanted into the prepared cartilage defect (Fig. 17.2). The patients followed the same specific rehabilitation program for a minimum of 6 months. Preoperative average values in the evaluated scores were significantly improved to final follow-up ($p < 0.001$). Patients younger than 45 years and those with smaller or single lesions showed better outcomes. MRI showed good stability of the implant and complete filling of the defect in 80% of patients, and hyaline-like cartilage was found in the histological analysis of the biopsied tissue. Second-look arthroscopies in seven knees revealed a smooth, newly formed intact tissue continuous with the healthy cartilage in all the patients; no hypertrophy was identified. Four patients consented for a concomitant biopsy which was taken from regenerated tissue at the site of the treated chondral lesion; good histological findings were reported for the four specimens analyzed, which presented with many hyaline-like cartilage features. No adverse reactions or postoperative complications were noted.

Clinical outcomes of cartilage repair using hyaluronic acid-based scaffold embedded with bone marrow aspirate concentrate (HA-BMAC) at a medium-term follow-up of 5 years have demonstrated this technique to be a promising treatment option in a wide range of lesion sizes [22]. The physical properties of the HA-BMAC graft allows for reliable arthroscopic implantation in select cases [48]. In cases of osteochondritis dissecans lesions of the knee that require reconstitution of subchondral bone, the HA-BMAC graft may be combined with a morselized bone graft inlay, to perform repair of the osteochondral unit by a technique described by Sadlik as biologic inlay osteochondral reconstruction (BIOR) [37].

Conclusion

OCD is a condition that continues to pose a dilemma for the orthopaedic surgeon, with regard to timely diagnosis and the selection of appropriate treatment. No one single technique has been deemed applicable for all stages of presenting OCD. Recent techniques with new biomaterials have shown good medium-term results, although greater lengths of follow-up are necessary to more accurately determine the durability of such treatment.

References

1. Aglietti P, Buzzi R, Bassi FB, Fioriti M. Arthroscopic drilling in juvenile osteochondritis dissecans of the medial femoral condyle. Arthroscopy. 1994;10:286–91.
2. Aglietti P, Ciardullo A, Giron F. Results of arthroscopic excision of the fragments in the treatment of osteochondritis dissecans of the knee. Arthroscopy. 2001;17:741–6.
3. Anderson AF, Pagnani M. Osteochondritis dissecans of the femoral condyles: long term results of excision of the fragment. Am J Sports Med. 1997;25:830–4.
4. Anderson AF, Richards D, Pagani MJ, Hovis WD. Antegrade drilling for osteochondritis dissecans of the knee. Arthroscopy. 1997;13:319–24.
5. Bates JT, Jacobs Jr JC, Shea KG. Emerging genetic basis of osteochondritis dissecans. Clin Sports Med. 2014;33(2):199–220.
6. Bradford G, Svendsen R. Synovitis of the knee after intraarticular fixation with Biofix: report of two cases. Acta Orthop Scand. 1992;63:680–1.
7. Cahill BR. Osteochondritis dissecans of the knee: treatment of juvenile and adult forms. J Am Acad Orthop Surg. 1995;3:237–47.
8. Cain EL, Clancy W. Treatment algorithm for osteochondral injuries of the knee. Clin Sports Med. 2001;20:321–42.
9. Caffey J, Madell S, Royer C, Morales P. Ossification of the distal femoral epiphysis. J Bone Joint Surg Am. 1958;40:647–54.
10. Campbell CJ, Ranawat C. Osteochondritis dissecans: the question of etiology. J Trauma. 1966;6:201–21.
11. Chiroff RT, Cooke C. Osteochondritis dissecans: a histologic and microradioographic analysis of surgical excised lesions. J Trauma. 1975;15:689–96.
12. Fairbank HA. Osteochondritis dissecans. British J Surg. 1933;21:67–82.
13. Filardo G, Kon E, Di Martino A, Busacca M, Altadonna G, Marcacci M. Treatment of knee osteochondritis dissecans with a cell-free biomimetic osteochondral scaffold clinical and imaging evaluation at 2-year follow-up. Am J Sports Med. 2013;41(8):1786–93.
14. Fisher AG. A study of loose bodies composed of cartilage and bone occurring in joints. With special reference to their aethiology and pathology. British J Surg. 1921;8:493–523.
15. Frederico DJ, Lynch J, Jokl P. Osteochondritis dissecans of the knee: a historical review of etiology and treatment. Arthroscopy. 1990;6:190–7.
16. Freidrichs MG, Greis P, Burks RT. Pitfalls associated with fixation of osteochondritis dissecans fragments using bioabsorbable screws. Arthroscopy. 2001;17:542–5.
17. Gardiner TB. Osteochondritis dissecans in three members of one family. J Bone Joint Surg Br. 1955;37:139–41.
18. Garrett JC. Osteochondritis dissecans. Clin Sports Med. 1991;10:569–93.
19. Garrett JC, Kress K, Mudano M. Osteochondritis dissecans of the lateral femoral condyle in the adult. Arthroscopy. 1992;8:474–81.

20. Gobbi A, Chaurasia S, Karnatzikos G, Nakamura N. Matrix-induced autologous chondrocyte implantation versus multipotent stem cells for the treatment of large patellofemoral chondral lesions: a nonrandomized prospective trial. Carcinogenesis. 2015;6(2):82–97.
21. Gobbi A, Scotti C, Karnatzikos G, Mudhigere A, Castro M, Peretti GM. One-step surgery with multipotent stem cells and Hyaluronan-based scaffold for the treatment of full-thickness chondral defects of the knee in patients older than 45 years. Knee Surg Sports Traumatol Arthrosc. 2016;14:1–8.
22. Gobbi A, Whyte GP. One-stage cartilage repair using a hyaluronic acid-based scaffold with activated bone marrow-derived mesenchymal stem cells compared with microfracture: five-year follow-up. Am J Sports Med. 2016;44:2846–54.
23. Green WT, Banks H. Osteochondritis dissecans in children. J Bone Joint Surg Am. 1953;35:26–47.
24. Guhl JF. Arthroscopic treatment of osteochondritis dissecans. Clin Orthop Relat Res. 1982;167:65–74.
25. Guzzo RM, Gibson J, Xu RH, Lee FY, Drissi H. Efficient differentiation of human iPSC-derived mesenchymal stem cells to chondroprogenitor cells. J Cell Biochem. 2013;114(2):480–90.
26. Hayashi D, Guermazi A, Kwoh CK, et al. Semiquantitative assessment of subchondral bone marrow edema-like lesions and subchondral cysts of the knee at 3T MRI: a comparison between intermediate-weighted fat-suppressed spin echo and Dual Echo Steady State sequences. BMC Musculoskelet Disord. 2011;12:198.
27. Hefti F, Beguiristain J, Krauspe R, et al. Osteochondritis dissecans: a multicenter study of the European Pediatric Orthopedic Society. J Pediatr Orthop B. 1999;8:231–45.
28. Johnson LL, De Lano MC, Spector M. The biological response following autogenous bone grafting for large-volume defects of the knee: index surgery through 12 to 21 Years' follow up. Carcinogenesis. 2012;3(1):86–99.
29. Kocher MS, Micheli L, Yaniv M, et al. Functional and radiographic outcomes of juvenile osteochondritis dissecans of the knee treated with transarticular drilling. Am J Sports Med. 2001;29:562–6.
30. Konig F. Ueber freie Körper in den Gelenken. Deutsche Zeitschr Chir. 1888;27:90–109.
31. Linden B. The incidence of osteochondritis dissecans in the condyles of the femur. Acta Orthop Scand. 1976;47:666–7.
32. Mubarak SJ, Carroll NC. Familial osteochondritis of the knee. Clin Orthop. 1979;140:131–6.
33. Peterson L, Minas T, Brittberg M, Lindhal A. Treatment of osteochondritis dissecans of the knee with autologous chondrocyte transplantation: results at two to ten years. J Bone Joint Surg Am. 2003;85:17–24.
34. Ribbing S. The hereditary multiple epiphyseal disturbance and its consequences for the aetiogenesis of local malacias-particularly the osteochondritis dissecans. Acta Orthop Scand. 1955;24:286–99.
35. Robertson W, Kelly BT, Green DW. Osteochondritis dissecans of the knee in children. Curr Opin Pediatr. 2003;15:38–44.
36. Rogers WM, Gladstone H. Vascular foramina and arterial supply of the distal end of the femur. J Bone Joint Surg Am. 1950;32:867–74.
37. Sadlik B, Gobbi A, Puszkarz M, Klon W, Whyte GP. Biologic inlay osteochondral reconstruction: arthroscopic one-step osteochondral lesion repair in the knee using morselized bone grafting and hyaluronic acid-based scaffold embedded with bone marrow aspirate concentrate. Arthrosc Tech. In press 2016. doi: 10.1016/j.eats.2016.10.023.
38. Schenck Jr RC, Goodnight JM. Osteochondritis dissecans. J Bone Joint Surg Am. 1996;78:439–78.
39. Schwarz C, Blazina ME, Sisto DJ, Hirsh LC. The results of operative treatment of osteochondritis dissecans of the patella. Am J Sports Med. 1988;16:522–9.
40. Smet AA, Ilahi OA, Graf BK. Untreated osteochondritis dissecans of the femoral condyles: prediction of patient outcome using radiographic and MR findings. Skelet Radiol. 1997;26(8):463–7.
41. Smillie IS. Treatment of osteochondritis dissecans. J Bone Joint Surg Br. 1957;29:248–60.
42. Stougart J. Familial occurrence of osteochondritis dissecans. J Bone Joint Surg Br. 1964;46:542–3.
43. Stougart J. The hereditary factor in osteochondritis dissecans. J Bone Joint Surg Br. 1961;43:256–8.
44. Sudo K, Kanno M, Miharada K, Ogawa S, Hiroyama T, Saijo K, Nakamura Y. Mesenchymal progenitors able to differentiate into osteogenic, chondrogenic, and/or adipogenic cells in vitro are present in most primary fibroblast-like cell populations. Stem Cells. 2007;25(7):1610–7.
45. Twyman RS, Desai K, Aichroth PM. Osteochondritis dissecans of the knee: a long term study. J Bone Joint Surg Br. 1991;73:461–4.
46. Wall EJ, Polousky JD, Shea KG, Carey JL, Ganley TJ, Grimm NL, Jacobs JC, Edmonds EW, Eismann EA, Anderson AF, Heyworth BE, Lyon R, Murnaghan ML, Nissen C, Weiss J, Wright R, Myer GD. Novel radiographic feature classification of knee osteochondritis dissecans: a multicenter reliability study. Am J Sports Med. 2015;43:303–9.
47. Wall E, Von Stein D. Juvenile osteochondritis dissecans. Orthop Clin North Am. 2003;34(3):341–53.
48. Whyte GP, Gobbi A, Sadlik B. Dry arthroscopic single-stage cartilage repair of the knee using a hyaluronic acid-based scaffold with activated bone marrow-derived mesenchymal stem cells. Arthrosc Tech. 2016;5:e913–8.
49. Wilson JN. A diagnostic sign in osteochondritis dissecans of the knee. J Bone Joint Surg Am. 1967; 49-A:477–80.
50. Wright RW, McLean M, Matava MJ. Osteochondritis dissecans of the knee: long term results of excision of the fragment. Clin Orthop Relat Res. 2004;424: 239–43.
51. Wu JZ, Herzog W, Hasler EM. Inadequate placement of osteochondral plugs may induce abnormal stress strain distributions in articular cartilage – finite element stimulations. Med Eng Phys. 2002; 24:85–97.

Knee and Tibial Fractures

18

Luís Silva, Ricardo Varatojo, Camila Cohen,
and Philippe Neyret

Contents

L. Silva (✉)
Clínica do Dragão, Espregueira-Mendes Sports Centre - FIFA Medical Centre of Excellence, Porto, Portugal

Dom Henrique Research Centre, Porto, Portugal

ULS-Guarda, Guarda, Portugal
e-mail: luisduartesilva1985@gmail.com

R. Varatojo
Head of the Knee and Ankle Surgery, Arthroscopy and Sports Trauma Unit, Orthopedic Center, Hospital Cuf Descobertas, Lisbon, Portugal
e-mail: jose.varatojo@jmellosaude.pt

C. Cohen
Department of Orthopedics and Traumatology, Faculty of Medical Sciences, Santa Casa of São Paulo, São Paulo, Brazil

Physician of the Cohen Institute, Orthopedics, Rehabilitation and Sports Medicine, São Paulo, Brazil
e-mail:camilacohen@kaleka.com.br

P. Neyret
Centre Albert Trillat – Hôpital de la Croix-Rousse, 69004 Lyon, France
e-mail: philippe.neyret@chu-lyon.fr

J. Espregueira-Mendes et al. (eds.), *Injuries and Health Problems in Football*,
DOI 10.1007/978-3-662-53924-8_18

According to a study performed by the Fédération Internationale de Football Association (FIFA), there are approximately 265 million active football players worldwide, a number which is constantly increasing, making it the world's most popular sport [1].

Football is considered a physically demanding and highly competitive sport, associated with highly athletic and financial expectations [2]. In light of these high expectations, there is an equally high intensity on the competitive sports, resulting in a consequently increased risk for sports-related injuries, with an estimated incidence of 8.5 injuries per 1000 playing hours and an average of 1.3 injuries per player within each season [3–5].

Football has been reported as the most common sport in the world, where fractures frequently occur [6]. Despite the high number of epidemiology studies on sports-related injuries, little attention has been paid on the etiopathogeny, suitable treatment, prognosis, and prevention of lower extremity fractures [7]. The most common injuries, accounting for 50% to 80% of all injuries, usually involve minor trauma, including muscle sprains, ligament strains, and contusions [7, 8]. Nevertheless, given to high impact nature of sports, such as football more severe injuries may occur, such as fractures [9]. Around 20% of the football injuries are fractures [10]. In this sense, the lower extremity is the most affected, in most cases caused by tackles [8].

Regarding youth sports, about 10% of all athletes' exposures to injury are fractures, with an overall rate of 1.82 fractures per 10,000 exposures. The lower leg accounts for about 10% of all sport-related fractures, and the proportion of fracture injury is inversely correlated with the athlete's age [11].

When focusing tibial and fibular fractures, Boden et al. [7] retrospectively reviewed 31 football players who have sustained a traumatic fracture of the lower leg. From all lower limb fractures, 15 involved both the tibia and fibula, 11 only the tibia, and 5 only the fibula, which most of them occurred in young, competitive athletes during game situations. Tibial and fibular fractures are majorly caused by a direct-impact trauma, such as a miskick or slide tackles, where the high kinetic energy is rather transmitted to the opponent's lower leg and not to the ball. When the tibial fractures were concurrent with fibular ones, major complications were present in 50% of the players and the return to sports averaged 40 weeks. This fact suggests that lower leg fractures are serious injuries, often requiring prolonged recovery time. In addition, Robertson et al. [12] in their study reported 367 football-related fractures, with a total of 117 fractures occurring in the lower limbs, which 18 were in the tibial diaphysis, 4 in the distal tibia, 4 in the fibula, 2 in the patella, and 2 on the proximal tibia. The mean time of return to sports was 26 ± 22 weeks in the players with lower limbs injuries, where the tibial diaphysis was responsible, in a rate of 20%, for the highest morbidity in not returning to football. These trauma injuries can often lead to kinesiophobia that is defined as "excessive, irrational, and debilitating fear of physical movement and activity resulting from a feeling of vulnerability to painful injury or re-injury" [13].

Fracture of the tibial plateau has also a considerable incidence in impact sports, including football [14]. These fractures have many different patterns of occurrence from undislocated split fractures and slightly/severely displaced depression fractures to more complex and comminuted fractures with severe destruction of the joint lines and cartilage lesions. In this sense, these are considered serious injuries once the majority of players are not able to return to their previous competitive level which can result in a premature career ending [15].

More uncommonly avulsions of the tibial tuberosity may occur, which account for only 3% of tibial fractures [16]. They are usually unilateral; however, it can also occur bilaterally [17]. Another uncommon injury of the tibia is the Segond fracture that is a small vertical avulsion of the lateral aspect of the proximal tibia, distal to the tibial plateau. It is usually caused by internal rotation forces of the knee coupled with varus stress while the knee flexed [18]. This fracture is generally correlated with intra-articular knee damage. The most commonly concomitant intra-articular injuries reported include the anterior cruciate ligament tear (75 to 100% of cases), meniscal tears (66 to 75%), instability or damage of the posterolateral corner of the knee, and, in most rare cases, rotatory knee instability (6 to 13%) [19].

The shin guard appears into the football game as an attempt to reduce and prevent abrasions, contusions, and fractures of the lower extremity. Though, these can only offer protection against lower extremity minor injuries [7]. Shin guards are usually required, and it is estimated to reduce the impact trauma, through up to 60% of deceleration of the impact and up to 20% reduction on the energy absorbed by the leg [20]. Several studies have showed that regardless using a shin guard, a fracture may still occur [7, 8]; nevertheless, in some cases, they may aid to prevent fractures [7, 8].

Acute compartment syndrome is a possible complication when considering tibial fractures, commonly associated with low-energy injuries, which can lead to potentially severe consequences [21]. These authors found that tibial fractures have a statistically significant association with the acute compartment syndrome in football players.

18.1 Distal Femur

18.1.1 Introduction

Distal femur fractures are rare in football, and there are only few reports in the literature regarding this theme [14, 22].

Typically these fractures occur in two distinct populations in young patients secondary to high-energy trauma and in the elderly from minor trauma [23].

Since it is a relatively atypical situation, only general principles will be addressed.

There is no universally accepted classification, and the most important feature of the classification systems is the distinction between extra-articular, intra-articular, and isolated condylar lesion [24].

18.1.2 Clinical Presentation

Severe pain, swelling, and a variable degree of deformity are present. In the young population and since it is a fracture associated with high-energy trauma, other severe injuries can be present. Special attention should be addressed to the neurovascular status of the limb, and careful evaluation should be performed [23–25].

18.1.3 Imaging Studies

In most cases, anteroposterior and lateral radiographs of the knee and distal femur are sufficient to perform a correct diagnosis. Computed tomography (CT) scans are performed is the presence of complex intra-articular fractures and osteochondral lesions. Magnetic ressonance imaging (MRI) can be performed if ligament or meniscal injuries are suspected [23–25].

18.1.4 Treatment

Conservative treatment has very few indications, and most of them are nondisplaced or incomplete fractures and those patients that are not fit for surgery because of medical comorbidities. The treatment consists of a hinged knee brace for nondisplaced fractures and a cast for 6–12 weeks for displaced fractures [24, 26].

Surgical treatment is applied in most fractures and the surgical approach most commonly used is the lateral. Several methods of fixation can be used such as retrograde nailing, screws, plates, skeletal traction, and external fixators (for temporary or definitive treatment) according with the type of fracture [23–26].

18.1.5 Prognosis

Regarding the conservative treatment, the results are considered to be poor particularly in the cases of prolonged immobilization [26].

Surgical treatment has a good to excellent result in most of the cases with a high percentage of patients that can walk without aids and 110 to 120 degrees of flexion. Infection, nonunion, malunion, knee stiffness, and hardware failure are some of the complications described in the literature [27].

18.2 Patella

18.2.1 Introduction

Patellar fractures are a rare event in football and represent a small percentage of fractures in this population. The literature is poor in what concerns at the description of specific fracture types in football. The main mechanisms of injury are direct, indirect, or a combination of both. Direct injuries can be of low or high energy, but obviously in most sports like football, they are of low energy. Indirect injuries are those caused by a forced contraction of the quadriceps with a knee in flexed position. The classification more commonly used in patellar fractures is descriptive (nondisplaced, displaced, transverse, comminuted, vertical, marginal, and osteochondral). In order for a patellar fracture to be considered displaced, the fragments should have more than 3 mm of separation or more than 2 mm of articular incongruity [23, 24, 27].

18.2.2 Clinical Presentation

The main characteristic is anterior knee pain of acute onset with a variable degree of inability to extend the knee actively. Hemarthrosis, pain at the fracture site during palpation, and a palpable defect are also consistent findings. Stability tests of the knee must be performed since anterior cruciate ligament (ACL) injury can be present [23, 24, 27].

18.2.3 Imaging Studies

Plain radiographs of the knee in lateral, anteroposterior, and axial patellofemoral views are generally the only exams necessary for the diagnosis. Contralateral knee imaging should be obtained in order to exclude anatomic variants such as a bipartite or tripartite patella [23, 24].

18.2.4 Treatment

Nonoperative management can be proposed only if there is no extensor mechanism disruption, less than 2 mm of articular incongruity and less than 3 mm of fracture fragment separation [28].

The patient is maintained in partial weight bearing with crutches and a hinged knee brace is applied. The rehabilitation period is divided in periods of 2 weeks: first two, the knee is in full extension; from the second to the fourth week, flexion from 0 to 45 degrees is allowed; from fourth to sixth week, flexion 0 to 90 degrees; and the two following weeks, full motion is allowed. Full weight bearing is allowed at week 8. A regular radiological assessment, lateral, anteroposterior, and axial patellofemoral views, is performed. Return to competition may vary between 6 to 12 weeks; however, residual deficits of the knee may persist, which will affect the sports participation [29, 30].

Surgical management is required to those patients with more than 2 mm of articular incongruity, more than 3 mm of fracture fragment separation, and osteochondral fracture with loose bodies (addressed in other chapter), and extensor mechanism compromise (loss of active extension) causes and treatment are also addressed in another chapter. Several methods of internal fixation have been described: a figure-of-eight tension wire with two k-wires, modified tension band with cannulated screws, and interfragmentary screws without tension banding. The longitudinal approach is more commonly used by the author [23, 24, 27]. The rehabilitation will depend on the type of osteosynthesis used. In case of a figure-of-eight tension wire with two k-wires, immediate mobilization can be performed.

18.2.5 Prognosis

The literature is poor regarding the prognosis of this pathology in football players, but in general population, the prognosis is very good with an overall satisfaction in both conservative and surgical treatment. Return to sports after surgery can occur at 10 weeks but is dependent to the rehabilitation [31]. Approximately in 15% of the cases, symptomatic hardware can be a complication and removal might be necessary as described in a related article [32]. Some complications mentioned are infection, nonunion, knee stiffness, and painful retained hardware [23] (Figs. 18.1 and 18.2).

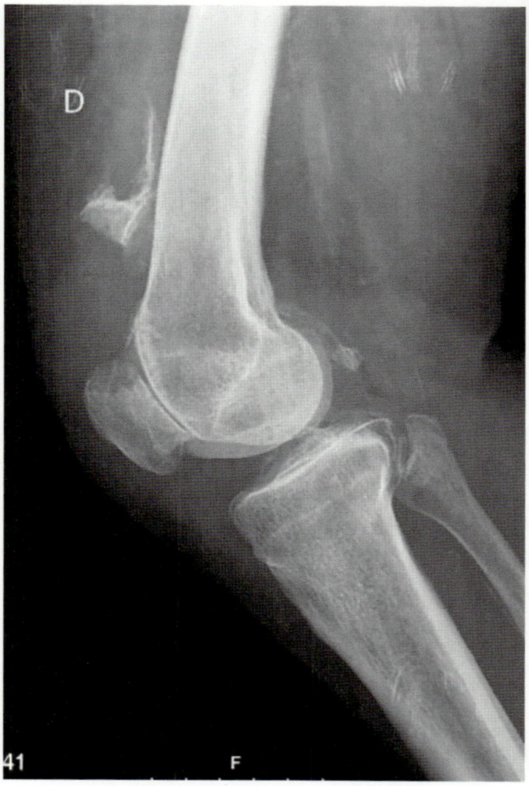

Fig. 18.1 Radiographs on AP view of the knee (patellar fracture)

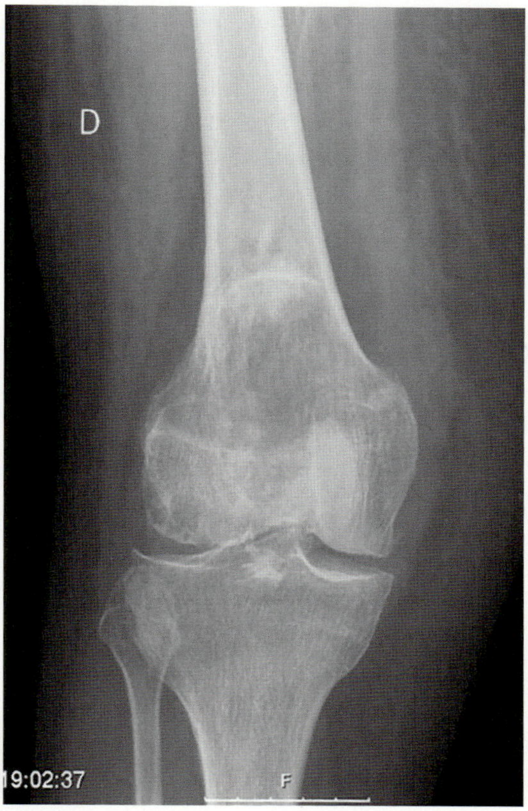

Fig. 18.2 Radiographs on lateral view of the knee (patellar fracture)

18.3 Tibial Spine Avulsion Fractures

18.3.1 Introduction

This type of fractures occurs by forced flexion or hyperextension with internal rotation of the tibia [26]. They are common in pediatric population 8–13 years and related to sports in contrast with the adult population; here these fractures are related to traffic accidents [33–36]. The classification system that is more commonly used is the Mayer and McKeever since 1959 [35] with the following types: I, undisplaced; II, partially displaced fracture; IIIA, completely displaced fragment; and IIIB, completely displaced fragment and rotated; Later Zariczynj [37] included type IV, complete displacement with comminution. In children cartilaginous tibial eminence fracture can occur, which are very often misdiagnosed. Nevertheless, there is a good prognosis even after misdiagnosis and treatment of the non-union, which may be due to the low-energy mechanism of injury and low rate of associated lesion. In this sense, the surgical treatment plays a crucial role because when the patient is exposed to the conservative treatment, the non-union might expose to ACL involution [38] (Fig. 18.3).

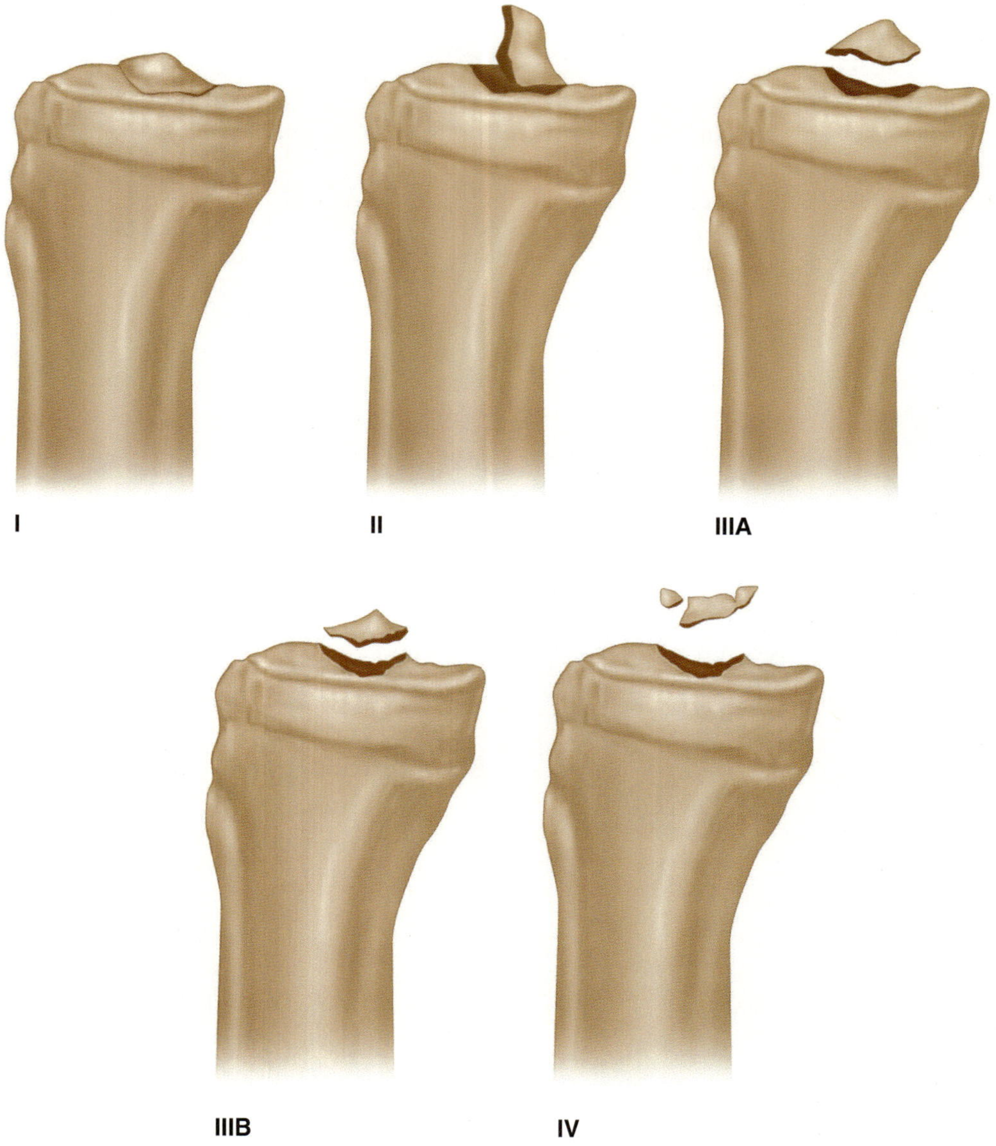

Fig. 18.3 Mayer and McKeever's classification modified by Zariczynj based on avulsion fracture of the tibial eminence: treatment by open reduction and pinning [37] and fracture of the intercondylar eminence of the tibia [35]

18.3.2 Clinical Presentation

Knee pain and hemarthrosis are present, and drainage of the hemarthrosis can be performed in order to relieve symptoms. Entrapment of soft tissue (such as the anterior horn of the lateral meniscus) can also occur [39].

18.3.3 Imaging Studies

The initial study is made by anteroposterior and true lateral radiographs. CT scans are obtained to obtain a better characterization of the degree of communication. MRI can be obtained for more information about the soft tissue structures [40, 41].

18.3.4 Treatment

Type I is treated with a long leg cast immobilization for 4–6 weeks with follow-up radiographs every 2 weeks [42].

In type II the treatment is controversial and can be conservative or surgical depending on the surgeon opinion [26, 42].

Type III/IV is managed surgically with arthroscopy. The more common methods of fixation are by a cannulated screw or by tensioning the fragment with a wire and then passing it through two tibial tunnels drilled to that purpose [26, 42]. Weight bearing is allowed with a pair of elbow crutches with early range of motion [43–45].

18.3.5 Prognosis

The prognosis for surgical treatment is considered very good [42]. Several complications such as residual laxity, growth deformity, and arthrofibrosis are described [39, 42].

18.4 Tibial Plateau Fractures

18.4.1 Introduction

This type of fractures is rarely associated with noncontact sports and can be considered an uncommon knee injury; they are usually related with high-impact incidents such as car accidents [23, 46]; however, there are some reports in amateur football that report this type of fracture as one of the most common in the inferior limb [14]. The fracture usually occurs with a varus or valgus force coupled with axial loading [23]. The classification of these fractures is mainly by the Schatzker classification (six types) that is pathoanatomic and suggests treatment strategies [24, 47, 48] (Fig. 18.4).

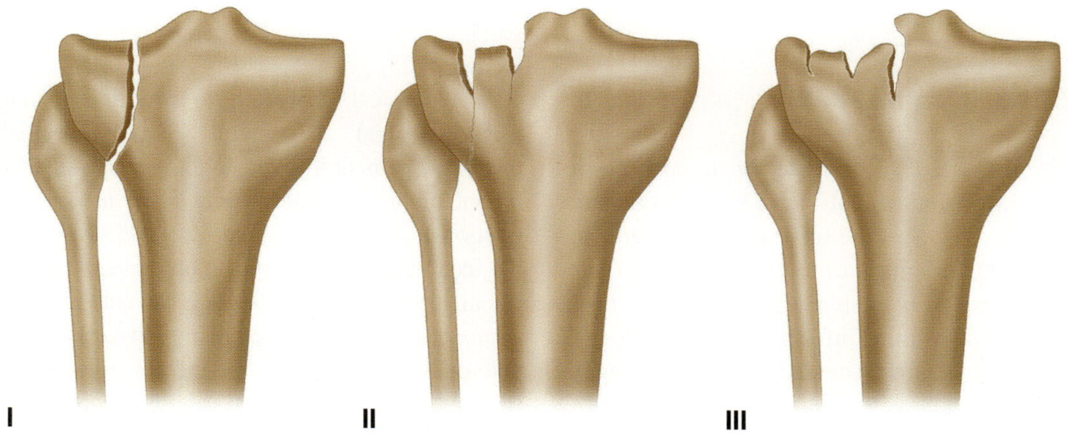

Fig. 18.4 Schatzker classification based on the tibial plateau fracture. The Toronto experience [48]

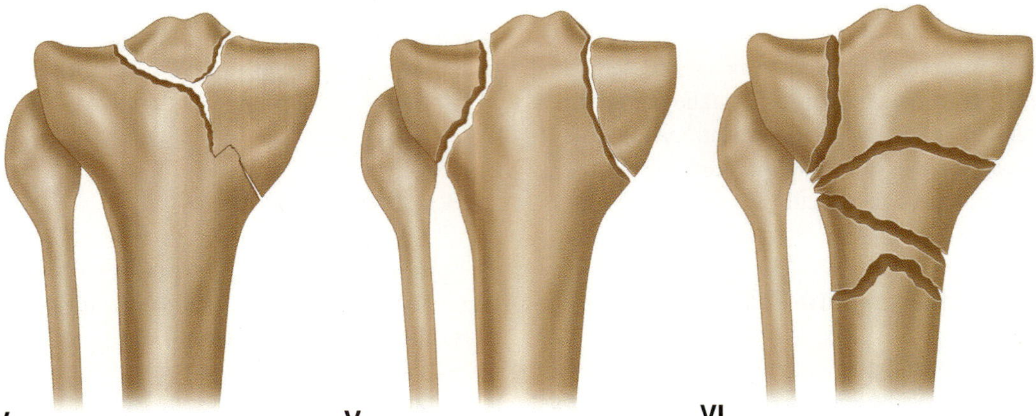

Fig. 18.4 (continued)

18.4.2 Clinical Presentation

The inability to continue to play immediately after this injury is mentioned in a case report of a tibial plateau fracture [46]. In hemarthrosis, a painful knee and inability to bear weight are typical findings [23].

Neurovascular examination and assessment for meniscal or ligament injury remain a key aspect in the evaluation of these fractures [23].

Compartment syndrome can occur but is more common in high energy fractures [23, 24].

Several associated lesions can occur to the meniscus and cruciate or collateral ligaments [23, 24].

18.4.3 Imaging Studies

The initial study is made by anteroposterior (10–15 degree caudal view) and lateral radiographs. CT scans are obtained to obtain a better characterization of the fracture pattern and for preoperative planning. MRI can be obtained for more information about the soft tissue structures (meniscus and ligaments) [23, 24].

18.4.4 Treatment

The conservative treatment can be performed in nondisplaced or minimal displaced fractures; other situations that are also managed by nonoperative treatment but that aren't related to this book are elderly patients or patients with severe medical problems. The patient is kept in a cast brace with non-weight bearing for 4–8 weeks and progressive weight bearing until 12 weeks [3, 7].

Obvious concerns exist to this kind of treatment due to the problem of the long period of immobilization in athletes.

Operative treatment is indicated with vascular injury, compartment syndrome, fractures, open fractures, displaced unstable fractures, and with a variable degree of articular depression <2 mm to 1 cm [23–25].

The surgical goals are to restore articular surface, tibial alignment, and associated menisco-ligament injuries. In this sense, preserving the menisci is fundamental. There are several fixation methods such as plates, screws, and external fixators, and their application depends on the fracture pattern. There are also several surgical approaches such anterolateral, posteromedial, anteromedial, posterolateral, and combined anterior and posteromedial that are used accordingly with the fracture pattern. Arthroscopy has several applications such as soft tissue lesion visualization, joint lavage, osteochondral fragment removal, reduction assistance, or other lesion repair. Weight bearing starts at 8–12 weeks after surgery [24, 25].

18.4.5 Prognosis

Excellent results have been reported with conservative treatment [24, 46].

The results with surgical treatment are largely dependent on the fracture pattern.

Several complications can occur such as infection, arthrofibrosis, malunion, or nonunion [23–25].

It is important to mention that most of the results are referent to non-athletes, and in the literature, the results for this type of population are not favorable like it was demonstrated in a paper where the majority of athletes did not return to the previous level with the authors referring that for competitive sports this can be a career-ending lesion [15] (Figs. 18.5, 18.6, and 18.7).

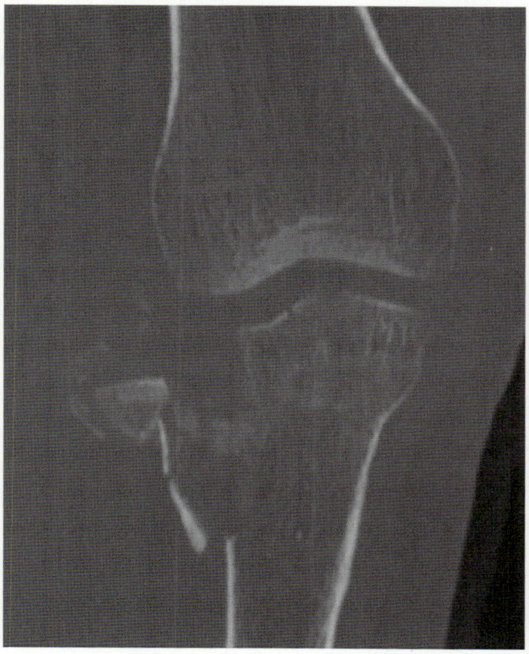

Fig. 18.5 CT scan on coronal view of the knee (tibial plateau fracture)

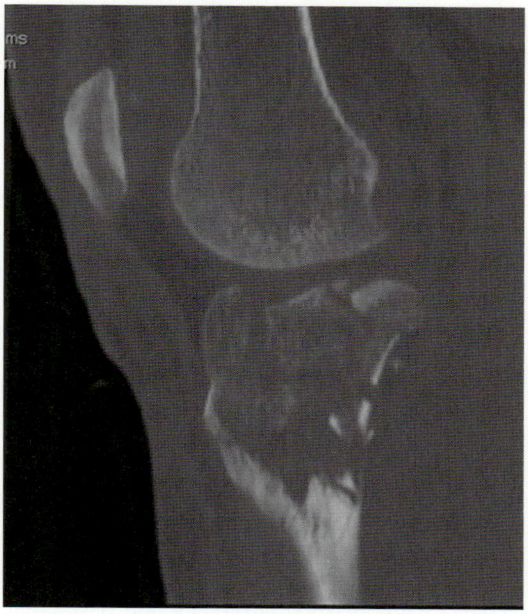

Fig. 18.6 CT scan on sagittal view of the knee (tibial plateau fracture)

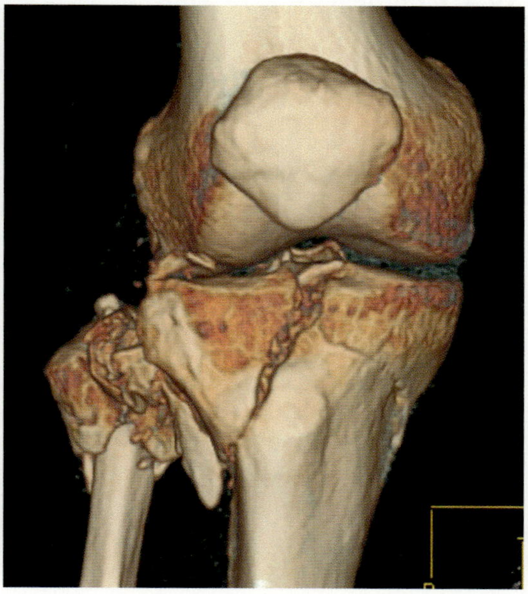

Fig. 18.7 CT reconstruction (tibial plateau fracture)

18.5 Tibial Tubercle

18.5.1 Introduction

This injury occurs mainly in the adolescent population just before the skeletal maturations occurs. It comprises 3% of tibial fractures and results from a vigorous contracture of the quadriceps, and it is typically an injury that occurs in males [16, 49, 50].

Initial classification was proposed by Watson-Jones [51] in three types and later revised by Ogden (subtypes A and B) in order to account the degree of displacement and comminution [52].

Type I consists of a fracture through the tubercle, type II in fracture at the level of the tibial physis, and type III in a fracture that extends into the joint.

More recently a rare type IV fracture was described, and it consists of a fracture that extends posteriorly through the physis [53] and a type V that consists of a type IV and IIIB, creating a Y configuration [50].

18.5.2 Clinical Presentation

An audible pop at the time of the injury may be heard. Acute pain, swelling, and tenderness characterize the presentation. The ability to extend the knee against gravity is variable but weakness is a constant finding. It is important to perform a meticulous knee examination to exclude other injuries such as meniscal or ligament tears [20, 49, 54].

18.5.3 Imaging Studies

Lateral, anteroposterior, and oblique radiographs are required. MRI is rarely necessary, only if associated injuries are suspected [54].

18.5.4 Treatment

Conservative treatment is proposed for the type I fractures and for IB or IIA that can be reduced anatomically with a long leg or cylinder cast.

Surgical treatment, open reduction and internal fixation with fluoroscopy, is reserved for types IB and IIA that can't be reduced, and for types IIB, III, IV, and V, the use of screws with or without washers, tension band wiring, and repair of periosteum are described in the literature. Arthroscopic-assisted techniques are important particularly in type III fractures to assess and repair any intra-articular pathology such as meniscal tear or osteochondral injury. In type V the epiphyseal and metaphyseal fractures should be treated independently. Immobilization is required after surgical treatment for 4–6 weeks [54, 55].

18.5.5 Prognosis

The prognosis is excellent and the main concerns should be addressed to the eventuality of a compartment syndrome. Loss of motion and patellar malposition have also been reported. Return to sports can be expected from 8–22 weeks depending if the treatment is conservative or surgical and the type of fracture [54, 55].

18.6 Segond Fracture

18.6.1 Introduction

Segond fracture avulsion was described in 1879 by Dr. Paul Segond; it is located at the lateral aspect of proximal tibia immediately distal to the plateau [56, 57]. The mechanism of injury is tibial internal rotation and varus stress [19, 57].

It is associated with ACL tears (75%–100%), meniscal tears (66%–75%), avulsion fracture of the intercondylar eminence, and other injuries

[19, 57–59]. Association between ACL injury and Segond fracture may be different in skeletally immature patients [60].

18.6.2 Clinical Presentation

In the acute setting, pain, edema, hemarthrosis, and muscle spasm are usually present, and special tests for ACL tear can be present and positive [19, 61, 62]. Pain on the proximal-lateral tibial plateau has been also described [61].

18.6.3 Imaging Studies

Initial studies consist of knee radiographs; anteroposterior is the best view for the lesion [63].

Since this pathology is associated almost always with other lesions, MRI should be performed [61].

18.6.4 Treatment

Since there are several associated lesions to Segond fracture, a personalized treatment should be performed [59] (described in other chapters).

18.6.5 Prognosis

Has stated before a broad spectrum of associated lesions exist with a variety of treatments performed according with each type making the prognosis associated with the concomitant injuries.

18.7 Tibia/Fibula Shaft Fractures

18.7.1 Introduction

These fractures constitute the most frequent among long bones to be fractured, and reports suggest also an elevated percentage when compared with other fractures among football players [14, 23]. In a paper, approximately 46% of the fractures are from both bones and about 34% from the tibia alone [7]. Usually the fractures are divided into high energy and low energy with the ones resulting from sports activities belonging to the last group [23, 24]. The classification systems have presented poor sensitivity, interobserver reliability, and reproducibility, and by this reason adopting a descriptive can be used (displacement, angulation, shortening, rotation, configuration, anatomic location, fragment number, and position; open or closed) [23].

18.7.2 Clinical Presentation

Pain and soft tissue swelling are characteristic; special attention should be made to the neurovascular status of the limb, to the condition of the soft tissue, and also to the possibility of compartment syndrome [23, 24].

18.7.3 Imaging Studies

Simple radiographic evaluation with anteroposterior and lateral views including the knee and ankle joints is required [23].

18.7.4 Treatment

Nonoperative treatment can be performed with a long leg cast near 0° for approximately 3–6 weeks (and full weight bearing in some cases at 2 weeks); by the end of this period, a fracture brace or patellar bearing cast is applied. In this sense, more than 50% cortical contact, less than 1 cm of shortening, less than 10 degrees of rotation or anterior/posterior angulation, and less than 5 degrees of varus/valgus are acceptable. Several factors can influence the time to union and so this time can be from 12 to 20 weeks [23, 24].

Surgical options include intramedullary nailing, plates and screws, and external fixation. In a study of Boden and coworkers the majority of athletes with fracture of both bones underwent intramedullary nailing [7]. When considering athletes, regarding the post-surgery rehabilitation, the early mobilization of the knee plays a key role.

Surgical complications may appear, majorly due to surgical pitfalls. Therefore, two screws should be light fixated, oriented in spiral fractures rather than a nail or very long plates.

18.7.5 Prognosis

It is referred in the literature that the prognosis and return to play for football players correlated with the energy of trauma (more energy in cases of both bones fractured). The average time mentioned in the literature is 40.2 weeks for both bones, 35 for tibia fractures, and 18 for fibula fractures [7]. Several complications exist in both types of treatments such as malunion, nonunion, and neurovascular injury, but special attention should be taken care to knee pain associated with intramedullary nailing [23–25] (Figs. 18.8 and 18.9).

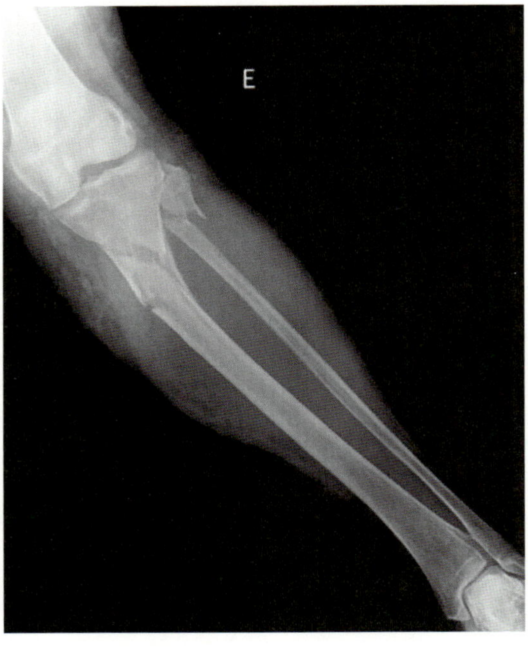

Fig. 18.8 Radiographs on AP view of tibia and fibula shaft fracture

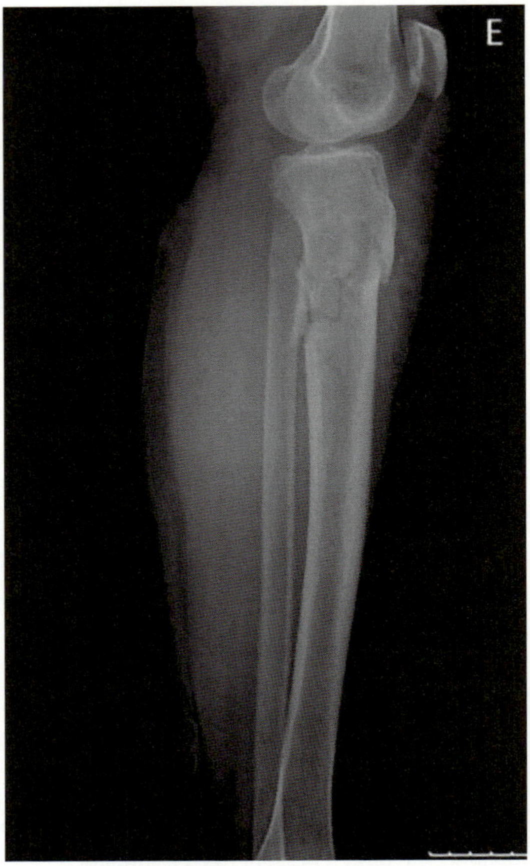

Fig. 18.9 Radiographs on lateral view of tibia and fibula shaft fracture

Conclusion

Fractures around the knee have a broad spectrum of consequences, and special attention should be taken in their prevention, diagnosis, and treatment since some can be career ending.

References

1. FIFA. Football worldwide 2000: official FIFA survey. 2000. http://www.fifa.com/mm/document/fifafacts/bcoffsurv/bigcount.statspackage_7024.pdf.
2. Vanlommel L, Vanlommel J, Bollars P, Quisquater L, Van Crombrugge K, Corten K, Bellemans J. Incidence and risk factors of lower leg fractures in Belgian soccer players. Injury. 2013;44:1847–50.
3. Hawkins R, Hulse M, Wilkinson C, Hodson A, Gibson M. The association football medical research programme: an audit of injuries in professional football. Br J Sports Med. 2001;35:43–7.

4. Hawkins RD, Fuller CW. An examination of the frequency and severity of injuries and incidents at three levels of professional football. Br J Sports Med. 1998;32:326–32.
5. Hawkins RD, Fuller CW. A prospective epidemiological study of injuries in four English professional football clubs. Br J Sports Med. 1999;33:196–203.
6. Court-Brown CM, Wood AM, Aitken S. The epidemiology of acute sports-related fractures in adults. Injury. 2008;39:1365–72.
7. Boden B, Lohnes JH, Nunley JA, Garrett Jr WE. Tibia and fibula fractures in soccer players. Knee Surg Sports Traumatol Arthrosc. 1999;7:262–6.
8. Cattermole H, Hardy J, Gregg P. The footballer's fracture. Br J Sports Med. 1996;30:171–5.
9. Gainor BJ, Piotrowski G, Puhl JJ, Allen WC. The kick: biomechanics and collision injury. Am J Sports Med. 1978;6:185–93.
10. Maehlum S, Daljord O. Football injuries in Oslo: a one-year study. Br J Sports Med. 1984;18:186–90.
11. Swenson DM, Henke NM, Collins CL, Fields SK, Comstock RD. Epidemiology of United States high school sports-related fractures, 2008–09 to 2010–11. Am J Sports Med. 2012;40(9):2078–84.
12. Robertson GA, Wood AM, Bakker-Dyos J, Aitken SA, Keenan AC. The epidemiology, morbidity, and outcome of soccer-related fractures in a standard population. Am J Sports Med. 2012;40:1851–7.
13. Kori S, Miller R, Todd D. Kinesiophobia: a new view of chronic pain behavior. Pain Management. 1990;3:35–43.
14. Goga I, Gongal P. Severe soccer injuries in amateurs. Br J Sports Med. 2003;37:498–501.
15. Kraus TM, Martetschläger F, Müller D, Braun KF, Ahrens P, Siebenlist S, Stöckle U, Sandmann GH. Return to sports activity after tibial plateau fractures 89 cases with minimum 24-month follow-up. Am J Sports Med. 2012;40:2845–52.
16. Hand W, Hand C, Dunn A. Avulsion fractures of the tibial tubercle. J Bone Joint Surg Am. 1971;53:1579.
17. Georgiou G, Dimitrakopoulou A, Siapkara A, Kazakos K, Provelengios S, Dounis E. Simultaneous bilateral tibial tubercle avulsion fracture in an adolescent: a case report and review of the literature. Knee Surg Sports Traumatol Arthrosc. 2007;15:147–9.
18. Cosgrave CH, Burke NG, Hollingsworth J. The Segond fracture: a clue to intra-articular knee pathology. Emerg Med J. 2012;29:846–7.
19. Campos JC, Chung CB, Lektrakul N, Pedowitz R, Trudell D, Yu J, Resnick D. Pathogenesis of the segond fracture: anatomic and MR imaging evidence of an iliotibial tract or anterior oblique band avulsion 1. Radiology. 2001;219:381–6.
20. Lees A, Cooper S. The shock attenuation characteristics of soccer shin guards. In: Atkinson G, Reilly T, editors. Sport leisure and ergonomics. London: Spon; 1995. p. 130–5.
21. Wind TC, Saunders SM, Barfield WR, Mooney III JF, Hartsock LA. Compartment syndrome after low-energy tibia fractures sustained during athletic competition. J Orthop Trauma. 2012;26:33–6.
22. Mabry LM, Ross MD, Abbott JL. Impaction fracture of the medial femoral condyle. J Orthop Sports Phys Ther. 2013;43:512.
23. Egol KA, Koval KJ, Zuckerman JD, Koval KJ. Handbook of fractures. 4th ed. Philadelphia: Wolters Kluwer/Lippincott Williams & Wilkins Health; 2010.
24. Rockwood CA, Green DP, Bucholz RW. Rockwood and Green's fractures in adults. 7th ed. Philadelphia: Wolters Kluwer/Lippincott Williams & Wilkins Health; 2010.
25. Canale ST, Beaty JH, Campbell WC. Campbell's operative orthopaedics. 12th ed. St. Louis/London: Mosby; 2012.
26. Espregueira-Mendes PP. O Joelho. Lousã: Lidel; 2006.
27. Wiesel SW. Operative techniques in orthopaedic surgery. Philadelphia: Lippincott Williams & Wilkins; 2011.
28. Bostrom A. Fracture of the patella. A study of 422 patellar fractures. Acta Orthop Scand Suppl. 1972;143:1–80.
29. Bharam S, Vrahas MS, Fu FH. Knee fractures in the athlete. Orthop Clin North Am. 2002;33:565–74.
30. Keeley A, Bloomfield P, Cairns P, Molnar R. Iliotibial band release as an adjunct to the surgical management of patellar stress fracture in the athlete: a case report and review of the literature. Sports Med Arthrosc Rehabil Ther Technol. 2009;1:15.
31. Hanel DP, Burdge RE. Consecutive indirect patella fractures in an adolescent basketball player. A case report. Am J Sports Med. 1981;9:327–9.
32. Smith ST, Cramer KE, Karges DE, Watson JT, Moed BR. Early complications in the operative treatment of patella fractures. J Orthop Trauma. 1997;11:183–7.
33. Kendall NS, Hsu SY, Chan KM. Fracture of the tibial spine in adults and children. A review of 31 cases. J Bone Joint Surg Br. 1992;74:848–52.
34. Gronkvist H, Hirsch G, Johansson L. Fracture of the anterior tibial spine in children. J Pediatr Orthop. 1984;4:465–8.
35. Meyers MH, Mc KF. Fracture of the intercondylar eminence of the tibia. J Bone Joint Surg Am. 1959;41-A:209–20. discussion 20-2
36. Meyers MH, McKeever FM. Fracture of the intercondylar eminence of the tibia. J Bone Joint Surg Am. 1970;52:1677–84.
37. Zaricznyj B. Avulsion fracture of the tibial eminence: treatment by open reduction and pinning. J Bone Joint Surg Am. 1977;59:1111–4.
38. Chotel F, Raux S, Accadbled F, Gouron R, Pfirrmann C, Berard J, Seil R. Cartilaginous tibial eminence fractures in children: which recommendations for management of this new entity? Knee Surg Sports Traumatol Arthrosc. 2015;24:688–96.
39. Coyle C, Jagernauth S, Ramachandran M. Tibial eminence fractures in the paediatric population: a systematic review. J Child Orthop. 2014;8:149–59.

40. Lafrance RM, Giordano B, Goldblatt J, Voloshin I, Maloney M. Pediatric tibial eminence fractures: evaluation and management. J Am Acad Orthop Surg. 2010;18:395–405.
41. Griffith JF, Antonio GE, Tong CW, Ming CK. Cruciate ligament avulsion fractures. Arthroscopy. 2004;20:803–12.
42. Bagaria V. Regional arthroscopy. INTECH. 2013; doi:10.5772/45960.
43. Reynders P, Reynders K, Broos P. Pediatric and adolescent tibial eminence fractures: arthroscopic cannulated screw fixation. J Trauma. 2002;53:49–54.
44. Shelbourne KD, Urch SE, Freeman H. Outcomes after arthroscopic excision of the bony prominence in the treatment of tibial spine avulsion fractures. Arthroscopy. 2011;27:784–91.
45. Patel NM, Park MJ, Sampson NR, Ganley TJ. Tibial eminence fractures in children: earlier posttreatment mobilization results in improved outcomes. J Pediatr Orthop. 2012;32:139–44.
46. Giulietti JA, Denegar CR, Harner CD. Tibial plateau fracture in a female soccer player: a case study. J Athl Train. 1994;29:32–5.
47. Schatzker J. Rationale of operative fracture care. Berlin: Springer-Verlag; 1988.
48. Schatzker J, McBroom R, Bruce D. The tibial plateau fracture. The Toronto experience 1968–1975. Clin Orthop Relat Res. 1979;138:94–104.
49. Pace JL, McCulloch PC, Momoh EO, Nasreddine AY, Kocher MS. Operatively treated type IV tibial tubercle apophyseal fractures. J Pediatr Orthop. 2013;33:791–6.
50. McKoy BE, Stanitski CL. Acute tibial tubercle avulsion fractures. Orthop Clin North Am. 2003;34:397–403.
51. Watson-Jones R. Fractures and Joint Injuries. 4th ed. Baltimore: Lippincott Williams & Wilkins; 1955.
52. Ogden JA, Tross RB, Murphy MJ. Fractures of the tibial tuberosity in adolescents. J Bone Joint Surg Am. 1980;62:205–15.
53. Ryu RK, Debenham JO. An unusual avulsion fracture of the proximal tibial epiphysis. Case report and proposed addition to the Watson-Jones classification. Clin Orthop Relat Res. 1985;194:181–4.
54. Current diagnosis & treatment in sports medicine. Lange medical book. New York: Lange Medical Books/McGraw Hill Medical Pub; 2007.
55. Frey S, Hosalkar H, Cameron DB, Heath A, David Horn B, Ganley TJ. Tibial tuberosity fractures in adolescents. J Child Orthop. 2008;2:469–74.
56. Segond P. Recherches cliniques et expérimentales sur les épanchements sanguins du genou par entorse. Prog Med. 1879;7:297–9. 319–21, 40–41
57. Goldman AB, Pavlov H, Rubenstein D. The Segond fracture of the proximal tibia: a small avulsion that reflects major ligamentous damage. AJR Am J Roentgenol. 1988;151:1163–7.
58. Felenda M, Dittel KK. Importance of the Segond avulsion fracture as a sign of complex ligamentous knee injury. Aktuelle Traumatol. 1992;22:120–2.
59. Zhao B, Ran X, Zhang M, He C, Jiang D. Surgical treatment of Segond fracture and complications. Zhongguo Xiu Fu Chong Jian Wai Ke Za Zhi. 2013;27:1045–9.
60. Luhmann SJ. Acute traumatic knee effusions in children and adolescents. J Pediatr Orthop. 2003;23:199–202.
61. Arneja SS, Furey MJ, Alvarez CM, Reilly CW. Segond fractures: not necessarily pathognemonic of anterior cruciate ligament injury in the pediatric population. Sport Health. 2010;2:437–9.
62. Fleming Jr RE, Blatz DJ, McCarroll JR. Lateral reconstruction for anterolateral rotatory instability of the knee. Am J Sports Med. 1983;11:303–7.
63. Gottsegen CJ, Eyer BA, White EA, Learch TJ, Forrester D. Avulsion fractures of the knee: imaging findings and clinical significance. Radiographics. 2008;28:1755–70.

Part V

Hip, Groin and Tigh Injuries

Groin Pain

19

Nuno Loureiro, João Pedro Araújo, Luís Simões, and Marco Fonseca

Contents

19.1 Introduction

Groin pain is a very common athletic complaint, but it poses a diagnostic and therapeutic challenge for team physicians, radiologists, consulting surgeons, athletic trainers, and athletes themselves [1]. This partly arises from the multiple anatomic structures in the hip and groin that are prone to injury. Furthermore, signs and symptoms of hip and groin disorders can mimic each other and can be similar to symptoms arising from more distant structures which make accurate diagnosis difficult. Between 2% and 8% of all athletic injuries involve the groin and mainly affect sports requiring rapid changes in direction, quick

N. Loureiro (✉)
Clinica do Dragão – Espregueira-Mendes FIFA Medical Centre of Excellence – FC Porto Dragão Stadium, Porto, Portugal

Paços Ferreira Football Club, Porto, Portugal

Medical Unit of Portuguese Cycling Federation, Lisbon, Portugal

Medical Olympic Committee of Portugal, Lisbon, Portugal
e-mail: nunoloureiro4@gmail.com

J.P. Araújo
Clinica do Dragão – Espregueira-Mendes FIFA Medical Centre of Excellence – FC Porto Dragão Stadium, Porto, Portugal

Al Jazira Football Club, Abu Dhabi, UAE
e-mail: joaopedroaraujo@gmail.com

L. Simões
Clínica Reequilibra, Coimbra, Portugal
e-mail: simasluis@gmail.com

M. Fonseca
Federação Portuguesa de Futebol, Cruz Quebrada- Dafundo, Portugal

Universidade do Porto, Porto, Portugal

Fisibarca – Clínica de Medicina Física e Reabilitação de Ponte da Barca, Viana do Castelo, Portugal
e-mail: maarku@gmail.com

J. Espregueira-Mendes et al. (eds.), *Injuries and Health Problems in Football*,
DOI 10.1007/978-3-662-53924-8_19

acceleration, kicking, and frequent side-to-side motions. In football, the incidence of groin injury has been estimated to be 10–18 per 100 football players per year. However, the definition and diagnostic criteria for groin pain in athletes are not clear, and in the literature, no consensus is provided [2]. Appropriate and successful conservative management relies upon precise clinical reasoning and decision making. Functional demands of the presenting sport must be understood in order to plan, guide, and progress rehabilitation so that the athlete returns to their optimal level and avoids reinjury.

Given the complexity and the difficulty in treating this condition, the athlete must be accompanied by a multidisciplinary team which should include sports medicine doctor, radiologist, physiotherapist, psychologist, and surgeon, among others.

19.2 Incidence of Groin Pain in Football

Groin injury/pain was a frequent occurrence in men's and women's senior football, comprising about 7–13% of all time-loss injuries, with a more than twofold higher rate identified in male compared with female players [3]. The nature of this injury is still poorly understood and reported (e.g., acute versus chronic, traumatic versus overuse, functional versus structural), so we believe that the incidence of groin injury/pain may be underestimated. Common sports associated with hip and groin injuries are those involving repetitive twisting, kicking, and turning movements which occur in american football, football, ice hockey, basketball, and tennis. In addition, sports that involve running with repetitive impact such as track and field are also affected by these injuries [4].

19.3 Risk Factors

It is difficult to compare the findings of risk factor studies because of the lack of a universal definition of groin injury/pain. Our perspective is that previous history of groin injury, altered biomechanics, playing at a higher level, muscle imbalances (mainly in the ratio hip abductor/adductor, core muscle weakness, as well as delayed onset of transversus abdominis), and errors in planning training are the main causes of groin injury/pain. Age, experience, and adductor length have still conflicting evidence in the literature [5].

Repetitive stressing of the musculotendinous structures has been proposed as one of the pathophysiological mechanisms of groin pain in football [6]. It has also been shown that the dominant leg was injured more frequently than the nondominant leg, suggesting that kicking may indeed be part of the problem [7].

19.4 Differential Diagnosis

There are many causes of groin pain, which are extensively referred in the literature. Causes of injuries and disorders include trauma, overuse, muscle strength and length abnormalities, endurance and coordination imbalances across the lumbopelvic region, decreased abdominal stability, inguinal wall weakness, and increased shear forces across the hemipelvis. Symptoms may originate from specific local structures (e.g., adductor tendons, hip joint) or may be referred from other structures (e.g., lumbar spine, sacroiliac joint, neural structures, abdominal viscera, knee joint) or can originate from other pathologies (e.g., rheumatic disorders). The pathology

Table 19.1 Causes of long-standing groin pain

Common	Less common	Not to be missed
Adductor related	Stress fracture	Slipped capital femoral epiphysis
Tendinopathy	Neck of femur	Perthes disease
Myofascial tightness	Pubic ramus	Intra-abdominal abnormality
Iliopsoas related	Acetabulum	Prostatitis
Neuromyofascial tightness	Nerve entrapment	Urinary tract infections
Tendinopathy	Obturator	Gynecological conditions
Bursitis	Ilioinguinal	Spondyloarthropathies
Abdominal wall related	Genitofemoral	Ankylosing spondylitis
Posterior inguinal wall weakness	Referred pain	Avascular necrosis of head of femur tumors
Tear of external oblique aponeurosis	Lumbar spine	Testicular
"Gilmore's sign"	Sacroiliac joint	Osteoid osteoma
Rectus abdominis tendinopathy	Apophysitis	
Pubic bone-related	Anterior superior iliac spine	
Pubic bone stress	Anterior inferior iliac spine (adolescents)	
Hip joint		
Chondral lesion		
Labral tear		

may be primary in origin or may be secondary due to a history of chronic injury. The variety of structures and potential causes of pain can make differential diagnosis a challenge for the clinician. Table 19.1 summarizes some common causes of groin injuries [8].

19.5 Clinical Overview

Due to the anatomical complexity of the region, there is often significant overlap in the signs and symptoms of different diagnoses of groin pain. Adding to this complexity, sportspeople often present with vague symptoms of insidious onset which allows them to continue to train and play with pain. As a result, athletic groin pain has a tendency to develop into a chronic presentation, and sportspeople can often return to sport before completing an adequate rehabilitation period [9].

19.5.1 Medical History

Usually the athlete cannot recall any acute incident, and it is often helpful to look into the activities the patient has been doing in the period preceding the injury as well as a how the symptoms developed.

A subjective assessment must include some themes:

- Type of sport: competitive level, main technical aspects of the sport, type of training, and any changes in training

- Detailed history of the condition: mechanism of injury, duration of symptoms, and previous successful or failed treatments
- Past medical history and medication: previous surgery, congenital hip disorders, degenerative joint disease, other medical conditions and red flags (e.g., history of cancer, weight loss, night pain), and current medication
- Aggravating and easing factors
- Patterns of pain: morning, daytime, and evening
- Current functional difficulties encountered by the athlete
- The athlete's goals for return to sport

Usually the athlete experiences an insidious onset of groin pain, usually felt proximally in one pubic bone, and/or one proximal adductor, but may also be centered on the lower abdomen. Pain starts in one region, unilateral, and then spreads to other regions becoming bilateral, aggravated by exercise, with activities like turning/twisting and kicking being the most challenging movements. The location of the pain in the early stages is important to determine the structure primarily affected. Pain usually presents initially following activity and is accompanied by stiffness in the next morning improving during the day. The ability to produce fast movements such as in sudden changes of direction, sprinting, and kicking is impaired and usually painful when the adductors and the iliopsoas muscles are involved. When the abdominal muscles are involved, strenuous sudden abdominal contractions such as coughing and sneezing can become painful. With the worsening of symptoms, pain appears earlier at the start of activity and does not slow down in the course of it. Nonsteroidal anti-inflammatory drugs (NSAIDs) tend to decrease pain but provide no cure.

19.5.2 Examination

Based on information gained in the subjective assessment, the physical examination is planned. The latter must be thorough and systematic to avoid misdiagnosis:

- Observation: Posture in sitting and standing, gait patterns from the frontal and sagittal plane, leg length discrepancies by observed or palpated differences in pelvic levels and skin creases, rotational differences between both legs, and muscle wasting
- Palpation: The exact site of symptoms should be identified by getting the patient to point to the most painful location. Accurate palpation of the symptomatic structures is essential to precisely pin-point structures at fault and to arrive at a diagnosis. For example, presence of the C sign usually indicates deep interior pain of the hip joint. Other structures that warrant palpation are the lumbar spine, sacroiliac joint, pubic symphysis, muscle bellies, lateral aspect of the greater trochanter, and trochanteric bursa. Bony pelvic landmarks such as the anterior superior iliac spine (ASIS), posterior superior iliac spine (PSIS), and iliac crest should be palpated for symmetry
- Range of motion tests: Any deviations from normal range of motion or changes in range between left to right side should be noted. Range of motion should be assessed in a consistent and reproducible manner (e.g., rotation can be measured in the seated position as the pelvis and hip are stabilized); abduction and adduction range can be measured by referencing the shaft of the femur to the midline of the pelvis. Any factors that may limit normal range of motion must be considered which can include capsuloligamentous, muscular, or articular causes
- Muscle testing: Manual muscle testing can be used to test the strength of the hip adductors and abductors, hip flexors and extensors, hip internal and external rotators, and knee extensors and flexors. However, the reliability of manual muscle testing has been found to be poor. Functional tests should also be considered for evaluation purposes. These may include squat, lunge,

single-leg dip, and hop tests where control, coordination, endurance, and any compensatory movement patterns are assessed. Isokinetic dynamometry testing can be used as an objective measure of hip strength. However further research is needed as there are a limited number of studies which address hip strength using isokinetic dynamometry

Assessment core stability of the deep abdominal and pelvic muscles, as well as adductor squeeze test performed with a dynamometer, has been shown to have good reliability and provide an objective measure which can be monitored or at least compared to a baseline in the event of an acute or gradual onset chronic injury [5].

A positive crossover sign means that the patient's typical groin pain is reproduced when one of the provocation tests (e.g., passive hip abduction, resisted hip adduction, resisted hip flexion in Thomas position) is performed on the contralateral side to the symptoms. A positive crossover functional impairment and the clinical implication is that the player is very unlikely to be able to run, train, or play.

19.6 Imaging

Following the history and physical examination, some musculoskeletal investigations such as ultrasound or MRI may be helpful in evaluating these athletes and ruling out other pathologies, although no radiographic study can rule out pubalgia syndrome. We can say that imaging chronic groin pain in athletes is a controversial topic. The insidious onset of symptoms is important as groin pain due to an acute muscular, tendinous, or osseous injury is easily visualized on imaging and generally carries a much better prognosis than chronic groin pain. Conventional X-rays and CT do not typically aid diagnosis as bone morphology does not correlate with symptoms, and as imaging techniques, they are insensitive to soft tissue changes and/or edema. Herniography and isotope bone scans are now rarely performed and have been superseded by high-resolution MRI. Diagnostic laparoscopy is not recommended.

Ultrasound has been used to detect inguinal hernias but it's use is controversial. Ultrasound can be helpful in the assessment of muscle and tendons. In terms of muscle injuries around the pelvis and hip, MRI can highlight disruption of musculotendinous margins and retracted muscle. MRI can differentiate between musculotendinous injuries and tendon avulsion injuries, which has an impact on management options and is the method of choice for studying this syndrome [10].

Though it should be noted that a high percentage of false-positive results are found in asymptomatic individuals, and the primary guidance in terms of treatment should be given by clinical findings.

Four findings were commonly reported in athletes with long-standing adductor-related or symphyseal groin pain: degenerative changes of the symphyseal joint, adductor muscle insertion pathology, pubic bone marrow edema, and secondary cleft signs. Their exact clinical relevance for treatment or prognosis remains unclear.

19.7 Treatment

19.7.1 Conservative Treatment and Rehabilitation

A few years ago, it was acceptable that treatment for groin pain was rest, electrotherapy, and stretching the most important muscle groups of the lower limbs. However this attitude resulted in recurrence of symptoms upon returning to sports. Compared with rest, active rehabilitation provides more than ten times the likelihood of successful pain-free return to sport [11].

In a recent study [12] that conducted a systematic review of treatment of groin pain in athletes, it was concluded that there is a moderate evidence for active physical training (consisting of adductor and abdominal strengthening and

Table 19.2 Domains and stages in the rehabilitation of pubalgia syndrome

Stages			Domains
Acute	Sub-acute	Chronic	
Trofic	Trofic	Trofic	Trofic
Osteoarticular	Osteoarticular	Osteoarticular	Osteoarticular
Neuromuscular	Neuromuscular	Neuromuscular	Neuromuscular
	Muscular	Muscular	Muscular
		Functional	Functional

coordination exercises) being superior to passive physical therapy modalities (consisting of laser, transverse frictions, adductor stretching, and electric nerve stimulation) for long-standing adductor-related groin pain.

It is very important to ensure that exercise is performed without pain, identify and reduce the sources of increased load on the pelvis, and make progressions in activity levels on the basis of regular clinical assessment.

When we plan a rehabilitation program for groin pain, we could consider three stages and five domains (Table 19.2).

During the acute phase, we must guide our treatment for trophic domains (pain relief and inflammatory response control), osteoarticular domain (correction alignments and relief capsuloligamentar tensions), and neuromuscular domain (improved motor control, timings, and activation sequences) (usually more than lack of strength, there is a lack of motor control, especially in the feedforward mechanism).

There are many forms of intervention for this syndrome, and the selection of the most appropriate will depend on the assessment and the primarily involved structures. It is not possible to create a standard treatment protocol but is intended to show some alternatives and the rationale for their use.

19.7.1.1 Acute Phase 1

To reduce pain, we can use medication, as well as auriculoacupuncture, mesotherapy, and electroacupuncture because of their important action to combat the trigger points and low pain threshold. The use of extracorporeal shock wave therapy (ESWT) can greatly assist the tendon turnover through a controlled low-grade inflammatory response, as well as the application of magnetotherapy and diathermy (initially pulsed) enhancing cellular tropism. The use of kinesio taping can also assist in controlling symptoms. The insoles may also be a giant ally, reminding the importance of correct biomechanics, posture alignment, and symmetry of the lower limbs.

19.7.1.2 Acute Phase 2

Manual therapy (massage, soft tissue mobilization, connective tissue techniques, myofascial release techniques, cranial sacral techniques, joint mobilizations and manipulations, visceral mobilizations, muscle energy techniques, and others) is important at this early stage, reducing pain, increasing range of motion, and improving relaxation of soft tissue and joint structures. Manual therapy may also hasten tissue healing, increase tissue extensibility, facilitate movement, and improve overall physical function. Stretching and core strengthening should start immediately as the symptoms permit. For this purpose, use low-impact exercises initially, and all exercises should be performed in the absence of pain.

19.7.1.3 Acute Phase 3

Exercise therapy is a key factor in rehabilitation of groin pain. At this stage exercise should be low impact and be primarily directed to the deepest and postural muscles, insisting on exercises that emphasize lumbopelvic stability, most of the time isometric at this level. The stabilizer (pressure biofeedback unit) and the fit reformer are two good working tools at this phase. The athletes can start training on bike, but care should be taken if there is contracture of the iliopsoas muscle.

19.7.1.4 Subacute Phase 1

In subacute phase the most important issue is to work the muscle and neuromuscular domains, considering that problems with other domains have become settled in the previous phase. The athlete may start running in a gravitational treadmill (Alter G), reducing the impact and allowing work components/motor patterns of running technique extremely important to maintain optimal neurophysiological process of recruitment of central pattern generators (functional units of the nervous system that program, start, and control the automatic activities). At this stage analytic muscle strengthening can be started and given priority to exercise in external arcs, in order to strengthen the connective tissue around the pelvic girdle and promote strengthening with range of motion gain in muscles that normally are shortened (we need to note that this is not a recipe, e.g., a trigger point usually leads to a decrease in muscle elongation); however, in muscles which are already very elongated, the presence of the triggers may be due to excessive strain due to stretching – in this case a good strategy to use is to reeducate the muscle concentrically (with prejudice we will be weakening collagen matrix despite relief from trigger point), and then we need to reeducate eccentrically within an intermediate external arc.

Muscle strength in closed kinetic chain is very good for increasing pelvic control, and a lot of studies show that when the strengthening of the gluteus medius is done in open kinetic chain, we can get a good range of recruitment of this muscle, as well as tensor fascia lata, which is an antagonist of the first in external rotation of coxofemoral – importance of external rotation on lower limb kinematics, correction of components of knee valgus. When this is done in closed kinetic chain, there is a decrease in tensor fascia lata activation compared with strengthening in open kinetic chain.

19.7.1.5 Subacute Phase 2

Eccentric strengthening of the muscles that insert or pass through the pelvic region to increase their stiffness should be initiated at this phase, thereby improving the stability, absorbency, orientation, and dispersion forces.

It is also advisable to start up with lower limb strengthening exercises primarily with co-contraction of the core muscles and hip adductors. For the core it is true that we can use this strategy in all stages of rehabilitation because physiologically it works this way, but for other joint complexes (like the knee), it may no longer be true, since it operates in reciprocal innervation mechanisms more than in co-contraction mechanisms.

19.7.1.6 Chronic Phase

At this stage we intend to focus more on the neuromuscular and functional domains. Thus, muscle strengthening can be associated with neuromotor control exercises.

Strengthening exercises should attempt to reproduce play motion components of the sports gesture and risk movements as well. At this stage the athlete can start with strengthening eccentric overload and focus particularly in exercises with pulleys and elastic/free weights to allow greater freedom of movement – the athlete must be able to "work with his body." At this stage think more about the recruitment of muscle chain than analytically muscle and progressions with core exercises must continue.

19.7.1.7 Return to Field

Stage 1 – Initiate with semi-static motor control exercises.

Stage 2 – Motor control and agility exercises that already do the transfer for some field exercises with the use of the ball.

Stage 3 – Increased demand from agility drills and readaptation to the sporting resture. Test the athlete in the most of the harmful components that trigger relapse, trying to recreate game situations, subjecting it to competitive stimulus, intensifying cardiorespiratory work, and preparing for the gradual return to work with the team.

19.7.1.8 Failure of Conservative Management

The most common reasons that can lead to failure of conservative therapy include:

- Incorrect diagnosis (hip joint pathology, hernia, stress fracture, referred pain)
- Inadequate period of rest
- Poor compliance
- Exercising into pain
- Inappropriate progressions
- Inadequate core stability
- Persistent lumbar intervertebral hypomobility
- Persistent adductor guarding

19.7.2 Surgical Treatment

As the long-standing groin pain is treated mostly with conservative treatment, surgical treatment is reserved for very specific and very few situations.

Surgery for long-standing athletic groin pain can be classified into open and laparoscopic techniques. The open technique can be a mesh repair (Lichtenstein) or a sutured repair (Shouldice). The suture repair can be "minimal," that is, plication of the transversus abdominis and fascia transversalis in a double layer and excision of the genital branch of the genitofemoral nerve (Muschaweck), anterior pelvic floor repair (Meyers), or darn reconstruction (Gilmore). Release of the adductor longus insertion onto the pubic bone ± release of the obturator nerve is often part of the groin reconstruction operation (Bradshaw). Laparoscopic repairs can be either transabdominal preperitoneal (TAPP), i.e., opening and closing peritoneum over a mesh repair, or totally extraperitoneal (TEP) repair performed without breaching the peritoneum by entering the retro-rectus space, preserving the parietal peritoneum and inserting mesh fastened with helical tacks, staples, or glue. Lloyd's release involves inguinal ligament tenotomy, i.e., taking the inguinal ligament attachment on the pubic tubercle and reinforcing the posterior inguinal canal wall with mesh.

Symptomatic labral tear of the hip joint is treated by arthroscopy and debridement as a separate preceding operation by an orthopedic specialist. Pubic bone stabilization with plate or screws is a rarely used surgical option because of the risk of stress fractures of the pelvis, but has been found successful in Welsh international rugby players in association with a soft tissue reconstruction [13]. We have some studies that point to indicate surgery for inguinal pathology and hip intra-articular injury.

The surgeon's choice of repair relies on his/her expertise as to whether to use an open or laparoscopic (TAPP or TEP) technique.

It was noted that the laparoscopic technique had a quicker recovery and return to sporting activity, but it was also accepted that the surgeon's relative expertise and experience in a particular technique was a major determining factor in the type of repair undertaken. Furthermore, there was no data from randomized controlled trials which suggests to any technique was superior [14].

Conclusion

Groin pain is an extremely common presentation in sports and exercise medicine, particularly in football, yet very poorly understood. One of the reasons is that the anatomy of the region is complex, and so the load in this region is extremely high in every sports that involve kicking and rapid change of direction. Sometimes long-standing groin pain starts with an acute partial tear of adductor longus muscle and represents a clinical challenge.

After identifying the main structures primarily involved through a very careful medical history, physical examination and confirmed or not by imagiologic study (in this case mainly MRI) it is outlined multimodal and multidisciplinary treatment plan and there must be a commitment from the athlete and a careful return to competition involving the coaching staff.

References

1. Omar I, Zoga A, Kavanagh E, Koulouris G, Bergin D, Gopez A, Morrison W, Meyers W. Athletic pubalgia and "sports hernia": optimal MR imaging technique and findings. Radiographics. 2008;28:1415–28.
2. Holmich P, Holmich L, Bjerg A. Clinical examination of athletes with groin pain: an intraobserver and interobserver reliability study. Br J Sports Med. 2004;38:446–51.
3. Waldén M, Hägglund M, Ekstrand J. The epidemiology of groin injury in senior football: a systematic review of prospective studies. Br J Sports Med. 2015;49:792–7.
4. Caudill P, Nyland J, Smith C, Yerasimides J, Lach J. Sports hernias: a systematic literature review. Br J Sports Med. 2008;42:954–64.
5. Quinn A. Hip and groin pain: physiotherapy and rehabilitation issues. Open Sports Med J. 2010;4: 93–107.
6. Ekberg O, Persson N, Abrahamsson P, Westlin N, Lilja B. Longstanding groin pain in athletes. A multidisciplinary approach. Sports Med. 1988;6:56–61.
7. Holmich P, Thorborg K, Dehlendor C, Krogsgaard K, Gluud C. Incidence and clinical presentation of groin injuries in sub-elite male soccer. Br J Sports Med. 2013;48:1245–1250.
8. Brukner P, Khan's K. Clinical sports medicine. 4th ed. NY, USA; McGraw-Hill Education - Europe: 2012. p. 548.
9. Domb B, Brooks A, Byrd J. Clinical examination of the hip joint in athletes. J Sport Rehabil. 2009;18:3–23.
10. Lischuk AW, Donates TM, Wong W, et al. Imaging of sports related hip and groin injuries. Sport Health. 2010;2:252–61.
11. Holmich P, Uhrskou P, Kanstrup I. Effectiveness of active physical training as treatment for longstanding adductor related groin pain in athletes: randomised trial. Lancet. 1999;355:439–43.
12. Server A, Eijck C, Beumer B, Holmich P, Weir A, de Vos R. Study quality on groin injury management remains low: a systematic review on treatment of groin pain in athletes. Br J Sports Med. 2015;49:813.
13. Garvey J. Surgical options for chronic groin pain in football players. Aspetar Sports Med J. 2013;2: 162–9.
14. Sheen A, Stephenson B, Lloyd D, Robinson P, Fevre D, Paajanen H, Beaux A, Kinsnorth A, Gilmore O, Bennett D, MacLennan I, Dwyer P, Sanders D, Kurzer M. Treatment of the sportsman's groin: British Hernia Society's 2014 position statement based on the Manchester Consensus Conference. Br J Sports Med. 2014;48:1079–87.

20 Femoroacetabular Impingement

André Sarmento, J. Cruz de Melo,
Alberto Monteiro, and Pieter D'Hooghe

Contents

A. Sarmento (✉) • A. Monteiro
Clínica do Dragão, Espregueira-Mendes Sports Centre - FIFA Medical Centre of Excellence, Porto, Portugal
e-mail: andresarmento1@gmail.com; albertohmonteiro@gmail.com

J.C. de Melo
Hospital da Luz Arrábida, Porto, Portugal
e-mail: ajcruzdemelo@gmail.com

P. D'Hooghe
Aspetar Hospital, Doha, Qatar
e-mail: Pieter.DHooghe@aspetar.com

20.1 Introduction

Femoroacetabular impingement (FAI) has been recently recognized as a cause for hip pain in adults particularly in young adults.

It has also been proposed that FAI may be an important underlying cause for early osteoarthritis of the hip.

For years, athletes would complain of groin pain, and its cause would remain unclear and for this reason untreated. Most of the times, it would be attributed to "pubalgia," a misnomer which literally means pain around the area of the pubic bone, and athletes would get treatment addressing the adductors, the rectus abdominis, or the abdominal wall which is only successful if the diagnosis was accurate. Patients with intra-articular problems would remain symptomatic. This would, oftentimes, lead to permanent disability not enabling the athlete to fulfill his or her potential or even cut short their career.

Ever since it was first described, FAI has been increasingly associated with hip and groin pain in athletes. Football, as a pivoting sport, places the hip at risk of hip injuries, and the number of players diagnosed with FAI has also increased. FAI is a syndrome caused by a femoral and acetabular mismatch. The understanding of the pathological alterations and its implications in hip kinematics is fundamental in interpreting the clinical picture, which can be varied, in order to ensure proper treatment. It is imperative to properly evaluate

J. Espregueira-Mendes et al. (eds.), *Injuries and Health Problems in Football*,
DOI 10.1007/978-3-662-53924-8_20

patients' complains and correlate them with their physical examination and imaging tools; otherwise follow-up can be undermined.

Treatment can be either conservative or surgical. Nonetheless, over the last years, the number of surgical procedures, both open and arthroscopic, to address the deformities which underlie FAI have increased dramatically. There have been numerous papers from several authors reporting on the results of surgical treatments most of which showing promising short to mid-term results. These have been supported by a high rate of returning to sports activities at the same level as prior to surgical intervention.

Results have been dependent on early detection and chondral damage at the time of surgical intervention. There are, at this time, however, no proof that treatment can avoid or even delay the development of hip arthritis. We are, nonetheless, optimistic regarding this last issue as we are on the verge of being able to address chondral damage as well as anatomic deformities.

20.2 Pathophysiology

Osteoarthritis of the hip can have numerous causes which include Legg-Calve-Perthes disease, slipped capital femoral epiphysis, avascular necrosis of the femoral head, inflammatory diseases, and dysplasia [1–9]. In the case of dysplasia, there is static overload over a small area of acetabular surface which leads to early degenerative changes in the hip joint, especially in the anterior region of the acetabulum [6–9].

There is a distinct group, nonetheless, one in which early osteoarthritis ensues even though they do not belong in any of the aforementioned groups. For these the cause of arthritis has remained unclear for years, and it was deemed as idiopathic osteoarthritis [10]. As early as 1976, Solomon claimed that <10% of osteoarthritis was idiopathic [9]. Ganz et al. [11] first coined the term femoroacetabular impingement to describe a condition in which subtle morphological changes in either the acetabulum of the femur or both under stresses over the physiologically tolerable would lead to damage in the labrum and cartilage leading to early arthritis. Ganz also claimed that arthritis would be attributed to anatomic abnormalities in over 90% of the cases [12]. However, this view that FAI may lead to arthritis is not shared by all authors.

Femoroacetabular impingement as defined by the US National Library of Medicine is a clinical entity in which a pathological mechanical process causes hip pain when morphologic abnormalities of the acetabulum and/or femur, combined with vigorous hip motion (especially at the extremes), lead to repetitive collisions that damage the soft tissue structures within the joint itself. So, there must be an anatomical abnormality, excessive motion which leads to abnormal contact between the acetabulum and femur, repetitive traumatic motion, and soft tissue damage. These can lead to pain defining the syndrome femoroacetabular impingement.

20.2.1 Mechanism and Types of Femoroacetabular Impingement

Stulberg et al. [3] first described the pistol grip deformity of the proximal femur (head and neck) which in their opinion would lead to early-onset osteoarthritis.

It was, however, Ganz et al. [11] who theorized over the mechanisms that would produce early degenerative changes.

Bedi et al. [13] showed that athletes with FAI exhibited larger amounts of biomarkers of cartilage degradation than a control group.

There are two main types of FAI: cam type and pincer type. However, most of the times, a coexistence of both mechanisms seems to occur.

20.2.1.1 Cam-Type Impingement

In this type of FAI, prominence of the anterolateral head and neck junction leads to abnormal contact with the acetabulum with motion especially flexion and internal rotation which will lead to chondral damage as well as tears in the chondrolabral junction and separation of the labrum. These changes often occur in the anterolateral

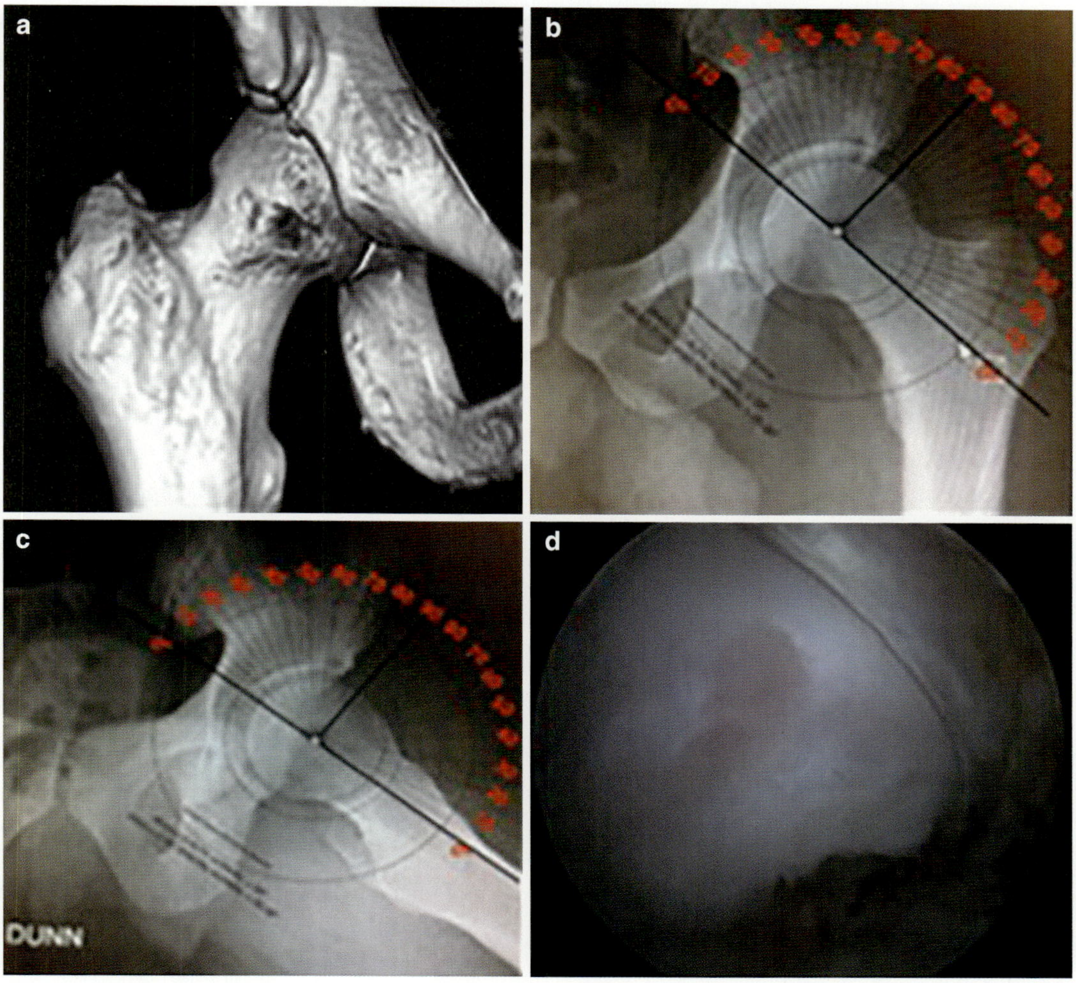

Fig. 20.1 Cam-type impingement. (**a**) Cam deformity as seen on CT scan; note prominence of anterior femoral neck (*arrow*); (**b** and **c**) cam deformity best evidenced on axial view (α where alpha angle can be measured); (**d**) cam-type deformity on arthroscopy showing chondral injury on impingement site

labrum and acetabulum [11, 14–16]. This is called cam-type impingement. In this type of impingement, the anatomical change occurs in the head and neck junction which leads to an increase in the alpha angle (Fig. 20.1). An angle over 55° is considered abnormal [15, 17]. In 2015, Wright et al. [18] concluded that an increase in the alpha angle is the only prognostic factor associated with the development of early osteoarthritis and labral tears.

The repetitive entering of the cam lesion on the hip joint results in cartilage injuries that can be as deep as 2 cm. With time, the femoral head can migrate into the defect.

These changes are more typical in young male adults, especially athletes. Males participating in certain sports appear to be at an increased risk for arthritis [19–27]. The current evidence supports the increased risk of cam deformity in athletes in hockey, basketball, and other jumping sports. Repetitive axial loading (jumping) or hip flexion (squatting) may stimulate anterolateral extension of the physis that ultimately results in bony overgrowth of the cam deformity.

20.2.1.2 Pincer-Type Impingement

On the other hand, pincer-type impingement is defined as an overcoverage of the anterior acetabulum, which with motion leads to abnormal contact between the acetabular rim and a normal femoral head and neck which leads to labral damage and eventually chondral damage. It is more typical of middle-aged women who participate in athletic activities. This type of impingement can derive from conditions such as *coxa profunda* or acetabular retroversion [4, 28, 29]. Labral damage is initially low; however with repeated contact, degenerative changes ensue with ganglion formation and rim ossification which in turn lead to further deepening of the acetabulum and worsening of the overcoverage. The levering of the femoral neck on the rim will lead to contact between the head and the postero-inferior acetabulum creating a countercoup lesion [12, 30].

20.2.1.3 Extra-articular Impingement

These are a variety of disorders which cause pain in the nonarthritic young patient especially in athletes.

Psoas impingement is first described by Heyworth in 2007 [31]. It is characterized by labral tears in the anterior region (3 o'clock position) of the acetabulum which is not typical of FAI. He noticed that by releasing the iliopsoas tendon, there would be an impingement-free range of motion. As supported by further studies, a tight iliopsoas tendon is responsible for anterior labrum tears.

Subspine impingement occurs between a prominent anteroinferior iliac spine (AIIS) and the femoral neck with extreme flexion [32, 33]. This prominence is associated with AIIS avulsion injuries which consolidated in inferior position.

Ischiofemoral impingement occurs because of a narrowing of the ischiofemoral space [34] with resultant impingement of the lesser trochanter on the ischial tuberosity.

Greater trochanteric pelvic impingement (GTPI) is generally a sequela of Perthes disease and takes place in extremes of abduction [35]·

20.2.2 Other Dynamic Causes of Hip Pain

Other dynamic causes of hip pain which must be considered when dealing with young adults with hip pain include true acetabular retroversion in which the anterior wall of the acetabulum is prominent while the posterior is shallow creating an anterior impingement in flexion, femoral retroversion which diminishes internal rotation [35, 36], and femoral varus which results in GTPI.

These conditions must be taken into account when dealing with the young adult with complains of hip pain once the treatment may be quite different.

20.3 Epidemiology

It is difficult to establish the true epidemiology of FAI. In fact, it is difficult, in the arthritic population, to distinguish pre-arthritic changes that might have led to arthritis from those secondary to arthritis itself. In fact, even in the young, there are many asymptomatic people who exhibit morphological abnormalities associated with FAI. Reichenbach et al. [37] reported on asymptomatic military recruits with a mean age of 19.9 years old in whom cam-type deformity is present in 24% of them. The same author, in a different study [38], also showed that the presence of cam deformity in asymptomatic hips was associated with magnetic ressonance imaging (MRI) evidence of labral lesions and herniation pits as well as a decrease in acetabular cartilage width. Hack et al. [39] showed a presence of imaging changes associated with FAI in 14% of asymptomatic people.

Frank et al. [40], in 2015, did a systematic review on prevalence of FAI imaging findings in asymptomatic volunteers. They showed that the cam-type deformity was present in 37% subjects and that the pincer type was present in 67% of subjects even though pincer-type deformity was more heterogeneously defined. The average alpha angle was 54° which is the borderline abnormal. Also, there was a 3:1 ratio in cam-type deformity when comparing athletes with nonathletes.

In particular, the athletic population seems to be particularly at risk of developing imaging characteristics of FAI as well as symptomatic impingement. There has been a great amount of work being done here. Nepple et al. [41] showed that, in the National Football League, players who have been previously evaluated for groin pain have evidenced signs of FAI in 94.3% of the players, most of the times mixed-type impingement. Also, males participating in certain sports activities show a higher probability of osteoarthritis later in life [19, 27]. Siebenrock et al. [42, 43] showed significantly greater prevalence of cam deformity (alpha angle >55) in elite basketball players (89%) compared with controls (9%). Philippon et al. [44] reported on a significantly higher prevalence of cam deformity among hockey players (75%) compared with skiers (42%). Agricola et al. [45] investigated elite football players and found a nonsignificant increase in prevalence of cam-type deformity in football athletes (26%) compared with controls (17%), whereas Johnson [46] did not show statistical difference between football players and control groups in both female and male population. In this way, there is a clear association between participation in sports activities especially basketball, hockey, and other jumping sports and the development of cam-type deformity. These sports might be linked to at-risk positions for stress to the proximal femoral physis [21, 24, 27, 47]. It is suggested that repetitive axial loading (i.e., jumping) or hip flexion (i.e., squatting) can stimulate anterolateral extension of the physis that ultimately results in bony overgrowth of the cam deformity.

Current literature shows a clear increase in prevalence of radiographic signs associated with hip impingement in athletes participating in high-intensity sports in adolescence, namely, cam-type impingement. Cam-type impingement is particularly associated with the development of labral and chondral injuries and the development of early arthritis. However, we cannot say at this time that engaging in sports will increase the likelihood of symptomatic hip disease or arthritis.

20.4 Clinical Features and Physical Examination

As previously stated, FAI imaging abnormalities will not suffice in making the diagnosis and treating the patient because these are very common in the general population. There must be a clear correlation between clinical picture and imaging before initiating the endeavor of treating an athlete suspected of suffering from FAI-related disability.

In order to evaluate the hip, one must be aware that there are many causes of groin pain both arising in the musculoskeletal system and in visceral organs. On the other hand, the athlete should be evaluated for coexisting disease, compensatory disease, or coincidences.

Coexisting diseases are common such as lumbar pathology where pain can be referred to buttocks or trochanteric region or athletic pubalgia with pain referred to the groin area. Athletic pubalgia and intra-articular problems coexist often [48, 49]. Increase pelvic motion puts greater stress in stabilizing structures. Athletic pubalgia is more associated with pain on palpation of the pubic rami, adductor, *and* rectus abdominis insertions and should not be aggravated by hip range of motion but by coughing or performing sit-ups.

As for compensatory diseases, athletes compensate for their joint disease in overloading surrounding hip structures leading to gluteal fatigue, trochanteric bursitis, and abductor pain or tears. These secondary pathologies have its origin, most of the times intra-articularly.

As for incidental findings, a snapping of the iliopsoas tendon is present in 10% of the population [50], and an asymptomatic one should not be confused with one that causes labral tears or even should not be treated in case of labral tears caused by conditions other than the snapping itself.

Pain in FAI usually begins gradually. Athletes might recall an inciting event, but most of the times there is not one. In one study [51], there was an average of 29.6 months between the onset of symptoms and surgery. Poor flexibility is usually present, but oftentimes it is not a problem because they can be compensated by lumbar or pelvic hyper mobility. Pain is usually located in the groin and radiates to the medial thigh. Athletes can exhibit the C sign of Byrd [52] with the hand cupped around the greater trochanter and gripping the fingers to the groin. Pain is worse with turning, twisting, pivoting, and ascending and descending inclined surfaces. Pain also aggravates with maximal flexion, and extending from this position is also uncomfortable. With advanced degenerative changes, symptoms may become constant. Snapping and clicking are also present in 25% of the patients operated for FAI [51].

Physical examination should begin on the standing position looking for pelvic asymmetry, spinal deformity, or limb length discrepancies. Gait should be evaluated. At least three to four walking strides should be visualized in order to distinguish normal gait from an antalgic one (generally with shorter steps) or a Trendelenburg-type gait because of abductor insufficiency [53]. Also, the patient should perform the single stance test whereby he stands on the affected leg and holds the other leg in about 45° hip flexion and 45° knee flexion. A positive test is a drop or shift on the contralateral pelvis of more than 2 cm.

Much of the exam takes place in the supine position.

Palpation of anterior and lateral structures can be performed as the anterior iliac spines, pubic symphysis, adductor tubercle, inguinal and abdominal regions as well as the trochanteric region.

ROM is evaluated. Internal and external rotations are measured with the hips at 90° of flexion. It can also be performed in the sited position where pelvis is stabilized at the ischial tuberosity. ROM should also be measured in the prone position and thus alter relative contributions of the ligamentous structures – flexion relaxed the iliofemoral ligament, but the main contributor to internal rotation is the ischiofemoral ligament [54]. ROM is dictated by a firm end point or pain.

Several provocative maneuvers can be performed. The dynamic external rotatory impingement test (DEXTRIT) is executed by instructing the patient to hold the contralateral leg eliminating lumbar lordosis and taking the affected leg to 90° and beyond and moving it through an arc of external rotation and abduction. The dynamic internal rotatory impingement test is similar except for the arc which is done in adduction and internal rotation. Both tests are positive with recreation of the patient's pain. The flexion/abduction/external rotation test (FABER) or Patrick test can elicit lumbar, sacroiliac, or posterior hip pain. The straight leg raise against resistance test (RSLR) also known as the Stinchfield test [55] evaluates flexors of the hip, namely, the iliopsoas and intra-articular problems. The passive supine rotation test (log roll) [52] assesses rotation of both hips noting differences of guarding and laxity. Pain or locking can elicit intra-articular or extra-articular pathology. The flexion/adduction/internal rotation (FADDIR) tests or impingement test [56] can be performed in the supine or lateral position. The affected leg is brought to 90° flexion, adduction, and internal rotation. Again, reproduction of the patient's pain indicates a positive test.

The lateral exam allows for inspection and palpation of the lateral structures (trochanteric region) as well as posterior iliac spines, iliac wing, and ischial tuberosity. Special tests can be performed as well. In the passive adduction tests, the examiner stands behind the patient and assesses adduction with the knee and hip in extension (contraction of the tensor fascia lata), with the hip in extension and the knee at 45° (contractures of the gluteus tendons), and with the hip in flexion, the knee in flexion, and the shoulders against the table (gluteus maximus contracture).

In the prone position, palpation of the posterior structures is possible, and the femoral neck version can be assessed with the Craig test [55]. The limb is rotated so that the lateral prominence of the greater trochanter is maximal. The angle between the leg (tibia) and a vertical line is indicative of femoral anteversion. ROM can also be assessed as well as contractures of the flexors by passively extending the hip.

Philippon et al. [51] showed that patients operated on by FAI had less mobility in all plains of motion versus the contralateral leg. Flexion was the more affected with a 9° side to side difference. The impingement test was present in 99% of patients. Abnormalities in the FABER test were also noted in 97% of the patients.

However, it must be noted that although most of these tests are quite sensible for hip pathology, their specificity is low. In a systematic review, Tijssen et al. [57] included 21 studies to evaluate their validity. All studies were either level IV or V. Many of the tests were object of previous studies, but results showed there was a lack of diagnostic accuracy. The authors found it difficult to interpret results as the variation of populations was high as well as there was a bias in population selection. In this way there was heterogeneity of results. For instance, the sensitivity of the anterior impingement test's varied from 0.59 to 0.99 and for the FABER test from 0.41 to 0.97. Also the positive predictive value and negative predictive values obtained are not applicable once the populations studied were at high suspicion of disease or even had labral tears and FAI confirmed and were not the general population. Burgess et al. [58] also concluded that there is too little information to draw a conclusion for clinical practice. Leibold et al. [59] referred that a negative result in the anterior impingement test, the flexion adduction axial compression test, and the Fitzgerald test provided the clinician confidence that labral pathology was absent. There is, however, to date, little evidence pertaining the accuracy and validity of most of the abovementioned tests.

20.5 MCDTs for Radiographic Evaluation

For athletes with suspected FAI, a true AP view of the pelvis and a lateral radiograph of the hip should be obtained. In the AP view, the coccyx should point to the symphysis with a distance of 1–2 cm between them, and obturator foramens should be symmetrical so that there is no rotation or pelvic tilt. It is of the upmost importance to obtain the adequate projection once variations in pelvic tilt can change our ability to ascertain acetabular version and coverage.

In the AP projection, the joint space, impingement, overcoverage, and other bony alterations that can be present are evaluated. Overcoverage of the anterior acetabulum is suggested by the crossover sign (the anterior wall of the acetabulum crosses the posterior wall) (Fig. 20.2) which should be distinguished from global overcoverage and acetabular retroversion indicated by the posterior wall sign (the posterior wall does not reach half of the femoral head).

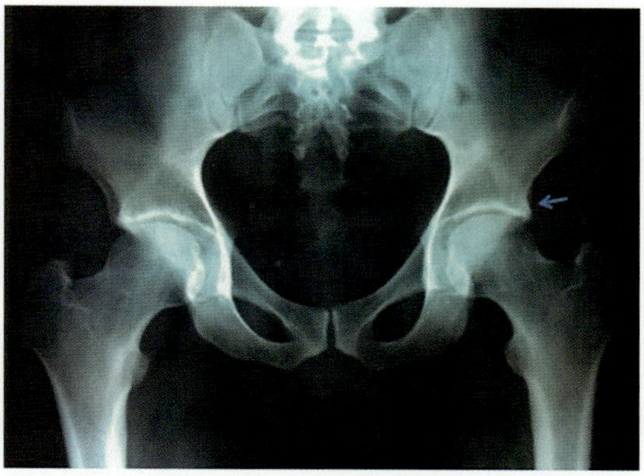

Fig. 20.2 Pincer-type impingement. Pelvis X-ray on AP views. Here, joint space and bone anomalies are evaluated. Focal (anterior) overcoverage is evidenced by the crossover sign evidenced on the left hip (*blue arrow*)

The sphericity of the femoral head should be evaluated in both the AP view as well as the lateral view which can be the 40° Dunn view or the frog lateral view. Both seem adequate in assessing the cam lesion [60, 61]. Herniation pits can be present at the head and neck junction indicating FAI. X-rays are extremely useful, but they depict a two-dimensional image when we are dealing with three-dimensional deformity.

Computed tomography (CT) scans can be used to further evaluate osseous anatomy at which it is much better than other imaging modalities. CT scans enable visualization of an os acetabulum otherwise not visible on MRI and can determine the degree of joint narrowing. Two-dimensional images obtained by CT scan underestimate the size of the cam lesion once it is necessary to bisect the apex of the lesion. So three-dimensional CT images are best to ascertain the morphology of the lesion both in the acetabulum providing additional information. In this way CT scans provide additional information as to the amount of resection necessary if surgical treatment is planned and for this reason can be an invaluable tool for preoperative planning.

MRI is a necessary exam when dealing with FAI and labral tears. High-resolution small-field images are necessary requiring at least a 1.5 T magnet with surface coils [62]. There is high sensitivity with conventional MRI to detect labral tears, but the ability to detect intra-articular cartilage damage associated with FAI is poor. If labral

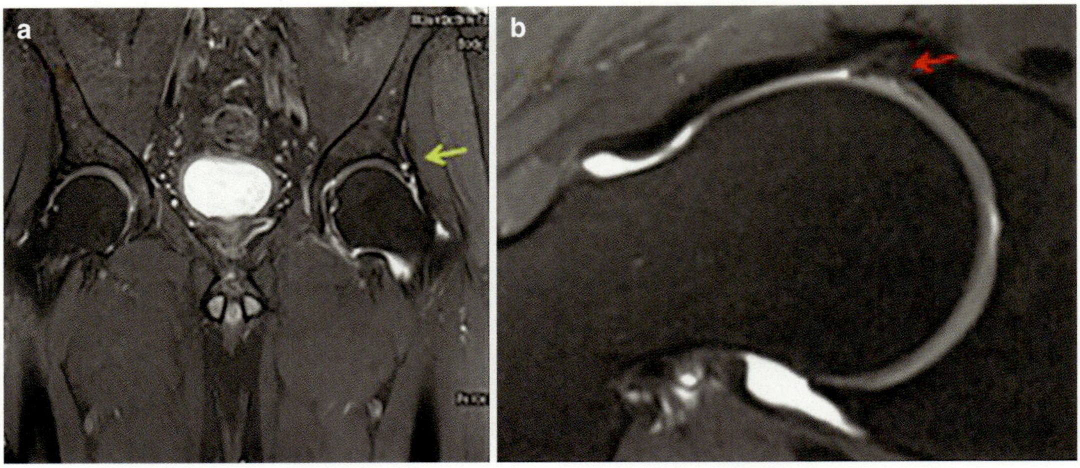

Fig. 20.3 MRI imaging in FAI. (**a**) MRI paralabral cyst which is indicative of a labral tear (*yellow arrow*); (**b**) MRI arthrogram showing an increase in alpha angle and labral degeneration (*red arrow*)

pathology is present, there is likely articular damage associated. Increased signal on T2-weighted images in anterior acetabulum wall is suggestive of articular damage. Also, increased activity within the herniation pit in the femoral neck may be associated with degenerative disease secondary to cam impingement. A paralabral cyst is pathognomonic for labral pathology, whereas subchondral cysts usually indicate articular pathology (Fig. 20.3a).

Also, MRI can be used to better define the alpha angle. This was first described by Notzli et al. [14] as the angle between a line from the center of the femoral head to the middle of the femoral neck and a second line between the center of the femoral and the point where the contour of the head and neck junction exceeds the radius of the femoral head. An angle over 55° is considered abnormal [17].

MRI can be performed as well with arthrography, whereby intra-articular contrast (gadolinium diethylenetriamine pentaacetate) is injected under fluoroscopy prior to image acquisition. MRI arthrograms (Fig. 20.3b) are very sensitive and specific for detecting labral tears and chondral injuries, but they lack the ability to detect undetached chondral separations [63]. A normal separation between the rim and the labrum can be evident which is different from a tear because its margins are smooth and it lacks the interdigitation of labral tissue. Anterior labral tears are more common.

Magnetic ressonance arthrography (MRA) has disadvantages as contrast injection does not allow for evaluation of effusion and can masquerade signal changes on osseous structures, so, ideally, sequences should be obtained prior and after contrast administration.

MRA also allows injection of a long-lasting anesthetic agent into the joint. The temporary relief of pain is a much important information as to whether the complaints actually come from inside the joint. If there is no pain relief, other causes for pain should be sought, once a poor relief of pain with surgical treatment for FAI can be expected [64].

Biochemical T2 mapping and dGEMRIC have been shown to improve accuracy in detecting chondral damage [65–68].

20.6 Nonsurgical Treatment

Pain in an athlete with FAI must be taken into consideration cautiously as it can be a sign of progressive articular damage. Many athletes exhibit great tolerance to pain, and this can postpone the awareness of the situation and further aggravate chondral damage.

It is, nonetheless, appropriate to perform a trial of conservative treatment initially, especially if symptoms are mild and stable. This includes activity modification which naturally includes restriction of athletic activities and nonsteroidal anti-inflammatory medications. For instance, squatting, which is part of most weight training programs associated with the majority of sports, can be quite deleterious for hips at risk and should be limited. Physical therapy aimed at improving range of motion and stretching is counterproductive as it exacerbates the impingement phenomenon and can increase symptoms. Initially, treatment should be oriented toward avoiding position which causes symptoms to exacerbate. Movement errors should be addressed afterward. Progressive strengthening in movements that mimic the athletes' activity is the final goal. This can be attained with several eccentric and concentric exercises. A maintenance program is ensued next, and follow-up prior to sports resuming is advised.

However, because of the high activity level of football athletes and personal ambitions, such treatment regimen usually fails to control symptoms. There is limited data concerning the results of nonsurgical treatment for FAI. Emara et al. [69] reported on 37 patients with cam-type FAI (mild deformity – alpha angle <60°) who were treated conservatively. At 2 years, 11% chose surgical intervention, and another 16% had recurrent symptoms. The 89% patients who chose not to have surgery exhibited an improvement in the mean Harris Hip Score of 19 points. Hunt et al. [70] reported on 17 patients treated conservatively – 6 (35.3%) improved modestly but did not require surgery. Patients who required surgery were more active than the group who did not ($p = 0.02$). Long-term results of patients treated conservatively are unknown.

Such patients, following conservative treatment, should be monitored closely as continued FAI can further cause damage to the hip joint, and surgery could be warranted.

20.7 Surgical Treatment

The ideal candidate for FAI surgery is one who exhibits classical symptoms (activity-related pain in the inguinal region that radiates to the trochanteric region), compatible physical examination (diminished internal rotations, positive provocative maneuvers), and typical radiographic morphology with concomitant labral tear on MRI and who failed conservative treatment and has a positive response to intra-articular anesthetic injection. Most of the times, not all these criteria are met. It is, in our view, imperative to exclude other causes for pain and to have positive response to intra-articular injection test.

The goal with surgical treatment is to address chondrolabral junction pathology as well as bone morphology abnormalities [11].

This can be achieved either through open – surgical dislocation or miniopen – or arthroscopic approaches. Open surgical dislocation was the initial description by Ganz et al. [71], whereas arthroscopic approach has gained recent popularity [72]. Surgical approach can be dictated by patients' characteristics and surgeon preference.

When dealing with cam-type deformity, the severity of the deformity is usually bigger on the anterosuperior head-neck junction which is easily accessible through arthroscopic approach. If this extends posteriorly to the retinacular vessels, it is not accessible arthroscopically to most surgeons. More complex proximal femur deformities can possibly be more easily corrected by open surgical dislocation.

The type of pincer deformity also dictates approach. Anterior overcoverage can be dealt with arthroscopic techniques. The amount of anterior and lateral resection should be noted preoperatively as not to create a dysplastic acetabulum. True acetabular retroversion which implies posterior undercoverage should be treated by an anteverting periacetabular osteotomy (PAO).

20.7.1 Open Treatment

20.7.1.1 Surgical Dislocation

Based on the detailed understanding of vascular supply to the femoral head (namely, the medial circumflex femoral artery and its lateral retinacular branches) and their protection throughout the procedure, the hip joint can be dislocated with minimal risk of necrosis. A trochanteric osteotomy is necessary but preserves muscular attachments of the gluteus medius muscles and the *vastus lateralis*. This is mobilized anteriorly allowing full access to the hip joint which allows the correction of bone deformities as well as addressing labral and chondral pathology. When dislocating the joint, the ligamentum teres is sectioned. Early studies showed moderate success as patients with arthritis were included. Ganz et al. [71] and Beck et al. [73] reported on initial results. At mean follow-up of 4.7 years, good to excellent results were evident in 13 of 19 patients. Arthritic changes, Tonnis grade 2 or higher, were associated with poorer results. Peters et al. [74] reported on 30 patients at mean follow-up of 2.7 years who improved their Harris Hip Score from 70 to 87 points with a conversion to total hip replacement of 13.3%. Espinosa [75] showed the importance of preserving the labrum when finding a rate of 28% excellent results in the group of simple debridement compared to 80% in the group where the labrum was fixed back to the acetabulum.

In athletes, Naal et al. [76] reported 96% returning to competitive level at follow-up, whereas Novais et al. [77], in the adolescent population, showed pain relief and increased activity level, after surgical dislocation for FAI treatment.

Major complications are rare. Osteonecrosis has not been reported. Trochanteric nonunion can rise up to 3% [71, 73, 74]. Trochanteric pain is common but often mild [78]. There has been a recent concern about *ligamentum teres* pathology. In fact, its reconstruction may be of clinical relevance. When performing surgical dislocation, an iatrogenic injury is performed. Once viewed as irrelevant, recently it has been demonstrated that instability symptoms may exist [79].

20.7.1.2 Miniopen Approach

An anterior approach through the Hueter's interval can be used to access the hip joint and effectively treat FAI. Ultimately, combination with arthroscopic tools is necessary to visualize the central compartment. In our view, it offers similar access to the arthroscopic approach and therefore can be used with the same indications by surgeons who are not trained in hip arthroscopy. There are numerous reports showing good results with this approach: Clohisy [80] showed a 25-point improvement in HHS, and Laude [81] found a 29.1-point improvement. Lincoln [82] found a 12-point improvement and an increase on the range of motion. Anterior miniopen approach also showed high prevalence of returning to sports with low complication rate [83] and with short recovery time.

20.7.2 Arthroscopic Treatment

Michael Burman [84] first described hip arthroscopy in 1931. Its widespread use in clinical practice begun only in the late 1970s. After the recognition of FAI, hip arthroscopy has evolved to address both femoral and acetabular morphological abnormalities, treating labral and chondral disease as well as numerous periarticular conditions which can be treated by hip arthroscopy. The limits of the deformities that can be corrected with hip arthroscopy continue unclear.

Hip arthroscopy is performed on traction table.

Typically two to three portals are used in hip arthroscopy: anterolateral, anterior or midanterior portal, and another accessory portal for anchor placement if necessary. The authors establishes an accessory anterolateral portal most of the time.

Some sort of capsulotomy is always necessary. An interportal capsulotomy might be enough to treat most labrum tears and perform femoral osteoplasty, but if the femoral deformity is large enough, a longitudinal capsulotomy may be performed as well. Capsular management has been under scrutiny in recent years. Hip capsule has been established as an important static stabilizer of the hip [85]. In early days, most capsules were not closed, but it is believed that this could lead to microinstability which can lead to further labral and chondral damage. So, presently, routine closure or placation of the capsule has been advocated by several authors [86, 87]. Nevertheless, results have been conflicting which is evidenced by studies showing no clinical difference between groups where capsule was closed and others where it has not [88]. There might be, however, the need for capsular plication if symptoms of instability ensue [89].

Femoral osteoplasty can be performed next to acquire a normal femoral neck offset according to preoperative planning and preserving femoral head vasculature (Fig. 20.4a) [90]. Studies have shown that arthroscopic correction can be as accurate as open correction [91]. Care must be taken not to perform femoral cortical notching as this can diminish the resistance to fracture [92].

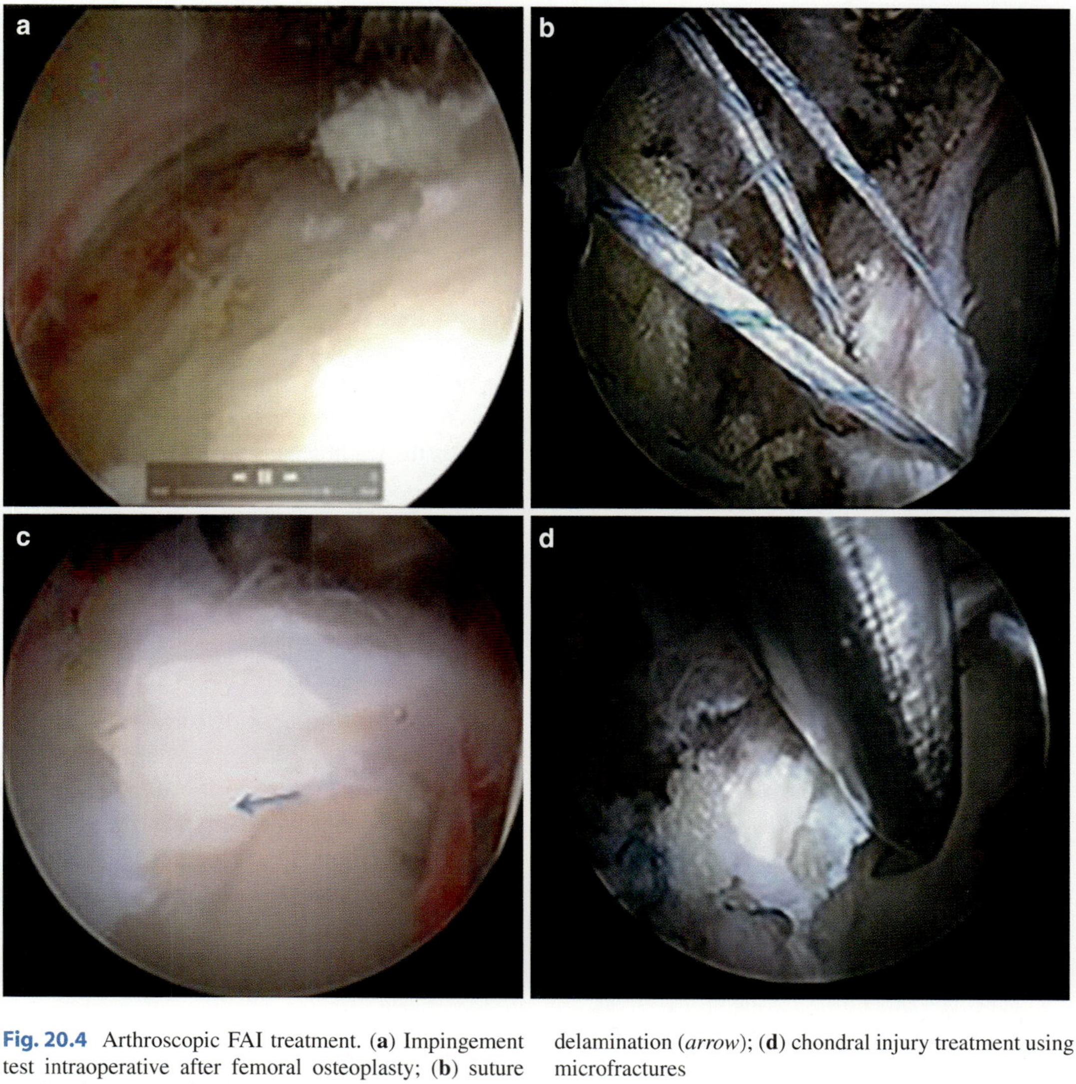

Fig. 20.4 Arthroscopic FAI treatment. (**a**) Impingement test intraoperative after femoral osteoplasty; (**b**) suture passing for labral refixation; (**c**) labral tear with chondral delamination (*arrow*); (**d**) chondral injury treatment using microfractures

Under traction, acetabular trimming is conducted to correct anterior and/or lateral overcoverage after labral detachment or not. Labral fixation (Fig. 20.4b) should be conducted as it is associated with superior results compared with simple debridement [75]. Chondral injury repair (Figs. 20.4c and 20.4d) is performed at this time which can vary from microfractures to fixation of chondral delamination with fibrin glue or chondrocyte transplantation.

After traction release, a verification of the absence of impingement is conducted. Radiographic intraoperative verification can be performed and can be used reliably [93].

Early outcomes for arthroscopic treatment of FAI reported success rates from 67% to 90% [94, 95]. Reported rates of conversion to total hip arthroplasty were 0–9% [96]. Byrd [97] presented a series of 44 athletes who underwent hip arthroscopy for labral tears: mean follow-up was 26 months. Most had labral tears ($n = 27$) or chondral damage ($n = 23$). Labral tears were addressed, but FAI was not. No statistical significance was shown. Guanche [98] reported on labral debridement and no FAI treatment on eight elite runners. WOMAC score was 94 at follow-up, and all returned to sporting activities. Recently, Philippon [99] reported on 45 athletes who underwent labral repair plus acetabular of femoral osteoplasty as necessary. Acetabular and femoral head chondral defects were managed either by chondroplasty or microfractures. Ninety-three percent were able to return to competitive sports. All three patients did not have previous severe osteoarthritic changes. Saw and Villar [100] presented a series of football players. Labrum was resected to a stable margin with five of six players returning to sports. Larson and Giveans [101] reported on 100 hip arthroscopies (96 patients). Labral debridement or repair was performed as well as addressing femoral and acetabular deformities. Patients with osteoarthritis Tonnis grade 3 were excluded. Outcomes were measured with the modified Harris Hip Score (MHHS) and SF-12. There was a significant improvement in all outcomes measured: ($p < 0.01$), MHHS (60.8 vs 82.7), SF 12 (60.2 vs 77.7), VAS (6.74 cm vs 1.88), and positive impingement test (100% vs 14%). Complications included heterotropic bone formation (six hips) and sciatic nerve neuropraxia (one hip). Conversion to total hip arthroplasty occurred in three patients.

Amenabar and O' Donnel [102] also reported on return to sports after hip arthroscopy for FAI in 36 Australian football players. At a mean of 52.5 months after surgery, all but one returned to competitive sport with an improvement in the MHHS from 83.6 to 98 ($p < 0.05$). Philippon et al. [103] evaluated the short-term return to play after microfractures were performed on high-level athletes for chondral damage in a series of 39 patients and compared them to a control group where no chondral treatment was deemed necessary. There were 30 out of 39 in the microfracture group who returned to play at the same level, and 79 out of 94 accomplished the same in the control group. They found no statistical difference in the short term.

Larson [104] evaluated patients with pubalgia symptoms associated with FAI and showed that addressing one pathology alone leads to a high rate of failure.

Cvetanovich et al. [105] researched on factors associated with revision hip arthroscopy and showed that undercorrection leading to persisting FAI was the leading cause.

20.7.3 Authors' Preferred Method of Treatment

A correct surgical indication and an optimal surgical technique are the keys for success.

It is possible to effectively correct the underlying deformities and address chondrolabral junction pathology in the majority of case with hip arthroscopy, so the latter is our favorite method of treatment.

Arthroscopy has the theoretical advantage (unproven) of faster recovery and return to sport. It is certainly less invasive. Obviously, it is imperative to recognize abnormalities that are not amenable to arthroscopic corrections and deal with them in the correct manner (osteotomy or surgical dislocation).

During arthroscopy, hypotensive anesthesia and an adequate fluid pump allow for good visualization with low fluid pressure avoiding compartment syndromes or abdominal extravasation of fluid. Also, traction time should be kept at the minimum possible to avoid complications such as neurologic palsies in the inferior limb and pudendal nerve.

The author approaches the hip and performs an interportal capsulotomy followed by a longitudinal limb if necessary (T-shape capsulotomy). The first author (AS) prefers approaching the hip from inside out, whereas the second author (CM) prefers to approach from outside in.

Correction of the deformities is carried out according to planning avoiding acetabular dysplasia and notching on the femoral neck but being careful not to undercorrect. Fluoroscopy can be used intraoperatively, but the author finds it seldom necessary.

The authors perform capsule closure systematically.

A rehabilitation protocol is started in the following day with restriction on mobility (external rotation and extension to facilitate capsular healing) and weight bearing (diminishing the theoretical risk of femoral neck fracture) for 4 weeks after which rehabilitation is allowed to progress.

Return to sport is allowed on an individual basis and taking into account the practice sport but not before 3 months after surgery.

Conclusion

Femoroacetabular impingement is a prevalent cause for hip and groin pain in athletes.

Diagnosis is challenging but with appropriate care, treatment results can be excellent.

References

1. Bombelli R. Osteoarthritis of the hip: pathogenesis and consequent therapy. Berlin: Springer-Verlag; 1976.
2. Elmslie RC. Aetiological factors in osteoarthritis of the hip. BMJ. 1933;1:1–3.
3. Stulberg SD, Cordell LD, Harris WH, Ramsey PL, MacEwen GD. Unrecognized childhood hip disease: a major cause of idiopathic osteoarthritis of the hip, in: the Hip: proceedings of the third meeting of the Hip Society. St. Louis: CV Mosby; 1975. p. 212–28.
4. Harris WH. Etiology of osteoarthritis of the hip. Clin Orthop Relat Res. 1986;213:20–33.
5. Reginster JY. The prevalence and burden of arthritis. Rheumatology (Oxford). 2002;41(suppl):3–6.
6. Murphy SB, Kijewski PK, Millis MB, Harless A. Acetabular dysplasia in the adolescent and young adult. Clin Orthop Relat Res. 1990;261:214–23.
7. Dora C, Zurbach J, Hersche O, Ganz R. Pathomorphologic characteristics of posttraumatic acetabular dysplasia. J Orthop Trauma. 2000;14:483–9.
8. Murray RO. The etiology of primary osteoarthritis of the hip. Br J Radiol. 1965;38:810–24.
9. Solomon L. Patterns of osteoarthritis of the hip. J Bone Joint Surg Br. 1976;58:176–83.
10. Flores RH, Hochberg MC. Definition and classification of osteoarthritis. In: Brandt KD, Doherty M, Lohmander LS, editors. Osteoarthritis. New York: Oxford Medical Publication/Oxford University press; 1998. p. 1–12.
11. Ganz R, Parvizi J, Beck M, Leunig M, Nötzli H, Siebenrock KA. Femoroacetabular impingement: a cause for osteoarthritis of the hip. Clin Orthop Relat Res. 2003;417:112–20.
12. Ganz R, Leunig M, Leunig-Ganz K, Harris WH. The etiology of osteoarthritis of the hip: an integrated mechanical concept. Clin Orthop Relat Res. 2008;466(2):264–72.
13. Bedy A, Lynch E, Enselman E, Davis M, De Wolf P, Makki T, Kelly B. Elevation in circulating biomarkers of cartilage damage and inflammation in athletes with femoroacetabular impingement. Am J Sports Med. 2013;41:2585.
14. Ito K, Minka II MA, Leunig M, Werlen S, Ganz R. Femoroacetabular impingement and the cam-effect: a MRI-based quantitative anatomical study of the femoral head-neck offset. J Bone Joint Surg Br. 2001;83:171–6.
15. Notzli HP, Wyss TF, Stoecklin CH, Schmid MR, Treiber K, Hodler J. The contour of the femoral head-neck junction as a predictor for the risk of anterior impingement. J Bone Joint Surg Br. 2002;84:556–60.
16. McCarthy JC, Noble PC, Schuck MR, Wright J, Lee J. The Otto E. Aufranc Award: the role of labral lesions to development of early degenerative hip disease. Clin Orthop Relat Res. 2001;393:25–37.
17. Tannast M, Siebenrock KA, Anderson SE. Femoroacetabular impingement: radiographic diagnosis – what the radiologist should know. AJR Am J Roentgenol. 2007;188(6):1540–52.
18. Wright AA, Naze GS, Kavchak AE, et al. Radiological variables associated with progression of femoroacetabular impingement of the hip: a systematic review. J Sci Med Sport. 2015;18(2):122–7.
19. Agricola R, Heijboer MP, Bierma-Zeinstra SMA, Verhaar JAN, Weinans H, Waarsing JH. Cam

impingement causes osteoarthritis of the hip: a nationwide prospective cohort study (CHECK). Ann Rheum Dis. 2013;72(6):918–23.
20. Clohisy JC. Radiographic structural abnormalities associated with premature, natural hip-joint failure. J Bone Joint Surg Am. 2011;93(suppl 2):3.
21. Klunder KB, Rud B, Hansen J. Osteoarthritis of the hip and knee joint in retired football players. Acta Orthop Scand. 1980;51(6):925–7.
22. Kujala UM, Kaprio J, Sarna S. Osteoarthritis of weight bearing joints of lower limbs in former e´lite male athletes. BMJ. 1994;308(6923):231–4.
23. L'Hermette M. Hip passive range of motion and frequency of radiographic hip osteoarthritis in former elite handball players. Br J Sports Med. 2006;40(1):45–9.
24. Lindberg H, Roos H, Gardsell P. Prevalence of coxarthrosis in former soccer players: 286 players compared with matched controls. Acta Orthop Scand. 1993;64(2):165–7.
25. Sankar WN, Nevitt M, Parvizi J, Felson DT, Agricola R, Leunig M. Femoroacetabular impingement: defining the condition and its role in the pathophysiology of osteoarthritis. J Am Acad Orthop Surg. 2013;21(suppl 1):S7–S15.
26. Schmitt H, Brocai DRC, Lukoschek M. High prevalence of hip arthrosis in former elite javelin throwers and high jumpers: 41 athletes examined more than 10 years after retirement from competitive sports. Acta Orthop Scand. 2004;75(1):34–9.
27. Shepard GJ. Ex-professional association footballers have an increased prevalence of osteoarthritis of the hip compared with age matched controls despite not having sustained notable hip injuries. Br J Sports Med. 2003;37(1):80–1.
28. Gekeler J. Coxarthrosis with a deep acetabulum. Z Orthop Ihre Grenzgeb. 1978;116:454–9.
29. Reynolds D, Lucas J, Klaue K. Retroversion of the acetabulum: a cause of hip pain. J Bone Joint Surg Br. 1999;81:281–8.
30. Ito K, Leunig M, Ganz R. Histopathologic features of the acetabular labrum in femoroacetabular impingement. Clin Orthop Relat Res. 2004;429:262–71.
31. Heyworth BE, Shindle MK, Voos JE, Rudzki JR, Kelly BT. Radiologic and intraoperative findings in revision hip arthroscopy. Arthroscopy. 2007;12:1295–302.
32. Hetsroni I, Larson C, Dela Torre K, Zbeda R, Magennis E, Kell B. Anterior inferior iliac spine deformity as an extraarticular source for hip impingement: a series of 10 patients treated with arthroscopic decompression. Arthroscopy. 2012;28:1644–53.
33. Hapa O, Bedi A, Gursan O, et al. Anatomic footprint of the direct head of the rectus femoris origin: cadaveric study and clinical series of hips after arthroscopic anterior inferior iliac spine/subspine decompression. Arthroscopy. 2013;29:1932–40.
34. Ali AM, Whitwell D, Ostlere SJ. Case report: imaging and surgical treatment of a snapping hip due to ischiofemoral impingement. Skeletal Radiol. 2011;40:653–6.
35. Dandachli W, Islam SU, Liu M, Richards R, Hall-Craggs M, Witt J. Three-dimensional CT analysis to determine acetabular retroversion and the implications for the management of femoro-acetabular impingement. J Bone Joint Surg Br. 2009;91:1031–6.
36. Yoo WJ, Choi IH, Cho TJ, Chung CY, Park MS, Lee DY. Out-toeing and in-toeing in patients with Perthes disease: role of the femoral hump. J Pediatr Orthop. 2008;28:717–22.
37. Reichenbach S, Jüni P, Werlen S, et al. Prevalence of cam-type deformity on hip magnetic resonance imaging in young males: a cross-sectional study. Arthritis Care Res. 2010;62(9):1319–27.
38. Reichenbach S, Leunig M, Werlen S, et al. Association between cam-type deformities and magnetic resonance imaging-detected structural hip damage: a cross-sectional study in young men. Arthritis Rheum. 2011;63(12):4023–30.
39. Hack K, Di Primio G, Rakhra K, Beaule PE. Prevalence of cam-type femoroacetabular impingement morphology in asymptomatic volunteers. J Bone Joint Surg. 2010;92:2436–44.
40. Frank J, Harris J, Erickson B, Slikker W, Bush-Joseph C, Salata M, Nho S. Prevalence of femoroacetabular impingement. Imaging findings in asymptomatic volunteers: a systematic review. Arthroscopy. 2015;6:1199–204.
41. Nepple J, Brophy R, Matava M, Wright R, Clohisy J. Radiographic findings of femoroacetabular impingement in National Football League Combine athletes undergoing radiographs for previous hip or groin pain. Arthroscopy. 2012;28(10):1396–403.
42. Siebenrock KA, Behning A, Mamisch TC, Schwab JM. Growth plate alteration precedes cam-type deformity in elite basketball players. Clin Orthop Relat Res. 2012;471(4):1084–91.
43. Siebenrock KA, Ferner F, Noble PC, Santore RF, Werlen S, Mamisch TC. The cam-type deformity of the proximal femur arises in childhood in response to vigorous sporting activity. Clin Orthop Relat Res. 2011;469(11):3229–40.
44. Philippon MJ, Ho CP, Briggs KK, Stull J, LaPrade RF. Prevalence of increased alpha angles as a measure of cam-type femoroacetabular impingement in youth ice hockey players. Am J Sports Med. 2013;41(6):1357–62.
45. Agricola R, Bessems JHJM, Ginai AZ, et al. The development of camtype deformity in adolescent and young male soccer players. Am J Sports Med. 2012;40(5):1099–106.
46. Johnson AC, Shaman MA, Ryan TG. Femoroacetabular impingement in former high-level youth soccer players. Am J Sports Med. 2012;40(6):1342–6.

47. Stull JD, Philippon MJ, LaPrade RF. "At-risk" positioning and hip biomechanics of the Peewee ice hockey sprint start. Am J Sports Med. 2011;39(1 suppl):29S–35S.
48. Meyers WC, McKechnie A, Philippon MJ, Horner MA, Zoga AC, Devon ON. Experience with "sports hernia" spanning two decades. Ann Surg. 2008;4:656–65.
49. Hammoud S, Bedi A, Magennis E, Meyres W, Kelly B. High incidence of athletic pubalgia symptoms in professional athletes with symptomatic femoroacetabular impingement. Arthroscopy. 2012;28(10):1388–95.
50. Byrd JWT. Evaluation and management of the snapping iliopsoas tendon. Instr Course Lect. 2006;55:347–55.
51. Philippon M, Maxwell R, Johnston T, Shencker M, Briggs K. Hip clinical presentation of femoroacetabular impingement knee surgery, sports traumatology. Arthroscopy. 2007;15:348.
52. Byrd JWT. Physical examination. In: JWT B, editor. Operative hip arthroscopy. 2nd ed. New York: Springer; 2005. p. 36–50.
53. Perry J. Gait analysis: normal and pathological function. Thorofare: SLACK; 1992.
54. Martin HD, Savage A, Braly BA, Palmer IJ, Beall DP, Kelly B. The function of the hip capsular ligaments: a quantitative report. Arthroscopy. 2008;24:188–95.
55. Reider B, Martel J. Pelvis, hip and thigh. In: Reider B, Martel J, editors. The orthopedic physical examination. Philadelphia: WB Saunders; 1999. p. 159–99.
56. Klaue K, Durnin CW, Ganz R. The acetabular rim syndrome. A clinical presentation of dysplasia of the hip. J Bone Joint Surg Br. 1991;73:423–9.
57. Tijssen M, Van Cingel R, Willemson L, Visser E. Diagnostics of femoroacetabular impingement and labral pathology of the hip: a systematic review of the accuracy and validity of physical tests. Arthroscopy. 2012;28(6):860–71.
58. Burgess RM, Rushton A, Wright C, Daborn C. The validity and accuracy of clinical diagnostic tests used to detect labral pathology of the hip: a systematic review. Man Ther. 2011;16:318–26.
59. Leibold MR, Huijbregts PA, Jensen R. Concurrent criterion related validity of physical examination tests for hip labral lesions: a systematic review. J Man Manip Ther. 2008;16:E24–41.
60. Clohisy JC, Nunley RM, Otto RJ, Schoenecker PL. The frog-leg lateral radiograph accurately visualized hip cam impingement abnormalities. Clin Orthop Relat Res. 2007;462:115–21.
61. Meyer DC, Beck M, Ellis T, Ganz R, Leunig M. Comparison of six radiographic projections to assess femoral head/neck asphericity. Clin Orthop Relat Res. 2006;445:181–5.
62. Byrd JWT, Jones KS. Diagnostic accuracy of clinical assessment, MRI, gadolinium MRI, and intraarticular injection in hip arthroscopy patients. Am J Sports Med. 2004;32(7):1668–74.
63. Leunig M, Podeszwa D, Beck M, Werlen S, Ganz R. Magnetic resonance arthrography of labral disorders in hips with dysplasia and impingement. Clin Orthop Relat Res. 2004;418:74–80.
64. Ayeni O, Farrokhyar F, Crouch S, Chan K, Sprague S, Bhandari M. Pre-operative intra-articular hip injection as a predictor of short-term outcome following arthroscopic management of femoroacetabular impingement. Knee Surg Sports Traumatol Arthrosc. 2014;22:801–5.
65. Bittersohl B, Hosalkar HS, Haamberg T, et al. Reproducibility of dGEMRIC in assessment of hip joint cartilage: a prospective study. J Magn Reson Imaging. 2009;30:224–8.
66. Miese FR, Zilkens C, Holstein A, et al. Assessment of early cartilage degeneration after slipped capital femoral epiphysis using T2 and T2* mapping. Acta Radiol. 2011;52:106–10.
67. Nishii T, Shiomi T, Tanaka H, Yamazaki Y. Loaded cartilage T2 mapping in patients with hip dysplasia. Radiology. 2010;256:955–65.
68. Pollard TC, McNally EG, Wilson DC, et al. Localized cartilage assessment with three-dimensional dGEMRIC in asymptomatic hips with normal morphology and cam deformity. J Bone Joint Surg Am. 2010;92:2557–69.
69. Emara K, Samir W, Motasem H, Ghafar KA. Conservative treatment for mild femoroacetabular impingement. J Orthop Surg (Hong Kong). 2011;19(1):41–5.
70. Hunt D, Prather H, Harris Hayes M, Clohisy JC. Clinical outcomes analysis of conservative and surgical treatment of patients with clinical indications of prearthritic, intra-articular hip disorders. PM & R. 2012;4(7):479–87.
71. Ganz R, Gill TJ, Gautier E, Ganz K, Krügel N, Berlemann U. Surgical dislocation of the adult hip: a technique with full access to the femoral head and acetabulum without the risk of avascular necrosis. J Bone Joint Surg Br. 2001;83(8):1119–24.
72. Colvin AC, Harrast J, Harner C. Trends in hip arthroscopy. J Bone Joint Surg Am. 2012;94(4):e23.
73. Beck M, Leunig M, Parvizi J, Boutier V, Wyss D, Ganz R. Anterior femoroacetabular impingement: part II. Midterm results of surgical treatment. Clin Orthop Relat Res. 2004;418:67–73.
74. Peters CL, Erickson JA. Treatment of femoro-acetabular impingement with surgical dislocation and débridement in young adults. J Bone Joint Surg Am. 2006;88(8):1735–41.
75. Espinosa N, Rothenfluh DA, Beck M, Ganz R, Leunig M. Treatment of femoro-acetabular impingement: preliminary results of labral refixation. J Bone Joint Surg Am. 2006;88(5):925–35.
76. Naal FD, Miozzari HH, Wyss TF, Nötzli HP. Surgical hip dislocation for the treatment of femoroacetabular

impingement in high-level athletes. Am J Sports Med. 2011;39(3):544–50.
77. Novais EN, Heyworth BE, Stamoulis C, Sullivan K, Millis MB, Kim YJ. Open surgical treatment of femoroacetabular impingement in adolescent athletes: preliminary report on improvement of physical activity level. J Pediatr Orthop. 2014;34(3):287–94.
78. Beck M, Büchler L. Prevalence and impact of pain at the greater trochanter after open surgery for the treatment of femoro-acetabular impingement. J Bone Joint Surg Am. 2011;93(suppl 2):66–9.
79. Phillips AR, Bartlett G, Norton M, Fern D. Hip stability after ligamentum teres resection during surgical dislocation for cam impingement. Hip Int. 2012;22(3):329–34.
80. Clohisy JC, Zebala LP, Nepple JJ, Pashos G. Combined hip arthroscopy and limited open osteochondroplasty for anterior femoroacetabular impingement. J Bone Joint Surg Am. 2010;92(8):1697–706.
81. Laude F, Sariali E, Nogier A. Femoroacetabular impingement treatment using arthroscopy and anterior approach. Clin Orthop Relat Res. 2009;467(3):747–52.
82. Lincoln M, Johnston K, Muldoon M, Santore R. Combined arthroscopic and modified open approach for cam femoroacetabular impingement: a preliminary experience. Arthroscopy. 2009;25(4):392–9.
83. Cohen S, Huang R, Ciccoti MG, Parvizi J. Treatment of femoroacetabular impingement in athletes using a mini-direct anterior approach. Am J Sports Med. 2012;40:1620.
84. Burman M. Arthroscopy or the direct visualization of joints. J Bone Joint Surg. 1931;13(4):669–94.
85. Telleria JJ, Lindsey DP, Giori NJ, Safran MR. A quantitative assessment of the insertional footprints of the hip joint capsular ligaments and their spanning fibers for reconstruction. Clin Anat. 2014;27:489–97.
86. Harris JD, Slikker III W, Gupta AK, McCormick FM, Nho SJ. Routine complete capsular closure during hip arthroscopy. Arthrosc Tech. 2013;2:e89–94.
87. Domb BG, Philippon MJ, Giordano BD. Arthroscopic capsulotomy, capsular repair, and capsular plication of the hip: relation to atraumatic instability. Arthroscopy. 2013;29:162–73.
88. Domb BG, Stake C, Finley Z, Baise R, Botser I. Two-year outcome of arthroscopic capsular repair of the hip: a prospective matched-pair controlled study. Orthop J Sports Med. 2013;1(4)(suppl 1).
89. Tindade C, Sawyer G, Fukui K, Briggs KK, Philippon MJ. Arthroscopic capsule reconstruction in the hip using iliotibial band allograft. Arthrosc Tech. 2015;4(1):e71–4.
90. Sussman P, Ranawat A, Kelly B. Vascular preservation during arthroscopic osteoplasty of the femoral head-neck junction: a cadaveric investigation. Arthroscopy. 2007;23(7):738–43.
91. Sussman P, Ranawat A, Kelly B. Arthroscopic versus open osteoplasty of the head-neck junction: a cadaveric investigation. Arthroscopy. 2007;23(12):1257–64.
92. Widjicks C, Balldin B, Jansen K, Stull J, LaPrade R, Philippon MJ. Cam lesion femoral osteoplasty: in vitro biomechanical evaluation of iatrogenic femoral cortical notching and risk of neck fracture. Arthroscopy. 2013;29(10):1608–14.
93. Ross J, Abedi A, Stone R, Enselman E, Leunig M, Kelly B, Larsson C. Intraoperative fluoroscopic imaging to treat cam deformities: correlation with 3-dimensional computed tomography. Am J Sports Med. 2014;42(6):1370–6.
94. Matsuda DK, Carlisle JC, Arthurs SC, Wierks CH, Philippon MJ. Comparative systematic review of the open dislocation, mini-open, and arthroscopic surgeries for femoroacetabular impingement. Arthroscopy. 2011;27(2):252–69.
95. Clohisy JC, St John LC, Schutz AL. Surgical treatment of femoroacetabular impingement: a systematic review of the literature. Clin Orthop Relat Res. 2010;468(2):555–64.
96. Stevens MS, Legay DA, Glazebrook MA, Amirault D. The evidence for hip arthroscopy: grading the current indications. Arthroscopy. 2010;26(10):1370–83.
97. Byrd JW, Jones KS. Prospective analysis of hip arthroscopy with 2-year follow-up. Arthroscopy. 2000;16:578–87.
98. Guanche CA, Sikka RS. Acetabular labral tears with underlying chondromalacia: a possible association with high-level running. Arthroscopy. 2005;21:580–5.
99. Philippon MJ, Schenker M, Briggs K, Kuppersmith D. Femoroacetabular impingement in 45 professional athletes: associated pathologies and return to sport following arthroscopic decompression. Knee Surg Sports Traumatol Arthrosc. 2007;15:908–14.
100. Saw T, Villar R. Footballer's hip: a report of six cases. J Bone Joint Surg Br. 2004;86:655–8.
101. Larson CM, Giveans MR. Arthroscopic management of femoroacetabular impingement: early outcomes measures. Arthroscopy. 2008;24:540–6.
102. Amenabar T, O' Donnel J. Return to sport in Australian Football League footballers after hip arthroscopy and midterm outcome. Arthroscopy. 2013;29(7):188–1194.
103. McDonald J, Mackenzie H, Philippon MJ. Return to play after hip arthroscopy with microfracture in elite athletes. Arthroscopy. 2013;29(2):330–5.
104. Larson C, Pierce B, Giveans R. Treatment of athletes with symptomatic intra-articular hip pathology and athletic pubalgia/sports hernia: a case series. Arthroscopy. 2011;27(6):768–75.
105. Cvetanovich G, Harris J, Erickson B, Bach B, Bush-Joseph C, Nho S. Revision hip arthroscopy: a systematic review of diagnoses, operative findings, and outcomes. Arthroscopy. 2015;31(7):1382–90.

Femur Fractures

21

Eurico Bandeira-Rodrigues, Sebastiano Vasta, José Carlos Leitão, and Joan Carles Monllau

Contents

E. Bandeira-Rodrigues (✉)
Hospital de Braga – Serviço de Ortopedia, Avenida José Moreira, 4715-243 Braga, Portugal
e-mail: eurico.rodrigues@hospitaldebraga.pt

S. Vasta
Università Campus Bio-Medico di Roma, Rome, Italy

J.C. Leitão
Hospital Geral de Santo António, Porto, Portugal

J.C. Monllau
Hospital del Mar; ICATME-Hospital Universitari Dexeus; Universitat Autònoma de Barcelona (UAB), Barcelona, Spain

21.1 Introduction

Femur fractures are a rare injury among players. They can be an easy to manage or devastating injury. They can be the result of two main causes: trauma or overuse.

21.1.1 Epidemiology

As femur is the strongest long bone in the human body, high-energy trauma will be needed for a fracture to occur. The distribution is not even in every player [1–3]. There is a relation to the age [4], the individual skills, and the environment. Match accounts for a higher incidence of lesions than training, probably because of the intensity differences. The second half or extension of a match is more related to injury, in relation to muscle fatigue. Reinjuries represent 12% of the total and are responsible for longer absence.

Femur fractures in children and young athletic population represent only 1% of all femur fractures. They represent the first peak in incidence,

J. Espregueira-Mendes et al. (eds.), *Injuries and Health Problems in Football*,
DOI 10.1007/978-3-662-53924-8_21

being elderly females with low-energy trauma the second and by far the greatest peak. Most of hospital admissions are from ages under 10, and there are only very rare traumatic fractures after the age of 14.

Overuse injuries occur at a rate of 19.9 per 10,000 persons per year [5], but they are more frequent in players than in the general population. That is the result of repetitive overload. Fracture results from a failed attempt of remodeling that is overcome by repetitive maximal load.

21.1.2 Differences Between Amateur and Professional Players

Amateur players do not have the same support in technical and health aspects. They neither have the same level of skills than professionals. These have constant medical support and benefit with both preventive action and optimized recovery. More skilled players will suffer less injuries [6]. Amateurs get injured most frequently during training sessions, and they have more severe [7] and recurrent injuries. Professionals get injured mostly during matches and less during training. Their injuries are less severe and are not as recurrent as for amateurs [8].

21.1.3 Age-Related Differences in Injuries

There are differences related to age in injuries [9]. Children's skeleton is immature, and fracture is more likely to occur with lesser-applied force [10]. The growth plates may be involved, with potential for growth disturbance as a result. Children suffer different injury patterns and treatment must differ from the adult's. To respect bone structures, mainly the growth plates, it must be adapted in order to avoid further damage.

Healing also has unique features in children. Callus formation and remodeling are very fast because of abundant vascularity and biologically active periosteum. In the shaft, anatomic reduction is not necessary to recover pre-injury function. Only alignment must be corrected. Even residual deformities will disappear by remodeling.

21.2 Traumatic Fractures

Traumatic fractures of the femur are rare comparatively to other football injuries. Amateur players suffer them more frequently than professionals. That is due to poorer technique. Children also suffer more fractures than adults due to the immaturity of their skeleton.

21.2.1 Mechanisms of Injury

Fracture can be the result of a force applied directly or indirectly. It occurs when the bone fails to dissipate or transmit a force that is applied to it. Such force exceeds its elastic resistance causing it to break. Some patterns are more related to a particular mechanism: transverse fracture is characteristic of a bending force; spiral fracture is related to twisting and oblique fracture to compression. There can be combinations of patterns.

Soft tissues around the bone also suffer that trauma. Fracture is not just bone damage. That is why many complications can associate to the fracture: wounds, infection, muscle, nerve, and/or vascular damage.

21.2.2 Diagnosis

Suspicion is fairly easy in the case of trauma. In fact, a fracture must always be ruled out. A good examination and imaging study are the best tools to have the diagnosis. It is important to understand how the trauma occurred as it will allow to a better recognition of injuries and treatment.

21.2.2.1 Signs and Symptoms

Of course, some deformities and some exposure wounds will leave no doubt. But the most frequent symptoms are acute pain and disability. Patients with proximal fracture will frequently present with shortening and external rotation. There will be no possibility to stand, walk, or even raise the limb.

21.2.2.2 Imaging Study

Most of fractures will be well defined using radiography. Proper study is directed to the limb segment involved. In the case of the femur, the hip, the shaft, and the knee, at least two perpendicular incidences will be needed, but other incidences may be needed in the case of some particular fracture cases.

CT scan is the best to diagnose fractures but will be needed rarely for diagnosis. It may be of the utmost importance to define articular fracture and for surgical planning.

Scintigraphy and MRI will have only a place in practice to diagnose stress fractures that can be difficult to observe at the onset of symptoms.

21.2.2.3 Classification

A classification system is a tool that is supposed to help physicians to describe fractures, define their severity, plan and orientate the treatment, and establish some form of prognosis. For each fracture, the ideal classification would have all these features, would be easy to use, and would not be intra- and interobserver variable. For each segment of the femur, there are multiple fracture classification systems to help the physicians, although most are not ideal.

21.2.3 Associated Injuries and Complications

21.2.3.1 Shock

The femur is very vascularized. Blood loss resulting from a femur fracture can be up to 1.5 L. The need for transfusion is up to 40% [11]. In the case of an open fracture, bleeding can be even more important.

21.2.3.2 Vascular Trauma

Large vessels can suffer laceration and a massive blood loss may result. These are rapidly life-threatening injuries. It is mandatory to apply some form of hemorrhage control, by direct pressure, packing, or some kind of tourniquet. In addition to this, emergent repair or angiographic sclerosis must be performed. As there may be the problem of limb ischemia, revascularization must be performed under a maximum of 6 h.

Small vessels can be involved causing avascular necrosis (AVN). That is the case of the femoral head in head and neck fractures. AVN will only have clinical manifestation months after the injury.

21.2.3.3 Deep Venous Thrombosis (DVT)/Pulmonary Embolism

This is more associated to the spine, pelvic, femur, and tibia fracture. The incidence can reach as high as 50%. Prophylaxis is indicated for femur trauma. The usual methods are compression and anticoagulation. With use of low molecular weight heparins, the incidence of DVT diminished to a rate of 11% [12].

21.2.3.4 Fat Embolism/Acute Respiratory Syndrome

The medullary canal is filled with bone marrow and fat. Fat can enter the bloodstream and create emboli that get trapped in the pulmonary vessels. Depending on the amount of pulmonary tissue excluded from circulation and therefore from gas exchange, the patient can be asymptomatic or suffer mild to severe respiratory distress.

21.2.3.5 Soft Tissue Damage

Open fractures have a great risk of necrosis and infection. That is directly related to the size of the wound and to the associated soft tissue injury. Open fracture wounds need debridement, dressing, and antibiotics. To help the healing, there may be the need for hyperbaric oxygen, vacuum-assisted closure, and/or reconstructive surgery.

Soft tissue injury may be less apparent but explains healing problems or delay related to high-energy trauma. Gustillo and Anderson [13] have developed a classification system that relates the kind of damage to the skin, the contamination, and the necrosis in the wound to the prognosis. Tscherne classification of closed fractures also indicates the severity grade of soft tissue injury.

21.2.3.6 Nerve Injury

Nerve damage is rare associated to femur fracture [14, 15]. Only in the case of fracture-dislocation of the femoral head, there is a 10% of sciatic nerve trauma [16].

21.2.3.7 Compartment Syndrome

The thigh contains three compartments: anterior, posterior, and adductor. Bleeding and edema cause the interstitial pressure to rise and cause vascular occlusion and ischemia to the muscles and the nerves.

The earliest sign is pain with passive stretch. A clinical suspicion can be verified using a device to measure the compartment pressure. It should not exceed 30 mmHg above the diastolic blood pressure. Late findings are paralysis and the absence of pulse. Long-term morbidity is present in 50% of cases with pain, decreased knee flexion, myositis ossificans, sensory deficits, and/or decreased strength.

Early diagnose and treatment with fasciotomy are the only possibility against irreversible damage to the muscles and nerves.

21.2.4 Specific Femur Fractures

21.2.4.1 Head Fractures

They are almost always associated to hip dislocation. The mechanism of injury is an axial load or avulsion by the ligamentum teres.

Being articular surface fractures, they need anatomical reduction and stable fixation. Because of the head's vascular anatomy, there is a risk of necrosis. The Pipkin classification states that fractures below the fovea have better prognosis. Fractures above the fovea or associated to neck fracture or dislocations have worse prognosis [17]. Indications for surgery are irreducible dislocation, displaced fracture, articular incongruence, and intra-articular loose fragment. The results are good to excellent in 47–83%. Late complications are AVN in 3–19% and osteoarthritis in 3–31% of the patients.

21.2.4.2 Neck Fractures

In the young, these usually are the result of axial loading. The morphology is more frequently vertically oriented, making them unstable. The soft tissue damage is usually greater because of the high energy involved. They can be present in 3–6% of femoral shaft fractures and therefore can be misdiagnosed.

Femoral neck fractures have a high risk of avascular necrosis, which is related to the stability and displacement of the fracture, as described by Garden (Fig. 21.1).

No matter how displaced the fracture, it is worth an osteosynthesis at these ages. The reduction, if needed, can be performed in an open or closed approach. Leadbetter has described the maneuver for closed reduction. It should be tried only once, in the operating room. It is performed under traction and by applying a sequence of flexion-adduction-extension-internal rotation. Open reduction is accomplished through anterior approach to preserve the vessels.

The most recommended type of fixation is compression screws (Fig. 21.2).

It has been demonstrated [18, 19] that they offer a lesser risk of failure when technique is well observed. Being intracapsular fractures, there is a great risk of pseudarthrosis. That can only be avoided with good anatomical or valgus reduction and stable compressive fixation. The screws need to be placed without any risk of vascularization damage by rotation of the femoral head and ideally in a number of 3. Varus fixation is related to postoperative displacement. Observing good technique is of utmost importance, for resistance to cyclic shearing forces. Entry point should be at or under the lesser trochanter level. Screws should stay 5 mm from chondral surface but should enter the denser subchondral bone. They should be placed near the cortical in the neck for increased stability.

The risk of AVN is 3–20%. Capsular decompression is to be considered.

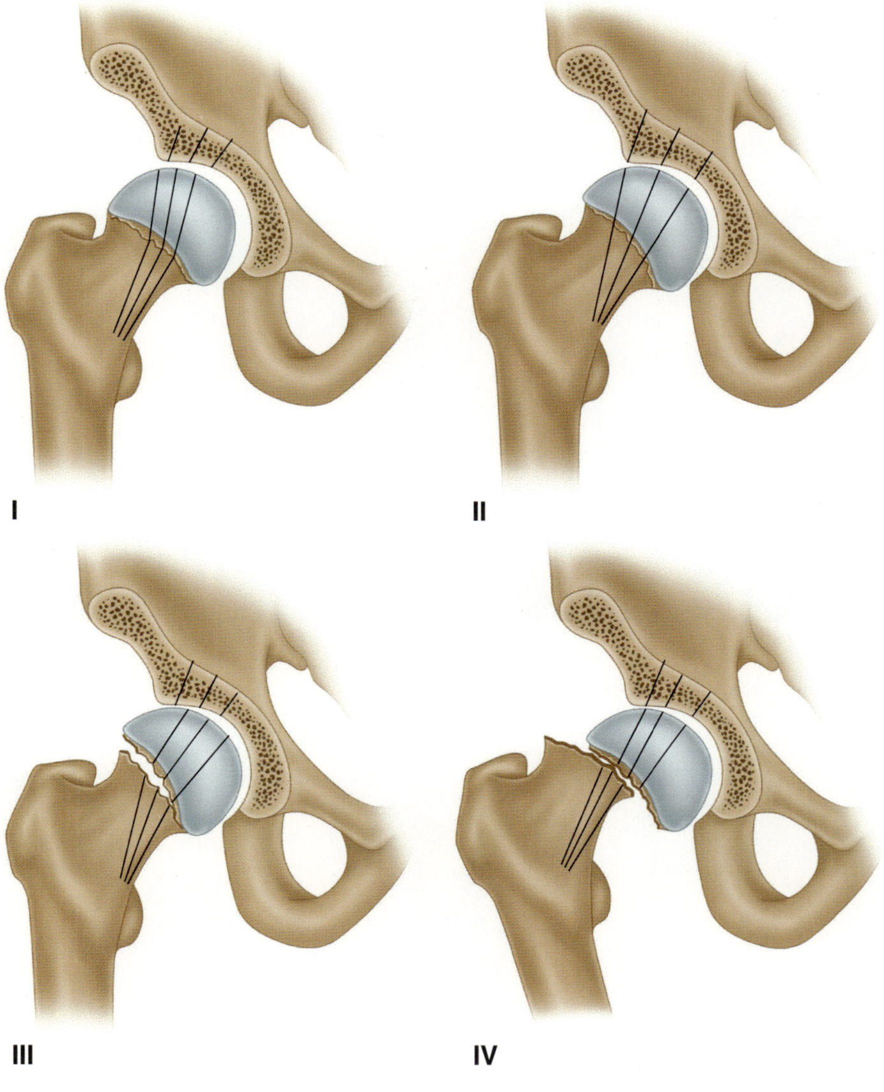

Fig. 21.1 Garden classification

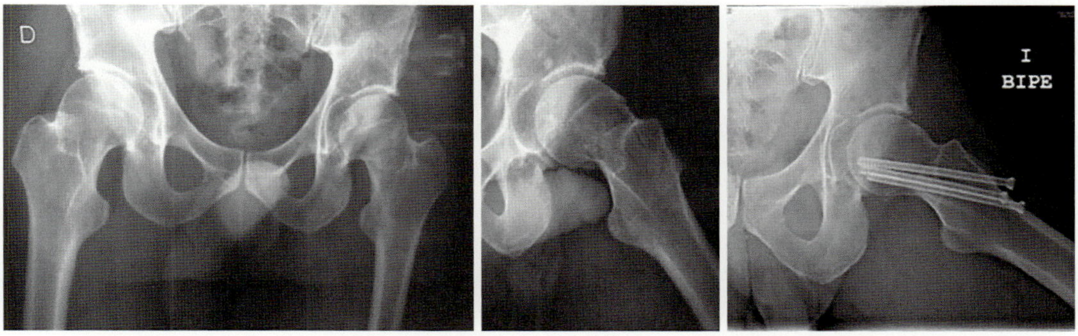

Fig. 21.2 Neck fracture from a fall during match in a 37-year-old professional goalkeeper. Treated with cannulated screws (Images from preop and 9-month post-op)

21.2.4.3 Pertrochanteric Fractures

The most frequent are intertrochanteric, but there can be fractures affecting only one trochanter (Fig. 21.3).

These extracapsular fractures do not put the femoral head vessels at risk and usually have a low risk of pseudarthrosis because they involve mostly cancellous bone. There are many classification systems, but the most important aspect is to determine if a fracture is stable or not. Evans classification describes progressive instability of intertrochanteric fractures (Fig. 21.4).

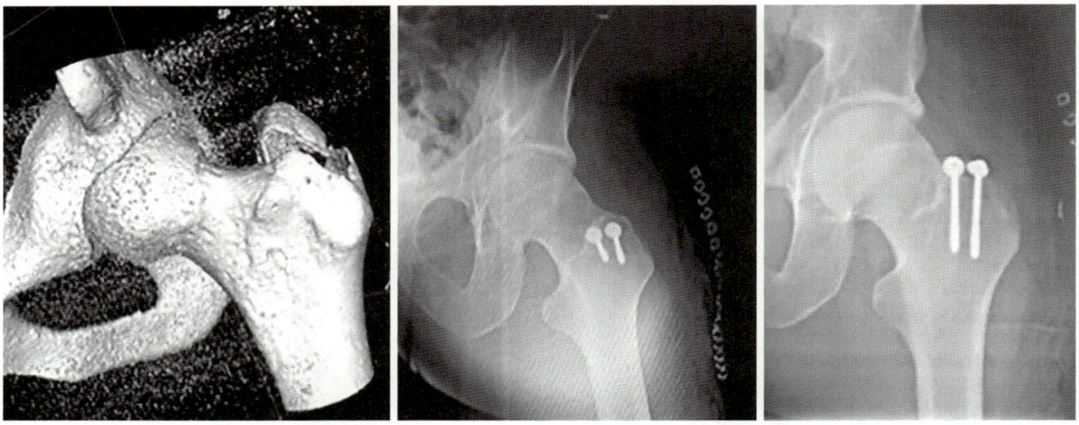

Fig. 21.3 Greater trochanter fracture from collision and forced abduction against resistance in a 27-year-old professional player (Images from preop and post-op)

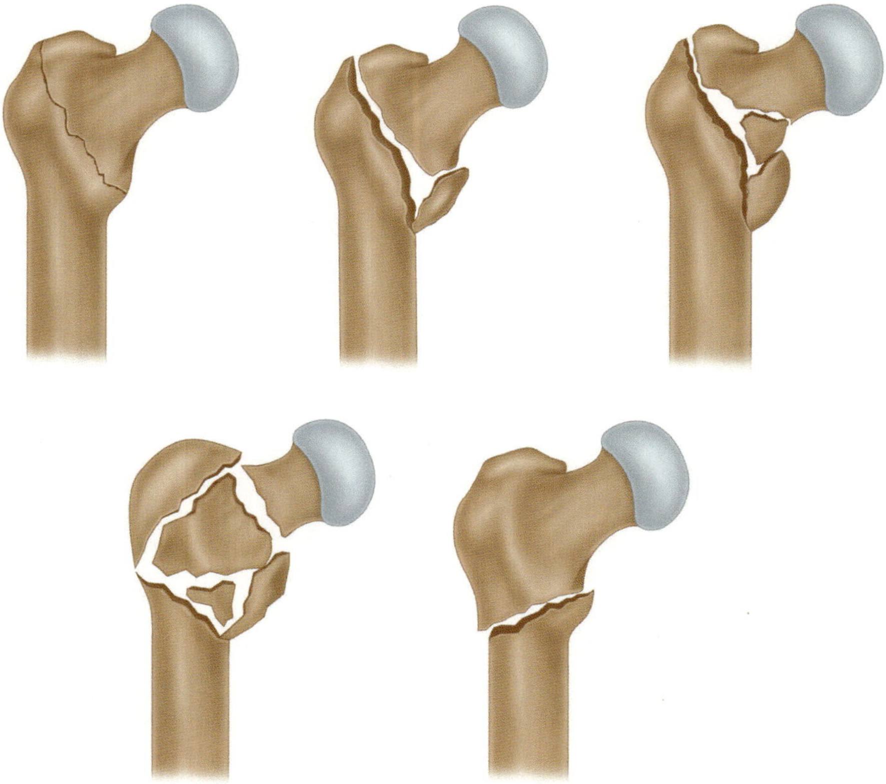

Fig. 21.4 Evans transtrochanteric fracture classification

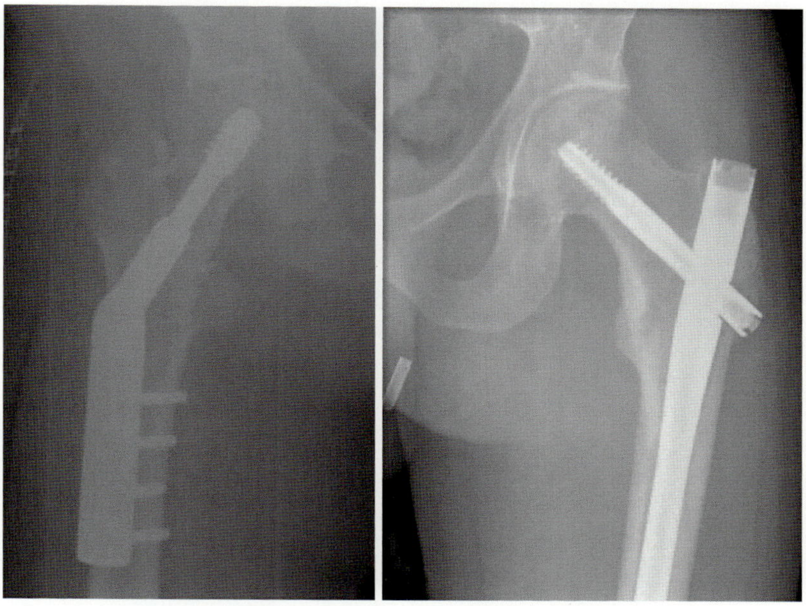

Fig. 21.5 Transtrochanteric fracture fixation with dynamic screw plate and nail

The usual types of fixation are sliding screw plates or nails (Fig. 21.5). Both have good results. The former have the need for more soft tissue dissection and are related to more blood loss during surgery but allow for intraoperative reduction of displaced fractures. Nails are placed closer to the mechanical axis and have smaller bending moments; they are associated to lesser blood loss during surgery, but they need a good closed reduction on the fracture table to ensure a good result.

21.2.4.4 Subtrochanteric Fractures

Subtrochanteric fractures are considered difficult to treat. The iliopsoas exerts a strong force that displaces the fracture in the three planes. This makes it more challenging to reduce and realign. The treatment often requires the combination of transtrochanteric with shaft fixation methods.

21.2.4.5 Shaft Fractures

Shaft fractures are the most frequent femur fractures in players, especially under the age of 20. They are associated to significant blood loss, and they need immediate stabilization to avoid serious complications such as shock, fat embolism, and eventually death. Thomas splints, or other traction splints, are all temporary stabilization devices that can be used before definitive treatment. External fixation is recommended for open fractures or in the case of a delay of internal fixation surgery, whatever the reason.

There are three main types of fractures: spiral, oblique, and transverse. They can present with variable degrees of comminution.

Being extra-articular fractures, they do not need anatomical reduction, just alignment and rotational deformity restoration. They will benefit from stable relative fixation, which allows for micromotion, such as nailing. This is probably the best choice of treatment (Fig. 21.6).

Using plates is an alternative, but they imply more tissue aggression. They should be placed as bridge plates to avoid losing the hematoma and the biologic local response to bone fracture. If used, they should be used percutaneously as an ideal procedure.

Open fractures need a different approach. The need for early stabilization remains the same. Surgical debridement is mandatory. Reaming of the medullary canal is not recommended, and internal fixation may need delaying for better local and skin conditions.

21.2.4.6 Supracondylar, Intercondylar, and Unicondylar Fractures

These are discussed in the chapter related to knee fractures.

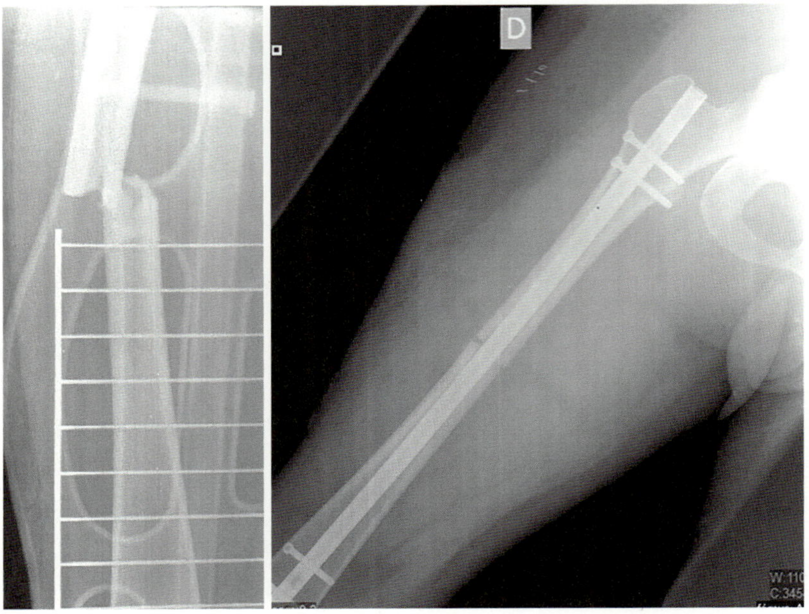

Fig. 21.6 Shaft fracture in a 32-year-old female professional resulting from direct blunt trauma during match (Images of preop and post-op)

21.2.5 Rehabilitation

Physical therapy is focused on early mobilization and gait resumption. A program will begin in immediate postoperative period.

In the first 4 weeks, many modalities can be used. Faradic stimulation will help in pain management, swelling control, and muscle reeducation. Gentle passive mobilization, active isodynamic, and isometric exercises of the muscles around the hip, knee, and ankle can begin: stretching of the hamstrings, gastrocnemius, and soleus; strengthening of the quadriceps; straight leg raise in four planes; ankle dorsiflexion; and plantar flexion, eversion, and inversion.

In the second phase (4–8 weeks), there will be progress in strengthening exercises, balance, and proprioceptive and gait retaining activities. For this, the criteria for progression are minimal effusion, 50% weight bearing, and fair grade strength of hip abductors and quadriceps. Fitting with stationary bicycle and pool therapy can begin.

After 8 weeks, progressing is depending on full weight bearing without assistive devices, no effusion, and strength of the hip abductors and quadriceps. Strengthening exercises gradually increase in effort and resistance. The same happens for balance, proprioception, and gait training activities. Fitness condition exercises gradually progress to regain pre-injury state. This can take up to 18 weeks.

21.3 Fractures in Children

Most of sport-related lesions in children are minor and self-limiting. So, children and youth sports are safe. But fractures may occur. Femur fractures are the least seen among others. This is related to the amount of energy necessary to cause fracture. It is, after all, the strongest of bones.

Risk factors are training in poor environment, improper footwear, and improperly supervised high-resistance training [20]. Although boys are predominant in football, it is the leading sport for injuries in girls. Amenorrheic anorectic females are at risk due to reduced bone density. To help reduce the risk of injury, cross-training and gradual schedule changes are good practices.

21.3.1 Children's Bone

There are many differences between children and adult bone healing. Because of a more biologically active periosteum, bone healing is faster.

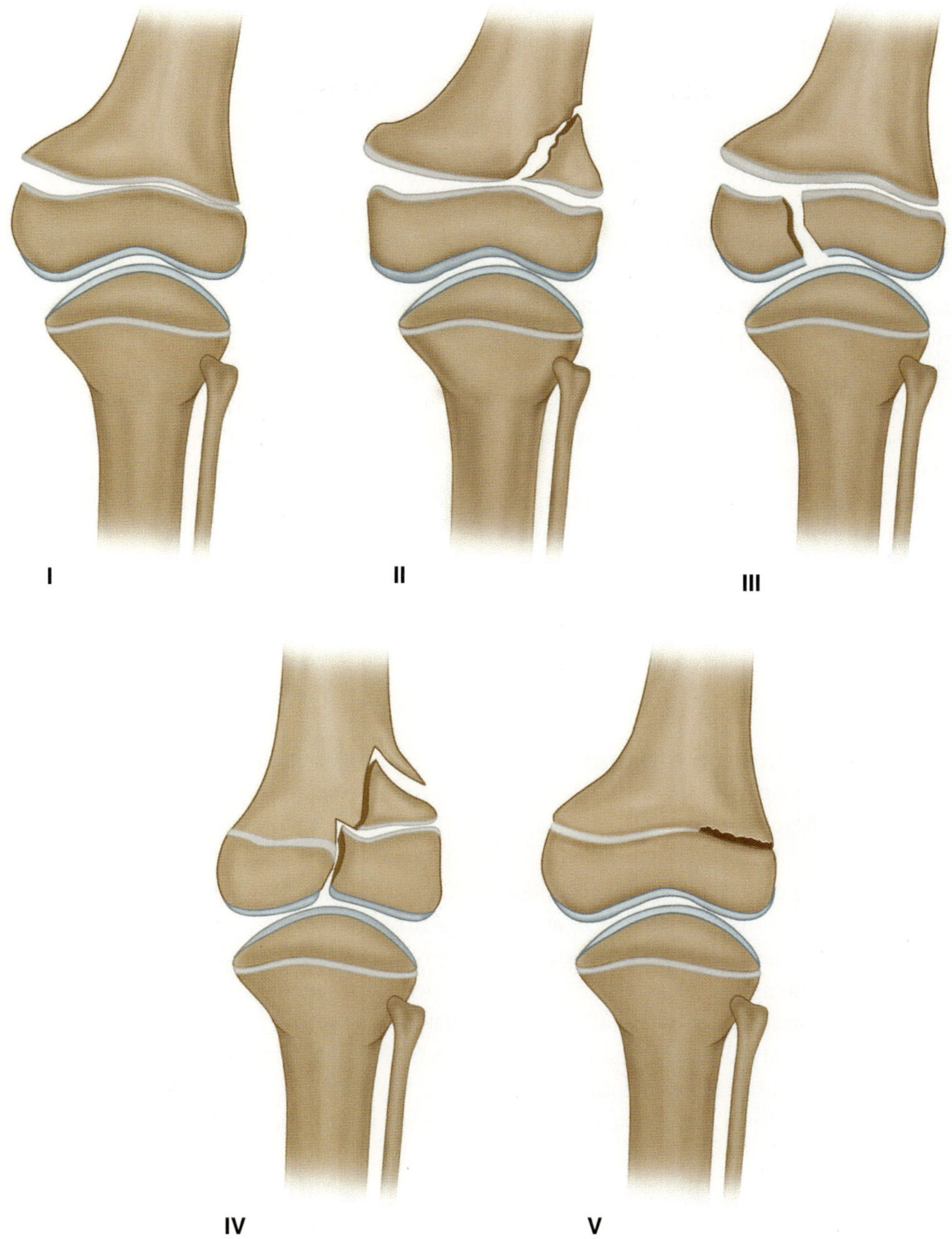

Fig. 21.7 Salter-Harris classification

Callus forms rapidly and there is a great potential for remodeling. Deformities resulting from malunion will often disappear with remodeling, excepting for rotational deformity. That means anatomic reduction is not necessary, and other forms of treatment are possible.

There are problems exclusive to children, such as overgrowth, causing limb length discrepancy. Deformities resulting from fractures at ossification centers or growth plates will progress with age. In growth plate trauma, some sort of growth disturbance might be expected, such as limb length inequality or angular deformity.

Salter and Harris have proposed a classification system that relates patterns of fracture with the risk of complications to the growth (Fig. 21.7).

Treatment can be conducted conservatively in many cases. When surgery is needed, it must be modified to avoid injury to ossification centers and growth plates.

21.3.2 Fractures of the Diaphysis

Femoral shaft fractures account for 1–2% of all pediatric fractures.

Because of the great remodeling potential children have, there is a place for conservative treatment. As long as there is no rotational deformity, the bone will heal well in the vast majority of the cases. Deformity resulting from malunion of displaced ends and limb length discrepancy will recover by remodeling. But that potential for full recovery decreases with age, and surgery will become necessary for comfort, to help faster mobility, and to avoid bad outcome.

Overgrowth after a fracture, causing length discrepancy, is a rare complication.

21.3.3 Fractures Through the Growth Plates, the Epiphysis, and the Apophysis

Growth plate injury can cause permanent and developing deformities. If growth stops at an entire growth plate, there will be a shortened limb. It will not grow as fast or as much as the contralateral. Or it may not grow at all. If the growth disturbance only affects a part of the growth plate, there will be an angular deformity. The affected part will be in the concave side of the deformity.

21.3.3.1 Traumatic Physeal Fracture of the Femoral Head

The femoral head represents less than 1% of all pediatric fractures.

The femoral head contributes for 30% of the length of the femur and 13% of the limb. Damage to the head causes shortening as well as articular damage.

The head is a structural weak area that can fail when subjected to strong shear forces.

21.3.3.2 Fracture Through the Greater Trochanter

The greater trochanter is a traction apophysis that contributes to the growth of the neck. Injury to this apophysis will cause it to be shortened and can cause coxa valga. Overgrowth will cause coxa vara and diminished distance between the trochanter and the joint.

21.3.3.3 Fracture of the Distal Epiphysis of the Femur

The distal epiphysis is responsible for 70% of the femur growth. Any disturbance in growth will produce a very important range of deformities.

21.3.4 Treatment

21.3.4.1 Proximal Fractures

They are classified according to Delbet:

- Type I (transepiphyseal)
- Type II (transcervical)
- Type III (cervicotrochanteric)
- Type IV (pertrochanteric)

All fracture types I and II and displaced fracture types III and IV are best treated with internal fixation (pins, Kirschner wires, or preferably cannulated screws) to prevent malunion and nonunion. Although there is still debate on the subject, some advocate capsulotomy to evacuate hematoma and reduce the risk of avascular necrosis.

21.3.4.2 Shaft Fractures

As proposed by Greene [21], the algorithm of treatment would be based on the age, stability, and severity of the trauma (Table 21.1).

21.3.4.3 Distal Fractures

Anatomic reduction is very important for a good result. All displaced fractures should be treated operatively and stabilized with fixa-

Table 21.1 Children femoral shaft fracture treatment algorithm

Age	Fracture	Treatment	Comment
6–11 year	Low energy/stable	Spica cast	Lesser remodeling potential than younger children Operative stabilization indicated for early mobilization Flexible intramedullary nailling preferred
	High energy/unstable	Traction followed by spica cast Internal fixation	
>11 year	Stable or unstable	Internal fixation	Limited remodeling potential Operative treatment preferred Need for restoration of length and alignment Avoid nailing through piriformis fossa due to risk of necrosis
	Comminuted, compound	Internal fixation External fixator?	

tion. Undisplaced fractures have a considerable risk for displacement, and surgery is advised.

21.3.4.4 Postoperative Management

A cast or a splint is necessary to protect and add stability to hip fractures, flexible nailing of the shaft, or to distal fractures.

Partial weight bearing is allowed after 2–3 weeks. Percutaneous pins or wires can be removed after 4 weeks. Casts can be removed with clinical and radiologic evidence of bony union.

21.4 Stress Fractures

21.4.1 Pathophysiology

Stress fractures account for 2% of all injuries in football. For example, 9 of the 24 players in US 1994 World Cup team have a history of stress fracture [22]. Femur stress fractures occur due to fatigue [23] and have a completely different pathophysiology than insufficiency fractures. Fatigue results in repetitive overload of the healthy bone with normal elastic resistance.

In response to repetitive load, microdamage occurs [24], and the bone attempts to remodel. Osteoblasts start producing new bone. Osteoclasts also participate in the process of remodeling. As loads become repetitive, multiple remodeling sites become active at the same time. As a result, bone resistance diminishes. The continuous addition of more microdamage sites ends with a crack and its propagation. Children can also have stress fractures.

Stress fractures should not be mistaken for pathologic fractures. Stress fractures occur in the healthy bone only. In insufficiency or pathologic fractures, normal stress causes damage on the bone with deficient elastic resistance. In that case, the bone is not healthy for some reason, and treatment should address not only the fracture but also the underlying disease (nutritional deficit, endocrine disease, neoplastic tissue). In children, the most frequent causes are osteogenesis imperfecta, aneurysmal bone cyst, unicameral bone cyst, non-ossifying fibroma, and generalized osteopenia due to neuromuscular disorders [25].

21.4.2 Risk Factors

In general, there are other risk factors: caloric restriction, decreased bone density, muscle weakness, leg-length differences, genetics, female sex, white ethnicity, low body weight, lack of weight-bearing exercise, intrinsic and extrinsic mechanical factors, amenorrhea, oligomenorrhea, decreased testosterone level in males, inadequate calcium and caloric intake, and disordered eating.

In football, the main reason for stress fracture is overtraining. The other factors are training on hard ground, poor shoe design, training errors, and lack of recovery after exercising. In professional leagues, there are well-planned strategies to avoid overuse injury.

21.4.3 Diagnosis

21.4.3.1 Signs and Symptoms

Early diagnosis can be difficult as there is unspecific groin pain. But the player feels a painful limitation that can progress until that they cannot run. Usually, resting is enough for the pain to stop.

21.4.3.2 Imaging Study

It is frequent that x-ray does not show any fracture as it may be incomplete and undisplaced.

Therefore, computed tomography, scintigraphy, and magnetic resonance imaging (MRI) are preferred for the diagnosis of stress fracture, because they have higher sensitivity.

Scintigraphy has low specificity and is not necessary if there is access to MRI.

MRI is highly sensitive and specific, avoids the use of ionizing radiation, and allows for better visualization of the medullary bone and for bone edema around the fracture site (Fig. 21.8).

21.4.4 Treatment

21.4.4.1 Conservative

There are very little indications for conservative treatment of a femur fracture. Some stress fractures can have a good outcome with load restriction only. The fracture that benefits from conservative treatment is an incomplete fracture, located on a compression-loaded cortex, not resulting of insufficiency. Unfortunately, a great pressure is put on the physician, related to the need to return to sports rapidly, making this option even more rare than the opportunity to use it. In such cases, surgery will not make the bone heal faster, and it is not always exempt from complications.

Weight-bearing restriction with crutches is the most important measure. Short-and long-term results are favorable [26]. Early rehabilitation is related to better outcome.

21.4.4.2 Surgical

Most of the fractures have a surgical indication, and the few fractures that had indication for conservative treatment are operated as discussed above. Undisplaced fractures on tension side of the femur must be fixated because of an elevated risk of displacement.

The fixation methods are the same that for trauma fractures. Supplementation on calcium and D-vitamin are usual in stress context.

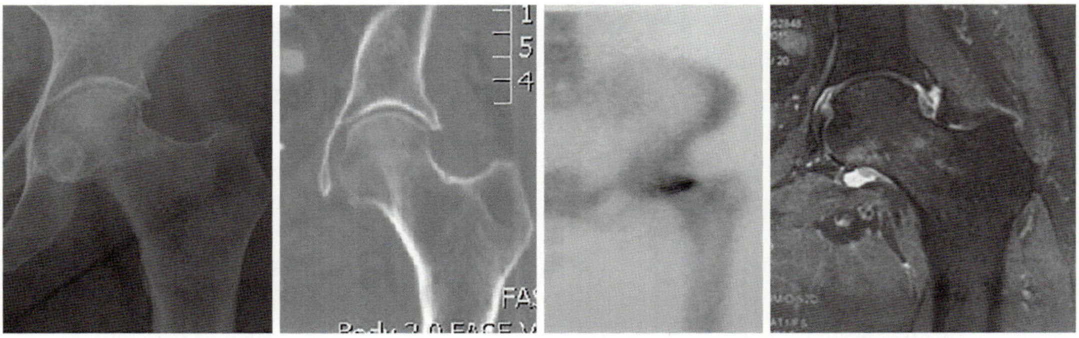

Fig. 21.8 Stress fracture: x-ray, CT, scintigraphy, and MRI

21.4.5 Rehabilitation

The primary focus of rehabilitation is the return to premorbid state.

In the case of nonsurgical treatment, therapy will focus on rest and modifying any training errors. To maintain fitness of the athlete, exercise of the non-affected extremities can be done. Muscle strengthening without weight bearing on the fracture side can be accomplished. Gait and anatomic abnormalities that could have predisposed to fracture must be evaluated. Once acute pain is relieved, strengthening exercises for hip stabilizers can be initiated. The main objective is to restore hip range of motion. When the patient is pain-free, weight bearing is gradually initiated. Weekly x-ray imaging supervision is performed until full weight bearing without any pain.

Running is started when the patient is completely pain-free. Time and distance are slowly increased. Any symptom of pain should indicate for rest. Progressive return to prior level is time dependent on symptoms.

Patients treated with surgery must rest for healing to progress. But early mobilization is related to faster recovery. Strengthening of muscles is important for stability and for gait. The most important are the gluteus medius, gluteus maximus, iliopsoas, adductors, quadriceps, and hamstrings. After gait has been normalized, eccentric muscle strengthening and sport-specific activities are then progressed.

Removal of implants may be needed to allow for full recovery.

References

1. Tourny C, Sangnier S, Cotte T, Langlois R, Coquart J. Epidemiologic study of young soccer player's injuries in U12 to U20. J Sports Med Phys Fitness. 2014;54:526–35.
2. Ekstrand J, Hägglund M, Waldén M. Injury incidence and injury patterns in professional football: the UEFA injury study. Br J Sports Med. 2011;45:553–8.
3. O'Hata HN, Kohno T, Morikawa T, Seki J. A 15-year prospective epidemiological account of acute traumatic injuries during official professional soccer league matches in Japan. Am J Sports Med. 2012;40:1006–14.
4. Weiss RJ, Montgomery SM, Al Dabbagh Z, Jansson KA. National data of 6409 Swedish inpatients with femoral shaft fractures: stable incidence between 1998 and 2004. Injury. 2009;40:304.
5. Niva MH, Kiuru MJ, Haataja R, Pihlajamäki HK. Fatigue injuries of the femur. J Bone Joint Surg Br. 2005;87:1385–90.
6. Poulsen TD, Freund KG, Madsen F, Sandvej K. Injuries in high-skilled and low-skilled soccer: a prospective study. Br J Sports Med. 1991;25:151–3.
7. Goga IE, Gongal P. Severe soccer injuries in amateurs. Br J Sports Med. 2003;37:498–501.
8. van Beijsterveldt AMC, Stubbe JH, Schmikli SL, van de Port IGL, Backx FJG. Differences in injury risk and characteristics between Dutch amateur and professional soccer players. J Sci Med Sport. 2014;18:145–9.
9. Esquivel AO, Bruder A, Ratkowiak K, Lemos SE. Soccer-related injuries in children and adults aged 5 to 49 years in US Emergency Departments from 2000 to 2012. Sports Health. 2015;7:4.
10. Ogden JA. Injury to the immature skeleton. In: Touloukian R, editor. Pediatric trauma. 2nd ed. New York: John Wiley & Sons; 1990.
11. Lieurance R, Benjamin JB, Rappaport WD. Blood loss and transfusion in patients with isolated femur fractures. J Orthop Trauma. 1992;6:175–9.
12. Stannard JP, Lopez-Ben RR, Volgas DA, Anderson ER, Busbee M, Karr DK, McGwin Jr GR, Alonso JE. Prophylaxis against deep-vein thrombosis following trauma: a prospective, randomized comparison of mechanical and pharmacologic prophylaxis. J Bone Joint Surg Am. 2006;88:261–6.
13. Gustilo RB, Anderson JT. Prevention of infection in the treatment of one thousand and twenty-five open fractures of long bones: retrospective and prospective analyses. J Bone Joint Surg Am. 1976;58:453–8.
14. Takami H, Takahashi S, Ando M. Sciatic nerve injury associated with fracture of the femoral shaft. Arch Orthop Trauma Surg. 1999;119:103–4.
15. Martins RS, Bastos D, Siqueira MG, Heise CO, Teixeira MJ. Traumatic injuries of peripheral nerves: a review with emphasis on surgical indication. Arq Neuropsiquiatr. 2013;71:811–4.
16. Cornwall R, Radomisli TE. Nerve injury in traumatic dislocation of the hip. Clin Orthop Relat Res. 2000;377:84–91.
17. Droll KP, Broekhuyse H, O'Brien P. Fracture of the femoral head. J Am Acad Orthop Surg. 2007;15:716–27.

18. Bonnaire FA, Weber AT. Analysis of fracture gap changes, dynamic and static stability of different osteosynthetic procedures in the femoral neck. Injury. 2002;33:C24–32.
19. Swiontkowski MF, Hansen ST. Percutaneous Neufeld pinning for femoral neck fractures. Clin Orthop. 1986;206:113–6.
20. Shanmugam C, Maffulli M. Sports injuries in children. Br Med Bull. 2008;86:33–57.
21. Greene WB. Displaced fractures of the femoral shaft in children. Unique features and therapeutic options. Clin Orthop Relat Res. 1998;353:86–96.
22. Knapp TP, Mandelbaum BR. Stress fractures. In http://www.ussoccer.com/ stories/2014/03/17/11/28/stress-fractures-can-be-a-concern-for-soccer-players. Accessed 11 June 2015.
23. Knapp TP, Mandelbaum BR, Garrett Jr WE. Why are stress injuries so common in the soccer player? Clin Sports Med. 1998;17:835–53.
24. Pepper M, Akuthota V, McCarty EC. The pathophysiology of stress fractures. Clin Sports Med. 2006;25:1–16.
25. Loder RT, O'Donnell PW, Feinberg JR. Epidemiology and mechanisms of femur fractures in children. J Pediatr Orthop. 2006;26:561–6.
26. Pihlajamäki HK, Ruohola J-P, Weckström M, Kiuru MJ, Visuri TI. Long-term outcome of undisplaced fatigue fractures of the femoral neck in young male adults. J Bone Joint Surg Br. 2006;88:1574–9.

Part VI

Spine and Head Conditions

First Aid and Cares in Spine Trauma

22

Luís Silva, J.M. Pinto de Freitas, and Jorge Mineiro

Contents

L. Silva (✉)
Clínica do Dragão, Espregueira-Mendes Sports Centre - FIFA Medical Centre of Excellence, Porto, Portugal

Dom Henrique Research Centre, Porto, Portugal

ULS-Guarda, Guarda, Portugal
e-mail: luisduartesilva1985@gmail.com

JM.P. de Freitas
Coordinator of the Orthopedic and Traumatology, Unit of the Lusíadas Hospital in Porto, Porto, Portugal

J. Mineiro
Hospital CUF Descobertas, Lisboa, Portugal
e-mail: jmineiro@netcabo.pt

22.1 First Aid and Cares in Spine Trauma

This chapter is divided into two parts, the first will address the clinical approach in general spine trauma and the second will report special conditions in sport trauma.

22.1.1 Spinal Column

The spinal column is composed by 7 cervical, 12 thoracic, and 5 lumbar vertebrae, the sacrum, and the coccyx [1–3].

The cervical spine has been considered the most vulnerable to sustain an injury due to its high mobility and exposure to external events. Once below C3 level, the spinal canal diameter is smaller; injuries to the vertebral column are more prone to happen [3, 4].

The thoracic spine, due to its movement restrictions and rib cage support, has a lower incidence of fractures, the most common is the wedged compression fracture [2, 5]. The thoracolumbar junction due to its characteristics is more susceptible to injuries [5].

22.1.2 Vertebral-Medullary Trauma

The cervical spine is the most affected spinal region, counting with a total of 55% of all

J. Espregueira-Mendes et al. (eds.), *Injuries and Health Problems in Football*,
DOI 10.1007/978-3-662-53924-8_22

vertebral-medullary injuries. The following 45% are correspondingly distributed by the thoracic, thoracolumbar, and lumbosacral spine [6].

When a vertebral-medullary injury is suspected, the initial approach should always include the airway and cervical assessment. The clinician should be careful in cases which the trauma can become a life-threatening situation to the athlete [6]:

- Neurogenic shock – interruption of descending sympathetic enervation to the heart and vasomotor tone, resulting in bradycardia and hypotension. The athlete becomes hypotensive. The treatment can include atropine and vasopressors
- Spinal shock – associated with the immediate loss of the reflexes and flaccidity. After the injury is installed, the hyperreflexia will occur

When evaluating these patients, the clinician should be aware of the mechanism of injury, once it will further help in the evaluation of suspected injuries [2, 4]. Special attention must be paid to lesions above the clavicles [6].

When assessing spinal cord injuries, it is important to evaluate both sides of the body, and attention must be directed to the following three tracts [3, 5]:

- The corticospinal tract: controls the motor power on the same side of the body, assessed by voluntary muscle contractions or involuntary response to painful stimuli
- Spinothalamic tract: transmits pain and temperature sensation to the contralateral side of the body, assessed by a light touch
- Dorsal columns: control proprioception, vibration, and light touch sensations on the same side of the body, assessed by position sense of toes/fingers or vibration

In addition, each nerve root dermatome and myotome should be examined [5].

22.1.3 On-Field Emergency

Following a traumatism, the player's assessment should be done the most accurate and quickly as possible. A systematic approach is required in order to save lives but also determine the player's degree and extent of injury and prevent subsequent complications [6–8].

In case of cervical trauma, the most important procedures in the field are to identify potential injuries, protect the cervical spine, maximize the respiratory and hemodynamic status, and provide a safe and fast transportation of the athlete. Therefore, the clinician should immobilize the cervical spine with a cervical collar, lateral immobilizers, and spine board with strappings (Fig. 22.1).

In cases when the clinician does not have the adequate equipment with him, he should place his hands in both sides of the head preventing any head movement [6]. Moreover, the spine board and strappings are used when a spine injury is suspected independently of the level of injury and transport is required.

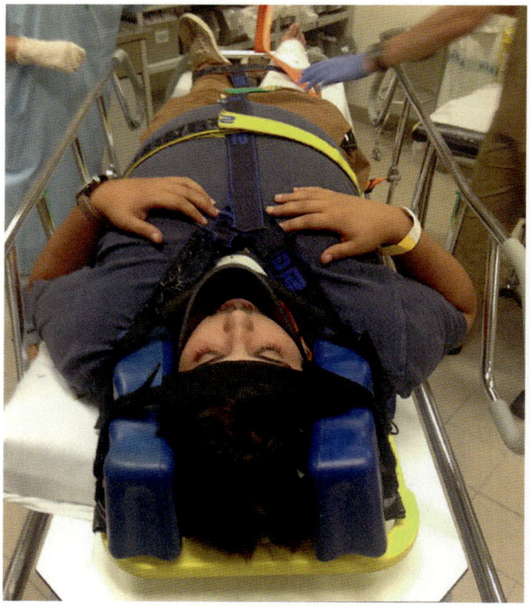

Fig. 22.1 Example of a patient on top of a spine board, immobilized with a cervical collar and lateral immobilizers

Since sport trauma occurs so unpredictable and fast, the mechanism of injury may not be so clear to the clinician. Independently of the cause, when assessing any critical patient, the clinician should start by the ABCDE approach, where each item should be assessed before passing to the next one [5, 6]:

A. = Airway maintenance and cervical spine protection
B. = Breathing and ventilation
C. = Circulation with hemorrhage control
D. = Disability/neurological status
E. = Exposure/environmental control

22.1.3.1 Airway Maintenance Cervical Spine Protection

The airway can be compromised by a primary injury, usually by a trauma incident, or by a secondary injury, which can result to a decreased conscious level, and can be evaluated through Glasgow Coma Scale [9].

When assessing or treating problems related to the airway, four options may be available [6]:

1. Airway clearance techniques
2. Basic airway aids
3. Advanced airway aids
4. Airway surgery

Within the airway clearance techniques, there are two major ones. The jaw-thrust maneuver is made every time a cervical injury is suspected. The clinician may approach the airway with manual inline stabilization or neck immobilizers without losing the control of the cervical spine [6, 8, 10]. If cervical trauma is excluded, the clinician may opt for extension of the head while lifting the chin. If these techniques do not clear the airways, then airway aids must be used [6, 8].

In regard to the airway aids, in more simple cases, it may be used with the Guedel pattern airway. It is inserted into the airways, which will further help to prevent the tongue from covering the epiglottis and maintain or open the patient's airways [6, 8]. It has the advantage to be easy to apply. However, if applied incorrectly, it can result in vomit reflex. As an alternative, or in combination, a nasopharynx tube can be used, which will facilitate the air flux within the pharynx. If fracture of the skull base is suspected, the nasopharynx tube should not be used because, if inserted incorrectly, it can worsen the condition. In more complicated cases, advanced airway aids are required. The endotracheal intubation is still the gold standard to assure airway security; however it requires domain over technique and a progressive learning curve. The laryngeal mask can further help the basic aids to protect the airway against secretions and is an adequate option to secure the airway function when an endotracheal intubation is not possible. If none of the above is functioning or possible to perform, surgical intervention will be required [6].

22.1.3.2 Breathing and Ventilation

It is crucial to assess the thoracic movements, hear the player's respiratory sounds, and palpate the thoracic anatomical structures, searching for asymmetries or anomalies [5, 6]. Special caution should be taken if the player presents dyspnea and/or tachypnea, in which case the problem may be associated with an airway commitment. Nonetheless, if the inadequate airway is caused by a pneumothorax or tension pneumothorax, using an intubation with a vigorous bag-mask ventilation can lead the player to even further deterioration [5]. Special attention must be taken in regard to the tension pneumothorax that can be a life-threatening condition due to a "one-way valve" mechanism from a perforated lung or penetration on the chest wall. This condition usually presents tracheal deviation, diminished or absent breath sounds unilaterally, hyperresonance on percussion, hypotension, and pulse rate more or equal to 140 beats per minute. Emergency treatment can be performed by chest decompression using an intravenous 14G catheter over a 3–6 cm needle at the second intercostal space, in the midclavicular line just on the superior border of the third rib. A sudden rush of air or aspirating free air into the syringe means that the needle is in the pleural space. The needle is then removed and the catheter left in place [11, 12].

22.1.3.3 Circulation with Hemorrhage Control

Hemorrhage has been considered as one of the main causes of preventable death [5]. Therefore, reassuring the patient circulation is essential to decide if the vital organs are being correctly perfused and to exclude a potential internal hemorrhage. In this sense, it is important to check for the player's paleness, localized pain, and/or possible internal or external bleeding and assess the cardiac frequency, the capillary filling, the arterial pressure, and the glycemia. It is also important to check for abdominal hematomas or other trauma secondary signs, pelvic instability, and femur fractures [3–6].

22.1.3.4 Disability: Neurological Status

It should perform a basic neurologic evaluation in order to confirm the suspicion of cranial and vertebral injury. Hence, it is necessary to assess the player's status of consciousness [8], the condition of the pupils, and the any lateralizing signs [5]. The first can be accomplished through Glasgow Coma Scale [9] or simply by a scoring system:

1. The player is totally conscious and responsive
2. The player gives verbal responses
3. The player gives physical feedback to painful stimuli
4. The player does not give any verbal or motor responses to painful stimuli

Regarding the condition of the pupils, it should assess the size, symmetry, and reaction to stimuli. In addition, it is also important to assess the mobility and sensibility of the upper and lower limbs and search for any lateralizing signs [5, 6].

22.1.3.5 Exposure/Environmental Control

The patient should be undressed to further assess the extent of the trauma and check for further missing details. However, trauma patients usually have loss of temperature. Therefore, as soon as the examination is finished, it is essential to warm the patient in order to prevent hypothermia [13].

22.2 Management of Most Common Spinal Injuries

In this second part of the chapter, some of the most common spinal injuries in sports will be addressed.

22.2.1 Cervical Strains

Cervical strains affect the musculotendinous part of the neck and are the most common sports neck injuries. The more usual mechanisms of injury are overuse syndrome or whiplash of the head and are commonly secondary to high-velocity contact sports [6, 14].

Prevention is a difficult task, once most of neck injuries are traumatic. Nevertheless, isometric and eccentric exercises of the neck muscles may provide some muscular reactive protection. In addition, good technical skills and good head and neck control, associated with proper muscular strength, are critical for preventing neck injuries [14, 15].

This injury can occur after a head trauma, compelling the muscles, which are already contracted, to an eccentric load. Cervical tenderness and limited range of motion are the typical complains. After the trauma and before the player is allowed to return to competition, it is very important to perform a neurologic examination and to observe a practically pain-free range of motion since this injury is often responsible for an early and forced substitution of the player. Ice may be applied while examining the patient [14, 15].

Radiographs are indicated and important to rule out fractures and dislocations when neck pain persists. Anteroposterior and lateral radiographs and, in some cases, flexion/extension are necessary. The last one may turn out to be hard to obtain in the acute setting and sometimes can only be performed after 2–3 weeks. Magnetic resonance imaging (MRI) may be required in more particular situations [6, 14].

The conservative treatment is followed in practically all cases. In this sense, a cervical collar can be used for a period of 7–10 days. Ice, anti-inflammatory medication, neuromuscular electrical stimulation, isometric strengthening, and mobilization exercises should be included into the treatment program. If the diagnosis cannot be initially confirmed, secondary imaging studies should be performed [14, 15].

22.2.2 Stinger

Stinger is characterized by pain or paresthesia in a superior limb after an impact on the neck or shoulder. It is differentiated from a radiculopathy once it only involves a single dermatome [6, 14].

The main mechanisms of injury are neck flexion to the contralateral side with the shoulder in downward displacement, which will stretch the brachial plexus and compress the nerve roots through head rotation to the affected side [16]. In many occasions, the player needs to hold the affected arm with the uninjured one, once it can have a severe mobility impairment [14].

It is imperative to perform a careful neurologic examination. Inspection, palpation, and assessment of cervical spine range of motion are also mandatory. The clavicle, glenohumeral, and acromioclavicular joints should be properly examined since associated injuries may be present [14]. Two key aspects are important to be kept in mind: the symptoms can resolve within minutes and motor weakness may appear days or hours after the trauma [6, 14, 17].

In most cases, cervical radiographs are sufficient to exclude other conditions. Electromyography is rarely indicated, and MRI is indicated when a nerve root or spinal cord lesion is suspected [17].

This condition is considered benign, and the main goal should be to restore neck motion and strengthening of upper extremity muscles [17]. Return to sports is allowed after full symptomatic recovery [14].

22.2.3 Spinal Cord Neuropraxia

Spinal cord neuropraxia requires careful initial steps of evaluation, and it is almost exclusive of the American football players and surfers. Nevertheless, it can also occur in other sports, like football [14, 18]. In most of the patients, a cervical stenosis may exist, leading to spinal cord compression as the neck is hyperextended. The result of this injury is temporary paralysis with full recovery of function. Neck pain is usually not present, but a spectrum of neurological manifestations may occur, including numbness, tingling, loss of muscular strength, or even complete paralysis. Initial evaluation and management must strictly follow the principles described previously.

This injury is classified according to the duration that the symptoms last [14, 19]:

- Grade I – symptoms resolve in 15 min
- Grade II – from 15 min to 24 h
- Grade III – over 24 h

Imaging examination should include cervical spine radiographs and MRI. Rehabilitation is performed aiming a pain-free range of motion, with complete recovery of the normal neurological status. Surgical management in this condition is reserved for special cases, with few reports in the scientific literature [6, 14].

Criteria to participate in collision activities were proposed by Torg and Ramsey-Emerhein [20] in those with cervical spine stenosis (developmental). These criteria are described in Table 22.1.

Table 22.1 Criteria to participate in collision activities in those with cervical spine stenosis (developmental), according to Torg and Ramsey-Emerhein [21, 22]

Criteria	Recommendation
Asymptomatic athlete with a Torg ratio under or equal to 0.8	No contraindication
One episode of cervical cord neurapraxia and Torg ratio under or equal 0.8	Relative contraindication
Athletes with over one episode of cervical cord neurapraxia with intervertebral disk disease and/or cervical spondylosis	Relative contraindication
Spinal cord defect or edema demonstrated on MRI in an athlete with one or more episodes	Relative/absolute contraindication
Documented episode of cervical cord neurapraxia with ligamentous instability (neurological symptoms lasting more than 36 h) and/or multiple episodes	Absolute contraindication

"Torg ratio": ratio of the diameter of the cervical canal to the width of cervical body on the X-ray lateral view [21, 22]

References

1. Standring S. Gray's anatomy: the anatomical basis of clinical practice. Expert consult – online and print 40e. Elsevier; 2008.
2. Dutton M. Dutton's orthopaedic examination evaluation and intervention. New York: McGraw Hill Professional; 2012.
3. Van De Graaff KM, Brown W. Human anatomy. Dubuque: Wm. C: Brown Publishers; 1992.
4. Moore KL, Dalley AF, Agur AM. Clinically oriented anatomy. Baltimore: Lippincott Williams & Wilkins; 2013.
5. ACSCT ACoSCoT. Advanced trauma life support student course manual. Chicago: American College of Surgeons; 2012.
6. Pessoa P, Jones H. Traumatologia desportiva. Lisbon: Lidel – edições técnicas, lda; 2014.
7. Mohammad A, Branicki F, Abu-Zidan FM. Educational and clinical impact of Advanced Trauma Life Support (ATLS) courses: a systematic review. World J Surg. 2014;38:322–9.
8. Ripoll P, Prado M, Zapata F, Pereira H, Gómez Á. Football medicine: immediate action guide for coaches and referees. Sport Clinic Rippol y de Prado; 2014.
9. Teasdale G, Jennett B. Assessment of coma and impaired consciousness. a practical scale. Lancet. 1974;2:81–4.
10. Austin N, Krishnamoorthy V, Dagal A. Airway management in cervical spine injury. Int J Crit Illn Inj Sci. 2014;4:50–6.
11. Eckstein M, Suyehara D. Needle thoracostomy in the prehospital setting. Prehosp Emerg Care. 1998;2:132–5.
12. Jain DG, Gosavi SN, Jain DD. Understanding and managing tension pneumothorax. J Indian Acad Clin Med. 2008;9:42–50.
13. Søreide K. Clinical and translational aspects of hypothermia in major trauma patients: from pathophysiology to prevention, prognosis and potential preservation. Injury. 2014;45:647–54.
14. McMahon PJ. Current diagnosis & treatment in sports medicine, Lange medical book. New York: Lange Medical Books/McGraw Hill Medical Pub; 2007.
15. Gallucci J. Soccer injury prevention and treatment: a guide to optimal performance for players, parents and coaches. New York: Demos Medical Publishing LLC; 2014.
16. Kelly JD, Aliquo D, Sitler MR, Odgers C, Moyer RA. Association of burners with cervical canal and foraminal stenosis. Am J Sports Med. 2000;28:214–7.
17. Feinberg JH. Burners and stingers. Phys Med Rehabil Clin N Am. 2000;11:771–84.
18. Bernsen HJ, Koetsveld A, Frenken CW, van Norel GJ. Neuropraxia of the cervical spinal cord following cervical spinal cord trauma: a report of five patients. Acta Neurol Belg. 2000;100:91–5.
19. Torg JS. Cervical spinal stenosis with cord neurapraxia and transient quadriplegia. Sports Med. 1995;20:429–34.
20. Torg JS, Ramsey-Emrhein JA. Suggested management guidelines for participation in collision activities with congenital, developmental, or postinjury lesions involving the cervical spine. Med Sci Sports Exerc. 1997;29:S256–72.
21. Torg JS, Pavlov H. Cervical spinal stenosis with cord neurapraxia and transient quadriplegia. Clin Sports Med. 1987;6:115–33.
22. Torg JS, Pavlov H, Genuario SE, Sennett B, Wisneski RJ, Robie BH, Jahre C. Neurapraxia of the cervical spinal cord with transient quadriplegia. J Bone Joint Surg Am. 1986;68:1354–70.

Low Back Pain

23

Rui Rocha, Ana Margarida Fernandes,
and António Oliveira

Contents

R. Rocha (✉)
Clínica do Dragão, Espregueira-Mendes Sports Centre – FIFA Medical Centre of Excellence, Porto, Portugal

Department of Orthopaedic Surgery, Centro Hospitalar Gaia/ Espinho, Vila Nova de Gaia, Portugal
ruimiguelreisrocha@gmail.com

A.M. Fernandes
Clínica do Dragão, Espregueira-Mendes Sports Centre – FIFA Medical Centre of Excellence, Porto, Portugal
ana.margarida.ssf@hotmail.com;
ana.margarida.ssf@gmail.com

A. Oliveira
Orthopaedic Department, Centro Hospitalar do Porto, Porto, Portugal
afonsecaoliveira1@gmail.com

J. Espregueira-Mendes et al. (eds.), *Injuries and Health Problems in Football*,
DOI 10.1007/978-3-662-53924-8_23

23.1 Introduction

Low back pain (LBP) is a common entity in the general population and causes significant disability when occurs. There is a lifetime incidence of 60–90% of LBP, but only 4% of these patients will need surgical intervention [1–4]. LBP is a symptom with multiple diagnostic possibilities. More often there is no correlation between the pain and an anatomical abnormality, which is a challenge to the physician. History of past events of LBP reflects a risk factor for recurrence of the condition [5–7].

Back pain in competitive active athletes is also a common feature, with an estimate prevalence related to sport ranging between 1% and 30% [8, 9]. LBP is the most common cause of lost playing and training time in professional players [8, 10]. Most episodes of LBP are of low intensity, and the professional athlete will continue to compete despite the discomfort [11]. Players rarely report the condition, so the prevalence may be higher, and most of the times the adequate treatment and rehabilitation will not be completed.

Although most LBP are non-specific and mechanical in nature, athletes are often at special risk because top-level sports require repetitive exercises with high loads, most often from an early age. Football players are prone to the same prevalence of LBP as other sports. There are no exhaustive and prospective randomised studies in the literature specifically for football players. But it is known that the duration of training, it's intensity, variety and the lack of rest are factors that are related to LBP in every sport, including football.

The aetiology and management of LBP depend on age and the presence of red flags in the history and physical examination. The most common back pain infirmities affecting athletes can be prevented by recognising epidemiologic patterns and implementing treatment plans accordingly. The majority of the cases are self-limiting and respond well to conservative treatment. But there are a number of disorders that will need a more exhaustive evaluation and management.

23.2 General Approach

LBP is a common symptom but never a diagnosis. Traditionally LBP is considered to be acute or chronic in nature. Epidemiological studies suggest that we cannot consider LBP as a stagnant entity and should not be categorised simply as acute or chronic. LBP oscillates over time with recurrences and exacerbations and should not be considered self-limiting. The natural history of LBP in football athletes is most probably no different. Sport participation in the general population contributes to less frequent episodes of LBP. This is true until the appearance of LBP. From that moment on, sport activities might increase the severity of pain and its recurrence [12].

It is uncommon that LBP is severe enough to prevent a football player from competing or from surrendering his place in the team. Despite this, in one study on elite football players, LBP was reported as the most common overuse injury [13]. Professional football players cannot stop participating in the game despite their lesions or pain. The career will be in danger, and the financial support of the club and the sponsors should not be neglected. These side effects mean that the management of athletes with LBP constitutes a challenge for the clinician.

23.2.1 History and Physical Examination

It is important to consider an extensive differential diagnosis list in order to avoid missing less frequent pathologies. The athlete's age, being familiar with the sport (in this case football), and the potential injury mechanisms for LBP that could occur in that context are also important. The most common cause of LBP is non-specific soft tissue injuries, but the physician must be alert in the younger athletes to the occurrence of spondylolysis/spondylolisthesis, hyperlordosis syndrome and intervertebral disc-related back pain. Adult athletes with LBP have greater risk of disc-related back pain than non-specific mechanical back pain.

Key information is determinant in order to reach a diagnostic, including mechanism of injury or the provocative incident, the site of pain, pain referral or irradiation and associated symptoms. The severity, progression of the pain, quality of pain, aggravating and relieving factors and movements, previous history of LBP or other back injuries and treatment methods used must be scrutinised.

History must identify potential red flags, these are conditions that may be present and indicate more serious pathology. The presence of these red flags in acute LBP suggests the need for further investigation and specialist referral as part of the overall strategy. If there are no red flags present, it is safe to comfort the patient and move ahead with the diagnostic possibilities. The red flags in history or physical findings are major trauma with possible fracture; fever or chills, recent bacterial infection or immunosuppression with possible infection; history of cancer, weight loss, pain at multiple sites, pain that worse at rest or at night, failure to improve with treatment or pain that persists 4–6 weeks; severe or progressive sensory alteration or weakness; bladder or bowel dysfunction; and evidence of neurological deficit in legs or perineum. It is important to exclude fractures, rheumatological or inflammatory diseases, infections and tumours.

Another type of flags, the yellow flags, may require the need to address psychosocial factors. These are psychosocial indicators suggesting increased risk of progression to long-term distress, disability and pain. They can relate to the patient's beliefs, emotions, behaviours, family and workplace. Future research is mandatory to investigate the relevance of these issues in athletic population.

The most common sport-related diagnoses, especially in young athletes, are sprains and strains, disc-related back pain, spondylolysis, spondylolisthesis, stress fractures and atypical Scheuermann's kyphosis.

Following history taking, physical examination should be equally detailed and incorporate range of motion assessment, palpation and traditional orthopaedic and neurological testing procedures to inform if further investigation is required. The activity that reproduces pain should be evaluated. Lumbar flexion stresses the anterior spine with multiple possible pathologies: disc pathology, epiphyseal injury and Scheuermann disease. Lumbar extension exercises hurt the posterior spine with possible spondylolysis/spondylolisthesis, facet pathology, hyperlordosis syndrome or lumbar muscle strain.

23.2.2 Investigation

A broad investigation is not necessary for all athletes with back pain. In fact, plain radiographs are usually unnecessary in the initial evaluation of the player. In the setting of an acute traumatic event, radiographic studies must be obtained. Much controversy exists surrounding the utility of plain films, computed tomography (CT), magnetic resonance imaging (MRI) and bone scintigraphy in the evaluation of sports-related spine injuries [14]. Radiographs demonstrate spinal deformities, instabilities and spondylolisthesis. MRI scans show vertebral discs, infections, tumours and the spinal cord. CT scans illustrate fractures and bone abnormalities. Bone scans can demonstrate suspected infection, inflammatory disease, tumours or stress and lytic pathologies. Laboratory tests may be helpful with certain diagnoses such as infection, inflammatory conditions and malignancy.

The physician must be conscious of specific signs that warrant further investigation. Diagnostic imaging should be used in an evidence-based and targeted fashion. When red flags are present, imaging studies are mandatory and are tailored to the situation, the history and the physical examination.

23.2.3 Management

It is important for the physician to address the cause of LBP, in order to establish the appropriate rehabilitation therapy [15]. Many athletes need to change training plans, sometimes even the technique of playing the sport.

The guidelines to be used in athletes are the same developed for the general population. Research and scientific evidences are required for the athletic population, and football is not an exception. The McGill [15] recommendations on how to reduce the risk of low back injuries in athletes are very useful in the daily train.

Evidence supports the principles to modify activity, remain active and replace aggravating activities for non-aggravating actions – relative rest [16, 17]. The recommendations include avoid end range of spine mobility in the first training days, spare the spine from full lateral bend, full flexion or extension and full rotation. Warm up is essential; the reduction of reaction moments and full contact is advisable. Management also includes modifications in training [18], because most LBP in athletes is likely to result from repetitive trauma and fatigue from the monotonous and cyclic overuses situations in training. Discussions should be made with coaching staff to develop a period of relative rest and activity modification, and, if relevant, technique adjustment is made to prevent the cycle of recurrent exacerbation and chronic pain.

Management of other specific pathologies is discussed ahead.

23.3 Non-specific Injuries

23.3.1 Soft Tissue Injuries

LBP in the athlete results almost always from a soft tissue insult. The soft tissue can be muscle, ligaments or fasciae tissue. The anatomy of an athlete's spine is no different from that of the nonathlete. When the back is submitted to stress forces, the physiology and biomechanical principles that rule general population are the same for football players. Lumbar muscle sprains and strains are common, moreover if we are dealing with inadequately conditioned athletes or in the beginning of the season, after a period with less activity. Abrupt changes in the training programme can also lead to episodes of LBP.

Sprain is a ligamentous injury, while a strain affects a muscle, tendon or musculotendinous junction. In sprains, some individual fibres of the spinal ligaments may be hurt, but the continuity of the ligament is maintained. Keene [19] concluded that the most commonly affected ligament in lumbar spine is the interspinous.

Strains occur by interruption of muscle fibres within the muscle belly or in the musculotendinous junction. Pain is more severe 24–48 h after injury and is associated with muscle spasm that may be localised latter to a trigger point [19]. Repeated muscle strains have asymptomatic periods between crises. Chronic strains are characterised by continued pain attributable to muscle injury. Nadler et al. [11] in their article show that athletes with lower extremity acquired ligamentous laxity or overuse and may be at risk for the development of noncontact LBP during athletic competition.

The physician must distinguish between adolescent and adult players. Younger players are characterised by unique conditions that can lead to conditions different from that in the adult athletes. In the growing period, there are anatomic and physiologic changes in the spine that represent different patterns of LBP. Hyperlordotic LBP is the second most common cause of back pain in the adolescents [20, 21]. Another juvenile characteristic is that, during growth, axial skeleton tends to develop more quickly than the surrounding fascia and muscles. This will cause pathologic stiffness and rigidity resulting in LBP. There are extrinsic kinetic forces leading to LBP like ground reactive forces, collision and fast changes in muscular dynamic. The intrinsic forces are also important because spinal mobility depends on pelvic flexibility and synchronisation of trunk muscle activation. These intrinsic biomechanical defects include iliopsoas inflexibility, abdominal weakness, thoracolumbar fascia tightness, femoral anteversion and genu recurvatum. Iliopsoas inflexibility increases lumbar lordosis and shear forces to the intervertebral disc. Understanding intrinsic defects and considering their interaction with sport-specific forces can help to anticipate possible injuries and predict rehabilitation.

These problems are studied by a throughout history and physical examination. Most of the times, the player does not remind the traumatic episode, and when the symptoms start, they are typified by lumbar muscle spasm and local tenderness provoked by bending, twisting and weight bearing, without radiculopathy. When the cause of LBP is a spasm of the lumbosacral fascia extending to the tensor fascia lata, the pain can radiate to the hips.

Physical signs may include local bruising and swelling or a spasmodic scoliosis. When the traumatic event is violent, the physician should consider underlying fractures or renal damage, particularly if haematuria is present.

In these patients with no red flags, no specific imaging is necessary. Conservative treatment with a rehabilitation program addressed to specific problems, as well as symptomatic treatment with ice or heat, depending on the timing of the injury, and occasionally deep tissue massage. It is important to improve strength of core musculature, flexibility and overall range of motion (ROM). Ninety percent of back pain resolves within 10 weeks of initial symptoms. The player who suffered low back pain or strain can return to sport when symptom-free, and full ROM is obtained. A wider investigation is needed if the symptoms persist with adequate treatment for more than 2 weeks.

23.4 Spondylolysis and Spondylolisthesis

Spondylolysis is a defect within the bone of the posterior part of the vertebral neural arch. It can develop at various locations, but the most common region affected is the isthmus of the bone between the cephalad and caudal articular processes – pars interarticularis. It is most frequently affected at L healing and bone union. A positive CT scan L5 (85–95% of cases) and L4 (5–15%). Forty percent of athletes with back pain lasting for more than 3 months have defects of the pars interarticularis in the lumbar spine. Though there may be many contributing factors: hyperlordosis, pre-existing dysplasia, iliopsoas inflexibility, thoracolumbar fascial tightness and abdominal weakness, the aetiology of isthmicspondylolysis is not well known. It is thought to be a stress fracture caused by repetitive loading or bony impingement of the pars of L5 sheared by inferior articular process of L4 and superior articular process of S1. The injury can occur without a precipitating trauma, but the trauma event can be present. The lesion can lead to the development of an anterolisthesis, which is the anterior slippage of a vertebral body on the one just below.

Most of the cases remain asymptomatic and may not be diagnosed until adulthood. Twenty-five percent of the symptomatic cases are linked with spondylolisthesis. The prevalence of spondylolysis in the adolescent athletes is estimated to be near 23%, but this figure has abundant variability in the literature. Sports requiring hyperextension movements of low back have proven to be a risk factor for the development of spondylolysis [22, 23].

The natural history has been an issue of controversy in the literature, but we know that a bilateral pars defect will develop symptomatic progression only in a few cases. Unilateral pars defects are not connected spondylolisthesis or incapacity [24].

23.4.1 Clinical Presentation

Most cases are asymptomatic. About one quarter of symptomatic cases are associated with spondylolisthesis. There are three classic patients at presentation: female, hyperlordotic and hypermobile; male, hypomobile/inflexible with tight paraspinal musculature; or someone new to a sport, deconditioned with poor core [24–26].

Low back pain is the main symptom. If the pain radiates, it does so to the buttocks or the back of the thigh and is more commonly from hamstring tightness than from radiculopathy. Pain is aggravated by extension of the lumbar spine, which is often triggered during examination (add side bending to affected side – Kemp test). The Stork test has low specificity and low sensitivity [27–29].

Inspection can demonstrate exaggerated lumbar lordosis from increased sacral inclination without a slip or from a spondylolisthetic deformity. With higher-grade spondylolisthesis, the buttocks can appear heart shaped, and a midline step-off between the spinous processes can be palpated. Point tenderness on palpation of the affected spinous process can be present in cases of spondylolysis alone. Straight-leg raising can demonstrate hamstring tightness, and generally it does not reproduce radicular pain. Neurologic examination usually reveals normal findings.

23.4.2 Imaging

Imaging of an athlete with suspected spondylolysis begins with a series of plain radiographs. Anteroposterior, lateral and both right and left oblique views must be obtained. Twenty percent of the defects are unilateral and will be missed without both oblique radiographs. Eighty-five percent of the defects are appreciable on the oblique view. But radiographs can miss occult and early stress lesions [30].

When plain radiographs of a patient with persistent symptoms reveal negative findings, a bone scan, CT scan or a magnetic resonance imaging scan can be made. We still don't have a consensus on imaging, radiation exposure in the adolescent and growing technology helping magnetic resonance imaging to potentially become a more sensitive option.

Single-photon emission computed tomography (SPECT) has high sensitivity and can localise the lesion, make early diagnosis of active lesions, differentiate between acute and chronic non-union and make correlation between pain and aetiology. The cons are poor specificity, radiation exposure (even so less than the computed tomography scan) and intravenous injection and can't detect alone a chronic non-union.

CT scan is the most sensitive and specific independent imaging modality to determine a complete or incomplete pars fracture. It can help stage the chronicity of the lesion (wide/sclerotic – chronic; narrow/non-corticated margins – acute). It can evaluate bone healing and surgical planning. The disadvantage is radiation exposure.

MRI scan is reliable for early stress lesions, for acute and complete lesions and for chronic ones. It has the advantage of the absence of radiation and the visualisation of other possible causes of low back pain. It has lower sensitivity for incomplete fractures. The existence of a high-signal change in the adjacent pedicle, on a T2-weighted MRI scan, is found to be a good predictor of bony union [31].

Negative CT scan and positive SPECT show a stress response pre-lysis with good prognosis for healing and bone union. A positive CT scan and a negative SPECT show a non-union of a chronic lesion [31] (Fig. 23.1).

23.4.3 Proposed Imaging Protocol

Lumbar radiographs (anteroposterior, lateral and both oblique views)

If negative: MRI for initial screen

Localised CT scan for positive spondylolysis on MRI (staging the lesion) or for symptoms prevailing with normal MRI

If all negative: SPECT

23.4.4 Conservative Management

The majority of athletes with spondylolysis or pars stress reactions respond well to non-operative treatment. Yet, the return to sport will be difficult, and, in most cases, the future performance will be affected by the underlying disease. Clinical decisions made with players presenting with spondylolysis and spondylolisthesis include apprehension for the future progression of the

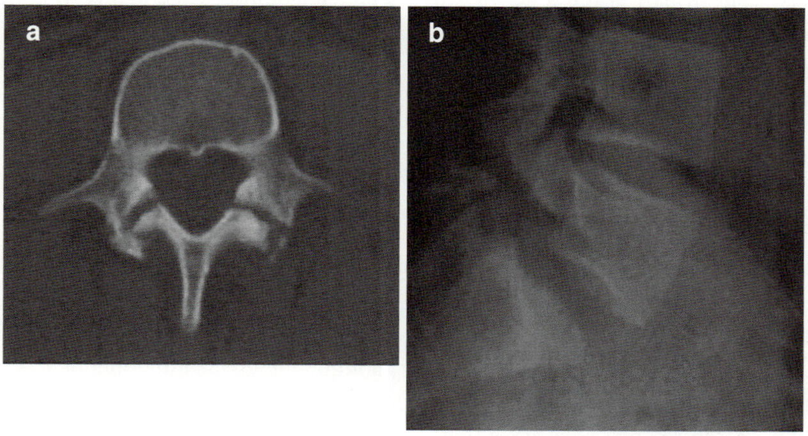

Fig. 23.1 (**a**) CT scan with bilateral spondylolysis (**b**) lateral radiographic study with L5-S1 spondylolisthesis

spondylolisthesis and issues concerning pain. In the acute setting, treatment includes rest from sport, stop repetitive extension/rotation activities and analgesic drugs. Achieve pain-free before initiating physical rehabilitation, and institute a return to play transition. Some authors advocate physical rehabilitation before pain-free.

The role and best type of external immobilisation continues to be debated. Controversy exists if the brace is to be used and the same applies to the type of brace. We still do not know unquestionably if the responsibility for the clinical improvement is the immobilisation or the forced compliance with activity restriction that works well in the pathology. Most authors defend bracing the acute lesions, but not the chronic ones. The objective is to limit hyperextension of the lumbar spine. There are many types of braces: thoraco-lumbar-sacral orthosis (TLSO) or Boston brace antilordotic, lumbar-sacral orthosis (LSO) antilordotic and corset/soft brace. The duration of immobilisation is another controversial subject. Authors defend 2–6 months brace 23 h a day. However the majority of authors have agreed that athletes can return to play when they are pain-free, regardless the time that has passed since the beginning of the symptoms or whether there is radiographic evidence of pars healing.

Bony stimulation is another option considered if the athlete has pain and no healing at 4 months treatment.

The authors defend return to sport after a short period of rest and brace, with transition when pain-free to physical rehabilitation for 1 month. Initial activities must be focused on core muscle strengthening and lower limb flexibility. Surgical excellent results mean that if pain persists after 1 month, the authors consider surgical treatment as a good option.

23.4.5 Surgical Treatment

Several operative treatments have been performed for patients who do not respond quickly to conservative treatment or who have a developing progressive spondylolisthesis.

The best techniques for surgical treatment are controversial in their use and can be separated in three categories: direct repair of spondylolysis when there is no slippage or a grade 1 slippage without disc pathology, decompression alone when there is just radiculopathy in an older patient and decompression and in situ fusion or reduction and fusion.

There are many techniques for pars repair; the authors' technique consists of iliac autograft and temporary fixation with transpedicular screws when there is a pars defect without spondylolisthesis or a pars defect with grade 1 spondylolisthesis with no disc disease. The screws are taken 1 year after the first procedure, and the results are excellent with full return to sport without physical limitations in most circumstances. When the disc is affected with spondylolysis or grade 1 spondylolisthesis, the authors use minimally invasive transforaminal interbody fusion (MIS TLIF). For grade 2 or more, the authors proceed to reduction and 360° fusion or in situ fusion without reduction (Fig. 23.2).

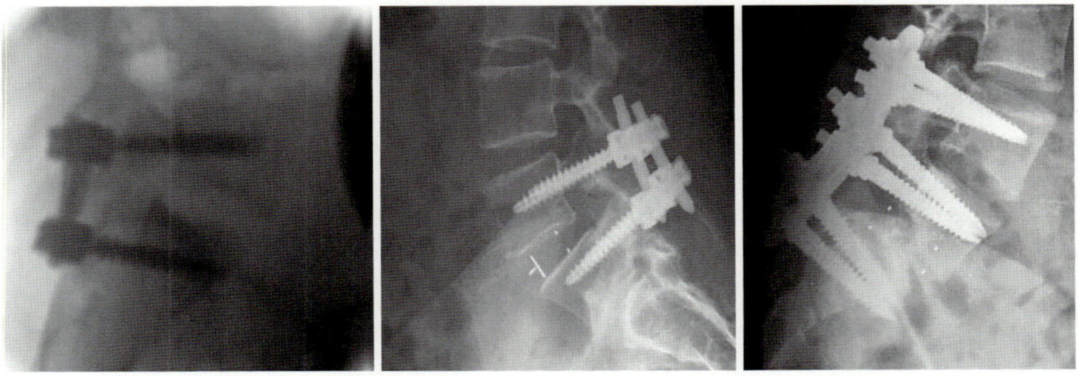

Fig. 23.2 (**a**) Iliac autograftand temporary fixation (**b**) MIS TLIF, (**c**) reduction and fixation

23.5 Lumbar Disc Disease and Lumbar Disc Herniation

The aetiology of degenerative disc disease is multifactorial, including genetic predisposition, occupational/leisure physical loading, ageing, smoking and anthropomorphic factors [32, 33]. While current research places genetic factors with the principal role, it is known that elite athletes experience greater forces on the lumbar spine over prolonged, repetitive and consisting training periods.

Intervertebral discs have an important biomechanical role within the spine, as they permit motion between the spinal segments while diffusing compressive, sliding and torsional forces [34]. The deterioration of the disc can decrease its ability to resist to extrinsic forces, as they are no longer transmitted proportionally and are strongly associated with LBP. Disc degeneration involves structural disruption as well as cell-mediated changes in composition.

Discs have a tendency to degenerate earlier than other musculoskeletal structures, with adolescents presenting signs between the ages of 11 and 16 years [35]. It is particularly susceptible in exercises with repetitive flexion, or hyperflexion, combined with lateral bending or rotation [36]. When these movements are combined with axial compression, there is a distress of the internal structure of the disc.

The posterolateral annulus fibrosus is the weakest area of the intervertebral disc and is the most susceptible area to herniation of the nucleus pulposus (HNP). HNP results from repetitive torsional forces with lumbar flexion. Acute HNP accounts for approximately 10% of back pain in adolescent athletes.

Participation in sports appears to be a risk factor for the development of disc degeneration. Disc degeneration appears to be influenced by the type and intensity of the sport. Football players showed disc degeneration almost exclusively in L4 to S1 levels [37].

23.5.1 Clinical Presentation

Axial discogenic pain is difficult to diagnose. The exact correlation between a degenerated disc and LBP remains vague. High rates of radiographic findings of degenerated discs in asymptomatic patients are evidence against a required relationship in the general population.

The pathogenesis of disc pain is explained only partially by the mechanical pressure of the disc protrusion. Symptoms of acute disc herniation may occur with minimal disc changes visualised by MRI. Secreted cytokines, such as phospholipase A2 and nitric oxide that stimulate inflammation at the dorsal root ganglion, have been identified. The nucleus pulposus itself may be a direct neurotoxin to the dorsal root ganglion.

Herniated discs in adolescent athlete tend to be more centrally located, with a smaller volume of extruded disc than encountered in adult athletes. Patients may present with tension signs of sciatica, but many athletes will present with non-specific buttock, low back or posterior thigh pain, neurogenic scoliosis and hamstring tightness. Examination usually reveals decreased lumbar motion, a positive straight-leg raise test and possibly a decrease in reflexes or strength.

Cauda equine syndrome is an infrequent but significant clinical entity in patients with back pain. Although it typically presents in more acute fashion with the characteristic findings of saddle paraesthesia, bowel or bladder incontinence or retention, and occasional radiculopathy at the lower lumbar levels, back pain also can be one of the findings. Cauda equine syndrome is a surgical emergency.

Disc herniation regularly is managed successfully with a multidisciplinary approach. Physical therapy is initiated with an extension-based stabilisation programme when the patient is able to support it. Therapy includes a trunk and pelvic flexibility and isometric strengthening programme. The pain management service assists with medication, such as the tricyclic antidepressants, neuroleptic agents and epidural corticosteroids. Surgical management is necessary only for cauda equine syndromes, a progressive neurologic deficit, and refractory pain.

Athletes with disc herniation may return to competition when they have attained a full range of motion, strength and sport-specific attention to technique.

23.5.2 Diagnostic Imaging

Typically, plain anteroposterior and lateral radiographs are used in the initial assessment of discogenic pain. Flexion and extension lateral radiographs can be used to show mobility across the lumbar segment or instability. The cost/utility of additional radiation has caused its clinical usefulness to be questioned [38].

Plain radiograph can show decrease in disc space height initially and osteophyte formation with disease evolution. Lundin proposed that the radiographic finding that most strongly correlated with LBP was decreased disc space height [39]. Additionally, the greater the number of levels involved, the more likely the athlete was to have had LBP. Plain radiographs may be normal in cases of lumbar disc herniation, although a lateral lumbosacral view may demonstrate a non-specific slight reduction in disc space height.

MRI is the imaging study of choice to study the disc and is highly sensitive to degenerative changes such as loss of signal intensity on T2-weighted images, annular tears, high-intensity zones and associated bone marrow vertebral endplate changes defined as Modic [40]. The clinical significance of Modic changes is controversial. Sword et al. [41] found that decreased signal intensity within the disc correlated with LBP in athletes and in nonathletes. Abnormal vertebral configuration with an increased anteroposterior diameter correlated with the occurrence of LBP. MRI is also the most sensitive test for detecting herniation and nerve root compression [42].

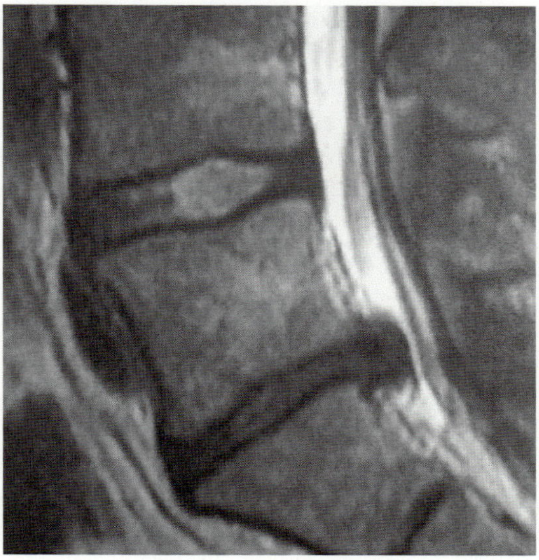

Fig. 23.3 Disc herniation with discopathy

Discography is another possible method to identify LBP of discogenic origin. The reproduction of a patient's typical LBP with discography suggests that leakage of intradiscal fluid or annular distension is involved in the production of back pain (Fig. 23.3).

23.5.3 Non-operative Treatment

Non-operative modalities are the pillars of treatment of discogenic LBP in the athlete. Several rehabilitation protocols have been suggested specifically for this condition. Cooke's five-stage protocol [43] is one of the most used and is composed of stage I early protected mobilisation, stage II dynamic spinal mobilisation, stage III spine safe strengthening and conditioning training, stage IV return to sports and stage V maintenance programme.

Each athlete has a unique clinical picture, and the recovery pattern will depend on the personalised rehabilitation programme.

Lumbar disc herniation has a rehabilitation protocol which is similar to that of discogenic back pain, and the return to sports activity happens when the athlete is free of symptoms. Ninety percent of the athletes with disc herniation improve with non-operative treatment. Therapy goals are always pain reduction and decreasing the length of symptomatic episodes.

23.5.4 Operative Treatment

Indications for operative treatment of lumbar discopathy are the source of controversial discussions in the literature. The traditional operative indications are mechanical LBP correlated with positive findings on imaging, continuous symptoms for at least 6 months despite active non-operative treatment and localised midline spinal tenderness that corresponds to the radiographic level of the disease [8]. Surgical treatment is either total disc replacement or lumbar fusion. The authors do not recommend surgical treatment for disc disease without herniation. Surgical treatment of disc disease has inconstant clinical outcomes in the literature for the general population. In high-level athletes, there are few reports concerning operative treatment for discopathy. The authors do not support surgical treatment in discogenic back pain.

Disc herniation indications for surgery are more consensual than the ones for discopathy alone. Progressive neurological deficit and radicular pain that does not respond to conservative treatment are the two main indications, and the results in athletes are excellent in terms of return to play and elimination of radiculopathy.

23.6 Another Causes of Vertebral Pain

23.6.1 Vertebral Growth and Stress Fractures

Adolescent spine is susceptible to injury because of the areas of growth cartilage and undeveloped ossification centres. In the junction between the vertebral body and the apophysis in the outer annulus fibrosus, there is a fragile link of force transfer which can lead to vertebral endplate fractures. The symptoms, when the avulsed fragment invades the spinal canal, are similar to the central herniated disc.

Stress fractures result from repeated submaximal loads causing fatigue of the bone structures. These fractures happen when the stress implicated in the bone is greater than the capacity of the bone to heal. Bone turnover depends on genetic, hormonal, mechanical and nutritional factors. The repetitive microdamage and the incapacity to keep appropriate skeletal repair (fatigue reaction or fracture) are characteristics of stress fractures in the athlete.

Specifically in football players, stress fractures occur almost always in lower extremities, with the majority occurring in the fifth metatarsal. Nevertheless, stress fractures of the spine can happen and lead to an inconclusive diagnostic. Stress fractures of the sacrum are an infrequent cause of LBP in athletes. Their prevalence is unknown. Such fractures are more common in female athletes, but they have been reported in male athletes as well.

Plain radiographs are usually normal, and the most common method for diagnosis of this stress fractures is bone scintigraphy, which can detect the fracture as early as few days after it occurs. MRI is not as sensitive as bone scan; however, it does enable to exclude other possible causes of pain. CT scan is another possibility with good accuracy in the literature detecting stress fractures.

Treatment should pass for a period of rest and physical rehabilitation; sometimes surgical treatment is required.

23.6.2 Bertolotti's Syndrome

Bertolotti's syndrome (BS) affects 4–8% of the population. This syndrome is characterised by the presence of a transitional vertebra, which represents an incomplete segmentation of the lower lumbar and upper sacral vertebrae. The vertebra can have a large transverse process on one side resulting in conflict with the sacrum or the ilium. This situation per se can cause lumbar pain. At the same time, there is an altered motion at the lumbosacral articulation which can cause L4-L5 disc disease with possible irritation of L5 nerve root and consequently radicular pain. The bony lumbar extension to de sacrum or ilium can form a pseudarthrosis. Players can suffer from this syndrome, which may simulate spondylolysis.

The initial treatment consists of calming the inflammation, which can be attainable with rest and an orthosis. Rehabilitation with physical therapy must be done, and sport-specific training is necessary.

23.7 Scheuermann Disease

Scheuermann disease (SD) is a form of osteochondrosis of the spine and is characterised by increased kyphosis of the thoracic spine in association with structural deformity of the vertebral elements. The disorder is sometimes painful during its relative acute phase and can cause significant truncal deformity that may be progressive.

In defining SD, the subgroup described as lumbar Scheuermann's or type II must be acknowledged and constitute the cause of some LBP in athletes. This condition, most commonly seen in athletically active adolescent males or those involved in heavy lifting, presents with localised back pain and radiographic vertebral changes at the thoracolumbar junction and is not typically associated with significant clinical kyphosis. The Schmorl's nodes and endplate irregularity may be so severe that SD can be confused with infection, tumour or other conditions.

Both classic and atypical SD are associated with back pain. Unlike classic thoracic Scheuermann's kyphosis, the treatment of lumbar SD is not controversial, as its course is nonprogressive and its symptoms resolve with rest, activity modification and time.

23.7.1 Tumours, Infections and Primary Inflammatory Conditions of the Lumbar Spine

These conditions are rare in the athlete, but should be suspected when patients manifest unusual symptoms such as nonmechanical pain, night pain or constitutional symptoms (loss of weight, poor appetite or cachexia). A thorough history will often lead the physician to the diagnosis of these more uncommon conditions. The identification of the condition is generally difficult and requires a high level of suspicion. For this reason, a significant delay often occurs between the first symptoms and diagnosis.

The most expected benign spine tumours in children and adolescent players include osteoid osteoma, osteoblastoma and aneurysmal bone cysts. Malignant neoplasms include osteosarcoma and Ewing's sarcoma. Malignant metastatic lesions are more common in adults as opposed to primary spine tumours. Leukaemia and lymphoma can occur in both adolescent and adult athletes.

Discitis is a diagnosis more common in the paediatric athlete than the adult one. Adult athletes are susceptible to vertebral osteomyelitis and soft tissue abscesses.

Spondyloarthropathies typically begin in adolescence and affect the spine, hips, knees and feet. Recent data in the rheumatologic literature allow earlier identification of these patients. Effective medication can alter the disease progression, making prompt diagnosis important. All patients should be asked four questions [44, 45]: (1) Does the morning back stiffness last over 30 min? (2) Does the back pain awaken the patient during the second period of sleep? (3) Does the pain alternate from one buttock to the other? (4) Does rest relieve the pain? If two out of these four questions are positive, there is a 70% sensitivity and 81% specificity for inflammatory back pain [44]. History is much more accurate than laboratory testing in diagnosing these patients. C-reactive protein has only 53% sensitivity and 70% specificity in spondyloarthropathies. HLA-B27 is not generally helpful because it has high positivity in the general population [46].

Workup for all of these conditions involves imaging scans and laboratory data and a multidisciplinary approach.

23.8 Non-orthopaedic Causes of Low Back Pain

The clinician must be aware of pain referred to the low back from other areas of the body such as the hip, the pelvis or the viscera. Renal disorders, bowel pathology or reproductive organ disease may present as LBP. The possibility of these disorders should be kept in mind in the patient whose diagnosis remains elusive. Referral to other specialists may be necessary if these conditions are suspected.

Conclusion

LBP in the football player is a common condition with multiple possible aetiologies. The prevalence is unknown because most athletes don't report the complaint in order to keep on playing. The management of LBP depends ultimately of the clinical history and physical examination, with special attention to the presence of red or yellow flags. Non-specific soft tissue injuries constitute the majority of the LBP and respond well to conservative treatment. Other common cause of LBP in football players is spondylolysis/spondylolisthesis, which can be treated with conservative methods for a short period with transition to surgical treatment if pain persists. The repair of the defect and provisional fixation showed excellent results in athletes. Discogenic pain is another common cause of LBP and is treated with conservative rehabilitation protocol. Symptomatic disc herniation is treated in most cases with conservative methods, but the surgical treatment is an option. Other causes of LBP are less common, but the physician must have a high suspicion in the presence of unusual symptoms.

References

1. Frymoyer JW, Pope MH, Clements FH, et al. Risk factors in low back pain: an epidemiologic survey. J Bone Joint Surg Am. 1983;65:213–8.
2. Frymoyer JW, Cats-Baril WL. An overview of the incidences and costs of low back pain. Orthop Clin North Am. 1991;22:263–71.
3. Svensson HO, Anderson JB, Johanson S. A retrospective study of low-back pain in 38- to 64- year old women: frequency of occurrence and impact on medical services. Spine. 1988;13:548–52.
4. Volkenberg HA, Haanen HCM. The epidemiology of low back pain. In: White III AA, Gordon SL, editors. Symposium on Idiopathic LBP. St Louis: CV Mosby; 1982. p. 9.
5. Biering-Sorensen F. Physical measurements as risk indicators for low-back trouble over a one-year period. Spine. 1984;9:106–19.
6. Harber P, Pena L, Hsu P, Billet E, Greer D, Kim K. Personal history, training, and worksite as predictors of back pain of nurses. Am J Ind Med. 1994;25:519–26.
7. Harraby MRI, Neergard K, Hesselsoe G, Kjer J. Are radiologic changes in the thoracic and lumbar spine of adolescents risk factors for low back pain in adults? A 25- year prospective cohort study of 640 schoolchildren. Spine. 1995;20:2298–302.
8. Bono CM. Current concepts review: low back pain in athletes. J Bone Joint Surg Am. 2004;86:392–6.
9. Tall RL, DeVault W. Spinal injury in sport: epidemiologic considerations. Clin Sports Med. 1993;12:441–7.
10. Bernstein RM, Cozen H. Evaluation of back pain in children and adolescents. Am Fam Physician. 2007;76:1669–76.
11. Nadler SF, Wu KD, Galski T, Feinberg JH. Low back pain in college athletes. A prospective study correlating lower extremity overuse or acquired ligamentous laxity with low back pain. Spine. 1998;23:828–33.
12. Jacob T, Baras M, Zeev A, Epstein L. Physical activities and low back pain: a community based study. Med Sci Sports Exerc. 2004;36:9–15.
13. Walden M, Hagglund M, Ekstrand J. UEFA Champions League study: a prospective study of injuries in professional football during the 2001–2002 season. Br J Sports Med. 2005;39:542–6.
14. Hollenberg GM, Beitia AO, Tan RK, Weinberg EP, Adams MJ. Imaging of the spine in sports medicine. Curr Sports Med Rep. 2003;2:33–40.
15. McGill SM. Kinetic potential of the lumbar trunk musculature about three orthogonal orthopaedic axes in extreme postures. Spine. 1991;16:809–15.
16. Koes BW, van Tulder MW, Ostelo R, Kim Burton A, Waddell G. Clinical guidelines for the management of low back pain in primary care: an international comparison. Spine. 2001;26:2504–13.
17. Arnau JM, Vallano A, Lopez A, Pellise F, Delgado MJ, Prat N. A critical review of guidelines for low back pain treatment. Eur Spine J. 2006;15:543–53.

18. Baranto A, Andersen TI, Sward L. Preventing low back pain. In: Bahr R, Engebretsen L, editors. Sports injury prevention. Chapter 8. Blackwell Publishing; 2009.
19. Keene JS, Drummond DS. Mechanical back pain in the athlete. Compr Ther. 1985;11:7–14.
20. d'Hemecourt PA, Gerbino II PG, Micheli LJ. Back injuries in the young athlete. Clin Sports Med. 2000;19:663–79.
21. Micheli LJ, Wood R. Back pain in young athletes: significant differences from adults in causes and patterns. Arch Pediatr Adolesc Med. 1995;149:15–8.
22. Kraft DE. Low back pain in the adolescent athlete. Pediatr Clin North Am. 2002;49:643–53.
23. Sassmannshausen G, Smith BG. Back pain in the young athlete. Clin Sports Med. 2002;21:121–32.
24. Beutler WJ, Fredrickson BE, Murtland A, Sweeney CA, Grant WD, Baker D. The natural history of spondylolysis and spondylolisthesis. 45-year follow-up evaluation. Spine. 2003;28:1027–35.
25. McCleary MD, Congeni JA. Current concepts in the diagnosis and treatment of spondylolysis in young athletes. Curr Sports Med Rep. 2007;6:62–6.
26. Congeni J. Evaluating spondylolysis in adolescent athletes. J Musculoskelet Med. 2000;17:123–9.
27. Kobayashi A et al. Diagnosis of radiographically occult lumbar spondylolysis in young athletes by magnetic resonance imaging. Am J Sports Med. 2013;41:169–76.
28. Masci L et al. Use of the one-legged hyperextension test and magnetic resonance imaging in the diagnosis of active spondylolysis. Br J Sports Med. 2006;40:940–6.
29. Sundell C-G et al. Clinical examination, spondylolysis and adolescent athletes. Int J Sports Med. 2013;34:263–7.
30. Leone A et al. Lumbar spondylolysis: a review. Skeletal Radiol. 2011;40:683–700.
31. Hollenberg GM et al. Stress reactions of the lumbar pars interarticularis: the development of a new MRI classification system. Spine. 2002;27:181–6.
32. Patel AA, Spiker WR, Daubs M, Brodke D, Cannon-Albright LA. Evidence for an inherited predisposition to lumbar disc disease. J Bone Joint Surg Am. 2011;93:225–9.
33. Hangai M, Kaneoka K, Hinotsu S, Shimizu K, Okubo Y, Miyakawa S, et al. Lumbar intervertebral disk degeneration in athletes. Am J Sports Med. 2009;37:149–55.
34. Leone A, Guglielmi G, Cassar-Pullicino VN, Bonomo L. Lumbar intervertebral instability: a review. Radiology. 2007;245(1):62–77.
35. Boos N, Weissbach S, Rohrbach H, Weiler C, Spratt KF, Nerlich AG. Classification of age-related changes in lumbar intervertebral discs: 2002 Volvo Award in basic science. Spine. 2002;27:2631–44.
36. Smeal WL, Tyburski M, Alleva J, Prather H, Hunt D. Conservative management of low back pain, part I. Discogenic/radicular pain. Dis Mon. 2004;50:636–69.
37. Videman T, Sarna S, Battie MC, Koskinen S, Gill K, Paananen H, Gibbons L. The long-term effects of physical loading and exercise lifestyles on back-related symptoms, disability, and spinal pathology among men. Spine. 1995;20:699–709.
38. Hammouri QM, Haims AH, Simpson AK, Alqaqa A, Grauer JN. The utility of dynamic flexion-extension radiographs in the initial evaluation of the degenerative lumbar spine. Spine. 2007;32:2361–4.
39. Lundin O, Hellstrom M, Nilsson I, Sward L. Back pain and radiological changes in the thoraco-lumbar spine of athletes. A long-term follow-up. Scand J Med Sci Sports. 2001;11:103–9.
40. Modic MT, Steinberg PM, Ross JS, Masaryk TJ, Carter JR. Degenerative disk disease: assessment of changes in vertebral body marrow with MR imaging. Radiology. 1988;166(1Pt1):193–9.
41. Sward L, Hellstrom M, Jacobsson B, Nyman R, Peterson L. Disc degeneration and associated abnormalities of the spine in elite gymnasts. A magnetic resonance imaging study. Spine. 1991;16:437–43.
42. Lively MW, Bailes Jr JE. Acute lumbar disk injuries in active patients: making optimal management decisions. Phys Sportsmed. 2005;33:21–7.
43. Cooke PM, Lutz GE. Internal disc disruption and axial back pain in the athlete. Phys Med Rehabil Clin N Am. 2000;11:837–65.
44. Braun J, Inman R. Clinical significant of inflammatory back pain for diagnosis and screening of patients with axial spondyloarthritis. Ann Rheum Dis. 2010;69:1264–8.
45. Yu DT. Diagnosis and differential diagnosis of ankylosing spondylitis in adults. http://www.uptodate.com/index. Published 15 June 2009.
46. Braun J, Bollow M, Remlinger G, et al. Prevalence of spondyloarthropathies in HLA-B27 positive and negative blood donors. Arthritis Rheum. 1998;41:58–67.

Brain Concussion in Football

24

Basil Ribeiro and Bruno Carvalho

Contents

B. Ribeiro (✉)
Sports Medicine, Rio Ave FC, Performance and Health Unit of the Portuguese Federation of Football, Vila Nova de Gaia, Portugal
e-mail: basil@sapo.pt

B. Carvalho
Neurosurgery Department, Centro Hospitalar S. João, Porto, Portugal

Key Messages

- Know the risk factors for sport-related concussion
- Use standardized assessment tools (SCAT3) and know "red flag" symptoms (ACSM)
- Remove the athlete from play
- Return to play is prohibited until the player is asymptomatic and off of medication
- Follow a graduated return to play protocol (no activity, light aerobic exercise, sport-specific exercise, noncontact training drills, full contact practice, return to play) (4th ICCS)
- Primary prevention (rules, equipment, athletes, coaches) and secondary prevention (appropriate return to play management) measures are essential to reduce the incidence and morbidity of brain concussion
- Second impact syndrome must be avoided at all cost since it is a potential fatal event

J. Espregueira-Mendes et al. (eds.), *Injuries and Health Problems in Football*,
DOI 10.1007/978-3-662-53924-8_24

24.1 Introduction

The name is football, but a lot of actions are done with the head. Concussion in sports, and in football in particular, is a serious and very frequent traumatic event. According to FIFA, 13% of all injuries sustained at FIFA World Cups™ involve the head and neck. Almost one in seven of those injuries resulted in concussion [1]. In a German study, published in 2011, 108 (23.9%) injuries were related to the head [2]. It is gaining increased awareness in sports and media, but also in schools. Although it is self-limited, it has a significant impact on sports participation and on adolescent's participation in school and social activities. It can result from a direct or indirect blow to the head or neck, where shear forces are applied to the brain. Immediately a neurometabolic cascade of events develops, leading to cellular energy crisis in the brain. The injured brain is now vulnerable to additional injury during the recovery phase that can last from some hours to several days. During this period another trauma to the head can deadly result in the second impact syndrome. The brain concussion is characterized by several symptoms, the most frequent is headache, and neurocognitive deficits can be identified as well. Since it is a functional injury, the magnetic ressonance imaging (MRI) and the computed tomography (CT) scan are normal, but some new technology can help on the diagnosis. The return to school or to sports is an issue that deserves a lot of attention, a very careful evaluation should be performed, and only the symptom-free player or student, and without any neurocognitive deficits, is allowed to return to the previous level of activity. There are tools that can help either in the diagnosis or in the decision to return to game. However, there should be a continuous vigilance/monitoring of the athlete or of the student during this returning period [3–8].

24.2 Definition

There are several definitions of brain concussion or mild traumatic brain injury (MTBI) for some authors [9, 10]. Others consider concussion as a subset of MTBI [5, 7], including those that participated on the 4th International Conference on Concussion in Sport held in Zurich, November 2012 [11]. The Centers for Disease Control and Prevention (CDC) defines a concussion as "a complex pathophysiologic process affecting the brain, induced by traumatic biomechanical forces secondary to direct or indirect forces to the head" [9]. It is a disturbance in brain function caused by a direct or indirect force to the head that results in a variety of nonspecific signs and/or symptoms, most of the times without loss of consciousness [12, 13]. Also, it can be defined as an immediate, short-lived transient disturbance in brain function, rather than a structural injury, and is the less severe of the traumatic brain injuries [5], followed by physical, cognitive, emotional symptoms and sleep disturbance [7]. It is caused by direct or indirect force to the head or to the neck [7, 10], resulting from a shear stress to brain [4, 10]. It is a shake of the brain inside the skull [7, 10]. The disturbance of brain function is associated with normal head CT and MRI findings, because there is no structural damage to the brain tissue or blood vessels [9], but some neurons can be damaged with consequences on the synaptic transmission of information inside the brain [10].

The adolescent age group is more vulnerable to brain injuries of all severity levels than adults. Traumatic injury to the developing brain may lead to long-lasting changes in cognitive potential, perhaps even with little evidence of an initial deficit [14]. A study has investigated the relationship between age at injury [before age 7 ($n = 16$) or after age 7 ($n = 20$)] and recovery following pediatric head injury. Children were evaluated at 4 months and 2 years post-head injury. Results revealed that children who sustained head injury prior to 7 years of age performed poorly than did those injured at or after age 7 and that recovery profiles following head injury were associated with age at injury. However, children injured later in childhood showed recovery consistent with that described in adult head injury [15], and there is still a protracted recovery from concussion in high school athletes [16].

24.3 Incidence

Concussions occur in all sports with the highest incidence in american football, hockey, rugby, football, and basketball [5]. It is estimated that as many as 3.8 million concussions occur in the USA per year during competitive sports and recreational activities, but 50% of the concussions are not reported [5]. The number of head injuries is probably underestimated due to the fact that the player is afraid of being prevented from returning to play [2].

It is a huge public problem, since in the USA approximately 1.6–3 million concussions occur annually [10]. On a recent paper, it is referred that more than 300,000 sports-related concussions occur every year in all sports at all levels of competition [6]. In the USA, the incidence rates for college athletes range from 5 to 7.9%, and approximately 8.9% of all high school athletic injuries are concussions [10]. Concussions result in more than 100,000 emergency department (ED) visits for children and adolescents each year [7]. A critical literature review of sport concussion by gender revealed that, after evaluating multiple years of concussion data in comparable sports, female athletes may be at greater risk for concussion than their male counterparts [2, 17]. Although younger athletes often have a greater incidence of concussion with longer recovery time frames [2, 18], children are not frequently diagnosed with concussions because rarely is anyone on hand to diagnose the injury and young players seldom report symptoms [19]. A prospective 11-year study evaluated the incidence and relative risk of concussion in 12 high school boys' and girls' sports between academic years 1997–1998 and 2007–2008 [20]. There were 2651 concussions in 10 926 892 athlete exposures, with an incidence rate of 0.24 per 1000, with boys' sports accounted for 53% of athlete exposures and 75% of all concussions. Football accounted for more than half of all concussions, with the highest incidence rate (0.60). Girls' football had the most concussions among the girls' sports and the second-highest incidence rate of all 12 sports (0.35), and they also roughly had twice the concussion risk of boys. The authors concluded that the concussion rate increased over time in all 12 sports and that it might be due to actual increased occurrence or greater coding sensitivity with widely disseminated guidance on concussion detection and treatment [20]. The condition might still be underdiagnosed because young athletes do not have the cognitive capacity to recognize their symptoms as being connected to trauma and also they do not realize they should inform an adult [19].

24.4 Pathophysiology

Direct overt impact on the head is not always necessary to cause a brain concussion. Trauma to the brain can result from a rapid acceleration or deceleration, with change in the head's velocity, and this can cause detrimental effects in the brain tissue [13, 21]. Acceleration and deceleration forces shake the brain inside the skull, setting off a cascade of neurometabolic changes occurring right after the head trauma, causing functional changes [6, 22, 23]. There is a neurological "software" problem rather than a "hardware" problem [7], although some microscopic changes do occur [21]. The forces applied to the brain generate a chemical cascade in the brain, where ionic imbalances, energy depletion, synaptic dysfunction, and neuronal injury/loss develop [14, 23]. Cell ion channel dysfunction, increased extracellular potassium and glutamate, activation of N-methyl-D-aspartate receptors, neuron depolarization, glial activation, altered brain glucose metabolism, and release of excitatory amino acids are involved [6, 7]. Furthermore, there is release of glutamate, efflux of potassium, and influx of calcium, leading to an increase of energy consumption in order to restore homeostasis. The temporary less efficient anabolic metabolism consumes more glucose, which will be depleted (and more is needed), but the delivery is compromised by the decrease in cerebral blood flow [3, 7]. If physical or cognitive activity becomes excessive, the cycle of inadequate metabolism and energy is perpetuated, and symptoms worsen [7]. The calcium itself jeopardizes the energetic metabolism at the mitochondrial level, and it facilitates the cell death as well [3, 14]. Although the increase in the calcium level lasts for 2 days, the energy production problem can last for 10 days [3]. Also, intra-axonal calcium flux has been shown to disrupt neurofilaments and microtubules, impairing posttraumatic neural connectivity [14]. Intracellular magnesium levels are also reduced after concussion and remain low for up to 4 days, and decreased magnesium levels may lead to neuronal dysfunction via multiple mechanisms [14]. In summary, there are several metabolic, hemodynamic, structural, and electric changes that alter normal cerebral function [23].

24.5 Risk Factors

The type of sport itself may be a risk factor. Football is also played with the head, and almost 2% of the injuries sustained at FIFA World Cups™ resulted in concussion [1]. Contact and collision sports are those where contusions occur most often. Also, the rules of the game and the protective equipment have also a role to play (see Prevention). Under the suggestion of the medical committee, FIFA changed the rules and now hardly penalizes the elbow contusions on the opponent player.

Risk factors for sport-related concussion [5]:

- A history of concussion is associated with a higher risk of sustaining another concussion, particularly within 10 days after initial concussion [24]
- A greater number, severity, and duration of symptoms after a concussion are predictors of a prolonged recovery
- In sports with similar playing rules, the reported incidence of concussion is higher in female athletes than in male athletes
- Certain sports, positions, and individual playing styles have a greater risk of concussion
- Youth athletes may have a more prolonged recovery and are more susceptible to a concussion accompanied by a catastrophic injury
- Pre-injury mood disorders, learning disorders, attention-deficit disorders (ADD/ADHD), and migraine headaches complicate diagnosis and management of a concussion

24.6 Diagnosis/Sideline Evaluation

It is definitely the most difficult medical evaluation on the injured athlete during a sports event due to the lack of specificity and paucity of signs and symptoms. Besides, that particular sports environment might create more pressure during those very few minutes of examination, with several thousands of spectators around, with national or international broadcast and the coach steering at the doctor waiting for information. On top of this, there is a conscious player "feeling good" that wants to go back to the game without being aware of his brain dysfunction. It is very difficult to make a timely diagnosis [25]. Robert Cantu states that it is easy to recognize a head trauma if the athlete loses conscience, but it is far more difficult when that does not happen and only a transitory change of the alertness exists. In more than 90% of the cases, there is no loss of conscience, and only a short period of posttraumatic amnesia or loss of the normal state of alertness exists [26].

The sideline evaluation should be based on recognition of injury and assessment of symptoms, cognitive and cranial nerve function, and balance. Some signs and symptoms may be delayed, and it is advised to keep the athlete out of participation when there is any suspicion of injury [25]. However, the sideline assessment of concussion in the athlete is very difficult to perform, due to the sensitivity and specificity of the sideline assessment tools [25]. For some people, especially nonmedical persons (parents, coaches, teachers), the diagnosis might not be so obvious, and if there is any doubt after a head trauma, the athlete must be removed from the training or game [10, 13].

It is fundamental to be aware of the mechanism of the injury, and a temporal relationship must be established [4]. Was there a fall over his/her head? Or a trauma from the opponent's elbow, head, or stick? Did he hit the goal or the wall of the gym? Then, it is important to see if the athlete stays on ground or soon after he got up, although this is not very important for the diagnosis.

A trauma to the head must be considered an emergent medical situation, where brain concussion might be present. The ABC (airway, breathing, circulation) of the basic life support must be started without delay. The signs and symptoms are nonspecific, the athlete may present a wide variety of symptoms, the headache is the most common [10], and they can last from minutes to months and even longer in a small number of cases [9]. Also very often reported are dizziness, confusion, and disorientation [10]. In less than 10% [10] to 20% of the cases, there is loss of conscience [9], and 95% of concussed athletes wake up in seconds or minutes [19], which means the doctor, rarely, finds an athlete unconscious when he reaches the injured player. Other somatic and cognitive symptoms/signs are present [4]. Also, a trauma to the head might cause injury to the brain and to the cervical spine, and the initial evaluation should also include the examination of the neck in order to exclude any spine injury [4]. Palpation of the spinous process of the cervical spine must be performed, and, at the same time, paresthesia symptoms in the extremities must be ruled out. However, caution with the mobilization of the neck must not be forgotten until a spinal injury has been excluded [10].

According to SCAT3 [12], concussion should be suspected in the presence of:

- Symptoms (e.g., headache)
- Physical signs (e.g., unsteadiness)
- Impaired brain function (e.g., confusion)
- Abnormal behavior (e.g., change in personality)

The American College of Sports Medicine (ACSM) describes the "red flag" symptoms after brain trauma that needs emergency care [13]:

- Increasing confusion or headaches
- Vomiting, double vision, or unequal pupils
- Irritability or behavior change
- Drowsiness or fading in and out of consciousness

Again, the ACSM divides the symptoms in four categories [13]:

- Physical symptoms – headaches, nausea, dizziness, vision or balance problems, sensitivity to light or noise
- Cognitive symptoms – feeling mentally slow or foggy, trouble concentrating, trouble remembering
- Emotional symptoms – irritability, sadness, nervousness, feeling more emotional than usual
- Sleep-related symptoms – sleeping more or less than usual, drowsiness, trouble falling asleep

By personal experience during 2 years with several cases of brain concussion in a first Portuguese football league revealed that the symptoms/signs found on the pitch right after the head trauma were:

- Headache
- Confusion, disorientation, fogginess
- Unsteadiness
- Vision disturbance – black spot (one player)

No cases of loss of consciousness, vomiting, or other usually described signs/symptoms were reported. In some cases the symptoms were very subtle, and the personal awareness for this situation might have helped to recognize the brain concussion.

A systematic review of 5437 abstracts and 1362 full-text publications, where only twenty-six studies met all criteria required to be used in the analysis, revealed that the prevalent and consistent indicators of concussion were the following [27]:

- Observed and documented disorientation or confusion immediately after the event
- Impaired balance within 1 day after injury
- Slower reaction time within 2 days after injury
- Impaired verbal learning and memory within 2 days after injury

There is a battery of tests to check any disturbance, such as neuropsychological tests and postural stability tests [4, 5, 28], but concussion is still a clinical diagnosis [5, 17]. CT and MRI are usually normal, but the functional MRI (fMRI) or the diffusion tensor imaging (DTI) may help in the diagnosis of sports-related concussion. These tools are only used in research studies and are not available in the clinical setting [6, 9, 13, 21]. At the microscopic level, the examination of brain tissue from primates exposed to concussion revealed axonal shear strain on autopsy. Shear strain injury is observed as the tearing or stretching of axons, but is totally useless in the clinical setting [21].

A subcommittee of the American Academy of Neurology graded symptom checklists, and the Standardized Assessment of Concussion, neuropsychological assessments, and the Balance Error Scoring System are the tools to investigate the concussion [24], but the capacity of neuropsychological tests to detect deficits suggestive of concussion is of doubt [27]. The magnetic resonance spectroscopy and diffusion tensor imaging prove to be effective clinical tools for both prognostic and treatment parameters [23].

In order to help the medical evaluation and the decision making, a group of medical experts gather together in Zurich (November 2012) and produced a very useful tool to deal with the brain concussion.

24.6.1 SCAT3

The SCAT3 [12] is a standardized tool to be used by medical professionals in the evaluation of injured athletes with brain concussion. It is applied to athletes older than (and including) 13 years old. For ages 12 and under, there is the Child SCAT3. For nonmedical professionals the Concussion Recognition Tool should be used. The testing performed on the beginning of the season gives baseline values to be compared with post-injury test scores. The authors advise that the SCAT3 should not be used solely to make or to exclude the diagnosis of concussion in the absence of clinical evaluation and an athlete with a normal SCAT3 can have a brain concussion. Instructions to conduct the questions and the tests are included.

It is stated in SCAT3 that "if any of the following signs are observed after a direct or indirect blow to the head, the athlete should stop participation, be evaluated by a medical professional and should not be permitted to return to sport the same day if a concussion is suspected:

- Any loss of consciousness
- Balance or motor incoordination (stumbles, slow / labored movements, etc.)
- Disorientation or confusion (inability to respond appropriately to questions)
- Loss of memory
- Blank or vacant look
- Visible facial injury in combination with any of the above"

And, "any athlete with a suspected concussion should be:

- removed from play
- medically assessed
- monitored for deterioration (i.e., should not be left alone) and
- should not drive a motor vehicle until cleared to do so by a medical professional

No athlete diagnosed with concussion should be returned to sports participation on the day of injury."

Similar considerations were proposed by the American Medical Society for Sports Medicine Position Statement about the concussion in sport [5]:

- "Any athlete suspected of having a concussion should be stopped from playing and assessed by a licensed healthcare provider trained in the evaluation and management of concussions
- Recognition and initial assessment of a concussion should be guided by a symptoms checklist, cognitive evaluation (including orientation, past and immediate memory, new learning and concentration), balance tests and further neurological physical examination
- Balance disturbance is a specific indicator of a concussion, but not very sensitive
- Imaging is reserved for athletes where intracerebral bleeding is suspected
- There is no same day RTP (Return-To-Play) for an athlete diagnosed with a concussion
- Athletes suspected or diagnosed with a concussion should be monitored for deteriorating physical or mental status"

Table 24.1 Glasgow Coma Scale (best eye, verbal and motor response)

Best eye response (e)	
No eye opening	1
Eye opening in response to pain	2
Eye opening to speech	3
Eyes opening spontaneously	4
Best verbal response (v)	
No verbal response	1
Incomprehensible sounds	2
Inappropriate words	3
Confused	4
Oriented	5
Best motor response (m)	
No motor response	1
Extension to pain	2
Abnormal flexion to pain	3
Flexion/withdrawal to pain	4
Localizes to pain	5
Obeys commands	6
Glasgow Coma Score (e + v + m)	*15*

The SCAT3 also includes the evaluation of the Glasgow Coma Scale (best eye, verbal and motor response) that should be recorded for all athletes with subsequent deterioration [12] (Table 24.1).

The Maddocks score results from the answers of five questions, and it helps only on the sideline diagnosis of concussion. The best response of the player is recorded, and the correct answer receives one point (maximum 5 points). The questions are:

- What venue are we at today?
- Which half is it now?
- Who scored last in this match?
- What team did you play last week/game?
- Did your team win the last game?

The SCAT3 also includes instructions for the follow-up and serial testing, and that includes:

- Questions about the background
- Symptom evaluation, with 22 questions, rated from zero to six according the intensity (none, mild, moderate, severe)
- Cognitive and physical evaluation (Standardized Assessment of Concussion – SAC)
  - Orientation
  - Immediate memory
  - Concentration (digits backward and month in reverse order)
- Neck examination
- Balance examination
- Coordination examination
- SAC delayed recall

On the last page of the SCAT3 document, a special alert is included about signs or problems that can arise during the coming hours or days, in which case the player has to contact a doctor or go to a hospital:

- Have a headache that gets worse
- Drowsy or can't be awakened
- Can't recognize people or places
- Have repeated vomiting
- Behave unusually or seem confused
- Is very irritable
- Have seizures
- Have weak or numb arms or legs
- Are unsteady on their feet
- Have slurred speech

24.7 Treatment

According to the American Medical Society for Sports Medicine, the care of these athletes is ideally performed by healthcare professionals with specific training and experience in the assessment and management of concussion [4]. In general, there is no specific treatment for concussion, but for children and adolescents, a more conservative approach should be considered [4], and children and adolescents who sustain a concussive brain injury should be closely monitored over time for the later appearance of neurobehavioral abnormalities [14].

The treatment is rest and vigilance until symptoms resolve and medically cleared. The rest should be physical and mental as well. It is wisely advised that after brain injury/concussion, there should be cognitive rest along with physical rest [4, 12, 13, 22]. The complete rest must be respected in the 24–48 h after the concussion

[12]. There shall be special caution with the medication: sleeping pills, aspirin, anti-inflammatory drugs, and sedating pain killers shall not be prescribed, and alcohol is not permitted [12]. Paracetamol is allowed for the headache. Sometimes the player during the recovery period might still complain of dizziness, neck pain, and headaches, attributed to cervical spine and vestibular system involvement, justifying cervical spine and balance treatments [6].

Students with a concussion must be restricted from physical activity, sports, or playground activity in order to protect the student-athlete from sustaining another blow to the head with already more vulnerable brain and because physical activity can cause symptoms to worsen during the early stages of recovery [7]. The goal is to limit cognitive activity to a level that is tolerable and that does not exacerbate or cause the reemergence of symptoms [22]. Any mental exercise should be avoided in order to prevent any excessive strain on the neurometabolic processes in the brain [3] and that includes, but is not limited to, playing video/computer games; watching movies/TV; using the computer, the tablet, or the mobile phone; reading or writing; listening to loud music; making crosswords; and any activity that requires processing speed, new learning retention, and working memory [4, 13, 22]. Symptom exacerbation follows cognitive activity (cognitive exertion effect) [22] and that is why the cognitive rest during the period of recovery after a brain injury has been considered important [7, 29]. The increased cognitive activity is associated with longer recovery from concussion [30].

24.8 The Recovery/the Prognosis

The medical team is always asked about the moment the player is coming back to sports, and predicting a prognosis would be very helpful. However, the recovery time is highly variable, ranges from days to weeks, and is not easily predicted at the time of injury [31]. It is important to have meaningful return-to-play criteria [21], and, fortunately, in 80–85% of athletes, brain dysfunction resolves within 10 days [6]. Most people with concussion will recover in 7–14 days [13]. American football players who sustained a concussion recovered the performance of the uninjured controls within 5 to 10 days after injury [21]. The cognitive performance deficits in concussed athletes may persist up to 7 [27, 31] and even to 14 days in some cases [31].

However, some athletes may be symptomatic for longer periods, and caution and good follow-up must be implemented. A systematic review of the highest quality literature about concussion was published in 2014 [27], and the answers to the question "What are the most common signs, symptoms, and neurologic and cognitive deficits within three months after a potential concussive event?" revealed:

- The prevalence of loss of conscience ranged from 1% to 14.3% (evidence from 10 studies)
- The prevalence of posttraumatic amnesia ranged from 2% to 29.7% (evidence from seven studies)
- The prevalence of retrograde amnesia ranged from 7.4% to 53.3% (evidence from five studies)
- The prevalence of disorientation/confusion ranged from 18% to 44.7% (evidence from three studies)

The recovery from the concussion varies among the athlete-students. The capacity to read without headache or reduced concentration can last for 30 min for some, and others will experience fatigue only after 15 min, but the tolerance for a cognitive activity is expected to increase as the recovery proceeds [22]. One week of cognitive and physical rest was enough to return to baseline on the neurocognitive assessment [22], but the patients involved on more cognitive activity after a concussion took longer time to recover [24]. Naomi J. Brown et al. [30] conducted a prospective cohort study of patients who presented to a Sports Concussion Clinic within 3 weeks of injury to determine the effect of cognitive activity level on duration of post-concussion symptoms. Thirty-five patients were included in the study (mean age of participants was 15 years), 19% reported a loss of consciousness, and 37% reported amnesia at the time of injury. The authors concluded that the increased cognitive activity is associated with longer recovery from concussion.

The neurocognitive test results and the self-reported symptom data had prognostic value in determining time to clinical recovery, and headache symptoms were associated with longer time to clinical recovery [32]. The study by Lau, B. C. et al. [33] investigated cutoff scores in neurocognitive testing and symptom clusters that predict protracted recovery from concussions in high school athletes. A computer-based neurocognitive test battery (Immediate Post-Concussion Assessment and Cognitive Testing) was applied on the first 48-h post-concussion and then before return to play. Athletes were classified as protracted recovery (>14 days) or short recovery (≤14 days). The authors concluded that there are numerical thresholds for clinicians to predict which concussed athletes will have a protracted recovery [33], and this information can be given to the coach. In the study of Iverson G, [34], "within 72 hours after injury, athletes with complex concussions performed poorly on neuropsychological testing and reported more symptoms than those with simple concussions. Athletes with complex concussions who were slow to recover were 18 times more likely to have three unusually low neuropsychological test scores than those with simple concussions." This case-control study included high school football players, all completed a computerized neuropsychological screening evaluation within 72 h of injury, and they were clinically followed until they recovered and were cleared to return to play. Another cohort study (level of evidence grade 2) was undertaken to determine which on-field signs and symptoms were predictive of a protracted (≥21 days) versus rapid (≤7 days) recovery after a sports-related concussion [35]. The sample included 107 male high school football athletes who completed computerized neurocognitive testing within an average 2.4 days after injury, and the results showed that dizziness at the time of injury was associated with a 6.34 odds ratio of a protracted recovery from concussion. Surprisingly, the remaining on-field signs and symptoms were not associated with an increased risk of protracted recovery in the current study [35].

The return to academic activities should gradually be increased, the amount of the time related to mental activities is progressive and accordingly to the symptoms, and usually in a period of 10 days, one has resumed the normal academic life [3]. Besides cognitive rest, physical rest is important, and the player is not allowed to train, to play, or to travel for a competition [6]. However, as soon the athlete starts to experience symptoms related to the concussion, he should stop the mental activities and get in cognitive rest once again [3].

Several criteria should be met to determine the endpoint of recovery [7]:

- Return of neurocognitive functioning to pre-injury levels
- Return of balance function to pre-injury levels
- Absence of symptoms (or return to pre-injury levels) when the individual is at rest
- Absence of symptoms when the individual engages in physical or cognitive activity

24.9 Return to School

Return to school after a concussion is a significant aspect of concussion management and requires an evidence-based, practical set of guidelines [9] because most children and adolescents look physically normal after a concussion and school officials often fail to recognize the need for academic or environmental adjustments [29]. Concussion recovery is variable [4], and athletes' concern is related to the return-to-play moment and to the repeated concussions that might cause structural injuries to the brain [19]. However, similar concern must also be directed to the return to school and to the academics activities, because these involve activity on a debilitated brain, and physical activity and cognitive activity are sources of neurometabolic demand on the brain, which will delay the recovery from the concussion [7, 22]. The individual's sensitivity to physical and cognitive exertion before taking a decision must be considered [7], and the student-athletes should return to their academic and sports activities smoothly and safely [3].

Reduced workload and extended time for tests while recovering from a concussion must be considered to the returning student [5]. Symptom checklists; neuropsychological tests, which are more sensitive for subtle cognitive impairment than clinical exam [5]; and postural stability tests are tools that have been used to monitor recovery [4] and to decide the moment to get back to the nonrestricted full play [3]. However, the athlete must be asymptomatic at "rest," and no symptoms are elicited by either cognitive activity or physical activity before return-to-sports participation is considered. A graded physical and cognitive activity progression is implemented [22].

There is a discussion about the routine use of baseline neuropsychological testing in order to better interpret the post-concussion scores. A subcommittee of the American Academy of Neurology is in favor of a baseline testing, especially because in some people the neurocognitive testing results might be compromised (previous concussion, for instance) [24]. Also, the National Collegiate Athletic Association (NCAA) from the USA recommends baseline assessments for student-athletes that should include the search for symptoms, balance and cognitive assessments, and neuropsychological tests. Other authors state that there is insufficient evidence to recommend the widespread routine use of baseline neuropsychological testing, although they recognize the great clinical value of this tool to evaluate the concussion [12]. Neurocognitive assessment is very important in concussion management, even in those cases without baseline assessment, and it is another tool to help to make a decision [3], together with the assessment of the symptoms and other cognitive and balance evaluation, such as those indicated in SCAT3 [12]. Besides, it seems that neurocognitive assessments may be more sensitive to recovery than symptoms alone in concussion management [5, 28], although the information gathered from the analysis of the symptoms must be considered of high value.

The timing for the neurocognitive assessment has been considered, and it has been suggested to be performed 72 h after the concussion [29], because it can provide more information in relation to analysis only of the symptoms, like a protracted recovery [5, 28, 29, 32, 33], although the ideal timing, frequency, and type of neuropsychological testing have not yet been determined [5]. However, most concussions can be managed appropriately without the use of neuropsychological testing, and it should not be used in isolation [5]. At 72-h post-concussion, the analysis might indicate the need for more time to recover and to postpone the return to school and the need for more cognitive (and physical) rest [3]. Any increase on both physical and mental activities will increase the metabolic activity of the brain and it will delay the recovery [9, 22].

24.10 Return to Play

The strong desire of the athletes to compete and to return to play might induce the sports community to minimize the seriousness of injuries and to promote a too early return [22]. The gradual return-to-play protocol for sports activity begins after complete resolution of symptoms during physical rest and no symptom return with cognitive exertion [5, 7, 13]. However, during this period the player must continuously be monitored for signs and symptoms of deterioration [10]. The premature return to sports is dangerous, not only because the decreased reaction time could increase the risk of injury but also the athlete can suffer another concussion leading to the second impact syndrome (see below) [5, 7]. The nonelite athlete may not have the same resources available as the elite athlete, and he/she will generally be managed more conservatively [32]. Younger athletes are often managed with less expertise and with limited resources [32]. There should be medical clearance to allow the player to get back to training and competition [5, 6], and caution and systematic evaluation should be undertaken before returning athletes with concussion to competition. Sole reliance on the self-report of the athlete may be inadequate [16].

Progression is the rule, and the athlete should gradually increase both the physical and the contact demands [5]. However, the player must step back on his physical preparation whenever the symptoms reappear, because this is a signal that the brain's dysfunctional neurometabolism is being pushed beyond its tolerable limits [22], and the athlete should revert back to the previous asymptomatic stage and resume the progression after 24 h [10].

The player can do aerobic exercise (AE) at intensity between 80% and 90% of the target heart rate, 20 min/day, and the target HR can be increased by 5–10 bpm every 1–2 weeks depending on individual recovery rate. When athletes can exercise at their usual perceived exertion in competition for 20 min without symptom exacerbation, they are physiologically recovered [6].

According the First International Conference on Concussion in Sport, Vienna 2001, the gradual return to play in sports takes place in five progressive steps [36], with careful monitoring for return of any post-concussive symptoms at each stage:

- 1st step – Light physical activity not involving any jarring of the head (e.g., walking, elliptical, or stationary bicycle) for relatively short periods of time
- 2nd step – Increase in the intensity and duration of activity with the introducing movement such as jogging and sport-specific drills
- 3rd step – Increase of the intensity and duration of physical activity incorporating movement in all three planes (forward-backward, side to side, and up and down)
- 4th step – Participation in controlled scrimmages or other supervised contact play
- 5th step – Participation in full contact competition

According to SCAT3, the returning of the athletes to play should follow a stepwise supervised program, with stages of progression [12]. An example is given (there should be at least 24 h (or longer) for each stage and if symptoms recur) (Table 24.2).

Table 24.2 Example of a stepwise supervised program that return-to-play athletes should follow

Rehabilitation stage	Functional exercise at each stage of rehabilitation	Objective of each stage
No activity	Physical and cognitive rest	Recovery
Light aerobic exercise	Walking, swimming or stationary cycling keeping intensity, 70% maximum predicted heart rate. No resistance training	Increase heart rate
Sport-specific exercise	Skating drills in ice hockey, running drills in football. No head impact activities	Add movement
Noncontact training drills	Progression to more complex training drills, e.g., passing drills in football and ice hockey. May start progressive resistance training	Exercise, coordination, and cognitive load
Full contact practice	Following medical clearance participate in normal training activities	Restore confidence and assess functional skills by coaching staff
Return to play	Normal game play	

The American College of Sports Medicine proposes the following schedule [13]:

- Day 1 – Low level of activity (walking, slow jogging)
- Day 2 – Increased the intensity of jogging, running, or biking
- Day 3 – Heavy noncontact activity, including sprinting
- Day 4 – Contact activity in controlled practice situation
- Day 5 – Full participation

24.11 Prevention

All sports-related concussions cannot be prevented [6], and there is no unfailing method to prevent a concussion from occurring [10]. Secondary prevention may be possible by appropriate return-to-play management. Understanding the mechanism of head trauma in football is a good tool to implement some prevention measures. In a retrospective study, a questionnaire was applied to 451 players from the German Football Association, with a history of injury, where they described the accident and the playing situation. For head injuries, head on head was the most common mechanism of injury in duels (41.4%), and upper extremity (elbow) to head only led to injury in 26.4% of cases. These results were similar to others indicated in the same paper [2]. Certainly these studies helped FIFA to penalize now the use of the elbow as an offending agent with a yellow card.

Prevention can be set at four levels:

- Rules alterations have been proposed to change the incidence of brain concussions. The strike of the elbow on the opponents face is now not allowed in football. Modifying the rules of play would be necessary to reduce the incidence of head trauma 2, and enforcement of the fair play is also welcomed
- The athletic equipment should meet recommended standards for safety. A properly fitted mouthguards may reduce the severity and incidence of cerebral concussion for specific mechanisms of injury [21], although there is no current evidence that mouthguards can reduce the severity of or prevent concussions. In American football, the helmets should be inspected, reconditioned, or replaced every year to ensure they meet safety standards [10], but, again, evidence has not shown reduction of the incidence and severity of concussions
- Athletes should know the rules and avoid unnecessary physical contacts that can jeopardize their and the opponent's health. In American football, proper training for contact on the sports field is also essential, and avoidance of spearing (using the head to tackle) will help a lot. Football players have to use proper form to head the football ball, to develop strong neck muscles, and they should tense them before heading the ball. This will help to dissipate the energy from the head to the torso and reduce the velocity change of the head [10, 21]. Some football organizations recommend not introducing heading until at least age 10 [19]
Ice hockey is a game with risks of injury, brain concussion included, and efforts have been made to prevent the injuries. Player-to-player contact contributes with 50% of head impacts in male and female leagues, followed by contact with boards and ice. Extrinsic and intrinsic risk factors must be considered for prevention. The helmets effectively decrease the impact energy, although they don't prevent the brain concussion. Again, there is no scientific evidence to guarantee the usefulness of the mouthguards. On the other hand, not infrequently, helmets and mouthguards are not worn according the manufacturers' instructions [6]
- Coaches have also a role as far as prevention is concern. Teaching the proper techniques and avoiding some risks behaviors are in their hands

24.12 FIFA and UEFA Legislation

In September 2014, both UEFA and FIFA created legislation about brain concussion in football, giving the attending doctor more time to make the medical assessment on the pitch. Now, in case of a potential brain concussion after head or cervical trauma, the team doctor has 3 min to complete an on-pitch evaluation of the injured player. He can take longer whenever the player must be treated or immobilized for transportation. The referee must be informed of this suspected incident of concussion. Now, the player can only proceed in the game after being cleared up by the team physician, which is the only person capable of such decision. No one else, coach or member of the board, is allowed to interfere with the return-to-play decision. FIFA states, that "the referee will only allow the injured party to continue playing with the authorisation of the team doctor, who will have the final decision" [37].

24.13 The Second Impact Syndrome (SIS)

This syndrome occurs when the player receives a second head injury while still symptomatic from a previous head injury [13, 19, 38, 39]. The symptoms from the first head injury still persist. Even a relatively mild impact, which can occur from days to weeks following the first head trauma on a dazed player, can cause this syndrome [38, 39]. There should be a lot of attention to a concussed player, because he/she is more susceptible to a second concussion with permanent sequela [40], and the SIS is the worst acute outcome, with 50% mortality and 50% morbidity rates [19]. It is a rare condition, with only a few cases worldwide identified each year [19], but a study published in 2000 revealed that 38% of the American football players suffering of SIS were playing while still symptomatic from a prior head injury sustained during that season 38, which justifies more awareness after the first brain concussion. The Center for Disease Control reports an average of 1.5 deaths per year from sports concussions, and in most cases, a concussion, usually undiagnosed, had occurred prior to the final one [39].

It was first described in 1973 by Richard Schneider in two young athletes who experienced initial concussive syndromes and subsequently died after a relatively minor second head injury. Later, in 1984, this condition was described as the second impact syndrome on a 19-year-old college football player who suffered a head injury with brief loss of consciousness, returned to play, reported a headache, and died 4 days later. Further investigation didn't reveal any space-occupying hematoma, but an extensive cerebral edema [40].

According to Robert Cantu [38], usually after the second impact, that can be minor and on the chest, the player does not have loss of conscience, but appear stunned, may stand on his feet for a while and quite suddenly collapses to the ground, and become semi-comatose with rapidly dilating pupils, loss of eye movement, and respiratory failure.

The pathophysiology underlining the SIS is related to brain swelling, consistent with dysautoregulation [38], which causes cerebral edema, increased intracranial pressure, and subsequent brain herniation, leading to collapse and death within minutes [38, 39]. The patient is unconscious within a minute due to rapid brain swelling linked to a loss of autoregulation of the brain, making SIS especially serious [19] that can be fatal [13]. Also, the concept of post-concussive vulnerability, with worsening metabolic changes within the cell [5], along with the several metabolic, hemodynamic, structural, and electric changes that alter normal cerebral function after the first impact can increase the brain's vulnerability to repeat injury and long-term disability [8].

According to Robert Cantu, the acute CT findings include the engorged hemisphere, with initial preservation of gray-white matter differentiation. There is abnormal mass effect and midline shift (i.e., the imaging definition of "cerebral hyperemia"). The basal cisterns and cerebral sulci are completely effaced, and the brainstem is distorted. None of patients included in their study had concomitant intra-axial injury (e.g., contusion or traumatic axonal injury) [38].

24.14 The New Concussion Consensus

On October 2016, in Berlin, it was held The 5th International Consensus Conference on Concussion in Sport. It is estimated that the new consensus will be released on February 2017 (on-line version) and the printing version on May 2017 [41].

References

1. FIFA collaborative project investigates the issue of concussion in football (FIFA.com). 12 Aug 2014 – News. http://www.fifa.com/development/news/y=2014/m=8/news=fifa-kooperationsprojekt-zum-thema-gehirnerschutterung-im-fussball-24199-2420132.html
2. Kolodziej M, Koblitz S, Nimsky C, Hellwig D. Mechanisms and consequences of head injuries in soccer: a study of 451 patients. Neurosurg Focus. 2011;31(5):E1.
3. Hall E, Ketcham C, Crenshaw C, Baker M, McConnell J, Patel K. Concussion management in collegiate student-athletes. Clin J Sport Med. 2015;25(3):291–6.
4. Scorza KA, Raleigh MF, O'Connor FG. Current concepts in concussion: evaluation and management. Am Fam Physician. 2012;85(2):123–32.
5. Harmon K, Drezner J, Gammons M, Guskiewicz K, Halstead M, Herring S, Kutcher J, Pana A, Putukian M, Roberts W. American medical society for sports medicine position statement. Clin J Sport Med. 2013;23(1):1–18.
6. Smith A, Stuart M, Dodick D, Roberts W, Alford P, Ashare A, Aubrey M, et al. Ice Hockey Summit II: zero tolerance for head hits and fighting. PM&R. 2015;7(3):283–95.
7. Sady M, Vaughan C, Gioia G. School and the concussed youth: recommendations for concussion education and management. Phys Med Rehabil Clin N Am. 2011;22(4):701–19.
8. ACSM Policy brief: youth sport concussion. http://www.acsm.org/docs/other-documents/Concussion%20Policy%20Brief.pdf. Accessed on June 2015.
9. Grady M, Master C, Gioia G. Concussion pathophysiology: rationale for physical and cognitive rest. Pediatr Ann. 2012;41(9):377–82.
10. Covassin, T., Elbin, R. Sport-related concussions. ACSM. 2012. https://www.acsm.org/access-public-information/articles/2012/01/13/sport-related-concussions. Accessed on June 2015.
11. McCrory P, Meeuwisse W, Aubry M, Cantu B, Dvorak J, Echemendia R, Engebretsen L, Johnston K, Kutcher J, Raftery M, Sills A. Consensus statement on concussion in sport – the 4th international conference on concussion in sport held in Zurich, November 2012. Clin J Sport Med. 2013;23(2):89–117.
12. SCAT3 – Sport concussion assessment tool – 3rd edition. Consensus statement on concussion in sport – the 4th international conference on concussion in sport held in Zurich, November 2012. http://www.rugby.com.au/Portals/18/Files/Administration/Policy%20Register/Policies/SCAT3%20%E2%80%93%20Sport%20Concussion%20Assessment%20Tool.pdf.
13. ACSM. Concussion in sports. https://www.acsm.org/docs/brochures/concussion-in-sports.pdf. Accessed on June 2015.
14. Giza C, Hovda D. The new neurometabolic cascade of concussion. Neurosurgery. 2014;75:S24–33.
15. Anderson V, Moore C. Age at injury as a predictor of outcome following pediatric head injury: a longitudinal perspective. Child Neuropsychol. 1995;1(3):187–202.
16. Field M, Collins M, Lovell M, Maroon J. Does age play a role in recovery from sports-related concussion? A comparison of high school and collegiate athletes. J Pediatr. 2003;142(5):546–53.
17. Dick R. Is there a gender difference in concussion incidence and outcomes? Br J Sports Med. 2009;43(Suppl_1):i46–50.
18. Putukian M, Aubry M, McCrory P. Return to play after sports concussion in elite and non-elite athletes? Br J Sports Med. 2009;43(Suppl_1):i28–31.
19. Nowinski C. Hit parade: the future of the sports concussion crisis. Cerebrum. 2013 Jan–Feb;2013:2. http://www.ncbi.nlm.nih.gov/pmc/articles/PMC3600860/.
20. Lincoln A, Caswell S, Almquist J, Dunn R, Norris J, Hinton R. Trends in concussion incidence in high school sports: a prospective 11-year study. Am J Sports Med. 2011;39(5):958–63.
21. Barth JT, Freeman JR, Broshek DK, Varney RN. Acceleration-deceleration sport-related concussion: the gravity of it all. J Athl Train. 2001;36(3):253–6.
22. McLeod TCV, Gioia GA. Cognitive rest: the often neglected aspect of concussion management. Athl Ther Today. 2010;15(2):1–3.
23. Barkhoudarian G, Hovda D, Giza C. The molecular pathophysiology of concussive brain injury. Clin Sports Med. 2011;30(1):33–48.
24. Giza C, Kutcher J, Ashwal S, Barth J, Getchius T, Gioia G, et al. Summary of evidence-based guideline update: evaluation and management of concussion in sports: report of the guideline development subcommittee of the American Academy of Neurology. Neurology. 2013;80(24):2250–7.
25. Putukian M, Raftery M, Guskiewicz K, Herring S, Aubry M, Cantu R, Molloy M. Onfield assessment of concussion in the adult athlete: table 1. Br J Sports Med. 2013;47(5):285–8.
26. Cantu R. Preface. Clin Sports Med. 1998;17(1):xi–xii.
27. Carney N, Ghajar J, Jagoda A, Bedrick S, Davis-O'Reilly C, du Coudray H, et al. Concussion guidelines step 1. Neurosurgery. 2014;75:S3–S15.
28. Johnson E, Kegel N, Collins M. Neuropsychological assessment of sport-related concussion. Clin Sports Med. 2011;30(1):73–88.
29. Halstead M, McAvoy K, Devore C, Carl R, Lee M, Logan K. Returning to learning following a concussion. Pediatrics. 2013;132(5):948–57.
30. Brown N, Mannix R, O'Brien M, Gostine D, Collins M, Meehan W. Effect of cognitive activity level on duration of post-concussion symptoms. Pediatrics. 2014;133(2):e299–304.

31. McClincy M, Lovell M, Pardini J, Collins M, Spore M. Recovery from sports concussion in high school and collegiate athletes. Brain Inj. 2006;20(1):33–9.
32. Lau B, Lovell M, Collins M, Pardini J. Neurocognitive and symptom predictors of recovery in high school athletes. Clin J Sport Med. 2009;19(3):216–21.
33. Lau B, Collins M, Lovell M. Cutoff scores in neurocognitive testing and symptom clusters that predict protracted recovery from concussions in high school athletes. Neurosurgery. 2012;70(2):371–9.
34. Iverson G. Predicting slow recovery from sport-related concussion: the new simple-complex distinction. Clin J Sport Med. 2007;17(1):31–7.
35. Lau B, Kontos A, Collins M, Mucha A, Lovell M. Which on-field signs/symptoms predict protracted recovery from sport-related concussion among high school football players? Am J Sports Med. 2011;39(11):2311–8.
36. Aubry M, Cantu R, Dvorak J, Graf-Baumann T, Johnston K, Kelly J, Lovell M, McCrory P, Meeuwisse W, Schamasch P. Summary and agreement statement of the 1st International Symposium on Concussion in Sport, Vienna 2001. Br J Sports Med. 2002;36(1):6–10.
37. FIFA. http://www.fifa.com/development/news/y=2014/m=9/news=fifa-s-medical-committee-proposes-new-protocol-for-the-management-of-c-2443024.html. Accessed on July 2014.
38. Cantu R, Gean A. Second-impact syndrome and a small subdural hematoma: an uncommon catastrophic result of repetitive head injury with a characteristic imaging appearance. J Neurotrauma. 2010;27(9):1557–64.
39. American Association of Neurological Surgeons. Patient information: concussion. http://www.aans.org/Patient%20Information/Conditions%20and%20Treatments/Concussion.aspx. Accessed on July 2015.
40. Wetjen N, Pichelmann M, Atkinson J. Second impact syndrome: concussion and second injury brain complications. J Am Coll Surg. 2010;211(4):553–7.
41. Concussion Sport Group. 2016. http://concussion-consensus.com/Berlin_Concussion_Consensus.pdf.

Face Trauma

25

Rui Pratas and Victor Hugo

Contents

25.1 Epidemiology

Cerulli et al. [1] examined all cases of sports-related maxillofacial trauma that required operative intervention over a 5-year period and found that the sport involved was football in 73.9% of cases.

A 7-year prospective cohort study [2] of 23 Union of European Football Associations teams found that lower extremity injuries were the most frequent (87%), with head injuries making up only 2% of the total.

On the other hand, a 6-year prospective cohort study of 20 Fédération Internationale de Football Association tournaments [3] reveals a head/neck injury rate significantly greater than that found in the Union of European Football Associations study. However, only 3% of these injuries were fractures, with the vast majority being contusions or lacerations (78%).

Kolodziej et al. [4] retrospectively reviewed 451 players from the German Football Association who had suffered injuries during football games. The head was affected in 23.9% of cases, and the areas most frequently involved were the facial and occipital regions.

Correa et al. [5] analyzed 113 first division matches of the Brazilian Football League in 2009, finding that in 84.1% of games, at least 1 craniofacial region-related incident happened, with a mean of 2.0 per match.

R. Pratas (✉) • V. Hugo
Clínica do Dragão - Espregueira-Mendes Sports Centre, FIFA Medical Centre of Excellence, Porto, Portugal
e-mail: rmgpratas@gmail.com

J. Espregueira-Mendes et al. (eds.), *Injuries and Health Problems in Football*,
DOI 10.1007/978-3-662-53924-8_25

Giannotti et al. [6] analyzed hospital admissions due to football trauma from the Canadian Hospitals Injury Reporting and Prevention Program, finding that male gender, playing unorganized football, football outside school premises, playing during the summer/fall, and having multiple body injuries, increased the likelihood of hospital admission.

Due to exposure and the lack of protection for the face, the occasional maxillofacial trauma sustained during football games often entails serious facial injuries requiring hospital admissions and invasive procedures.

In comparison with other sports (rugby, American football, etc.) where physical contact occurs more frequently and the higher incidence of traumatic events justifies the use of protective measures, football is not a particularly violent sport. In fact, the low incidence of fractures, severity of the lesions, and discomfort caused by possible protective masks make their routinely use unjustified in football players.

25.2 Causes

Maxillofacial traumas in football are caused by violent impacts between players that take place mainly when the ball is played with the forehead. The zygomatic and nasal regions are mainly involved. It can be an elbow-head impact or a head-head impact. Most studies reveal that elbow-head impact is the most frequent [1].

25.3 Nasal Trauma

Nasal injuries can include bleeding, septal hematomas, and/or nasal fractures.

25.3.1 Epistaxis

Nose bleeding (epistaxis) is one of the most frequent problems due to facial trauma. It may be mild with spontaneous resolution or severe with the need of hospitalization. For protection of every athlete, it is important that the player with epistaxis stays outside the game field until bleeding stops.

Most cases of simple epistaxis involve disruption of the Kiesselbach's plexus in the anterior chamber of the nose. This is usually expediently controlled with direct pressure (i.e., pinching the nares together during 2–5 min.) and/or the application of a vasoconstrictive spray/drop (oxymetazoline or phenylephrine) and/or local application of ice. In some cases, additional anterior nasal packing with a hemostatic Gelfoam will be necessary.

Brisk nasopharyngeal bleeding may occur from disruption of the sphenopalatine artery as it enters the lateral wall of the nasal cavity. This posterior epistaxis requires nasal packing with materials that can produce more compression into the nose, and in rare cases it may be necessary a bleeding control in an operating room.

25.3.2 Septal Hematoma

Septal hematomas deserve special attention because of their potential for perichondral injury and subsequent necrosis. A septal hematoma appears as a purple, grapelike swelling from the nasal septum. It may develop minutes or hours after the facial trauma. The athlete may feel a unilateral or bilateral nasal obstruction and is mandatory a prompt treatment in order to avoid further important complications. Incision and drainage followed by anterior nasal packing may prevent the possibility of septal necrosis, infection, impaired breathing, and altered cosmetic.

25.3.3 Nasal Fractures

The common perception of the broken nose as innocuous may account for its high rate of undertreatment. However, a poorly managed acute nasal fracture leads to chronic nasal deformities and, sometimes, breathing difficulties that may impair the performance of competitive athletes.

Nasal fractures account for approximately 50% of sports-related facial fractures; 15% of those fractures are recurrent. Because of its prominent location on the face, the nose is the most commonly fractured facial structure in football.

Nasal bones are thicker superiorly near the radix and thinner and more prone to fractures inferiorly as they approach the "keystone" area. Fractures in this region were often accompanied by nasal bleeding.

25.3.3.1 Examination and Diagnosis

The diagnosis of a nasal fracture is made clinically. The most common findings in a nasal fracture include epistaxis, swelling and tenderness of the nasal dorsum, bruising around the eyes, and an obvious nasal deformity. Palpation of the nasal bones can demonstrate mobility, irregular surface, or crepitus. If the injured athlete reports a nasal obstruction during inspiration, the examiner should strongly consider a nasal/septal fracture or dislocation.

The intranasal examination should be conducted under proper lighting with a nasal speculum. The examiner can spray the intranasal structures with a vasoconstrictor such as phenylephrine or oxymetazoline if that would allow for better visualization.

During a football match, a diagnosis of an unstable nasal fracture is an indication for the athlete to stop playing.

25.3.3.2 Treatment

The indications for treatment of nasal/septal injuries by a physician are persistent bleeding and obvious external nasal deformity. Any open wounds must be treated with copious irrigation, and to minimize swelling, ice can be used. Swelling that occurs over time obscures the deformity and makes acute closed reduction difficult. If swelling has also occurred, waiting at least 4–7 days for the swelling to subside before treating the nasal fracture is prudent [7].

Treatment can be limited to a simple closed reduction of the nasal bones using topical and local anesthesia or can be a more involved open reduction of a fractured or severely dislocated septum and/or nasal dorsum in the operating room. The realigned septum or nasal bones are then splinted externally and internally. The splints are usually removed in 7–10 days.

Carefully consider the decision to return the athlete to competition and the need for nasal protection. The nasal bones generally heal sufficiently within 4–8 weeks, allowing the athlete to return to competition in contact sports. If the athlete resumes competition soon after repair, it is strongly recommended that he or she use a protective facial device of sufficient strength to prevent further injury.

References

1. Cerulli G, Carboni A, Mercurio A, Perugini M, Becelli R. Soccer-related craniomaxillofacial injuries. J Craniofac Surg. 2002;13:627–30.
2. Ekstrand J, Hägglund M, Waldén M. Injury incidence and injury patterns in professional football: the UEFA injury study. Br J Sports Med. 2011;45:553–8.
3. Fuller CW, Junge A, Dvorak J. A six year prospective study of the incidence and causes of head and neck injuries in international football. Br J Sports Med. 2005;39:i3–9.
4. Kolodziej MA, Koblitz S, Nimsky C, Hellwig D. Mechanisms and consequences of head injuries in soccer: a study of 451 patients. Neurosurg Focus. 2011;31:E1.
5. Correa MB, Knabach CB, Collares K, Hallal PC, Demarco FF. Video analysis of craniofacial soccer incidents: a prospective study. J Sci Med Sport. 2012;15:14–8.
6. Giannotti M, Al-Sahab B, McFaull S, Tamim H. Epidemiology of acute soccer injuries in Canadian children and youth. Pediatr Emerg Care. 2011;27:81–5.
7. Rohrich RJ, Adams Jr WP. Nasal fracture management: minimizing secondary nasal deformities. Plast Reconstr Surg. 2000;106:266–73.

Ophthalmic Lesions in Football

26

Luís Torrão

Contents

Every year > 600,000 sports- and recreation-related eye injuries occur [1]. About 42,000 of these are of a severity that requires emergency room attention, with roughly 13,500 of these resulting in permanent loss of sight. Emergency rooms in the USA treat a sports-related ocular injury every 13 min. Playing games are responsible for anywhere between 10% and 20% of all ocular injuries.

Football ocular injury is an important eye health problem in Europe and probably worldwide.

Closed globe injuries account for most sports-related eye injuries. The anterior segment is the portion of the eye most frequently damaged by blunt trauma, and hyphaema is the most common mode of clinical presentation [2]. The extent of ocular damage depends on the size, hardness, and velocity of the blunt object, and the force imparted directly to the eye. A direct blow to the globe from a blunt object smaller than the eye's orbital opening causes rapid anteroposterior compression and dilation of the middle of the globe, transmitting a great force to the internal ocular structures. A blunt object larger than the orbital opening (> 5 cm in diameter) exerts force on the floor of the orbit or the medial wall, resulting in fractures of the thin bones. This 'pressure-release valve' may prevent rupture of the globe; however, there is a high incidence of occult internal ocular injuries [3].

Examples of blunt injuries include orbital blowout fracture, orbital and lid contusions, iris

L. Torrão
Clínica do Dragão, Espregueira-Mendes Sports Centre – FIFA Medical Centre of Excellence, Porto, Portugal
e-mail: ltorrao@gmail.com

J. Espregueira-Mendes et al. (eds.), *Injuries and Health Problems in Football*,
DOI 10.1007/978-3-662-53924-8_26

injury, traumatic iritis, subconjunctival haemorrhage, hyphaema, retinal haemorrhage, commotio retinae, vitreous haemorrhage, choroidal rupture, retinal tears, and retinal detachment.

Open-globe injuries are relatively uncommon. Such injuries range from mild abrasions to serious lacerations.

26.1 Mechanism of Injury

Although there are differences between the opening of the bony orbit (1.461.6 in.) and the diameter of a standard football ball (8.6 in.), the laboratory experiments carried out confirmed that football balls deform significantly on impact, allowing a small "knuckle" of the ball to enter the orbit and impact the globe. Still more, it was proved that the football ball is unique among the sports balls tested: orbital penetration is lower, but the time in the orbit is longer, and during rebound a secondary suction effect is produced on the orbital contents. The expansion of the eyeball perpendicular to the direction of impact has been proposed as the major cause of the contusion injuries [4].

The assumption that when a large object such as a football ball hits the eye, more energy is directly transmitted to the exposed temporal retina while the nasal retina is protected by the nose could explain the predilection of football eye injury lesions to the superotemporal quadrant [5]. Vitreous haemorrhage was the posterior segment injury found in the highest percentage (50%) [6]. Firm attachments of the vitreoretinal base in young population probably are responsible for these haemorrhages.

The need for protective eyewear in football remained far less clear than for other sports. Probably collisions with other players, resulting in a finger in the eye, a head or elbow or knee in the eye, etc., are the biggest ocular safety risks in football. The ball is large and moves at high rates of speed, so it could cause serious ocular trauma, corneal abrasion, hyphaema, detached retina, etc. This is 'just part of the game' to a large extent. There are rules to protect players from opponents' feet and knees going above waist level. Protective goggles with polycarbonate lenses might add a little more security to a monocular player. Quick reflexes and reaction time are probably the best defence for all ocular safety risks.

Even though the incidence of an eye injury to any given player in one football game is quite small, the large number of worldwide football players makes this relatively small risk to a given individual an injury occurrence problem for society [7]. Retinal breaks are the most frequent diagnosis in follow-up period [8].

In most cases (80%), retinal tears caused by football balls were associated with retinal detachment, which may reveal that much more energy transmits to the retina than estimated [6].

Choroidal rupture is a common finding in smaller ball traumas (paint ball, tennis, golf) rather than football-related ones. It is most temporally located near macula and resulted in poor visual outcome. This finding may reveal that orbital penetration secondary to football ball is deeper than estimated [6].

26.2 Football Eye Protector

If protective devices are necessary, then performance standards must be written to ensure that the protective devices will meet the visual requirements of the game while reducing the probability of injury to a specified level [7]. The majority of sports eyewear standards written in the USA comes under the jurisdiction of ASTM (American Society for Testing and Materials, http://www.astm.org/), a non-profit corporation organised, as early as 1898, for the development of voluntary standards arrived at by consensus, with strict guidelines for due process, among all interested parties [9].

There are recommendations for ASTM F803 for subjects who require prescription lenses, for functionally one-eyed athletes and for those who have had refractive surgical procedures that weaken the eye [10]. The use of protective eyewear in football was popularised by a well-known professional player of the Dutch national team, Edgar Davids.

References

1. Goldstein MH, Wee D. Sports injuries: an ounce of prevention and a pound of cure. Eye Contact Lens. 2011;37:160–3.
2. American Academy of Pediatrics, Committee on Sports Medicine and Fitness and American Academy of Ophthalmology, Eye Health and Public Information Task Force. Protective eyewear for young athletes. Ophthalmology. 2004;111:600–3.
3. Vinger P, Duma S, Crandall J. Baseball hardness as a risk factor for eye injuries. Arch Ophthalmol. 1999;117: 354–8.
4. Schepens CL. Contusion trauma. In: Schepens CL, Hartnett ME, Hirose T, editors. Retinal detachment and allied diseases, vol. 1. Philadelphia: WB Saunders; 1983.
5. Capão-Filipe JA. Soccer (football) ocular injuries: an important eye health problem. Br J Ophthalmol. 2004;10:159–60.
6. Gökçe G, Ceylan OM, Erdurman FC, Durukan AH, Sobacı G. Soccer ball related posterior segment closed-globe injuries in outdoor amateur players. Ulus Travma Acil Cerrahi Derg. 2013;19:219–22.
7. Vinger PF, Capão-Filipe JA. The mechanism and prevention of soccer eye injuries. Br J Ophthalmol. 2004;88:167–8.
8. Capão-Filipe JA, Rocha-Sousa A, Falcão-Reis F, Castro-Correia J. Modern sports eye injuries. Br J Ophthalmol. 2003;87:1336–9.
9. Vinger PF. The eye and sports medicine. In: Tasman W, Jaeger EA (eds) Duane's clinical ophthalmology, vol. 5. Philadelphia: JB Lippincott; 1994, pp 1–103.
10. Alphonse VD, Kemper AR. Literature review of eye injuries and eye injury risk from blunt objects. Brain injuries and biomechanics symposium, Washington DC; April 3, 2013.

ColorADD: Color Identification System for Color-Blind People

27

Miguel Neiva

Contents

M. Neiva
Ashoka Fellow, Porto, Portugal

Miguel neiva design studio, Porto, Portugal
e-mail: coloradd@gmail.com

27.1 Introduction to the Colorblindness Problem

Colorblindness is the common denomination to a congenital alteration related to the incapability to distinguish several colors of the spectrum due to a visual deficiency (Fig. 27.1).

These people have a normal vision relatively to the other characteristics which compose it, even though the deficiency hampers or even makes it impossible for those afflicted to perform certain everyday social and professional tasks. Colorblindness affects approximately 350 million people – 10% of the world's population – and it's a handicap usually of genetic origin associated to a flaw in the X chromosome. Because of this, 98% of color-blind people are male.

The first symptoms of colorblindness are detected at school age due to the difficulty in interpreting drawings and maps and identifying colored pencils. Later in life a color-blind person is prohibited of performing certain jobs, while some professions will bring added difficulties. Similarly, managing daily routine poses problems, as well as, for instance, buying and choosing wardrobe as well as using maps and signs to provide orientation. Even while accessing the Internet, some texts can become illegible due to the use of certain colors.

Some companies have started creating web pages which can be seen correctly and easily by all. This has been possible due to the rising awareness that color-blind people represent a high percentage of the world population [1–3].

J. Espregueira-Mendes et al. (eds.), *Injuries and Health Problems in Football*,
DOI 10.1007/978-3-662-53924-8_27

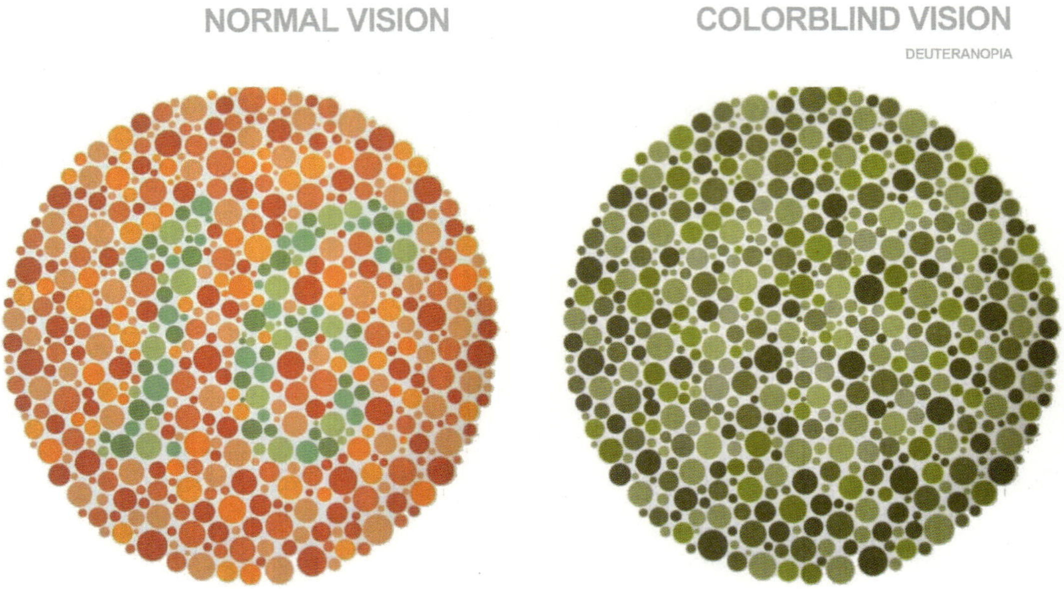

Fig. 27.1 Color-blind vision

27.2 Objectives and Methodologies

Once the problem had been identified, its extent and impact on the subjects was evaluated. On a first phase of the study, a sample of color-blind people was identified and presented with a questionnaire. Its purpose was to identify the main difficulties of the respondents concerning their colorblindness and the processes and methods used by them to lessen and overcome these obstacles.

The collected information was treated and analyzed. Based on these results, a conceptual basis was defined, capable of constituting a universal method of graphic color identification, easy to comprehend and memorize [4].

27.3 Materials and Methods

Using primary colors, represented through simple symbols, the system was constructed through a process of logical association and direct comprehension, allowing its rapid inclusion in the "visual vocabulary" of the user. This concept makes additive color a mental game, which lets the colorblind relate the symbols among each other and with the colors they represent, without having to memorize them individually.

The system proposed is based on the search of the pigment color, using as basis the primary colors – blue (cyan), red (magenta), and yellow its additive secondary colors (Fig. 27.2) and not the light color (RGB) – because the color-blind person does not possess the correct vision of the colors nor a tangible knowledge of how their addition works.

Each primary color of the code is associated to a graphic form (Fig. 27.3) which represent red, yellow, and blue; from these three forms the code is developed.

Two additional forms were added representing black and white (Fig. 27.3); in conjunction with the other elements, they represent lighter or darker tons of the colors.

The secondary colors can be formed using the basic forms as if "mixing" the primary pigments themselves (Fig. 27.4), making their perception and subsequently the composition of a color pallet easy [5, 6].

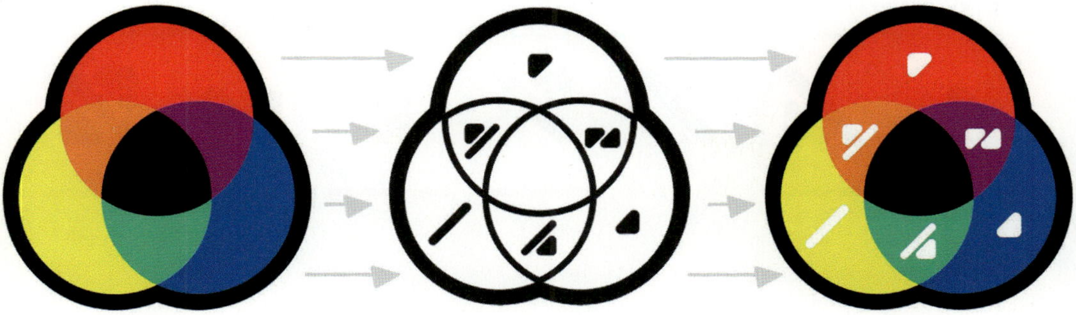

Fig. 27.2 Primary color addition – pigment colors

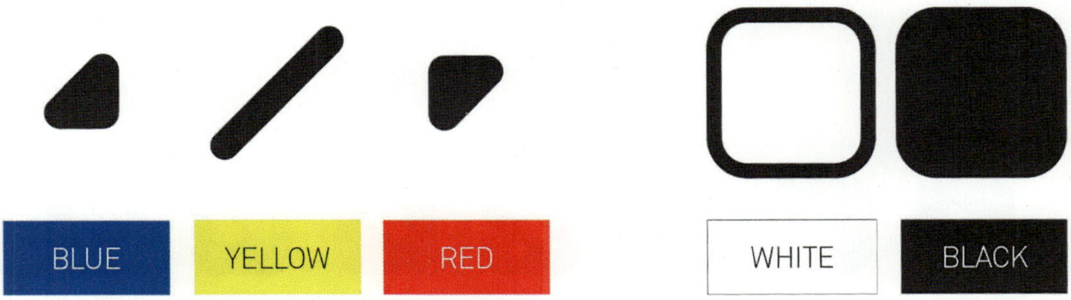

Fig. 27.3 Graphic symbols for three primary pigment colors and *white* and *black*

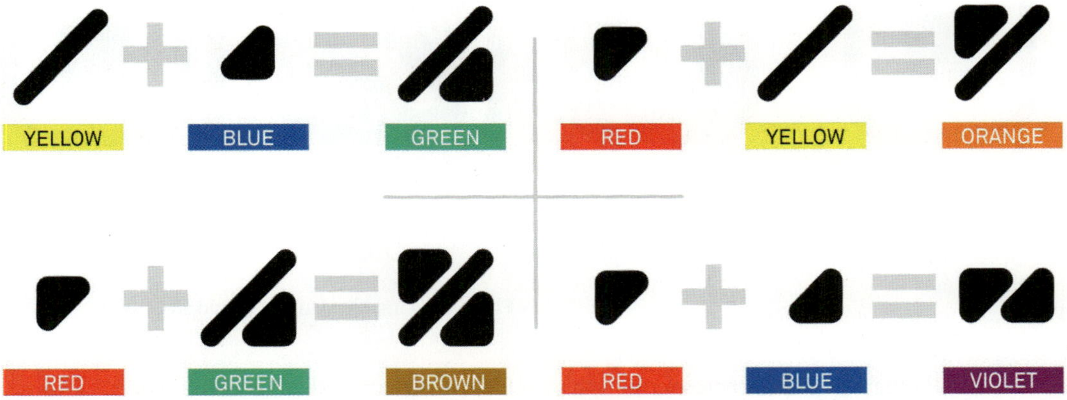

Fig. 27.4 Graphic symbols – three primary colors and their addition

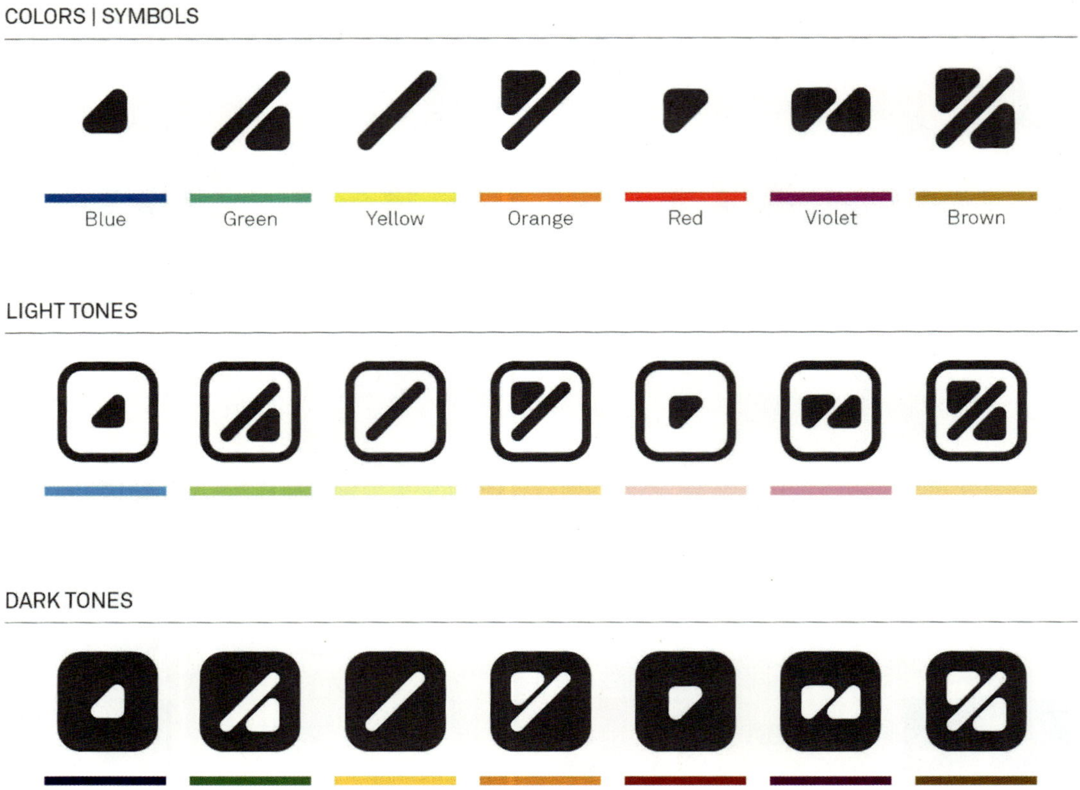

Fig. 27.5 Graphic representation of color addition with dark and light

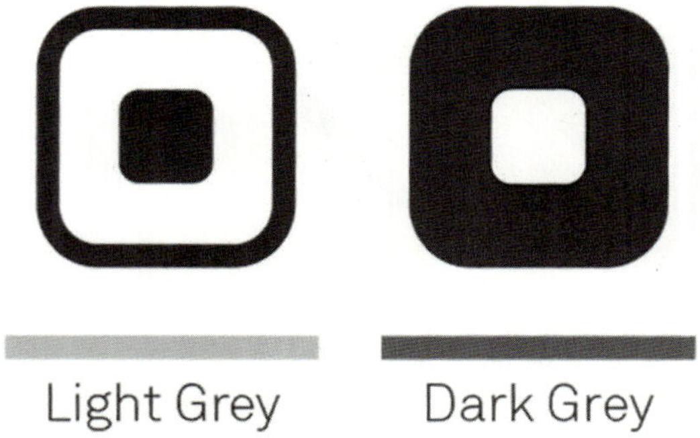

Fig. 27.6 Graphic symbols – tons of gray

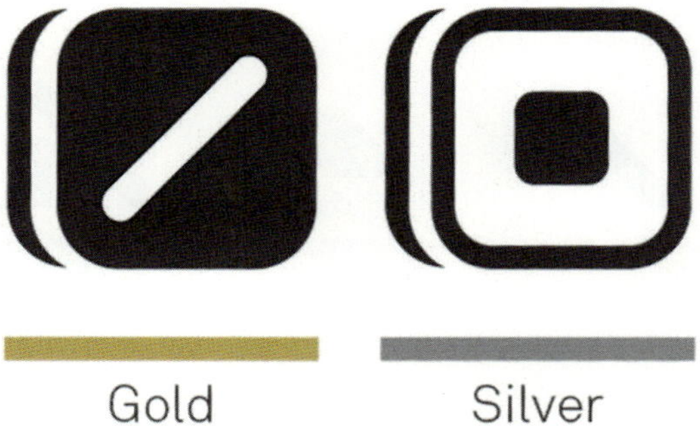

Fig. 27.7 Graphic symbols – gold and silver

By associating the icons representing white and black to define darker and lighter tones to the three basic forms and their additions, a wide palette is constructed as observed in Fig. 27.5.

Conventional color designations were attributed to the additions and other combinations of colors, especially those used in apparel.

Grey was divided into two tones: light grey and dark grey (Fig. 27.6). The importance of gold and silver in clothes implies the creation of a specific icon. Considering the logic of the codes' construction, these colors are represented by the combination of the dark yellow and the element representing shine to define gold; light grey with the same element identifies silver (Fig. 27.7).

The totality of the code, represented in Fig. 27.8, covers a considerable number of colors and can be easily conveyed through information posted at the sales point, on web sites, or the product itself (Fig. A) [7–9].

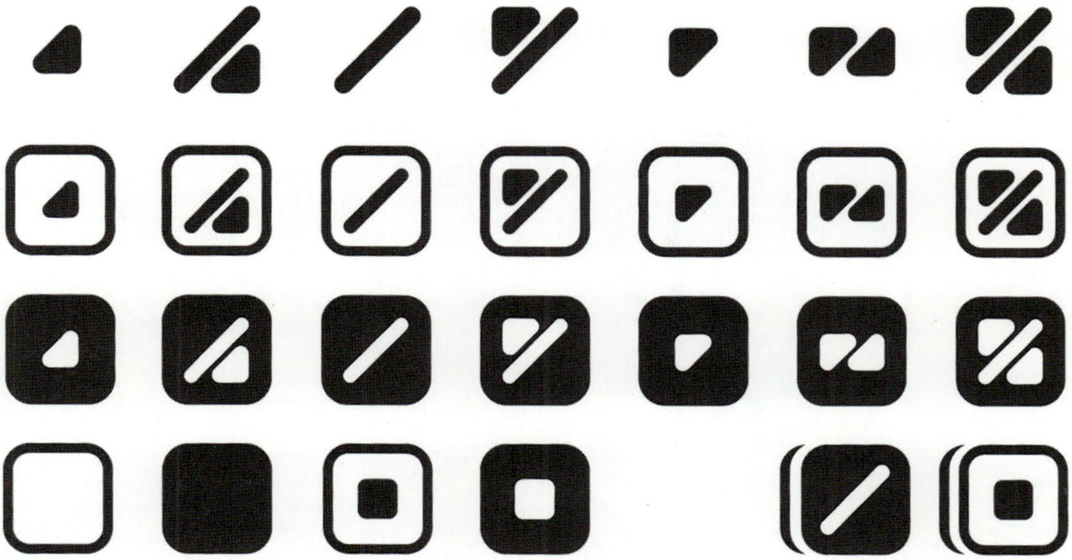

Fig. 27.8 Monochromatic graphic code

27.4 Results

The application of the system is transversal to all the areas of the global society, regardless of their geographical localization, culture, language, and religion, as well as to all the socioeconomic aspects.

27.4.1 School and Stationery

It is at school age that usually appear the first and sometimes traumatic situations and difficulties caused by the wrong color identification.

The inclusion of the system in the school and stationery leads to inclusion (Figs. 27.9 and 27.10), allowing the color-blind kid a perfect integration, with no doubts and shames.

27.4.2 Sports and Sportive Activities

In all sportive activities, especially those played in group, color has a decisive role – it helps in differentiating teams, players, contestants, etc. In fact, color in sports is so relevant that, during the Football World Championship in South Africa, the ball initially proposed was orange – this fact prevented color-blind people from distinguishing the ball from the grass, and, after some official requests, the ball was changed into a white one, thus allowing everyone to see the match in equal conditions (Fig. 27.11).

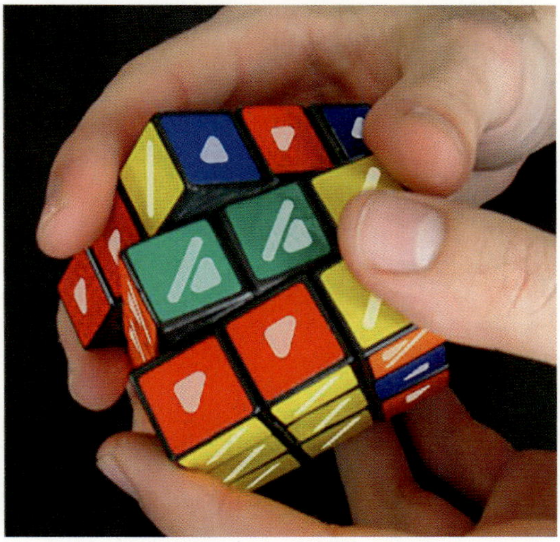

Fig. A A more colorful “Rubik Cube”

Also in sport competitions and events, color is an important element, not only to identify the physical space of the event but also to permit identifying the different teams/countries

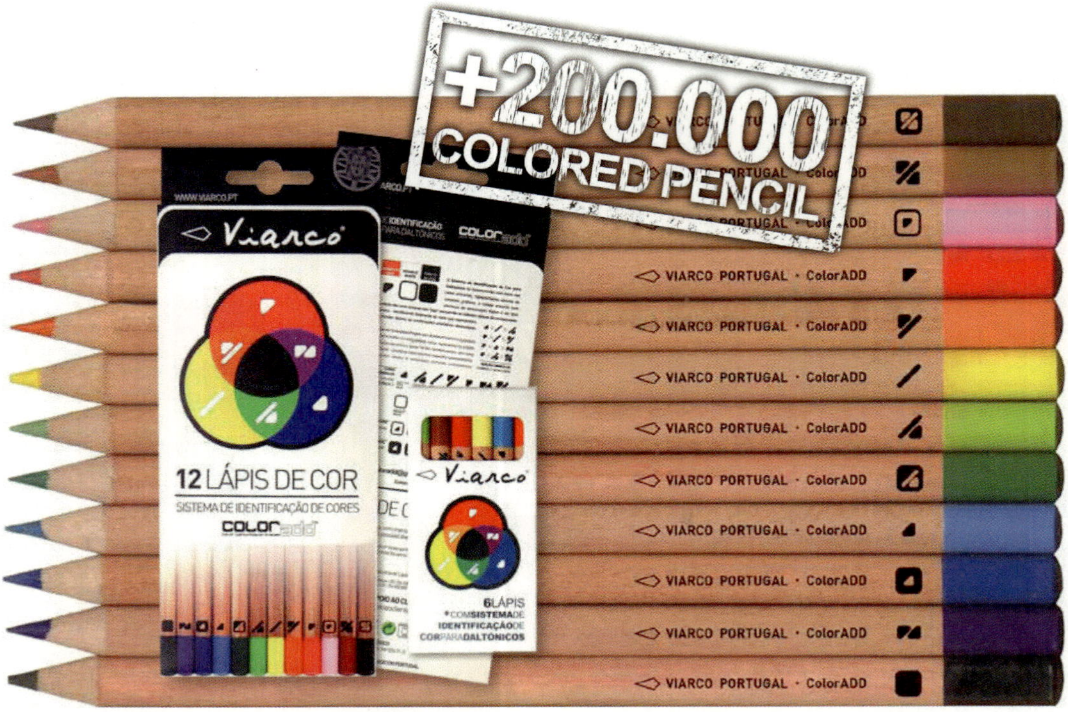

Fig. 27.9 School material (real implementation)

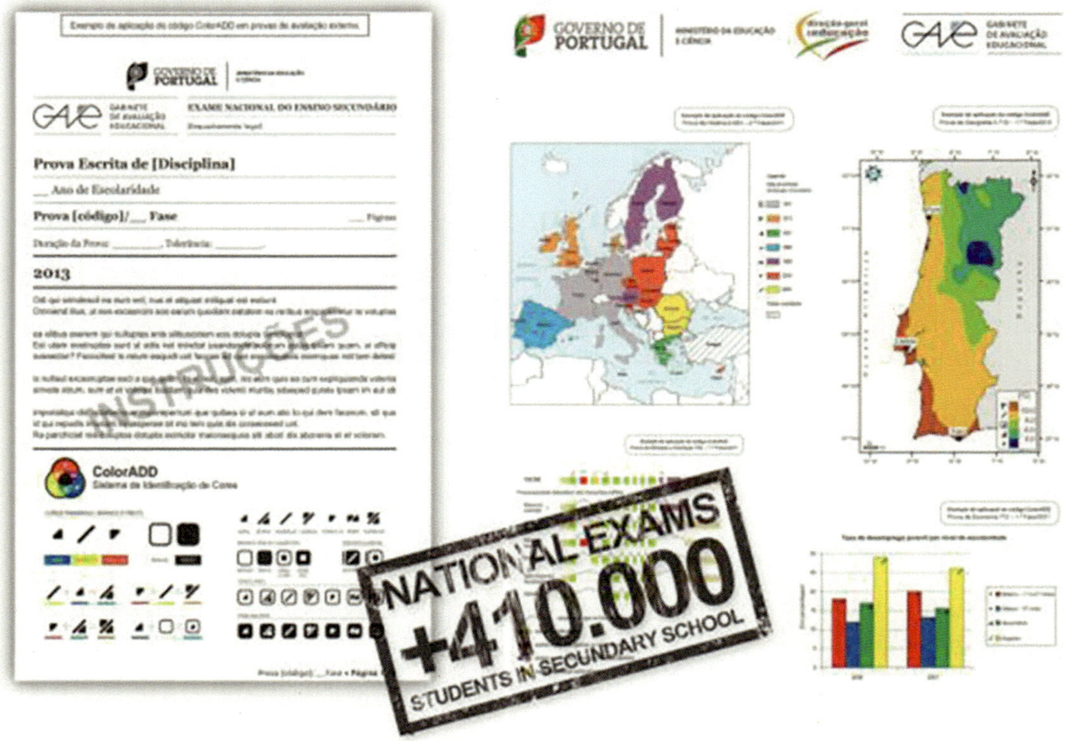

Fig. 27.10 National exams (real implementation)

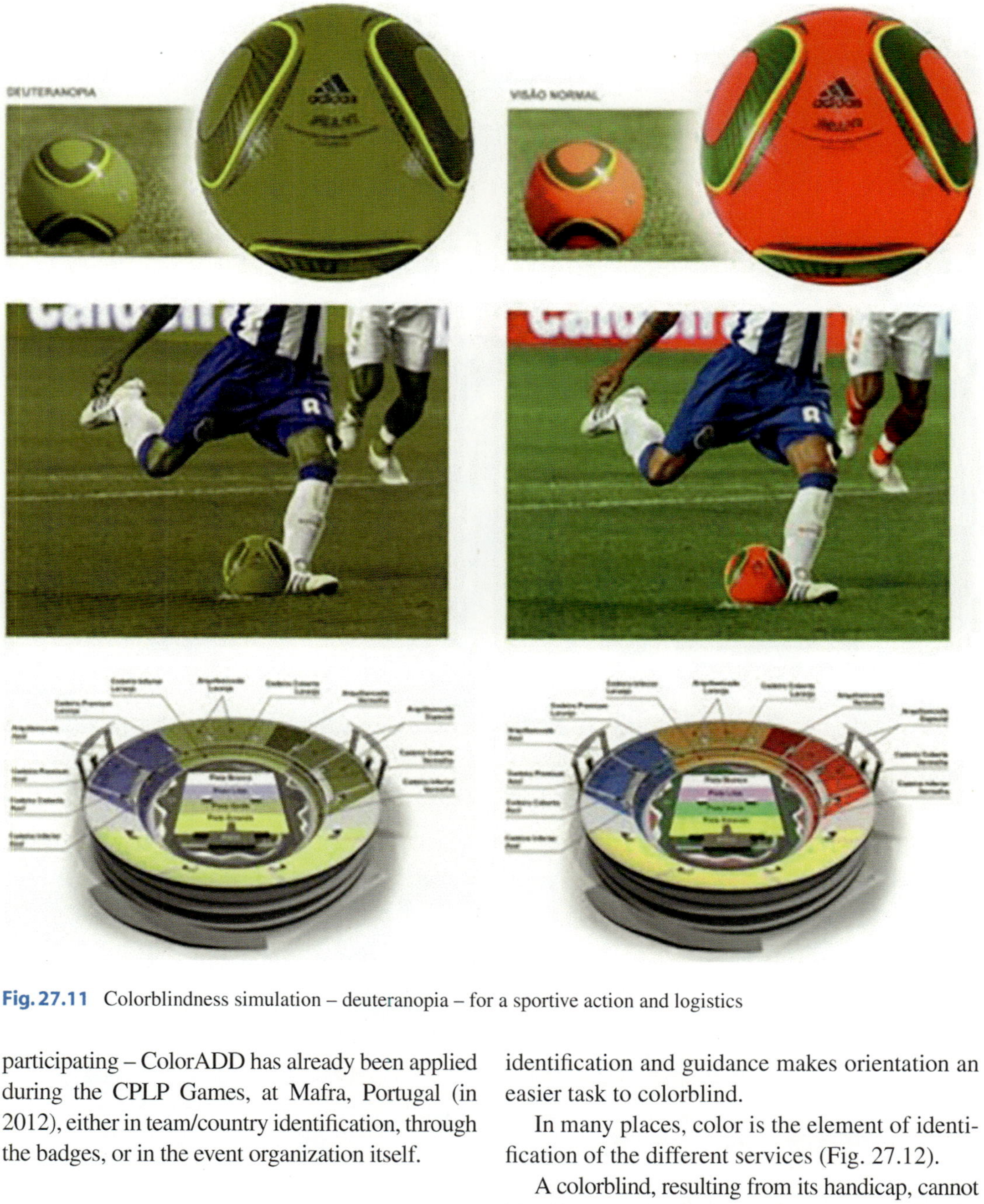

Fig. 27.11 Colorblindness simulation – deuteranopia – for a sportive action and logistics

participating – ColorADD has already been applied during the CPLP Games, at Mafra, Portugal (in 2012), either in team/country identification, through the badges, or in the event organization itself.

27.4.3 Health and Services

The selection of patients at hospitals is made through color. At the ER, an evaluation of the grade of "gravity" of a patient is carried out, and a bracelet corresponding to a certain grade of priority is provided.

The inclusion of the system in hospital services and spaces where color is an element of identification and guidance makes orientation an easier task to colorblind.

In many places, color is the element of identification of the different services (Fig. 27.12).

A colorblind, resulting from its handicap, cannot identify the color and its meaning. Also, many medicines have color as an identifying factor (Fig. 27.13).

27.4.4 Transports

The Metro system maps are a different context but equally valid on what concerns the use of the color identification code, in this case to individualize the different transit lines (Fig. 27.14).

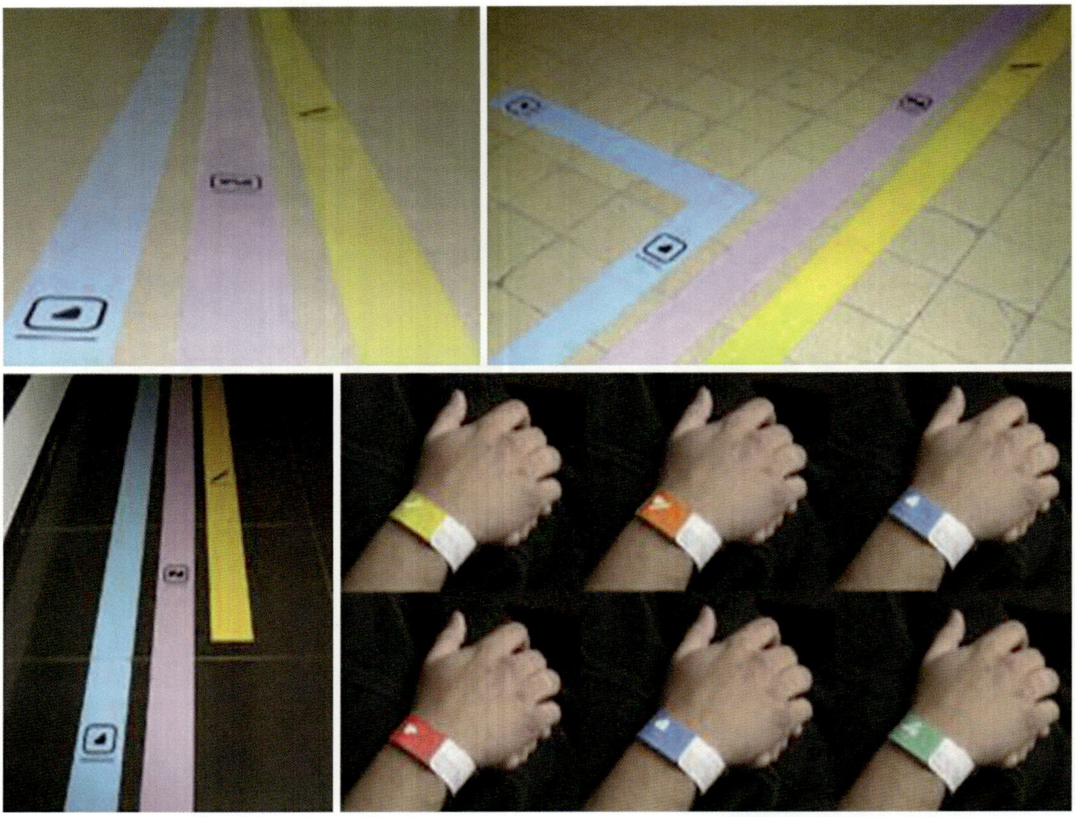

Fig. 27.12 Heath and hospitals (real implementation)

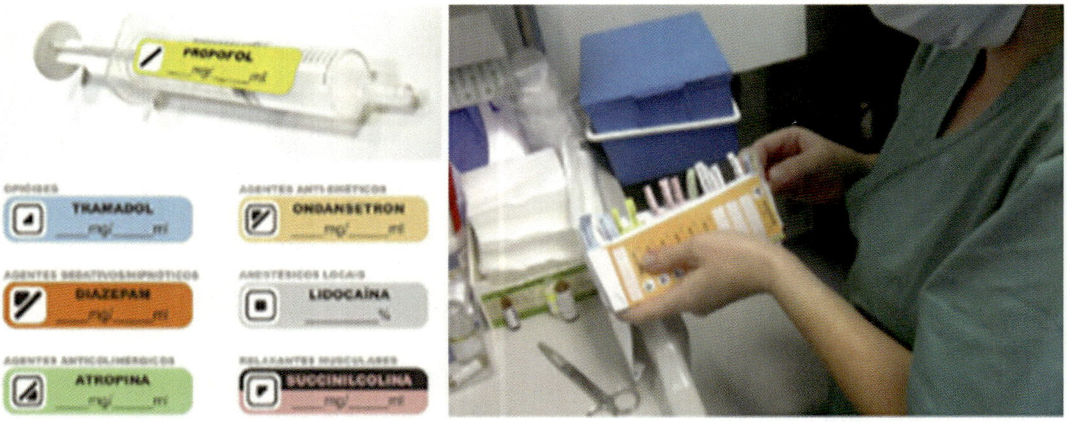

Fig. 27.13 Heath and hospitals (real implementation)

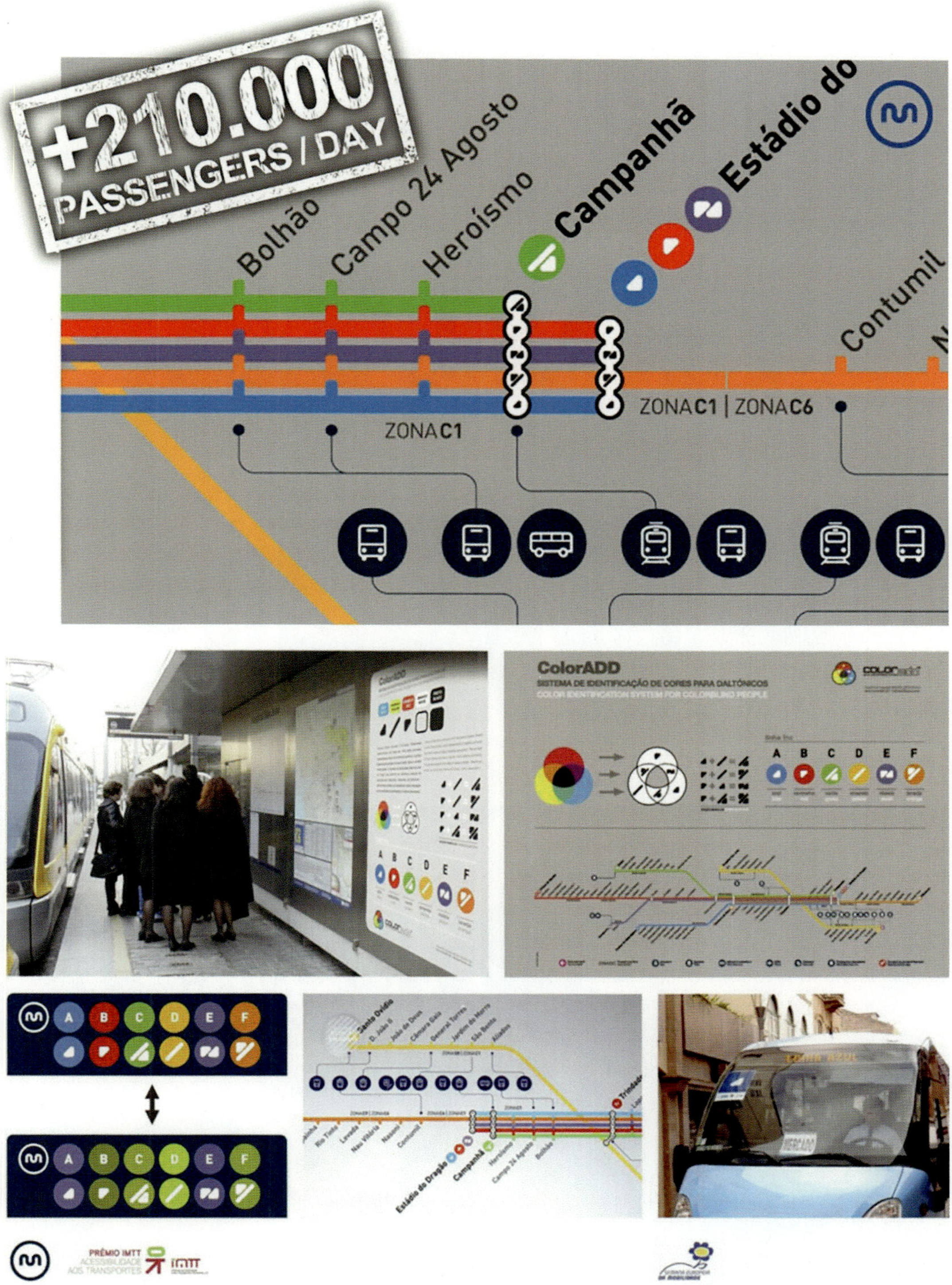

Fig. 27.14 Porto Metro map (real implementation)

27.4.5 Clothing and Textiles

The developed code can be applied in multiple contexts in which color is important. One of the most relevant fields of application is in apparel, and the color identification symbols can be applied to tags or integrated into the clothes themselves, similarly to maintenance and care information. The simple and stylized graphics and its monochromatic nature reduce the production cost of the labels in paper or cardboard, textile, or stamp (Fig. 27.15) and other implementation in cross sector (Fig. 27.16).

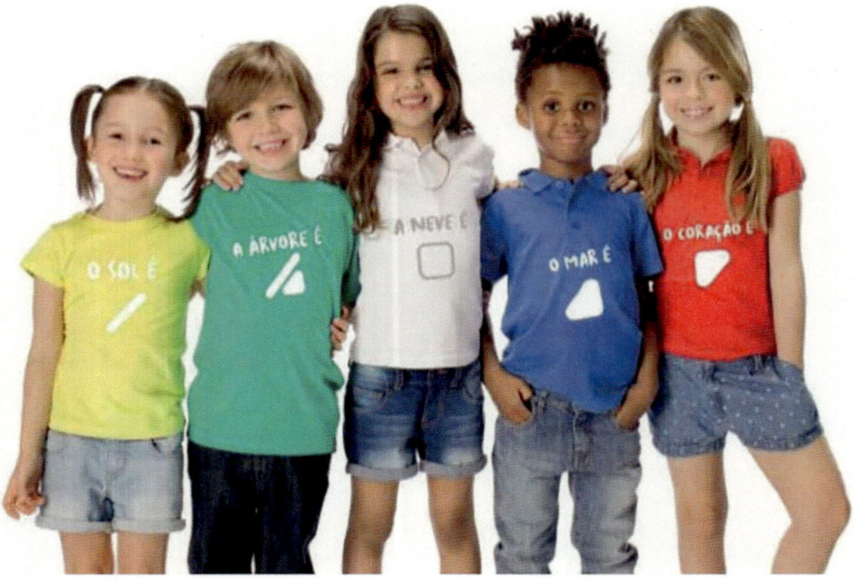

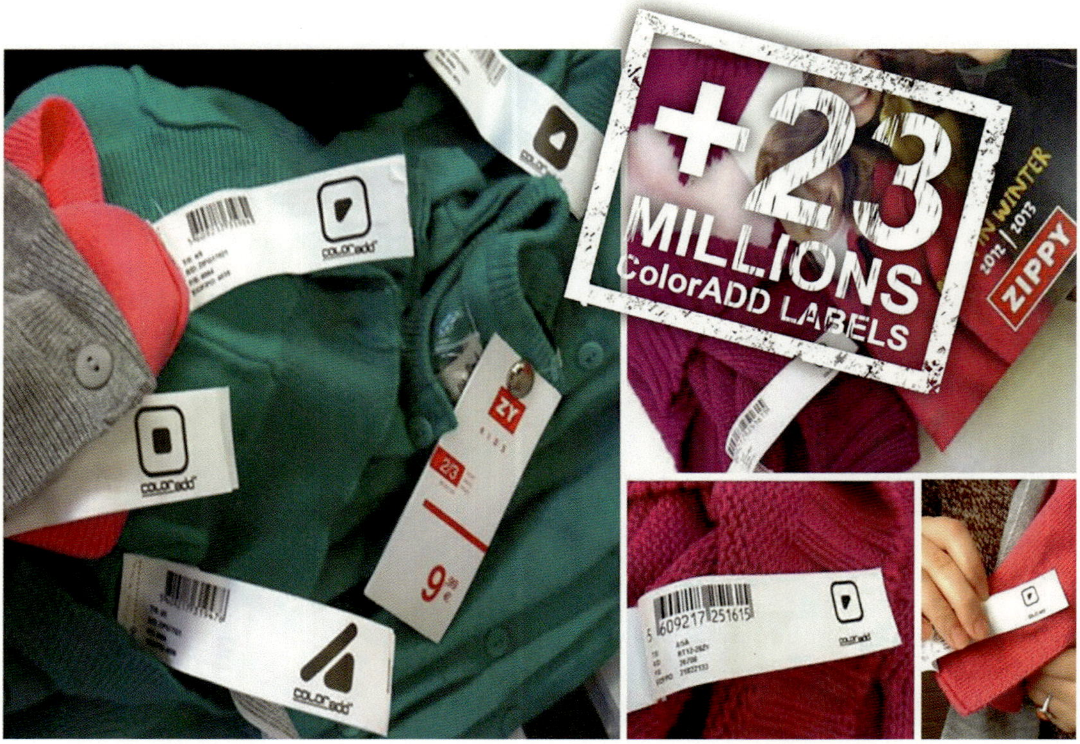

Fig. 27.15 Application clothing tags (real implementation)

27.4.6 ColorADD in Other Sectors

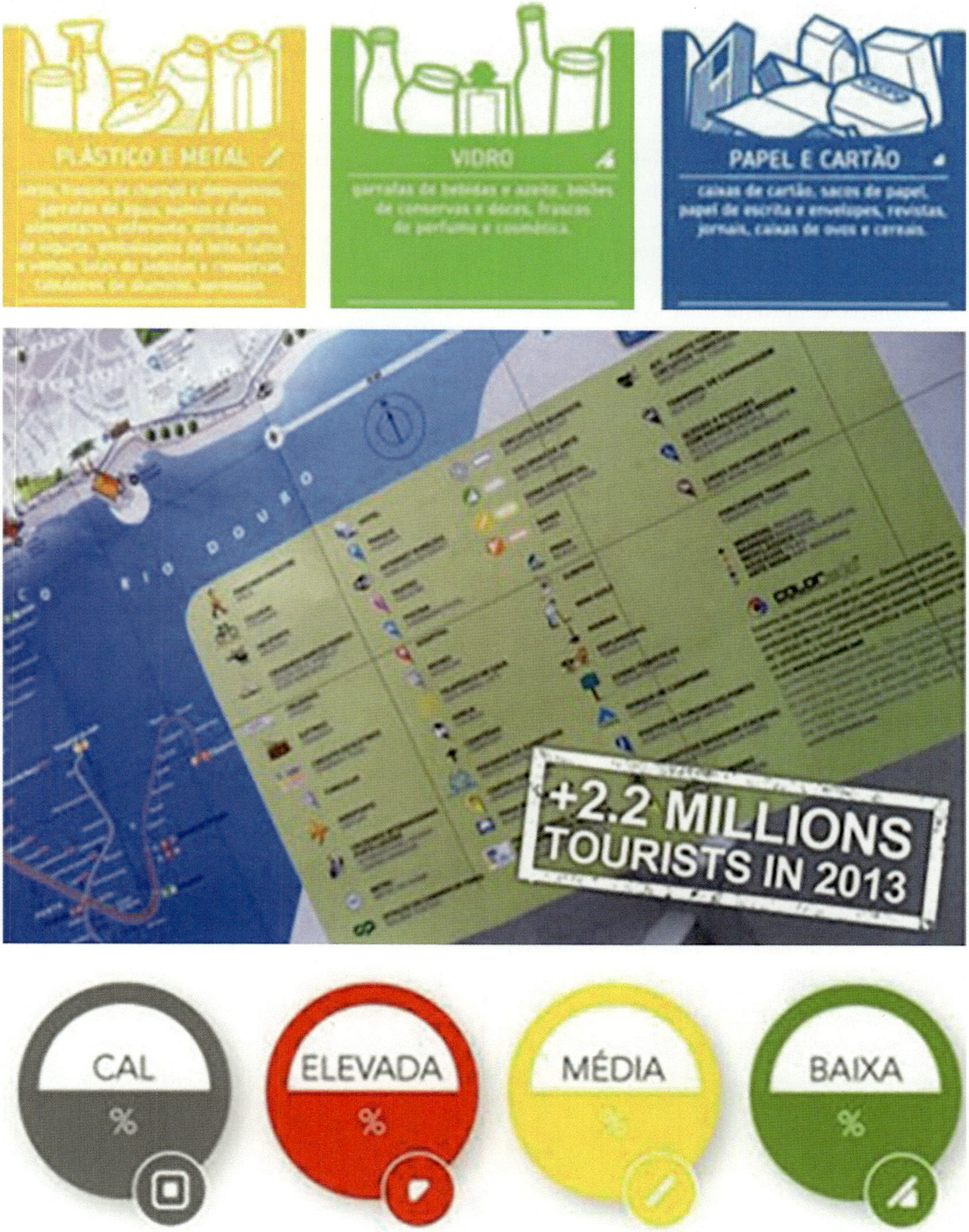

Fig. 27.16 Examples of different areas where the code is already in use: Recycling bins, City maps and Nutricional traffic light

Conclusion

Each day society grows more individually centered. Each person, sometimes, becomes totally dependent on itself, and asking for another person's help, besides creating some frustration and feelings of dependence, is not always even possible.

The "wrong" interpretation of colors can harbor insecurity in social integration of the individual whenever the projected personal "image" is a key factor in rendering judgment.

The color identification system, aimed at colorblind, can be greatly beneficial to a group which represents such a significant percentage of the population. Its use, given the characteristics of the system, means a practically insignificant cost, and its adoption by the industry and society can improve the satisfaction and well-being of a group of individuals whose particular vision characteristics deprive them of a fully independent and quiet everyday experience of choosing the right color.

References

1. Goldman L, Ausiello DC. Textbook of medicine. 22nd ed. Philadelphia: WB Saunders; 2004. p. 2410.
2. Yanoff M, Duker JS, Augsburger JJ, et al. Ophthalmology. 2nd ed. St. Louis: Mosby; 2004. p. 34.
3. Lanthony P. Science et Vie, nr. 216, September 2001.
4. Hogg A, Vaughan GM. Social psychology. 2nd ed. Sydney: Prentice Hall; 1998.
5. Arnhein R. Arte e Percepção Visual. São Paulo: Ed. Livraria Pioneira Editora; 1982.
6. Worsley P. Introdução à Sociologia. Lisboa: Publicações Dom Quixote; 1993.
7. Dubois B. Compreender o Consumidor. Lisboa: Publicações Dom Quixote; 1993.
8. Frutigier A. Signos, Símbolos, Marcas y Señales. Barcelona: Ed. Gustavo Gili; 1981.
9. Learch E. Cultura e Comunicação, Edições 70. Lisboa; 1993

Part VII

Upper Limb Injuries

28 Acute Fractures of the Upper Limb

Carina Cohen, Horácio Sousa, Nuno Sevivas, and Guillermo Arce

Contents

The frequency of football injuries reported in medical literature is estimated to be approximately 10–35 per 1000 playing hours. During football tournaments injuries of the lower extremity are almost ten times more common than upper extremity lesions. However, shoulder lesions are seldom seen if we consider the total of injuries reported [1]. In the FIFA World Cup, one of the most popular sporting events, a total of 104 injuries were reported: lower extremity accounted to 65.4%, followed by head/neck in 18.3%, upper extremity 9.6% (10 reports), and trunk in 6.7% [2].

Moreover, if we consider a total of 3944 injuries reported from 1546 matches in the World Football Tournaments (1998–2012), most injuries affected lower extremity (n = 2706, 70%), followed by injuries to the head and neck (n = 577, 15%), trunk (n = 302, 8%), and upper

C. Cohen (✉)
Shoulder and Elbow division of CETE (Centro de Traumatologia do Esporte), UNIFESP (Universidade Federal de São Paulo), São Paulo, Brazil

Instituto Cohen, São Paulo, Brazil

Hospital Israelita Albert Einstein, São Paulo, Brazil
e-mail: cacohen18@gmail.com

H. Sousa
Department at Clinica da Sé, Madeira University, Funchal, Madeira, Portugal
e-mail: horaciosousa@netmadeira.com

N. Sevivas
Life and Health Sciences Research Institute (ICVS), School of Health Sciences, University of Minho, Campus de Gualtar, 4710-057 Braga, Portugal

ICVS/3B's – PT Government Associate Laboratory, Braga/Guimarães, Portugal

Orthopaedics Department, Hospital de Braga, Braga, Portugal

Clínica Espregueira-Mendes, FIFA Medical Centre of Excellence, Estádio do Dragão, Porto, Portugal
e-mail: nunosevivas@gmail.com

G. Arce
Department of Orthopaedic Surgery, Instituto Argengino de Diagnóstico y Tratamiento, Buenos Aires 1425, Argentina
e-mail: guillermoarce8@gmail.com

J. Espregueira-Mendes et al. (eds.), *Injuries and Health Problems in Football*,
DOI 10.1007/978-3-662-53924-8_28

extremity (n = 269, 7%) [3]. Although shoulder injuries are relatively rare, once they occur, they produce a significant functional impairment that can limit performance since football is a demanding activity, in relation to increased velocity of playing and blocking and frequency of field hitting, especially for goalkeepers.

In general, traumatic dislocation of acromioclavicular and glenohumeral joints are the most frequent lesions of the upper extremity in football, but fractures may also happen and are the most common injury of the forearm and the second most common injury to the wrist [4].

Along this chapter we focus on the acute upper extremity fractures that might be seen in football. They usually occur during falls onto an outstretched arm (FOOSH), and goalkeepers may also be injured during collisions when attempting to catch the ball.

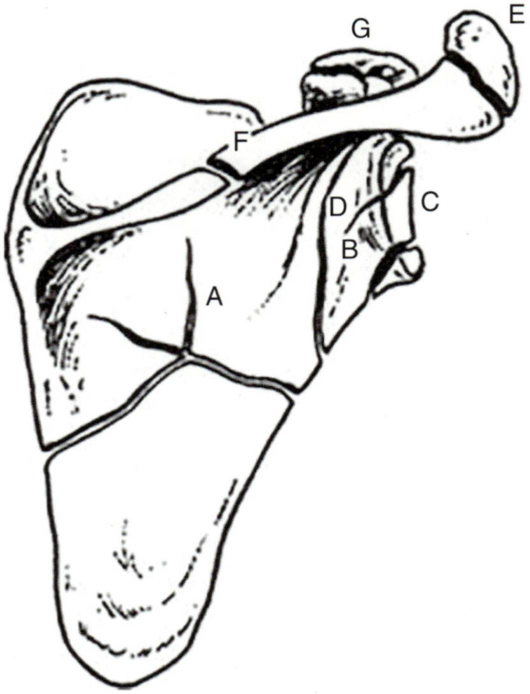

Fig. 28.1 Anatomic classification (Zdravkovic and Damholt) (**a**) scapula body, (**b**, **c**) glenoid, (**d**) scapula neck, (**e**) acromion, (**f**) scapula spine, (**g**) coracoid
Type I: Scapula body
Type II: Apophyseal fractures, including the acromion and coracoid
Type III: Fractures of the superolateral angle, including the scapular neck and glenoid

28.1 Scapular Fractures

Scapular fractures are rare, accounting for 3–5% of shoulder girdle fractures and 1% of all fractures [5]. Scapular fractures generally result from injury force through either direct impact or lateral compressive injury but can also be caused by indirect forces via axial transmission through the humerus or secondary to muscular or ligamentous traction. In football they are very uncommon since they usually result from high-impact trauma and are associated with serious bony or soft tissue injuries in 80–95% of cases, including pneumothorax, hemothorax, pulmonary injuries, and spinal injuries. Fractures are classified according to the anatomic area and are grouped into intra-articular glenoid fossa and rim, extra-articular glenoid neck, acromion, coracoid, and scapular body (Fig. 28.1).

More than 90% of scapular fractures are nondisplaced or minimally displaced and do well with conservative management; however, a specific subset of fractures may lead to poor outcomes after conservative treatment.

28.1.1 Intra-Articular Glenoid Fractures

Intra-articular glenoid fractures generally occur by transmission of force through the humeral head to the glenoid cavity. They are classified according to the Ideberg system with the Goss modification, which includes six fracture types (Fig. 28.2).

Type I fractures are true glenoid rim fractures, but types II–VI are glenoid fossa fractures with varying extension through the scapular body. Glenoid fractures with minimal displacement and angulation are treated conservatively in 90% of cases. [6].

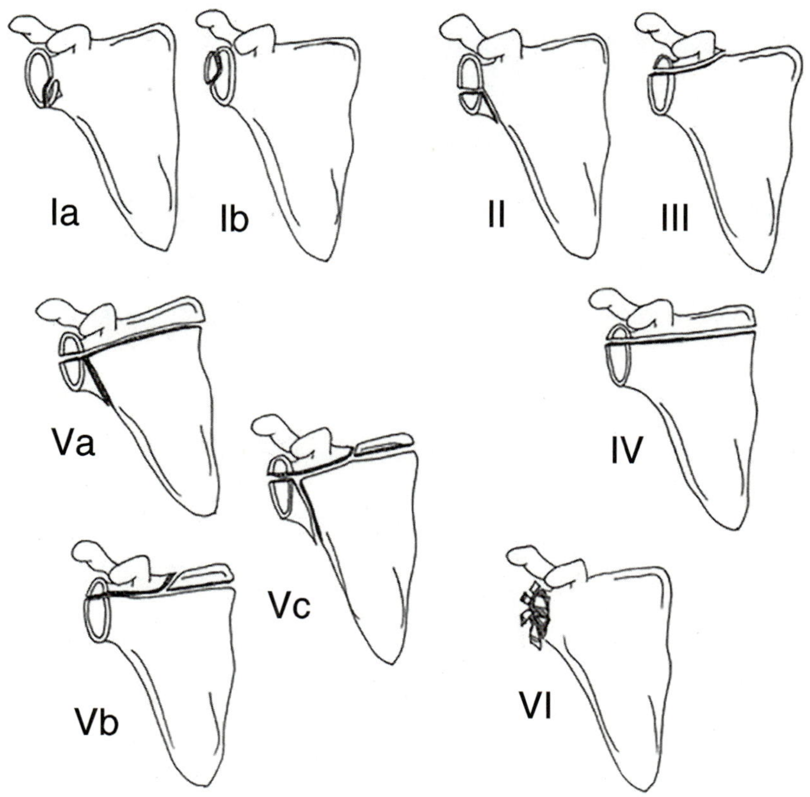

Fig. 28.2 Ideberg classification. (**Ia**) Anterior rim fracture. (**Ib**) Posterior rim fracture. (**II**) Fracture through glenoid exiting scapula laterally. (**III**) Fracture through glenoid exiting scapula superiorly. (**IV**) Fracture through glenoid exiting scapula medially. (**Va**) Combination of types II and IV. (**Vb**) Combination of types III and IV. (**Vc**) Combination of types II, III, and IV. (**VI**) Severe comminution

28.1.2 Extra-Articular Neck Fracture

Glenoid neck fractures are extra-articular, but the mechanisms are similar to that of intra-articular glenoid fractures, most commonly involving humeral head impact on the glenoid after direct lateral impact or a FOOSH injury. They can be classified into two main categories: Type I fractures, nondisplaced which respond to nonsurgical treatment, generally treated symptomatically with early range-of-motion exercises. Type II injuries involve greater than 1 cm of translational fragment displacement or more than 40° of angular displacement and most often require surgical repair. Anatomic neck fractures are inherently unstable and require surgical fixation. Surgical neck fractures can be unstable when they are associated with a clavicular fracture or with coracoclavicular and coracoacromial ligament disruption. This situation denominated by “floating shoulder” compels surgical repair. Internal fixation of the clavicular fracture generally results in adequate stabilization for healing of the glenoid fracture.

28.1.3 Scapular Body Fracture

Approximately 50% of scapular fractures involve the scapular body. The mechanisms include direct impact onto the scapula and sudden muscular contraction. These fractures respond well to conservative management and are usually treated nonsurgically in the acute phase. Operative fixation is rarely indicated, with non-operative measures generally effective. Open reduction may be considered when neurovascular compromise is present and exploration is required. Nonunion or malunion is uncommon but may require delayed surgical fixation if symptomatic, particularly with fragment displacement of greater than 10 mm or if impingement symptoms are present.

Fig. 28.3 Kuhn classification
Type I acromion fractures are nondisplaced and include Type IA (avulsion) and Type IB (complete fracture)
Type II fractures are displaced laterally, superiorly, or anteriorly, but they do not reduce the subacromial space
Type III fractures cause a reduction in subacromial space (Modified from Kuhn et al. [7])

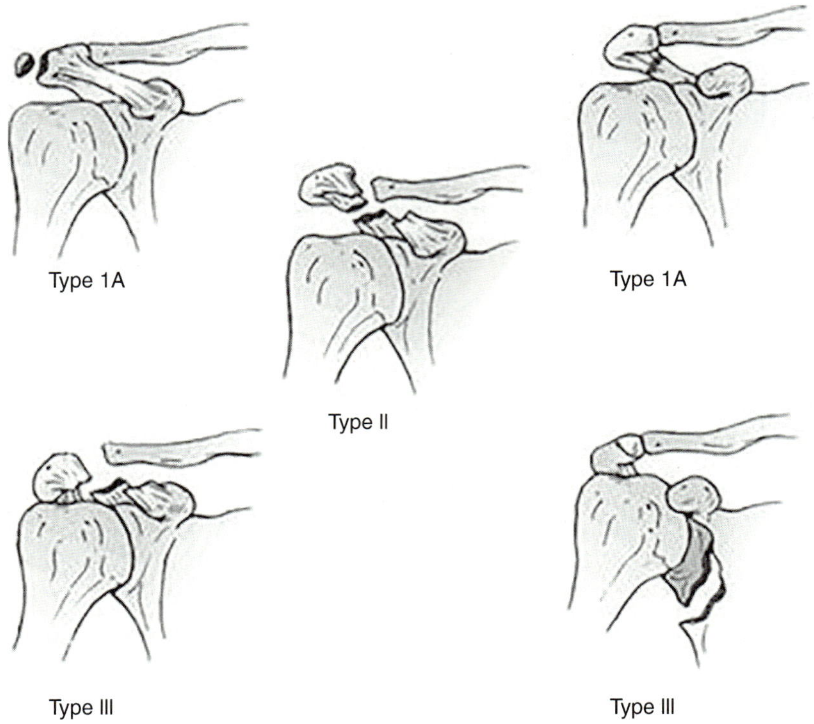

28.1.4 Acromion Fracture

Fractures of the acromion are very rare and most often occur due to a lateral impact, a direct strike to the top of the shoulder, or, rarely, impact after superior humeral subluxation. They are classified with the Kuhn system into three types (Fig. 28.3).

Type I and minimally displaced type II fractures can be managed with immobilization. Surgical fixation is recommended for markedly displaced types II and III to reduce the acromioclavicular joint and prevent nonunion, malunion, impingement, or rotator cuff injury. Os acromiale must first be ruled out, as well as concomitant rotator cuff injuries. When displaced, acromion fractures lead to subacromial impingement; therefore, they need reduction and fixation by dorsal tension band wiring.

28.1.5 Coracoid Fracture

Coracoid fractures may appear in football injuries as injury mechanisms include a direct blow to the shoulder from a lateral impact, muscle avulsion, direct humeral head impact during anterior shoulder dislocation, and a variant of acromioclavicular joint separation. They are classified into two types with the Ogawa system. Type I fractures are proximal, and type II fractures are distal to the coracoclavicular ligament insertion. There is no clear consensus about the treatment of coracoid process fractures, but nondisplaced and minimally displaced fractures are most commonly type II and can be treated conservatively. Type I fractures are more likely to be markedly displaced. When associated with acromioclavicular separation, displaced acromial fracture, clavicular fracture, or glenoid fracture, these combinations commonly require surgical treatment. Complete third-degree acromioclavicular separation accompanied by a significantly displaced coracoid fracture is an indication for open reduction and internal fixation of both injuries.

28.2 Clavicle Fractures

Clavicular fractures represent approximately 2–4% of all fractures and 35–45% of shoulder girdle injuries [8]. The most common mechanism is fall onto lateral aspect of shoulder that generates compression of shoulder girdle, which translates into compression and distraction at clavicular shaft, resulting in clavicular fracture and tear of conoid ligament. Less common mechanisms are direct impact on the shaft and indirect FOOSH mechanisms. Patients usually present with splinting of the affected extremity, with the arm adducted across the chest and supported by the contralateral hand to unload the injured shoulder.

A careful neurovascular examination is necessary to assess the integrity of neural and vascular elements lying posterior to the clavicle. Most brachial plexus injuries are associated with proximal third clavicle fractures.

The proximal fracture end is usually prominent and may tent the skin. Assessment of skin integrity is essential to rule out open fracture. Up to 9% of patients with clavicle fractures have additional fractures, most commonly rib fractures.

Clavicular fractures are classified according to the Allman system. Group I involves the middle third of the clavicle and comprises approximately 80% of clavicle fractures. Group II (15%) involves the distal clavicle, and Group III (5%) involves the proximal clavicle.

28.2.1 Middle Third (Midshaft) Clavicle Fracture

More than 75–80% of clavicle fractures occur in the midshaft region. Displaced and shortened fractures of the mid-third of the clavicle are common in the young, athletic populations and are frequently high-energy sports injuries. It is this subgroup of patients with displaced and shortened midshaft fractures of the clavicle that often requires operative fixation.

In 2005, Zlowodzki et al. [9] found increasing age, fracture displacement, female gender, and fracture comminution to be associated with the development of nonunion and long-term sequelae after non-operative treatment. In 2006, Nowak et al. [10] found predictable risk factors including lack of osseous contact at fracture site, a transverse fracture, and increasing age that may cause complications in fracture healing and overall recovery and were considered to be indications for operative treatment. Studies of midshaft clavicle fractures with substantial shortening have reinforced these biomechanical findings by demonstrating higher patient satisfaction and improved functional outcomes after operative treatment. The traditional conservative protocol provides positive results in more than 90% of athletes treated with a figure-8 sling [11]. However, recent reports have discussed decreased union rates of displaced midshaft clavicular fractures treated non-operatively. Closed treatment may lead to significant deficits, whereas surgical management results in an earlier and more reliable return to full function [11, 12].

Displaced fractures of clavicle with shortening of 15 mm or more have better results with surgery. Operative fixation allows earlier rehabilitation with a high level of patient satisfaction with respect to shoulder function. Pain relief is faster and there is no need to use shoulder wraps. Rigid internal fixation may also allow patients to return to activities earlier. Reconstruction plates can be contoured best to the three-dimensional anatomy of the clavicle.

Operative management of clavicular fractures includes external fixation, intramedullary fixation, and osteosynthesis with plate and screws (Figs. 28.4 and 28.5).

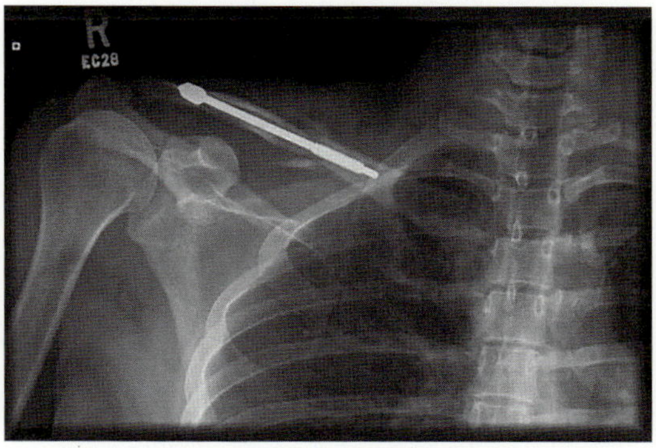

Fig. 28.4 Midshaft clavicle fracture with intramedullary fixation

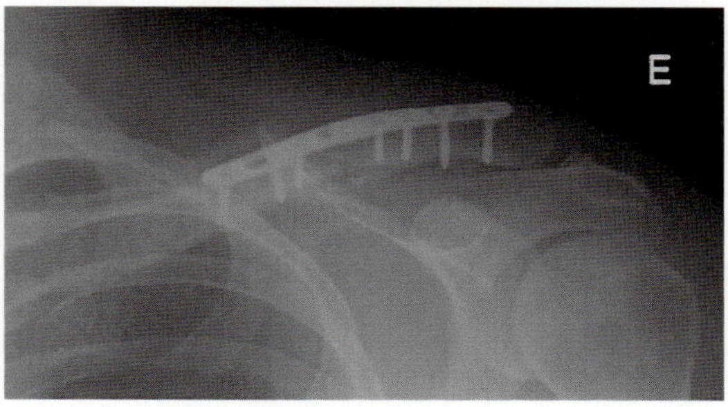

Fig. 28.5 Midshaft clavicle fracture fixed with plate and screws

With respect to displaced fractures, plating of 460 patients resulted in a nonunion rate of 2.2% compared with a nonunion rate of 15.1% in 159 patients treated non-operatively [13].

An athlete undergoing traditional treatment of a clavicular fracture would have been immobilized for 3–6 weeks before any range-of-motion exercises were started. However, in the past few years, more aggressive treatment protocols for clavicular fractures have become popular. Success rates of 94–100% with low rates of infections and complications have been reported with plate fixations of acute midshaft clavicular fractures [9]. Fixation with intramedullary nailing using titanium elastic nails has also evolved [13]. With surgical treatment and appropriate rehabilitation, athletes are able to return to competition at 6 weeks without compromising their health or safety [14, 15].

28.2.2 Distal Clavicle Fractures

The distal clavicle fractures (Group II of Allman) were divided into five subtypes according to the Neer classification modified by Craig [16]. Their classification is based on the location of the fracture in relation to the coracoclavicular ligament and their intactness (Fig. 28.6).

The Neer type I is a fracture lateral to the coracoclavicular ligament attachment, which has very minimal displacement. Type II is one which is medial to the ligament attachment. It is divided into IIA and IIB. In IIA both the conoid and the trapezoid ligaments are attached to the distal fragment, and in IIB the conoid is detached from the proximal fragment, while the trapezoid is attached to the distal fragment. Type III is one with intra-articular extension. Type IV occurs in

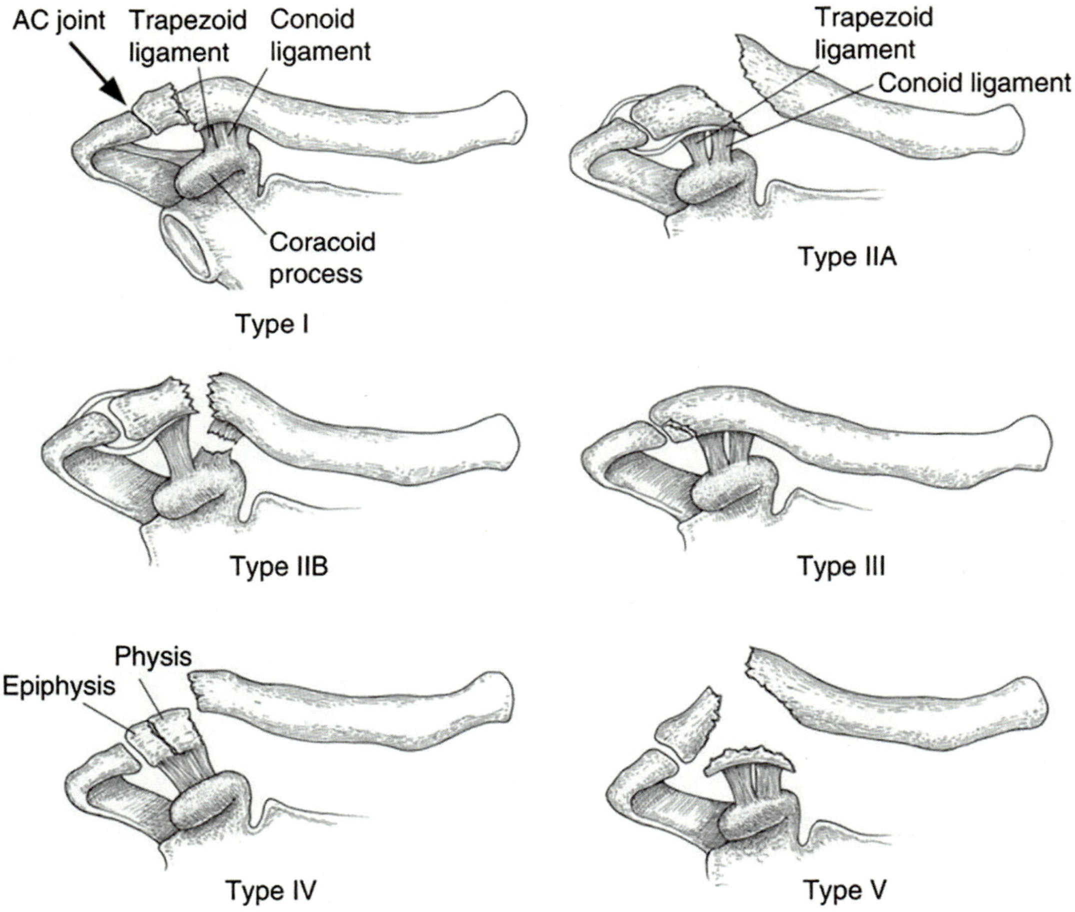

Fig. 28.6 Clavicle fractures Neer classification

children where a periosteal sleeve gets avulsed from the inferior cortex with the attached coracoclavicular ligament, and the medial fragment gets displaced upwards. Type V is similar to type II which involves an avulsion leaving behind an inferior cortical fragment attached to the coracoclavicular ligament. Types II and V are unstable, and there are many controversies about the best management.

The distal clavicle fractures accounts for 2.6–4% of the total adult fractures, more frequently seen in elderly females with osteoporotic bones than in young active adult. It can also happen as a football injury and may be remembered as differential diagnosis of acromioclavicular dislocations. Lateral end fracture constitutes 21–28% of all clavicle fractures, and of these 10–52% are displaced fractures. Till date there is no gold standard treatment recommendation for this injury. The unstable nature of these fractures makes them prone for nonunion and impeding normal shoulder function [17].

Treatment and outcome of the fracture of distal clavicle depends on displacement and injury to coracoclavicular ligament which makes the fracture unstable. Type 1 injuries are generally stable and not displaced and are managed conservatively with a sling to support the weight of the limb. Type 2 injuries are managed similarly but may lead to AC joint arthrosis which may deserve a distal clavicle resection. Type 4 is just a periosteal disruption in children, and bone fills the periosteal sleeve resulting in union and remodeling. The management of types 3 and 5 is the most controversial topic. Both being similar in instability and displacement can be considered together. Different treatment modalities are available for their management. Till date no gold standard technique has been described. The treatments available can be broadly divided into conservative management or rigid fixation such as osteosynthesis with locking plate (Fig. 28.7), hook plate fixation, fixation with a distal radius locking plate, coracoclavicular screws, or Knowles pin fixation. In addition, other treatment modalities are simple K-wire fixation, tension band wiring, suture anchors, vicryl tape, or Dacron arterial graft for coracoclavicular ligament reconstruction.

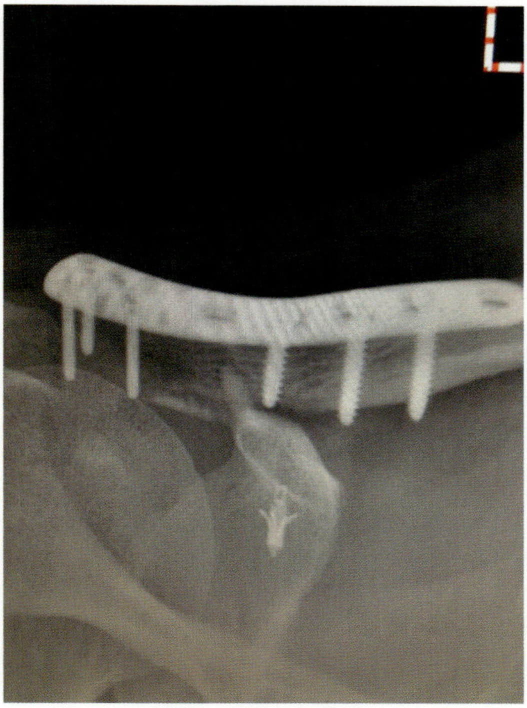

Fig. 28.7 Distal clavicle fixation with locking plate and suture anchors for coracoclavicular ligament reconstruction

28.2.3 Medial Clavicle Fractures

Fractures of the medial third of the clavicle are rare and constitute only 2–4% of all clavicle fractures [18]. These fractures have traditionally been treated non- operatively, even when they are significantly displaced with intervention classically being reserved for open fractures or fractures with neurovascular compromise [19].

However, non-operative treatment of these fractures can lead to poor functional outcomes and symptomatic, painful nonunions. Some studies reported an overall nonunion rate approaching 15%, and others stated that up to half of patients are symptomatic a year after injury [20]. Displaced fractures of the medial clavicle are uncommon. A fracture is considered to be displaced when displacement is more than 10 mm. Some authors have advocated non-operative treatment for these fractures; however, many case reports described complications when these fractures had been treated conservatively or missed [20]. When needed, the surgical treatment has demonstrated good results and full return to normal activities and sports. These goals are achieved after bone union which usually takes from 6 weeks to 4 months [21]. Oe et al. reported excellent functional outcomes for ten patients who underwent operative fixation of a displaced, periarticular medial-end clavicle fracture [22].

28.3 Proximal Humerus Fractures

Proximal humerus fractures are the seventh most frequent fracture in adults and the third in patients over 65 following wrist and femoral neck fractures. Approximately 5% of all fractures are fractures of the proximal humerus [23]. The mechanisms of these fractures can be classified as direct or indirect. The high impact during the football games leads to a higher proportion of direct fractures involving a direct impact along the shaft of the humerus in a traditionally high-energy non-axial force vector.

Although around 80% of the fractures may be treated conservatively, we have to consider the high demand and need of early return when treating football athletes. When surgical therapy is considered, early intervention can minimize the development of functional deficits, though the decision for surgical repair is also based on imaging findings, patient age, bone quality, rotator cuff status, fracture severity, and premorbid health [23].

The Neer classification remains the most commonly used system [24] and is based on six groups and four main fracture segments comprising the head, greater tuberosity, lesser tuberosity, and shaft (Fig. 28.8).

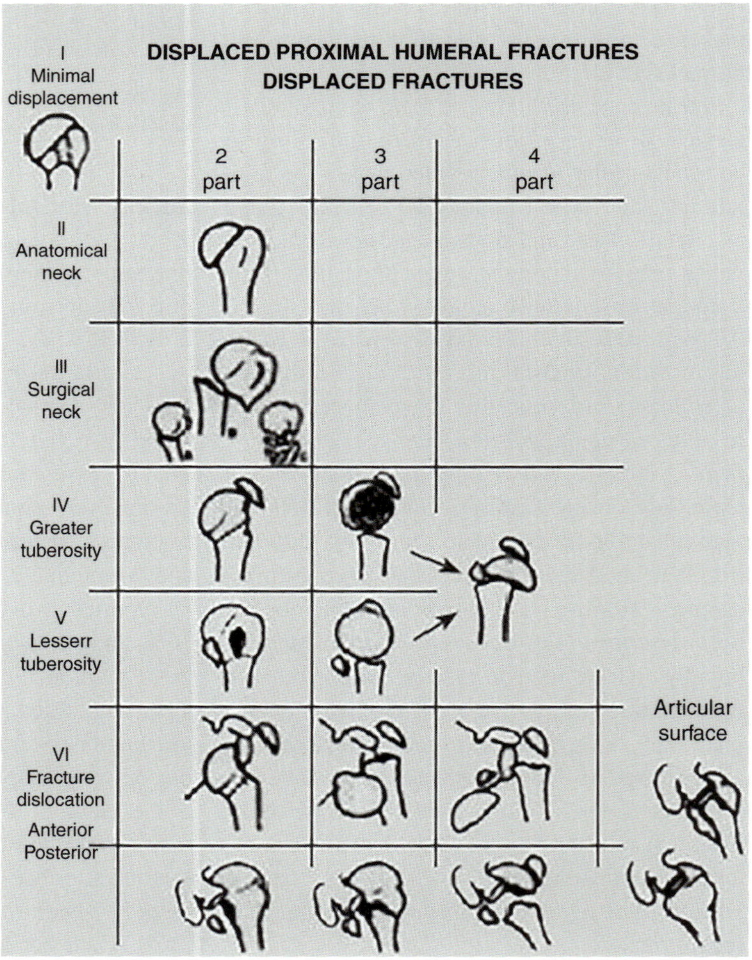

Fig. 28.8 Neer classification

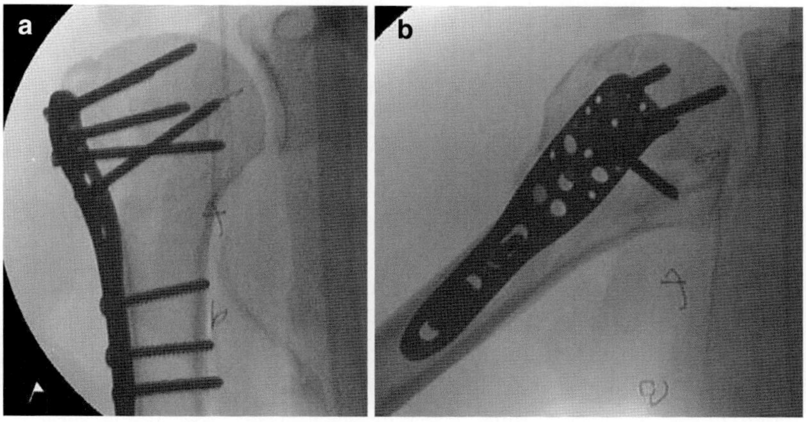

Fig. 28.9 Proximal humeral fixation with locking plate (**a**) Anteroposterior view (**b**) Anteroposterior view with internal rotation

Displacement is defined as more than 1 cm of translation or 45% of angulation. Group I includes all fracture configurations with minimum displacement and is treated conservatively. Group II includes two-part fractures of the anatomical neck with articular-segment displacement. Two-part fractures involving the surgical neck and lesser tuberosity can be treated conservatively if displaced less than 66% but are often best treated surgically. Treatment of two-part greater tuberosity fractures is often more aggressive, and surgery is usually recommended for fragment displacement greater than 3 mm in active younger patients, athletes, and people who engage in routine overhead activity. Group III comprises three types of displaced two-part surgical neck fractures with shaft displacement. Group IV consists of two- or three-part fractures with greater tuberosity displacement. Group V includes two- or three-part fractures with lesser tuberosity displacement. Groups IV and V merge in the four-part fracture where both tuberosities are displaced in addition to the head and shaft. Group VI comprises true fracture-dislocation of two-, three-, or four-part fractures with ligamentous injury and is subdivided into anterior and posterior dislocations of the glenohumeral joint and partial dislocations of the humeral head with articular surface fractures.

Conservative treatment generally consists of analgesia and a period of immobilization in a sling, followed by rehabilitation and physiotherapy. Complications encountered with closed treatment include malunion, subacromial impingement, avascular necrosis, shoulder pain, and stiffness secondary to osteoarthritis and rotator cuff deficiency. Most conservatively treated fractures will progress to full union with an estimated risk of nonunion between 1.1% and 10%.

The Neer three- and four-part fracture configurations are associated with less optimal results than one- or two-part fractures and fortunately are less common in younger patients. Seventy percent of all three- and four-part fractures are seen in patients aged over 60 years and 50% in patients aged over 70 years. With regards to the athletes, these fractures are best treated with open reduction and internal fixation (Fig. 28.9).

Operative interventions for the management of proximal humerus fractures may be generally classified into reconstructive procedures and prosthetic replacements. In high-demand young patients, reconstruction followed by close monitoring should be the first option. In the event of failure, early conversion to hemiarthroplasty remains a valuable alternative. Intraoperatively, the surgeon may find fractures that are not feasible for internal fixation, and they need to be converted to hemiarthroplasty. An adequate preoperative planning is necessary to be prepared for these demanding scenarios [25].

28.4 Humeral Shaft Fracture

Humeral shaft fractures account for about 5% of all fractures and are the third most common type of long bone fracture. They almost exclusively occur in young people following a high-energy trauma or older people following low-energy trauma. Many of these fractures are still being treated conservatively using functional (Sarmiento) bracing or a hanging arm cast. When these fractures are treated nonsurgically, union is obtained in an average of 10 weeks, making the humerus a well-suited bone for conservative treatment. This extended time usually is considered too long for athletes and young active people. Surgery allows them to quickly return to their activities. The goal of surgical treatment is to obtain anatomical reduction, while providing stability that allows for early mobilization of adjacent joints. It has its place in multi-fracture patients, open fractures, failed conservative treatment, and obese patients or those who refuse to comply with the inconveniences of conservative treatment with a hanging arm cast for 6 weeks, while accepting the risk associated with surgery (nonunion, secondary radial nerve palsy).

Surgical approaches to the humeral shaft include:

- Anterolateral approach: preferred for proximal third humeral shaft fractures. Radial nerve is identified in the interval between the brachialis and brachioradialis and traced proximally. This can be extended proximally to the shoulder or distally to the elbow
- Anterior approach: muscular interval between the biceps and brachialis muscles
- Posterior approach: provides excellent exposure to most of the humerus but cannot be extended proximally to the shoulder, muscular interval between the lateral and long heads of the triceps

When the surgical treatment is indicated, fixation can be obtained with a plate, intramedullary nailing, or an external fixator. The average nonunion rate in published studies was 4.4% for conservative treatment, 2.8% for plating, 6.3% for bundle nailing, 5.9% for locked IM nails, and 3.5% for external fixation [26].

- Plate and screw fixation of the fracture results in union in 11–19 weeks. This is associated with the best functional results. It allows direct fracture reduction and stable fixation of the humeral shaft without violation of the rotator cuff. A 4.5-mm dynamic compression plate with fixation of eight to ten cortices proximal and distal to the fracture is used. Lag interfragmentary compression screws should be utilized wherever possible. One should preserve soft tissue attachments to butterfly fragments
- Anterograde or retrograde locked intramedullary nailing requires knowledge of nailing techniques and regional anatomy to avoid the complications associated with the technique. Union is obtained in 10–15 weeks. It is preferably indicated for segmental fractures in which plate placement would require considerable soft tissue dissection, humerus fractures in extremely osteopenic bone, and pathologic humerus fractures. Antegrade humeral nailing is associated with a high incidence of postoperative shoulder pain (Fig. 28.10)

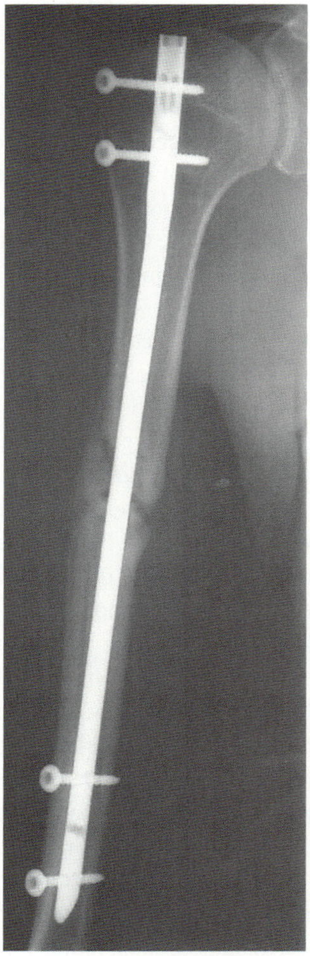

Fig. 28.10 Humeral shaft fixation (A) anterograde intramedullary interlocked nailing

- External fixation: indicated for infected nonunions, burn patients with fractures, or open fractures with extensive soft tissue loss. Complications include pin tract infection, neurovascular injury, and nonunion

Conclusion

The treatment of fractures in athletes needs a comprehensive approach. The first step is pain control, followed by the correct treatment option and lastly the recovery of motion, strength, and neuromuscular control. Sport-specific functional rehabilitation is very important and has to be tailored to each athlete. Special attention should be given on neuromuscular control of the kinetic chain, starting from core stability and progressing from the proximal to the distal segment. The kinetic chain as the main power generator for the upper limb must be recovered. The last phase and one of the most important is the on-field rehabilitation to give the footballer full skill control and self-confidence in playing. The complete process of functional recovery including surgery and rehabilitation takes the injured players 2–6 months out of the game depending on the severity of the lesion and individual factors.

References

1. Longo UG, Loppini M, Berton A, Martinelli N, Maffulli N, Denaro V. Shoulder injuries in soccer players. Clin Cases Miner Bone Metab. 2012;9:138–41.
2. Junge A, Dvořák J. Football injuries during the 2014 FIFA World Cup. Br J Sports Med. 2015;49:599–602.
3. Junge A, Dvorak J. Injury surveillance in the World Football Tournaments 1998–2012. Br J Sports Med. 2013;47:782–8.
4. Halpern B, Thompson N, Curl WW, Andrews JR, Hunter SC, Boring JR. High school football injuries: identifying the risk factors. Am J Sports Med. 1987;15:316–20.
5. Goss TP, Owens BD. Fractures of the scapula. In: Rockwood CA, editor. The shoulder. Philadelphia: Saunders/Elsevier; 2009. p. 333–80.
6. Goss TP. Fractures of the glenoid cavity. J Bone Joint Surg Am. 1992;74:299–305.
7. Kuhn JE, Blasier RB, Carpenter JE. Fractures of the acromion process: a proposed classification system. J Orthop Trauma. 1994;8(1):6–13.
8. Khan LA, Bradnock TJ, Scott C, Robinson CM. Fractures of the clavicle. J Bone Joint Surg Am. 2009;91:447–60.
9. Zlowodzki M, Zelle BA, Cole PA, Jeray K, Mckee MD. Evidence-based orthopaedic trauma working group. Treatment of midshaft clavicle fractures: systematic review of 2144 fractures: on behalf of evidence-based orthopaedic trauma working group. J Orthop Trauma. 2005;19:504–7.
10. Nowak J, Holgersson M, Larsson S. Can we predict long term sequelae after fractures of the clavicle based on initial findings? A prospective study with nine to ten years of follow up. J Shoulder Elbow Surg. 2004;13:479–86.
11. Robinson CM, Court-Brown CM, McQueen MM, Wakefield AE. Estimating the risk of nonunion following nonoperative treatment of a clavicular fracture. J Bone Joint Surg Am. 2004;86:1359–65.
12. Hill JM, McGuire MH, Crosby LA. Closed treatment of displaced middle-third fractures of the clavicle gives poor results. J Bone Joint Surg Br. 1997;79:537–9.
13. Smekal V, Irenberger A, Struve P, Wambacher M, Krappinger D, Kralinger FS. Elastic stable intramedullary nailing versus non- operative treatment of displaced midshaft clavicular fractures: a randomized, controlled, clinical trial. J Orthop Trauma. 2009;23:106–12.
14. Choudhari P, Chhabra. Displaced mid-shaft clavicle fractures: a subset for surgical treatment. Malays Orthop J. 2014;8:1–5.
15. Meisterling SW, Cain EL, Fleisig GS, Hartzell JL, Dugas JR. Return to athletic activity after plate fixation of displaced midshaft clavicle fractures. Am J Sports Med. 2013;41:2632–6.
16. Craig EV. Fractures of the clavicle. In: Rockwood Jr CA, Matsen III FA, editors. The shoulder. Philadelphia: WB Saunders; 1990. p. 367–401.
17. Sambandam B, Gupta R, Kumar S, Maini L. Fracture of distal end clavicle: a review. J Clin Orthop Trauma. 2014;5:65–73.
18. Postacchini F, Gumina S, De Santis P, Albo F. Epidemiology of clavicle fractures. J Shoulder Elbow Surg. 2002;11:452–6.
19. Throckmorton T, Kuhn JE. Fractures of the medial end of the clavicle. J Shoulder Elbow Surg. 2007;16:49–54.
20. Jain S, Monbaliu D, Thompson JF. Thoracic outlet syndrome caused by chronic retrosternal dislocation of the clavicle. Successful treatment by transaxillary resection of the first rib. J Bone Joint Surg Br. 2002;84:116–8.
21. Sidhu VS, Hermans D, Duckworth DG. The operative outcomes of displaced medial-end clavicle fractures. J Shoulder Elbow Surg. 2015;24:1728–34.
22. Oe K, Gaul L, Hierholzer C, Woltmann A, Miwa M, Kurosaka M, Buehren V. Operative management of periarticular medial clavicle fractures-report of 10 cases. J Trauma. 2011;72:E1–7.
23. Bohsali KI, Wirth MA. Fractures of the proximal humerus. In: Rockwood CA, Matsen FA, Wirth MA, Lippitt SB, editors. The shoulder. 4th ed. Philadelphia: Saunders/Elsevier; 2009. p. 455–97.

24. Neer II. CS. Displaced proximal humeral fractures. Part 1. Classification and evaluation. J Bone Joint Surg Am. 1970;52:1077–89.
25. Vachtsevanos L, Hayden L, Desai AS, Dramis A. Management of proximal humerus fractures in adults. World J Orthop. 2014;5:685–93.
26. Paris H, Tropiano P, Clouet D'Orval B, Chaudet H, Poitout D-G. Fractures diaphysaires de l'humérus: ostéosynthèse systématique par plaque: résultats anatomiques et fonctionnels d'une série de 156 cas et revue de la littérature. Rev Chir Orthop. 2000;86: 346–59.

Traumatic Lesions of the Elbow and Wrist

29

Ricardo Bastos, Miguel Trigueiros, Nuno Sevivas, and Luigi Pederzini

Contents

R. Bastos, MD, PhD (✉)
Fluminense Federal University, Niterói, Rio de Janeiro, Brazil

Dom Henrique Research Centre, Porto, Portugal

Clínica do Dragão, Espregueira-Mendes Sports Centre - FIFA Medical Centre of Excellence, Estádio do Dragão, Porto, Portugal

M. Trigueiros
Orthophysiatrics department HSA_CHP Porto, Pathology of the Hand/Wrist and Elbow Unit, Porto, Portugal

Hospital de Santa Maria, Porto, Portugal

Invited professor at the Sports Medicine Postgraduation, Faculdade de Medicina Universidade do Porto, Porto, Portugal

N. Sevivas
Life and Health Sciences Research Institute (ICVS), School of Medicine, University of Minho, Campus de Gualtar, 4710–057 Braga, Portugal

ICVS/3B's - PT Government Associate Laboratory, Braga/Guimarães, Portugal

Orthopaedics department, Hospital de Braga and Hospital Privado de Braga, Braga, Portugal

Clínica do Dragão, Espregueira-Mendes Sports Centre - FIFA Medical Centre of Excellence, Estádio do Dragão, Porto, Portugal

L. Pederzini, MD
Orthopaedic and Arthroscopic Department, New Sassuolo Hospital, via F. Ruini, 2, 41049 Sassuolo, Modena, Italy

29.1 Introduction

Football is a sport characterized by physical contact, which explains the high rate of musculoskeletal injuries in players described in the literature. The most common injuries are lower limb injuries (69–88%) [1–4], but there has also been a recent increase in the rate of upper limb injuries associated with football [5, 6]. A small but significant proportion of injuries occur in the upper limb (6%), a large percentage of which affect goalkeepers (often in the thumb, 9%) [7]. Among the other players, however, there is a disturbing incidence of acute traumas due to falls. These injuries tend to affect the elbows, wrists, and hands and are sustained predominantly by players in the full-back, center-forward, and center-half positions. Outfield players are prone to acute lesions (bruises, lacerations, and sprains), whereas fractures and dislocations are less common. Despite its grass covering, the football field is hard. Players sometimes fall from a height of 2–3 m directly onto the ground and often use the upper limbs to deaden the impact.

J. Espregueira-Mendes et al. (eds.), *Injuries and Health Problems in Football*, DOI 10.1007/978-3-662-53924-8_29

These falls can be very traumatic. The upper limb receives all of the axial forces, causing indirect traumas with resultant injuries to the shoulder, elbow, and wrist. As mentioned above, although not common, fractures and dislocations are possible. These injuries must be diagnosed quickly as they represent a serious risk to the player.

This chapter discusses the main injuries involving the elbow and wrist encountered in football players.

29.2 Traumatic Lesions of the Elbow

The most common traumatic lesions of the elbow are sprains. Serious injuries due to contact with the ground are unlikely, and football players do not wear the elbow pads used in other sports. However, there are rare instances of capitulum humeri lesions due to abnormal falls with the hand in a defensive attitude, as well as isolated olecranon fractures.

29.2.1 Elbow Dislocation

29.2.1.1 Anatomy

The elbow may be described as a "modified hinge" joint (ginglymotrochoid) composed of three articulations: ulnohumeral (hinge), radiohumeral (rotation), and proximal radioulnar (rotation). The bone structure associated with the ligament complex, tendons, and muscles gives the joint excellent stability.

29.2.1.2 Mechanism of Injury

Posterior dislocation is the most common type of elbow injury. These injuries occur due to contact with an opponent when running or to a fall after heading the ball. There are three possible mechanisms of dislocation:

1. Levering force that unlocks the olecranon, combined with loading that causes complete dislocation
2. Direct injury to the elbow, although dislocation is often caused indirectly by a fall onto the palm of the hand with the arm extended and retroposed; the combination of elbow extension, arm abduction, and forearm supination results in soft tissue injury to the capsule, collateral ligaments, and musculature (posterior type dislocation)
3. Direct force at the posterior forearm, with the elbow in the flexed position (anterior type dislocation). Deformity, functional impairment, and pain require radiographic confirmation and immediate dislocation reduction

29.2.1.3 Diagnosis

Elbow dislocation is often evident on inspection. Deformity, pain, and functional impairment indicate dislocation, but confirmation is required by radiography (anteroposterior and lateral views). Oblique views are helpful to determine periarticular bone fragments.

Magnetic resonance imaging (MRI) and computed tomography (CT) scans can be indicated in cases of articular fractures, osteochondral fragments, and for evaluation of the interosseous membrane.

29.2.1.4 Classification

Based on the relationship between the radius and ulna and the distal humerus, dislocations can be classified as posterior, posterolateral (90% of dislocations), posteromedial, lateral, medial, anterior, or divergent (rare).

29.2.1.5 Associated Injuries

As mentioned above, the elbow is a very stable joint due to the particular characteristics of its bone structure, ligaments, tendons, and muscle. A dislocation caused by a fall requires application of a major levering force, which often leads to serious associated injuries that must be screened for rapid diagnosis and treatment. These injuries can be neurological, vascular, or fractural.

1. Vascular

The brachial artery is at risk in falls. During dislocation, collateral circulation is often disrupted; prompt recognition of this is essential.

Radial and brachial pulses must be investigated, and closed reduction to reestablish perfusion is indicated.

In cases of suspected vascular injury, angiography to identify the lesion may be needed, and arterial reconstruction with reverse saphenous vein graft should be considered.

2. Neurological

The median nerve can be injured by stretching or entrapment following closed reduction. Ulnar and anterior interosseous nerves may also be affected. Neurological deficits at the time of the injury should be observed, and spontaneous recovery may be expected. Any decline in nerve function after reduction should be explored and decompressed as necessary.

3. Fractural

Associated fractures are not rare. Several bone complexes, including the radial read (5–11%), medial or lateral epicondyle (12–24%), and coronoid process (5–10%), can be subject to fracture.

29.2.1.6 Treatment

Elbow dislocation is highly traumatic for the athlete, as well as team supporters and anyone else witnessing the event. This is a very painful and disabling lesion, necessitating removal of the player from the field regardless of their importance to the team and match situation. A reduction maneuver should never be performed before proper clinical and radiological evaluation. Dislocation reduction on the field is a "shot in the dark," because there is no way to predict associated fractures, or nerve and vascular injuries. The player must be removed from the field after temporary immobilization. Radiological and clinical evaluations are required before any reduction maneuver, which should be performed under intravenous sedation or general or regional anesthesia. The elbow is flexed during distal traction (posterior dislocation). Reassessment of neurovascular status, range of motion (ROM), and stability is required, and postreduction radiography is mandatory.

29.2.1.7 Postreduction Management

After evaluation of stability, a posterior splint at 90° with loose circumferential wraps can be used, and a return of gentle ROM is associated with better results. Prolonged immobilization leads to unsatisfactory results and larger flexion contracture.

A hinged elbow brace allowing a stable arc of motion is applied in cases of instability without associated fractures.

Full recovery of motion and strength requires 3–7 months.

29.2.1.8 Complications

Complications include recurrent pain, loss of extension, neurological/vascular injuries, instability and redislocation, ectopic calcification, heterotopic bone or myositis ossificans, and compartment syndrome (Volkmann's contracture).

29.3 Traumatic Lesions of the Wrist

The wrist and its many bones are common sites of sprains, lunate dislocations, and scaphoid fractures, usually due to falling with the hand in a defensive attitude. Distal radius fractures are serious but uncommon lesions that are related to falls in which the hand is in a flexed or extended position.

29.3.1 Distal Radius Fractures

29.3.1.1 Anatomy

The metaphysis of the radius is composed primarily of cancellous bone with thin cortices. Eighty percent of the radial load is supported by the distal radius, with the remaining 20% supported by the ulna and triangular fibrocartilage complex. These anatomical characteristics render the radius susceptible to fractures if subjected to axial and shear forces.

29.3.1.2 Mechanism of Injury

Distal radius fractures are usually due to falling with the hand in a defensive attitude. The fracture will show different characteristics depending on the hand position (flexed, extended, pronated, or supinated). The most common mechanism of injury is falling with the hand at 40–90° extension. Biomechanically, injuries may be characterized by bending (metaphysis fail in tension – Colles' and Smith's fractures), compression (fracture of the articular surface with impaction of subchondral and metaphyseal bone – "die-punch" fracture), avulsion fracture, shearing (fracture of the articular surface – Barton's fracture), or any combination of the above.

29.3.1.3 Clinical Evaluation

Distal radius fracture is characterized by pain, swelling, and bruising of the wrist.

29.3.1.4 Radiographic Evaluation

Normal radioulnar and radiocarpal joints have a number of characteristics that must be well understood to analyze a radiograph.

1. Radial inclination: average = 23° (range: 13–30°)
2. Radial length: average = 13 mm (range: 8–18 mm)
3. Volar tilt: average = 11°(range: 1–21°)
4. Ulnar variance: 0–2 mm

Radiological evaluation consists of four views:

1. Posteroanterior view
2. Lateral view
3. Oblique with 45°pronation (evaluation of the radial styloid)
4. Oblique with 45°supination (dorsomedial cortex)

29.3.1.5 Fracture Patterns

Colles' Fracture

Colles' fracture accounts for more than 90% of distal radius fractures. The original description was of extraarticular fracture. The mechanism of injury involves falling on a hyperextended, radially deviated wrist with the forearm in pronation.

Smith's Fracture

Smith's fractures occur due to falling with the wrist flexed and the forearm fixed in supination.

Barton's Fracture and Smith II Fracture

Barton's fracture and Smith II fracture, which involve subluxation of the wrist, are caused by falling on the extended wrist with the forearm fixed in pronation. Barton's fracture is intra-articular and can be classified as dorsal or volar, depending on the hand position; volar Barton's fracture is the most common type.

Radial Styloid Fracture

Eponyms: "chauffeur's fracture," "backfire fracture," "Hutchinson's fracture"

The mechanism of injury in radial styloid fracture is compression of the scaphoid against the styloid with the wrist in dorsiflexion and ulnar deviation, causing an avulsion fracture.

Lunate Die-Punch Fracture

These are fractures of the pyramidal fossae caused by an axial force.

29.3.1.6 Associated Injuries

Scapholunate ligament: 30%

Lunotriquetral ligament: 15%

Median nerve compression

29.3.1.7 Treatment

In cases of injury to football players, a number of factors must be taken into consideration before choosing the best treatment. One such factor is the necessity of returning to sport. Therefore, surgical management is often preferred. Internal fixation with plates allows direct fixation of articular fragments, early mobilization, and satisfactory ROM and eliminates the need for plaster immobilization or casts.

29.3.1.8 Closed Reduction Maneuver and Immobilization

Closed reduction may be attempted immediately for pain relief and temporary immobilization. This procedure is performed in two steps. First, light traction is applied by hand, to exacerbate the mechanism of fracture and deformity, to produce a levering force with the bone cortex acting as a pivot. Then, movement opposite to the fracture mechanism is affected. Immobilization is performed with the wrist at 30° flexion.

29.3.2 Other Injuries of the Wrist

29.3.2.1 Scaphoid Fracture

The scaphoid is the most commonly fractured carpal bone.

The mechanism of injury involves falling on the outstretched hand, which imposes a force of extension, ulnar deviation, and intercarpal supination.

Other possible sites of injury include the hook of hamate, capitate fractures, and carpal dislocations.

Conclusion

Injury to the upper limb in football is uncommon, accounting for approximately 6% of all injuries. The most common mechanism of injury involves falling over with the arm in a defensive position, which can lead to indirect fracture or dislocation. Direct traumas are rare. Elbow dislocation represents an emergency situation that requires immediate reduction under anesthesia immediately after radiological and clinical evaluation.

Distal radius fracture is a serious injury that must be treated by an orthopedic surgeon. Surgical treatment should be considered even in cases of stable fracture to allow a rapid return to sport.

References

1. Cohen M, Abdalla RJ, Ejnisman B, Amaro JT. Lesões ortopédicas no futebol. Revista Brasileira de Ortopedia (São Paulo, Dez). 1997;32(12):940–4.
2. Silva AA. Estudo epidemiológico das lesões no futebol profissional e propostas de medidas preventivas. In: I Premio INDESP de literatura desportiva, vol. 2. Brasília; 1999.
3. Sizínio H. Ortopedia e traumatologia: princípios e prática. 3rd ed. Porto Alegre: Artmed; 2003.
4. Bulhões JRS, Simão AP, Pinto KNZ, Navega MT, Rosa SMGM, Avaliação Isocinética da Performace Funcional dos Músculos Quadríceps e Isquiotibiais de Jogadores Profissionais de Futebol. Fisioterapia Brasil; Volume 8; Número 1;p. 04–8; jan/fev. 2007.
5. Schmith-Olsen S, Jorgensen U, Kaalund S, Sorensen J. Injuries among young soccer players. Am J Sports Med. 1991;19:273–5.
6. Volpi P. Soccer injury epidemiology. J Sports Traumatol. 2000;22:123–31.
7. Hunt M, Fulford S. Amateur soccer: injuries in relation to field position. Br J Sports Med. 1990; 24:4–265.

Shoulder Instability

30

Nuno Gomes, Nuno Sevivas, Pietro Randelli,
and Marc Safran

Contents

N. Gomes (✉)
Hospital Forças Armadas – Polo do Porto,
Av. Boavista, 4050-112 Porto, Portugal

Hospital CUF Porto, Estrada da Circunvalação
14341, 4100-180 Porto, Portugal
e-mail: andresampaio@yahoo.com

N. Sevivas
Life and Health Sciences Research Institute (ICVS),
School of Health Sciences, University of Minho,
Campus de Gualtar, 4710-057 Braga, Portugal

Orthopaedics Department, Hospital de Braga,
Braga, Portugal

Clínica do Dragão, Espregueira-Mendes Sports
Centre - FIFA Medical Centre of Excellence, Porto,
Portugal

ICVS/3B's–PT Government Associate Laboratory,
Braga/Guimarães, Braga, Portugal
e-mail: nunosevivas@gmail.com

30.1 Introduction

Shoulder injuries in football are a lot less common than those involving the lower limb, due to the characteristics of the game, with more than four out of five injuries located in the lower extremities [1–5].

Medical reports from the Olympics and FIFA tournaments [6–12] have shown that the rate of shoulder injuries is low, ranging from 2% to 13% [11]: 3.8% at the 2004 Olympic games in Athens [10] and 4.4% during the Euro 2004 [9].

The consequences of an injury to the shoulder vary based on the specific injury or the player's position, whether he is a goalkeeper or a field player. Unlike for the lower extremity, little has been published regarding the incidence, nature, and time loss for injuries to the upper limb in football.

Ekstrand et al. [1] prospectively studied 57 male European elite football teams over a 10-year period from 2001 to 2011, registering 11,750 injuries. Out of this total, 355 (3%) affected the upper

P. Randelli
Dipartimento di Scienze Biomediche per la Salute,
Università degli Studi di Milano, Milan, Italy

U.O. Ortopedia 2, IRCCS Policlinico San Donato,
Milan, Italy
e-mail: pietro.randelli@unimi.it

M. Safran
Professor of Sports Medicine and Arthroscopy,
Department of Orthopaedic Surgery, Stanford School
of Medicine, Stanford, CA, 94063 USA
e-mail: msafran@stanford.edu

J. Espregueira-Mendes et al. (eds.), *Injuries and Health Problems in Football*,
DOI 10.1007/978-3-662-53924-8_30

extremities and nearly half of these (197, 1.7%) involved the shoulder girdle/clavicle. In general, a football team with 25 players can expect 1-2 upper extremity injuries each season, as compared to 40–45 injuries to the lower extremity.

The same author defined a severe injury as one where an athlete misses more than 28 days. Ekstrand et al. [2] reported that for the most common injuries in football, those involving the hip and groin, only 11% were classified as severe, resulting in greater than 28 days of absence from play. On the other hand, however, those authors reported that 28% of shoulder injuries were severe, stressing the epidemiologic importance of shoulder lesions despite its overall low incidence.

Specific to upper extremity injuries, Ekstrand et al. [1] found that the two most common injuries (25% altogether) were acromioclavicular joint sprains and shoulder dislocations. The latter was associated with the longest time away from sport and the highest recurrence rate of the six most common injury types, with an average of 41 days of absence and 32% reinjury rate. The time away from full training and matches was twice as long for goalkeepers as for other position players, reflecting the importance of shoulder function for those. Almost one-third (32%) of shoulder dislocations were recurrent injuries, which seems to be high in such a population with access to the best rehabilitation care, suggesting a need for improved functional assessment before letting the athlete back to play after this injury.

Furthermore, Ekstrand found that 90% of upper limb injuries were traumatic, while only 10% derived from overuse, mainly affecting the rotator cuff.

Considering the player position, he also demonstrated what seemed obvious: upper limb injuries were five times more common in goalkeepers than in field players, which is in contrast with injuries overall. The percentage of all injuries that affected the upper extremity was consistently higher among goalkeepers (18%) compared to outfield players (2%) ($p < 0.005$), resulting in more days away from sport for the former. He noted that the consequences of upper limb injuries were more serious for goalkeepers, concluding that focusing on their prevention would be of significant benefit.

30.2 Shoulder Instability

Shoulder instability can present in different ways, and it is commonly accepted they fit into three different major patterns, based on their etiology and treatment:

1. TUBS: Traumatic, Unidirectional, associated with a Bankart lesion that frequently requires Surgery
2. AMBRI: Atraumatic, Multidirectional, usually Bilateral and requiring Rehabilitation or, when it fails, a surgical Inferior capsular shift
3. AIOS: Acquired Instability from Overstress, such as in the case of throwing athletes, usually requiring Surgery (also often called GUTS – Genetically predisposed, Unidirectional, micro-Traumatic, often requiring Surgery – by some authors)

This simple classification, however, does not cover all the pathological conditions related to shoulder instability. In order to fill this gap, Kuhn et al. in 2010 [13, 14] developed the FEDS system, an acronym that stands for Frequency, Etiology, Direction, and Severity of the instability, the four elements it considers. The proceedings of the ISAKOS Upper Extremity Committees 2009–2013 [15] further added the anatomic lesions as another element and proposed the modified FEDS classification for shoulder instability (Table 30.1). It is a very comprehensive system that aims gathering all types of instability but still needs definitive validation.

Instability from overuse is classically associated with overhead activity and that is why most literature on shoulder lesions in sports refer to those activities where overhead motion and shoulder injuries are more common, such as American football or baseball, with less attention to football. Shoulder instability in overhead athletes can be considered unique entities among shoulder lesions and have therefore deserved a particular attention from researchers, many of whom from countries where overhead sports are more popular than football. We believe that shoulder instability in the setting of football demands specific concentration as well.

The game of modern football has been characterized by increasing intensity and a growing number of legal and illegal physical contact, where

Table 30.1 The modified FEDS classification for shoulder instability [15]

Direction	Etiology	Severity	Frequency	Anatomic lesion[a]
Anterior	Traumatic	Pain[b]	Single episode	Capsule
Posterior	Required reduction	Subluxations	2–5 times	Labrum
Inferior	Never required reduction	Dislocations	>5 times	Bone
	Atraumatic	Locked	Locked	
	Involuntary			
	Positional			
	Habitual			
	Repetitive microtrauma[b]			

[a]As determined by either preoperative imaging studies (CT arthrogram, MRI, etc.) or intraoperative findings. A capsular lesion is diagnosed only if there are no labral avulsions or glenoid bone defects associated with the instability
[b]Only applicable to shoulder instability in the overhead and throwing athlete

tackling and collisions are common – factors leading to an increase in traumatic injuries [6]. As a result, though football has not classically been considered a collision sport, it clearly is a contact sport. As such shoulder instability in this environment fits in the traumatic category in its large majority.

30.3 The Emergency Setting

The approach to a case of shoulder instability in football obviously depends on the setting – including player position, whether it is a first-time or recurrent dislocation, time in the season, etc. Literature is scarce on this subject, and, as far as our research could find, it is nearly nonexistent concerning the emergency setting, with no clear guidelines for treatment.

A comprehensive search using PUBMED with the words "shoulder," "dislocation," "prehospital," and "treatment" identified only four articles: one clinical case [16], two similar reports on interscalene brachial plexus block [17, 18], and a recent study on the management of shoulder dislocation in the prehospital environment [19]. The latter is, in fact, the only one that is close to addressing that major question that may arise with any club's medical team when a sportsman with a shoulder dislocation is sustained during a match or training session: should the shoulder be reduced immediately (on the sideline or in the training room) or should that be done in a hospital environment by an orthopedic surgeon, after an X-ray evaluation to rule out a fracture and confirm the diagnosis?

The reality is that the prehospital treatment of shoulder dislocations is influenced by a few unfavorable factors [19]. The incidence is low among all sports emergencies, meaning its treatment is not routine and only a few physicians have the clinical expertise for the best approach. These observations lead to the question whether prehospital reduction of a dislocated shoulder is absolutely necessary or not.

Helfen et al. [19], in an assessment of 70 patients that were subject to prehospital reduction by emergency physicians in 16 rescue stations in Germany and Austria over 12 months, concluded that such reduction is possible but not obligatory. The knowledge and skill to perform the reduction was acceptable among all physicians regardless of the medical speciality – most were surgeons or anesthesiologists but also internists and general practitioners – although the surgeons were the quickest. Further, there were no documented neurovascular lesions resulting from the attempts and all identified neurological deficits recovered after reduction. The authors found these to be clear arguments in favor of the effectiveness of prehospital reduction by any doctor.

Guidelines for the best technique are lacking, but recommendations from the British College of Emergency Medicine in 2014 [20] suggest that the first attempt of reduction should be within 2 h (75%) and 3 h (90%) of arrival. One should bear in mind these consensus-based standards include pain management and an X-ray within 60 min. of arrival to the emergency department, conditions not necessarily met during a match or training session. However, the bottom line is reduction should take place as fast as possible as delays to first reduction attempt either from the time of injury or within the ED are associated with lower reduction success rates due to muscle spasms and pain [21,

22] and also with potential sequelae. Particularly in one of this chapter's author's experience, the ability to reduce the shoulder is much easier in the first few minutes after dislocation, frequently not requiring pain medication to relax the patient, a finding also supported by the literature [21]. There are no strict criteria for a mandatory reduction in the prehospital setting so it seems clear that good common sense must prevail. Each situation should be evaluated individually, regarding factors like the expertise of the clinician to attempt the reduction as well as the number of assistants available, patient's condition and presentation, time available, and the distance to an emergency department, where both imaging evaluation and medication for pain and relaxation are available. Furthermore, suspicion of the diagnosis must be high enough, as in a recurrent dislocation case, and the medical team must feel comfortable and be skilled enough to go for a gesture that can be potentially harmful. As with any medical decision-making, final decision to advance belongs to the medical team after considering all these variables.

Closed reduction of a dislocation can be achieved in several ways, and no specific technique can be recommended as superior for prehospital use, as the ability to perform it is more important than the method used. Classical techniques include Kocher, Hippocratic, Stimson's, and Milch, and many others are variations of these. Methods can be classified according to whether leverage, scapular manipulation, or traction is employed. Traction can be further subdivided according to where the arm is placed while traction is applied.

30.3.1 Leverage Techniques

30.3.1.1 Kocher's Method

This classic, time-tested technique is noted to be relatively painless and excludes traction, using leverage alone:

> Bend the affected arm at 90° at the elbow, adducted against the body; the wrist and the point of the elbow can be grasped by the surgeon. Slowly externally rotate between 70–85° until resistance is felt. In a conscious patient, take plenty of time gradually rotating, and try to distract the patient with conversation and then continue. Lift the externally rotated upper arm in the sagittal plane as far forward as possible then internally rotate the shoulder as this brings the patient's hand towards the opposite shoulder.

The humeral head should then slip back into place. However, complications can occur with this technique, namely, when traction is applied or the procedure is carried out hastily, tearing of the subscapularis, spiral fracture of the humerus or even damage to the axillary vein, and associated death have been reported (Fig. 30.1) [23].

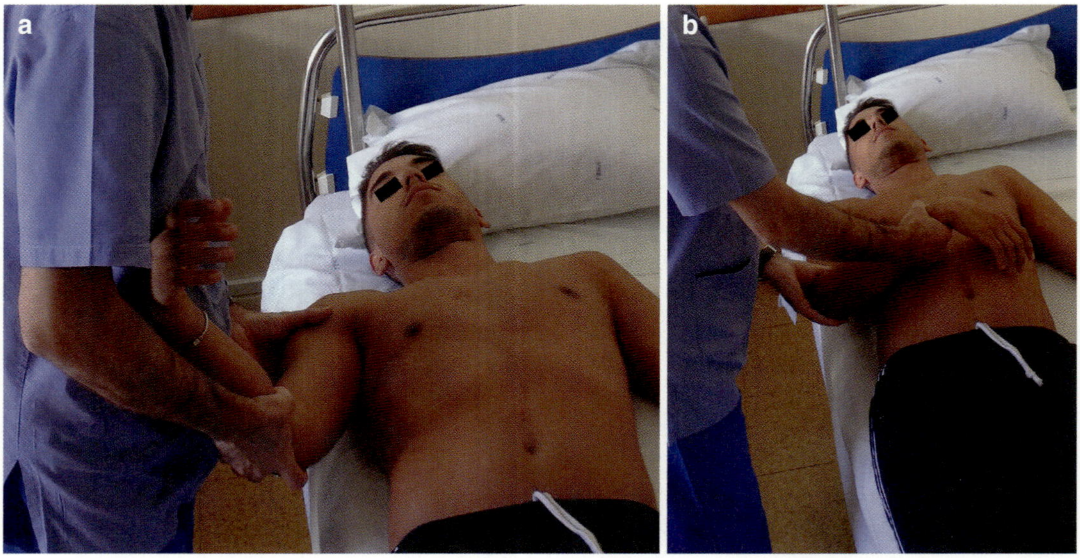

Fig. 30.1 (**a**) Kocher's method. Lift in the sagittal plane the adducted arm in external rotation; (**b**) Slow internal rotation brings head back into place

Performing just the first part of this technique, i.e., gently externally rotating the arm without lifting it, may sometimes be enough as the shoulder is usually reduced by the time the arm is in the coronal plane, especially when performed within the first half hour after dislocation. This is named the *external rotation method* and has recently been found to be an easier and less painful technique when performed without anesthesia and compared to the Milch Technique [50].

30.3.1.2 Milch Technique

This can be performed with the patient in a supine or prone position. Despite adaptations over the years, the original description uses leverage alone, and the rationale behind it is the same as the Kocher method, except that the arm is placed in abduction and not in adduction.

The physician holds the affected shoulder with his hand, bracing his fingers against the humeral head to keep it displaced and steady. Next the surgeon's other hand gently abducts and externally rotates the patient's arm into an overhead position, while fixing the humeral head so that it does not move from its dislocated position. The surgeon now gently pushes the humeral head back into the glenoid fossa with his thumb (Fig. 30.2) [24].

30.3.2 Traction Techniques

30.3.2.1 Hippocratic Method

The physician grasps the hand and forearm, with his heel placed gently in the axilla acting as a fulcrum. Traction is then applied while the arm is adducted until the reduction and a "pop" is felt. A potential complication is damage to the axillary nerve from the foot in the axilla (Fig. 30.3) [24].

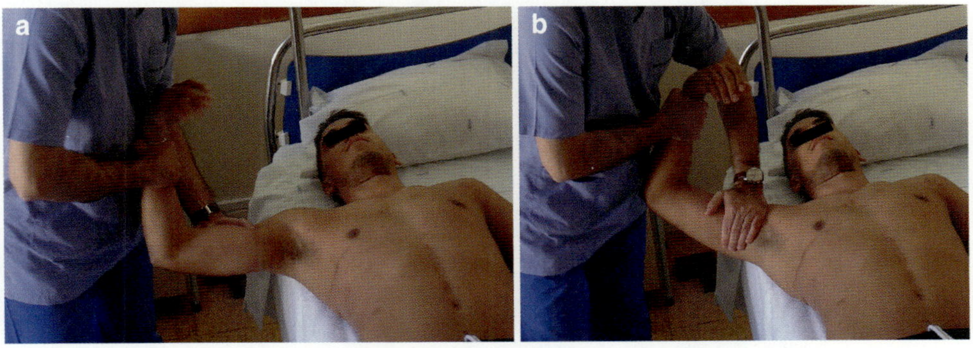

Fig. 30.2 (**a**) Milch technique. Gentle abduction and external rotation; (**b**) in an overhead position, gently push head into glenoid fossa

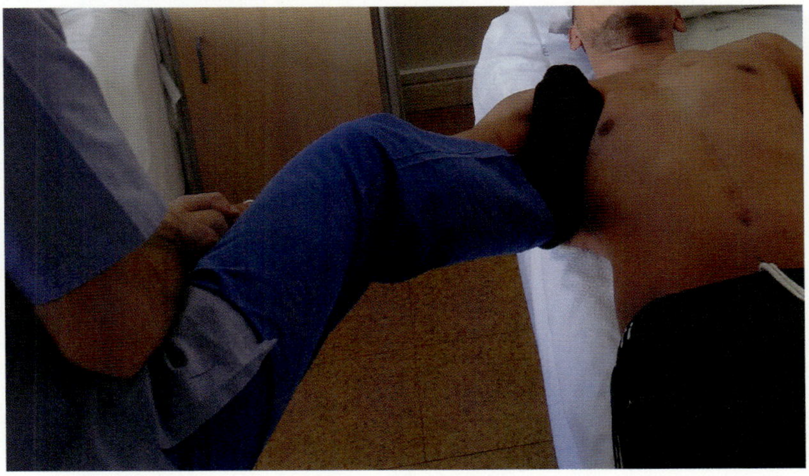

Fig. 30.3 Hippocratic method

30.3.2.2 Stimson's Method

The patient is prone on a table with the affected arm hanging down in forward flexion and with a 5 kg weight applied to the wrist. A preliminary analgesic is usually required, and muscle fatigue and ultimate relaxation will eventually lead to the reduction of the dislocation.

30.3.2.3 Matsen's Traction-Countertraction

This is one of the author's preferred methods, and, again, variations of the original technique have been described. Traction is applied to the affected arm with the shoulder in slight abduction, while an assistant applies firm countertraction to the chest using a folded sheet. The elbow is flexed at 90° to help rotate the shoulder internally and externally to unhinge the dislocated humeral head, while a second sheet, tied loosely around the physician's waist and looped over the patient's forearm provides adequate traction. In the author's experience, this same maneuver can be done with an extended elbow, with similar success and less discomfort for the patient (Fig. 30.4).

30.3.2.4 Spaso Technique

Another of the author's preferred method, like the previous one, can be performed with the patient lying supine on the ground. The affected arm is grasped by the wrist or distal forearm and lifted vertically with gentle traction. The shoulder is then externally rotated, and reduction usually occurs spontaneously or by pushing the humeral head into position while maintaining traction (Fig. 30.5).

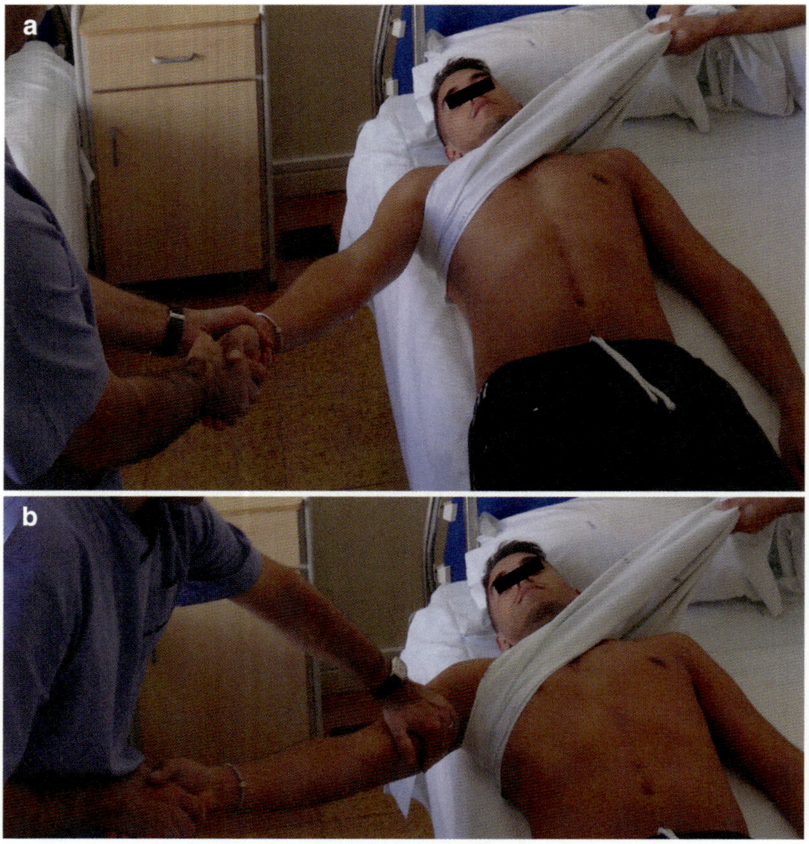

Fig. 30.4 (**a**) Matsen's traction-countertraction; (**b**) gently push head back into the glenoid fossa if reduction has not yet been felt

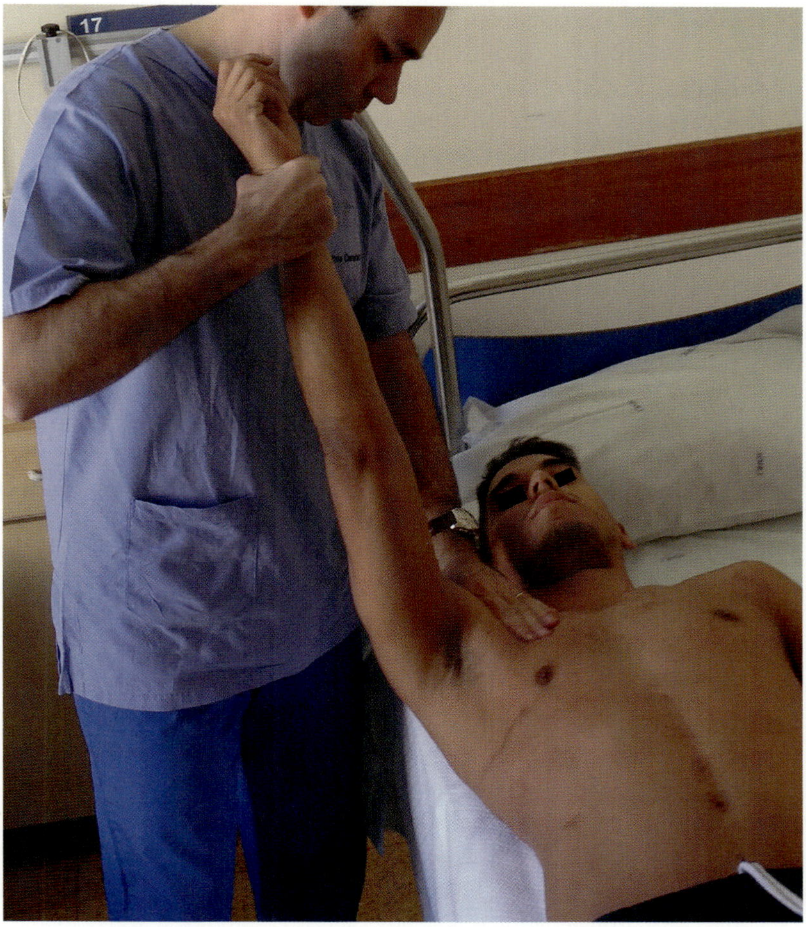

Fig. 30.5 Spaso technique. Gentle vertical traction and external rotation

30.3.3 Scapular Manipulation

This starts with the patient prone with the affected arm hanging over the edge of the table, with traction resulting from a weight attached to the wrist just like the Stimson's method. As the patient begins to relax, reduction is then attempted by pushing on the tip of the scapula medially, with rotation of the superior aspect of the scapula laterally [25].

30.4 Management of Shoulder Instability After Reduction

Management of a patient with shoulder instability is based on the prognosis expected for that particular situation. That is to say, regardless of the functional capacity of the joint and symptoms of that patient, which must be, of course, taken into consideration for decision as well, one must assume each individual will have a certain risk of recurrence. So the greatest challenge of dealing with traumatic anterior instability, namely, after a first event, is deciding which patient may benefit from surgical intervention. Variability among the reports of long-term follow-ups does not provide the clinician the exact recurrence rate for a given patient, but it is clear that younger (under 25) males involved in contact or overhead sports have the highest recurrence rates when treated non-operatively, approaching 100% in some series [26–33]. Success of the treatment, whether it is surgical or conservative, depends on several factors such as patient's age, activity level, arm dominance, sex, specific sport, pattern of instability, tissue and bone quality, timing, patient expectations, and also surgeon factors, whose level of expertise has certainly its weight.

It is also evident that there is more to successful treatment of shoulder instability than simply avoiding recurrence. Sachs and colleagues showed that patients that cope with instability (and do not achieve early stability) have lower functional outcome scores than those who undergo surgical stabilization of their Bankart lesion. This suggests that while avoidance of recurrence is mandatory, each patient's ability to deal with sport, other daily activities, and emotional aspects of the injury also factor into successful recovery [29, 34].

In order to provide the best outcome information for operative versus non-operative treatment for different individuals, Mather and colleagues [33] designed a decision analysis model using the Western Ontario Shoulder Instability score as the primary outcome measure, with secondary outcome measures including risk at one year and overall instability, stability at 10 years, and risks of future surgery and of revision surgery. All the data used were from levels I and II studies only. The goal is to develop a tool that provides with more information regarding potential surgical outcomes based on individual data, by entering information into the model using a computer program. For example, the decision analysis model shows that an 18-year-old male treated conservatively has a 77% risk of recurrent dislocation within the first year and only a 32% chance of having a stable shoulder at 10 years. When treated operatively, that rate drops to 17%. It is a system that should provide personalized patient care, allowing various factors to help the best decision for each patient.

The goal of the treatment is to have the athlete back to competition safely and fit; however, there is often pressure to shorten the period of absence from competition. Decision-making must take several things into consideration, and a few aspects should be verified before returning to play after an instability event, including symmetric or near normal pain-free range of motion and strength, ability to perform sport-specific skills, and the absence of subjective or objective instability [26, 35]. Timing within the season is also of major importance for the decision on how to manage each particular case, as surgery will take the athlete from competition for a relatively long period. This time away from sports after surgery must be weighed against a shorter time away with non-operative treatment, though there are other risks involved, including recurrence and more time-out. If surgical intervention is planned, ideally it should take place when the 4–6 months of expected convalescence does not affect the athlete's season [22], or even more in the case of overhead athletes. In the author's experience, this time planning should not rule out the possibility of having the field football player back to game sooner, if recovery allows it. Factors such as being a recurrent versus first-time dislocator, having had failed prior treatments or not, and the severity of instability at time of evaluation help to guide decisions [36].

30.4.1 Evaluation

The football player will often report an acute traumatic event, either initial or recurrent, usually noting a force to the upper arm directed from anterior to posterior while the arm is in abduction and external rotation.

Others may not describe a dislocation event but rather episodes where the arm feels "dead," heavy or weak, or a sharp posterior pain in a forced overhead position, which should raise suspicion for shoulder subluxation or an underlying diagnosis of "multidirectional" instability if there is no history of injury. The latter will often present with bilateral shoulder symptoms and/or generalized laxity and, according to the latest trends in defining the type of instability, would be better off classified according to the direction of instability with most symptoms, eliminating the concept of "multidirectional" [13–15].

In the acute setting, a patient with a dislocation will usually present with the arm in adduction and internal rotation held by the opposite hand for comfort, and an asymmetry of the deltoid contour and/or prominence of the acromion may be obvious (Fig. 30.6). A search for acute neurovascular deficits is mandatory.

In those patients who present after relocation, physical examination should address both shoulders, looking for asymmetries in the range of motion, muscle atrophy, or nerve injuries. The most common complication is the axillary nerve injury, leading to numbness over the lateral shoulder, and when presentation is delayed, there may be visible deltoid atrophy. However, suprascapular nerve traction with external rotation dysfunction and long thoracic nerve injury with scapular winging have also been reported. In those with prior open surgery, it is important to test subscapularis function as failure of a prior repair may occur [36, 37].

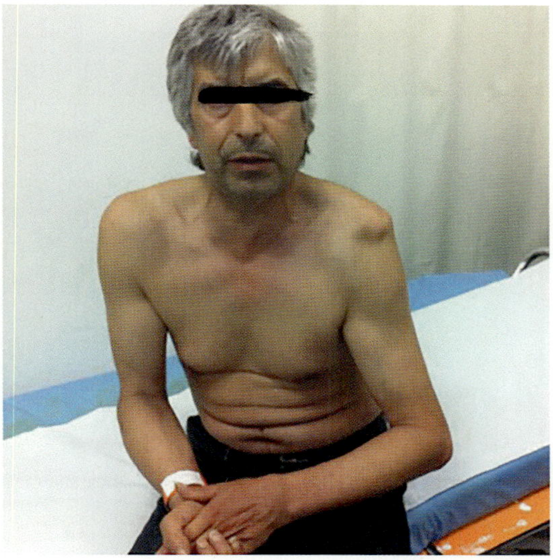

Fig. 30.6 Anterior dislocation of left shoulder

Evaluation of the shoulder stability comprises two components: quantification of passive translation between the humeral head and the glenoid fossa – laxity, a sign – and reproduction of the symptoms of subluxation and apprehension by placing the shoulder under stress – instability, a symptom. Several special tests may be used to characterize the instability pattern, allowing the identification of its direction and magnitude. Again, this chapter will focus on the posttraumatic anterior instability.

30.4.1.1 Load and Shift Tests or Anterior and Posterior Drawer Tests

Laxity is often difficult to assess and requires experience. These tests may be performed with the patient sitting and then supine (after Gerber-Ganz). The amount of translation observed can be asymptomatic or symptomatic, suggesting instability (which is symptomatic laxity) in this case.

While one of the examiner's hands stabilizes the scapula, the other holds the humeral head. By pushing the humerus against the glenoid, the humeral head is usually centered in its concentric position within the glenoid, allowing an appropriate starting position. Then an anterior and posterior force on the humeral head is performed to evaluate translation of the head (Fig. 30.7) [38].

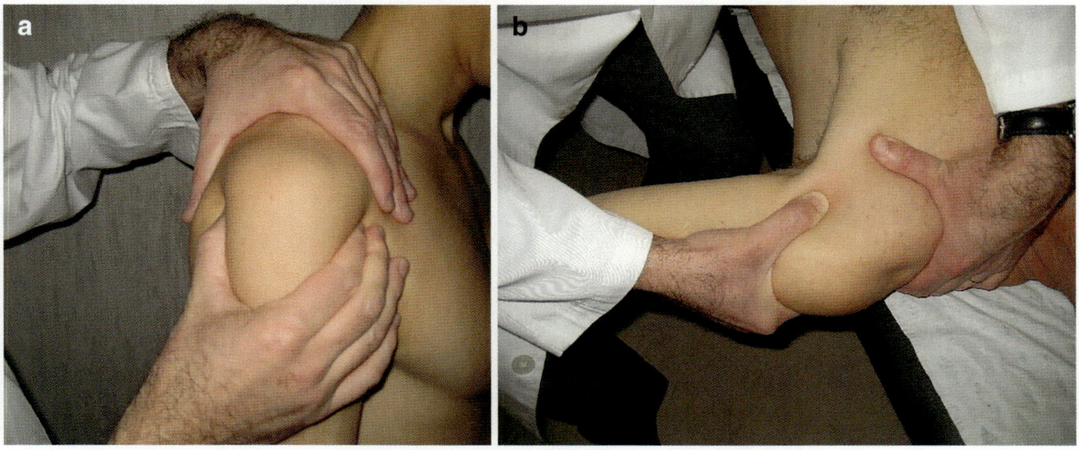

Fig. 30.7 (**a**) Drawer test sitting [38]; (**b**) Drawer test supine [38]

30.4.1.2 Sulcus Sign

Sulcus sign measures inferior glenohumeral laxity and is often present in patients with generalized laxity at risk for instability in more than one direction. It is usually performed with the patient in the sitting position: the limb is held at the elbow, and inferior traction is applied to the arm in neutral rotation. An augmentation of the space between the acromion and the humeral head, with a sulcus noted below the acromion, is quantified but is only considered abnormal in the symptomatic patient [39]. The same test is performed with the arm in 25–30° of external rotation, and persistence of the sign suggests incompetence of the superior glenohumeral ligament and rotator interval, while its elimination suggests competence of the pulley structures.

30.4.1.3 Gagey Hyperabduction Test

The examiner is behind the seated patient and passively elevates the arm in the coronal plane, while forcing the top of the shoulder downwards (Fig. 30.8) [38]. The patient must be totally relaxed, elbow flexed at 90° and forearm horizontal. Hyperabduction of 105° or a difference of 15° to the opposite shoulder suggests hyperlaxity with a lesion of the IGHL (inferior glenohumeral ligament) that should be addressed if surgery is considered.

30.4.1.4 Apprehension and Jobe Relocation Tests for Anterior Instability

The former may be performed with the patient seated or supine. Guarding or apprehension as the shoulder is taken to increasing abduction and external rotation indicates a positive test (Fig. 30.9) [38]. Pain without apprehension is not considered a positive test but may indicate more subtle anterior instability and posterosuperior impingement.

The relocation test, described by Jobe, is performed with the patient supine and by applying a posteriorly directed force on the humeral head with the arm in the apprehension position. Disappearance of symptoms produced by the apprehension test with this maneuver and immediate return of apprehension as that force is released is considered a positive test, with high

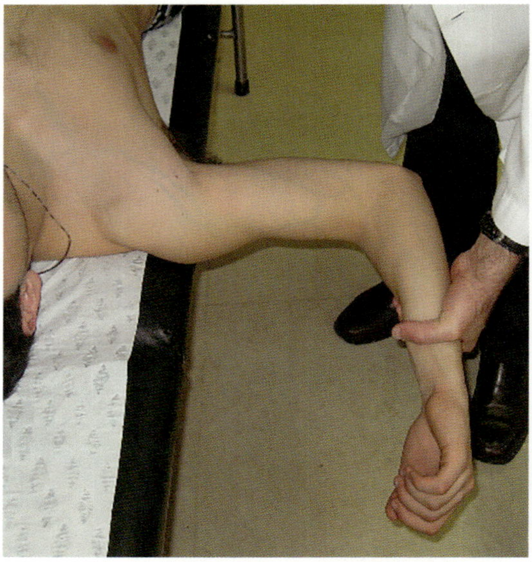

Fig. 30.9 Apprehension test in the supine position allows more relaxation and support of the scapula against the table [38]

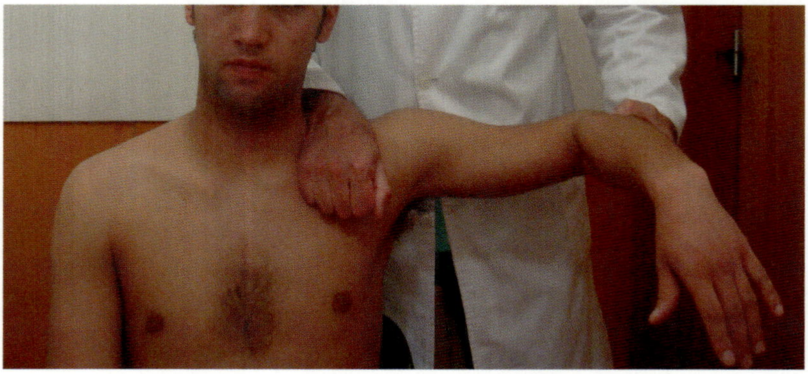

Fig. 30.8 O. Gagey hyperabduction test [38]

positive and negative predictive values (Fig. 30.10) [26] [38].

Radiographic evaluation should start with quality plain X-rays. True AP in internal and external rotation, scapular Y, and axillary views can confirm reduction and may reveal any bone loss that may contribute to instability (Fig. 30.11). However, the CT scan is widely accepted as the gold standard for preoperative assessment of glenoid or humeral head bone loss due to its high accuracy in detecting fracture fragments (Fig. 30.12). A CT scan associated with arthrography will allow evaluation of soft tissue lesions as well (Fig. 30.13). It is a common option for many surgeons, especially those in countries where access to MRI is or was subject to restrictions.

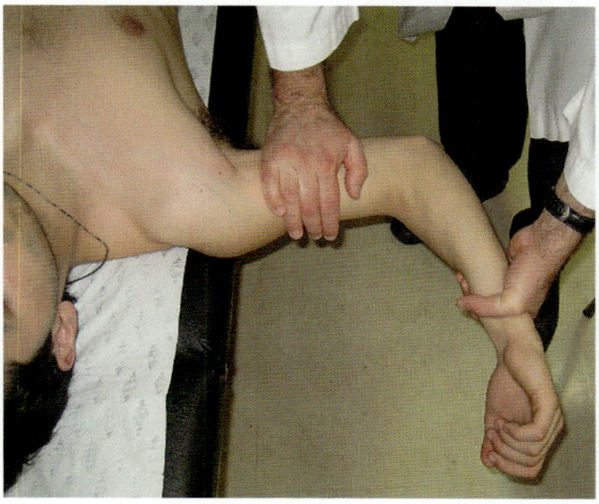

Fig. 30.10 Jobe relocation test [38]

On the other hand, the detail of soft tissue provided by the MRI is unmatched (Fig. 30.14). Considering that its capacity to evaluate bone defects has also been shown to be very high with the newest scanners, it is most surgeons' first choice for the evaluation of shoulder instabilities. Arthrography can further be added to the MRI in order to enhance its sensitivity for the detection of soft tissue lesions but with a few setbacks: increasing costs, more time-consuming, iatrogenic risks, and discomfort for the patient, not to mention a potential limited availability. An MRI done in the acute phase, with hemarthrosis functioning as contrast, or having the patient move the shoulder intensely right before the exam to force detachment of any eventual adhesions of the capsulolabral structures (author's personal impression, with no scientific evidence) may improve the quality of the exam and eventually turn the arthrography unnecessary.

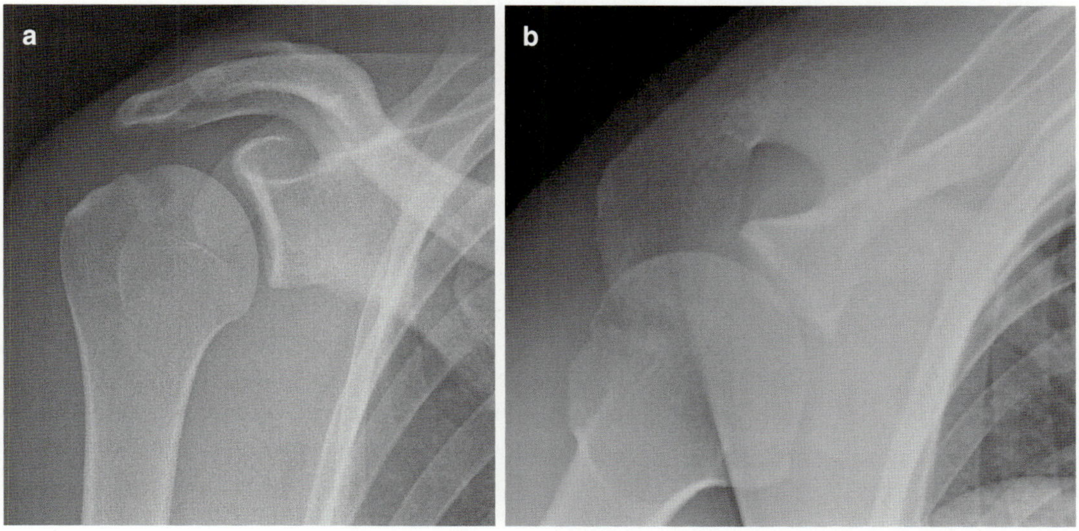

Fig. 30.11 (**a**) AP view and (**b**) axillary view X-Rays evidencing bony depression on the posterosuperior area of the humeral head, the Hill-Sachs lesion

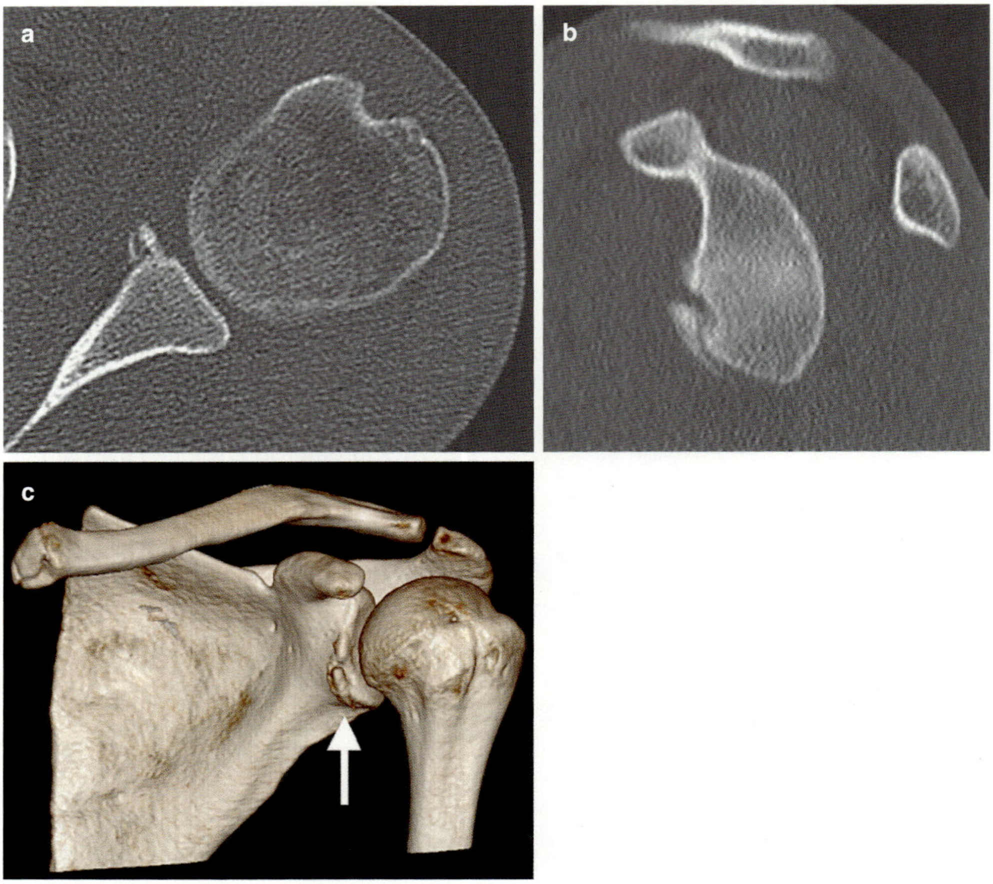

Fig. 30.12 Bony Bankart on CT scan. (**a**) Axial cut; (**b**) sagittal cut; (**c**) 3D reconstruction

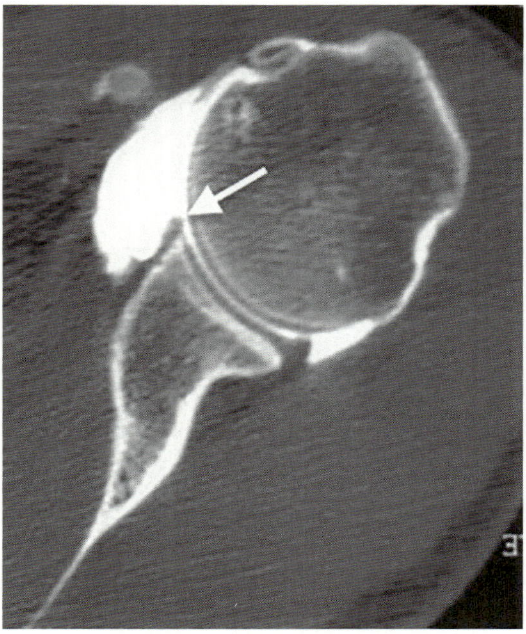

Fig. 30.13 Arthro-CT. Anterior labrum Bankart lesion variant

30.4.2 Treatment

30.4.2.1 Conservative Treatment

A classical and common option for the acute first-time dislocator is non-operative management. However, there is increasing evidence that it is associated with a higher recurrence rate and that quality of life is improved with surgical treatment in the young athletic population [27, 40, 41, 51].

However, conservative treatment remains an acceptable alternative in the non-overhead athlete with desire to return to sport in season, as long as the patient is able to perform sport-specific drills without pain or instability, has full range of motion and good strength, has no or minor osseous lesions, or refuses surgery. Relative and absolute contraindications to non-operative treatment should be considered (Tables 30.2 and 30.3), taking into account these criteria are based on lower levels of evidence and expert opinion, since no

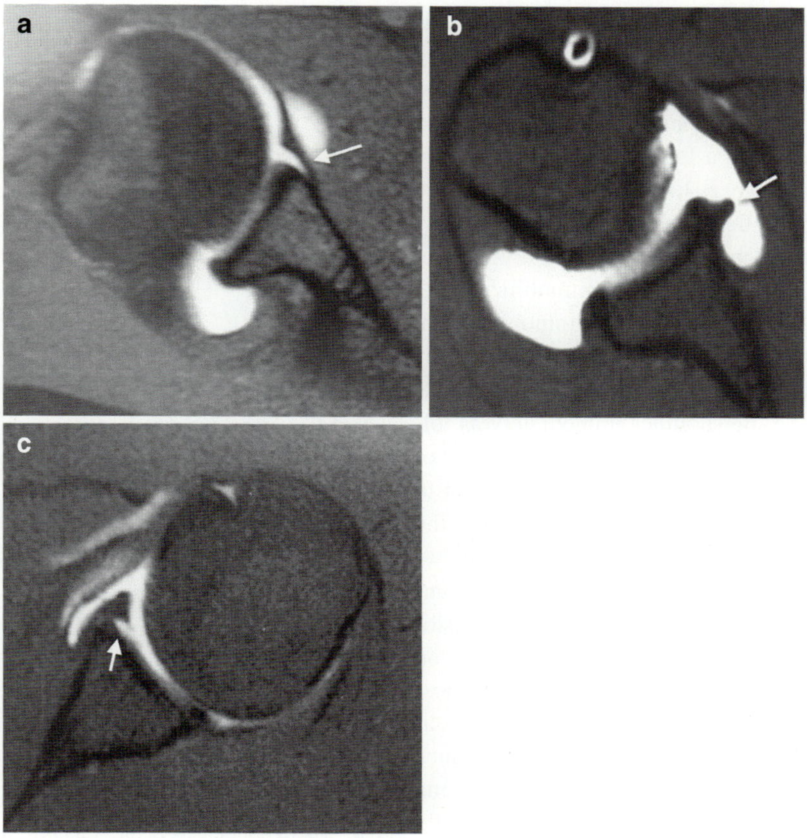

Fig. 30.14 Arthro-MRI after anterior shoulder dislocations. (**a**) Anterior labrum periosteal sleeve avulsion (ALPSA) lesion; (**b**) chronic ALPSA lesion; anterior labrum has healed more medially on the glenoid neck; (**c**) glenolabral articular disruption (GLAD) lesion, with associated cartilage damage

Table 30.2 Contraindications to non-operative in-season management of anterior shoulder instability

Dominant arm in a throwing or overhead athlete
Failure of non-operative treatment/brace wear/previous surgery
Recurrent dislocator
Large or engaging Hill-Sachs lesion
Glenoid bone loss greater than 20–25%

Table 30.3 Absolute indications for early in-season surgery [26]

Associated injuries, fractures
Rotator-cuff tear involving > 50% thickness
Glenoid osseous defect > 25%
Humeral head articular surface osseous defect > 25%
Irreducible dislocation
Failed trial of rehabilitation
Inability to tolerate shoulder restrictions
Inability to perform sport-specific drills without instability

well-designed studies exist [42]. Additionally, counseling with the patient is mandatory, as this could be a temporary measure with surgery planned after the season due to the risk of redislocation.

Non-operative treatment may include a brief period of immobilization, physical therapy, and bracing. Buss [43] studied 30 athletes with in-season dislocation and found 26 returned to play and completed the season without even a short period of immobilization. However, 37% experienced at least one additional instability episode, and 12 required surgical stability later on, but this study indicates that even for contact athletes, non-operative treatment can still allow the completion of a season with an absence from sports of an average 10 days.

Type and duration of immobilization is still subject to debate. Current standard continues to immobilize the shoulder in internal rotation with an adducted arm. However, Itoi [44, 45] and colleagues have challenged this by demonstrating better reduction of the labral detachment with the shoulder in adduction and external rotation and an association with a lower recurrent instability rate. On the other hand, others [46] have attempted to duplicate the results of Itoi's study without success, possibly due to the low patient compliance of wearing a bulky immobilizer.

With regard to the duration of immobilization, several authors have found no difference in recurrence rates between using a sling for 3–4 weeks and mobilizing the shoulder immediately as tolerated [26, 28]. In fact, after recurrent episodes of dislocation, there is limited interest or reason to immobilize the shoulder. In such cases, it is the authors' opinion to let the shoulder move freely.

Regardless of immobilization or not, recommendations for rehabilitation following a dislocation are fairly consistent. It must focus on having the player back to sports as soon as possible but also on the prevention of recurrent instability episodes, of paramount importance especially with goalkeepers. Cryotherapy and early initiation of ROM exercises are generally the initial steps of non-operative management. Once the patient has achieved near full range of motion, progressive strengthening exercises are introduced, focusing the dynamic shoulder stabilizers, with increasing resistance aiming symmetric shoulder and scapular strength. Core stability and prevention of glenohumeral internal rotation deficit (GIRD) with appropriate stretching must also be addressed. Sport-specific exercises, including plyometrics and focus on proprioception, are then added until the athlete has no complaints of instability [36, 43].

Bracing for return to play has not been shown to decrease recurrence rate [26], but the rationale behind it is the contribution to a better joint proprioception with improvement of the sense of stability, helping with return to sports. Bracing can range from simple neoprene sleeves to motion-limiting supports that limit abduction, extension, and external rotation in adjustable degrees (Fig. 30.15), which, for obvious reasons, are better tolerated by collision athletes than by overhead athletes.

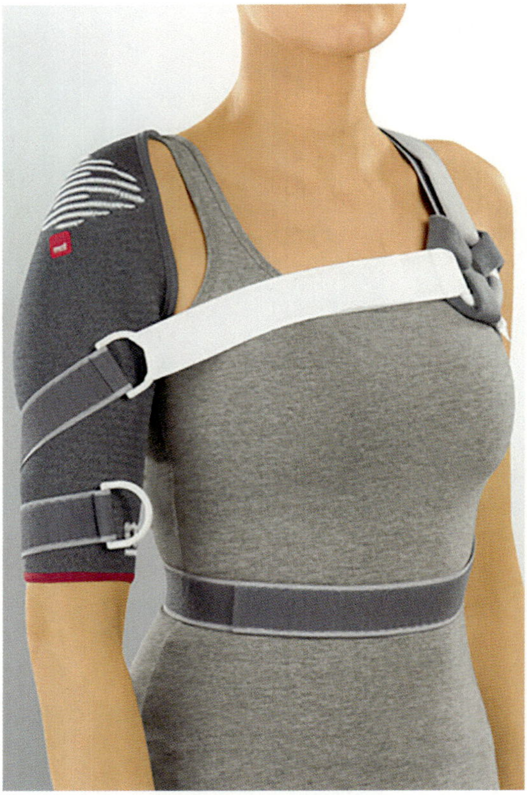

Fig. 30.15 Shoulder joint support with movement restricting function (Omomed by MEDI® – authorized)

30.4.2.2 Surgery: Anatomical Versus Nonanatomical Repair

Proceeding to surgery is not a straightforward decision for most first-time dislocators. The concern is that recurrent instability events risk further damage to the joint or acute neurovascular injury. That being so, it is largely accepted today that those at a higher risk of recurrence should undergo surgery following the first event [27, 40, 41].

The next big question is the best timing for surgery during the season. Deciding for early surgery within the season should be based on the relative contraindications for non-operative treatment (Table 30.2), complemented by absolute indications for surgery as outlined by Owens (Table 30.3) [26]. Multiple shoulder dislocations during the season and age under 20 are relative criteria that would push gray-zone cases toward surgery.

Arthroscopic Bankart repair (Fig. 30.16) and the open Latarjet bone block procedure (Fig. 30.17) are widely considered mainstays for surgical treatment of recurrent anterior shoulder instability, with similar results in carefully selected patients. Choosing between the two depends mainly on the surgeons' preference or training rather than on published evidence.

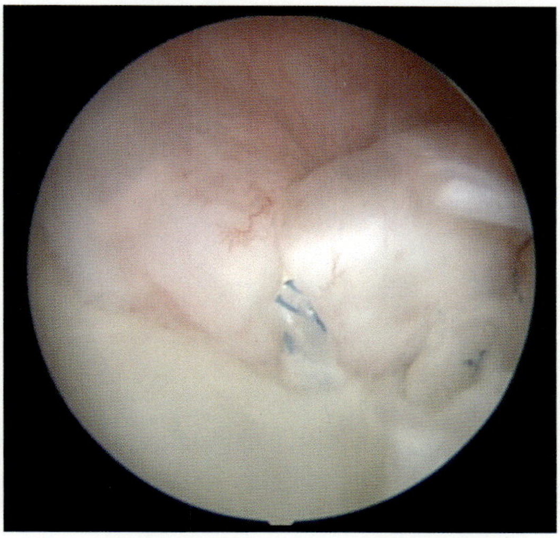

Fig. 30.16 Low-profile labral repair with all-soft knotless #1 suture anchors

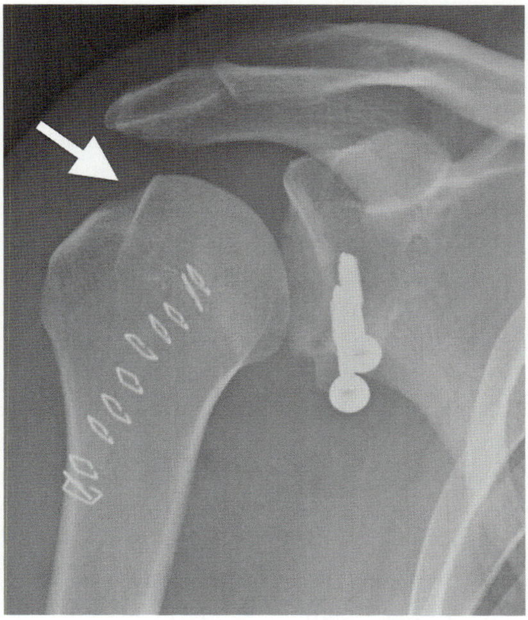

Fig. 30.17 Post-op X-ray; Bristow-Latarjet and evident Hill-Sachs lesion on the humeral head (*arrow*)

Balg and Boileau in 2007 [47] described the instability severity index score (ISIS) as a method to identify patients who will develop recurrent instability after an arthroscopic Bankart procedure and who would be better served by an open operation. Despite its limitations, this score identifies important risk factors: patient age under 20 years at the time of surgery, involvement in competitive or contact sports or those involving forced overhead activity, shoulder hyperlaxity, a Hill-Sachs lesion present on an anteroposterior radiograph of the shoulder in external rotation, and/or loss of the sclerotic inferior glenoid contour. At that time, the authors argued that those with a score over six points would be better served with a Bristow-Latarjet procedure, due to an unacceptable recurrence risk of 70% ($p < 0.001$) following an arthroscopic Bankart repair. Further evidence from the same clinical center and from previous reports comparing open Bankart and Bristow-Latarjet procedures [48] demonstrate greater success of the bone block over the anatomical capsulolabral repair. Those authors ultimately suggest an isolated arthroscopic Bankart repair should only be used in carefully selected patients with an ISIS of 3 or less.

On the other hand, Larrain et al. [49] evaluated rugby players that underwent arthroscopic stabilization after careful selection. Exclusion criteria were humeral bony deficiencies greater than one-fourth of the articular humeral head, bony glenoid deficiencies of more than 25%, capsular laxity with poor tissue quality, and humeral avulsion of the glenohumeral ligament (HAGL). They reported good or excellent results in 94.8% of the acute instability group and in 91.6% of the recurrent instability group. Similar results published by others and the fact that new arthroscopic stabilizing procedures have been described in the last decade, such as the Hill-Sachs remplissage (Fig. 30.18), capsular shift, Latarjet (Fig. 30.19) or Bankart, and bone block simultaneously, which aim to repair different lesions at the same time, should allow one to accept that an "a la carte" approach may lead to lower recurrence

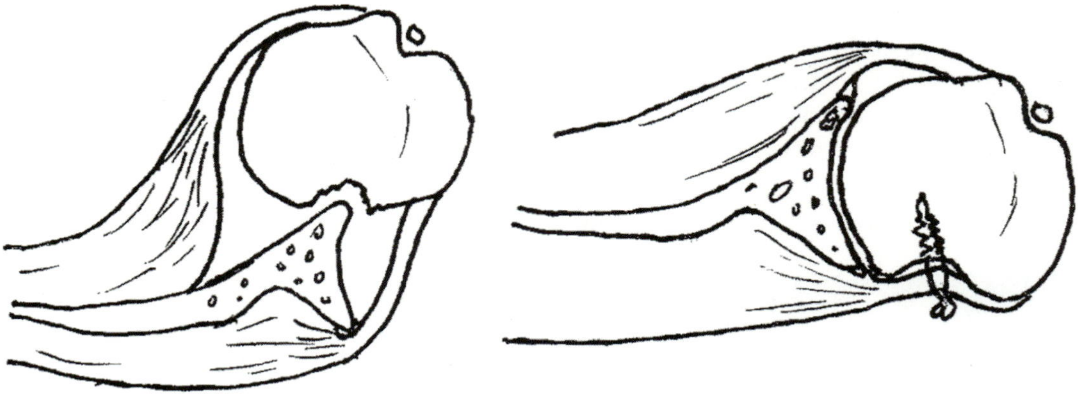

Fig. 30.18 Remplissage. Posterior capsulotenodesis on the Hill-Sachs lesion. Prevents redislocation by filling the humeral head bone defect that may engage on the anterior rim of the glenoid

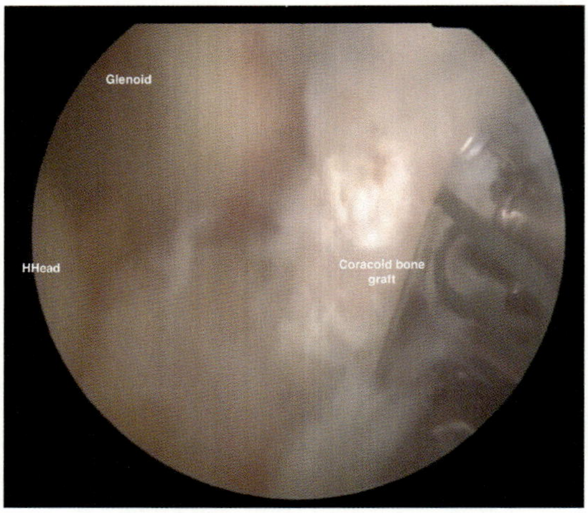

Fig. 30.19 Coracoid graft fixation in arthroscopic Latarjet procedure

rates and less residual apprehension in the near future in similar high-risk groups.

Nevertheless, the authors believe, supported by current evidence and their expertise, that in the specific population addressed here, with such important risk factors, the Bristow-Latarjet, open or arthroscopic, would be the correct procedure to consider in most cases, although the arthroscopic anatomical repair has its place. Reasoning for favoring the Bristow-Latarjet is that the procedure is less dependent on the need for correction of all associated lesions and therefore more tolerant of such lesions that in fact may be left uncorrected and contribute to failure, than an arthroscopic anatomical repair.

30.4.2.3 Prevention

As with any other injury, the first measure to avoid injury is prevention. The FIFA 11+ program is geared toward preparing the athletes' bodies for the rigors of playing football – refer to Chap. 49 . A fit athlete will be less prone to injuries, including those of the shoulder. However, a specific approach to the shoulder is important to minimize the risks to this joint.

Preseason screening of athletes can help prevent common sports injuries to the shoulder. This should include, in the case of football and shoulder instability, assessment and management of core and scapular stability, joint flexibility, rotator-cuff control, and general strength. The objective is to identify and correct shoulder asymmetries and imbalances, namely, of the scapula (dyskinesis) and the rotator cuff, which are of primary importance in maintaining the humeral head centered on the glenoid. Often overlooked in athletes is the muscular imbalance between the front and back of the shoulder, as many often overwork and build up the muscles they can see at the front, such as pectoralis major, anterior deltoids, and upper trapezius, leaving their lower trapezius, rhomboids, serratus, posterior rotator cuff, and posterior deltoids underdeveloped.

In the case of the recurrent dislocator, prevention may not be as straightforward. Longer lay-off periods after injury, using stabilizing braces, and strengthening of the scapular and glenohumeral stabilizers, all should contribute to minimize the risk of recurrence. However, these are the athletes where the management is so controversial, as discussed above. In fact, surgery might actually be the best prevention.

References

1. Ekstrand J, Hägglund M, Törnqvist H, Kristenson K, Bengtsson H, Magnusson H, Waldén M. Upper extremity injuries in male elite football players. Knee Surg Sports Traumatol Arthrosc. 2013;21:1626–32.
2. Ekstrand J, Hägglund M, Waldén M. Injury incidence and injury patterns in professional football – the UEFA injury study. Br J Sports Med. 2011;45:553–8.
3. Árnason Á, Gudmundsson Á, Dahl HA, Jóhannsson E. Soccer injuries in Iceland. Scand J Med Sci Sports. 1996;6:40–5.
4. Waldén M, Hägglund M, Ekstrand J. UEFA Champions League study: a prospective study of injuries in professional football during the 2001–2002 season. Br J Sports Med. 2005;39:542–6.
5. Árnason A, Tenga A, Engebretsen L, Bahr R. A prospective video-based analysis of injury situations in elite male football: football incident analysis. Am J Sports Med. 2004;32:1459–65.
6. Longo UG, Loppini M, Berton A, Martinelli N, Maffulli N, Denaro V. Shoulder injuries in soccer players. Clin Cases Miner Bone Metab. 2012;9(3):138–41.
7. Junge A, Dvorak J, Graf-Baumann T. Football injuries during the World Cup 2002. Am J Sports Med. 2004;32(1 Suppl):23S–7S.
8. Dvorak J, Junge A, Grimm K, Kirkendall D. Medical report from the 2006 FIFA World Cup Germany. Br J Sports Med. 2007;41(9):578–81.
9. Waldén M, Hägglund M, Ekstrand J. Football injuries during European Championships 2004–2005. Knee Surg Sports Traumatol Arthrosc. 2007;15(9):1155–62.
10. Junge A, Langevoort G, Pipe A, Peytavin A, Wong F, Mountjoy M, et al. Injuries in team sport tournaments during the 2004 Olympic Games. Am J Sports Med. 2006;34(4):565–76.
11. Junge A, Dvorak J, Graf-Baumann T, Peterson L. Football injuries during FIFA tournaments and the Olympic Games, 1998–2001: development and implementation of an injury-reporting system. Am J Sports Med. 2004;32(1 Suppl):80S–9S.
12. Junge A, Engebretsen L, Mountjoy ML, Alonso JM, Renström PA, Aubry MJ, et al. Sports injuries during the Summer Olympic Games 2008. Am J Sports Med. 2009;37(11):2165–72.
13. Kuhn JE. A new classification system for shoulder instability. Br J Sports Med. (2010);44(5):341–346.
14. Kuhn JE, Helmer TT, Dunn WR, Throckmorton VTW. Development and reliability testing of the frequency, etiology, direction, and severity (FEDS) system for classifying glenohumeral instability. J Shoulder Elbow Surg. 2011;20(4):548–56.
15. Shea KP. ISAKOS Consensus Shoulder Instability Classification System. In: Arce G, et al., editors. Shoulder concepts 2013: consensus and concerns: ISAKOS; Springer: Berlin Heidelberg; 2013. p. 29–34.
16. Lee AJ, Hardy PJ, Kitchen E, Shahane S. Luxatio erecta: a prehospital challenge in patient packaging. Emerg Med J. 2009;26(10):745–6.
17. Lagrabette JF, Minville V, Colombani A, Bounes V, Fourcade O. Interscalene brachial plexus block for glenohumeral luxation in prehospital medicine. Ann Fr Anesth Reanim. 2008;27(4):338–40.
18. Gros T, Delire V, Dareau S, Sebbane M, Eledjan JJ. Interscalene brachial plexus block in prehospital medicine. Am Fr Anesth Reanim. 2008;27(10):859–60.
19. Helfen T, Ockert B, Pozder P, Regauer M, Haasters F. Management of prehospital shoulder dislocation: feasibility and need of reduction. Eur J Trauma Emerg Surg. 2016;42(3):357–62.
20. Clinical Standards for Emergency Medicine from the College of Emergency Medicine. 2014. Available from www.rcem.ac.uk. Accessed 10 July 2015.
21. Kanji A, Atkinson P, Fraser J, Lewis D, Benjamin S. Delays to initial reduction attempt are associated with higher failure rates in anterior shoulder dislocation: a retrospective analysis of factors affecting reduction failure. Emerg Med J. 2016;33(2): 130–3.
22. Wang RY, Arciero RA. Treating the athlete with anterior shoulder instability. Clin Sports Med. 2008;27:631–48.
23. Kirker JR. Dislocation of the shoulder complicated by rupture of the axillary vessels. Repeat of a case. J Bone Joint Surg. 1952;34B:72–3.
24. McRae R. Pocketbook of orthopaedics and fractures. 2nd ed. New York: Churchill Livingstone Elsevier; 2006. p. 276–80.
25. Kothari RU, Dronen SC. Prospective evaluation of the scapular manipulation technique in reducing anterior shoulder dislocation. Ann Emerg Med. 1992;21:1349–52.
26. Owens BD, Duffey ML, Nelson BJ, et al. The incidence and characteristics of shoulder instability at the United States Military Academy. Am J Sports Med. 2007;35(7):1168–73.
27. Kirkley A, Werstine R, Ratjek A, Griffin S. Prospective randomized clinical trial comparing the effectiveness of immediate arthroscopic stabilization versus immobilization and rehabilitation in first traumatic anterior dislocations of the shoulder: long-term evaluation. Arthroscopy. 2005;21(1):55–63.

28. Hovelius L, Eriksson K, Fredin H, Hagberg G, Hussenius A, Lind B, Thorling J, Weckström J. Recurrences after initial dislocation of the shoulder. Results of a prospective study of treatment. J Bone Joint Surg Am. 1983;65(3):343–9.
29. Siparsky PN, Taylor DC. Acute traumatic anterior shoulder instability: surgical management for the first-time dislocator. In: Brockmeier SF, et al., editors. Surgery of shoulder instability: ISAKOS; Springer: Berlin Heidelberg; 2013. p. 1–22.
30. Handoll HH, Almaiyah MA, Rangan A. Surgical versus non-surgical treatment for acute anterior shoulder dislocation. Cochrane Database Syst Rev. 2004;(1):CD004325.
31. Hovelius L, Augustini BG, Fredin H, Johansson O, Norlin R, Thorling J. Primary anterior dislocation of the shoulder in young patients. A ten-year prospective study. J Bone Joint Surg Am. 1996;78(11):1677–84.
32. Jakobsen BW, Johannsen HV, Suder P, Søjbjerg JO. Primary repair versus conservative treatment of first-time traumatic anterior dislocation of the shoulder: a randomized study with 10-year follow-up. Arthroscopy. 2007;23(2):118–23.
33. Mather 3rd RC, Orlando LA, Henderson RA, Lawrence JT, Taylor DC. A predictive model of shoulder instability after a first-time anterior shoulder dislocation. J Shoulder Elbow Surg. 2011;20(2):259–66.
34. Sachs RA, Lin D, Stone ML, Paxton E, Kuney M. Can the need for future surgery for acute traumatic anterior shoulder dislocation be predicted? J Bone Joint Surg Am. 2007;89(8):1665–74.
35. McCarty EC, Ritchie P, Gill HS, McFarland EG. Shoulder instability: return to play. Clin Sports Med. 2004;23(3):335–51, vii–viii.
36. Cavagnaro MA, Cohen SB. Management of shoulder instability in the collision athlete. In: Brockmeier SF, et al., editors. Surgery of shoulder instability: ISAKOS; Springer: Berlin Heidelberg; 2013. p. 23–35.
37. Piasecki DP, Verma NN, Romeo AA, Levine WN, Bach Jr BR, Provencher MT. Glenoid bone deficiency in recurrent anterior shoulder instability: diagnosis and management. J Am Acad Orthop Surg. 2009;17:482–93.
38. Gomes N. Exame clínico da cintura escapular. In: Cartucho A, Espregueira-Mendes J, editors. O Ombro. Lisboa: Ed Lidel; 2009. p. 29–50.
39. Gaskill TR, Taylor DC, Millett PJ. Management of multidirectional instability of the shoulder. J Am Acad Orthop Surg. 2011;19:758–67.
40. Randelli P, Taverna E. Primary anterior shoulder dislocation in young athletes: fix them! Knee Surg Sports Traumatol Arthrosc. 2009;17:1404–5.
41. Postacchini F, Gumina S, Cinotti G. Anterior shoulder dislocation in adolescents. J Shoulder Elbow Surg. 2000;9(6):470–4.
42. Ward JP, Bradley JP. Decision making in the in-season athlete with shoulder instability. Clin Sports Med. 2013;32:685–96.
43. Buss DD, Lynch GP, Meyer CP, Huber SM, Freehill MQ. Nonoperative management for in-season athletes with anterior shoulder instability. Am J Sports Med. 2004;32(6):1430–3.
44. Itoi E, Hatakeyama Y, Sato T, Kido T, Minagawa H, Yamamoto N, et al. Immobilization in external rotation after shoulder dislocation reduces the risk of recurrence. A randomized controlled trial. J Bone Joint Surg Am. 2007;89(10):2124–31.
45. Itoi E, Sashi R, Minagawa H, Shimizu T, Wakabayashi I, Sato K. Position of immobilization after dislocation of the glenohumeral joint: a study with use of magnetic resonance imaging. J Bone Joint Surg Am. 2001;83(5):661–7.
46. Liavaag S, Brox JI, Pripp AH, Enger M, Soldal LA, Svenningsen S. Immobilization in external rotation after primary shoulder dislocation did not reduce the risk of recurrence: a randomized controlled trial. J Bone Joint Surg Am. 2011;93(10):897–904.
47. Balg F, Boileau P. The instability severity index score. A simple pre-operative score to select patients for arthroscopic or open shoulder stabilisation. J Bone Joint Surg Br. 2007;89-B:1470–7.
48. Bessière C, Trojani C, Carles M, Mehta SS, Boileau P. The open latarjet procedure is more reliable in terms of shoulder stability than arthroscopic bankart repair. Clin Orthop Relat Res. 2014;472(8): 2345–51.
49. Larrain MV, Montenegro HJ, Mauas DM, Collazo CC, Pavón F. Arthroscopic management of traumatic anterior shoulder instability in collision athletes: analysis of 204 cases with a 4- to 9-year follow-up and results with the suture anchor technique. Arthroscopy. 2006;22(12):1283–9.
50. Sapkota K, Shrestha B, Onta PR, Thapa P. Comparison between external rotation method and Milch method for reduction of acute anterior dislocation of shoulder. J Clin Diagn Res. 2015;9(4):RC01–3.
51. Robinson CM, Howes J, Murdoch H, Will E, Graham C. Functional outcome and risk of recurrent instability after primary traumatic anterior shoulder dislocation in young patients. J Bone Joint Surg Am. 2006;88(11):2326–36.

31 Overuse Injuries of the Goalkeeper

Nuno Sevivas, Mustafa Karahan, Carlos Vilela, and António Cartucho

Contents

N. Sevivas (✉)
Life and Health Sciences Research Institute (ICVS), School of Medicine, University of Minho, Campus de Gualtar, 4710-057 Braga, Portugal

ICVS/3B's – PT Government Associate Laboratory, Braga/Guimarães, Portugal

Orthopaedics Department, Hospital de Braga and Hospital Privado de Braga, Braga, Portugal

Clínica do Dragão – Espregueira-Mendes Sports Centre, FIFA Medical Centre of Excellence, Porto, Portugal
e-mail: nunosevivas@med.uminho.pt

M. Karahan
Acibadem University, Istanbul, Turkey
e-mail: drmustafakarahan@gmail.com

C. Vilela
Orthopaedics Department, Hospital de Guimarães, Guimarães, Portugal
e-mail: vilela.carlos@sapo.pt

A. Cartucho
Orthopaedics Department, Hospital Cuf Descobertas, Lisboa, Portugal
e-mail: a.cartucho@netcabo.pt

31.1 Introduction

Football is a very popular sport with more than 260 million active practitioners worldwide [1], and its practice puts in risk the players of every age, at all playing levels and field positions, to an injury. Due to the way football is played, the injury incidence is higher in the lower than in the upper extremity [2], but goalkeepers (GK), however, due to the specificity of this job, are prone to upper-extremity injury, with a five times higher incidence compared to outfield players [3].

An overuse injury has been defined as a pain syndrome of the musculoskeletal system with insidious onset caused by repeated microtrauma and without a single traumatic, identifiable event responsible for the injury [4, 5]. This type of injury occurs gradually over time, when the repetition of the exercise can cause a consequent injury of the involved tissue that exceeds the natural capacity to heal. The spectrum of diseases depends on the specificity of the exercise involved that applies the same stress to specific areas of the human body causing an imbalance between work/injury and recovery.

The injury may appear as consequence of overtraining, repetitive actions, or inadequate periods of rest that prevents the organism to recover adequately from the stress.

The football GK is a specific tactical position that requires performing strenuous actions during practice sessions and competitive games [6]. It has

J. Espregueira-Mendes et al. (eds.), *Injuries and Health Problems in Football*, DOI 10.1007/978-3-662-53924-8_31

been observed that GK presents higher lactate dehydrogenase (LDH) and IL-6 than players occupying other tactical positions, leading to the conclusion that this specific job can cause more inflammation and muscle damage than other positions [7].

31.2 Epidemiology

Football is a lower-limb-dominant sport, and so it is not surprising that the incidence of upper-limb injuries is less frequent and it is also a less frequent concern than in sports like rugby or volleyball [8, 9]. Moreover, only 10% of upper-extremity injuries are related to repeated microtrauma and are by definition really overuse injuries. Among these non-acute traumatic injuries, approximately one third of all lesions affect the rotator cuff [3].

GK had a significantly higher incidence of upper-extremity injuries compared to outfield players (0.8 vs. 0.16 injuries/1000 h, RR 5.0, 95% CI 4.0–6.2, $p < 0.001$). Of all injuries registered among them, 18% affected the upper extremities, and its prevalence per season was consistently higher among GK than to outfield players (10–25% vs. 2–5%). These upper-extremity lesions in GK were also related with more layoff days and missed matches or training sessions [3].

31.3 Etiology and Pathomechanics

31.3.1 Shoulder

Shoulder injuries are 3.3% of all injuries reported in football players. When one considers the field position, GK do not suffer from minor trauma injuries as their midfield partners but are more likely to be injured from high-energy events. The most common overuse goalkeeper lesions are rotator cuff tendinopathy and partial or complete rotator cuff tears with an incidence of 50% of all lesions in this population, in contrast to 12% in the outfield players. Superior labrum anterior to posterior (SLAP) lesions and Bankart lesions are the most common ligamentous lesions, and humeral avulsion glenohumeral ligament (HAGL) and anterior labral periosteal sleeve avulsion (ALPSA) are seldom verified.

- *Treatment*

For treatment strategy reasons, shoulder lesions in football goalkeepers may be classified as major (bony Bankart, ALPSA, rotator cuff tear, and HAGL) and minor (undisplaced labral tear, cuff tendinopathy, and partial rotator cuff tears). If the last may be managed during season and if necessary operated near its end, the first must be address as soon as possible in order to avoid extension of the lesions and to recover the player early next season.

31.3.1.1 Cuff Tendinopathy and Partial Rotator Cuff Tears

Cuff tendinopathy and partial-thickness tears occur mainly on the supraspinatus tendon. Symptoms arise from mechanical impairment with adaptive response of the shoulder girdle, from inflammatory changes and involvement also of the long head of the biceps. Clinical diagnosis may be confirmed by magnetic ressonance imaging (MRI) allowing also to classify the tear as articular (AT), bursal (BT), or intratendinous (IT) [10].

- *Conservative Treatment*

Physiotherapy, anti-inflammatory drugs, and subacromial injections are all included as conservative treatment strategies of subacromial tendonitis. The objectives are to diminish the inflammatory response and to regain shoulder girdle normal biomechanics. Corticoid subacromial injections should be avoided. Growth factors have been proved to ameliorate pain and inflammatory signs of patients operated on for rotator cuff tears [11, 12]. Based on these results, authors propose to manage, during the season, patients that are still able to play and suffer from cuff tendonitis or partial rotator cuff tears, recurring to growth factors in subacromial injection.

Patients with degenerative partial-thickness tears due to impingement are treated similarly to those with rotator cuff tendinopathy and subacromial bursitis. Local rest, application of cold or heat, massage, nonsteroidal anti-inflammatory medication for a short period of time, modification of activities, gentle exercises for anterior and posterior capsular stretching, and later, muscle strengthening for the rotator cuff and the periscapular musculature to restore the mechanical balance [13]. Subacromial or intra-articular corticosteroid injections can also be used judiciously, depending on the location of the tear for those patients with persistent symptoms unresponsive to other means of pain reduction.

Pain and loss of active elevation have been identified as poor prognostic factors for successful conservative treatment [14]. Most bursal tears (BTs) respond poorly to conservative treatment [15]. Once the vicious circle of subacromial impingement has been established and/or the tear is deep, conservative treatment is rarely helpful. Early surgical intervention should be considered when the severe clinical manifestations and if imaging suggests a BT diagnosis [16]. In most cases, 3 months of conservative treatment are sufficient to assess the clinical improvement achievable without surgery. A fast therapeutic response predicts better outcomes and strength usually is difficult to improve [10, 17]. In other hand, conservative treatment consistently alleviated the pain and improved the range of motion.

- *Operative Treatment*

Timing for surgical treatment is crucial in sports. Degenerative partial tears that become symptomatic during the season may be treated conservatively, and return to play may be decided according to symptom control and functional recovery. Traumatic acute partial tears may also be conservatively controlled during the season. Nevertheless anterior supraspinatus and superior subscapularis tear as they interfere with the bicipital pulley, and BTs are more difficult to deal by conservative measures.

Surgical treatment is performed arthroscopically. This technique allows the surgeon to inspect all the shoulder and to take the right measures based on the clinical history and exam supported by complementary exams. For diagnosis confirmation, a systematic inspection and palpation of the joint and bursal sides of the cuff should be performed. Joint side fraying should be debrided, the extent of the lesion measured and a suture marker passed. Then a bursal side inspection should be performed, with bursectomy and quality assessment of the bursal side of the tendon. If an intratendinous lesion is suspected, thinning of the cuff, bulging and pressing the tendon with a probe on elevation or rotation of the arm can give the location of the lesion. Additionally, using the shaver can put the lesion in sight.

Treatment of most symptomatic partial tears should be directed toward a primary diagnosis such as an impingement syndrome or instability, with treatment of the partial tear itself being considered a part of a broader problem. Nevertheless, in traumatic lesions, the rotator cuff lesion is the cause of the dynamic impairment and consequently of the secondary inflammatory process of the bursa and the long head of the biceps (LHB). In this case, repair of the structural problem is the key.

Arthroscopy might be performed on a "beach chair" or lateral decubitus position depending on the training and preferences of the surgeon. Through a posterior portal, an articular side inspection is performed. The quality of the supraspinatus should be accessed, fraying should be debrided, and the presence of associated lesions should be noted. Very often a superior labrum lesion is present. Normally, a Snyder type 1 lesion resulting from vertical dynamic instability of the humeral head and only a debridement should be considered (Fig. 31.1). In other rare cases with type 2 or 3 SLAP lesions, the stability of the fragments and of the LHB should be accessed in order to decide whether to repair the lesion or perform a biceps tenodesis. In this specific

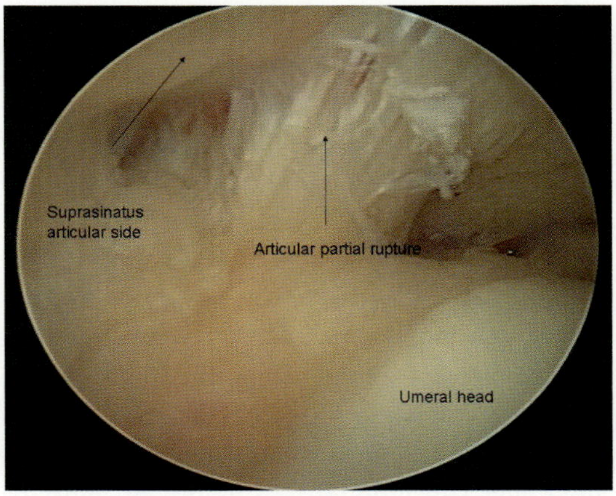

Fig. 31.1 Articular partial tear

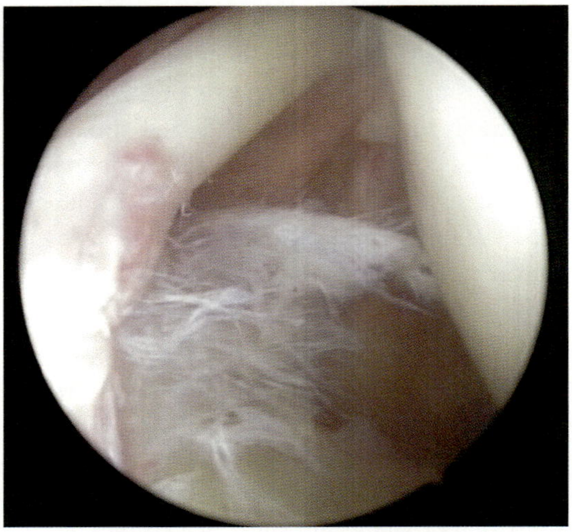

Fig. 31.2 Long head of the biceps (LHB) tenosynovitis and fraying associated to biceps Instability

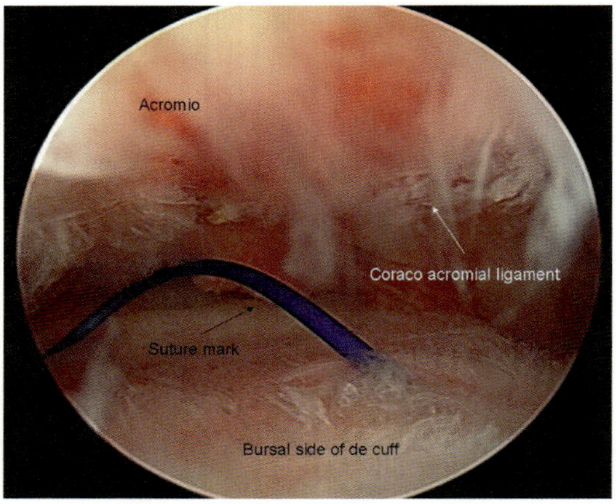

Fig. 31.3 Subacromial view

population our method of choice is to suprapectoraly fixate the LHB with an interference screw. After debriding, the extent of the lesion should be measured and marked. Care should be taken to access the integrity of the biceps posterior pulley and biceps stability (Fig. 31.2).

At the subacromial space, a careful but complete bursectomy should be performed and the suture marker identified. The quality of the tendon on the bursal side should be accessed, and indirect signs of impingement like fraying of the coracoacromial arch should be noted (Fig. 31.3). If the tear is 7 mm or less deep, debridement alone and subacromial decompression must be considered associated with stabilization of the LHB if necessary. If the tear is deeper than 7 mm, a repair using a suture anchor should be performed.

The surgeon must decide whether to do a trans-tendon repair or to remove the remaining tissue and treat the rupture as a complete tear. Some authors believe that the remaining cuff tissue in continuity is of poor quality, which increases the likelihood of postoperative pain and retear [18]. If completion of the rupture has been decided, configuration of the fixation, such as single-row, double-row, or transosseous equivalent, should be designed according to the extent of the tear, tissue quality, and elasticity.

Surgical approach results for partial-thickness supraspinatus tears have been extensively reported [18–21]. For instance, Park showed that surgical repair yields 93% of all patients with good or excellent results, and 95% demonstrated satisfactory outcome with regard to pain reduction and functional outcome.

Subscapularis tendon tears are less common than supraspinatus tears but more prone to cause significant disability, producing an unbalanced shoulder and originating an unstable LHB by lesion of the anterior pulley. Lesions may be classified according to Lafosse et al. [22], and the ruptured tendon should be repaired to the bone, using, for example, suture anchors. According to the same author, arthroscopic repair of subscapularis isolated tears can yield marked improvements in shoulder function and pain reduction.

31.3.1.2 Total Rotator Cuff Tears

Total rotator cuff tears in this young and sporty population must be surgically approached as soon as possible. Supraspinatus is more frequently involved. Arthroscopic treatment and repair using suture anchors is the "gold standard." The use of single-row, double-row, or transosseous equivalent has been a matter of discussion. In order to decide the best type of tendon repair, the surgeon might have taken into consideration the young age and sport activity of this population, the type of tear, and the quality of the tendon.

31.3.1.3 Labral Tears

Four types of superior labrum anterior to posterior (SLAP) lesions were initially described according to Snyder et al. [23]. However in the last years, several classifications have reported an increasing number of different types of SLAP lesions. The clinical usefulness of these last is not well established [23, 58].

As said previously, undisplaced tears of all the glenoid quadrants may be dealt conservatively during the season, and if signs of instability subside, they can be surgically repaired at the end of the season.

Surgical repair is accomplished arthroscopically, and stabilization can be done repairing the labrum using suture anchors. However, some authors prefer to treat SLAP 2 lesions with a LHB tenodesis in order to obtain a better control of pain and functional impairment [24]. This method may also be applied to type 3 and 4 lesions that involve the LHB or turn this structure instable. Tenodesis should be performed with a strong primary stabilization method, and an interference screw is a good option for this high-demanding population [25].

31.3.2 Elbow

The elbow joint is a trochoginglymoid joint, between the humerus, radius, and ulna, with two degrees of freedom [26]. Stability is provided by a complex and interrelated structure of bony and ligamentous anatomy, and the restraints are often classified as either primary or secondary. The primary stabilizers are the anterior bundle of the medial collateral ligament (MCL), the ulnohumeral joint congruency, and the lateral collateral ligament (LCL) complex, and the secondary stabilizers are the anterior joint capsule, the forearm musculature, and radial head [27–29].

The LCL is a complex of ligaments, composed of four distinct structures: the annular ligament, radial collateral ligament (RCL), accessory lateral collateral ligament, and lateral ulnar collateral ligament (LUCL) [30]. The LUCL in particular has been credited with a great clinical significance as a constraint against posterolateral rotatory instability and its reconstruction after lesion is advised [31, 32].

The MCL has anterior, posterior, and transverse bundles [33, 34] where the former originating in the medial epicondyle and inserting into the medial aspect of the coronoid process is the primary restraint to valgus and internal rotation [35, 36].

The muscles around the elbow joint are dynamic constraints, which help to provide stability [29, 37, 38]. The wrist extensors originate from the lateral epicondyle of the humerus, whereas the flexors originate from the medial epicondyle.

31.3.2.1 Epicondylar Pain

Epicondylar pain is a frequent complaint that commonly is referred to as tennis elbow (in the lateral side) and golfer's elbow (in the medial side). These entities are overuse injuries related to sport activities where repetitive movements and micro traumatisms of the wrist flexor and extensor tendons are thought to be the mechanism for injury. Moreover, repetitive movements with eccentric contraction (muscle-tendon unit lengthening while contracting) increase susceptibility to epicondylitis [39].

Despite the name suggesting inflammation as the origin of the pathology, the hallmark of this disease is microvascular damage, degenerative cellular processes, and disorganized healing, and so "tendinosis" is considered a more appropriate name for this clinical entity. Moreover, histologic examination of the extensor carpi radialis brevis (ECRB) in lateral epicondylitis has demonstrated chronic degeneration with few inflammatory cells, many immature fibroblasts, disorganized vascular elements, and disorganized collagen [40].

Overall, lateral epicondylitis is 7–10 times more common than medial epicondylitis [41].

Clinically, the elbow pain at the lateral or medial side that can radiate a few centimeters down the forearm according to the group of tendons affected is usually the presenting complaint. It has an insidious onset that is worsened with activity and relieved by rest. Patients may also feel weakness in the hand or difficulty carrying items.

Physical examination is important to confirm the diagnosis and exclude other differential diagnoses affecting the cervical spine, shoulder, elbow, and wrist. Tenderness in the lateral epicondyle and the origin of the wrist extensor muscles is suggestive of lateral epicondylitis and pain more distally located, approximately 5 cm from the lateral epicondyle is suggestive of a posterior interosseous nerve syndrome. Palpation of the medial aspect of the elbow aids diagnosing medial epicondylitis, an ulnar nerve entrapment, a MCL sprain, or a combination of the three entities. Palpation of the medial epicondyle and muscle bellies of the wrist flexor tendons elicits tenderness in a case of medial epicondylitis. In the wrist, pain with resisted wrist extension is suggestive of lateral epicondylitis and pain with resisted wrist flexion is suggestive of medial epicondylitis.

Epicondylitis is a clinical diagnosis, but imagiological examinations (e.g., X-ray, ultrasonography, or MRI) are used after a failure of conservative therapy to rule out other clinical entities [39]. Even though a radial nerve entrapment can be a dynamic situation, electromyography studies are used to help identifying this condition [42].

The treatment is summarized in the acronym PRICEMM (*p*rotection, *r*est, *i*ce, *c*ompression, *e*levation, *m*edication, *m*odalities) [39]. *Protection* means that overuse activity that resulted in tendon injury should be avoided to stop the vicious cycle and to prevent further damage. Relative *rest* is important because some therapeutic exercise can help healing the damaged tendon. *Ice* massage can assist in pain control. A counterforce elbow strap for *compression* approximately 2 cm below the painful epicondyle can help offload the proximal tendon during wrist extension or flexion. The effectiveness in pain control can be evaluated during the clinical examination, asking the patient to perform the movements that elicit pain (e.g., wrist or finger extension) and feel if the manual compression by the examinator's hand decreases the visual analog scale (VAS) for pain.

Medications are used only for pain control. Physical therapy modalities, such as electrical stimulation, phonophoresis, and iontophoresis, are effective in assisting on pain control but are unable to correct the underlying tendinosis. To accomplish this, stretching and strengthening exercises are performed on the flexor-pronator group or the extensor-supinator group according the affected tendons. Progression to eccentric exercises is the goal, because this is thought to reestablish normal tendon architecture [43].

A corticosteroid injection is frequently used and safe for trial in refractory cases of epicondylitis and can relieve pain of neurogenic origin [44]. However the natural course of the disease may be unaltered or potentially worsened by this intervention [39]. Moreover, in professional practitioners, its use must be communicated in advance for the Doping Control Commission to avoid legal problems for the athlete.

Autologous blood injections and platelet-rich plasma (PRP) injections have been used to treat epicondylitis, and the results are promising but inconsistent [45, 46]. The rationale for its use is the hypovascular and noninflammatory nature of epicondylitis. Both autologous blood injections and PRP injections are thought to use platelet-derived growth factors and angiogenic mediators to aid in the healing response by recruiting vascularity to the damage tissue [47].

Extracorporeal shock wave therapy (ECSWT) has been used in refractory cases, and the procedure uses acoustic waves to treat tendinosis. The mechanism of action is thought to be related to the activation of the inflammatory cycle, release of local growth factors, and the recruitment of appropriate stem cells to the affected area [48]. However a systematic review of ECSWT concluded that there was little to no benefit from this procedure in the treatment of lateral elbow pain [49].

When conservative treatment fails to improve the symptoms, then surgery is advised. Releases of the tendon origins by percutaneous, open, or arthroscopic means are proposed surgical options in recalcitrant cases. All methods have good results in pain relief, but if posterior interosseous nerve compression is associated, then the open approach offers the opportunity to associate the decompression of the nerve in the same procedure.

31.3.2.2 UCL Injury

Ulnar collateral ligament (UCL) injury may be acute or chronic, and the latter is associated with movements like throwing a ball with the hand, which is a typical action of GK when passing the ball to teammates. The classic presentation is medial elbow pain worsened during throwing maneuver, and physical exam can often diagnose this entity with the "milking" maneuver. To confirm the diagnosis, radiography, which may be normal initially, may demonstrate changes associated with chronic laxity and valgus extension overload. Medial joint opening >2 mm on valgus views is consistent with instability. MRI is the gold standard diagnosing UCL sprain or tearing with 100% sensitivity for complete tears of the anterior band of the UCL. However, MRI has a low sensitivity (14%) for partial-thickness tears, whereas magnetic ressonance imaging (MRA) has a sensitivity of 86% and specificity of 100% for partial tears [50].

Physical therapy, evaluation of throwing mechanics, and a hinged elbow brace are part of the conservative treatment. Persistent valgus instability after 6 months of nonsurgical management may indicate a need for surgical intervention with anterior bundle UCL reconstruction, often using palmaris longus autograft, to restore valgus stability [51]. In addition, UCL calcification or tears typically require surgical intervention, again via UCL reconstruction [52].

31.3.2.3 Osteochondritis Dissecans (OCD) of the Capitellum

Repetitive impact injuries to the elbow of GK caused by the ball hitting the fully extended distal part of a forearm have been well described [53, 54]. It is supposed that elbow valgus loading is the likely cause of such impact injuries to the elbow [55].

OCD of the capitellum is a flap of cartilage typically with a bone attached that is lifted off its underlying bony bed (Fig. 31.4) and can result also from that repetitive valgus force applied to the capitellum [56]. The valgus loads at the time of ball blockade during the ball hitting and mechanical mismatch between the central radial head and lateral capitellum could be considered as the reason for the disease. Although the OCD is primarily a disorder of adolescents, adults can also develop the problem, and incomplete cure of acute elbow injuries may result in OCD due to inadequate treatment [54].

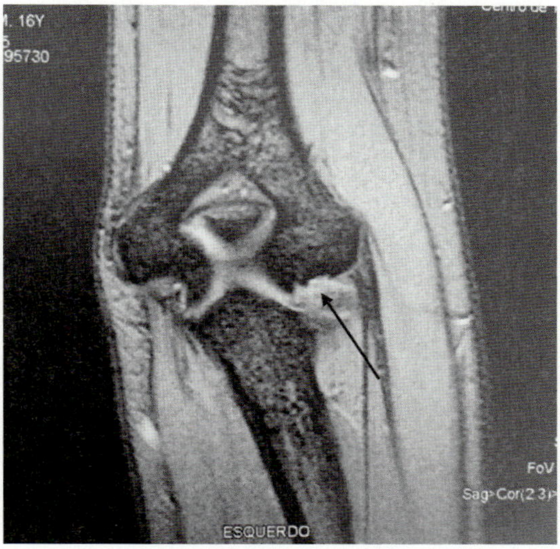

Fig. 31.4 Osteochondritis Dissecans (OCD) of the Capitellum (*arrow*)

Radiographically, localized fragmentation of the capitellum may be seen, possibly with progression to loose body formation and, on MRI, demonstrates low T1 signal intensity in the early phase. MRA is the preferred modality to evaluate articular cartilage as well as for the presence and stability of loose bodies [50].

Nondisplaced stable fragments can be treated conservatively until symptoms subside. Surgical intervention might improve clinical pain, but pediatric athletes may never return to their presurgical competitive level [50, 57].

Conclusion

Sports practice became common in the general population, and both children and the elderly more often maintain this practice on a regular basis where football is probably the most popular and practiced worldwide.

Shoulder overuse lesions of the GK predominantly involve the rotator cuff. Cuff tendinopathy associated with impingement syndrome and partial rotator cuff tears may be treated conservatively. Complete rotator cuff tears should be operated on as soon as possible, and arthroscopy is the preferred method allowing a rationale strategy and treating associated lesions. Instable and symptomatic labral lesions should be treated arthroscopically using suture anchors, and SLAP lesions might benefit of LHB tenodesis instead of repair in athletes from the third decade of life.

GK with elbow or wrist pain warrant clinical examination and further evaluation with imagiological studies to establish the correct diagnosis. Conservative treatment based on rest, specific sportive technique evaluation, and correction and rehabilitation is usually the first step. However, if the patient does not improve, then he/she may benefit from surgical intervention followed by a specific program of protection and rehabilitation.

Knowledge of the technical specificity of the GK, most frequent associated overuse injuries and a proper diagnostic and therapeutic approach, allows returning the athlete to the playing field while minimizing long-term adverse outcomes. It is important to emphasize that the sport practice should be resumed only after the subsidence of the symptoms.

References

1. FIFA Big Count 2006: 270 million people active in football http://www.fifa.com/mm/document/fifafacts/bcoffsurv/bigcount.statspackage_7024.pdf.
2. Ekstrand J, Gillquist J. Soccer injuries and their mechanisms: a prospective study. Med Sci Sports Exerc. 1983;15:267–70.
3. Ekstrand J, Hagglund M, Tornqvist H, Kristenson K, Bengtsson H, Magnusson H, Walden M. Upper extremity injuries in male elite football players. Knee Surg Sports Traumatol Arthrosc. 2013;21:1626–32.
4. Hagglund M, Walden M, Bahr R, Ekstrand J. Methods for epidemiological study of injuries to professional football players: developing the UEFA model. Br J Sports Med. 2005;39:340–6.
5. Fuller CW, Ekstrand J, Junge A, Andersen TE, Bahr R, Dvorak J, Hagglund M, McCrory P, Meeuwisse WH. Consensus statement on injury definitions and data collection procedures in studies of football (soccer) injuries. Br J Sports Med. 2006;40:193–201.
6. Ziv G, Lidor R. Physical characteristics, physiological attributes, and on-field performances of soccer goalkeepers. Int J Sports Physiol Perform. 2011;6:509–24.
7. de Moura NR, Borges LS, Santos VC, Joel GB, Bortolon JR, Hirabara SM, Cury-Boaventura MF, Pithon-Curi TC, Curi R, Hatanaka E. Muscle lesions and inflammation in futsal players according to their tactical positions. J Strength Cond Res. 2013;27:2612–8.
8. Ekstrand J, Hagglund M, Walden M. Injury incidence and injury patterns in professional football: the UEFA injury study. Br J Sports Med. 2011;45:553–8.
9. Hart D, Funk L. Serious shoulder injuries in professional soccer: return to participation after surgery. Knee Surg Sports Traumatol Arthrosc. 2015;23:2123–9.
10. Ellman H. Diagnosis and treatment of incomplete rotator cuff tears. Clin Orthop Relat Res. 1990;254:64–74.
11. Randelli PS, Arrigoni P, Cabitza P, Volpi P, Maffulli N. Autologous platelet rich plasma for arthroscopic rotator cuff repair. A pilot study. Disabil Rehabil. 2008;30:1584–9.
12. Randelli P, Arrigoni P, Ragone V, Aliprandi A, Cabitza P. Platelet rich plasma in arthroscopic rotator cuff repair: a prospective RCT study, 2-year follow-up. J Shoulder Elbow Surg. 2011;20:518–28.
13. Kuhn JE. Exercise in the treatment of rotator cuff impingement: a systematic review and a synthesized evidence-based rehabilitation protocol. J Shoulder Elbow Surg. 2009;18:138–60.
14. Yamaguchi K, Tetro AM, Blam O, Evanoff BA, Teefey SA, Middleton WD. Natural history of asymptomatic rotator cuff tears: a longitudinal analysis of asymptomatic tears detected sonographically. J Shoulder Elbow Surg. 2001;10:199–203.
15. Hawkins RH, Dunlop R. Nonoperative treatment of rotator cuff tears. Clin Orthop Relat Res. 1995;321:178–88.
16. Cordasco FA, Backer M, Craig EV, Klein D, Warren RF. The partial-thickness rotator cuff tear: is acromioplasty without repair sufficient? Am J Sports Med. 2002;30:257–60.
17. Bokor DJ, Hawkins RJ, Huckell GH, Angelo RL, Schickendantz MS. Results of nonoperative management of full-thickness tears of the rotator cuff. Clin Orthop Relat Res. 1993;294:103–10.
18. Porat S, Nottage WM, Fouse MN. Repair of partial thickness rotator cuff tears: a retrospective review with minimum two-year follow-up. J Shoulder Elbow Surg. 2008;17:729–31.
19. Park JY, Chung KT, Yoo MJ. A serial comparison of arthroscopic repairs for partial- and full-thickness rotator cuff tears. Arthroscopy. 2004;20:705–11.
20. Weber SC. Arthroscopic debridement and acromioplasty versus mini-open repair in the management of significant partial-thickness tears of the rotator cuff. Orthop Clin North Am. 1997;28:79–82.
21. Weber SC. Arthroscopic debridement and acromioplasty versus mini-open repair in the treatment of significant partial-thickness rotator cuff tears. Arthroscopy. 1999;15:126–31.
22. Lafosse L, Jost B, Reiland Y, Audebert S, Toussaint B, Gobezie R. Structural integrity and clinical outcomes after arthroscopic repair of isolated subscapularis tears. J Bone Joint Surg Am. 2007;89:1184–93.

23. Nam EK, Snyder SJ. Diagnosis and treatment of superior labrum anterior and posterior (SLAP) lesions. Am J Sports Med. 2003;31:798–810.
24. Boileau P, Parratte S, Chuinard C, Roussanne Y, Shia D, Bicknell R. Arthroscopic treatment of isolated type II SLAP lesions: biceps tenodesis as an alternative to reinsertion. Am J Sports Med. 2009;37:929–36.
25. Boileau P, Krishnan SG, Coste JS, Walch G. Arthroscopic biceps tenodesis: a new technique using bioabsorbable interference screw fixation. Arthroscopy. 2002;18:1002–12.
26. Morrey BF, Sanchez-Sotelo J. The elbow and its disorders. Philadelphia: WB Saunders Company; 2009.
27. McKee MD, Schemitsch EH, Sala MJ, O'Driscoll SW. The pathoanatomy of lateral ligamentous disruption in complex elbow instability. J Shoulder Elbow Surg. 2003;12:391–6.
28. Morrey BF, An KN. Stability of the elbow: osseous constraints. J Shoulder Elbow Surg. 2005;14: 174S–8S.
29. Tarassoli P, McCann P, Amirfeyz R. *Complex* instability of the elbow. Injury. 2013;48:568–77.
30. Reichel LM, Milam GS, Sitton SE, Curry MC, Mehlhoff TL. Elbow lateral collateral ligament injuries. J Hand Surg Am. 2013;38:184–201.
31. O'Driscoll SW, Bell DF, Morrey BF. Posterolateral rotatory instability of the elbow. J Bone Joint Surg Am. 1991;73:440–6.
32. O'Driscoll SW, Morrey BF, Korinek S, An KN. Elbow subluxation and dislocation. A spectrum of instability. Clin Orthop Relat Res. 1992;280:186–97.
33. Morrey BF, An KN. Functional anatomy of the ligaments of the elbow. Clin Orthop Relat Res. 1985;201:84–90.
34. Floris S, Olsen BS, Dalstra M, Sojbjerg JO, Sneppen O. The medial collateral ligament of the elbow joint: anatomy and kinematics. J Shoulder Elbow Surg. 1998;7:345–51.
35. Regan WD, Korinek SL, Morrey BF, An KN. Biomechanical study of ligaments around the elbow joint. Clin Orthop Relat Res. 1991;271:170–9.
36. Morrey BF, Tanaka S, An KN. Valgus stability of the elbow. A definition of primary and secondary constraints. Clin Orthop Relat Res. 1991;265:187–95.
37. Safran MR, Baillargeon D. Soft-tissue stabilizers of the elbow. J Shoulder Elbow Surg. 2005;14: 179S–85S.
38. An KN, Hui FC, Morrey BF, Linscheid RL, Chao EY. Muscles across the elbow joint: a biomechanical analysis. J Biomech. 1981;14:659–69.
39. Pitzer ME, Seidenberg PH, Bader DA. Elbow tendinopathy. Med Clin North Am. 2014;98:833–49, xiii.
40. Kraushaar BS, Nirschl RP. Tendinosis of the elbow (tennis elbow). Clinical features and findings of histological, immunohistochemical, and electron microscopy studies. J Bone Joint Surg Am. 1999;81:259–78.
41. Leach RE, Miller JK. Lateral and medial epicondylitis of the elbow. Clin Sports Med. 1987;6:259–72.
42. Lubahn JD, Cermak MB. Uncommon nerve compression syndromes of the upper extremity. J Am Acad Orthop Surg. 1998;6:378–86.
43. Stanish WD, Rubinovich RM, Curwin S. Eccentric exercise in chronic tendinitis. Clin Orthop Relat Res. 1986;208:65–8.
44. Ljung BO, Alfredson H, Forsgren S. Neurokinin 1-receptors and sensory neuropeptides in tendon insertions at the medial and lateral epicondyles of the humerus. Studies on tennis elbow and medial epicondylalgia. J Orthop Res. 2004;22:321–7.
45. Peerbooms JC, Sluimer J, Bruijn DJ, Gosens T. Positive effect of an autologous platelet concentrate in lateral epicondylitis in a double-blind randomized controlled trial: platelet-rich plasma versus corticosteroid injection with a 1-year follow-up. Am J Sports Med. 2010;38:255–62.
46. Suresh SP, Ali KE, Jones H, Connell DA. Medial epicondylitis: is ultrasound guided autologous blood injection an effective treatment? Br J Sports Med. 2006;40:935–9.
47. Bales CP, Placzek JD, Malone KJ, Vaupel Z, Arnoczky SP. Microvascular supply of the lateral epicondyle and common extensor origin. J Shoulder Elbow Surg. 2007;16:497–501.
48. Thiel M. Application of shock waves in medicine. Clin Orthop Relat Res. 2001;387:18–21.
49. Buchbinder R, Green SE, Youd JM, Assendelft WJ, Barnsley L, Smidt N. Systematic review of the efficacy and safety of shock wave therapy for lateral elbow pain. J Rheumatol. 2006;33:1351–63.
50. Paz DA, Chang GH, Yetto Jr JM, Dwek JR, Chung CB. Upper extremity overuse injuries in pediatric athletes: clinical presentation, imaging findings, and treatment. Clin Imaging. 2015;39:954–64.
51. Conway JE. Arthroscopic repair of partial-thickness rotator cuff tears and SLAP lesions in professional baseball players. Orthop Clin North Am. 2001;32:443–56.
52. Safran MR. Ulnar collateral ligament injury in the overhead athlete: diagnosis and treatment. Clin Sports Med. 2004;23:643–63.
53. Tyrdal S, Bahr R. High prevalence of elbow problems among goalkeepers in European team handball – 'handball goalie's elbow'. Scand J Med Sci Sports. 1996;6:297–302.
54. Rod E, Ivkovic A, Boric I, Jankovic S, Radic A, Hudetz D. Acute hyperextension/valgus trauma to the elbow in top-level adult male water polo goalkeepers: a cause of osteochondritis dissecans of the capitellum? Injury. 2013;44(Suppl 3):S46–8.
55. Akgun U, Karahan M, Tiryaki C, Erol B, Engebretsen L. Direction of the load on the elbow of the ball blocking handball goalie. Knee Surg Sports Traumatol Arthrosc. 2008;16:522–30.
56. Jobe FW, Nuber G. Throwing injuries of the elbow. Clin Sports Med. 1986;5:621–36.
57. Kobayashi K, Burton KJ, Rodner C, Smith B, Caputo AE. Lateral compression injuries in the pediatric elbow: Panner's disease and osteochondritis dissecans of the capitellum. J Am Acad Orthop Surg. 2004;12:246–54.
58. Maffet MW, Gartsman GM, Moseley B. Superior labrum-bicepcs tendon complex lesion of the shoulder. Am J Sports Med. 1995;23:93–8.

Part VIII

Muscle Injuries in the Lower Limb

Epidemiology, Risk Factors, and Prevention

32

Paulo Barreira, João Pedro Araújo, Ruben Ferreira, and Nuno Loureiro

Contents

32.1 Introduction

Muscle injuries are the number one problem for football players and medical and technical staffs, representing an average of 35% of all injuries in football. Besides that, this kind of injury also represents the one causing more match and training absences, showing the importance to understand it [1, 2].

Although it has been always a relevant issue in football teams, only in 2001 football injuries started to be conveniently studied by Ekstrand et al. [1, 2] in a study using the clubs participating in the Europe Champions League. This was the first football injuries' epidemiological study performed in a large scale that provided football professionals with an injury profile of such an amazing sport [1, 2].

Later on, and in order to specifically study muscle injury behavior in football, Ekstrand et al. presented us with another large-scale

P. Barreira (✉)
Physiotherapist (PhD)/Osteopath, Football Medicine®, Al Jazira SC, Abu Dhabi, UAE
e-mail: paulobarreiragmr@gmail.com

J.P. Araújo
Clínica do Dragão, Espregueira-Mendes Sports Centre – FIFA Medical Centre of Excellence, Porto, Portugal

Football Medicine, Medical Department, Al Jazira Football Club, Abu Dhabi, UAE
e-mail: joaopedroaraujo@gmail.com

R. Ferreira
Physiotherapist, Football Medicine®, Al Jazira SC, Abu Dhabi, UAE
e-mail: rubenferreira88@gmail.com

N. Loureiro
Medical Director of Paços Ferreira FC, Paços de Ferreira, Portugal

Medical Director of Portuguese Cycling Federation and Medical Committee of the Portuguese Olympic Committee, Paços de Ferreira, Portugal

Clínica do Dragão, Espregueira-Mendes Sports Centre - FIFA Medical Centre of Excellence, Porto, Portugal
e-mail: nunoloureiro4@gmail.com

J. Espregueira-Mendes et al. (eds.), *Injuries and Health Problems in Football*,
DOI 10.1007/978-3-662-53924-8_32

epidemiological study, becoming the most important study among this issue [1, 2].

That particular study had a significant importance once it showed football community the relevance of the injuries throughout the season, revealing the number of absences to trainings and matches and highlighting the importance of adopting more efficient prevention strategies.

The best prevention program will be the one that is able to control or decrease the greatest number of injury risk factors of each player. This way, to successfully implement a muscle injury prevention program, sports professionals must, first, have knowledge about its risk factors, being able to screen it, and then have strategies to reduce it.

This chapter's goal is to give the reader an overview regarding football muscle injury epidemiology and identify its risk factors to ultimately able sports professionals to wisely develop a muscle injury prevention program with a wide approach.

32.2 Epidemiology

As mentioned above, the studies performed by Ekstrand et al. [1, 2] became the reference in what concerns to muscle injuries' epidemiology in football. Considering that, this chapter will focus on Ekstrand's research, clarifying the reader about this issue [1, 2].

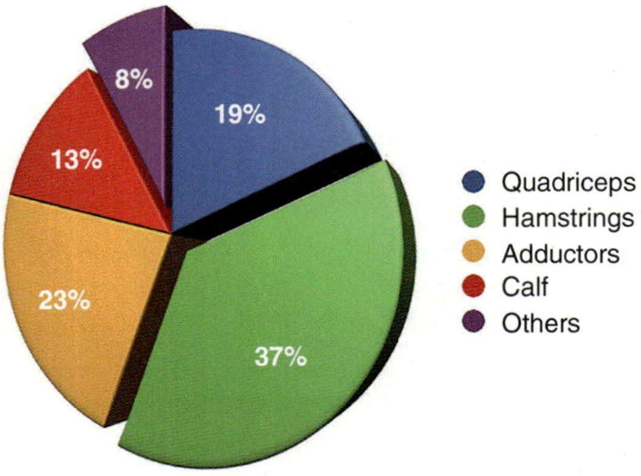

Fig. 32.1 Muscle injuries incidence distribution in football (Adapted from Ekstrand et al. (2011))

32.2.1 Incidence

Muscle injuries occupy the first position among football injuries' incidence; however, its distribution within lower limb muscles is not homogeneous, neither its injury mechanism [1, 2].

Muscle injuries may be classified as direct or indirect, resulting from a contusion or a strain, respectively, being 95% of them due to an indirect mechanism (e.g., sprinting, kicking) [1–3].

As shown in Fig. 32.1, the hamstrings are the most injured muscles in football, counting 37% of them and 12% of all injuries in football, being the biceps femoris the most commonly implicated portion [4].

Besides having a lower incidence, there are some other muscle injuries that might occur in professional football practice (e.g., rectus abdominis strain); however, its incidence is considerably lower than the muscle mentioned above, once all other muscles' injuries represent only 8% of all muscle injuries in football [1, 2].

32.2.2 Injury Mechanism

As mentioned before, most of the muscle injuries in football are muscle strains due to an indirect mechanism.

This kind of injury happens usually on the myotendinous junction where the muscle fibers converge and the forces tend to be more tangential in this place, turning it more prone to injury during eccentric efforts when the connective tis-

Table 32.1 Typical injury mechanism of the most frequently injured muscles in football

Muscle group	Typical injury mechanism
Hamstrings	Sprinting (Biceps Femoris)
	Stretching (Semimembranous)
Quadriceps	Shooting (Rectus Femoris)
	Sprinting
Groin	Changing Direction
	Shooting
	Stretching
Calf	Acceleration/Deceleration

sue is heavily tensioned. Besides that, the myotendinous junction is also a less irrigated tissue, which may contribute also to the injury risk at this location. However, muscle strains may also occur in myofascial location or, less often, being an intramuscular injury [5].

Although the typical injury mechanism of each of the most frequently injured muscles in football is different (e.g., groin muscle group while changing direction), it usually happens during an eccentric effort, when the muscle is elongating at the same time it is contracting (e.g., hamstrings slowing down the thigh and leg while sprinting) or in the transition between the eccentric and concentric phase of the movement [6].

Table 32.1 represents the most frequently injury mechanism for each muscle group in football.

32.2.3 Severity

According to Ekstrand et al. [1, 2] studies, in general, a professional football team can expect around 58% of the muscle injuries will result in an absence of more than 1 week, whereas 11% of the muscle injuries will be able to be classified as severe once it will cause a period of training and match absence of more than 4 weeks.

Quadriceps strains were the injuries that caused longer absence periods of around 17 days on average, followed by calf muscles (15 days), hamstrings (14 days), and groin strains (13 days).

32.2.4 Recurrence

Besides not being statistically different between them, quadriceps and groin muscle group are the ones with higher recurrence rate (17%), followed by hamstrings (16%) and calf (13%), leading to higher absence periods than the index injury [1, 2].

32.3 Risk Factors

Nowadays, the term "injury prevention" is one of the most mentioned in sports environment. Injuries may lead to decreased competitive performance, reducing players' availability to train and play. That is the reason why epidemiology and risk factors identification have a considerable importance once it will give us the lead to decrease injury risk.

There are two kinds of risk factors, *non-modifiable* and *modifiable*. The first ones are related with race, age, or weather, for instance, those are the ones that, besides being important, sports professionals are not able to interfere on it.

On the other hand, modifiable risk factors identification has a significant importance to sports professionals once, addressing them, professionals might be able to decrease injury risk – strength, range of motion, and motor control are examples of this category.

Longitudinal studies have been helping sports community to better understand muscle injuries' risk factors in football; however, there is still some conflict in literature when trying to quantify the strength of each risk factor identified [7].

Considering the continuously high recurrence of muscle injuries besides all the efforts made in order to prevent it, sports professionals should consider that not all risk factors are identified still, a fact that can be leading us to an ineffective approach regarding the modifiable risk factors [8].

Figure 32.2 represents a hierarchy relative to the existing level of evidence regarding each muscle injury risk factor [7, 9–15]. On the bottom of the pyramid are seen two levels of muscle injury risk factors that have a significant amount of evidence to be considered as a risk factor for the most relevant football muscle injuries, followed by the intermediate level which represents risk factors that are important and gather a considerable amount of evidence in some of the more common football muscle injuries; and, on the top of the pyramid are represented the muscle injuries' risk factors that, besides being clinically significant for sports professionals, there is still some controversy regarding its strength as a muscle injury risk factor taking in consideration the small amount of and ambiguous studies outcomes.

32.4 Prevention

Considering the importance of muscular strength as a risk factor in hamstring injuries, the normalization of eccentric strength and

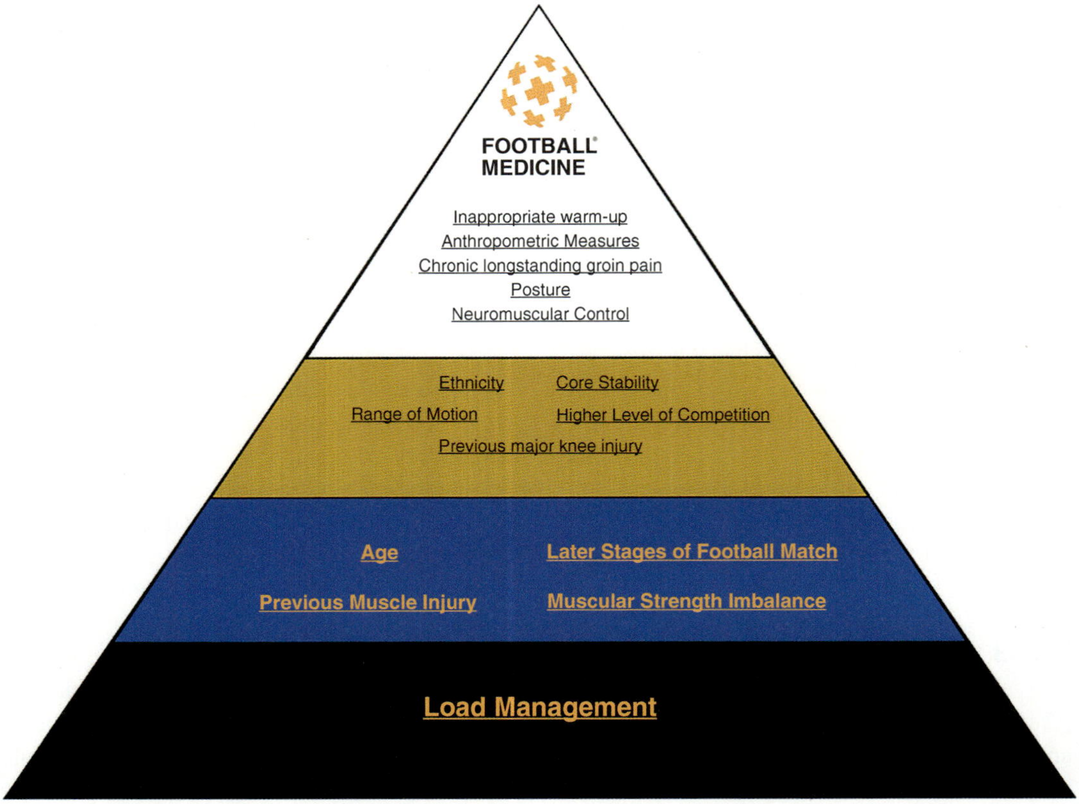

Fig. 32.2 Muscle injury risk factors pyramid

functional ratios between/in both sides are of significantly importance when trying to prevent its strain [16]. However, muscle injuries are multifactorial, with modifiable/non-modifiable risk factors and some others that might be still unknown – considering the consistent significant incidence and recurrence of muscle injuries in football throughout the years – which means that, regardless all the efforts, prevention strategies are tools that might allow us to *decrease* the injury risk, but will not assure that injuries will not happen [8].

Muscle injuries' risk factors assessment should be done during the preseason screening and monitored systematically during the season (see Chap. 34 in this book), in order to:

1. Assess injury prevention program's efficiency to solve/decrease the risk factors throughout the season
2. Make sure those players that did not have a specific risk factor in preseason do not develop it during the season (e.g., strength deficit due to inappropriate training, injuries, and pain-related inhibitory processes)

Figure 32.2 shows the injury risk factors that should be assessed and controlled during the season in order to establish athlete's muscle injury risk profile, being able to develop an individualized injury prevention program addressing those risk factors.

Muscle injury prevention programs' aim is to decrease/eliminate or manage the know injury risk factors of each athlete, focusing especially on the modifiable ones. However, some non-modifiable risk factors might be addressed indirectly. Considering "age" as a risk factor for hamstring muscle strains, besides not being able to modify it, but knowing that hamstring strains usually happen

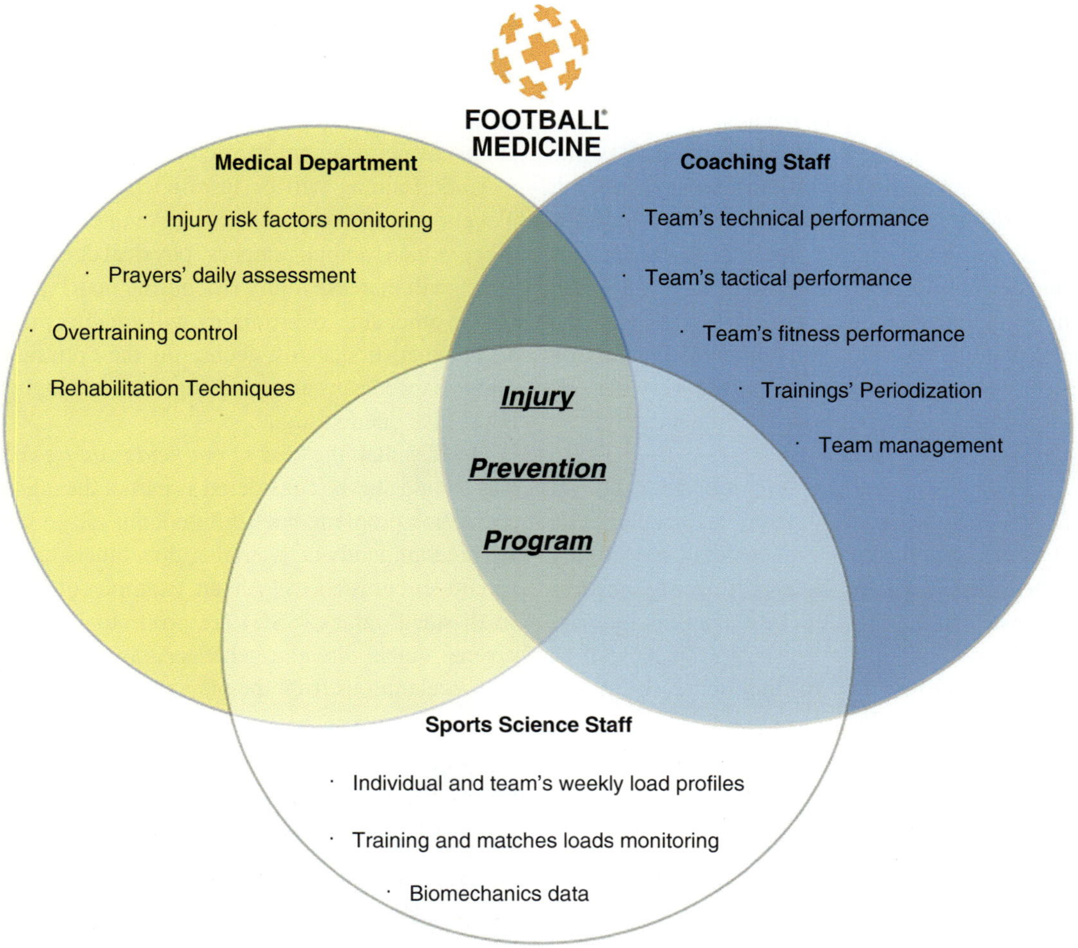

Fig. 32.3 Injury prevention program planning dynamic

while performing a high-speed run or a sprint [4], sports professionals can control player's very high intensity (VHI) distance during trainings, in order to decrease its risk of injury due to its intrinsic factor "age" that cannot be modified, avoiding an overload. This example highlights the importance of training load monitoring and also the need to create cutoffs on players' training load goals considering their injury risk factors and athlete's individual fitness performance profile.

Traditionally, the term "injury prevention program" was intuitively connected with gym/field routines contemplating strength, flexibility, and motor control exercises. Nowadays, the term "injury prevention program" must be seen with a broader view, engaging medical, sports science, and technical staffs in order to develop individual and team strategies to prevent injuries through trainings and load management (e.g., avoid overload and recovery strategies), individualized exercise prescription (e.g., normalize left hamstring eccentric strength), and rehabilitation techniques (e.g., improve left dorsiflexion lunge score).

Considering Fig. 32.3 is possible to understand that injury prevention goes far beyond a traditional gym workout. Injury prevention starts before any training, from the moment players' complaints are heard to discuss their availability to train or not and can go as far as individual out-field training modification according to players' complaints and physical data from the previous trainings.

Every injury prevention program should contemplate at least the below mentioned interventions.

32.4.1 Load Management

32.4.1.1 Training Periodization

Stress Versus Recovery Periods

Recovery is most likely as important as the stimulus given by the training session, once it will be the recovery periods that will allow athletes body to improve their physical performance. Important physiological event will happen during those periods, allowing the accommodation and adaptation to the training loads, which will not happen if recovery periods are not respected, having a detrimental effect on physical performance [10].

Studies suggest that the muscle needs at least 48 h to recover from a mechanically stressful stimulus. This means that, before that time, muscle will be underperforming, absorbing less load that it would be expecting, increasing the risk of joint overuse injuries as well as muscle injuries due to the decrease in the strength levels [17].

Considering those points, training periodization should be planned carefully in order to allow muscle adaptation after heavy load stimulus. Besides that, players should be monitored regarding their recovery status, which can be done using scales/questionnaires, implementing recovery strategies whenever possible.

32.4.1.2 Training Load Quantification

As mentioned above, players' subjective fatigue perception is important for decision-making regarding their availability to train. However, objective data is considerably important once it will allow us to quantify and compare training loads between sessions. Figure 32.4 as a GPS monitoring system to monitor training load.

GPS Monitoring [9]

- VHI
- Accelerations/decelerations
- Running symmetry
- Team and players' profiles
- Weekly load increments

32.4.1.3 Undertraining Versus Overtraining

Training loads should be monitored carefully in order to avoid undertraining or overtraining situations, reaching an *optimal load* instead [10, 17].

Undertraining will be insufficient to develop players' physical capabilities or even not be able to reproduce football matches' physical demands, which will increase injury risk during match play. On the other side, overtraining will conduct players to exhaustion status, decreasing their physical performance levels and exposing them to a higher injury risk due to fatigue.

Besides that, the *kind of out-field training volume* should also be considered as part of the injury prevention program, once different muscle groups are predominantly active rather than others under certain circumstances. As an example of that, small-sided games (SSG) are prone to promote several quick direction changes, accelerations, and decelerations from the players, however with

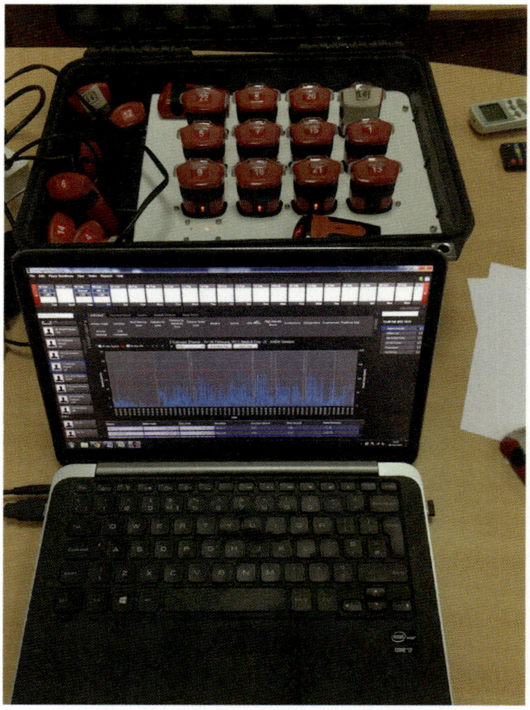

Fig. 32.4 GPS monitoring system with player's training raw data

a considerable moderated maximum speed. On the other hand, exercises in a wider space (50 m length) will be more prone to promote higher speeds, increasing players VHI distance content during the training session.

Considering this, SSG may be more specific to load muscle groups in the groin area as well as quadriceps femoris and calf muscles, once they have a tight relationship with acceleration and deceleration abilities, as well as with changing direction, while exercises in a wider space can preferentially load the hamstrings once its work is more demanding when players get closer to 80% of their maximum speed, which will only be possible to achieve when playing in spaces with bigger lengths than in the SSG.

Those finding must warn football professionals regarding the importance of training variability in terms of exercises and its volume, once they may increase the risk of injury, both due to overtraining or undertraining.

32.4.2 Strength

Football players should have a gym routine in order to correct their strength deficits or maintain their strength levels in case they are balanced.

It is clear that the most important kinds of strength training for football are the *maximum strength* and *power strength* trainings, which can be done combined or separately, according to team schedules [18].

Some considerations should be taken when planning strength program to *prevent injuries*:

- Muscle recovery from a high-load stimulus (e.g., match or hard training) takes at least 48 h [17]
- Maximum strength program is better applied in the end of the training session rather than before it, once that strategy will avoid outfield training with muscular fatigue (see Fig. 32.5 as an example of strength exercise with eccentric phase focus)
- 1–2 times per week, considering team match fixtures [18]

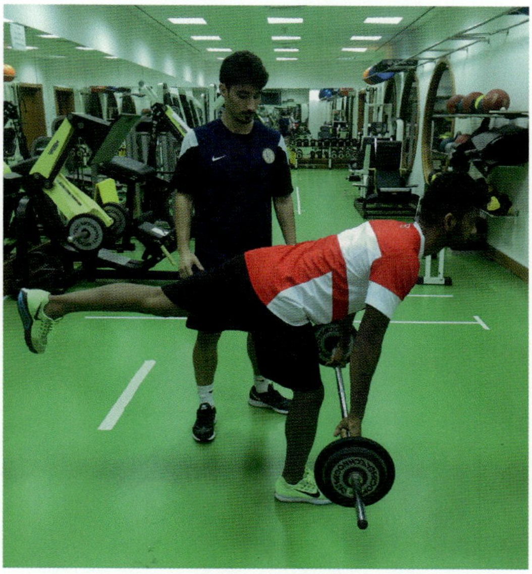

Fig. 32.5 Single-leg Romanian dead lift

32.4.3 Flexibility and Range of Motion (ROM)

Flexibility and ROM imbalances detected during the preseason screening should be corrected either through manual therapy (see Fig. 32.6) or therapeutic exercise and then maintained as a workout routine.

Besides that, stretching routines might be also implemented as a recovery strategy in the day after high-load sessions, avoiding stiffness complains.

32.4.4 Motor Control

Players should have a motor control program in order to:

1. Re-educate movement patterns and correct motor control imbalance (see "running man" exercises in exercise in Fig. 32.7)
2. Improve motor control levels with more challenging tasks, considering football players' needs in terms of decelerating, side cutting, turning, landing, shooting, and running "economy."

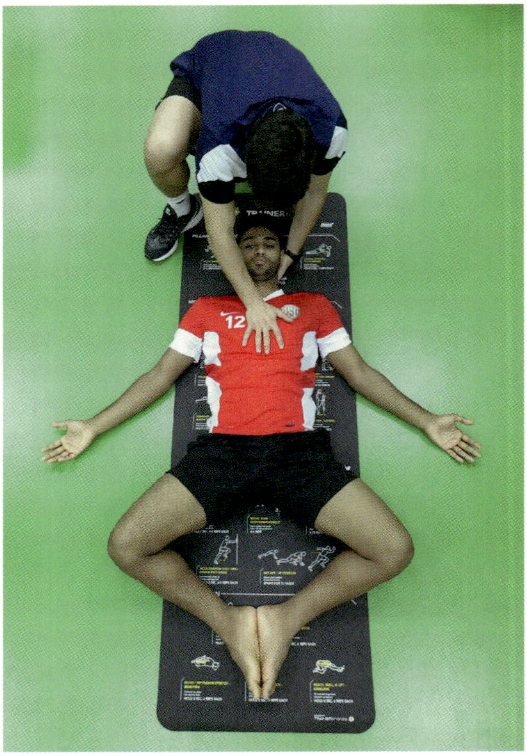

Fig. 32.6 Anterior muscle chain stretch

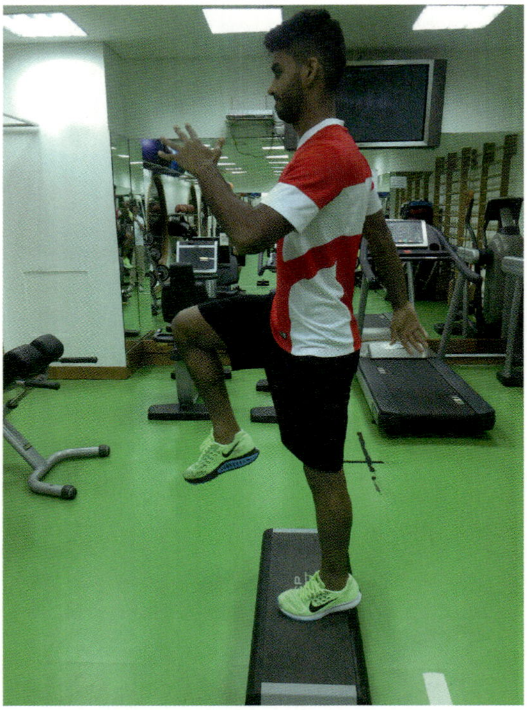

Fig. 32.7 Running man exercise

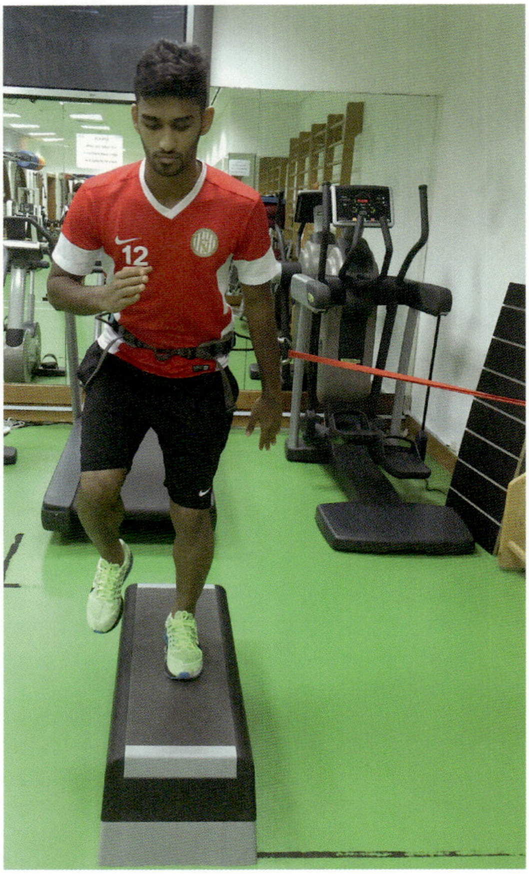

Fig. 32.8 Low-load lateral traction

Figure 32.8 show an example of exercise involving lateral traction and balance exercise

As discussed in Chap. 34, core stability should be considered as part of the motor control; however, when dealing with its improvement, clinicians should consider the rule of the 48 h for muscle recovery.

Conclusion

Muscle injury knowledge is one of the most important subjects for football professionals to be aware once, due to its relatively high incidence and long absence periods, it can have detrimental effects on team's performance.

Epidemiological studies have been helping us to better understand the circumstances of muscle injury occurrence in order to turn football professionals able to develop better and more efficient injury prevention programs. Those programs should involve medical, coaching, and sports science staffs in order to collect the valuable information of each other regarding players' conditions and demands for training. This highlights the importance of a systematic, individual, and meticulous screening in order to reveal player's individual injury risk factors.

Injury prevention programs will have better results if they target to decrease or eliminate muscle injury risk factors of each player, rather than being a nonspecific program. Training loads should be monitored carefully in order to optimize this program.

References

1. Ekstrand J, Hägglund M, Waldén M. Epidemiology of muscle injuries in professional football (soccer). Am J Sports Med. 2011;39(6):1226–32.
2. Ekstrand J, Hägglund M, Waldén M. Injury incidence and injury patterns in professional football – the UEFA injury study. Br J Sports Med. 2011;45(7): 553–8.
3. Mueller-Wohlfahrt H-W, Haensel L, Mithoefer K, Ekstrand J, English B, McNally S, et al. Terminology and classification of muscle injuries in sport: the Munich consensus statement. Br J Sports Med. 2013;47:342–50.
4. Ekstrand J, Healy JC, Waldén M, Lee JC, English B, Hägglund M. Hamstring muscle injuries in professional football: the correlation of MRI findings with return to play. Br J Sports Med. 2011; 46(2):1–6.
5. Järvinen T, Järvinen T, Kääriäinen M, Kalimo H, Järvinen M. Muscle injuries: biology and treatment. Am J Sports Med. 2005;33(5):745–64.
6. Petersen J, Holmich P. Evidence based prevention of hamstring injuries in sport. Br J Sports Med. 2005;39: 319–23.
7. Freckleton G, Pizzari T. Risk factors for hamstring muscle strain injury in sport: a systematic review and meta-analysis. Br J Sports Med. 2013;47:351–8.
8. Ekstrand J, Waldén M, Hägglund M. Hamstring injuries have increased by 4% annually in men's professional football, since 2001: a 13-year longitudinal analysis of the UEFA Elite club injury study. Br J Sports Med. 2016;50(12):731–7.
9. Colby M, Dawson B, Heasman J, Rogalski B, Gabbett T. Accelerometer and GPS-derived running loads and injury risk in elite Australian footballers. J Strength Cond Res. 2014;28(8):2244–52.
10. Gabbett TJ. The training-injury prevention paradox: should athletes be training smarter and harder? Br J Sports Med. 2016;50(5):273–80.
11. Gabbett TJ, Ullah S. Relationship between running loads and soft-tissue injury in elite team sport athletes. J Strength Cond Res. 2012;26(4):953–60.
12. Hägglund M, Waldén M, Ekstrand J. Risk factors for lower extremity muscle injury in professional soccer: the UEFA injury study. Am J Sports Med. 2013;41(2): 327–35.
13. Ibrahim A, Murrell G, Knapman P. Adductor strain and hip range of movement in male professional soccer players. J Orthop Surg. 2007;15(1):46–9.
14. Mendiguchia J, Alentorn-Geli E, Idoate F, Myer GD. Rectus femoris muscle injuries in football: a clinically relevant review of mechanisms of injury, risk factors and preventive strategies. Br J Sports Med. 2012;47(6):359–66.
15. Rogalskia B, Dawsona B, Heasman J, Gabbett TJ. Training and game loads and injury risk in elite Australian footballers. J Sci Med Sport. 2013;16(6):499–503.
16. Croisier JL, Ganteaume S, Binet J, Genty M, Ferret JM. Strength imbalances and prevention of hamstring injury in professional soccer players: a prospective study. Am J Sports Med. 2008;36(8):1469–75.
17. Bishop PA, Jones E, Woods AK. Recovery from training: a brief review. J Strength Cond Res. 2008; 22(3):1015–24.
18. Turner AN, Stewart PF. Strength and conditioning for soccer players. Strength Cond J. 2014;36(4):1–13.

Muscle Injury Classification

33

Xavier Valle, Johannes L. Tol, Bruce Hamilton, and Ricard Pruna

Contents

X. Valle (✉) • R. Pruna
Medical Department, FC Barcelona, Barcelona, Spain
e-mail: xavier.valle@fcbarcelona.cat

J.L. Tol
Department of Sports Medicine, Aspetar, Doha, Qatar

The Sports Physician Group, Department of Sports Medicine, OLVG-West, Amsterdam, The Netherlands

Academic Center for Evidence Based Sports Medicine, Academic Medical Center, Amsterdam, The Netherlands

B. Hamilton
High Performance Sport NZ, Millenium Institute of Sport and Health, Auckland, New Zealand

High Performance Centre, Health Consortium of Terrassa, Barcelona, Spain

The muscle extracellular matrix (ECM) is a complex and interconnected structure [1–3] where the muscle fibers are embedded. This structure is mechanically interconnected [4], so the forces generated by actin-myosin interaction will be transmitted to the net of connective tissue. This connective tissue net structure and its role in force generation and transmission is a key factor in muscle injury signs, symptoms, and prognosis [5].

Magnetic resonance imaging [6–15] (MRI) and ultrasound [16–18] (US) are needed to describe with accuracy muscle injuries, especially the location, size, and tendon involvement. Several parameters regarding the size of muscle injury and the tendon involvement could be associated with the severity of the injury.

When there are no findings on MRI and US, another condition must be considered, but recently the concept of grade 0 muscle injury has been developed [15, 19]. It represents a muscle injury which is undetectable with current imaging modalities [20, 21]. This injury grade has been associated with a quicker return to sport, and, therefore, it is of relevance in a grading system.

33.1 Previous Classifications

Several grading and classification systems for muscle injuries [18, 22–27], for specific muscles [28, 29], or group of muscles [30–32], have been

J. Espregueira-Mendes et al. (eds.), *Injuries and Health Problems in Football*,
DOI 10.1007/978-3-662-53924-8_33

published during the last century. New proposals have recently been published: one imaging-based which introduced injury anatomical description (US and MRI) [33], another which is focused on the location of the injury and its relation to the tendon and fascia [34], and lastly, the third which combines clinical signs and imaging [19] (Table 33.1). In recent years, functional assessment [31]

Table 33.1 Summary of the muscle classification system

Mechanism of injury (M)	Locations of injury (L)	Grading of severity (G)	Number of muscle reinjuries (R)
Hamstrings direct injuries			
T (direct)	*P* Injury located in the proximal third of the muscle belly *M* Injury located in the middle third of the muscle belly *D* Injury located in the distal third of the muscle belly	0–3	0 First episode 1 First reinjury 2 Second reinjury and so on
Hamstrings indirect injuries			
I (indirect) plus subindex *s* for stretching type or subindex *p* for sprinting type	*P* Injury located in the proximal third of the muscle belly. The second letter is a subindex p or d to describe the injury relation with the proximal or distal MTJ, respectively *M* Injury located in the middle third of the muscle belly, plus the corresponding subindex *D* Injury located in the distal third of the muscle belly, plus the corresponding subindex	0–3	0 First episode 1 First reinjury 2 Second reinjury and so on
Negative MRI injuries (location is pain related)			
N plus subindex *s* for indirect injuries stretching type or subindex *p* for sprinting type	*N* p proximal third injury *N* m middle third injury *N* d distal third injury	0–3	0 First episode 1 First reinjury 2 Second reinjury and so on
Grading of injury severity			
0	When codifying indirect injuries with clinical suspicion but negative MRI, grade 0 injury is codified. In these cases the second letter describes the pain locations in the muscle belly		
1	Hyperintense muscle fiber edema without intramuscular hemorrhage or architectural distortion (fiber architecture and pennation angle preserved). Edema pattern: interstitial hyperintensity with feathery distribution on FSPD or T2 FSE+ STIR images		
2	Hyperintense muscle fibers and/or peritendon edema with minor muscle fiber architectural distortion (fiber blurring and/or pennation angle distortion) ± minor intermuscular hemorrhage, but no quantifiable gap between fibers. Edema pattern, same as for grade 1		
3	Any quantifiable gap between fibers in craniocaudal or axial planes. Hyperintense focal defect with partial retraction of muscle fiber ± intermuscular hemorrhage. The gap between fibers at the injury's maximal area in an axial plane of the affected muscle belly should be documented. The exact % CSA should be documented as a subindex to the grade		
r	When codifying an intra-tendon injury or an injury affecting the MTJ or intramuscular tendon showing disruption/retraction or loss of tension exists (gap), a superscript (r) should be added to the grade		

MRI magnetic resonance imaging, *FSPD* fat sat proton density, *FSE* fast spin echo, *STIR* short tau inversion recovery, *CSA* cross-sectional area and clinical evaluation [19] have also been considered as prognostic factors [35].

The best classification should be reproducible, capable of distinguishing between different categories, easy to remember, and related to the prognosis.

33.2 New Proposal "MLG-R"

Our proposal describes the injury based on mechanism "M," location "L," and its relation with the muscle tendon junction (MTJ) and connective tissue evaluation, grading by imaging description "G," and, finally, reinjury "R." This classification system is summarized in Tables 33.2, 33.3, and 33.4. Imaging diagnosis techniques, both MRI and US, are essential in correctly describing the injury [36]. US is capable of providing a description of the location [37, 38], but the best description will be based on the MRI features of the muscle injury [39–41]. This classification has been designed for hamstrings because it is the most frequently injured muscle group in almost all sports worldwide. In the future, another muscles and special situations must be considered. The specific muscle that has been injured should also be named.

The main goal would be to group the injuries by severity and further try to link with different management protocols and therapies. An easy, useful and reliable classification would allow monitoring of each injury with any therapy protocol and its progression [42]. With an acronym, we offer the possibility of describing the injury, the mechanism, the location, and chronological evolution. It is easy to use, avoiding confusing terminology and allowing communication among medical staff; and its flexible structure will permit to incorporate new knowledge in the future.

Table 33.2 Summary of the "MLG-R" classification system (part 1)

Mechanism	Location	Grade	Reinjury
T (direct)	*p* Injury located at the proximal third of the muscle belly		
	m Injury located at the middle third of the muscle belly		
	d Injury located at the distal third of the muscle belly		
	Hamstrings indirect injuries		
I plus subindex S for *Indirect* injuries *Stretching* type, or subindex P for *Sprinting* type.	*P* Injury located at the proximal third of the muscle belly. The second letter has a subindex p or d describe the injury relation with the proximal or distal MTJ.		
	M Injury located at the middle third of the muscle belly, plus the corresponding subindex.		R0 1st episode R1 1st reinjury R2 2nd reinjury ..and so on.
	D Injury located at the distal third of the muscle belly, plus the corresponding subindex.	See below	
	Rectus Famoris indirect injuries		
I Indirect injuries	*P* Injury located at the proximal third of the muscle belly. The second letter has a subindex P or D to describe the injury relation with the proximal or distal MTJ.		
	M Injury located at the middle third of the muscle belly, plus the corresponding subindex.		
	D Injury located at the distal third of the muscle belly, plus the corresponding subindex.		

Table 33.3 Summary of the "MLG-R" classification system (part 2)

G (Grade)

- 0 When codifying indirect injuries with clinical suspicion but *negative MRI,* we will codify a Grade 0 injury. In this cases the second letter will describe the pain locations at the muscle belly.
- 1 Hyperintense oedema without intramuscular haemorrhage or architectural distortion *(fibres architecture and penation angle preserved)*. Oedema pattern: interstitial hyperintensity with f eathery distribution on FSPD or T2 FSE+ STIR images.
- 2 Hyperintense oedema with small +/– intramuscular/intermuscular haemorrhage or architectural distortion (*fibres architecture or penation angle distortion*); but no quantifiable gap between fibres. Oedema pattern: interstitial hyperintensity plus feathery distribution on FSPD or T2 FSE+ STIR images.
- 3 Hyperintense hemorrhage with *quantifiable gap between fibres* in craniocaudal or axial planes. Interstitial hyperintensity with focal hyperintensity representing hemorrhage in muscle belly +/– intramuscular fluid. Hyperintense focal defect with partial retraction of muscle fibers. We will record the gap between fibers at the injury's maximal area, in an axial plane of the affected muscle belly.
- When codifying an injury affecting the MTJ or intramuscular *tendon* showing *disruption/retraction or loss of tension exist* (gap), we have to add a superscript (r) to the grade.

Table 33.4 Summary of the "MLG-R" classification system: Indirect injuries codification

Indirect injuries codification			
Mechanisme	Location (PAIN RELATED)	Grade	Reinjury
N (Negative MRI injuries) plus subindex S for Indirect injuries Stretching type, or subindex P for Sprinting type.	N p proximal third injury		R0 1st episode
	N m middle third injury	0 negative MRI	R1 1st reinjury
	N d distal third injury		R2 2nd reinjury
			..and so on.

References

1. Passerieux E, Rossignol R, Letellier T, Delage J. Physical continuity of the perimysium from myofibers to tendons: involvement in lateral force transmission in skeletal muscle. J Struct Biol. 2007;159:19–28.
2. Huijing PA. Epimuscular myofascial force transmission: a historical review and implications for new research. International society of biomechanics Muybridge award lecture, Taipei, 2007. J Biomech. 2009;42:9–21.
3. Stecco C, Gagey O, Macchi V, Porzionato A, De Caro R, Aldegheri R, Delmas V. Tendinous muscular insertions onto the deep fascia of the upper limb. First part: anatomical study. Morphologie. 2007;91:29–37.
4. Gillies AR, Lieber RL. Structure and function of the skeletal muscle extracellular matrix. Muscle Nerve. 2011;44:318–31.
5. Kjær M, Magnusson P, Krogsgaard M, Møller JB, Olesen J, Heinemeier K, Hansen M, Haraldsson B, Koskinen S, Esmarck B. Extracellular matrix adaptation of tendon and skeletal muscle to exercise. J Anat. 2006;208:445–50.
6. Schneider-Kolsky ME, Hoving JL, Warren P, Connell DA. A comparison between clinical assessment and magnetic resonance imaging of acute hamstring injuries. Am J Sports Med. 2006;34:1008–15.
7. Askling CM, Tengvar M, Saartok T, Thorstensson A. Acute first-time hamstring strains during high-speed running a longitudinal study including clinical and magnetic resonance imaging findings. Am J Sports Med. 2007;35:197–206.
8. Askling CM, Tengvar M, Saartok T, Thorstensson A. Proximal hamstring strains of stretching type in different sports injury situations, clinical and magnetic resonance imaging characteristics, and return to sport. Am J Sports Med. 2008;36:1799–804.
9. Slavotinek JP, Verrall GM, Fon GT. Hamstring injury in athletes: using MR imaging measurements to compare extent of muscle injury with amount of time lost from competition. AJR Am J Roentgenol. 2002;179:1621–8.
10. Ekstrand J, Healy JC, Waldén M, Lee JC, English B, Hägglund M. Hamstring muscle injuries in professional football: the correlation of MRI findings with return to play. Br J Sports Med. 2012;46:112–7.

11. Connell DA, Schneider-Kolsky ME, Hoving JL, Malara F, Buchbinder R, Koulouris G, Burke F, Bass C. Longitudinal study comparing sonographic and MRI assessments of acute and healing hamstring injuries. AJR Am J Roentgenol. 2004;183:975–84.
12. Gibbs N, Cross T, Cameron M, Houang M. The accuracy of MRI in predicting recovery and recurrence of acute grade one hamstring muscle strains within the same season in Australian rules football players. J Sci Med Sport. 2004;7:248–58.
13. Koulouris G, Connell DA, Brukner P, Schneider-Kolsky M. Magnetic resonance imaging parameters for assessing risk of recurrent hamstring injuries in elite athletes. Am J Sports Med. 2007;35:1500–6.
14. Cross TM, Gibbs N, Houang MT, Cameron M. Acute quadriceps muscle strains magnetic resonance imaging features and prognosis. Am J Sports Med. 2004;32:710–9.
15. Verrall GM, Slavotinek JP, Barnes PG, Fon GT, Esterman A. Assessment of physical examination and magnetic resonance imaging findings of hamstring injury as predictors for recurrent injury. J Orthop Sports Phys Ther. 2006;36:215–24.
16. Koulouris G, Connell D. Imaging of hamstring injuries: therapeutic implications. Eur Radiol. 2006;16:1478–87.
17. Bianchi S, Martinoli C, Waser N, Bianchi-Zamorani M, Federici E, Fasel J. Central aponeurosis tears of the rectus femoris: sonographic findings. Skeletal Radiol. 2002;31:581–6.
18. Takebayashi S, Takasawa H, Banzai Y, Miki H, Sasaki R, Itoh Y, Matsubara S. Sonographic findings in muscle strain injury: clinical and MR imaging correlation. J Ultrasound Med. 1995;14:899–905.
19. Mueller-Wohlfahrt H-W, Haensel L, Mithoefer K, Ekstrand J, English B, McNally S, Orchard J, van Dijk CN, Kerkhoffs GM, Schamasch P. Terminology and classification of muscle injuries in sport: the Munich consensus statement. Br J Sports Med. 2013;47:342–50.
20. Meyer RA, Prior BM. Functional magnetic resonance imaging of muscle. Exerc Sport Sci Rev. 2000; 28:89–92.
21. Cermak NM, Noseworthy MD, Bourgeois JM, et al. Diffusion tensor MRI to assess skeletal muscle disruption following eccentric exercise. Muscle Nerve. 2012;46:42–50.
22. O'Donoghue DH. Treatment of injuries to athletes. Philadelphia/London: W.B. Saunders; 1962.
23. Ryan AJ. Quadriceps strain, rupture, and Charlie horse. Med Sci Sports. 1969;1:106–11.
24. Peetrons P. Ultrasound of muscles. Eur Radiol. 2002;12:35–43.
25. Stoller DW. Magnetic resonance imaging in orthopaedics and sports medicine. 2Bde. San Francisco, California, USA: Wolters Kluwer Health; 2007.
26. Smart M. The principles of treatment of muscles and joints by graduated muscular contractions. Oxford: Oxford University Press, Humphrey Milford, [Oxford, Printed by John Johnson]; 1933.
27. Ciullo J, Zarins B. Biomechanics of the musculotendinous unit: relation to athletic performance and injury. Clin Sports Med. 1983;2:71.
28. ElMaraghy AW, Devereaux MW. A systematic review and comprehensive classification of pectoralis major tears. J Shoulder Elbow Surg. 2012;21:412–22.
29. Connell DA, Potter HG, Sherman MF, Wickiewicz TL. Injuries of the pectoralis major muscle: evaluation with MR imaging. Radiology. 1999;210:785–91.
30. Jackson DW, Feagin JA. Quadriceps contusions in young athletes relation of severity of injury to treatment and prognosis. J Bone Joint Surg Am. 1973;55:95–105.
31. Malliaropoulos N, Papacostas E, Kiritsi O, Rad P-M, Papalada A, Gougoulias N, Maffulli N. Posterior thigh muscle injuries in elite track and field athletes. Am J Sports Med. 2010;38:1813–9.
32. Cohen SB, Towers JD, Zoga A, Irrgang JJ, Makda J, Deluca PF, Bradley JP. Hamstring injuries in professional football players magnetic resonance imaging correlation with return to play. Sports Health. 2011;3:423–30.
33. Chan O, Del Buono A, Best TM, Maffulli N. Acute muscle strain injuries: a proposed new classification system. Knee Surg Sports Traumatol Arthrosc. 2012;20:2356–62.
34. Pollock N, James SL, Lee JC, Chakraverty R. British athletics muscle injury classification: a new grading system. Br J Sports Med. 2014;48:1347–51.
35. Warren P, Gabbe BJ, Schneider-Kolsky M, Bennell KL. Clinical predictors of time to return to competition and of recurrence following hamstring strain in elite Australian footballers. Br J Sports Med. 2010;44:415–9.
36. Woodhouse JB, McNally EG. Ultrasound of skeletal muscle injury: an update. In Seminars in ultrasound, CT and MRI. Elsevier; 2011. pp 91–100.
37. Bianchi S, Martinoli C. Ultrasound of the musculoskeletal system. Berlin: Springer; 2007.
38. Stoller DW. Magnetic resonance imaging in orthopaedics and sports medicine. Philadelphia: Lippincott Williams & Wilkins; 2007. p. 1112.
39. Slavotinek JP. Muscle injury: the role of imaging in prognostic assignment and monitoring of muscle repair. Semin Musculoskelet Radiol 2010;14(2): 194–200. DOI: 10.1055/s-0030-1253160.
40. Verrall G, Slavotinek J, Barnes P, Fon G, Spriggins A. Clinical risk factors for hamstring muscle strain injury: a prospective study with correlation of injury by magnetic resonance imaging. Br J Sports Med. 2001;35:435–9.
41. Comin J, Malliaras P, Baquie P, Barbour T, Connell D. Return to competitive play after hamstring injuries involving disruption of the central tendon. Am J Sports Med. 2013;41:111–5.
42. Tol JL, Hamilton B, Best TM. Palpating muscles, massaging the evidence? An editorial relating to 'Terminology and classification of muscle injuries in sport: the Munich consensus statement'. Br J Sports Med. 2013;47:340–1.

Diagnosis and Management of Muscle Injuries

34

Ricard Pruna and Matilda Lundblad

Contents

As a result of the frequency of muscle injuries, many are treated clinically in the absence of confirmatory imaging. However, the clinical appearance is not always clear, and determining the optimal treatment for an injury can be difficult. Imaging can help to confirm both the presence and extent of muscle injury, and the typical modalities used include magnetic resonance imaging (MRI) and ultrasound (US) [1].

The clinical appearance of a skeletal muscle injury depends on the severity of the injury and, in part, on the nature of the resulting haematoma [2]. Detailed history of the injury mechanism and preceding history in combination with careful examination are essential in making a correct diagnosis. A critical goal of the history and examination is to differentiate between those players with injuries possibly requiring surgical treatment and those players with non-surgical injuries.

R. Pruna MD, PHD
HMO FC Barcelona. FIFA Medical Center of Excellence, AV. Once de Setiembre S/N 07890, St Joan Despi. Barcelona, Spain
e-mail: ricard.pruna@fcbarcelona.cat

M. Lundblad MD
Department of Orthopaedics, Sahlgrenska University, Gothenburg, Sweden
e-mail: matildalundblad@gmail.com

J. Espregueira-Mendes et al. (eds.), *Injuries and Health Problems in Football*, DOI 10.1007/978-3-662-53924-8_34

An appropriate history should incorporate the following components:

Regarding the general player history:
Has the player suffered similar injuries before? (Some muscle injuries have a high reinjury rate, players may report a previous injury, often near the current place of injury [3])
Is he/she susceptible to injuries?
Is the player using any medications?
Regarding the mechanism of injury:
What was the trauma mechanism? (A direct blow to the muscle or an indirect mechanism)
During work, training or competition?
When did it start? Date and relationship with the sports session (beginning, middle or the end of the session)
How did it start (Suddenly, gradually, progressively)
Any audible pop or snapping sensation with the onset of pain [4]
Regarding the initial progress:
Was the player able to continue or was he forced to stop?
How was the player treated following the immediate injury?
How has the pain progressed over time?

Physical examination involves the inspection and palpation of the injured area, as well as testing the function of the injured muscles both with and without external resistance. A bilateral comparison should always be performed. The physical examination is performed to determine the location (muscle, tendon or fascia) and the injury severity.

For injuries involving the intramuscular tendon, a 'battery' of tests which incorporate measures of function, strength and range of motion may provide an acceptable estimate of rehabilitation duration [5]. Specifically, a past history of hamstring strain and being unable to walk at a normal pain-free pace [6].

For injuries to the proximal free tendon, the amount of impairment identified from these tests is not predictive of the recovery time needed to return to pre-injury level [7]. We recommend that specific measures be used during the examination of all acute muscle injuries, at the very least to serve as a baseline from which progress can be assessed.

Muscle examination should include:

Inspection	Looking for ecchymosis or deformities on the muscle belly profile
Palpation	Useful for identifying the specific region/muscle injured through pain provocation, as well as the presence or absence of a palpable defect in the musculotendinous junction
Strength assessment	Through manual resistance applied distally to the injury site. Due to the changes in musculotendon length that occur with joint positions, multiple test positions are used to assess isometric strength and pain provocation. It is important to note that pain provocation with this assessment is as relevant as noting weakness
Range of motion	Tests should consider joints at either end of the injury site. For hamstring injuries, passive straight leg raise (hip) and active and passive knee extension test (knee) (AKET, PKET) are commonly used to estimate hamstring flexibility and maximum length [8]. Pain and discomfort during testing are key considerations when performing and evaluating these tests
Muscle length	The extent of joint motion available should be based on the onset of discomfort or stiffness reported by the player. In the acutely injured athlete, tests are often limited by pain and may not provide a valid assessment of musculotendon extensibility
Pain provocation manoeuvres	It has been suggested that players with a biceps injury would feel more pain during stretching than contraction (on VAS), while those injured in SM or ST will have more pain during contraction than stretching

VAS visual analogue scale; *SM* semimembranosus; *ST* semitendinosus

34.1 Imaging of Muscle Injury

Unless an avulsion fracture with bony fragment or apophyseal fracture in a skeletally immature individual is suspected, the value of plain radiographs is limited [9]. On the other hand, MRI and US are able to describe the location (which muscle and tissue), the injury size and the lesion nature (oedema, haemorrhage) as depicted by echotexture and signal intensity, respectively [10].

Both imaging modalities are useful in identifying muscle injuries when oedema and haemorrhage are present [11]. As a result of its cost-effectiveness, US has been traditionally the imaging system of choice for clinical diagnosis of muscle injuries. However, it has the disadvantage of being radiologist's experience dependent.

US is a dynamic and interactive examination, allowing 'echopalpation' of painful areas which complements the clinical examination. US also enables the monitoring of progress and can guide the evacuation of fluid collections, as such it is of great help in topographic diagnosis. However, MRI is considered superior for evaluating injuries to deep portions of muscles [12], or, when a previous injury is present as residual scarring, it could be misinterpreted in an US image as an acute injury.

Due to its increased sensitivity in highlighting subtle oedema, measuring the size of injury (length and cross-sectional area) is probably more accurate with MRI.

MRI is believed by some doctors to be useful in prognosticating return to play (RTP) with MRI grading associated with lay-off times after injury [13].

On the other hand, some studies concluded that there is currently no strong evidence for any MRI variable to predict the time to RTP after an acute hamstring injury due to considerable risks of bias in the studies [14].

Hamstring muscle injuries are the very well documented in the literature, and MRI provides very specific anatomical and pathological information. MRI can sensitively evaluate the relative involvement of tendons, fascia and muscle contractile tissue [15]. MRI has demonstrated to be more accurate than US in the evaluation of proximal hamstring injuries, and it can assess the degree of tendon retraction, which has proved to be an important element of preoperative planning in proximal hamstring ruptures or avulsions [16]. Whereas MRI correctly identified all avulsion cases, US identified only 58% of hamstring avulsions despite the examination being performed by experienced musculoskeletal operators [17].

In distal hamstring injuries, US could better detect injuries as a result of the more superficial anatomy of the distal hamstring tendons [10]. With injuries near the groin area or close to the myotendinous junction, MRI has also demonstrated its superiority over US [11].

The limited availability and high costs of MRI may restrict the use of this modality for routine assessment of injuries among junior and amateur athletes. Schneider-Kolsky et al. showed that MRI was not required for estimating the duration of rehabilitation for an acute minor hamstring injury in professional football players. However, a positive MRI result appeared useful as a predictor of duration of rehabilitation in severe hamstring injuries and also that MRI was helpful in the planning of surgical interventions [5].

34.1.1 Routine MRI Protocol

As an absolute minimum, each MRI examination should generally include at least two orthogonal planes and pulse sequences. In addition to the requisite axial plane, the long-axis plane is generally sagittal (when evaluating abnormalities at the anterior or posterior aspect of an extremity) or coronal (when evaluating abnormalities at the medial or lateral aspect of an extremity). At least one of these pulse sequences should use a fat-suppression technique [18].

34.2 Initial Management of a Suspected Muscle Injury

In Table 34.1, the most appropriate timing for carrying out complementary investigations is highlighted. Real utilization will depend on the physician and athlete preference, funding and the availability of resources.

34.2.1 Management of a Muscle Injury

(*) For follow-up of the functional recovery and sometimes to help to decide return to play:

- *At muscle:* Tensiomyography, electromyography and strength tests

Table 34.1 Summary of methodology diagnosing muscle injuries and timing

Timing		**Clinical history**	**Physical exam**	**US**	**MRI**	**Treatment**
Initial acute phase	Immediate	X	X		Could be made anytime	Rest Ice Compression Elevation Analgesia
	12 h		X	X		
	24 h		X	X		
	48 h		X	X		
					Functional tests (*)	
Subacute and functional phase	First week	Monitoring players' feelings	X	x	To evaluate how the progression of loads are assumed	Rehabilitation Progressive protocol
	Weekly		X	X		
	Return to play		X	X		
Timing		**Clinical history**	**Physical exam**	**US**	**MRI**	**Treatment**
Initial acute phase	Immediate	X	X		Could be made anytime	Rest Ice Compression Elevation Analgesia
	12 h		X	X		
	24 h		X	X		
	48 h		X	X		
					Functional tests (*)	
Subacute and functional phase	First week	Monitoring players feelings	X	x	To evaluate how the progression of loads are assumed	Rehabilitation Progressive protocol
	Weekly		X	X		
	Return to play		X	X		

The significance of * means functional tests according each professional, but we propose GPS technology to assess all of them.

- *At player:* GPS, HR and self-administered scales during and after the rehabilitation sessions on field

Immediately Once injury is suspected through observation of the injury occurring, questioning of the player about their general history regarding the mechanism of injury, and the initial progress (see above.) A structured physical examination based on inspection, palpation, strength assessment, range of motion and post-injury muscle length without pain or stiffness (see above). When the injury is not obvious or significant 'strain' early detailed diagnosis may not be easy. It is important and necessary to observe the injury for several hours to note its progression as well as carrying out the appropriate complementary tests.

12 Hours An ultrasound study at this early stage does not allow for an accurate diagnosis of minor muscular injuries, but may detect the more severe grade II injuries.

24 Hours Most specialists in MRI agree that this is the most appropriate time to establish a clear diagnosis and prognosis. It is important that the personnel who interpret the MRI have experience in this type of injury. It has been suggested that after an injury of the proximal musculotendinous junction of the biceps femoris muscle, the following parameters are prognostic for the return to competition and the risk of reinjury [19]:

- Total length of the injury
- Distance between the ischiatic tuberosity and the proximal ending of the injury
- Cross-sectional area of affected muscle [20]

48 Hours This has been determined to be the optimum time to establish an accurate diagnosis and prognosis when using US alone.

Tensiomyography evaluates the involuntary contractibility of the muscle belly, and it is influenced by the viscoelastic properties of the muscle. While there is little scientific evidence for this methodology, further research should support a role for it in monitoring the functional recovery with US and strength test [21].

Conclusion

When a typical history of muscle contusion or muscle strain is followed by local pain, swelling and/or distal ecchymosis, the diagnosis of a muscle injury may be apparent. The grade of injury and which muscle is injured, particularly if the athlete is unable to walk at a normal pace pain-free within 24 h of injury, may all be relatively straightforward. On the other hand, haematomas that are small in size and those injuries deep within the muscle belly can be more difficult to diagnose clinically, but the imaging modalities (ultrasonography and MRI) provide useful means to delineate injury details.

MRI can accurately confirm or exclude a muscle injury and is able to provide a very detailed characterization of the lesion, even with the risk of being considered somewhat oversensitive at times. The clinical diagnosis of muscle injury is sufficient in most cases, but US can be considered a valid first-line tool if a more exact characterization of the injury is desired. MRI might be of value when there is a clear discrepancy between the clinical symptoms, the physician's findings, and/or the US finding.

References

1. Armfield DR, Kim DH-M, Towers JD, Bradley JP, Robertson DD. Sports-related muscle injury in the lower extremity. Clin Sports Med. 2006;25:803–42.
2. Kalimo H, Rantanen J, Järvinen M. Muscle injuries in sports. Baillieres Clin Orthop. 1997;2:1–24.
3. Heiderscheit BC, Sherry MA, Silder A, Chumanov ES, Thelen DG. Hamstring strain injuries: recommendations for diagnosis, rehabilitation, and injury prevention. Orthop Sports Phys Ther. 2010;40:67–81.
4. Askling CM, Tengvar M, Saartok T, Thorstensson A. Proximal hamstring strains of stretching type in different sports injury situations, clinical and magnetic resonance imaging characteristics, and return to sport. Am J Sports Med. 2008;36:1799–804.
5. Schneider-Kolsky ME, Hoving JL, Warren P, Connell DA. A comparison between clinical assessment and magnetic resonance imaging of acute hamstring injuries. Am J Sports Med. 2006;34:1008–15.
6. Warren P, Gabbe BJ, Schneider-Kolsky M, Bennell KL. Clinical predictors of time to return to competition and of recurrence following hamstring strain in elite Australian footballers. Br J Sports Med. 2010;44:415–9.
7. Askling C, Saartok T, Thorstensson A. Type of acute hamstring strain affects flexibility, strength, and time to return to pre-injury level. Br J Sports Med. 2006;40:40–4.
8. Reurink G, Goudswaard GJ, Oomen HG, Moen MH, Tol JL, Verhaar JA, Weir A. Reliability of the active and passive knee extension test in acute hamstring injuries. Am J Sports Med. 2013;41:1757–61.
9. Clanton TO, Coupe KJ. Hamstring strains in athletes: diagnosis and treatment. J Am Acad Orthop Surg. 1998;6:237–48.
10. Koulouris G, Connell D. Imaging of hamstring injuries: therapeutic implications. Eur Radiol. 2006;16: 1478–87.
11. Connell DA, Schneider-Kolsky ME, Hoving JL, Malara F, Buchbinder R, Koulouris G, Burke F, Bass C. Longitudinal study comparing sonographic and MRI assessments of acute and healing hamstring injuries. Am J Roentgenol. 2004;183:975–84.
12. Koulouris G, Connell D. Hamstring muscle complex: an imaging review 1. Radiographics. 2005;25:571–86.
13. Hallén A, Ekstrand J. Return to play following muscle injuries in professional footballers. J Sports Sci. 2014;32:1–8.
14. Reurink G, Brilman EG, Vos R-J, Maas M, Moen MH, Weir A, Goudswaard GJ, Tol JL. Magnetic resonance imaging in acute hamstring injury: can we provide a return to play prognosis? Sports Med. 2014;45:133–46.
15. Bencardino JT, Mellado JM. Hamstring injuries of the hip. Magn Reson Imaging Clin N Am. 2005;13:677–90.
16. Comin J, Malliaras P, Baquie P, Barbour T, Connell D. Return to competitive play after hamstring injuries involving disruption of the central tendon. Am J Sports Med. 2013;41:111–5.
17. Koulouris G, Connell D. Evaluation of the hamstring muscle complex following acute injury. Skeletal Radiol. 2003;32:582–9.
18. Boutin RD, Fritz RC, Steinbach LS. Imaging of sports-related muscle injuries. Radiol Clin. 2002;40:333–62.
19. Orchard J, Best TM. The management of muscle strain injuries: an early return versus the risk of recurrence. Clin J Sport Med. 2002;12:3–5.
20. Orchard J, Best TM, Verrall GM. Return to play following muscle strains. Clin J Sport Med. 2005;15:436–41.
21. Hunter AM, Galloway SD, Smith IJ, Tallent J, Ditroilo M, Fairweather MM, Howatson G. Assessment of eccentric exercise-induced muscle damage of the elbow flexors by tensiomyography. J Electromyogr Kinesiol. 2012;22:334–41.

35 Conservative Treatment

Luis Til, Paulo Barreira, João Pedro Araújo,
Nuno Loureiro, and Stefano Della Villa

Contents

35.1 Initial Management and Decision-Making on Muscle Injuries

When a typical history of muscle contusion or muscle strain is followed by local pain, swelling and/or distal ecchymosis, the diagnosis of a muscle injury may be apparent. The grade of injury and what muscle is injured, particularly if the athlete is unable to walk at a normal pace pain-free within 24 h of injury, may all be relatively straight forward. On the other hand, hematomas that are small in size and those injuries deep within the muscle belly can be more difficult to diagnose clinically, but the imaging modalities (ultrasonography and magnetic ressonance imaging (MRI)) provide useful means to delineate injury details [1].

MRI can accurately confirm or exclude a muscle injury, and is able to provide a very detailed characterisation of the lesion, even with the risk of being considered somewhat oversensitive at times. The clinical diagnosis of muscle injury is sufficient in most cases, but US can be considered a valid first-line tool if a more exact characterisation of the injury is desired. MRI might be of value when there is a clear discrepancy between the clinical symptoms, the physician's findings and/or the US finding [2].

The most appropriate timing for carrying out complementary investigations is highlighted in Table 35.1. Real utilisation will depend on the

L. Til (✉)
Barcelona Medical Services, FIFA Medical Center of Excellence, Avda. Onze de Setembre s/n St Joan Despí, 08970 Barcelona, Spain
e-mail: lluis.til@fcbarcelona.ca

P. Barreira
Physiotherapist (PhD)/Osteopath, FootballMedicine®, Al Jazira SC, Abu Dhabi, UAE
e-mail: paulobarreiragmr@gmail.com

J.P. Araújo
Clínica do Dragão, Espregueira-Mendes Sports Centre – FIFA Medical Centre of Excellence, Porto, Portugal

Medical Department, Al Jazira Football Club, Dubai, UAE
e-mail: joaopedroaraujo@gmail.com

N. Loureiro
Clínica do Dragão, Espregueira-Mendes Sports Centre – FIFA Medical Centre of Excellence, Porto, Portugal
e-mail: nunoloureiro4@gmail.com

S. Della Villa
Isokinetic Medical Group, v. Casteldebole 8/4, 40132 Bologna, Italy
e-mail: s.dellavilla@isokinetic.com

J. Espregueira-Mendes et al. (eds.), *Injuries and Health Problems in Football*,
DOI 10.1007/978-3-662-53924-8_35

Table 35.1 Management of a muscle injury from muscle injury clinical guidelines FCB-Aspetar Jan 2015

		Clinical history	Physical exam	US	MRI	Treatment
Initial acute phase	Immediate	X	X		Could be made anytime	Rest Ice Compression Elevation Analgesia
	12 h		X	X		
	24 h		X	X		
	48 h		X	X		
					Functional tests	
Subacute and functional phase	First week	Monitorise players' feelings	X	X	To evaluate how the progression of loads are assumed	Rehabilitation progressive protocol
	Weekly		X	X		
	Return to play		X	X		

physician and athlete preferences, funding and the availability of resources. Immediately, once injury is suspected through observation of the injury occurring, questioning of the player regarding the mechanism of injury, and the initial progress, a structured physical examination based on inspection, palpation, strength assessment, range of motion and post-injury muscle length without pain or stiffness. When the injury is not an obvious or significant 'strain', early detailed diagnosis may not be easy. It is important and necessary to observe the injury for several hours to note its progression as well as carrying out the appropriate complementary tests.

An ultrasound study 12 h after the injury does not allow for an accurate diagnosis of minor muscular injuries but may detect the more severe grade II injuries. Twenty-four hours after could be the most appropriate time to establish a clear diagnosis and prognosis. For instance, in an injury of the proximal musculotendinous junction of the biceps femoris muscle, the following parameters are prognostic for the return to competition and the risk of reinjury [3]: total length of the injury, distance between the ischiatic tuberosity and the proximal ending of the injury, the cross-sectional area of affected muscle [4]. The optimum time to establish an accurate diagnosis and prognosis when using US alone is 48 h after. Immediately after the injury, compression, ice and non-painful movements are encouraged. As soon as a normal gait (pain-free) and a normal posture are achieved, the rehabilitation protocol has to be started [5].

Tensiomyography evaluates the involuntary contractibility of the muscle belly, and it is influenced by the viscoelastic properties of the muscle. While there is little scientific evidence for this methodology, further research should support a role for it in monitoring the functional recovery with US and strength test [6].

35.2 Rehabilitation Programmes

Rehabilitation protocols designed for muscle injuries should be built on the scientific knowledge about the injury and the therapeutic options we have to treat them. The knowledge about muscle injuries would include muscle injury biology; muscle group anatomy, structure, histology and function; types and mechanisms of injury; injury risk factors; reinjury risk factors; etc. The biology of healing a muscle injury is a reparative process [7] with the formation of a scar [8]. The healing process of a skeletal muscle injury is divided into three phases: destruction, repair and remodelling, ending with a new myotendinous junction (MTJ) between the repaired myofibers [9, 10]. The optimal healing process is characterised by stimulating regeneration and minimising reparation, so the smallest scar possible.

There is no clear evidence regarding the use of medications [11], cooling [12] or platelet-rich plasma [13] with limited impact on return to play (RTP) or reinjury statistics. Several protocols have been published to treat hamstring muscle injuries (HMIs) using stretching exercises [14], balance [15], eccentric exercises [16, 17] and different combinations [18–20]. Although the aetiology of HMIs is multifactorial, most rehabilitation

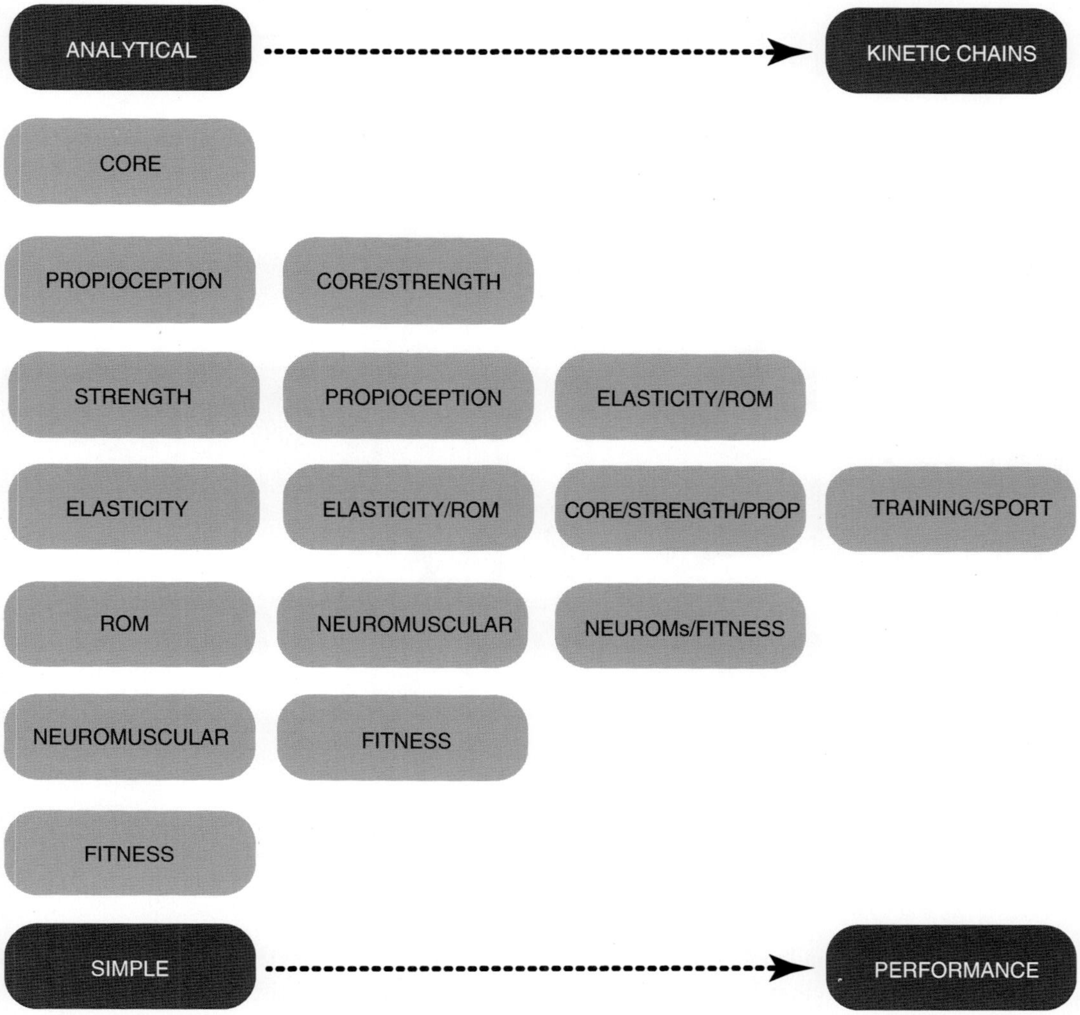

Fig. 35.1 Rehabilitation protocol for HMIs

programmes focus on just one or two factors [21]. Our purpose is to design and develop a criteria-based rehabilitation programme with clear objective progression criterion for each phase and RTP. The main of knowledge about muscle injuries has been reached about hamstring and rectus femoris injuries, so the process for a rehabilitation protocol for HMIs has been described (Fig. 35.1).

Many exercises to achieve a global approach to the injury have been used, with the aim of correcting and reducing the biomechanical disorders, which influence the progression of injury [22, 23]. We will include exercises or programmes showing effectiveness as treatments for HMIs or reducing the risk of injury to lower extremities such as proprioception or neuromuscular exercises [24]. To design an exercise standard offers the option of adapting the protocol to the patient's physical condition, sport or the available equipment. Exercises will progress from single, basic, low demanding to more complex and combined, until accomplished exercises reproduce sport movements.

The design of exercises will be completed keeping in mind hamstring anatomy and function, injury mechanism, etc. in order to target the muscle and location we need to treat [25, 26]. It is also important to design the exercises focusing not only on contraction type and load; ROM, uni-bilateral exercises in open-closed kinetic chain,

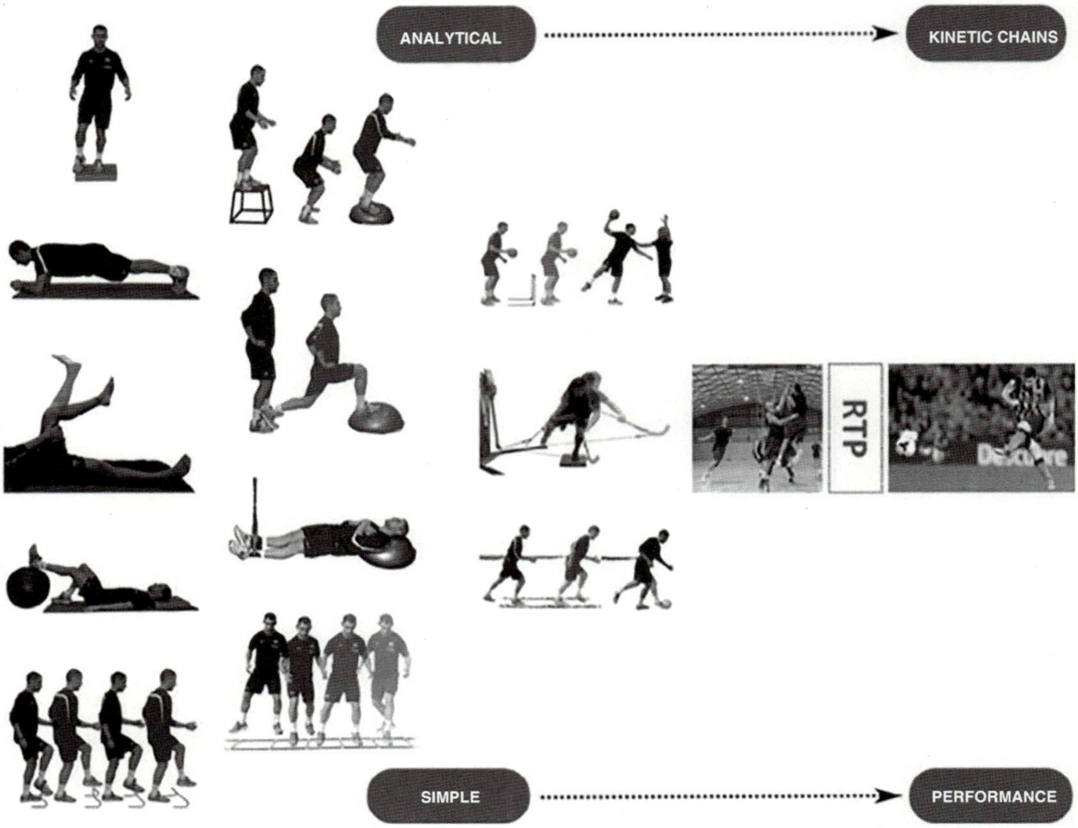

Fig. 35.2 Representation of the typical design of exercises.

hip- or knee-dominant and multi-joint movement exercise and length of the movement need to be taken into account [27, 28] (Fig. 35.2).

The concept of elongation stress on hamstrings (ESH) has recently been introduced and aims to assess hamstring elongation. This is achieved by subtracting the knee flexion angle from the hip flexion angle [29]. The more positive the ESH is, the more stress on hamstrings and the opposite. Therefore, we can use the ESH as a criterion to objectively monitor hamstring stretch progression during.

About the strength, the load for an exercise is a key point in a training programme, and as muscle injury rehabilitation is a training programme, if loads are not appropriated correctly, we will not be able to achieve our goals. Hamstrings' peak torque (PT) angle shifts to longer muscle length after eccentric training, and as more elongate is the muscle during eccentric work, the higher is the shift in the PT angle [30]. This shift in hamstrings' PT angle has been also reported after concentric exercises, but only when performed at long lengths [31]. Eccentric lengthening exercises have shown good results in HMIs rehabilitation; we purpose to perform all strength exercises at longer length possible in order to correct PT angle during the whole rehabilitation process. About the quantification and progression of strength exercises, isometric, concentric and eccentric exercises will overlap during the protocol, with part of the strength work performed at long lengths [32, 33] (Table 35.2).

As RTP decisions should be taken based on specific criteria including assessment tests to confirm recovery, we applied this concept to the whole rehabilitation protocol.

When all functional phase criteria are achieved, strength, flexibility, fitness and core stability will be normalised, but this does not mean that the athlete's performance is also recovered. Based on our experience with elite athletes,

Table 35.2 Exercise design criteria from muscle injury clinical guidelines FCB-Asper Jan 2015

	Acute phase	Subacute phase	Functional phase
Proprioception	Static movement and progress to low unstable dynamic Light instability exercises (soft mat) Knee flexion 0–30°	Moderate reactive movement Increase instability (bosu, balance board, etc.) Knee flexion 45°	Intense reactive movement Unstable surface Knee flexion 90°
Core	Static exercises on stable surface	Dynamic exercises from stable surface and progress to one unstable point	Dynamic exercises on two unstable points Standing exercises reproducing functional movements
Flexibility and ROM	Stretch with ESH <45 avoiding pain	Stretch with ESH <70° avoiding pain	No limit
Strength and power	Isolated knee flexion or hip extension exercises and progressing to combined exercises Closed kinetic chain exercises (first bipodal, second unipodal) Starting with isometric and progressing to concentric and finally to eccentric exercises (progressing in muscle length, without pain or discomfort)	In ESH progress in analytic movements, length, velocity and load to the maximum effort Open kinetic chain exercises Increase combined movement demands	No limit Progress in length, join velocity, load and complexity Horizontal strength application exercises
Neuromuscular and fitness	Start on pool and soft surfaces (to reduce eccentric contraction) Walking on the treadmill and progress to Vmax 8 km/h, 5 % slope	Start on soft surface and progress to hard Run on the treadmill and progress to 70 % of his maximal speed, 3 % slope	Hard surface Progress to his maximal speed, flat and negative slope

Table 35.3 Goal and test to progress in treatment of HMIs from muscle injury clinical guidelines FCB-Aspetar Jan 2015

	Acute phase	Subacute phase	Functional phase
Pain and posture	No pain and maintain neutral spine position during exercises	No pain and no tilting pelvis and spine position during exercises	
Strength	Isometric knee flexion 50 % of previous data or uninjured leg Isometric hip extension 50 % of previous data or uninjured leg	Isometric knee flexion 90 % of previous data or uninjured leg Isometric hip extension 90 % of previous data or uninjured leg	Isometric knee flexion no asymmetry Isometric hip extension no asymmetry
ROM	Full knee and hip isolated tested ROM	Less than 10 % asymmetry in AKET test[a] Less than 10 % asymmetry in active hip flexion test	No asymmetry in AKET test[a] No asymmetry in active hip flexion test
Specific exercises		Deep squat test Single leg squat Runner pose test In-line lunge test	

[a]AKET (active knee-extension test [14])

we recommend that the athlete has to accomplish a normal week training of at least four sessions without pain, discomfort or 'fear' [34]. During this week, performance can be monitored for normality by GPS and heart rate data; this performance control should be extended to competitions after RTP. Obviously, before starting normal training, there will be a progression in exercise demands, physically and technically, to go from individual to team training (Table 35.3).

References

1. Boutin RD, Fritz RC, Steinbach LS. Imaging of sports-related muscle injuries. Radiol Clin N Am. 2002;40:333–62.
2. Reurink G, Brilman EG, de Vos RJ, Maas M, Moen MH, Weir A, Goudswaard GJ, Tol JL. Magnetic resonance imaging in acute hamstring injury: can we provide a return to play prognosis? Sports Med. 2015;45:133–46.
3. Orchard J, Best TM. The management of muscle strain injuries: an early return versus the risk of recurrence. Clin J Sport Med. 2002;12:3–5.
4. Orchard J, Best TM, Verrall GM. Return to play following muscle strains. Clin J Sport Med. 2005;15:436–41.
5. Kwak H-S, Lee K-B, Han Y-M. Ruptures of the medial head of the gastrocnemius ("tennis leg"): clinical outcome and compression effect. Clin Imaging. 2006;30:48–53.
6. Hunter AM, Galloway SD, Smith IJ, Tallent J, Ditroilo M, Fairweather MM, Howatson G. Assessment of eccentric exercise-induced muscle damage of the elbow flexors by tensiomyography. J Electromyogr Kinesiol. 2012;22:334–41.
7. Järvinen TA, Järvinen TL, Kääriäinen M, Kalimo H, Järvinen M. Muscle injuries biology and treatment. Am J Sports Med. 2005;33:745–64.
8. Silder A, Thelen DG, Heiderscheit BC. Effects of prior hamstring strain injury on strength, flexibility, and running mechanics. Clin Biomech. 2010;25:681–6.
9. Järvinen TA, Järvinen TL, Kääriäinen M, Äärimaa V, Vaittinen S, Kalimo H, Järvinen M. Muscle injuries: optimising recovery. Best Pract Res Clin Rheumatol. 2007;21:317–31.
10. Silder A, Heiderscheit BC, Thelen DG, Enright T, Tuite MJ. MR observations of long-term musculotendon remodeling following a hamstring strain injury. Skeletal Radiol. 2008;37:1101–9.
11. Robinson M, Hamilton B. Medical interventions in the management of hamstring muscle injury. Eur J Sport Sci. 2014;14(7):743–51.
12. Bleakley C, Glasgow P, Webb M. Cooling an acute muscle injury: can basic scientific theory translate into the clinical setting? Br J Sports Med. 2012; 46:296–8.
13. Andia I, Sánchez M, Maffulli N. Platelet rich plasma therapies for sports muscle injuries: any evidence behind clinical practice? Expert Opin Biol Ther. 2011;11:509–18.
14. Malliaropoulos N, Papalexandris S, Papalada A, Papacostas E. The role of stretching in rehabilitation of hamstring injuries: 80 athletes follow-up. Med Sci Sports Exerc. 2004;36:756–9.
15. Kraemer R, Knobloch K. A soccer-specific balance training program for hamstring muscle and patellar and achilles tendon injuries an intervention study in premier league female soccer. Am J Sports Med. 2009;37:1384–93.
16. Schmitt B, Tim T, McHugh M. Hamstring injury rehabilitation and prevention of reinjury using lengthened state eccentric training: a new concept. Int J Sports Phys Ther. 2012;7:333–41.
17. Askling CM, Tengvar M, Thorstensson A. Acute hamstring injuries in Swedish elite football: a prospective randomised controlled clinical trial comparing two rehabilitation protocols. Br J Sports Med. 2013;47(15):953–9.
18. Sherry MA, Best TM. A comparison of 2 rehabilitation programs in the treatment of acute hamstring strains. J Orthop Sports Phys Ther. 2004;34:116–25.
19. Silder A, Sherry M, Sanfilippo J, Tuite M, Hetzel S, Heiderscheit B. Clinical and morphological changes following 2 rehabilitation programs for acute hamstring strain injuries: a randomized clinical trial. J Orthop Sports Phys Ther. 2013;43(5):284–99.
20. Heiderscheit BC, Sherry MA, Silder A, Chumanov ES, Thelen DG. Hamstring strain injuries: recommendations for diagnosis, rehabilitation and injury prevention. J Orthop Sports Phys Ther. 2010;40:67.
21. Mendiguchia J, Brughelli M. A return-to-sport algorithm for acute hamstring injuries. Phys Ther Sport. 2011;12:2–14.
22. Mendiguchia J, Alentorn-Geli E, Brughelli M. Hamstring strain injuries: are we heading in the right direction? Br J Sports Med. 2012;46:81–5.
23. Frohm A, Heijne A, Kowalski J, Svensson P, Myklebust G. A nine-test screening battery for athletes: a reliability study. Scand J Med Sci Sports. 2012;22:306–15.
24. Cameron ML, Adams RD, Maher CG, Misson D. Effect of the HamSprint Drills training program on lower limb neuromuscular control in Australian football players. J Sci Med Sport. 2009;12:24–30.
25. Kubota J, Ono T, Araki M, Torii S, Okuwaki T, Fukubayashi T. Non-uniform changes in magnetic resonance measurements of the semitendinosus muscle following intensive eccentric exercise. Eur J Appl Physiol. 2007;101:713–20.
26. Mendiguchia J, Garrues MA, Cronin JB, Contreras B, Los Arcos A, Malliaropoulos N, Maffulli N, Idoate F. Nonuniform changes in MRI measurements of the thigh muscles after two hamstring strengthening exercises. J Strength Cond Res. 2013;27:574–81.
27. Guex K, Millet GP. Conceptual framework for strengthening exercises to prevent hamstring strains. Sports Med. 2013;43(12):1207–15. doi:10.1007/s40279-013-0097-y.
28. Malliaropoulos N, Mendiguchia J, Pehlivanidis H, Papadopoulou S, Valle X, Malliaras P, Maffulli N. Hamstring exercises for track and field athletes: injury and exercise biomechanics, and possible implications for exercise selection and primary prevention. Br J Sports Med. 2012;46:846–51.
29. Guex K, Gojanovic B, Millet GP. Influence of hip-flexion angle on hamstrings isokinetic activity in sprinters. J Athl Train. 2012;47:390–5.
30. Guex K, Degache F, Gremion G, Millet GP. Effect of hip flexion angle on hamstring optimum length after a single set of concentric contractions. J Sport Sci. 2013;31:1545–52.

31. Blazevich AJ, Cannavan D, Coleman DR, Horne S. Influence of concentric and eccentric resistance training on architectural adaptation in human quadriceps muscles. J Appl Physiol. 2007;103:1565–75.
32. Schache AG, Dorn TW, Blanch PD, Brown NA, Pandy MG. Mechanics of the human hamstring muscles during sprinting. Med Sci Sports Exerc. 2012; 44:647–58.
33. Chumanov ES, Heiderscheit BC, Thelen DG. The effect of speed and influence of individual muscles on hamstring mechanics during the swing phase of sprinting. J Biomech. 2007;40:3555–62.
34. Ardern CL, Taylor NF, Feller JA, Webster KE. A systematic review of the psychological factors associated with returning to sport following injury. Br J Sports Med. 2013;47:1120–6.

Surgical Treatment of Muscle Injuries

36

Jordi Puigdellívol, Ricard Pruna, Luis Til,
Daniel Medina, Pedro Luís Ripoll,
and João Espregueira-Mendes

Contents

36.1 Introduction

Operative treatment is seldom considered in the treatment of muscle injuries, including hamstring strains, and the phrase "muscle injuries heal without intervention" could be used as a guiding principle [14, 28].

However, there are certain highly specific indications in which surgical intervention might actually be beneficial for severe muscle injuries, even in the absence of an evidence-based treatment protocol.

These indications include an athlete with a complete (grade III) rupture of a muscle with few or no agonist muscles, a tear (grade II) if more than half of the muscle is torn, or a large intramuscular hematoma [1, 17].

Many authors claim that surgery has no place due to the lack of firm evidence, while some surgeons believe surgical treatments with postoperative rehabilitation protocols should be considered

J. Puigdellívol (✉) • R. Pruna • L. Til • D. Medina
FC Barcelona Medical Services, FIFA Medical Center of Excellence, Avda. Onze de Setembre s/n St Joan Despí, 08970 Barcelona, Spain
e-mail: jordipg33@gmail.com

P.L. Ripoll
Ripoll y De Prado Sport Clinic, FIFA Medical Center of Excellence, Paseo de la Habana, 43, Madrid 28026, Spain

J. Espregueira-Mendes
Clínica do Dragão, Espregueira-Mendes Sport Center, FIFA Medical Center of Excellence, Porto, Portugal

Dom Henrique Research Centre, Porto, Portugal

3B's Research Group–Biomaterials, Biodegradables and Biomimetics, University of Minho, Headquarters of the European Institute of Excellence on Tissue Engineering and Regenerative Medicine, AvePark, Parque de Ciência e Tecnologia, Zona Industrial da Gandra, 4805-017 Barco, Guimarães, Portugal

ICVS/3B's–PT Government Associate Laboratory, Braga/Guimarães, Portugal

Orthopaedics Department of Minho University, Minho, Portugal

J. Espregueira-Mendes et al. (eds.), *Injuries and Health Problems in Football*,
DOI 10.1007/978-3-662-53924-8_36

Table 36.1 Authors' recommended surgical treatment algorithm for muscle injuries

Type of Injury	Muscle	Part of Muscle	Tendon	Treatment
Tendon bone detachment desinserctions	Quadriceps	Rectus Femoris Proximal	Direct head	Surgical reattachment
			Indirect head	Small gap conservative Large gap surgical
			Direct + Indirect	Surgical
	Hamstrings	Proximal	Biceps Femoris Long Head and/or Semitendinosus (Common tendon)	Surgical
			Semimembranosus	Conservative, if there are persisting symptoms after 4 m: surgical reattachment must be considered
		Distal	All (rare)	Surgical reattachment must be considered
	Adductors	Not included in this project by different approaches between FCB group (this injury is a progression of groin pain could be treated with tenotomy) and Turku group (the acute injuries could be treated with surgical reattachment)		
Bine avulsions	Quadriceps	Proximal	ASIS or AIIS	Conservative : unless > 2cm
		Distal	Patellar avulsion	Surgical : (except non displaced)
	Hamstrings	Proximal	Ischial tuberosity	Gap < 2cm conservative Larger gaps : surgical
		Distal	All (rare)	Surgical reattachment must be considered
Muscle injuries at the myotendinous junction, when the main tendon is evolved at less than 7cm from bone origin, with loss of tension of the rest of the tendon		Quadriceps & Hamstrings	< 2 cm from bone insertion	Reattachment to the bone and liberate tension at MTJ
			2 – 7 cm from bone insertion	Surgical treatment: Anatomical Repair with minimally invasive approach

Muscle Injuries Clinical Guide 3.0 FC Barcelona, January 2015

if a patient complains of chronic pain (more 4–6 months) in a previously injured muscle, especially if the pain is accompanied by a clear extension deficit [13].

In these chronic cases, scar tissue formation and adhesions restricting the movement should be suspected, and surgical release of adhesions can be considered (Table 36.1).

36.2 Proximal Hamstring Injuries

The incidence of hamstring muscle injuries has been estimated to be 3.0–4.1 hamstring strains per 1000 h of match play and 0.4–0.5 per 1000 h of training [2]. The prevalence of complete proximal hamstring ruptures has been estimated to be 9% of all by MRI-evaluated hamstring injuries [3].

Most authors advocate that only in the presence of a complete rupture of the proximal attachment of the musculotendinous complex (Fig. 36.1) should surgical repair be considered [27]. More assertive recommendations have recently been made [8] suggesting that a pure isolated biceps femoris and semitendinosus conjoint tendon avulsion should be repaired in active patients.

Nowadays with elite athletes, according to the common guidelines, acute complete proximal hamstring avulsions/ruptures with loss of function (grade III) should be operated on as soon as posible. In cases where only one of them is torn, the controversy persists. Cohen and Bradley [5] suggested surgical treatment when two out of three hamstring tendons are ruptured at the ischial tuberosity. For athletes, more aggressive recommendations with reattachment of isolated tendon avulsions (BF/ST/SM) can be found [21].

In partial proximal hamstring tears, surgical treatment should be considered since in most of these cases, excellent or good results can be expected after surgical repair [19] (Fig. 36.2).

36.3 Proximal Hamstring Avulsion Fracture

In adolescents, apophyseal avulsions at sites of proximal hamstring muscle insertions are occasionally seen [30]. Operative treatment has been recommended if the displacement of the avulsed fragment is 2 cm or more [16, 32]. Suggested even more is active operative treatment, and recommended is early surgical fixation if the fracture displacement is more than 1 cm [10]. Dissection was carried down to the gluteal fascia, with care to avoid the posterior femoral cutaneous nerve,

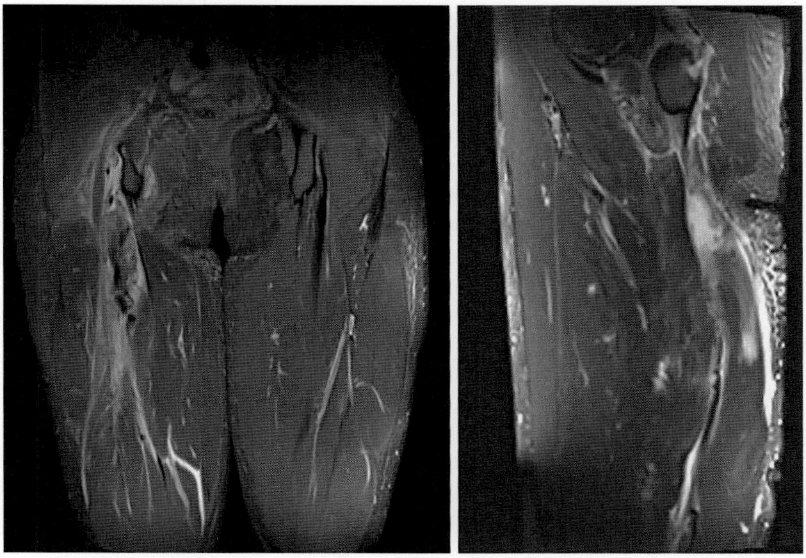

Fig. 36.1 Magnetic resonance image showing T2-weighted coronal and sagittal views, a complete rupture of the proximal attachment of the hamstring musculotendinous complex

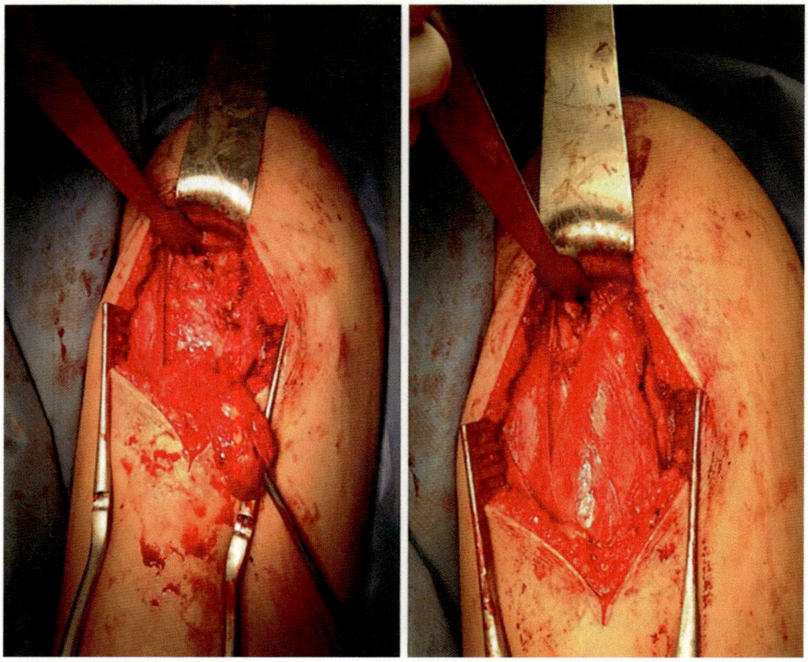

Fig. 36.2 Surgical reattachment with three anchors in ischial tuberosity

which crosses the hamstring from lateral-proximal to medial- distal and can cause hypoesthesia to the posterior thigh when damaged.

36.4 Central Tendon Hamstring Injuries

Hamstring injuries that disrupt the central tendon enclosed within the muscle belly require a longer recovery time than those injuries involving only muscle, epimysial fascia, or the musculotendinous junction. When injury involves the enclosed central portion of the tendon (Fig. 36.3), the distinction between injury to the hamstring muscle and injury to the hamstring tendon is underappreciated as being a distinct entity. Central tendon disruption was identified in 45% of the biceps femoris injuries and in none of the injuries to the other two muscles [6].

The long time in recovering and a high reinjury rate, the surgical treatment, in our opinion, should be considered, giving tension to the tendon amb reinforcement with anchors in ischial tuberosity. Other authors [33], prior to surgery, use ultrasound transducer placed at the muscle-tendon junction to locate the injury site and metallic anchor loaded with a metallic wire placed in the identified lesion site. Excision of the scar tissue, including the torn portion of the tendon, was then performed and tension-free suturing of the belly remnant of the biceps femoris to the adjacent semitendinosus.

Due to the low incidence of proximal hamstring avulsions, most published reports are retrospective case studies with limited numbers of patients. Technical notes on endoscopical repair have recently been published [7]. These less invasive techniques could have some advantages with minimal disruption of normal anatomy and improved visualization with possible decreased neurovascular complications and decreased bleeding, but it involves some technical challenges of passing and shuttling the suture for repair and increased operative time. This arthroscopic repair would be done to avoid scarring and ischiofemoral impingement on the nerve.

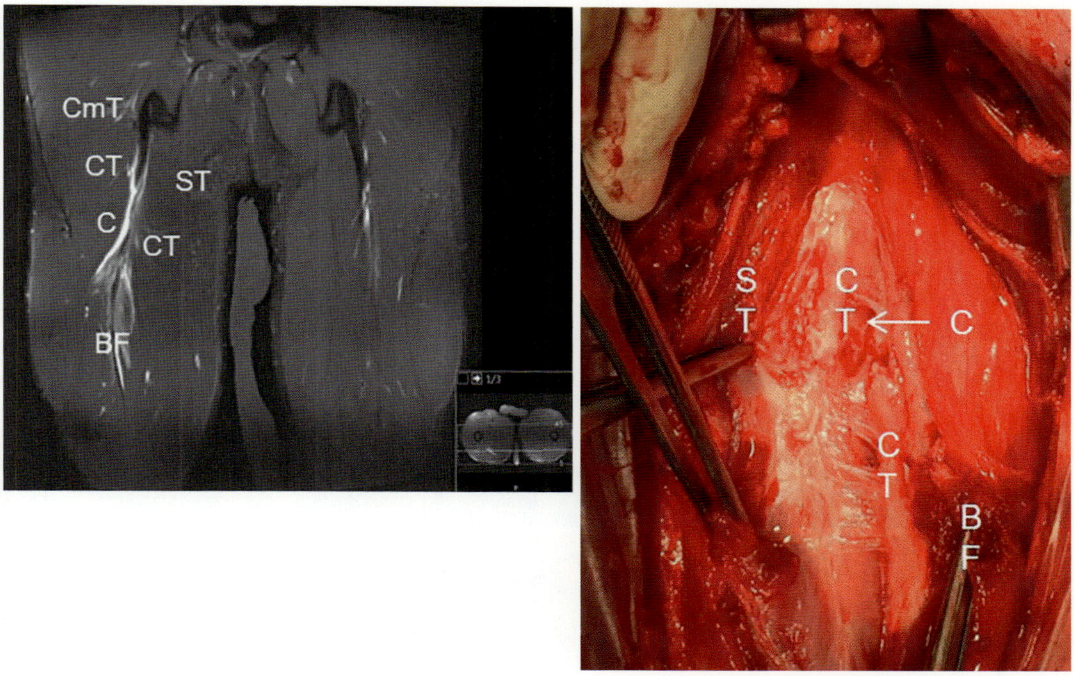

Fig. 36.3 MRI musculotendinous biceps femoris grade 2 injury, showing the disruption and loss of tension in the central tendon. Intraoperative view. *CmT* common tendon, *CT* central tendon, *ST* semitendinosus, *BF* biceps femoris, *C* cavity

36.5 Distal Hamstring Injuries

Distal hamstring injuries are rare and usually associated with severe traumas to the knee joint or with other traumatic musculotendinous injuries around the knee [4, 18]. However, isolated distal hamstring tendon avulsions have also been described [24, 31, 35], and operative treatment for these has been recommended (Fig. 36.4).

36.6 Rectus Femoris Injury

Muscle strains, including grade III avulsion injuries, are often treated nonoperatively [25]. The surgical treatment of a complete tendon avulsion in professional players allow an anatomic repair and return to full activities following rehabilitation.

Proximal avulsions of the rectus femoris muscle at the anterior inferior iliac spine (AIIS) are uncommon. They have been described in adolescent and young individuals, as well as in sports such as sprinting and kicking the ball.

The footprint may have anatomical variations. More common are the acute total avulsion tears (Fig. 36.5) [11, 12]. The mechanical strength of suture anchors has been found to be equal to fixation through bone tunnels [22]. Ten proximal rectus femoris tears [9] have been reported and treated surgically (Fig. 36.6) in professional football players. The author's method is reattached to the direct head and secured with bone suture anchors.

Although these proximal ruptures are well described, we have found only one report of a complete rupture of the direct head of the rectus femoris muscle at the musculotendinous junction [34] (Fig. 36.7).

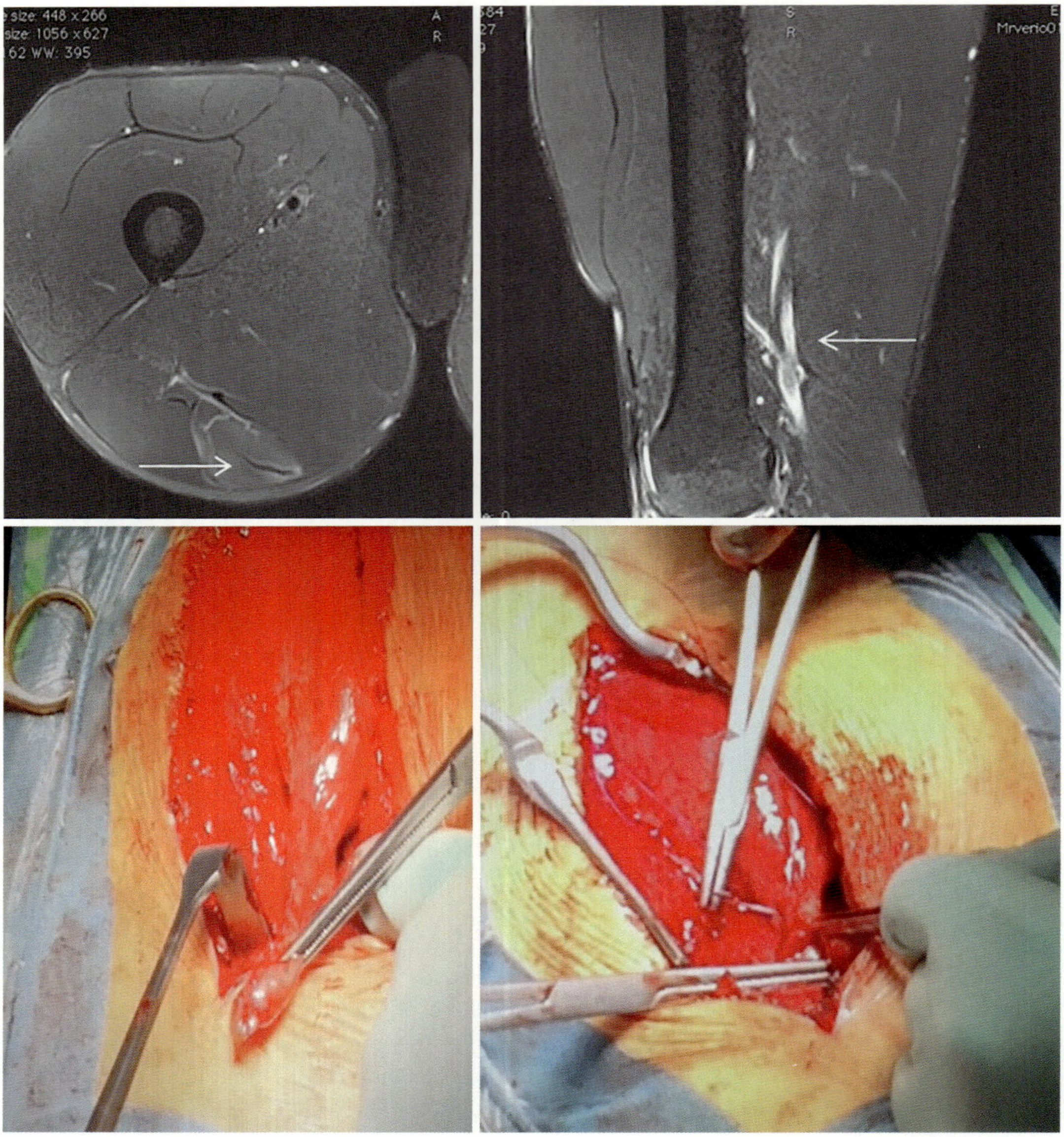

Fig. 36.4 MRI of distal hamstring injury (*white arrow*). Intraoperative views of semitendinosus distal rupture sutured to the adjacent semimembranosus distal tendon, in professional football player

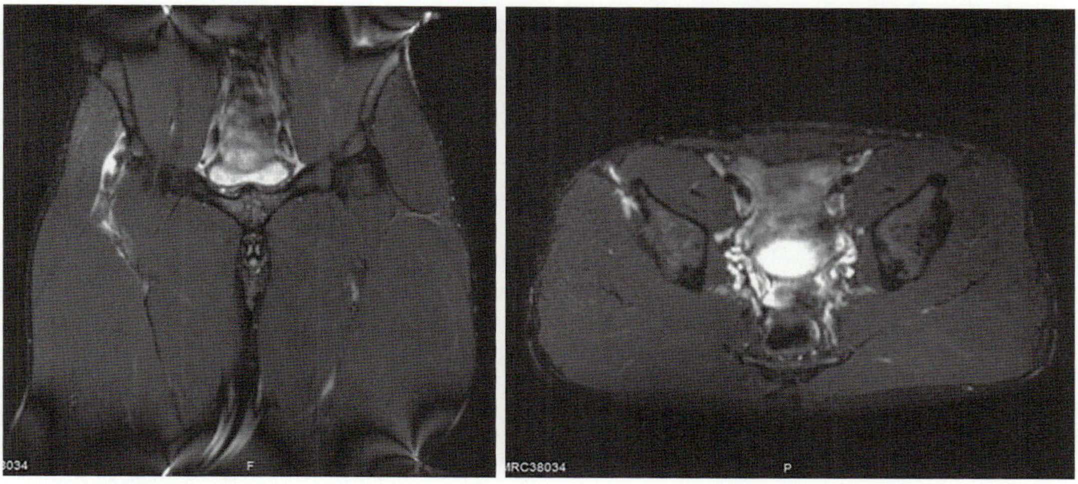

Fig. 36.5 MRI views of proximal rectus femoris avulsion

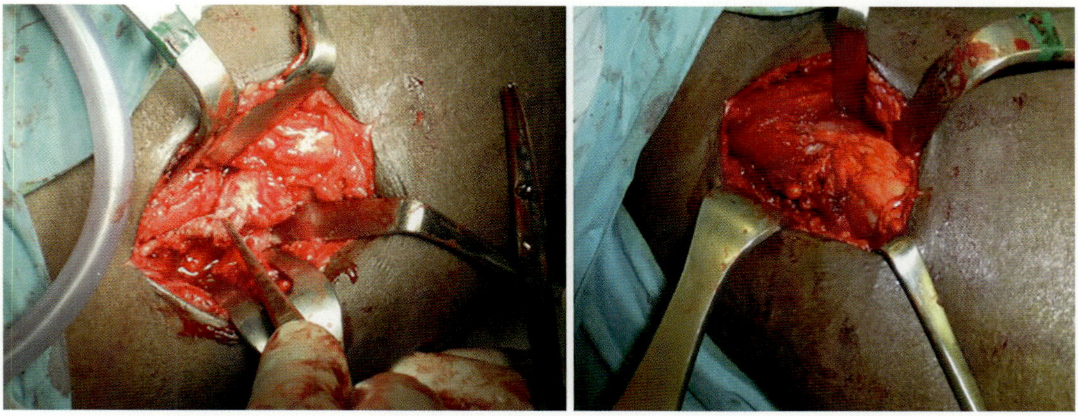

Fig. 36.6 Intraoperative views, reattachment in AIIS of the direct head of his rectus femoris with two anchors

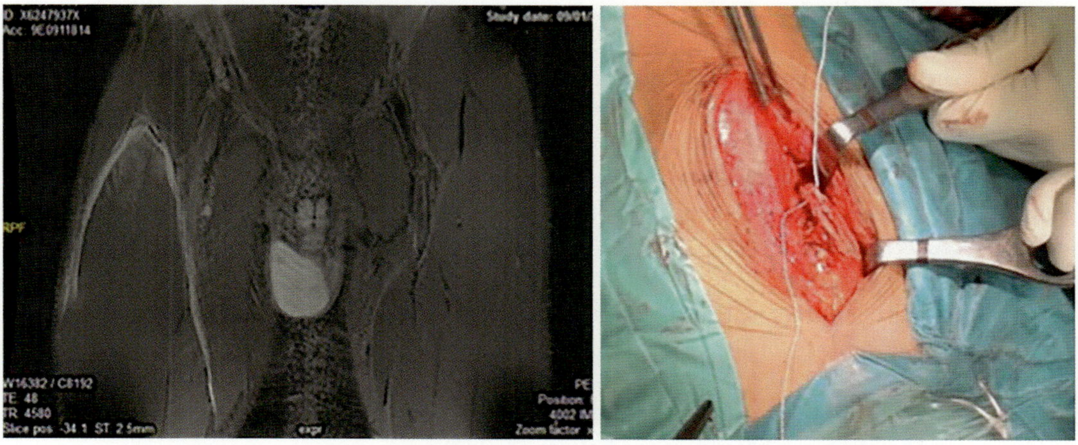

Fig. 36.7 Coronal MRI T2-weighted image. Intraoperative view of rectus femoris tendon secured with No. 2 FiberWire (Arthrex Inc., Naples, Florida), in professional football player

36.7 Chronic Injuries

Surgery should be considered if the symptoms (pain, weakness, and loss of function) persist longer than 6 months, which is the time expected for healing.

It has been shown that an athlete is unlikely to return to the previous level of sporting activity after complete proximal hamstring rupture unless treated surgically. On the other hand, no differences between early and late repairs have been identified with regard to functional outcome or return to sport. In elite athletes, early surgical refixation of complete proximal hamstring ruptures is recommended.

The surgical procedure may include excision of adhesions, fasciectomies, and tendon bone reattachments. Occasionally retracted muscles can be reattached to the bone by using a tension-free autograft augmentation reattachment with fascia lata autograft [20] or Achilles allograft [26].

It has been shown that an athlete is unlikely to return to the previous level of sporting activity after complete proximal hamstring rupture unless treated surgically. On the other hand, no differences between early and late repairs have been identified with regard to functional outcome or return to sport [15]. The ischial nerve should be freed from adhesions.

Tendinopathy is a clinical condition characterized by activity-related pain and impaired performance, focal tendon tenderness and swelling, and intratendinous imaging changes [23].

Proximal hamstring tendinopathy may be resistant to conservative treatment. In such cases, surgery seems to be a good option, and satisfactory results can often be expected [29].

Heterotopic calcification could be an expression of chronic tendinopathy. Calcification of the proximal rectus femoris tendon has also been described, although rarely, following avulsion (with or without bony fragment) or tendon rupture (partial or complete) of the rectus femoris origin in young people, especially in kicking athletes and in football players.

A similar condition has been described after an avulsion of the AIIS. The healing process could lead to an extra bony mass extending inferiorly and resulting in a prominent AIIS that eventually will impinge on the femoral neck when the hip is flexed over 90 This has been referred to as iliac spine impingement, AIIS impingement, or subspine impingement.

Calcification of the rectus femoris tendon has been traditionally addressed by local injection of anesthetic and corticosteroids or by open excision of the lesion through an anterior (Smith-Petersen) approach. Hip arthroscopy has been proposed, with satisfactory outcomes, as a less invasive surgical alternative for both conditions [36].

Symptomatic chronic myofascial injuries in rectus femoris distal, gastrocnemius, and soleus can be affected that could be treated by excision of scar tissue.

36.8 Postoperative Rehabilitation

Postoperative hamstring surgery rehabilitation is guided by the diagnosis, the surgical procedure, and the patient's progress. We recommend an elastic bandage for 1–2 weeks postoperatively without immobilization, casts, or orthoses.

During the first 2–4 weeks, light touch weight-bearing is allowed with gradual progression to full weight-bearing at the end of six weeks. After 3–4 weeks, light pool training including swimming is allowed, and after 4–6 weeks, cycling is allowed. The range of motion exercises start during this phase, but stretching exercises of the hamstrings should be avoided during the first 4 weeks. Progressing to running and more active muscle training is advised 2–4 months after the operation depending on the patient's progress.

In rectus femoris surgery, passive range of motion was initiated for the patient's hip for 4 weeks, with weight-bearing (as tolerated) in a knee brace locked in extension. Eccentric exercises were allowed 6 weeks after surgery, jogging and running 8 weeks after surgery and was cleared for full sport activity within 3–4 months.

References

1. Almekinders LC. Results of surgical repair versus splinting of experimentally transected muscle. J Orthop Trauma. 1991;5:173–6.
2. Arnason A, Andersen T, Holme I, et al. Prevention of hamstring strains in elite soccer: an intervention study. Scand J Med Sci Sports. 2008;18:40–8.
3. Birmingham P, Muller M, Wickiewicz T, et al. Functional outcome after repair of proximal hamstring avulsions. J Bone Joint Surg Am. 2011;93:1819–26.
4. Clanton T, Coupe K. Hamstring strains in athletes: diagnosis and treatment. J Am Acad Orthop Surg. 1998;6:237–48.
5. Cohen S, Bradley J. Acute proximal hamstring rupture. J Am Acad Orthop Surg. 2007;15:350–5.
6. Comin J, Malliaras P, Baquie P, et al. Return to competitive play after hamstring injuries involving disruption of the central tendon. Am J Sports Med. 2012;41:11–5.
7. Domb BG, Linder D, Sharp KG, et al. Endoscopic repair of proximal hamstring avulsion. Arthrosc Tech. 2013;2:e35–9.
8. Folsom GJ, Larson CM. Surgical treatment of acute versus chronic complete proximal hamstring ruptures: results of a new allograft technique for chronic reconstructions. Am J Sports Med. 2008;36:104–9.
9. García V, Duhrkop D, Seijas R, et al. Surgical treatment of proximal ruptures of the rectus femoris in professional soccer players. Arch Orthop Trauma Surg. 2012;132:329–33.
10. Gidwani S, Bircher M. Avulsion injuries of the hamstring origin – a series of 12 patients and management algorithm. Ann R Coll Surg Engl. 2007;89:394–9.
11. Hsu J. Proximal rectus femoris avulsions in National Football League kickers: a report of 2 cases. Am J Sports Med. 2005;33:1085–7.
12. Irmola T, Heikkilä J, Orava S, et al. Total proximal tendon avulsion of the rectus femoris muscle. Scand J Med Sci Sports. 2007;17(4):378–82.
13. Jarvinen T. Muscle injuries: biology and treatment. Am J Sports Med. 2005;33:745–64.
14. Järvinen T, Järvinen T, Kääriäinen M, et al. Muscle injuries: optimising recovery. Best Pract Res Clin Rheumatol. 2007;21:317–31.
15. Klingele KE, Sallay PI. Surgical repair of complete proximal hamstring tendon rupture. Am J Sports Med. 2002;30:742–7.
16. Kujala U, Orava S. Ischial apophysis injuries in athletes. Sports Med. 1993;16:290–4.
17. Kujala U, Orava S, Järvinen M. Hamstring injuries. Sports Med. 1997;23:397–404.
18. LaPrade R, Terry G. Injuries to the posterolateral aspect of the knee: association of anatomic injury patterns with clinical instability. Am J Sports Med. 1997;25:433–8.
19. Lempainen L. Surgical treatment of hamstring injuries and disorders – the clinical spectrum from chronic tendinopathy to complete rupture [Academic dissertation]. Finland: University of Turku; 2009.
20. Lempainen L, Sarimo J, Orava S. Recurrent and chronic complete ruptures of the proximal origin of the hamstring muscles repaired with fascia lata autograft augmentation. Arthroscopy. 2007;23:441–5.
21. Lempainen L, Banke I, Johansson K, et al. Clinical principles in the management of hamstring injuries. Knee Surg Sports Traumatol Arthrosc. 2015;23:2449–56.
22. Lighthart W, Cohen D, Levine R, et al. Suture anchor versus suture through tunnel fixation for quadriceps tendon rupture: a biomechanical study. Orthopedics. 2008;31(5):441.
23. Maffulli N. Overuse tendon conditions: time to change a confusing terminology. Arthroscopy. 1998;14:840–3.
24. Mann G, Shabat S, Friedman A, et al. Hamstring injuries. Review. Orthopedics. 2007;30:536–40.
25. Mendiguchia J, Alentorn-Geli E, Idoate F, et al. Rectus femoris muscle injuries in football: a clinically relevant review of mechanisms of injury, risk factors and preventive strategies. Br J Sports Med. 2013;47:359–66.
26. Murray P, Lowe W. Achilles allograft reconstruction of a chronic complete proximal hamstring rupture. Knee Surg Sports Traumatol Arthrosc. 2009;17:1360–3.
27. Orava S, Kujala U. Rupture of the ischial origin of the hamstring muscles. Am J Sports Med. 1995;23:702–5.
28. Petersen J, Hölmich P. Evidence based prevention of hamstring injuries in sport. Br J Sports Med. 2005;39:319–23.
29. Puranen J, Orava S. The hamstring syndrome: a new diagnosis of gluteal sciatic pain. Am J Sports Med. 1988;16:517–21.
30. Rossi F, Dragoni S. Acute avulsion fractures of the pelvis in adolescent competitive athletes: prevalence, location and sports distribution of 203 cases collected. Skeletal Radiol. 2001;30:127–31.
31. Sebastianelli W, Hanks G, Kalenak A. Isolated avulsion of the biceps femoris insertion. Clin Orthop Relat Res. 1990;259:200–3.
32. Servant C, Jones C. Displaced avulsion of the ischial apophysis: a hamstring injury requiring internal fixation. Br J Sports Med. 1998;32:255–7.
33. Sonnery-Cottet B, Daggett M, Gardon R et al. Surgical management of recurrent musculotendinous hamstring injury in professional athletes. Orthop J Sports Med. 2015;3(10):108.
34. Straw R. Surgical repair of a chronic rupture of the rectus femoris muscle at the proximal musculotendinous junction in a soccer player. Br J Sports Med. 2003;37:182–4.
35. Werlich T. Die isolierte Bizepssehnenruptur am Kniegelenk. Unfallchirurg. 2001;104:187–90.
36. Zini R, Panasci M, Papalia R et al. Rectus femoris tendon calcification: arthroscopic excision in 6 top amateur athletes. Orthop J Sports Med. 2014;2(12):227.

Criteria in Return to Football

37

Luis Serratosa, Hélder Pereira, João Pedro Araújo, Rogério Pereira, and Nuno Loureiro

Contents

37.1 Introduction

Muscle injury is one of the major problems in football, representing one third of all time-loss injuries (one fourth of total injury absence) in male professional players and up to 23% of all injuries at the amateur level [1–3]. Injuries to the major muscle groups of the lower limb (adductors, hamstrings, quadriceps and calf) account for more than 90% of all muscle injuries in professional football [1]. Besides its high incidence and great efforts in trying to improve prevention strategies, our understanding of mechanisms and risk factors is still limited, and the truth is that reported injury and reinjury rates have not decreased in the last decades [4, 5].

L. Serratosa (✉)
Ripoll & De Prado Sport Clinic, FIFA Medical Centre of Excellence, Murcia, Spain

Hospital Universitario Quironsalud Madrid, Madrid, Spain
e-mail: lserratosa62@gmail.com

H. Pereira
Ripoll & De Prado Sport Clinic, FIFA Medical Centre of Excellence, Murcia, Spain

3B's Research Group–Biomaterials, Biodegradables and Biomimetics, University of Minho, Headquarters of the European Institute of Excellence on Tissue Engineering and Regenerative Medicine, AvePark, Parque de Ciência e Tecnologia, Zona Industrial da Gandra, 4805-017 Barco/Guimarães, Portugal

ICVS/3B's–PT Government Associate Laboratory, Braga/Guimarães, Portugal

Orthopedic Department, Centro Hospitalar Póvoa de Varzim-Vila do Conde, Póvoa de Varzim, Portugal

J.P. Araújo
Clínica do Dragão, Espregueira-Mendes Sports Centre – FIFA Medical Centre of Excellence, Porto, Portugal

Medical Department, Al Jazira Football Club, Dubai, UAE

R. Pereira • N. Loureiro
Clínica do Dragão, Espregueira-Mendes Sports Centre – FIFA Medical Centre of Excellence, Porto, Portugal

J. Espregueira-Mendes et al. (eds.), *Injuries and Health Problems in Football*,
DOI 10.1007/978-3-662-53924-8_37

Reinjuries are sure among the major concerns among players and sports medicine practitioners who will almost always need to engage in a risk-benefit analysis, when making return to play (RTP) decisions. The RTP concept refers to the time the athlete will be able to return to normal sports activity with a minimum risk of reinjury [6–8]. Thresholds for "acceptable level of risk" will be different for different individuals and will change depending on context [7]. Quite frequently and especially in professional sports, in important competitions and at certain parts of the season, both athletes and health professionals might feel pressured to accept a premature RTP with the consequent increased injury risk. As RTP decisions in muscle injuries are very much related with risk management, RTP decisions usually need of athletes and sports medicine professionals shared decision-making.

One of the most widely accepted risk factors for lower extremity muscle injury in football is a previous identical injury. Hägglund et al. [2] have reported reinjury rates of 21–30% in their sample of 2123 lower limb muscle injuries of the UEFA injury study, with 12–14% being early recurrences occurring within 2 months of RTP. The same authors [2] also reported higher quadriceps (68%) and calf (91%) injury rates with a history of previous injury to other lower limb muscle groups. In their prospective study including 32 hamstring injuries in Australian Rules footballers, Verrall et al. [9] found that together with previous posterior thigh injury, history of knee and groyne injury also increased the risk of hamstring injury. In addition, it is well known that reinjuries are usually more severe and cause longer absence than the index injury [1].

All these factors highlight the importance of previous injury history, objective measurements and individually tailored rehabilitation programmes aimed to develop the player's functional abilities, in order to make better and safer RTP decisions. But nowadays and in real life, the truth is that there is a lack of empirical evidence and consensus on which are the best criteria based on player's injury history, symptoms, physical and lab tests and psychological readiness, which should be used in RTP decisions [7]. Quite frequently and even at the elite level, RTP decisions in muscle injuries mainly rely on estimated (guessed) post-injury timeline, clinician's individual experience and player's subjective feelings. Objective and quantitative clinical and functional tests with the potential to identify neuromuscular and biomechanical deficits are therefore needed. These tests should be performed regularly and always consider the interrelationships between the measured variables (i.e. flexibility, joint mobility, strength, etc.) in order to determine when and how to progress through the phases of the rehabilitation programme [5]. Mendiguchia and Brughelli [10] propose an algorithm approach based on a multifactorial global analysis of the various risk factors related with hamstring injuries, through three basic phases (acute phase, subacute or regeneration phase and functional phase) which would hopefully decrease the risk of reinjury and lead to a more successful RTP (Fig. 37.1). More recently, Tol et al. [11] have also proposed a model with functional criteria-based progressions through a six-stage rehabilitation protocol. In these and other similar models, successful RTP in muscle injuries depends on every decision taken from the very beginning of the acute phase, because the athlete is not allowed to progress to the next phase until meeting specific criteria. More prospective interventional studies using these or similar types of systematic and individualized approach are needed to improve both our primary and secondary prevention strategies of muscle injuries in football.

a

Acute Phase		
Treatment	Timeline	Purpose
Immobilization	3 to 4 days	Decrease scar size, increase tensile strength and elasticity, and allow proper alignment for myofibril regeneration
RICE	Immediately and up to 24 hours	Reduce pain, bleeding and inflammation
Water Immersion	Days 2 to 4	Displacement of fluids from extremities to central cavities through hydrostatic pressure
SIJ Manipulation	Days 3 to 4	Re-establish lumbo-pelvic-hip and sacroiliac joint function

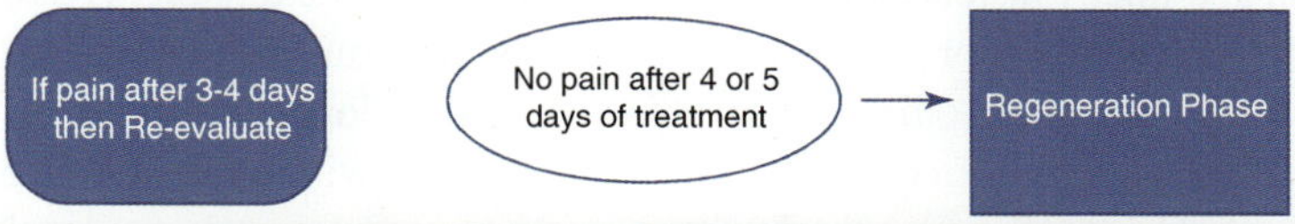

b

Regeneration Phase		
Variable	Test	Criteria for progression
Pain after injury	Prone with knee flexed to 15	No pain
Isolated strength at long muscle Lengths	Probe with knee flexed to 15	<10% asymmetry
Neural deficiencies	Slump test	No pain
Hamstring flexibility	Active knee extension (AKE) test	<10% asymmetry and <20
Hip flexor flexibility	Modified Thomas test (MTT)	>5 and symmetry below horizontal

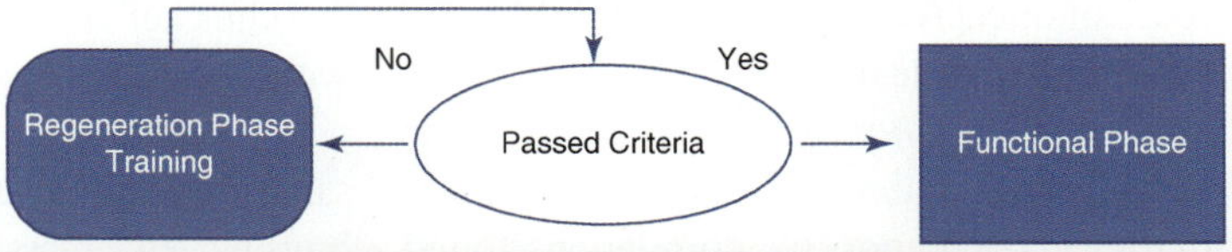

c

Functional Phase		
Variable	Test	Criteria for Progression
Optimum angle of peak torque	Isokinetic knee flexion at 60/second	<28 during knee flexion and <8 asymmetry between legs
Hip extension strength	Isokinetic hip extension at 60/second	<10% asymmetry between legs
Horizontal force during running	Non-motorized treadmill at 80% maximum running velocity	<20% asymmetry between legs
Magnetic Resonance Imaging (MRI)	Hamstring image	Edema size and/or length
Lumbar rotation stability	ASLR test	No Anterior Pelvic Tilt

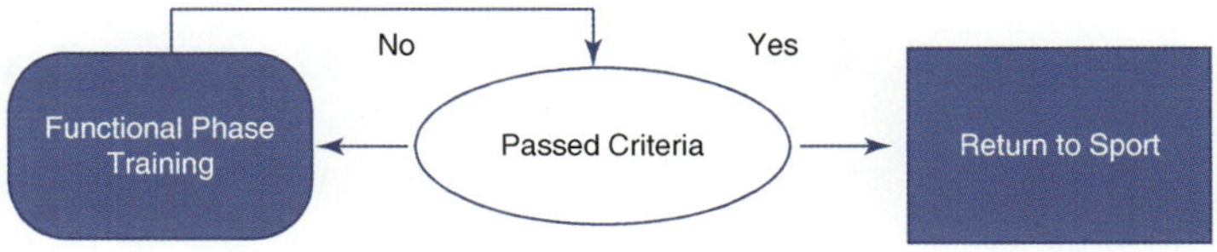

Fig. 37.1 The acute phase, subacute or regeneration phase and functional phase of the return-to-sport algorithm for hamstring injuries proposed by Mendiguchia and Brughelli [10] (Reprinted from a return-to-sport algorithm for acute hamstring injuries, by Mendiguchia and Brughelli [10]. Copyright [2010] by Elsevier Ltd. Reprinted with permission)

37.2 Clinical Examination

37.2.1 History

When dealing with muscle injuries, making an accurate diagnosis and determining injury severity needs of as much information as possible related with injury mechanism, affected muscles, anatomical location of the injury inside the muscle (myofascial, intramuscular, muscle-tendon junction, intra tendinous), size of the injury, tendon involvement and finally history of previous injuries in the lower limbs, groyne or low back. This information together with some other more subjective variables, such as pain, may be useful in guiding us through the rehabilitation programme.

The *injury mechanism* (sprinting, changing direction, kicking, dominant/non-dominant, stance/swing leg and trauma) may be one of the first aspects to consider. Muscle contusions usually need a shorter recovery period than the non-contact injuries, thought to be caused by lengthening beyond the optimal length of the activated muscles [12]. In a sample of 2003 thigh muscle injuries of the UEFA Elite League injury study, the mean lay-off time for indirect (strain) injuries was of 18.5 days, significantly longer than the 7 days of direct (contusion) injuries [13].

Lower limb muscle injuries have a high rate of recurrence, and *reinjuries* seem to cause up to 30% longer absence time than first-episode muscle injuries [1]. The positive correlations found between lower limb muscle injury incidence and previous lower limb muscle, knee or groyne injuries [2, 9, 14] could support the hypothesis of biomechanical changes and related post-injury inadequate compensations as the cause of further injuries. This highlights the importance for clinicians to investigate the player's injury history and regularly monitor those biomechanical alterations that could be related with previous injuries, before allowing players to RTP [2].

37.2.2 Physical Examination

The purpose of the first physical examination is to determine the location and severity of the injury. More than the length of the painful area, it has been suggested that it is the distance from the point of maximum *pain* to the proximal insertion that is associated with the absence period [15]. The more proximal the site of maximum pain, the greater the time needed to return to preinjury level [16].

Related with the lower limb affected muscle, quadriceps injuries are usually the ones requiring longer rehabilitation periods for RTP, while groyne muscle injuries cause the shorter absence [1, 3]. Injuries involving damage to the proximal free tendon [17, 18] or the central tendon of the muscle [19–22] are usually more severe and take longer for RTP. On the contrary, injuries located within the muscle belly, not involving the tendon or muscle-tendon junction, usually have a more benign prognosis and a shorter recovery period until RTP [23].

More than 1 day to walk pain-free has been shown to be associated with a longer (> 3 weeks) recovery period to RTP in hamstring injuries [24]. Symptoms that persist for more than 5 days might need considering more extensive tissue damage or intramuscular hematoma and most probably require special attention and a longer recovery [10].

Verrall et al. [25] found that patient reported pain and clinician's estimate of injury severity correlated with the RTP in 83 Australian Rules football players with posterior thigh injuries. A few years later, the same group of researchers [26] found that swelling, bruising, tenderness and pain on hamstring contraction in the initial clinical examination had no value in predicting the likelihood of reinjury in 30 hamstring injuries of Australian Rules footballers. Besides the above-mentioned conflicting findings, looking at early clinical signs and symptoms and continuous monitoring during the rehabilitation period is highly recommended. We still need further studies to confirm the validity of clinical findings for predicting the severity and prognosis of lower limb muscle injuries.

37.2.3 Core Stability

A lack of core stability has been widely considered as a risk factor for hamstring injuries [10]. It has been proposed that any *sacroiliac joint and/*

or pelvic dysfunction can affect hamstring mechanical behaviour, alter the load transfer from the spine to the legs and thereby increase the injury risk [10]. Correcting these alterations early in the acute phase may help in restoring the lumbopelvic function and lead to a more successful RTP in thigh muscle injuries.

Sherry and Best [27] found that a rehabilitation programme consisting of progressive agility and trunk stabilization exercises is more effective in promoting return to sports and preventing injury recurrence in athletes suffering an acute hamstring strain than a more traditional isolated hamstring stretching and strengthening programme. Although the morphological and neuromuscular factors were not measured, these results suggest that there may be a role for lumbopelvic neuromuscular control exercises in the prevention of hamstring injuries and reinjuries [28]. The lumbar muscles provide localized segmental control of the lumbar spine, and it has been shown that a smaller size (cross-sectional area) of the multifidus or quadratus lumborum muscles may be predictive of lower limb injury incidence in Australian Rules football players [29].

Abdominal and lumbar muscles may also be important in preventing quadriceps injuries. During kicking, abdominal muscles are necessary to reduce the quadriceps overload and help in controlling the lateral displacement of the trunk to the non-kicking side at foot-to-ball contact [30]. Kicking may also demand high levels of activation of the quadratus lumborum of the non-kicking side, to counteract torsion and side flexion moments [31]. Core stability exercises have therefore become an important part of most thigh injuries prevention and rehabilitation programmes and should be incorporated early in the subacute phase.

37.2.4 Flexibility and Range of Movement (ROM)

Despite conflicting data in the literature, it has traditionally been suggested that greater flexibility may reduce the risk of muscle injuries due to greater compliance of the passive components of the muscle-tendon unit, at least in sports involving bouncing and jumping activities with a high intensity of stretch-shortening cycles [32]. A few prospective studies have identified relationships between reduced hamstring flexibility and hamstring injuries [33–35] as well as between reduced quadriceps flexibility [35] or quadriceps asymmetries [36] and quadriceps injuries, in professional football players. Malliaropoulos et al. [37] found that knee active ROM deficit was correlated with recovery time in 165 track and field athletes with acute, first-time, unilateral posterior thigh muscle injuries. Recently, Moen et al. [38] reported that passive straight leg raise deficit was associated with time to RTP in 80 non-professional athletes with magnetic resonance imaging (MRI)-positive hamstring injuries. By contrast, Askling et al. [17] found no correlation between measures of hip flexion ROM and time to RTP of hamstring injuries, in 18 elite sprinters and 15 professional dancers. Part of the contradictory results might be related with the absence of gold standard methods for flexibility measurements and with difficulties in stabilizing the hip and lumbar spine in some of the most widely used tests, such as the sit-and-reach, straight leg raise and toe-touch test [39]. Hunter and Speed [40] recommend the active knee extension (AKE) test that measures hamstring flexibility at 90 degrees of hip flexion, but more dynamic tests such as the active hamstring flexibility test proposed by Askling et al. [41] might be more sensitive to detect differences not only in flexibility but also in insecurity before allowing the player to return to full training and competition.

Reduced hip flexors flexibility has also been identified as a risk factor for hamstring injuries. An increase in anterior pelvic tilt, due to tight hip flexors and limited hip extension, could cause excessive hamstring stretch in the opposite limb and thus increase the risk of hamstring injury [10, 42].

Hamstring and hip flexors flexibility exercises should be initiated soon after injury, but always trying to avoid an increase in neural tension and including dynamic and functional exercises that also involve hip stability and neuromuscular control [10].

There are a few reasons to support that achieving optimal levels of both quadriceps and hip flexors flexibility should be a cornerstone of any quadriceps prevention and rehabilitation programme in football players [31]. In the kicking action, the hip flexors generate greater hip flexion moment by using the stretch-shortening cycle. A lack of hip extension during the early swing phase due to a tight iliopsoas may require higher force generation from the rectus femoris and lead to overload and early fatigue during repetitive kicking sessions. Mechanical irritation of the femoral nerve due to a restricted psoas has also been suggested as a possible cause of rectus femoris injuries [31]. The modified Thomas test is recommended for quadriceps and hip flexors flexibility assessment during any thigh injury rehabilitation programme [43].

Decreased ROM of the hip has been suggested to be a risk factor for sports-related chronic groin pain in athletes [44]. A decrease in hip abduction [45] and internal-external rotation [46] ROM of the hip have both been reported to be correlated with occurrence of groyne strains in professional football players. Although more prospective studies are needed, interventions directed at players with limited hip ROM could lead to reduce *adductors* injury and reinjury incidence and should therefore be considered in any groyne muscle injury rehabilitation programme.

Lower limb muscle injuries are sure related with different joints and groups of muscles, so an analytic approach to flexibility assessment in such a complex system should be avoided. Testing should be ideally performed with dynamic tests and in all the involved muscles. We should be very careful when interpreting results from static measures and avoid generalizing to dynamic actions [5].

37.2.5 Strength

Decreased muscle strength and strength imbalances have long been proposed as related to increased risk of thigh muscle injuries. Reduced *hamstring* strength is commonly perceived to be a risk factor for hamstring injuries, most of which occur during the late swing [47] or early stance phase [48] of sprinting. Hamstring eccentric strength training has been shown to increase the optimum length of tension development [49] and decrease hamstring injury risk in professional and amateur football players [50–52].

Isokinetic strength testing is frequently used in football, but there is still lack of consensus regarding its usefulness in RTP decisions [53]. Peak torque at greater knee flexion angle (i.e. shorter optimum length) [12] and eccentric hamstring strength deficits compared to the uninjured side, as well as the ratios of concentric hamstring to concentric quadriceps strength and eccentric hamstring to concentric quadriceps strength, have been proposed as the most useful variables to predict hamstring injury risk [54, 55]. In a recent study in 52 professional male football players with MRI-positive hamstring injuries, Tol et al. [11] found that when compared with the uninjured leg, 67% of the clinically recovered players showed at least one hamstring isokinetic testing deficit of more than 10%. They concluded that normalization of hamstring isokinetic strength variables does not seem to be required for successfully completing a football-specific rehabilitation programme. Because of the low reinjury incidence, it was not possible to conclude if there was any association between isokinetic strength deficits and reinjury incidence. In their study with hamstring injuries in sprinters and dancers, Askling et al. [17] did not find any correlation between knee flexion isometric strength (measured in prone position and with knee extended) and time to RTP. Freckleton et al. [14] demonstrated a significant deficit in preseason single leg hamstring bridge scores on the right thigh of Australian Rules football players that subsequently sustained a right-sided hamstring injury. The lack of correlation between strength and time to RTP in some studies could probably be related with the fact that assessment was performed with non-functional tests that are very different from the football-specific demands. Hamstring strength should be tested and trained at long muscle lengths, with the hip and knee at functional angles and aiming to assess and improve strength, power and endurance.

Hamstring eccentric training may result in greater structural stability at longer muscle lengths and consequently may have interesting implications for injury prevention. Despite the demonstrated benefit of the Nordic hamstring exercise in several studies [50–52], there might be greater benefit by using more functional unilateral eccentric exercises that involve both hip and knee motion, similar to that needed for sprinting and other football activities [28, 56, 57]. An adequate progression would allow the player to include these exercises in the last stages of the rehabilitation programme.

During running, the *gluteus maximus* has a multifaceted role not only as a powerful hip extensor but also to control trunk flexion of the stance leg and decelerate the swing leg [58]. Gluteus maximus activity has been shown to be much greater during sprinting than during running [59]. Any alteration in gluteus maximus strength, endurance or activation pattern will place greater demand on the hamstrings and may therefore increase the injury risk of this muscle group. Sugiura et al. [60] reported that hamstring injuries in a group of elite sprinters were associated with reduced hip extensors concentric strength. Exercises aimed at teaching how to isolate gluteus maximus activation from hamstrings, and improving gluteus maximus strength and endurance, should be included already in the subacute phase of hamstring injuries rehabilitation programmes [10].

Quadriceps injuries are more common in the kicking leg, most probably related with a greater exposure to high-risk actions [2]. Both the iliopsoas and rectus femoris contribute to hip flexion, and the ability to generate a greater hip flexion moment is critical to achieve a high foot velocity during kicking [31]. A reduction in strength and/or activation of the iliopsoas in football players may result in overload and increased injury risk of the rectus femoris [31]. Achieving optimal and balanced levels of quadriceps and hip flexors strength at long muscle lengths should be considered as a priority in every prevention and rehabilitation programme of rectus femoris injuries.

Eccentric training of the quadriceps has been shown to increase the optimum length of the knee extensors in professional football players [49]. As muscle injuries are thought to occur when muscles are contracted beyond their optimal length [12], rectus femoris prevention and rehabilitation programmes should also include sport-specific eccentric exercises of the knee extensors, with distances (sprints and decelerations), velocities and directional components similar to the football movements [31]. These eccentric exercises aimed to increase the optimal length of the knee extensors should only be incorporated in the last part of the functional phase of the rehabilitation programme.

Weak *adductors* have been suggested to be a risk factor of groyne injuries in sports requiring side-to-side cuttings, quick accelerations and decelerations and sudden changes in direction. Professional ice hockey players were 17 times more likely to sustain an adductor muscle strain if their adductor strength was less than 80% of the abductor strength [61]. Engebretsen et al. [62] found that the risk for a new groyne injury (22/61 acute injuries) in football players (first, second and third Norwegian divisions) with weak adductors was four times the risk of players with normal strength. An intervention programme aimed at improving adductor's strength proved to be effective to prevent adductor injuries in professional ice hockey players [63]. Hip adductors/abductor strength assessment with hand-held dynamometer in the supine position has been shown to be a simple and reliable method [64], and athletes with an adduction-to-abduction strength ratio of less than 80% with this test have been considered as at risk [63]. Tyler et al. [63] propose a three-phase adductor muscle strain rehabilitation programme, progressing from submaximal isometric adduction exercises already in the acute phase to eccentric and sport-specific exercises in the last stages.

37.3 Muscle Mechanical Properties

Hamstrings play an important role in horizontal force production during the acceleration phase of sprint activities which are, with no doubt, essential in football performance. Forward orientation of ground reaction force (GRF) has been shown to be a stronger determinant of field sprint acceleration performance than the overall magnitude of vertical or resultant GRF [65]. Mendiguchia et al. [66] used a recently validated simple field method that only needs time and velocity measurements during a single sprint, to quantify both horizontal mechanical properties and performance measures in football players with a unilateral hamstring injury, during the entire acceleration phase of a 50 m sprint. Upon returning to sports, injured players were moderately slower, and their ability to produce a high level of horizontal force in the first metres of the acceleration phase was impaired, compared to the uninjured players. Within 2 months after returning to sports, the horizontal force production and acceleration capacity were both improved, which appears to indicate that the initial differences between injured and uninjured players were most probably related with the hamstring injury. Assessing and training horizontal force production during sprint running should therefore be recommended in both primary and secondary prevention of hamstring injuries. These more football-specific testing and training methods should be included in the last stages of the rehabilitation programme and could also be useful to monitor the mechanical imbalances during the early phase after injured players RTP.

37.4 Football-Specific Functional Testing

The last stages of any rehabilitation programme should include exercises mimicking sport-specific tasks. In the last three stages of a six-stage criteria-based standardized rehabilitation programme, Tol et al. [11] require the injured player to successfully complete a football-specific functional field test (FFT) that includes direction changes, sprints, jumps, (cross-) passes, shooting, interval running, one-on-one attacking and defence drills, mimicking muscle fatigue and competitiveness during football training and game situations.

In order to assess if the player has completed sufficient training to be prepared for competition, the model proposed by Blanch and Gabbett [67] that includes the acute-to-chronic workload ratio (training load for a given week compared to average of previous 4 weeks) in the RTP decision-making process could be a very useful tool to estimate the player's reinjury risk. The ratio can be calculated for any internal and external workload variable considered to be relevant for the player and specific injury (session minutes X self-reported RPE, total running volume, intensity of high-speed running, collisions, accelerations and decelerations, etc.). The model is hoped to become more accurate with more data overtime and even specific for the player who provides the data.

Any football player with a lower limb muscle injury should be able to complete a few training sessions with the team (not less than a week), with full functional ability and without limitations and/or symptoms, before being allowed for a gradual RTP.

37.5 Imaging Criteria

During the last decades, there have been several attempts to establish an evidence-based correlation between the imaging findings and clinical prognosis of muscle injuries. In the largest study analysing the relationship between MRI findings and RTP in professional football, Hallén and Ekstrand [3] analysed the MRI studies of 386 muscle injuries registered during the 2001–2013 UEFA Champions League study period. The authors concluded that radiological grading was associated with lay-off times after injury and could therefore be considered valuable for prognosticating time to RTP. Lay-off days were also related to the injured muscle, with groyne muscle injuries causing shorter median absence (9 days), compared to hamstring (13 days), quadriceps (12 days) and calf muscle (13 days) injuries. Among the limitations of this study, it should be noted that MRIs were analysed by several radiologists from different countries and that it included a heterogeneous group of muscle injuries and, most probably, many different treatment methods that could have sure influenced the lay-off times.

Reurink et al. [68] found that 89% of 53 MRI-positive (grade 1 and 2) non-contact hamstring injuries showed intramuscular increased signal intensity on fluid-sensitive sequences of the MRI at RTP. The authors concluded that normalization of the increased signal, which can take up to 6 months [69], does not seem required for successful RTP. Eighteen (34%) of the 53 injuries showed low-signal intensity on RTP, suggestive of newly developed fibrous tissue at the site of injury, but its clinical significance for reinjury risk could not be determined. After analysing 180 male athletes with acute onset posterior thigh pain, Wangensteen et al. [70] reported that the additional predictive value of MRI was negligible compared with baseline patient history and clinical examinational alone, concluding that there is no rationale for routine MRI after acute hamstring injury. In their recent systematic review of 12 studies (11 with a high risk of bias), Reurink et al. [71] concluded that there is currently no strong evidence for any MRI finding that gives a prognosis on the time to RTP after an acute hamstring injury. In their review, they just found moderate evidence for shorter time to RTP in injuries without hyperintensity on fluid-sensitive sequences and longer time to RTP associated with injuries involving the proximal free tendon.

Ultrasound (US) may be a very useful tool in assessing muscle injuries and is becoming increasingly popular in sports medicine. Compared to MRI, US is inexpensive, widely available and allows for dynamic imaging while mobilizing the injured limb. Main drawbacks are its operator dependency and reduced sensitivity when compared to MRI. Petersen et al. [72] investigated the US examinations of 51 hamstring injuries of Danish football players finding that neither the presence of sonographic findings nor the size of the findings was correlated with time to RTP and therefore concluded that the prognosis of hamstring injuries should not be guided by US findings alone.

RTP decisions exclusively based on US and MRI results are therefore not recommended and should always be taken in conjunction with information obtained from other objective clinical and functional tests. Hopefully in the future, advanced imaging techniques (diffusion tensor imaging, phosphorus MR spectroscopy, MR elastography) may provide with more precise information on muscle function, composition and microstructure and allow sports medicine practitioners to more accurately estimate the prognosis of lower limb muscle injuries [73].

37.6 Psychological Readiness

Psychological readiness is also an important aspect that should be considered in the muscle injuries RTP decision-making process. Motivation, confidence and low fear of reinjury are associated with a sooner RTP and greater likelihood of returning to the preinjury level of participation [74]. Fear seems to be a prominent emotional response at the time of RTP, but overall emotions become more positive as recovery and rehabilitation progress [74]. The sports medicine practitioner (sports physician, physiotherapist, athletic trainer) must provide the player with as much evidence-based information as possible, as well as with constant and true reassurance. In certain cases, probably more in reinjuries, help from a sports psychologist should be considered. All those involved in the rehabilitation process should work as a team, with similar objectives and providing the player with the same information. In professional sports, this might be quite frequently difficult to achieve because there are too many sources of information (sports medicine practitioners, fitness coaches, coaches, directors, agents, media, etc.). The Injury-Psychological Readiness to Return to Sport (I-PRRS) scale has been shown to be a valid and reliable tool to assess player's psychological readiness to RTP after injury [75].

Conclusion

Lower limb muscle injuries are one of the major problems in football. Besides its high incidence and great efforts in trying to improve prevention strategies, our understanding of mechanisms and risk factors is still limited, and reported injury and reinjury rates have not decreased in the last decades.

The biomechanical changes and related post-injury inadequate compensations caused by previous muscle, knee or groin injuries appear to increase the lower limb muscle reinjury risk.

Regular assessment of football players with lower limb muscle injuries should include objective and quantitative, clinical and functional tests with the potential to identify neuromuscular and biomechanical deficits. Our approach to lower limb muscle injuries should always consider the interrelationships between all the multiple risk factors (previous injury, core stability, flexibility, strength, etc.) involved in these complex injuries.

Successful RTP in lower limb muscle injuries depends on every decision taken from the early stages of the rehabilitation programme, in which progress through the different phases should only be allowed after meeting specific criteria.

RTP decisions exclusively based in imaging results are not recommended and should always be taken in conjunction with information obtained from other objective clinical and functional tests. Whenever possible, assessment should be performed with dynamic and football-specific functional tests.

In football, RTP decisions in muscle injuries are very much related with risk management and usually need of players and clinicians shared decision-making.

References

1. Ekstrand J, Hägglund M, Walden M. Epidemiology of muscle injuries in professional football (soccer). Am J Sports Med. 2011;39(6):1226–32.
2. Hägglund M, Walden M, Ekstrand J. Risk factors for lower extremity muscle injury in professional soccer: the UEFA Injury Study. Am J Sports Med. 2013;41(2):327–35.
3. Hallén A, Ekstrand J. Return to play following muscle injuries in professional footballers. J Sports Sci. 2014;32(13):1229–36.
4. Ekstrand J, Hägglund M, Kristenson K, Magnusson H, Walden M. Fewer ligament injuries but no preventive effect on muscle injuries and severe injuries: an 11-year follow-up of the UEFA champions league injury study. Br J Sports Med. 2013;47(12):732–7.
5. Mendiguchia J, Alentorn-Geli E, Brughelli M. Hamstring strain injuries: are we heading in the right direction? Br J Sports Med. 2012;46(2):81–5.
6. Clover J, Wall J. Return-to-play criteria following sports injury. Clin Sports Med. 2010;29(1): 169–175.
7. Creighton DW, Shrier I, Shultz R, Meeuwisse WH, Matheson GO. Return-to-play in sport: a decision-based model. Clin J Sport Med. 2010;20(5):379–85.
8. Orchard J, Best TM, Verrall GM. Return to play following muscle strains. Clin J Sport Med. 2005;15(6): 436–41.
9. Verrall GM, Slavotinek JP, Barnes PG, Fon GT, Spriggins AJ. Clinical risk factors for hamstring muscle strain injury: a prospective study with correlation of injury by magnetic resonance imaging. Br J Sports Med. 2001;35(6):435–9.
10. Mendiguchia J, Brughelli M. A return-to-sport algorithm for acute hamstring injuries. Phys Ther Sport. 2011;12(1):2–14.
11. Tol JL, Hamilton B, Eirale C, Muxart P, Jacobsen P, Whiteley R. At return to play following hamstring injury the majority of professional football players have residual isokinetic deficits. Br J Sports Med. 2014;48(18):1364–9.
12. Brockett CL, Morgan DL, Proske U. Predicting hamstring strain injury in elite athletes. Med Sci Sports Exerc. 2004;36(3):379–87.
13. Ueblacker P, Muller-Wohlfahrt HW, Ekstrand J. Epidemiological and clinical outcome comparison of indirect ('strain') versus direct ('contusion') anterior and posterior thigh muscle injuries in male elite football players: UEFA Elite League study of 2287 thigh injuries (2001–2013). Br J Sports Med. 2015;49(22):1461–5.
14. Freckleton G, Cook J, Pizzari T. The predictive validity of a single leg bridge test for hamstring injuries in Australian rules football players. Br J Sports Med. 2014;48(8):713–7.
15. Heiderscheit BC, Sherry MA, Silder A, Chumanov ES, Thelen DG. Hamstring strain injuries: recommendations for diagnosis, rehabilitation, and injury prevention. J Orthop Sports Phys Ther. 2010;40(2): 67–81.
16. Askling CM, Tengvar M, Saartok T, Thorstensson A. Acute first-time hamstring strains during high-speed running: a longitudinal study including clinical and magnetic resonance imaging findings. Am J Sports Med. 2007;35(2):197–206.
17. Askling C, Saartok T, Thorstensson A. Type of acute hamstring strain affects flexibility, strength, and time to return to pre-injury level. Br J Sports Med. 2006;40(1):40–4.
18. Askling CM, Tengvar M, Saartok T, Thorstensson A. Proximal hamstring strains of stretching type in different sports: injury situations, clinical and magnetic resonance imaging characteristics, and return to sport. Am J Sports Med. 2008;36(9):1799–804.
19. Balius R, Maestro A, Pedret C, Estruch A, Mota J, Rodriguez L, et al. Central aponeurosis tears of the

rectus femoris: practical sonographic prognosis. Br J Sports Med. 2009;43(11):818–24.
20. Comin J, Malliaras P, Baquie P, Barbour T, Connell D. Return to competitive play after hamstring injuries involving disruption of the central tendon. Am J Sports Med. 2013;41(1):111–5.
21. Cross TM, Gibbs N, Houang MT, Cameron M. Acute quadriceps muscle strains: magnetic resonance imaging features and prognosis. Am J Sports Med. 2004; 32(3):710–9.
22. Pedret C, Rodas G, Balius R, Capdevila L, Bossy M, Vernooij RW, et al. Return to play after soleus muscle injuries. Orthop J Sports Med. 2015;3(7):2325967115595802.
23. Garrett Jr WE, Califf JC, Bassett 3rd FH. Histochemical correlates of hamstring injuries. Am J Sports Med. 1984;12(2):98–103.
24. Warren P, Gabbe BJ, Schneider-Kolsky M, Bennell KL. Clinical predictors of time to return to competition and of recurrence following hamstring strain in elite Australian footballers. Br J Sports Med. 2010; 44(6):415–9.
25. Verrall GM, Slavotinek JP, Barnes PG, Fon GT. Diagnostic and prognostic value of clinical findings in 83 athletes with posterior thigh injury: comparison of clinical findings with magnetic resonance imaging documentation of hamstring muscle strain. Am J Sports Med. 2003;31(6):969–73.
26. Verrall GM, Slavotinek JP, Barnes PG, Fon GT, Esterman A. Assessment of physical examination and magnetic resonance imaging findings of hamstring injury as predictors for recurrent injury. J Orthop Sports Phys Ther. 2006;36(4):215–24.
27. Sherry MA, Best TM. A comparison of 2 rehabilitation programs in the treatment of acute hamstring strains. J Orthop Sports Phys Ther. 2004;34(3): 116–25.
28. Sherry MA, Best TM, Silder A, Thelen DG, Heiderscheit BC. Hamstring strains: basic science and clinical research applications for preventing the recurrent injury. Strength Cond J. 2011;33(3):56–71.
29. Hides JA, Stanton WR. Can motor control training lower the risk of injury for professional football players? Med Sci Sports Exerc. 2014;46(4):762–8.
30. Lees A, Nolan L. Three dimensional kinematic analysis of the instep kick under speed and accuracy conditions. In: Spinks W, Reilly T, Murphy A, editors. Science and football IV. London: E & FN Spon; 2002. p. 16–21.
31. Mendiguchia J, Alentorn-Geli E, Idoate F, Myer GD. Rectus femoris muscle injuries in football: a clinically relevant review of mechanisms of injury, risk factors and preventive strategies. Br J Sports Med. 2013;47(6):359–66.
32. Witvrouw E, Mahieu N, Danneels L, McNair P. Stretching and injury prevention: an obscure relationship. Sports Med. 2004;34(7):443–9.
33. Bradley PS, Portas MD. The relationship between preseason range of motion and muscle strain injury in elite soccer players. J Strength Cond Res. 2007; 21(4):1155–9.
34. Henderson G, Barnes CA, Portas MD. Factors associated with increased propensity for hamstring injury in English premier league soccer players. J Sci Med Sport. 2010;13(4):397–402.
35. Witvrouw E, Danneels L, Asselman P, D'Have T, Cambier D. Muscle flexibility as a risk factor for developing muscle injuries in male professional soccer players. A prospective study. Am J Sports Med. 2003;31(1):41–6.
36. Fousekis K, Tsepis E, Poulmedis P, Athanasopoulos S, Vagenas G. Intrinsic risk factors of non-contact quadriceps and hamstring strains in soccer: a prospective study of 100 professional players. Br J Sports Med. 2011;45(9):709–14.
37. Malliaropoulos N, Papacostas E, Kiritsi O, Papalada A, Gougoulias N, Maffulli N. Posterior thigh muscle injuries in elite track and field athletes. Am J Sports Med. 2010;38(9):1813–9.
38. Moen MH, Reurink G, Weir A, Tol JL, Maas M, Goudswaard GJ. Predicting return to play after hamstring injuries. Br J Sports Med. 2014;48(18): 1358–63.
39. Opar DA, Williams MD, Shield AJ. Hamstring strain injuries: factors that lead to injury and re-injury. Sports Med. 2012;42(3):209–26.
40. Hunter DG, Speed CA. The assessment and management of chronic hamstring/posterior thigh pain. Best Pract Res Clin Rheumatol. 2007;21(2):261–77.
41. Askling CM, Nilsson J, Thorstensson A. A new hamstring test to complement the common clinical examination before return to sport after injury. Knee Surg Sports Traumatol Arthrosc. 2010;18(12):1798–803.
42. Chumanov ES, Heiderscheit BC, Thelen DG. The effect of speed and influence of individual muscles on hamstring mechanics during the swing phase of sprinting. J Biomech. 2007;40(16):3555–62.
43. Harvey D. Assessment of the flexibility of elite athletes using the modified Thomas test. Br J Sports Med. 1998;32(1):68–70.
44. Verrall GM, Hamilton IA, Slavotinek JP, Oakeshott RD, Spriggins AJ, Barnes PG, et al. Hip joint range of motion reduction in sports-related chronic groin injury diagnosed as pubic bone stress injury. J Sci Med Sport. 2005;8(1):77–84.
45. Arnason A, Sigurdsson SB, Gudmundsson A, Holme I, Engebretsen L, Bahr R. Risk factors for injuries in football. Am J Sports Med. 2004;32(1 Suppl):5S–16S.
46. Ibrahim A, Murrell GA, Knapman P. Adductor strain and hip range of movement in male professional soccer players. J Orthop Surg (Hong Kong). 2007; 15(1):46–9.
47. Chumanov ES, Schache AG, Heiderscheit BC, Thelen DG. Hamstrings are most susceptible to injury during the late swing phase of sprinting. Br J Sports Med. 2012;46(2):90.
48. Orchard JW. Hamstrings are most susceptible to injury during the early stance phase of sprinting. Br J Sports Med. 2012;46(2):88–9.
49. Brughelli M, Mendiguchia J, Nosaka K, Idoate F, Arcos AL, Cronin J. Effects of eccentric exercise on

optimum length of the knee flexors and extensors during the preseason in professional soccer players. Phys Ther Sport. 2010;11(2):50–5.
50. Arnason A, Andersen TE, Holme I, Engebretsen L, Bahr R. Prevention of hamstring strains in elite soccer: an intervention study. Scand J Med Sci Sports. 2008;18(1):40–8.
51. Petersen J, Thorborg K, Nielsen MB, Budtz-Jorgensen E, Holmich P. Preventive effect of eccentric training on acute hamstring injuries in men's soccer: a cluster-randomized controlled trial. Am J Sports Med. 2011;39(11):2296–303.
52. van der Horst N, Smits DW, Petersen J, Goedhart EA, Backx FJ. The preventive effect of the nordic hamstring exercise on hamstring injuries in amateur soccer players: a randomized controlled trial. Am J Sports Med. 2015;43(6):1316–23.
53. Delvaux F, Rochcongar P, Bruyère O, Bourlet G, Daniel C, Diverse P, et al. Return-to-play criteria after hamstring injury: actual medicine practice in professional soccer teams. J Sports Sci Med. 2014;13(3): 721–3.
54. Croisier JL, Forthomme B, Namurois MH, Vanderthommen M, Crielaard JM. Hamstring muscle strain recurrence and strength performance disorders. Am J Sports Med. 2002;30(2):199–203.
55. Croisier JL, Ganteaume S, Binet J, Genty M, Ferret JM. Strength imbalances and prevention of hamstring injury in professional soccer players: a prospective study. Am J Sports Med. 2008;36(8):1469–75.
56. Brughelli M, Cronin J. Preventing hamstring injuries in sport. Strength Cond J. 2008;30(1):55–64.
57. Malliaropoulos N, Mendiguchia J, Pehlivanidis H, Papadopoulou S, Valle X, Malliaras P, et al. Hamstring exercises for track and field athletes: injury and exercise biomechanics, and possible implications for exercise selection and primary prevention. Br J Sports Med. 2012;46(12):846–51.
58. Lieberman DE, Raichlen DA, Pontzer H, Bramble DM, Cutright-Smith E. The human gluteus maximus and its role in running. J Exp Biol. 2006;209(Pt 11): 2143–55.
59. Bartlett JL, Sumner B, Ellis RG, Kram R. Activity and functions of the human gluteal muscles in walking, running, sprinting, and climbing. Am J Phys Anthropol. 2014;153(1):124–31.
60. Sugiura Y, Saito T, Sakuraba K, Sakuma K, Suzuki E. Strength deficits identified with concentric action of the hip extensors and eccentric action of the hamstrings predispose to hamstring injury in elite sprinters. J Orthop Sports Phys Ther. 2008;38(8):457–64.
61. Tyler TF, Nicholas SJ, Campbell RJ, McHugh MP. The association of hip strength and flexibility with the incidence of adductor muscle strains in professional ice hockey players. Am J Sports Med. 2001;29(2):124–8.
62. Engebretsen AH, Myklebust G, Holme I, Engebretsen L, Bahr R. Intrinsic risk factors for groin injuries among male soccer players: a prospective cohort study. Am J Sports Med. 2010;38(10):2051–7.
63. Tyler TF, Nicholas SJ, Campbell RJ, Donellan S, McHugh MP. The effectiveness of a preseason exercise program to prevent adductor muscle strains in professional ice hockey players. Am J Sports Med. 2002;30(5):680–3.
64. Thorborg K, Petersen J, Magnusson SP, Holmich P. Clinical assessment of hip strength using a handheld dynamometer is reliable. Scand J Med Sci Sports. 2010;20(3):493–501.
65. Morin JB, Edouard P, Samozino P. Technical ability of force application as a determinant factor of sprint performance. Med Sci Sports Exerc. 2011;43(9):1680–8.
66. Mendiguchia J, Samozino P, Martinez-Ruiz E, Brughelli M, Schmikli S, Morin JB, et al. Progression of mechanical properties during on-field sprint running after returning to sports from a hamstring muscle injury in soccer players. Int J Sports Med. 2014;35(8):690–5.
67. Blanch P, Gabbett TJ. Has the athlete trained enough to return to play safely? The acute: chronic workload ratio permits clinicians to quantify a player's risk of subsequent injury. Br J Sports Med. 2016;50(8):471–5.
68. Reurink G, Goudswaard GJ, Tol JL, Almusa E, Moen MH, Weir A, et al. MRI observations at return to play of clinically recovered hamstring injuries. Br J Sports Med. 2014;48(18):1370–6.
69. Sanfilippo JL, Silder A, Sherry MA, Tuite MJ, Heiderscheit BC. Hamstring strength and morphology progression after return to sport from injury. Med Sci Sports Exerc. 2013;45(3):448–54.
70. Wangensteen A, Almusa E, Boukarroum S, Farooq A, Hamilton B, Whiteley R, et al. MRI does not add value over and above patient history and clinical examination in predicting time to return to sport after acute hamstring injuries: a prospective cohort of 180 male athletes. Br J Sports Med. 2015;49(24):1579–87.
71. Reurink G, Brilman EG, de Vos RJ, Maas M, Moen MH, Weir A, et al. Magnetic resonance imaging in acute hamstring injury: can we provide a return to play prognosis? Sports Med. 2015;45(1):133–46.
72. Petersen J, Thorborg K, Nielsen MB, Skjodt T, Bolvig L, Bang N, et al. The diagnostic and prognostic value of ultrasonography in soccer players with acute hamstring injuries. Am J Sports Med. 2014;42(2): 399–404.
73. Crema MD, Yamada AF, Guermazi A, Roemer FW, Skaf AY. Imaging techniques for muscle injury in sports medicine and clinical relevance. Curr Rev Muscoskelet Med. 2015;8(2):154–61.
74. Ardern CL, Taylor NF, Feller JA, Webster KE. A systematic review of the psychological factors associated with returning to sport following injury. Br J Sports Med. 2013;47(17):1120–6.
75. Glazer DD. Development and preliminary validation of the injury-psychological readiness to return to sport (I-PRRS) scale. J Athl Train. 2009;44(2):185–9.

Part IX

Tendon Injuries in the Lower Limb

Epidemiology, Risk Factors and Prevention

38

Renato Andrade, Pedro Figueiredo, Parag Sancheti, Gino Kerkhoffs, and João Páscoa Pinheiro

Contents

38.1 Introduction

Injuries of the muscle-tendon complex are among the most common injuries sustained by football players.

Tendon injuries were ranked fifth after muscle injuries, joint injuries, contusions and low back pain in an analysis of 254 injuries of a top Italian football team [1]. In the 11-year follow-up of the UEFA Champions League Injury Study, the Achilles tendinopathy was the tenth most common injury, with a 0.2/1000 h injury rate and 4.2 injury burden (days absent/1000 h) [2].

Tendon injuries usually result from microtraumatic events and are more frequent in the tendons of powerful muscles. Taking into account the

R. Andrade (✉)
Faculdade de Desporto da Universidade do Porto, Porto, Portugal

Dom Henrique Research Centre, Porto, Portugal

Clínica do Dragão, Espregueira-Mendes Sports Centre – FIFA Medical Centre of Excellence, Porto, Portugal
e-mail: randrade@espregueira.com

P. Figueiredo
Centro Hospitalar e Universitário de Coimbra, Coimbra, Portugal

P. Sancheti
Sancheti Institute for Orthopaedics & Rehabilitation, Pune, India

G. Kerkhoffs
Department of Orthopedic Surgery, Academic Medical Center, University of Amsterdam, Amesterdam, Netherlands

Academic Center for Evidence based Sports medicine (ACES), Amesterdam, Netherlands

Amsterdam Collaboration for Health and Safety in Sports (ACHSS), AMC/VUmc IOC Research Center, Amesterdam, Netherlands

Team NL, NOC-NSF, Arnhem, Netherlands

J. Páscoa Pinheiro
Faculdade de Medicina, Universidade de Coimbra, Coimbra, Portugal

J. Espregueira-Mendes et al. (eds.), *Injuries and Health Problems in Football*,
DOI 10.1007/978-3-662-53924-8_38

lower limb, the most affected tendons in the lower limb are the adductor, proximal hamstrings, patellar and Achilles tendons. The repetitive submaximal abnormal loading leads to a disruption on repair chain by the tenocytes cells and results in collagen modification, fibre disorganisation and neovascularisation [3]. The initial clinical manifestations are delayed, and the tissue normalisation does not always immediately follow the symptomatic recovery. These facts predispose to an underdiagnosis and/or high recurrence rate (nearly 25% for patellar and Achilles tendon), due to early return to play in a professional environment [4].

In youth players, the skeletal maturity progression leads to different manifestations in the tendon-bone unit (osteochondrosis/tendinopathy). In this subgroup, a recent study indicated a relationship between injury occurrence and training time, match-play time and the chronologic age-skeletal age difference [5].

38.2 Epidemiology

38.2.1 Adductor Tendinopathy

The typical groin injury involves one or more muscle-tendinous structures in the groin region, usually including the adductors, the iliopsoas or the abdominals. Most epidemiological studies on groin injuries in the athletic population do not differentiate between anatomical structures. Therefore, the existing studies are difficult to compare, as injuries in the region are mainly reported as a groin injury/strain/tendinitis or likewise [6].

In male football, a prospective study of the elite teams in UEFA during seven seasons found a total of 628 hip/groin injuries, accounting for 12–16% of all injuries per season. The total injury incidence was 1.1/1000 h (3.5/1000 match hours and 0.6/1000 training hours). This means that a male professional football team will suffer an average of seven groin injuries per season, with more than half of them leading to at least 1 week injury time [7]. Groin injury appears to be more frequent among male footballers compared with their female counterparts regardless of the injury definition, study design, setting and playing level. In a recent review, the rates ranged from 0.2 to 2.1/1000 h in males and 0.1 to 0.6/1000 h in females, and the aggregated data indicated a 2.4 higher rate of groin injury in males. Possible reasons for this gender bias in groin injury rates might include both internal (e.g. differences in pelvic anatomy, muscle strength and force development, the occurrence of abdominal wall weakness/sportsman's hernia, etc.) and external factors (e.g. training and match load, playing intensity, etc.) [8].

38.2.2 Proximal Hamstrings Tendinopathy

The incidence of hamstring injuries among athletes varies based upon the definition used. The most common injury in football is thigh strain, typically affecting the hamstring muscle group. Thigh strain represents about 17% of all injuries, and a typical 25-player squad can expect ten thigh strains each season, with seven hamstring and three quadriceps strains [9].

Proximal hamstring tendon pathologic abnormalities are less common. These abnormalities are grouped clinically as "high hamstring tendinopathy", and patients usually present with subacute onset of deep buttock or thigh pain that is exacerbated by repetitive activity, such as long-distance running or football and often is aggravated by sitting [10–13].

Regarding the acute strain injuries, an observational study reported a single-season prevalence rate greater than 50% among elite football players. Recurrent hamstring injuries develop in more than 30% of athletes, which most occurred during the ensuing sporting season [14]. With regard to proximal hamstrings tendinopathy incidence, there is a lack of prospective epidemiology information in the current scientific literature. Currently, only a few studies are available [12, 13, 15].

38.2.3 Patellar Tendinopathy

About one-third of sports injuries that are treated at outpatient sports clinics involve the knee joint.

The most common knee disorders are Osgood-Schlatter disease and patellar tendinopathy. Martens et al. [16] found that football and volleyball were the sports in which two-thirds of all their patients with patellar tendinopathy were involved. The most common knee disorders were insertional tendinopathy at the lower pole of the patella (at the proximal end of the patellar tendon) or jumper's knee (20%), Osgood-Schlatter disease (10%) and patellar tendinopathy (6%) [17].

A recent study [18] in professional football players found that patellar tendon injuries represent 1.5% of all injuries, with an incidence of 0.12 injuries/1000 h and a season prevalence of 2.4%. Most injuries (60%) were minimal to mild (<8 days absence), and 19% were recurrent complaints. No difference in season prevalence or incidence was observed between teams playing on artificial turf and natural grass. High total exposure hours and increased body mass were significant risk factors for patellar tendon injury.

38.2.4 Achilles Tendinopathy

The most common clinical diagnosis of Achilles overuse injuries is tendinopathy of the main body of the tendon (55–65%), followed by insertional problems, such as retrocalcaneal bursitis and insertional tendinopathy (20–25%) [17].

The annual incidence of tendon ruptures in population is increasing with a peak incidence of 37 per 100.000 persons. A bimodal age distribution has been reported with the biggest incidence in the 30–39-year age group, mostly by sports-related reasons (73%) [19]. Achilles tendon ruptures have higher incidence in men, with a ratio 10:1 [9].

A recently published study of UEFA Champions League [20] showed that Achilles tendon disorders (tendinopathies and ruptures) accounted for 2.5% of all injuries and 3.8% of layoff times in male professional football players. A higher injury rate was found during the preseason compared with the competitive season, 0.25 vs. 0.18/1000 h. The mean layoff time for Achilles tendinopathies was 23 days, while a rupture of the Achilles tendon, on average, caused 161 days of absence. The mean age for Achilles tendon disorders was 27.2 ± 4 years, significantly older than the rest. Twenty-seven percent of all Achilles tendinopathies were reinjures. A higher reinjury risk was found after short recovery periods (31%) compared with longer recovery periods.

38.3 Risk Factors

Over the last few decades, due to the increasing demands on the intensity and frequency of training and matches in football, the tendon overuse injuries have emerged as an important clinical challenge to overcome. In this sense, the overuse injuries have been characterised by insidious onset without trauma, often due to an overextending of the musculoskeletal system tolerance through repetitive submaximal abnormal loading, resulting in injuries at the microscopic level [2, 21, 22].

More recently, the concept of "looking beyond the tendon" has been employed, providing a biomechanical approach to the intrinsic and extrinsic risk factors within the umbrella of tendinopathy [23]. In this sense, several clinical, biological and environmental features have been explored in the scientific literature as possible intrinsic (within the body) and extrinsic risk (outside the body) factors for sustaining a tendon injury. These can be further divided into modifiable or non-modifiable risk factors [24]. The intrinsic risk factors may predispose the football player to a specific injury, and the extrinsic risk factors will determine the susceptibility to sustain the injury (Fig. 38.1) [25–27]. Nonetheless, these risk factors will not directly cause an injury, but rather the occurrence of a specific inciting event (mechanism of injury) will determine the onset of the injury. In this sense, different categories of inciting events can be considered: playing situation, player and/or opponent behaviour, individual gross (whole body) and specific biomechanical characteristics [26, 27]. In which concerns the tendon injuries, these inciting events can happen suddenly (tendon ruptures), or occur due to a repetitive and systematic exposure to one or several risk factors, which is the case of the overuse injuries (tendinopathy).

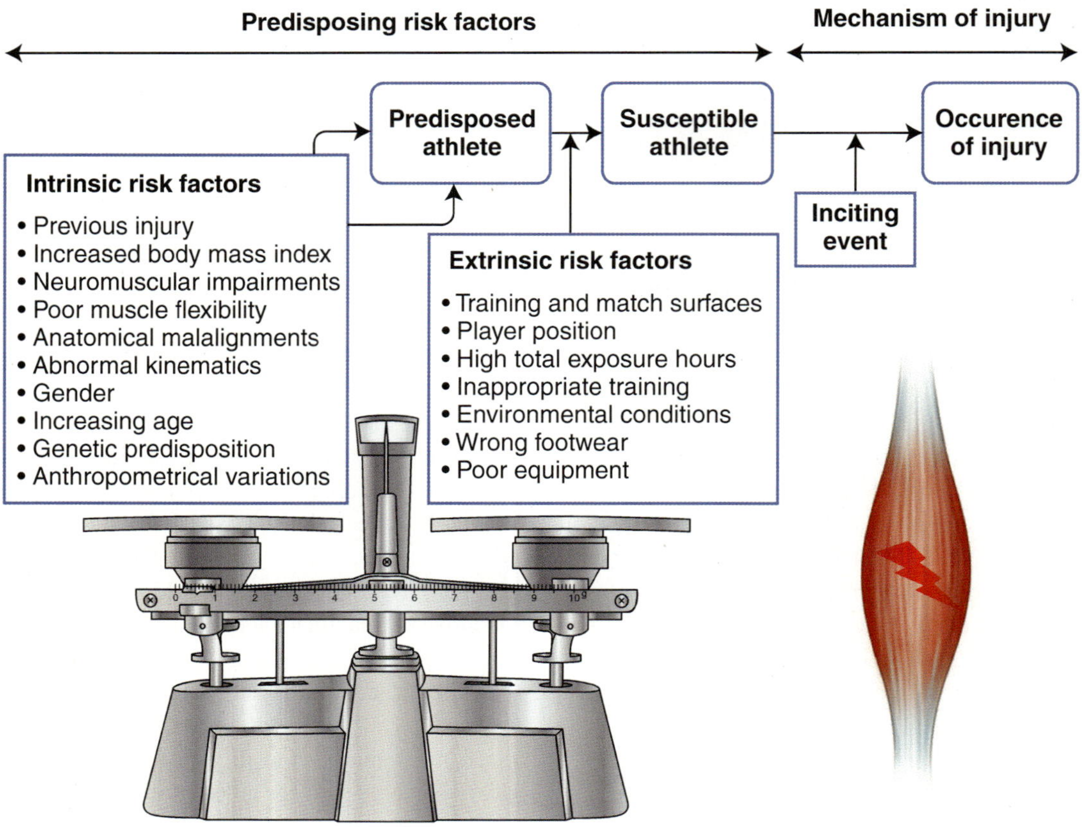

Fig. 38.1 Schematic injury causation model illustrating the relationship between the predisposing risk factors and the occurrence of injury (Adapted from Meeuwisse [28] and Bahr and Krosshaug [26])

Tendinopathy often leads to structural and functional dysfunction of the tendon, reflecting into pain over the tendon and subsequent altered biomechanics [29]. These movement dysfunctions, if not properly corrected, can further lead to the chronicity of the symptomatology [23]. Moreover, each individual athlete may display a unique cluster of risk factors, depending on the site and nature of the injury process [23, 29]. Nevertheless, it may also occur without any presence of overuse symptomatology whatsoever [30]. Thus, recognising and understanding the pathomechanics and clinical implications of these risk factors may further assist the clinicians in planning and implementing risk factor modifying prevention and treatment strategies.

38.3.1 Intrinsic Factors

The intrinsic risk factors are directly related to the individual characteristics; thus, its modifiability is often not possible. Nevertheless, knowledge regarding both modifiable and non-modifiable intrinsic risk factors may be used to target intervention measures in those at risk of sustaining a tendon injury. In this sense, several modifiable and non-modifiable intrinsic risk factors can be associated with the tendon injury.

38.3.1.1 Modifiable Intrinsic Risk Factors

The modifiable intrinsic risk factors are often related with biomechanical and structural deficits, which can be addressed in order to reduce the predisposition to the specific injury. Thus, many modifiable intrinsic risk factors can be taken into account: muscle imbalances or insufficiency [21, 23, 31–34], poor muscle flexibility [23, 34, 35], anatomical malalignments [21, 23], abnormal kinematics [22, 23, 32, 36–41], medication intake [42] and adiposity/elevated body mass index [23, 34, 43–45].

38.3.1.2 Non-modifiable Intrinsic Risk Factors

The most important non-modifiable intrinsic risk factor is the occurrence of previous tendon injury at the specific tendon. In addition, other non-modifiable intrinsic risk factors can be pointed out: gender [42, 44, 46–49], increasing age [23, 50–52], blood type O [53, 54], individual genetic predisposition [55–58], anthropometrical variations [31, 34, 44] and hypertension [42].

38.3.2 Extrinsic Risk Factors

Although some extrinsic risk factors can be modifiable, these depend upon external factors, which some of them can be due to random occasions (per example, environmental conditions of the training or match). Hence, the extrinsic risk factors related to tendon injury include training and match surfaces (turf or artificial turf) [21, 23, 59, 60], player position, high total exposure hours [31, 43, 61, 62], inappropriate training (volume, magnitude, speed of loading, frequency, inclination, fatigue, wrong sportive gesture, abrupt or acute modifications in amount or type of load) [21, 59], environmental conditions (in colder temperatures, the tendons become stiffer and with decreased blood supply) [21, 23, 63, 64] and wrong footwear and poor equipment available [21, 23]. In addition, excessive dietary intake of cholesterol has been pointed out as an extrinsic risk factor once it will result in accumulation of oxidised low density lipoprotein within the load-bearing areas of tendon, impairing the production of type I collagen and thus reducing the tendon energy storage capacity and strength [23].

38.3.3 Specific Risk Factors

38.3.3.1 Adductor Tendinopathy

During maximal effort football kick, the adductor longus seems to be at greater risk of injury in the swing phase, where eccentric active forces and stretching forces occur simultaneously [65–67]. Hence, by decreasing the demand on the adductor longus, it can reduce the risk of injury during cutting or other lateral change-of-direction manoeuvers [68]. Other factors seem to put the adductor tendon at risk of injury:

- Muscle imbalances at the symphysis pubis and surrounding pubic bone (specially between the adductors and rectus femoris) [69, 70]
- Decreased hip range of motion [69] or specially decreased hip extension range of motion [67]
- Reduced flexibility of the posterior chain muscles and/or iliopsoas muscle [71]
- Previous rectus abdominis tendinopathy [72]
- Lumbar hyperlordosis [71]
- Temporomandibular joint dysfunction and malocclusion [71]
- Altered lower limb kinematics (defects of plantar support) and sports particularities (sudden changes of direction, continuous acceleration and deceleration, sliding tackles and kicking) [71]
- Anthropometrical variations (marked asymmetry of lower limbs) [71] or female lower limb morphology and morphometric, such as the pelvis geometry and the knee valgus
- Incorrect training and equipment (unsuitable footwear, environmental weather, training and match surfaces and inappropriate training volume/loading) [71]

38.3.3.2 Proximal Hamstrings Tendinopathy

The scientific literature has few reports regarding the proximal hamstrings tendon pathology, also known as “high hamstring tendinopathy”, “hamstring syndrome”, “ischiatic intersection syndrome”, “hamstring enthesopathy” and “hamstring origin tendinopathy” [73–76]. It is often overlooked as a cause of chronic gluteal pain and includes tendon degeneration, partial tearing and peritendinous inflammatory reaction [15, 76]. Usually, these conditions present subacute onset of deep buttock and/or thigh pain, particularly at the ischial tuberosity, which can be exacerbated by repetitive activity and often is aggravated by sitting [10–13]. Little information is available about the risk factors for hamstrings proximal tendinopathy. In this sense, different possible risk factors can be pointed out:

- Muscle imbalances
- Eccentric hamstrings overload [15]
- Poor muscle flexibility
- Core weakness [76]
- Lumbopelvic dysfunction [76]
- Inadequate warm-up
- Previous hamstrings injury

38.3.3.3 Patellar Tendinopathy

Patellar tendinopathy seems to be consequent of a combination of different risk factors [22, 43]. Furthermore, it has been suggested that unilateral and bilateral patellar tendinopathies have a unique aetiology [31]. In this sense, the scientific literature has been suggesting different risk factors that may predispose the development of patellar tendinopathy:

- Male gender [44]
- High total exposure hours [61, 62]
- Altered lower limb kinematics (such as, high ankle inversion-eversion moments, high external tibial rotation and plantar flexion moments, large vertical ground reaction forces, deeper knee flexion angle and high rate of knee extensor moment development) and reduced muscle activity [37–39]
- Muscle imbalances (reduced eccentric strength) [31, 34]
- Poor muscle flexibility (quadriceps and hamstrings muscles) [34, 35]
- Anthropometrical variations (tibia length to stature ratio, waist to hip ratio, trunk lean to total lean) [31, 34]
- Elevated body mass index [77]

38.3.3.4 Achilles Tendinopathy

Achilles tendinopathy often occurs in athletes who systematically perform running and jumping as sportive actions, including the football [78]. Nevertheless, it specific cause still remains unclear [79]. Some authors have suggested a failed healing response as a major cause for the aetiology of Achilles tendinopathy [80, 81]. In this sense, many risk factors have been suggested to predispose to Achilles tendinopathy:

- Male gender [46–48]
- Increasing age [47, 50, 82]
- Individual genetic predisposition [56, 57]
- Medication intake (local or systemic steroid exposure or oestrogen supplementation) [42]
- Hypertension [42]
- Elevated body mass index [42, 77, 83]
- Foot posture (pes cavus valgus or pes planus varum) [82]
- Altered ankle kinematics (increase in eversion displacement of the subtalar joint) [40]
- Muscle imbalances or insufficiency [33, 84]
- Decreased environmental temperature may increase the viscosity of the lubricant, increasing the friction and risk of Achilles paratendinitis [63, 64]
- Sudden changes in the intensity of the training load, such as period of rest following the preseason, have been suggested due to the inability of the Achilles tendon to adapt fast enough to these changes [20, 85, 86]

38.4 Prevention

The cornerstone of every prevention program is to accurately identify the predisposing risk factors and modify them and, also prepare the players for the physical demands of their athletic competition. Hence, the sports medicine professionals should first establish the extent of the injury/deficit (incidence, severity, predisposing risk factors) and determine the cause and mechanism of the injury and then implement the preventive strategy and assess its effectiveness in a systematic fashion [26].

38.4.1 Modification of Risk Factors

It has been shown that athletes with tendinopathies related to an overused repetitive sportive gesture, such as jumping in the case of patellar tendinopathy, have also higher performance levels in this specific tasks (e.g. athletes with patellar tendinopathy often show better jumping performance than athletes without patellar tendinopathy) [45, 87]. Nevertheless, these motor control deficits should be properly approached because athletes with tendinopathy at a specific site have potentially increased risk of developing tendinopathy at other locations [88]. Furthermore, it has been shown that tendinopathy-associated motor and sensory (greater cortical inhibition [89]) impairments are often present bilaterally, even when the tendinopathy is presented unilaterally [90]. In addition, once most of lower limb activities are performed bilaterally and symmetrically, the uninjured side may be striving in order to protect the potential vulnerable tendon and stand the loads imposed by the athlete in demand for optional performance [88]. In this sense, the importance of the core and trunk muscles should not be overlooked, since these muscle play an important role in achieving the proper biomechanics and motor control and, therefore, should be included in the prevention program [91]. All these abovementioned considerations highlight the multifactorial nature of tendinopathy and stress the importance of correctly addressing and controlling the predisposing risk factors.

To design a particular prevention protocol, the clinician should take into account the location of the injured tendon as also the associated deficits. In this sense, addressing the associated strength kinematic abnormalities may play a crucial role in increasing the movement variability, reduce the risk of overuse tendon injury and, in addition, even improve the sports-specific gesture. Along this line, athletes with patellar tendinopathy often show altered landing patterns [92] as consequence of the protective strategies employed to avoid pain [88]. By increasing the movement variability in these athletes will fine-tune the load patterns and decrease the imposed load accumulation in the specific region of the tendon and consequently prevent the potential development of an overuse injury [92–94].

Another essential concept that needs to be properly understood and incorporated into the prevention planning rationale is the tendon biology. It is known that after maturation, tendons undergo biochemical, cellular, mechanical and pathological changes, leading to structural and functional deficits, diminished capacity to readapt to the environmental stress and loss of tissue homeostasis [52]. Moreover, the different tendons have also dissimilar biological characteristics, reflecting into different histopathological, pathomechanical and pathophysiological responses [23, 81, 95, 96]. In addition, within the tendinopathy umbrella, several terminologies can be used (tendinosis, tenosynovitis, paratenonitis), and, therefore, knowledge of these different terminologies is important to better address the preventive programs [23]. Along these lines, neuroplastic training has been proposed as a potential approach for the optimisation of the motor control and sensory neuroplasticity in athletes with tendinopathy [88].

Taking into account all the considerations exposed above, the clinician should be capable to plan a prevention program which includes all these features. Addressing predominantly the motor control and strength deficits, as well as several external factors (in particular, footwear and dietary modification), may determine the success of the preventive program. In this sense, these preventive features should be adapted and directed to the specific tendinopathy to further enhance its effectiveness. A suggested approach to the modifiable risk factors of the different lower limb tendinopathies (adductor, hamstrings, patellar or Achilles) is presented in Table 38.1.

38.4.2 Training System Particularities

Tendinopathy is caused by multiple factors and therefore should be address by a multidisciplinary team. In this sense, the medical team should work together to prevent and/or modify the different

Table 38.1 Potential control or interventional approaches for modifiable risk factors

Specific tendinopathy	Modifiable risk factor	Potential control or interventional approaches
Adductor tendinopathy	Altered lower limb kinematics [71]	N-M exercises targeted to correct kinematic deficits, particularly the plantar support and knee adduction/abduction moments
	Muscle imbalances [69, 70]	Muscular strengthening exercises targeting to correct muscle imbalances
	Decreased hip ROM [67, 69] and reduced flexibility of the posterior chain muscles and/or iliopsoas muscle [52]	Stretching exercises of the hip targeting the increase of range of movement
	Previous rectus abdominalis tendinopathy [72]	Rectus abdominalis strengthening exercises
Proximal hamstrings tendinopathy	Muscle imbalances	Muscular strengthening exercises targeting to correct muscle imbalances
	Eccentric hamstrings overload [15]	N-M exercises targeting the improvement of motor control and hamstrings correct contraction awareness
	Poor muscle flexibility	Stretching exercises of hamstrings targeting the increase muscle elasticity
	Core weakness [76] and lumbopelvic dysfunction [76]	Core static and functional exercises
	Previous hamstrings injury	Secondary prevention of hamstrings muscles through eccentric exercises and stretching of the thigh muscles
Patellar tendinopathy	Altered lower limb kinematics [37–39]	N-M exercises targeted to correct lower limb kinematic deficits and footwear modification
	Muscle imbalances [31, 34]	Muscular isotonic strengthening exercises targeting the hamstrings/quadriceps unilateral ratio normalisation and bilateral asymmetry (supervised by isokinetic evaluations)
	Poor muscle flexibility [34, 35]	Stretching exercises of quadriceps targeting the increase muscle elasticity
	Elevated body mass index [77]	Motorised physical exercise targeting weight loss and dietary counselling
Achilles tendinopathy	Altered ankle kinematics [40]	N-M exercises targeting ankle and foot posture correction, footwear modification and, eventually, sports taping limiting eversion of the foot
	Muscle imbalances or insufficiency [33, 84]	Muscular eccentric strengthening exercises targeting the plantar flexor muscles
	Elevated body mass index and hypertension [42, 77, 83]	Motorised physical exercise targeting weight loss and dietary counselling (lipid profile)

Legend: *N-M* neuromuscular, *ROM* range of movement

potential predisposing risk factors. Thus, the medical team should include all the sports medicine professionals that may play a role in the different aspects within the sports injury scope: sports medicine physician, physiotherapist, strength and conditioning trainer, radiologist, psychologist and nutritionist, among others.

In addition to the multidisciplinary approach, the prevention program should be customised to the specific tendinopathy and to the football player himself in order to address the different particularities inherent to each individual. Along this line, it is of upmost importance to adapt the prevention program in accordance to the player's current fitness status, level of competition and positional role in order to enhance the adherence and effectiveness of the program. Moreover, since female football has been fast growing worldwide (nearly 10% of total number of footballers), it is crucial to also know the specificities of the female player, such as hormonal particularities, sexual maturation and anthropometry [97]. In addition, it has been shown that female footballers have different football-specific biomechanical and skills

Table 38.2 Training tips and pearls

Tips and pearls
Avoid sudden changes in the training (intensity, frequency and type)
Caution upon in the choice/change of football boots (if needed ask for help)
Keep a healthy diet and control your body composition
Make sure there is no biomechanical and strength deficits
Remember that motor control deficits may persist after injury recovery
Adequate the training loads
Keep in mind that well-developed physical qualities may be part of the best prevention strategies
Identify the origin of the problem and try to fix it
Implement individualised and progression-based preventive programs

performance [98–102], highlighting the need to adapt the training loads and intensities to their physical demands and capacities [97].

A progression-based prevention program can help the players, once they start with easier exercises and progress to more complex ones as they improve the physical capabilities and skills. Training tips and pearls are described in Table 38.2.

Another important training particularities are the method of strengthening and the loads applied. In this sense, performing muscular assessment allows to tailor the prevention program to fit the needs of each individual athlete. At earlier stages more isometric exercises should be performed in order to initiate the muscle-tendon unit loading, and, as the program progresses, more isotonic exercises can be performed in order to increase the tolerance to higher loads, especially during eccentric exercises. Attention should be paid to excessive loads once these often lead to maladaptations within the tendon structure causing pain [103]. As the strength performance is balanced, high velocity exercises (such as jumping and landing, acceleration, deceleration and cutting/change-of-direction activities) may be incorporated to program aiming to replicate the high demands of football. In addition, exercises targeting motor control and football-specific skills should be implemented into the prevention program.

38.4.3 Clinical Follow-Up

The tendinopathy in the athlete is usually characterised by pain and impaired performance [104]. Nevertheless, when the symptomatology appears, the inflammation already may be present for a long time, as result of the repetitive loading placed in the tendon [105]. In addition, these injuries often result in prolonged periods of rehabilitation, leading to a delayed return to play [106]. Moreover, biomechanical and strength deficits may persist even after the player return to the competition [88]. Thus, continuous assessment follow-up plays a crucial role in keeping the player healthy and injury-free, ensuring his safe and best performance.

The history of previous injury is the most important predisposing risk factor [107, 108]. Hence, a complete and comprehensive anamnesis should be performed prior to the planning of the preventive program.

Movement analysis is a critical part of the clinical examination follow-up once it can detect motor control deficits that may be predisposing the athlete to tendinopathy. Thus, the athlete's quality of movement should be followed during his career in order to detect and correct eventual biomechanical deficits and enhance his performance. In this sense, the most important exercises to be evaluated during the movement analysis are the acceleration mechanics, cutting and pivoting exercises due to its frequency during the football game. In addition, landing mechanics may also be explored in order to investigate further deficits [109].

Functional testing may also play an important role in the identification of biomechanical deficits. In this sense, significant differences in hopping kinematics in athletes have been found [41, 110–112]. A set of hopping and agility functional tests can be performed in order to assess eventual biomechanical deficits: single-leg vertical hop test, single-leg hop test, triple hop test, crossover hop test, square hop test, side hop test, single-leg squat test, retro step-up test, 6-m timed hop test, agility T-test, slalom test and star excursion balance test, among others. A limb symmetry index of 85–90% has been recommended throughout the scientific literature for other conditions, which may also be applied to tendinopathies [113–116].

Continuous assessment of potential muscular and flexibility deficits may help clinicians to identify potential predisposing factors. Concerning the muscular deficits, these can be assessed through an isokinetic evaluation, and the unilateral (agonist/antagonist) and bilateral (injured/uninjured) muscular balance can be assessed and accordingly corrected [117]. In which concerns the flexibility deficits, it has also been shown that specific range of motion limitations can lead to particular tendinopathies, such as Achilles and patellar tendinopathies [118, 119].

38.4.4 Prevention Protocols

There is limited prospective evidence in which concerns the implementation of preventive protocols in football cohorts with tendinopathy. The most common approaches are eccentric strengthening and stretching exercises, core stability and football-specific proprioceptive training, preventive education and shoewear modification [120]. Nevertheless, the prevention programs should always be directed to the individual deficits of the football player and the identified predisposing risk factors and also prepare the football player's muscles and tendons to withstand the football-specific demands. In this sense, we suggest a couple of exercises that can be applied to prevent adductor (Fig. 38.2), proximal hamstrings (Fig. 38.3), patellar (Fig. 38.4) and Achilles tendinopathies (Fig. 38.5).

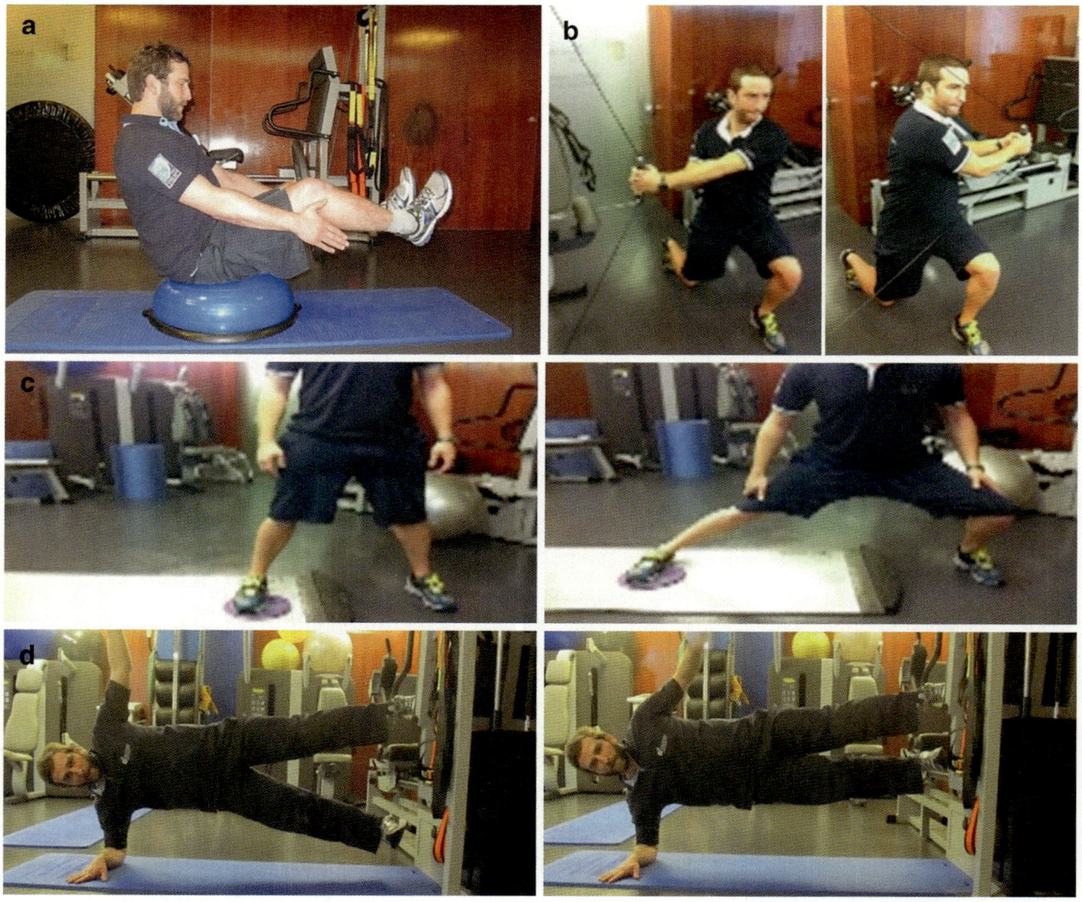

Fig. 38.2 Set of preventive exercises for adductors tendinopathy. (**a**) Core strengthening with lumbopelvic stabilisation – perform a bosu crunch, isometrically contracting your adductors with a pilates circle between your knees. (**b**) Oblique core functional exercises – perform diagonal functional movement (upper limbs) while maintaining your core isometrically contracted. (**c**) Lateral eccentric glide – lunge eccentrically sideways by sliding the foot in the gliding mat. (**d**) Copenhagen adduction – the downward leg is adducted until the feet touch each other and the body is in a straight line

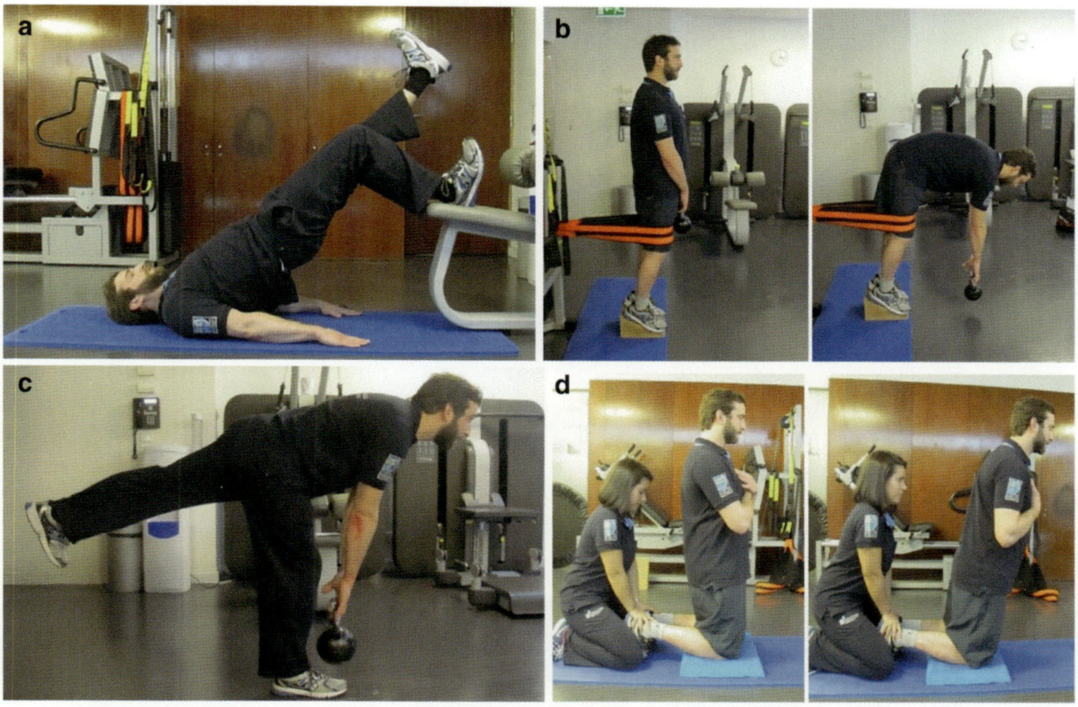

Fig. 38.3 Set of preventive exercises for proximal hamstrings tendinopathy. (**a**) Eccentric hamstrings bench exercise – while locking your calcaneus on a bench, raise your pelvis from the ground and slowly get back down eccentrically. (**b**) Eccentric hamstring exercise with Russian belt – lean slowly forward while holding a kettlebell with your lower limbs locked by a Russian belt. (**c**) Hamstrings diver – lean slowly forward holding a kettlebell while the static leg is performing the eccentric slowing down of the upper limb. (**d**) Nordic hamstrings exercise – lean slowly forward trying to maintain your hamstrings eccentrically holding your body as long as possible

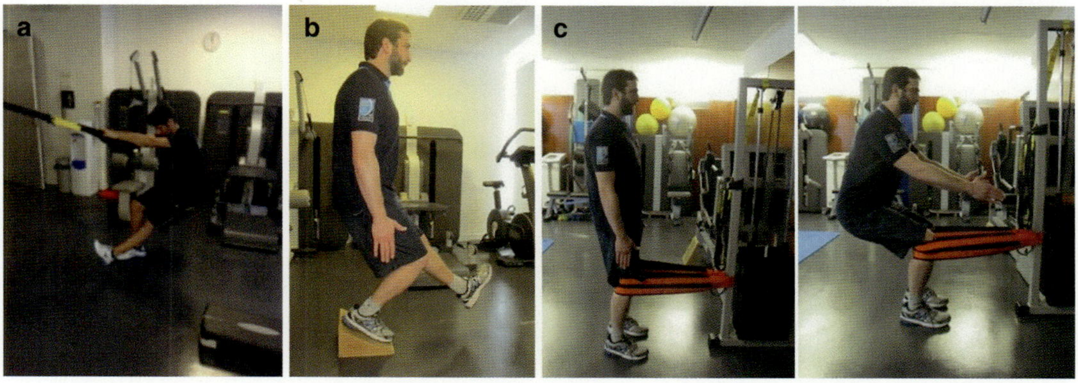

Fig. 38.4 Set of preventive exercises for patellar tendinopathy. (**a**) Eccentric lunges – perform eccentric unilateral lunges with your support leg extended with the help of TRX®. (**b**) Single-leg decline squat – perform a single-leg squat on top a 25° declined surface. (**c**) Eccentric squats – perform eccentric squats with the help of a Russian belt. (**d**) Instable bosu lunges – perform lunges on top of the bosu and unstable surfaces

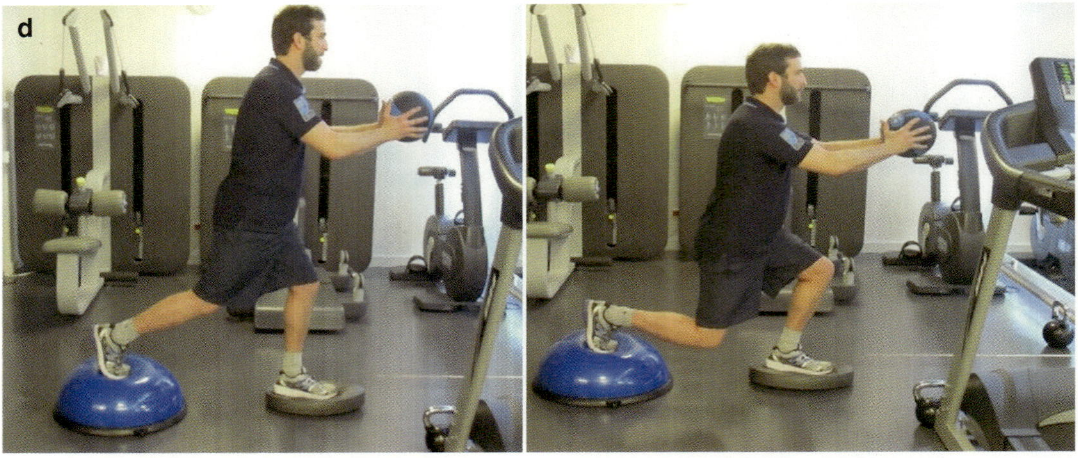

Fig. 38.4 (continued)

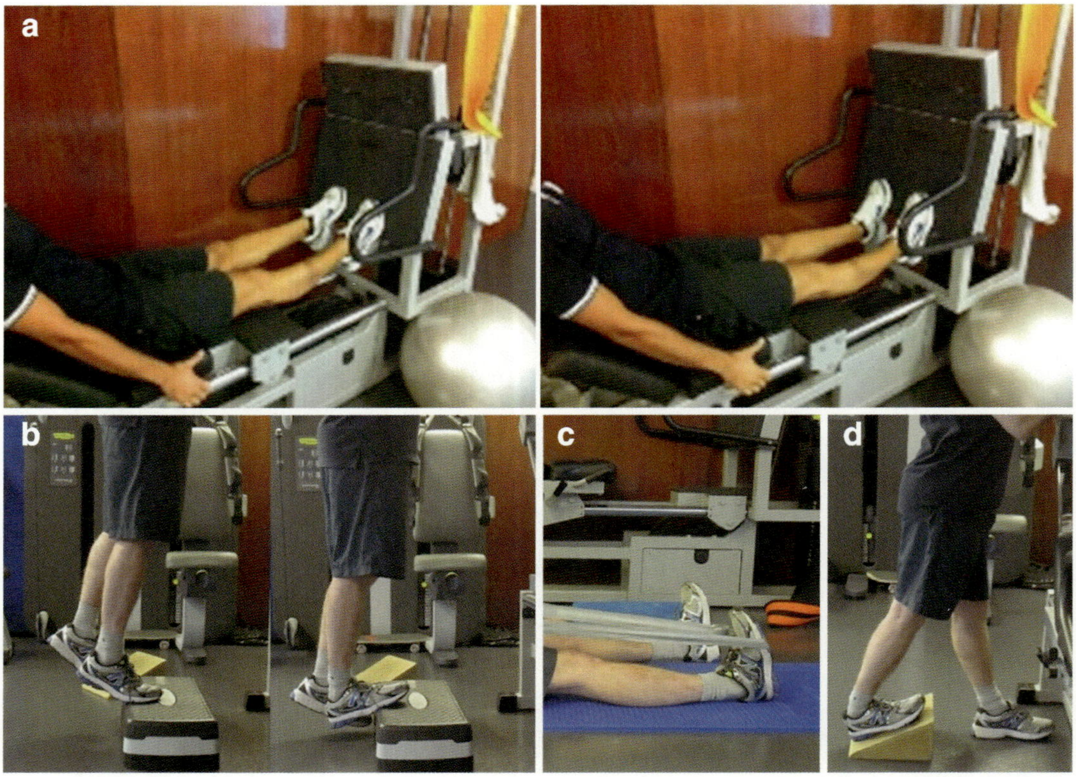

Fig. 38.5 Set of preventive exercises for Achilles tendinopathy. (**a** and **b**) Eccentric plantar flexors exercise – perform eccentric contraction of plantar flexors muscles with a leg press machine or with a step platform. (**c** and **d**) Plantar flexors stretching – stretch the plantar flexors muscles with an elastic band or with declined surface

References

1. Tavana R. Epidemiology of the muscular injuries in Italian soccer. The rehabilitation of sports and muscles and tendon injuries. Proceedings of XIII International Congress on Sports Rehabilitation and Traumatology; 2004, Milano.
2. Ekstrand J, Hägglund M, Kristenson K, Magnusson H, Waldén M. Fewer ligament injuries but no preventive effect on muscle injuries and severe injuries: an 11-year follow-up of the UEFA Champions league injury study. Br J Sports Med. 2013;47:732–7.
3. Maffulli N, King J, Helms P. Training in elite young athletes (the training of young athletes (TOYA) study): injuries, flexibility and isometric strength. Br J Sports Med. 1994;28:123–36.
4. Eirale C. Epidemiology in professional footballers. In: Volpi P, editor. Football traumatology: new trends. Cham: Springer; 2015. p. 3–9.
5. Malina RM. Maturity status and injury risk in youth soccer players. Clin J Sport Med. 2010;20:132.
6. Hölmich P, Thorborg K. Epidemiology of groin injuries in athletes. In: Diduch D, Brunt L, editors. Sports hernia and athletic pubalgia. New York: Springer; 2014. p. 13–21.
7. Werner J, Hägglund M, Waldén M, Ekstrand J. UEFA injury study: a prospective study of hip and groin injuries in professional football over seven consecutive seasons. Br J Sports Med. 2009;43:1036–40.
8. Waldén M, Hägglund M, Ekstrand J. The epidemiology of groin injury in senior football: a systematic review of prospective studies. Br J Sports Med. 2015. doi:10.1136/bjsports-2015-094705.
9. Ekstrand J, Hägglund M, Waldén M. Epidemiology of muscle injuries in professional football (soccer). Am J Sports Med. 2011;39:1226–32.
10. Zissen MH, Wallace G, Stevens KJ, Fredericson M, Beaulieu CF. High hamstring tendinopathy: MRI and ultrasound imaging and therapeutic efficacy of percutaneous corticosteroid injection. AJR Am J Roentgenol. 2010;195:993–8.
11. Young IJ, van Riet RP, Bell SN. Surgical release for proximal hamstring syndrome. Am J Sports Med. 2008;36:2372–8.
12. Lempainen L, Sarimo J, Mattila K, Vaittinen S, Orava S. Proximal hamstring tendinopathy results of surgical management and histopathologic findings. Am J Sports Med. 2009;37:727–34.
13. Cacchio A, Rompe JD, Furia JP, Susi P, Santilli V, De Paulis F. Shockwave therapy for the treatment of chronic proximal hamstring tendinopathy in professional athletes. Am J Sports Med. 2011;39:146–53.
14. Askling C, Karlsson J, Thorstensson A. Hamstring injury occurrence in elite soccer players after preseason strength training with eccentric overload. Scand J Med Sci Sports. 2003;13:244–50.
15. White KE. High hamstring tendinopathy in 3 female long distance runners. J Chiropr Med. 2011; 10:93–9.
16. Martens M, Wouters P, Burssens A, Mulier J. Patellar tendinitis: pathology and results of treatment. Acta Orthop Scand. 1982;53:445–50.
17. Paavola M, Kannus P, Järvinen M. Epidemiology of tendon problems in sport. In: Maffulli N, Renström P, Leadbetter W, editors. Tendon injuries: Springer; 2005. p. 32–9. http://link.springer.com/book/10.1007%2Fb137778
18. Hägglund M, Waldén M, Zwerver J, Ekstrand J. Epidemiology of patellar tendon injury in elite male soccer players. Br J Sports Med. 2011;45: 324.
19. Houshian S, Tscherning T, Riegels-Nielsen P. The epidemiology of Achilles tendon rupture in a Danish county. Injury. 1998;29:651–4.
20. Gajhede-Knudsen M, Ekstrand J, Magnusson H, Maffulli N. Recurrence of Achilles tendon injuries in elite male football players is more common after early return to play: an 11-year follow-up of the UEFA Champions League injury study. Br J Sports Med. 2013;47. doi:10.1136/bjsports-2013-092271.
21. Maffulli N, Wong J, Almekinders LC. Types and epidemiology of tendinopathy. Clin Sports Med. 2003;22:675–92.
22. Kannus P. Etiology and pathophysiology of chronic tendon disorders in sports. Scand J Med Sci Sports. 1997;7:78–85.
23. Scott A, Backman LJ, Speed C. Tendinopathy: update on pathophysiology. J Orthop Sports Phys Ther. 2015;45:833–41.
24. Reinking M. Tendinopathy in athletes. Phys Ther Sport. 2012;13:3–10.
25. Collins M, Raleigh SM. Genetic risk factors for musculoskeletal soft tissue injuries. In: Collins M, editor. Genetics and sports. Basel: Karger Publishers; 2009. p. 136–49.
26. Bahr R, Krosshaug T. Understanding injury mechanisms: a key component of preventing injuries in sport. Br J Sports Med. 2005;39:324–9.
27. Bahr R, Holme I. Risk factors for sports injuries – a methodological approach. Br J Sports Med. 2003;37:384–92.
28. Meeuwisse WH. Assessing causation in sport injury: a multifactorial model. Clin J Sport Med. 1994;4:166–70.
29. Macdermid JC, Silbernagel KG. Outcome evaluation in tendinopathy: foundations of assessment and a summary of selected measures. J Orthop Sports Phys Ther. 2015;45:1–34.
30. Ackermann PW, Renström P. Tendinopathy in sport. Sports Health. 2012;4:193–201.
31. Gaida J, Cook J, Bass S, Austen S, Kiss Z. Are unilateral and bilateral patellar tendinopathy distinguished by differences in anthropometry, body composition, or muscle strength in elite female basketball players? Br J Sports Med. 2004;38:581–5.
32. Grau S, Maiwald C, Krauss I, Axmann D, Janssen P, Horstmann T. What are causes and treatment strategies for patellar-tendinopathy in female runners? J Biomech. 2008;41:2042–6.

33. O'Neill S, Watson P, Barry S. 75 Plantarflexor muscle power deficits in runners with Achilles tendinopathy. Br J Sports Med. 2014;48:A49–A.
34. van der Worp H, van Ark M, Roerink S, Pepping G-J, van den Akker-Scheek I, Zwerver J. Risk factors for patellar tendinopathy: a systematic review of the literature. Br J Sports Med. 2011;45:446–452.
35. Witvrouw E, Bellemans J, Lysens R, Danneels L, Cambier D. Intrinsic risk factors for the development of patellar tendinitis in an athletic population a two-year prospective study. Am J Sports Med. 2001;29:190–5.
36. Abate M, Gravare-Silbernagel K, Siljeholm C, Di Iorio A, De Amicis D, Salini V, Werner S, Paganelli R. Pathogenesis of tendinopathies: inflammation or degeneration? Arthritis Res Ther. 2009;11:235.
37. Azevedo LB, Lambert MI, Vaughan CL, O'Connor CM, Schwellnus MP. Biomechanical variables associated with Achilles tendinopathy in runners. Br J Sports Med. 2009;43:288–92.
38. Richards DP, Ajemian SV, Wiley JP, Brunet JA, Zernicke RF. Relation between ankle joint dynamics and patellar tendinopathy in elite volleyball players. Clin J Sport Med. 2002;12:266–72.
39. Richards DP, Ajemian SV, Wiley JP, Zernicke RF. Knee joint dynamics predict patellar tendinitis in elite volleyball players. Am J Sports Med. 1996;24:676–83.
40. Ryan M, Grau S, Krauss I, Maiwald C, Taunton J, Horstmann T. Kinematic analysis of runners with Achilles mid-portion tendinopathy. Foot Ankle Int. 2009;30:1190–5.
41. Souza RB, Arya S, Pollard CD, Salem G, Kulig K. Patellar tendinopathy alters the distribution of lower extremity net joint moments during hopping. J Appl Biomech. 2010;26:249–55.
42. Holmes GB, Lin J. Etiologic factors associated with symptomatic achilles tendinopathy. Foot Ankle Int. 2006;27:952–9.
43. Crossley KM, Thancanamootoo K, Metcalf BR, Cook JL, Purdam CR, Warden SJ. Clinical features of patellar tendinopathy and their implications for rehabilitation. J Orthop Res. 2007;25:1164–75.
44. Lian ØB, Engebretsen L, Bahr R. Prevalence of jumper's knee among elite athletes from different sports a cross-sectional study. Am J Sports Med. 2005;33:561–7.
45. Lian Ø, Refsnes P-E, Engebretsen L, Bahr R. Performance characteristics of volleyball players with patellar tendinopathy. Am J Sports Med. 2003;31:408–13.
46. Åström M. Partial rupture in chronic Achilles tendinopathy: a retrospective analysis of 342 cases. Acta Orthop. 1998;69:404–7.
47. Åström M, Rausing A. Chronic Achilles tendinopathy: a survey of surgical and histopathologic findings mats. Clin Orthop Relat Res. 1995;316:151–64.
48. Knobloch K, Schreibmueller L, Meller R, Busch KH, Spies M, Vogt PM. Superior Achilles tendon microcirculation in tendinopathy among symptomatic female versus male patients. Am J Sports Med. 2008;36:509–14.
49. Ramos LA, Carvalho RT, Garms E, Navarro MS, Abdalla RJ, Cohen M. Prevalence of pain on palpation of the inferior pole of the patella among patients with complaints of knee pain. Clinics. 2009;64:199–202.
50. Birch H, Smith T, Tasker T, Goodship A. Age related changes to mechanical and matrix properties in human Achilles tendon. Transactions of the 47th annual meeting of the Orthpaedic research society, San Francisco, CA; 2001;713.
51. Sargon MF, Ozlu K, Oken F. Age-related changes in human tendo calcaneus collagen fibrils. Saudi Med J. 2005;26:425–8.
52. Tuite D, Renström P, O'brien M. The aging tendon. Scand J Med Sci Sports. 1997;7:72–7.
53. Jozsa L, Balint J, Kannus P, Reffy A, Barzo M. Distribution of blood groups in patients with tendon rupture. An analysis of 832 cases. J Bone Joint Surg Br. 1989;71:272–4.
54. Kujala U, Järvinen M, Natri A, Lehto M, Nelimarkka O, Hurme M, Virta L, Finne J. ABO blood groups and musculoskeletal injuries. Injury. 1992;23:131–3.
55. Magra M, Maffulli N. Genetics: does it play a role in tendinopathy? Clin J Sport Med. 2007;17:231–3.
56. Mokone GG, Gajjar M, September AV, Schwellnus MP, Greenberg J, Noakes TD, Collins M. The guanine-thymine dinucleotide repeat polymorphism within the tenascin-C gene is associated with Achilles tendon injuries. Am J Sports Med. 2005;33:1016–21.
57. Mokone G, Schwellnus M, Noakes T, Collins M. The COL5A1 gene and Achilles tendon pathology. Scand J Med Sci Sports. 2006;16:19–26.
58. Ribbans W, Collins M. Pathology of the tendo Achillis: do our genes contribute? Bone Joint J. 2013;95:305–13.
59. Ferretti A. Epidemiology of jumper's knee. Sports Med. 1986;3:289–95.
60. Sousa P, Rebelo A, Brito J. Injuries in amateur soccer players on artificial turf: a one-season prospective study. Phys Ther Sport. 2013;14:146–51.
61. Hägglund M, Zwerver J, Ekstrand J. Epidemiology of patellar tendinopathy in elite male soccer players. Am J Sports Med. 2011;39:1906–11.
62. Visnes H, Bahr R. Training volume and body composition as risk factors for developing jumper's knee among young elite volleyball players. Scand J Med Sci Sports. 2013;23:607–13.
63. Milgrom C, Finestone A, Zin D, Mandel D, Novack V. Cold weather training: a risk factor for Achilles paratendinitis among recruits. Foot Ankle Int. 2003;24:398–401.
64. Orchard JW, Waldén M, Hägglund M, Orchard JJ, Chivers I, Seward H, Ekstrand J. Comparison of injury incidences between football teams playing in different climatic regions. Open Access J Sports Med. 2013;4:251.

65. Friden J, Lieber RL. Structural and mechanical basis of exercise-induced muscle injury. Med Sci Sports Exerc. 1992;24:521–30.
66. Lieber RL, Friden J. Muscle damage is not a function of muscle force but active muscle strain. J Appl Physiol. 1993;74:520–6.
67. Charnock BL, Lewis CL, Garrett Jr WE, Queen RM. Adductor longus mechanics during the maximal effort soccer kick. Sports Biomech. 2009;8:223–34.
68. Chaudhari AM, Jamison ST, McNally MP, Pan X, Schmitt LC. Hip adductor activations during run-to-cut manoeuvres in compression shorts: implications for return to sport after groin injury. J Sports Sci. 2014;32:1333–40.
69. Orchard J, Read JW, Verrall G, Slavotinek JP. Pathophysiology of chronic groin pain in the athlete. Int J Sports Med. 2000;1:1–15.
70. Gilmore J. Groin pain in the soccer athlete: fact, fiction, and treatment. Clin J Sport Med. 1998;17:787–93.
71. Valent A, Frizziero A, Bressan S, Zanella E, Giannotti E, Masiero S. Insertional tendinopathy of the adductors and rectus abdominis in athletes: a review. Muscles Ligaments Tendons J. 2012;2:142.
72. Bouvard M, Dorochenko P, Lanusse P, Duraffour H. La pubalgie du sportif – stratégie thérapeutique: Revue de la littérature et proposition d'un protocole de rééducation. Journal de Traumatologie du Sport. 2004;21:146–63.
73. Puranen J, Orava S. The hamstring syndrome a new diagnosis of gluteal sciatic pain. Am J Sports Med. 1988;16:517–21.
74. Migliorini S, Merlo M, Pricca P. The hamstring syndrome. Clinical and diagnostic features, etiology, and surgical management. J Sports Traumatol Relat Res. 2000;22:86–92.
75. Koulouris G, Connell D. Hamstring muscle complex: an imaging review 1. Radiographics. 2005;25:571–86.
76. Fredricson M, Moore W, Guillet M, Beaulieu C. High hamstring injuries: etiology, diagnosis, and treatment. Phys Sports Med. 2005;33:32–43.
77. Gaida JE, Ashe MC, Bass SL, Cook JL. Is adiposity an under-recognized risk factor for tendinopathy? A systematic review. Arthritis Care Res (Hoboken). 2009;61:840–9.
78. Fredberg U, Bolvig L, Andersen NT. Prophylactic training in asymptomatic soccer players with ultrasonographic abnormalities in Achilles and patellar tendons the Danish super league study. Am J Sports Med. 2008;36:451–60.
79. Maffulli N, Sharma P, Luscombe KL. Achilles tendinopathy: aetiology and management. J R Soc Med. 2004;97:472–6.
80. Cook JL, Khan KM, Purdam C. Achilles tendinopathy. Man Ther. 2002;7:121–30.
81. Maganaris CN, Narici MV, Almekinders LC, Maffulli N. Biomechanics and pathophysiology of overuse tendon injuries. Sports Med. 2004;34:1005–17.
82. Pessoa P, Jones H. Traumatologia desportiva. Portugal: Lidel; 2014.
83. Frey C, Zamora J. The effects of obesity on orthopaedic foot and ankle pathology. Foot Ankle Int. 2007;28:996–9.
84. Mahieu NN, Witvrouw E, Stevens V, Van Tiggelen D, Roget P. Intrinsic risk factors for the development of Achilles tendon overuse injury a prospective study. Am J Sports Med. 2006;34:226–35.
85. Fredberg U, Stengaard-Pedersen K. Chronic tendinopathy tissue pathology, pain mechanisms, and etiology with a special focus on inflammation. Scand J Med Sci Sports. 2008;18:3–15.
86. Woods C, Hawkins R, Hulse M, Hodson A. The football association medical research programme: an audit of injuries in professional football – analysis of preseason injuries. Br J Sports Med. 2002;36:436–41.
87. Lian Ø, Engebretsen L, Øvrebø RV, Bahr R. Characteristics of the leg extensors in male volleyball players with jumper's knee. Am J Sports Med. 1996;24:380–5.
88. Rio E, Kidgell D, Moseley GL, Gaida J, Docking S, Purdam C, Cook J. Tendon neuroplastic training: changing the way we think about tendon rehabilitation: a narrative review. Br J Sports Med. 2016;50:209–215.
89. Weier AT, Pearce AJ, Kidgell DJ. Strength training reduces intracortical inhibition. Acta Physiol. 2012;206:109–19.
90. Heales L, Lim E, Hodges P, Vicenzino B. Sensory and motor deficits exist on the non-injured side of patients with unilateral tendon pain and disability – implications for central nervous system involvement: a systematic review with meta-analysis. Br J Sports Med. 2014;48:1400–6.
91. Malliaras P, Cook J, Purdam C, Rio E. Patellar tendinopathy: clinical diagnosis, load management, and advice for challenging case presentations. J Orthop Sports Phys Ther. 2015;45:1–33.
92. Edwards S, Steele JR, McGhee DE, Beattie S, Purdam C, Cook JL. Landing strategies of athletes with an asymptomatic patellar tendon abnormality. Med Sci Sports Exerc. 2010;42:2072–80.
93. James CR, Dufek JS, Bates BT. Effects of injury proneness and task difficulty on joint kinetic variability. Med Sci Sports Exerc. 2000;32:1833–44.
94. Bartlett R, Wheat J, Robins M. Is movement variability important for sports biomechanists? Sports Biomech. 2007;6:224–43.
95. Khan KM, Cook JL, Bonar F, Harcourt P, Åstrom M. Histopathology of common tendinopathies. Sports Med. 1999;27:393–408.
96. Michener LA, Kulig K. Not all tendons are created equal: implications for differing treatment approaches. J Orthop Sports Phys Ther. 2015;45:829–32.
97. Martínez-Lagunas V, Niessen M, Hartmann U. Women's football: player characteristics and demands of the game. J Sport Health Sci. 2014;3:258–72.

98. Sigward SM, Powers CM. Loading characteristics of females exhibiting excessive valgus moments during cutting. Clin Biomech (Bristol, Avon). 2007;22: 827–33.
99. Sakamoto K, Sasaki R, Hong S, Matsukura K, Asai T. Comparison of kicking speed between female and male soccer players. Procedia Eng. 2014;72:50–5.
100. Sakamoto K, Hong S, Tabei Y, Asai T. Comparative study of female and male soccer players in kicking motion. Procedia Eng. 2012;34:206–11.
101. Ball K. Loading and performance of the support leg in kicking. J Sci Med Sport. 2013;16:455–9.
102. Jones PA, Herrington LC, Graham-Smith P. Technique determinants of knee joint loads during cutting in female soccer players. Hum Mov Sci. 2015;42:203–11.
103. Davenport TE, Kulig K, Matharu Y, Blanco CE. The EdUReP model for nonsurgical management of tendinopathy. Phys Ther. 2005;85:1093–103.
104. Kaux J-F, Forthomme B, Le Goff C, Crielaard J-M, Croisier J-L. Current opinions on tendinopathy. J Sports Sci Med. 2011;10:238–53.
105. Rees JD, Stride M, Scott A. Tendons–time to revisit inflammation. Br J Sports Med. 2013. doi:10.1136/bjsports-2012-091957.
106. Rudavsky A, Cook J. Physiotherapy management of patellar tendinopathy (jumper's knee). J Physiother. 2014;60:122–9.
107. Gabbe BJ, Finch CF, Bennell KL, Wajswelner H. Risk factors for hamstring injuries in community level Australian football. Br J Sports Med. 2005;39:106–10.
108. Hutson M, Speed C. Sports injuries. New York: Oxford University Press; 2011.
109. Kulig K, Joiner D, Chang Y. Landing limb posture in volleyball athletes with patellar tendinopathy: a pilot study. Int J Sports Med. 2015;36:400–6.
110. Debenham JR, Travers MJ, Gibson W, Campbell A, Allison GT. Achilles tendinopathy alters stretch shortening cycle behaviour during a sub-maximal hopping task. J Sci Med Sport. 2016;19:69–73.
111. Van der Worp H, De Poel H, Diercks R, Van Den Akker-Scheek I, Zwerver J. Jumper's knee or lander's knee? A systematic review of the relation between jump biomechanics and patellar tendinopathy. Int J Sports Med. 2014;35:714–22.
112. Rosen AB, Ko J, Simpson KJ, Kim S-H, Brown CN. Lower extremity kinematics during a drop jump in individuals with patellar tendinopathy. Orthop J Sports Med. 2015;3:2325967115576100.
113. Rohman E, Steubs JT, Tompkins M. Changes in involved and uninvolved limb function during rehabilitation after anterior cruciate ligament reconstruction implications for limb symmetry index measures. Am J Sports Med. 2015;43:1391–8.
114. Adams D, Logerstedt D, Hunter-Giordano A, Axe MJ, Snyder-Mackler L. Current concepts for anterior cruciate ligament reconstruction: a criterion-based rehabilitation progression. J Orthop Sports Phys Ther. 2012;42:601–14.
115. Barber SD, Noyes FR, Mangine RE, Hartman W. Quantitative assessment of functional limitations in normal and anterior cruciate ligament-deficient knees. Clin Orthop Relat Res. 1990;255: 204–14.
116. Hildebrandt C, Müller L, Zisch B, Huber R, Fink C, Raschner C. Functional assessments for decision-making regarding return to sports following ACL reconstruction. Part I: development of a new test battery. Knee Surg Sports Traumatol Arthrosc. 2015;23:1273–81.
117. Croisier J-L, Ganteaume S, Binet J, Genty M, Ferret J-M. Strength imbalances and prevention of hamstring injury in professional soccer players a prospective study. Am J Sports Med. 2008;36: 1469–75.
118. Backman LJ, Danielson P. Low range of ankle dorsiflexion predisposes for Patellar Tendinopathy in junior elite basketball players a 1-year prospective study. Am J Sports Med. 2011;39:2626–33.
119. Rabin A, Kozol Z, Finestone AS. Limited ankle dorsiflexion increases the risk for mid-portion Achilles tendinopathy in infantry recruits: a prospective cohort study. J Foot Ankle Res. 2014;7:1–7.
120. Peters JA, Zwerver J, Diercks RL, Elferink-Gemser MT, van den Akker-Scheek I. Preventive interventions for tendinopathy: A systematic review. J Sci Med Sport. 2016;19:205–11.

Tendon Injuries in the Lower Limb Diagnosis and Classification

39

Lucio Ernlund and Lucas de A. Vieira

Contents

39.1 Introduction

Tendons are a specific dense regular connective tissue and bind muscles to bone acting as transducers of the muscle contraction to skeletal structures, allowing mobility and joint stability. In the tendinous tissue, two main types of fibroblasts are present. Tenoblasts are immature cells and tenocytes are mature tenoblast which synthesizes the extracellular matrix. In this matrix, there are collagen fibers arranged in regular arrays, and they account for 70–80% of the dry weight of a tendon. The type I collagen is the most common. These fibers of collagen are organized in bundles that are wrapped in the endotenon which in turn are enveloped by an epitenon, forming the actual tendon [1–3].

Tendon injuries are a common clinical condition both in sports and in the workplace. In professional football players, the most prevalent diagnoses are muscle-tendon injuries, and the lower limbs are the most common location of injury [4, 5]. Tendons subjected to the highest stresses, exposed to repeated strains and with less vascularization, are the most frequently damaged [2, 6, 7].

These injuries vary in a range of acute rupture to chronic tendinopathy. Acute tendon tears are derived from a traumatic event or a spontaneous rupture in a degenerate tissue, while chronic tendinopathy is due to overuse situation as in excessive sports activity [8, 9].

The most common tendon disorder is the tendinopathy (often called tendinitis or tendinosis), and the overuse may be considered the initial disease factor, which leads to small tendon injuries. As a result, the tissue fails to heal before further trauma occurs [3, 6, 10].

L. Ernlund (✉) • L.de A. Vieira
Knee and Shoulder Institute, Curitiba, PR 80240-021, Brazil
e-mail: ernlund@brturbo.com.br; lucasvieiracb@gmail.com

J. Espregueira-Mendes et al. (eds.), *Injuries and Health Problems in Football*,
DOI 10.1007/978-3-662-53924-8_39

Clinical status of tendinopathy is a combination of pain, swelling, and impaired performance. Tendon tears appear as sudden pain, deformity, and functional impotence [11, 12].

39.2 Diagnosis

39.2.1 Clinical Presentation

The chronic tendon degeneration is often clinically silent, and its only manifestation may be a consequent tear. Patients with acute tendon rupture have pain and joint movement dysfunction. A palpable gap and inability to move the joint against gravity and resistance of strength are found in the physical examination [2, 12].

About the tendinopathy, the clinical scenario is quite uniform. Patients complain of pain in the affected tendon area, sometimes insidiously during a sports practice, advancing to light activities, or the pain may even be present at rest. Local tenderness, swelling, and reduced articular range of motion could be shown. Some patients experience exacerbated symptoms despite a few alterations in imaging examinations, and the opposite can also occur. There is not always a correlation between the extents of anatomic injuries in displayed exams and clinical founds [2, 3].

Another condition in the physical examination is the lack of flexibility. This situation has been associated with tendinopathy in the lower limb. Range of movement is also important in the tendinopathy pathogenesis. Decreased ankle dorsiflexion increases the amount and rate of loading on Achilles and patellar tendons. There is sufficient evidence that overload is a critical factor in tendinopathy [13].

Pain in tendinopathy is resultant of a combination of mechanical and biochemical changes, which affected the local cells and peripheral nerves. Chemical irritants and neurotransmitters may generate pain in tendinopathy. Lactate levels increased, and presence of neurotransmitter glutamate and substance P has been described in tendinopathy [3, 7, 14].

39.2.1.1 Tendon Injuries Around the Hip

Calcific tendinitis in the lower limb is the most common in the gluteus medius tendon. It is the result of deposition of calcium phosphate crystals in the tendons or adjacent soft tissues. The patient, who usually is a 50-year-old female, has severe pain and motion limitations. Acute calcific tendinitis is often misdiagnosed [15].

Proximal hamstring tendinopathy is an overuse injury characterized by lower gluteal pain, especially during sports. The pain in the proximal posterior thigh appears and increases gradually, and continued exercises made the situation worse. It has been descripted especially in sprinters and middle- and long-distance runners [11].

Hamstring muscle and tendon injuries are common in sports requiring sprinting, acceleration, and kicking. The British Athletics Muscle Injury Classification is based on magnetic ressonance imaging (MRI) features and described the extent and the localization of the injuries. In grade 0 the imaging is normal, and in grade 1 there is a small tear to the muscle. In grade 2 it's about moderate injuries and grade 3 extensive tears to the muscle. In grade 4 injuries are complete tears to either the muscle or tendon. For grades 1–4 injuries, the suffix "a" denotes a myofascial injury in the peripheral aspect of the muscle; "b" an injury within the muscle belly, most commonly at the muscle-tendon junction; and "c" an injury which extends into the tendon. The most common site of muscle injury is at the muscle-tendon junction, and the injury within the tendon is associated with a poorer prognosis [16]. Brunker [17] shows that the slow stretch type of injury and injuries involving the central tendon both requires longer times to return to play, and Pollock et al. [18] report that hamstring injuries that extend into the tendon ("c") are more prone to re-injury and delay time to return to full training (Fig. 39.1).

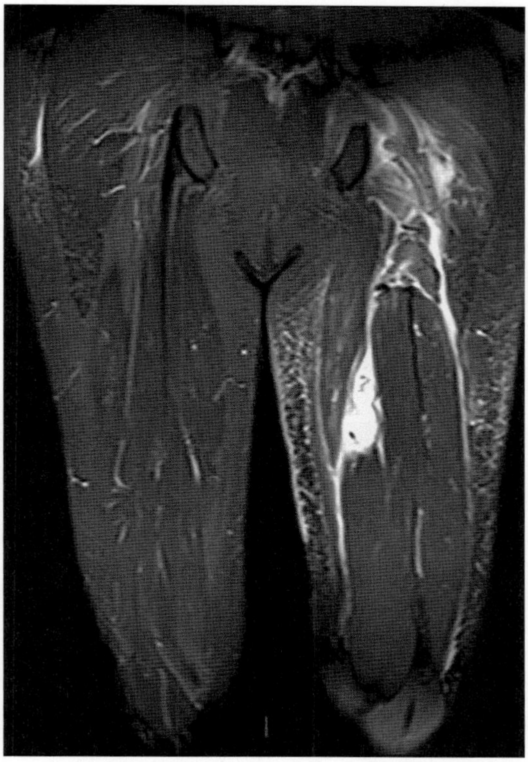

Fig. 39.1 Hamstring injury

39.2.1.2 Tendon Injuries Around the Knee

The main patellar pathology is proximal patellar tendinopathy, also known as jumper's knee. The patellar tendon is more vulnerable to overuse injuries than quadriceps tendon, particularly in adolescents and young adults [19, 20]. Patellar tendinopathy is a common cause of anterior knee pain, is involved with the overuse injury in sports, and is common among athletes in sports with prolonged repetitive stress of the knee extensor apparatus such as jumping (volleyball, basketball), kicking (football, american football), quick stops and starts (tennis, squash), and running [3]. Clinical symptoms may include pain, perceived swelling or fullness, and a sensation of "weakness" or "giving way" [21].

Hägglund et al. [22] published that patellar tendinopathy is a fairly common condition in elite football, and the recurrence rate is high (12–27%). High total amount of exposure was identified as a risk factor for patellar tendinopathy.

The extensor mechanism ruptures are rare injuries, which often occur through a degenerative tendon and produce painful and swollen knee. The patient has difficulty walking and cannot straighten their leg against gravity or resistance due the loss of extensor function. There may be a palpable defect in the suprapatellar or infrapatellar regions and an abnormal position of the patella. Hemarthrosis may or may not be present [23].

These injuries are produced by an eccentric contraction of the quadriceps muscle applied to the flexed knee. In young athletes, the typical mechanism is abrupt deceleration while running. In the elderly population, the most frequent mechanism is a sudden loss of balance that results in a fall on the fixed and flexed knee [20, 23].

Patellar tendon rupture can be the end stage of "Jumper's knee" due to the cumulative effect of repetitive trauma and microtearing of the tendinous fibers [21].

Quadriceps tendon tears are most common than patellar tendon ruptures and occur most often at the tendo-osseous junction. Usually the patient is around 40–60-year-old man, while the majority of patellar tears are seen at ages between 30 and 50 years. When a sudden flexion occurs in a normal bone, the tendons are susceptible to rupture, but if it is a osteoporotic bone, a patellar fracture might occur. Therefore, patellar and quadriceps tears are rare in woman, but patellar fractures are seen more commonly in them by which hormonal matters have more incidence of osteoporosis [9, 12, 24].

39.2.1.3 Tendon Injuries Around the Ankle

Achilles tendinopathy occurs both in sportspeople and sedentary people. Top level runners have an incidence of 7–9%, and sedentary lifestyle people have 30%. Pain, diffuse or localized swelling, and impaired performance of the Achilles tendon is seen in this clinical condition. Tendinopathy of the midportion of the tendon accounts for 55–65% of all injuries. In the beginning, pain occurs a short while after the end of the exercise. As the pathologic process progresses, pain may occur during the exercise and interferes with activities of daily living. Maffulli et al. [14] name that clinical examination is the best diagnostic tool. Location of pain from 2 to 6 cm above the insertion into the calcaneum and pain on palpation are reliable and accurate tests for diagnosis.

In an acute rupture of the Achilles tendon, the patients report that they thought that they had been struck by an object or kicked in the tendon area. An audible snap usually is reported too. These injuries are common in sports practice, and the patients may present pain, palpable gap, and Thompson signal besides being unable to bear weight and notice weakness.

Although they are common injuries and usually easy to diagnose, there are reports that 20% of cases are not diagnosed by the first examining physician. This indicates that a high index of suspicion is necessary because a neglected rupture will result in greater difficulty in treatment and rehabilitation [1, 14].

Ress et al. [13] cite that gender is a key genetic expression, and women develop less tendinopathy than men, but after the onset of menopause, they are also prone to Achilles tendon ruptures. Estrogen may protect tendons.

The tibialis posterior is the most powerful inverter of the foot and an important dynamic stabilizer of the foot arch. Traumatic injuries, such as lacerations or dislocation, are associated with ankle or calcaneal fracture. Tendinopathy of the tibialis posterior occurs frequently in runners and is associated with valgus flatfoot-pronation deformities [3].

Posterior tibialis tendon deficiency is a presentation of this tendinopathy. The incidence is higher in middle-aged women who have coexisting obesity. Pain around the posteromedial aspect of the ankle, fatigue or weakness of the foot and ankle, and difficulty in walking are seen, and it can lead to flatfoot deformity [25].

Tibialis anterior tendon rupture is an uncommon disorder. The main clinical presentation is an atraumatic rupture in a man over the age of 45 years due to an eccentric loading of a degenerated tibialis anterior tendon against a plantar flexed ankle. Traumatic injuries occur in a laceration or blunt trauma. Pseudotumor at the anteromedial aspect of the ankle, loss of the contour of the tibialis anterior tendon, and the use of the extensor halluces longus and extensor digitorum communis to dorsiflex the ankle are the physical findings [26].

Peroneal tendon injuries are a common cause of pain in the lateral aspect of the ankle. These injuries also vary from traumatic situation, like after ankle sprain, or degenerative chronic disorders, often in patients with predisposing structural components such as hindfoot varus, lateral ligamentous instability, an enlarged peroneal tubercle, and a symptomatic os peroneum. The clinical presentation is a patient with pain, weakness with hindfoot eversion, and unstable gait [27, 28] (Fig. 39.2).

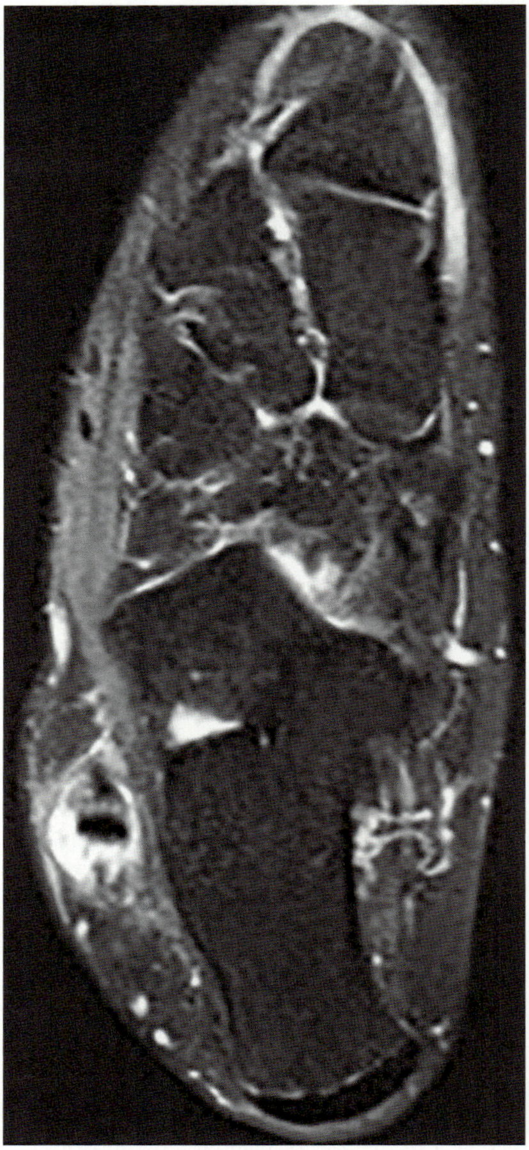

Fig. 39.2 Peroneal tenosynovitis

39.2.2 Imaging

The diagnosis of these lesions should always be based on the patient clinical condition. Imaging tests are used to confirm and describe these lesions, assisting in the therapeutic decision. Each exam has its indication and limitation, and in clinical practice they are completed. The radiographs are indicated in traumatic injuries to search for fractures that may be associated. In chronic cases, they can show tendinopathy alterations as osteophytosis. The MRI is useful for bone and soft tissue disorders. Ultrasonography (US) also can describe bone and soft tissue injuries in addition to revealing neovascularization in the pathologic tendon [20, 21, 29].

39.2.2.1 Radiography

Plain radiography is a fast and cost-effective way to identify a wide range of joint disorders. It is used to diagnose associated or incidental bony alteration [14, 20].

In the evaluation of extensor mechanism ruptures, the tendon may appear widened and indistinct, and a patellar displacement and avulsion fractures can be seen. So in a quadriceps tendon tear, the avulsion fragment originates from the patellar superior pole, and in a complete tear, the patella baja is seen. The opposite happens in the patellar tears. The patellar detachment is proximal and the avulsion fractures, which often are present, occur in the patellar lower pole [21, 30] (Fig. 39.3).

Pires Albuquerque et al. [9] described the radiographic analysis of tendon tears in the knee extensor mechanism. The most prevalent abnormality was suprapatellar osteophytes alone, followed by alterations of infrapatellar calcification, suprapatellar calcification, and supra- and infrapatellar osteophytes. The most rare abnormality seen was the infrapatellar osteophytes alone. This alteration can be identified before the tears and indicate a prevention measures (Fig. 39.4).

Radiographic of an Achilles tendon tear may show Kager's triangle loss of its regular configuration. When it occurs, calcaneal tuberosity avulsion fractures are possible evidence [1].

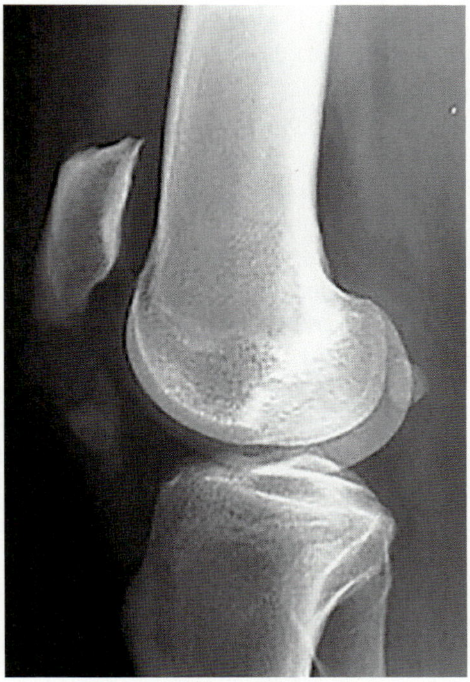

Fig. 39.3 Proximal patellar detachment in patellar tendon injury

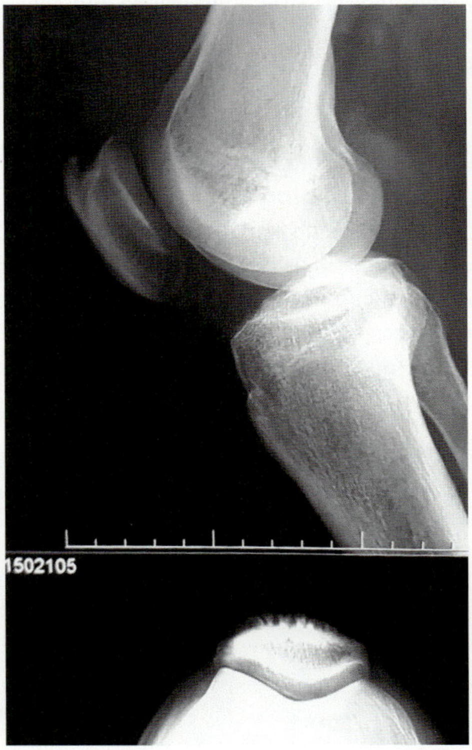

Fig. 39.4 Osteophyte suprapatelar in the quadriceps tendinopathy

Osteophytosis is a process of calcification and osseous metaplasia that occurs in chronic tendinosis. They also can be seen in plain radiography of the hip, knee, or foot and ankle with tendinopathy.

39.2.2.2 Ultrasonography

US is an important imaging method. It has a good cost-effectiveness, does not present a contraindication of radiation, and can be done in dynamic mode. However, the examination is operator dependent [14, 24].

Grayscale US is a conventional imaging technique that can show tendinopathy thickening and alterations in the tendon structure. In the tendon insertion on the bone, mucoide degeneration may be seen. Doppler sonography is another technique which is able to indicate the presence of neovessels in a degenerative tendon area. This neovascularization is frequent in patients symptomatic for pain [3].

There are indications of US such as in traumatic or non-traumatic and acute or chronic tendon injuries. The normal tendons appear hyperechoic (bright) on ultrasound although tendinopathy is a hypoechoic area. Rupture can be seen as an acoustic vacuum with thick and irregular edges [1, 24] (Fig. 39.5).

39.2.2.3 Magnetic Resonance Imaging

MRI is an excellent diagnostic tool to evaluate sports-related injuries involving the ligaments, tendons, menisci, osseous structures, and articular surfaces.

Knee disorders are the most frequent indications for MRI in the lower extremities. Routine protocols are sufficient for most pathologies of the extensor mechanism. Its integrity is best evaluated on T2-weighted sagittal MRI [20, 30, 31].

The quadriceps tendon is a multilaminar structure. Zeiss et al. [32] described the tendon as conjoined structure serving all the muscle groups combined; the most superficial layer arises from the rectus femoris muscle and the deepest layer from the vastus intermedius muscle. In this study, most tendons were composed by three layers, so that the intermediate layer is formed by the vastus lateralis and vastus medialis. Rarely cases where the tendon was seen as four thin layers or a convergence of all the layers like a single tendon band were found.

This laminated configuration is significant in the discrimination between partial and full tears. Discontinuity of any of these layers is consistent with a partial tear, and the insert of the rectus femoris tendon on the patellar superior pole is the most common site of disruption. A complete tendon rupture is seen when all layers tear and is associated with edematous tissue, hemorrhage, and retraction of the proximal fibers. The insertion of the quadriceps tendon at the patella upper pole is the typical area of rupture. In chronic overuse injury or tendinopathy of the quadriceps tendon, thickening and increased T2 signal are found in the MRI [20, 23, 31, 32] (Fig. 39.6).

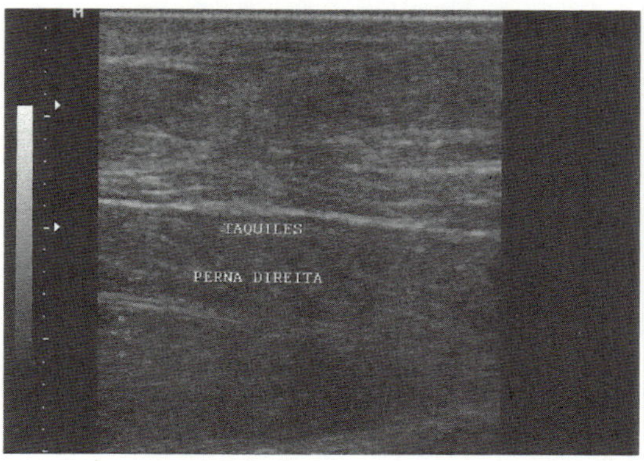

Fig. 39.5 Achilles tendon partial rupture

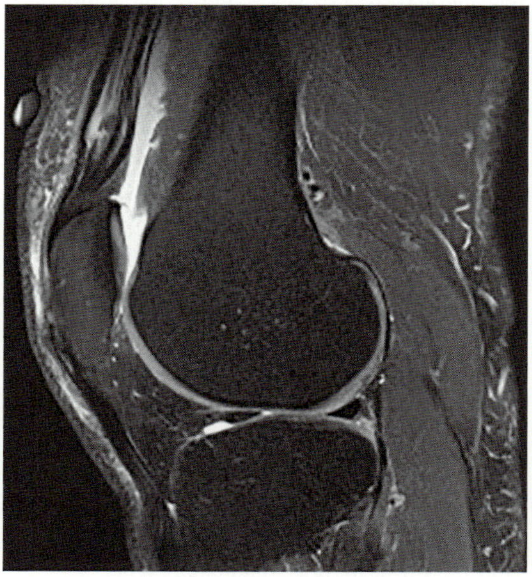

Fig. 39.6 Quadriceps tendon partial rupture

Unlike the quadriceps tendon, the patellar tendon is a solid tendon, and the MRI demonstrates homogenous low signal intensity, may have a convex anterior border, and should always have a well-defined posterior border [31]. Yun et al. [19] published that the increased signal of the proximal patellar tendon on T1-weighted image and fluid-sensitive MRI results from invaginating fat, vessels, and perivascular connective tissue. It is not pathological but a normal and common finding. Jumper's knee alterations in magnetic resonance imaging include a focal thickening of the proximal one-third of the tendon, an anterior-posterior diameter greater than 7 mm, and focal T2 hyperintensity located within the medial aspect of the tendon, near its patellar attachment. Others found indistinct posterior tendon border, edema in the adjacent Hoffa's fat pad, and bone marrow edema within the adjacent inferior pole of the patella [20, 21, 23, 30, 31] (Fig. 39.7).

In chronic or neglected cases, the entire length of the patellar tendon may be involved, and the MRI shows a fusiform thickening of the tendon with altered signal intensity [20].

An acute patellar tear may be partial or full thickness. Fluid signal within the expected location is an indication of partial patellar tendon rupture. In complete disruption, imaging shows discontinuity of the patellar tendon, retraction of its fibers, hemorrhage that can extend to the Hoffa's fat pad, and edema that can result in blurring of the posterior margin of the tendon [21, 31].

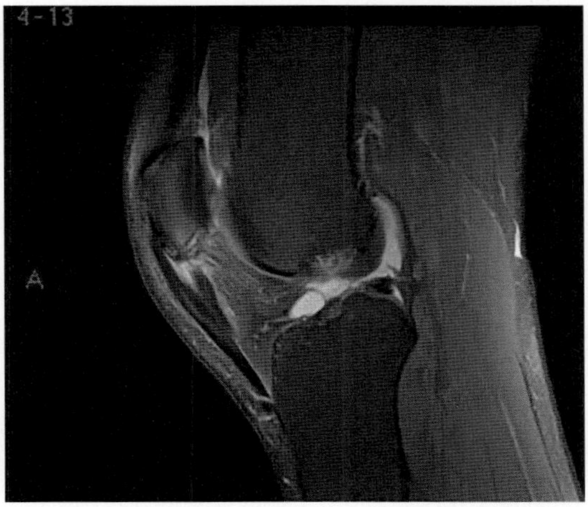

Fig. 39.7 Jumper's knee with partial patellar tendon rupture

MRI of the Achilles tendon is useful to evaluate the various stages of chronic degeneration and in differentiating between peritendinitis and tendinopathy because it provides information on the internal morphology of the tendon and the surrounding structures. In Achilles tendon tears, the indications of this study are for preoperative planning in ambiguous presentations and subacute or chronic injuries [14]. Garras et al. [33] show that in acute Achilles tendon ruptures, the physical examination findings were more sensitive than MRI, which is time-consuming and expensive and can lead to treatment delays.

39.3 Classification

There are a variety of diseases that are part of the spectrum of tendon injuries. These lesions vary in relation to their form of presentation, and they can be classified according to symptoms, imaging findings, histopathological process, evolution of time, causal factor, correlated risk factors, and other associated diseases or drugs.

Specific classifications for a given tendinopathy can become classical. However, other classifications, initially described for a condition, may be used to describe the pathological process in other tendon injuries.

Jumper's knee classic classification of Blazina et al. [34] as modified by Roels et al. [35] describes four phases of tendinopathy and their clinical repercussion in relation to pain and impaired performance:

Phase I: pain only after activity

Phase II: pain and discomfort during activity but does not interfere with participation

Phase III: pain both during and after participation, which interferes with competition

Phase IV: complete tendon disruption

Weinstabl et al. [36] identified four Achilles tendon injury categories according to MRI findings:

Group I: Inflammatory reaction. Tendon thickening without structural change

Group II: Degenerative change. Thickening of the tendon with longitudinally and centrally located image changes

Group III: Incomplete rupture. The thickening of the tendon with structural changes longitudinally and horizontally including the paratendon

Group IV: Complete rupture, visible discontinuity of the tendon

Based on the same injury categories reported by Weinstabl et al. [27], they describe a classification to peroneal tendon tears according to US and surgical criteria as grade 0 (normal), grade I (tendinosis), grade II (partial-thickness tear), or grade III (full-thickness tear).

39.3.1 About Histopathological Process

Tendinopathy is a pathological condition which etiology is overhead and overuse. It can cause partial injuries or even total tears on the damaged tissue. The process can be classified as tendinitis or tendinosis. Tendinitis is associated with acute lesions, and it is the degeneration caused by inflammatory microtears in the tendon tissue due to a tensile force too heavy or abrupt. Tendinosis occurs when the overload and overuse process is continuous, so there is no time for the healing response, leading to a collagen fiber degradation in a degenerative process. Despite tendinopathy, the tendons may suffer abrupt action of an external factor, such as a trauma, and suffering complete ruptures [2, 37, 38].

Historically, pain in tendinopathy has been attributed to the inflammatory process. However chronic tendinopathy does not reveal histopathological evidence of inflammation. Besides this, many intratendineous injuries detected by imaging are not painful. The roles of both the inflammation and the degeneration are a matter of debate, and the exact pathogenic mechanism is still unknown [3, 7].

Ress et al. [13] report that inflammation plays a role only in the initiation, but not in the propagation and progression of the disease process. Histologic studies show either absent or minimal inflammation, and they generally also show hypercellularity, a loss of the tightly bundled collagen appearance, an increase in proteoglycan content, and commonly neovascularization. So this has been named as a "failed healing response" [39].

Maffulli et al. [40] name that the term "tendinopathy" is a generic descriptor of the clinical conditions (both pain and pathological characteristics) associated with overuse in and around tendons. The histological descriptive terms "tendinosis" (a degenerative pathological condition with a lack of inflammatory change) and "tendonitis" or "tendinitis" (implying an inflammatory process) should be used only after histopathological confirmation.

39.3.2 About Evolution of Time

About disease timing, tendon pathology is classified as acute or chronic. These terms are common in the description of orthopedics injuries, and literature varies widely in their definitions. Flint et al. [41] conducted a study of these terminologies in sports injuries. Particularly concerning tendon injuries, the Achilles tendon rupture was evaluated. Acute Achilles tendon rupture was defined as less than 1 week from injury; chronic rupture is defined as greater than 4 weeks from injury.

In clinical practice, the definition between acute or chronic is more necessary in tendon ruptures than in tendinopathy, and it helps in planning treatment. In acute lesions the primary repair of damaged structures is possible, whereas in chronic lesions, or neglected ones, it may necessitate augmentation or reconstruction procedures of the damaged tendon.

39.3.3 About Causal Factor

The tendon's function is to transfer the force generated in muscle contraction to bony structures so that the movement occurs. The trauma, direct or indirect, on this muscle-tendon-bone unit or chronic overload of this structure may be the tendinopathy cause.

Injuries may be caused by intrinsic or extrinsic factors or even by a combination of these. In acute tears, the extrinsic factor is predominant, but probably, it is associated with previous degeneration pathology that reduces tensile strength predisposing to rupture [2, 7, 8].

39.3.3.1 Traumatic Tears

In the extensor mechanism ruptures, trauma plays an important role. Indirect trauma is a result of a sudden and eccentric contraction of the quadriceps muscle with the foot planted and the knee flexed. When compared to direct trauma, indirect trauma is twice as common in the quadriceps tendon injuries and three times more common in lesions of the patellar tendon. Indirect trauma usually leads to retinacula injuries and complete transection of the extensor mechanism, resulting in the inability to extend the knee. Direct trauma, such as a violent impact on taut tendon, may cause isolated rupture or be associated with complex knee injuries. The injured tendon conditions also have an importance in the genesis of rupture. Previous degeneration or hypovascularity areas can determine spontaneous ruptures [12, 23, 42].

39.3.3.2 Overuse Injuries

More than half of sports injuries are due to overuse. Similarly, main tendons of the musculoskeletal system are vulnerable to this overload. Tendinopathy is correlated with situations when there is an increase load on the tendon and its insertion, as repeated activity or physical stress. Tendon cells experience a great deal of load repetitions developing degenerative alterations and tendinopathy. Exercise-induced hyperthermia is also harmful to tendon tissue. Hypovascular tendon areas are more susceptible to the effects of this hyperthermia [1, 6, 13].

39.3.4 About Correlated Risk Factors

39.3.4.1 Extrinsic Factors

Specific situations can lead to overuse and result in tendinopathy. In the sports practice, training errors, changes in training routines, increased load, and muscle fatigue are extrinsic factors examples in tendinopathy genesis. Long distances, strong intensity, and poor running technique are correlated with pathology of the Achilles tendon. Frequency and intensity of training and activities with jumps are risk factors for patellar tendinopathy. Environmental conditions as wrong or defective equipment and footwear, cold weather during outdoor training, and hard or slanting superficies also are described as causal factor of tendinopathy [2, 3, 14, 22].

39.3.4.2 Intrinsic Factors

Intrinsic factors related to tendinopathy include genetic predisposition, age, body weight, and biomechanical irregularities, such as muscle imbalance. Individuals who are older, heavier, and male are more likely to develop tendon injuries [2, 6].

Besides age and obesity, dysfunctions of gastrocnemius-soleus, pes cavus, marked forefoot varus, and lateral ankle instability have also been described as risk factors for Achilles tendinopathy. Hyperpronation of the foot is a very prevalent alteration in this condition. In patellar tendinopathy, intrinsic factors are male gender, tall stature, high body mass, and reduced ankle dorsiflexion [7, 14, 22].

39.3.5 About Other Associated Diseases or Drugs

Many diseases are described as risk factors for tendon injuries. Chronic renal failure is classically correlated with the knee extensor mechanism tears. Autoimmune diseases, such as systemic lupus erythematosus, also are tendinopathy risk factors. In diabetes mellitus, advanced glycation end products, which are directly proportional to the level of blood glucose, act on the tendons causing degeneration and fibrotic tissue formation. Moreover, as well as hypertension, diabetes mellitus operates on tendon vascularization. The thyroid hormone is correlated with the synthesis of collagen. Hypothyroidism is also associated with tendinopathy and tendon injuries.

In general, conditions that alter the vasculature, nutrition, metabolism, and tendon structure will lead to tendinopathy [3, 12, 14, 20].

The use of medications also is a risk factor for tendon pathology. Balasubramaniam and Prathap [43] described tissue necrosis in calcaneal tendon of rats only 45 min after the local injection of hydrocortisone. It is known that steroids decrease collagen and matrix synthesis of the tendon tissue. The anti-inflammatory and analgesic action of this drug may mask symptoms of tendinopathy, and the patient continues to put strain on the injured tendon [1, 14].

Another kind of medicine that can induce tendon lesion is a fluoroquinolone. By inhibiting the tendon metabolism, tenocyte proliferation and collagen synthesis are reduced, leading to a mechanism that induces tendinopathy. This degenerated tendon can evolve to spontaneous ruptures, particularly in the elderly population [1, 7, 14, 44].

Acknowledgments The authors would like to thank Bruno Rick Ogata musculoskeletal radiologist from DAPI/Curitiba-Brazil for kindly providing images of this text.

References

1. Maffulli N. Current concepts review rupture of the achilles tendon. J Bone Joint Surg. 1999;81:1019–36.
2. Morais DS, Torres J, Guedes RM, Lopes MA. Current approaches and future trends to promote tendon repair. Ann Biomed Eng. 2015;43:2025–35.
3. Abate M, Silbernagel KG, Siljeholm C, di Iorio A, de Amicis D, Salini V, Werner S, Paganelli R. Pathogenesis of tendinopathies: inflammation or degeneration? Arthritis Res Ther. 2009;11:235–50.
4. Reis GF, Santos TR, Lasmar RC, Oliveira Júnior O, Lopes RF, Fonseca ST. Sports injuries profile of a first division Brazilian soccer team: a descriptive cohort study. Braz J Phys Ther. 2015;19:390–7.
5. Stubbe JH, van Beijsterveldt AM, van der Knaap S, Stege J, Verhagen EA, van Mechelen W, Backx FJ. Injuries in professional male soccer players in the Netherlands: a prospective cohort study. J Athl Train. 2015;50:211–6.
6. Xu Y, Murrell GA. The basic science of tendinopathy. Clin Orthop Relat Res. 2008;466:1528–38.
7. Sharma P, Maffulli N. Tendon injury and tendinopathy: healing and repair. J Bone Joint Surg. 2005; 87:187–202.
8. Muller SA, Todorov A, Heisterbach PE, Martin I, Majewski M. Tendon healing: an overview of physiology, biology, and pathology of tendon healing and systematic review of state of the art in tendon bioengineering. Knee Surg Sports Traumatol Arthrosc. 2015;23:2097–105.
9. Pires Albuquerque R, Campos ALS, dos Santos Neto JF, Karam E, Neves JG, Di Tullio P, et al. Radiographic analysis of factors predisposing toward tendon tears in the knee extensor mechanism. Rev Bras Ortop. 2014;49:374–8.
10. Andia I, Maffulli N. Muscle and tendon injuries: the role of biological interventions to promote and assist healing and recovery. Arthroscopy. 2015;33:999–1015.
11. Lempainem L, Sarimo J, Mattila K, Vaittinen S, Orava S. Proximal hamstring tendinopathy: results of surgical management and histopathologic findings. Am J Sports Med. 2009;37:727–34.
12. Negrin LL, Nemecek E, Hajdu S. Extensor mechanism ruptures of the knee: differences in demographic data and long-term outcome after surgical treatment. Injury. 2015;46:1957–63.
13. Ress JD, Maffulli N, Cook J. Management of tendinopathy. Am J Sports Med. 2009;37:1855–67.
14. Maffulli N, Via AG, Oliva F. Chronic Achilles tendon disorders: tendinopathy and chronic rupture. Clin Sports Med. 2015;34:607–24.
15. Park SM, Baek JH, Ko YB, Lee HJ, Park KJ, Ha YC. Management of acute calcific tendinitis around the hip joint. Am J Sports Med. 2014;42:2659–65.
16. Pollock N, James SLJ, Lee JC, et al. British athletics muscle injury classification: a new grading system. Br J Sports Med. 2014;48:1347–51.
17. Brukner P. Hamstring injuries: prevention and treatment – an update. Br J Sports Med. 2015;49: 1241–4.
18. Pollock N, Patel A, Chakraverty J, Suokas A, James SL, Chakraverty R. Time to return to full training is delayed and recurrence rate is higher in intratendinous ('c') acute hamstring injury in elite track and field athletes: clinical application of the British Athletics Muscle Injury Classification. Br J Sports Med. 2016;50:305–10.
19. Yun SJ, Jin W, Park YK, Kim GY, Yoon SH, Park SY, Lee JE, Park JS, Ryu KN. Increased signal intensity at the proximal patellar tendon: correlation between MR imaging and histology in eight cadavers and clinical MR imaging studies. Eur Radiol. 2015;25: 2976–83.
20. Skiadas V, Perdikakis E, Plotas A, Lahanis S. MR imaging of anterior knee pain: a pictorial essay. Knee Surg Sports Traumatol Arthrosc. 2013;21:294–304.
21. Samim M, Smitaman E, Lawrence D, Moukaddam H. MRI of anterior knee pain. Skelet Radiol. 2014;43:875–93.
22. Hägglund M, Zwerver J, Ekstrand J. Epidemiology of patellar tendinopathy in elite male soccer players. Am J Sports Med. 2011;39:1906–11.

23. Yu JS, Petersilge C, Sartoris DJ, Pathria MN, Resnick D. MR imaging of injuries of the extensor mechanism of the knee. Radiographics. 1994;14:541–51.
24. Mankad K, Hoey E, Grainger AJ, Barro DA. Trauma musculoskeletal ultrasound. Emerg Radiol. 2008;15:83–9.
25. Gluck GS, Heckman DS, Parekh SG. Tendon disorders of the foot and ankle, part 3: the posterior tibial tendon. Am J Sport Med. 2010;38:2133–44.
26. Sammarco VJ, Sammarco GJ, Henning C, Chaim S. Surgical repair of acute and chronic tibialis anterior tendon ruptures. J Bone Joint Surg Am. 2009; 91:325–32.
27. Grant TH, Kelikian AS, Jerebm SE, McCarthy RJ. Ultrasound diagnosis of peroneal tendon tears. J Bone Joint Surg. 2005;87:1788–94.
28. Roster B, Michelier P, Giza E. Peroneal tendon disorders. Clin Sports Med. 2015;34:625–41.
29. Suzue N, Matsuura T, Iwame T, Higashino K, Sakai T, Hamada D, et al. State-of-the-art ultrasonographic findings in lower extremity sports injuries. J Med Investig. 2015;62:109–12.
30. Ostlere S. The extensor mechanism of the knee. Radiol Clin N Am. 2013;51:393–411.
31. Sanders TG, Miller MD. A systematic approach to magnetic resonance imaging interpretation of sports medicine injuries of the knee. Am J Sports Med. 2005;33:131–48.
32. Zeiss J, Saddemi SR, Ebraheim NA. MR imaging of the quadriceps tendon: normal layered configuration and its importance in cases of tendon ruptures. AJR. 1992;159:1031–4.
33. Garras DN, Raikin SM, Bhat SB, Taweel N, Karanjia H. MRI is unnecessary for diagnosing acute achilles tendon ruptures. Clin Orthop Relat Res. 2012; 470:2268–73.
34. Blazina ME, Kerlan RK, Jobe FW, Carter VS, Carlson GJ. Jumper's knee. Orthop Clin North Am. 1973;4:665–78.
35. Roels J, Martens M, Mulier JC. Patellar tendinitis (jumper's knee). Am J Sports Med. 1978;6:362–8.
36. Weinstabl R, Stiskal M, Neuhold A, Aamlid B, Hertz H. Classifying calcaneal tendon injury according to mri findings. J Bone Joint Surg (Br). 1991;73:683–5.
37. Rodrigues MT, Reis RL, Gomes ME. Engineering tendon and ligament tissues: present developments towards successful clinical products. J Tissue Eng Regen Med. 2013;7:673–86.
38. Sharma P, Maffuli N. Biology of tendon injury: healing, modeling and remodeling. J Musculoskelet Neuronal Interact. 2006;6:181–90.
39. Maffulli N, Longo UG, Denaro V. Novel approaches for the management of tendinopathy. J Bone Joint Surg Am. 2010;92:2604–13.
40. Maffulli N, Khan KM, Puddu G. Overuse tendon conditions: time to change a confusing terminology. Arthroscopy. 1998;14:840–3.
41. Flint JH, Wade AM, Giuliani J, Rue JP. Defining the terms acute and chronic in orthopaedic sports injuries: a systematic review. Am J Sports Med. 2014; 42:235–41.
42. Yepes H, Tang M, Morris SF, Stanish WD. Relationship between hypovascular zones and patterns of ruptures of the quadriceps tendon. J Bone Joint Surg Am. 2008;90:2135–41.
43. Balasubramaniam P, Prathap K. The effect of injection of hydrocortisone into rabbit calcaneal tendons. J Bone Joint Surg. 1972;54:729–34.
44. Kupczik F, Vialle LRG, Nobre LO, Vieira LA, Fernandes AEO. Influence of ciprofloxacin on femoral fractures healing in rats. Acta Ortop Bras. 2009;17:228–31.

Nonsurgical Treatment

40

Pablo E. Gelber, Ferran Abat, Georgios Tzoanos, and Jón Karlsson

Contents

P.E. Gelber (✉)
Department of Orthopaedic Surgery, Hospital de la Santa Creu i Sant Pau, Universitat Autònoma de Barcelona, C/Sant Quintí 89, 08041 Barcelona, Spain
e-mail: personal@drgelber.com; pablogelber@gmail.com

F. Abat
Department of Sports Orthopaedics, ReSport Clinic, Passeig Fabra i Puig 47, 4th floor, 08030 Barcelona, Spain
e-mail: abat@resportclinic.com

G. Tzoanos
Tzoanos Sports Clinic, 18 Thiseos str, 71201 Heraklion, Crete, Greece
e-mail: tzoanos@hotmail.com

J. Karlsson
Department of Orthopaedics, Sahlgrenska University Hospital, Sahlgrenska Academy, Gothenburg University, Gothenburg, Sweden
e-mail: jon.karlsson@telia.com

40.1 Introduction

Despite the physiological adaptation of the tendons to different loads [1, 2], tendinopathy is a clinical problem of great magnitude, and it is growing in terms of prevalence [3]. Tendon injuries including tendinopathy represent approximately 50% of all sports injuries [3, 4]. The traditional description of "tendonitis" as an inflammatory process is now obsolete, as several publications [5, 6] have shown that the pathological process of the tendon is mainly degenerative (tendinosis). This is justified by the absence of inflammatory cells, the presence of areas of collagen degeneration, myxoid degeneration and an increase in ground substance and the condition is associated with the failure of the tendon repair process [5, 6].

Tendinopathy is characterised by prolonged pain and is often activity related. Athletes usually respond poorly to most conservative modalities. Different pathologies like tendinosis, paratendonitis, calcifications or partial ruptures are often found in the same tendon. This indicates that there is neither a single aetiology nor a single pathogenesis that is able to explain the tendon pain [7].

Most tendinopathies in the lower limbs involve the Achilles (Fig. 40.1) or patellar tendons

J. Espregueira-Mendes et al. (eds.), *Injuries and Health Problems in Football*,
DOI 10.1007/978-3-662-53924-8_40

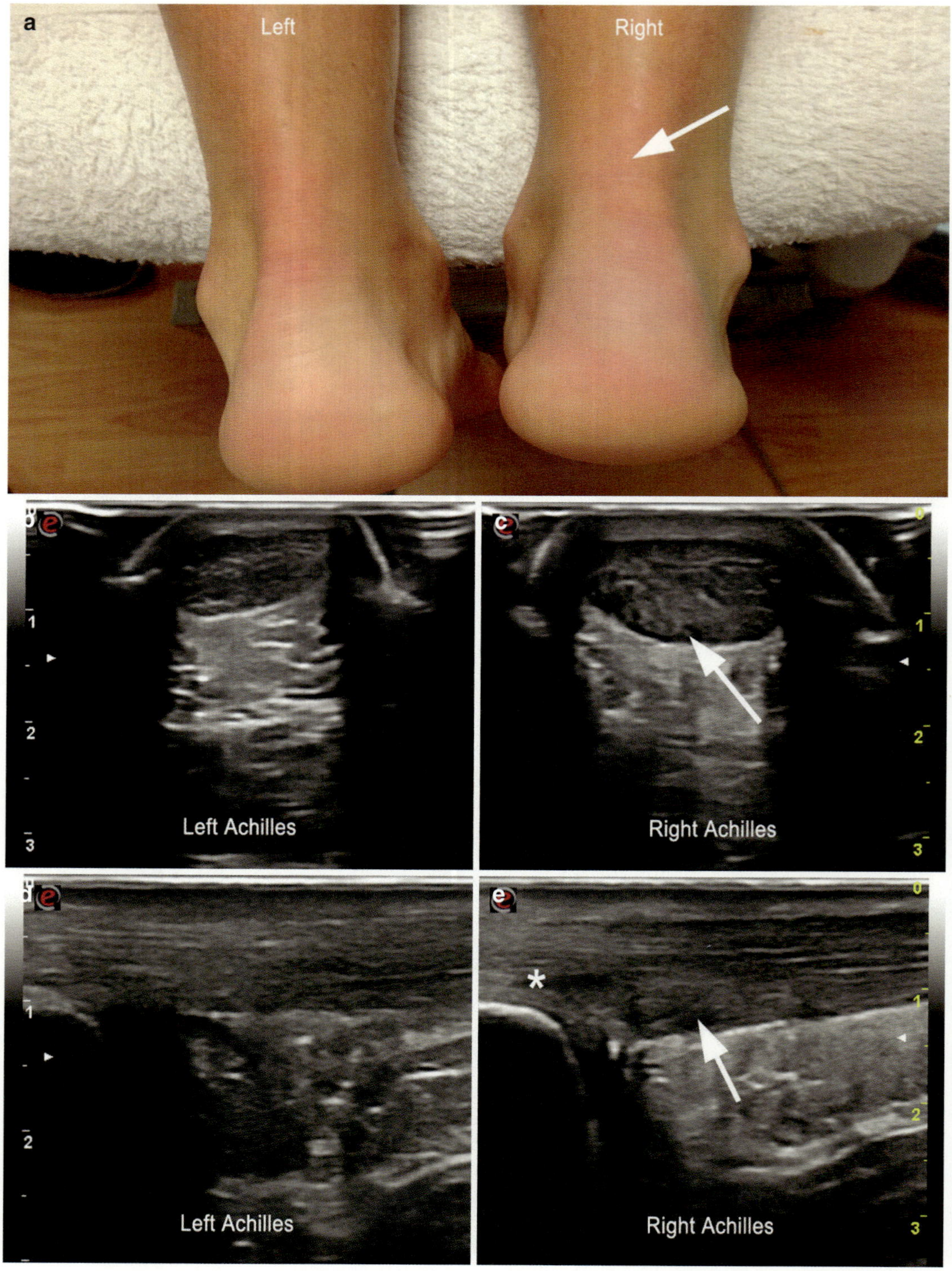

Fig. 40.1 Achilles tendinopathy. (**a**) Clinical aspect; difference between the thickened and swollen injured tendon (*right* side, *white arrow*) and the noninjured tendon (*left* side). (**b–e**) High-definition ultrasound study; transverse (**b, c**) and longitudinal views (**d, e**). US images revealed considerable thickening of the tendon (*white arrows*) in combination with hypoechoic zones (*)

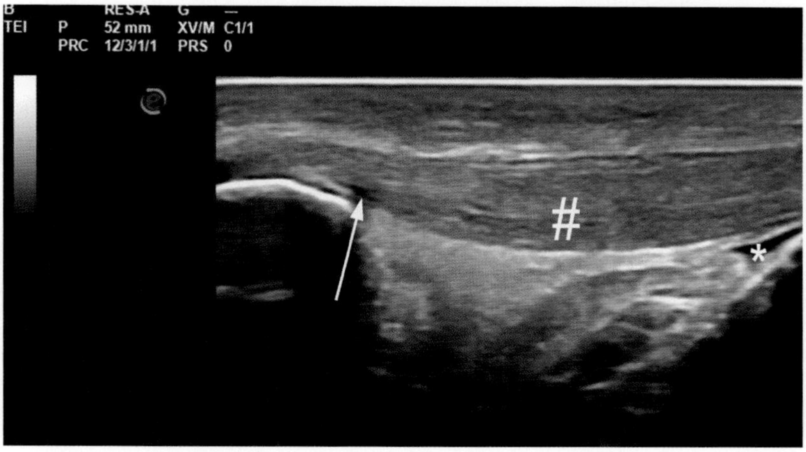

Fig. 40.2 High-definition ultrasound image showing patellar tendinopathy. Substantial tendon thickening was detected, with a width of 9.3 mm and hypoechoic zones (*arrow*)

(Fig. 40.2) [8]. Different studies [9–11] have reported a prevalence of patellar tendinopathy in football players of between 3% and 23%, with a recurrence rate as high as 20%. A similar scenario has been described for Achilles tendinopathy [12, 13].

Other tendinopathies in football players include the following:

- Proximal hamstring tendinopathy, which is localised in the lower gluteal area [14]. In some cases, an injury to the myotendinous union of the hamstring muscles may lead to a sciatic nerve irritation that can worsen the pain of the tendinopathy [15]
- Adductor longus tendinopathy resulting from rapid accelerations or decelerations, changes of direction and kicking [16]
- Injury to the flexor hallucis longus (FHL) related to overuse and in some cases related to trauma, such as an ankle sprain [17]

Tendinopathy is usually characterised by progressive tendon pain, tenderness to palpation, in combination with articular pain, which leads to the recurrent or long-standing impairment of athletic performance. A diagnosis can be made by ultrasound [18] and/or magnetic resonance imaging.

There are multiple therapeutic options for the treatment of tendon injuries [19]. Since the underlying pathology of chronic tendinopathy can be defined as a "defect healing response", the treatment should aim to stimulate the regeneration of the tendon, pain modulation and the restoration of normal biomechanics [19–21].

In this chapter, an update on the current conservative treatment of lower limb tendinopathies in football players is given.

Conventional conservative treatments have been used to reduce pain and inflammation [2, 10, 19–21]. This treatment includes rest and/or activity modification, cold, stretching, braces, physiotherapy and biomechanical correction. The treatment is usually given in the acute setting. However, these techniques do not restore the changes in the ultrastructure of the tendon [22–24], because the structuring and maturation of collagen fibres require mechanical stress, physiological stimulus and time.

40.2 Nonsteroidal Anti-inflammatory Drugs

The aim of nonsteroidal anti-inflammatory drugs (NSAIDs) is to reduce inflammation by inhibiting the synthesis of inflammatory factors (inflammatory cells, prostaglandins, interleukins and so on), and their use has been widespread in the management of tendinopathy for years [25, 26]. NSAIDs affect the activity of tenocytes and glycosaminoglycan synthesis [26]. A study showed that it is possible to block the release of prostaglandins by blocking the COX with NSAIDs, leading to a decrease in the cellular production of PGE2 [26].

40.3 Glucocorticoids

The literature suggests that the majority of patients may experience a short-term improvement in terms of pain and/or function. On the other hand, patients will face a high risk of relapse at midterm and side-effects that may even lead to a tendon rupture [27–29]. In addition, two recent systematic reviews reported poorer results after the use of glucocorticoids compared with no intervention or placebo treatment at medium- and long-term follow-ups [28, 29].

Despite the frequent use of corticosteroids to treat acute tendinopathies, scientific evidence reveals important damage to cellularity and tendon structure with these infiltrations [29].

40.4 Orthopaedic Support Devices

Orthopaedic devices (e.g. braces) are widely used in the conservative treatment of tendinopathy. However, there is no evidence to support their use [30]. The use of insoles in some cases of biomechanical imbalance might have a beneficial effect on the outcome of tendinopathies.

40.5 Eccentric Exercises

Eccentric exercise programmes have been proposed as a key element of rehabilitation after tendon injuries [31–35]. They are supposedly able to counteract the response of defect healing, by promoting the creation of collagen fibres within the tendon [9–12, 25]. The literature emphasises the importance of controlled balance to load [33, 35].

The "continuum" physiological model proposed by Cook et al. [7] in tendinopathy provides a basis for the protocol to be performed depending on the current clinical presentation. The protocol consists of 3 sets of 15 repetitions, performed twice a day, 7 days a week for 12 weeks.

An up-to-date study by Romero-Rodriguez et al. [35] demonstrated that eccentric overload using isoinertial training devices (Yoyo™) produces improved muscle function and pain reduction in patients with patellar tendinopathy.

40.6 Extracorporeal Shock Wave Therapy

Several clinical trials have evaluated the use of extracorporeal shock wave therapy (ESWT) for the treatment of patients with chronic tendinopathy, but the results have been inconsistent [36–40]. Multiple variables are associated with this therapy [41]:

- Type of shock wave generator (electrohydraulic, electromagnetic or piezoelectric)
- Wave type (radial or focal)
- Intensity (total energy per shock waves/session)
- Frequency
- Protocol of application and repetitions

One of the important effects of ESWT on tendinopathy that can produce an analgesic effect is the inhibition of nociception with the release of endorphins and an increase in the permeability of the cell membranes of neurons [40]. Evidence of the effectiveness of ESWT in the treatment of tendinopathy is inconsistent [38]. However, it is widely used after sports injuries. It appears that the combination of treatments may have a synergistic effect and lead to better results [40, 42]. A recent study revealed better results by combining ESWT and eccentric exercises than those obtained with eccentric exercises alone [42].

40.7 Sclerosing Injections

Based on the theory that neovascularisation is frequently observed in tendinopathies [43], the use of polidocanol (a vascular sclerosing agent) has been proposed [44]. Polidocanol is used to sclerose areas of increased intratendinous blood flow, which is sometimes called "neovascularisation". This can be observed [43] using high-resolution ultrasound with Doppler colour.

Some studies have reported beneficial effects from the use of polidocanol for patellar tendinopathy, tennis elbow or Achilles tendinopathy [44–46].

40.8 High-Volume Image-Guided Injection (HVIGI)

High-volume image-guided injection (HVIGI) is based on the injection of large volumes of saline solution, corticosteroids or anaesthetics that make the neovessels stretch, break or occlude [47, 48]. This occlusion or interruption of the neovessels may also affect their accompanying innervation [49, 50].

HVIGI with aprotinin produced a significant improvement in both pain and function in a 12-month short-term follow-up [50].

40.9 US-Guided Intratendon Application of Galvanic Current

In recent years, the ultrasound-guided intratendon application of galvanic current (Fig. 40.3) has been introduced. One of these techniques is intratissue percutaneous electrolysis (EPI®), which has become more relevant in the scientific literature [51–53], given the good results produced in the treatment of refractory tendon injuries in comparison with other previous nonsurgical treatments.

The application of ultrasound-guided intratissue percutaneous electrolysis produces a nonthermal electrochemical reaction centred on degenerated tissue (tendinosis). This produces a controlled local inflammatory reaction that may lead to the regeneration of damaged tissue [52]. Intratissue percutaneous electrolysis produces a localised organic reaction. The subsequent regeneration of the affected tissue is followed by the production of new immature collagen fibres that become mature by means of eccentric stimulus [51, 53]. This has shown beneficial effects in the short and long term in terms of pain and function.

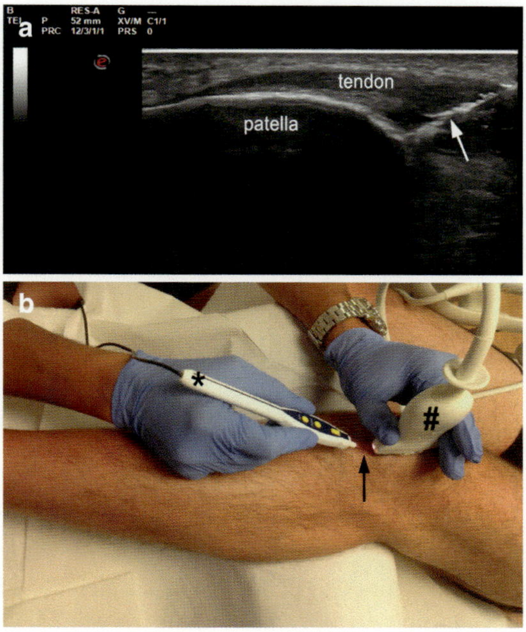

Fig. 40.3 (**a**) High-definition ultrasound during intratendon application of galvanic current. The arrow shows the hyperechogenic image produced by the 0.3 mm needle during the galvanic current flow. (**b**) Clinical application. Galvanic current device (*) and a 0.3 mm needle (*arrow*). A US device (#) during the procedure improved the accuracy and effectiveness of the technique

40.10 Platelet-Rich Plasma

Injections of platelet-rich plasma (PRP) have been used for the treatment of tendinopathy (Fig. 40.4). The aim of PRP treatment is to provide cellular and humoral mediators to induce healing in areas of degeneration [54]. PRP is a widespread treatment option for the treatment of chronic tendon injuries, and its beneficial effects have been demonstrated in several studies [55–58].

A recent experimental study showed that the use of PRP in tendinopathy produced an increase in fibroblasts and bone marrow stem cells. Cell proliferation was twice as high, and the PRP-treated group also showed a significant increase in type I and III collagen when compared with the control group [57]. Another in vitro study in humans showed that, following the application of PRP, there was increase in cellular proliferation, collagen production in tenocytes, an overexpression of the receptor of vascular endothelial

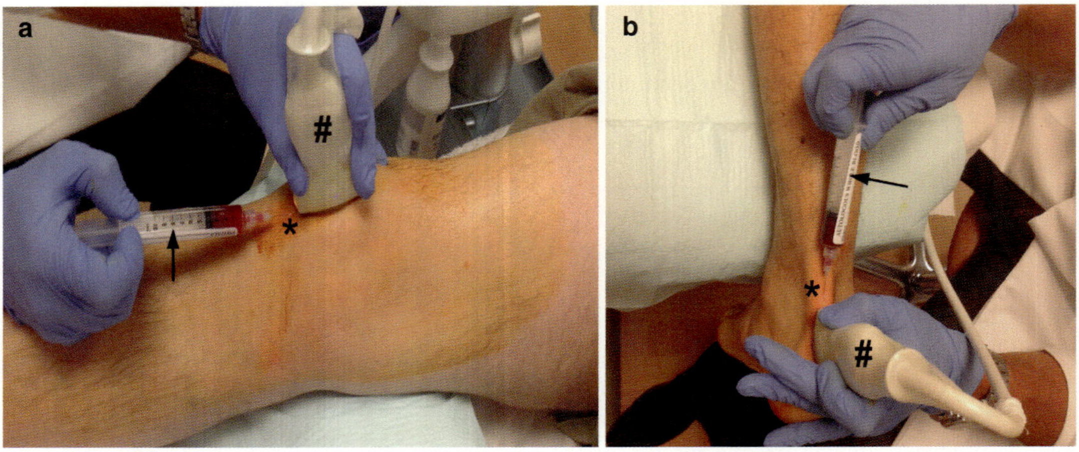

Fig. 40.4 Ultrasound-guided application of PRP (*arrow*) in a patellar (**a**) and in an Achilles tendon (**b**). Using a US-guided (#) technique allows for a more accurate placement of the PRP into the tendons (*)

growth factor-A (VEGF-A) and an increase in the concentration of transforming growth factor beta (TGF-B), indicating an increase in the production of type I and III collagen [58]. Despite these experimental findings, the huge differences between different techniques for preparing PRP should be highlighted [59]. This leads to different volumes and concentrations of platelets, preactivated or non-preactivated preparations, the presence of leukocytes and differences in the number of injections and the exact interval between injections [59]. With the current research, it is difficult to draw conclusions about the effectiveness of PRP treatment for tendinopathy [60].

40.11 Others Modalities

Other proposed treatments, such as ultrasound (US), deep transverse friction massage (DTFM) or acupuncture [31, 61, 62], have reported disappointing and widely questioned results. Finally, it has recently been proposed that adult stem cells would be good candidates for the regeneration of tendons [63]. It has been suggested that they differentiate into tenocytes and that they would subsequently be involved in the healing process by producing collagen and remodelling the extracellular matrix. Although in vitro research has produced encouraging results, this form of treatment is still the subject of research, and its clinical benefits remain uncertain.

Considering the various conservative treatment options that are available, an algorithm for the nonsurgical treatment of lower limb tendinopathies in football players is suggested (Fig. 40.5).

40.12 Discussion

Multiple techniques have been described for the treatment of lower limb tendinopathies/tendinosis and, although some of them [19, 51] are emerging as the most accepted treatment option, more randomized controlled trials (RCTs) are still needed clearly to establish the treatment protocol that is preferable. Although the authors suggest a treatment algorithm, there is insufficient evidence from high-level RCTs to draw any strong conclusions.

Doubts have mainly centred on the fact that there are few controlled prospective studies that analyse all the aspects of tendinosis and few studies that investigate the early stages of these processes and their healing mechanisms [5–7]. The exact mechanism by which tendinopathy develops in humans is not yet clearly understood. Despite its prevalence, the precise pathogenic mechanisms of tendinopathy are not clear [64].

One of the clinical effects that eccentric training might have in tendinopathy relates to pain modulation [32]. However, there is little evidence

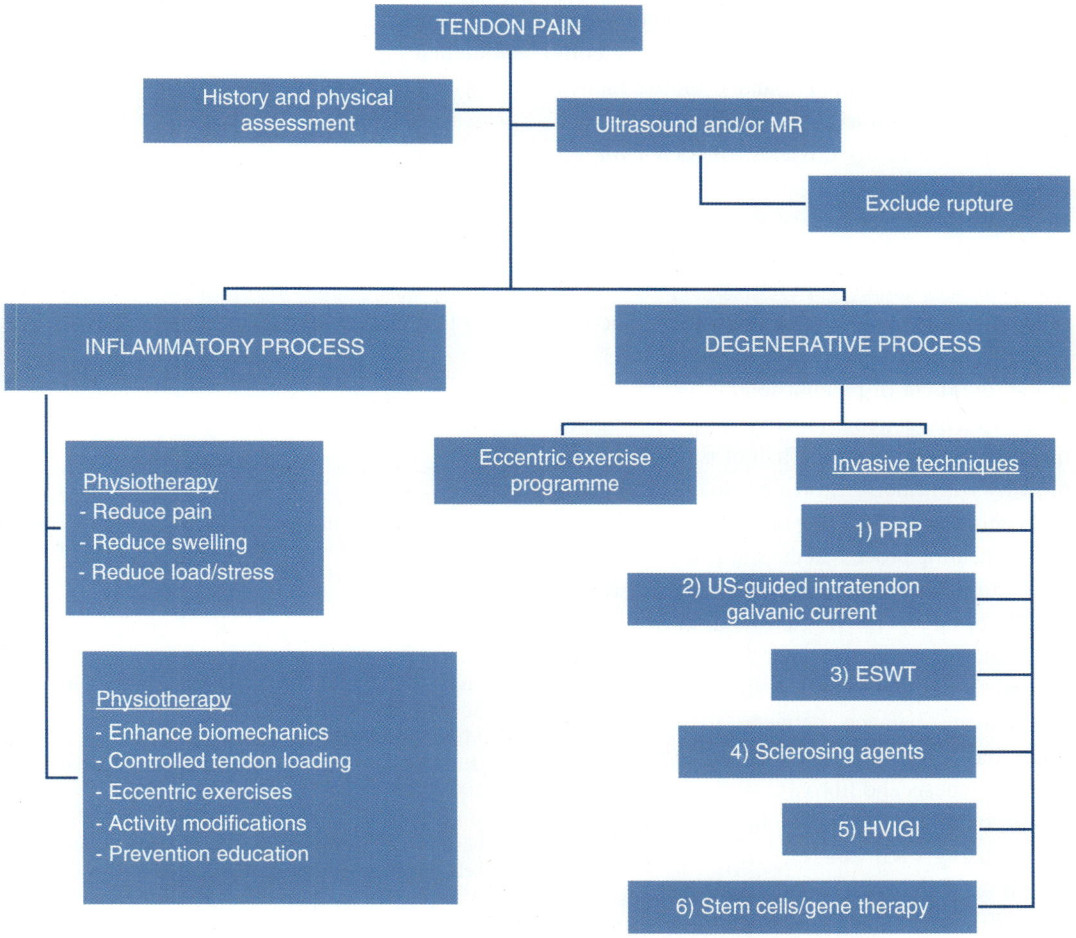

Fig. 40.5 Conservative management algorithm for lower limb tendinopathies

to suggest that isolated eccentric exercise reduces pain in tendinopathy compared with concentric exercise.

In the treatment of patellar tendinopathy, there is conflicting evidence that eccentric exercises are superior to other load programmes, such as eccentric-concentric exercises [65–67]. Eccentric work on an inclined plane did not improve functional outcomes when it was performed during a competitive season in volleyball [66]. In another study, continuous sporting activity did not compromise clinical outcomes at 12 months, as long as the sport was introduced incrementally, ensuring minimal pain during and after loading [67]. Further studies are needed to assess the unique effects of an eccentric strengthening programme. Eccentric loading should be considered in conjunction with concentric loading, rather than isolated eccentric loading, in Achilles and patellar tendinopathy. Patients with substantial muscle weakness may benefit from a programme of progressive eccentric-concentric loading [65]. On the other hand, maximum eccentric loading may be best for some groups of patients, as it enables adaptive changes in the tendon [34, 35].

Despite the fact that eccentric muscle training has become the dominant conservative strategy in treating Achilles and patellar tendinopathy, with great results in the majority of cases, some patients do not respond to this treatment [66].

Despite more than 15 years' experience of the use of intratissue percutaneous electrolysis and its widespread deployment in sporting clubs around the world, this technique has only become popular in recent years [51–53]. While this technique focused on biological tissue recovery, complementary functional and biomechanical recovery was obtained with eccentric exercise.

In terms of the effectiveness of ESWT for tendonitis, no conclusive results can be drawn, due to unclear clinical effectiveness [68, 69]. This is consistent with a recent study that showed that ESWT had no effect in athletes with patellar tendinopathy who compete actively [38]. There is currently controversy relating to the use of ESWT in the treatment of patellar tendinitis [38, 41], as well as Achilles tendinopathy [69]. The mechanisms of the therapeutic effect of ESWT in tendinopathy with calcification are also uncertain [40].

When using PRP, the aim is to enhance the natural healing process at the site of injury through the action of growth factors (PDGF, IGF-1, VEGF, bFGF, TGF-β1, EGF and so on) to promote matrix synthesis and the healing of the injured tissue [54–56, 70]. It should be noted that the delicate balance between these cytokines might have important implications in the control of angiogenesis and fibrosis.

Although many studies have reported good results using PRP [54–58, 71, 72], others have shown no differences in comparison with a placebo [73]. At the same time, many questions have been raised about the optimal concentration of platelets, the phase of the injury during which is it better to perform the infiltration or how it should be prepared.

The use of polidocanol is based on the theory that neovascularisation is associated with the mechanism underlying tendinopathy [43, 44]. However, it is unclear whether this is a causal agent in the pathophysiology of tendinopathy [6, 7]. In fact, these "neovessels" may be associated with the ingrowth of nerves in the areas of pathological tendons [43], and it is possible that these nerve fibres are the pain generators in chronic tendinopathy. A priori, polidocanol injections may not only sclerose the veins but may also eliminate the pain nerve fibres [44, 45]. Although polidocanol injections appear to provide pain relief, the role they may play in the ultimate tendon healing is unclear. Some studies associating sclerosing injections with eccentric training have shown a decrease in pain [45]. Nonetheless, further studies are needed to evaluate its safety (possible nerve damage), effectiveness, determination of the injection protocol (volume/concentration) and the combination with other therapies.

Some authors advocate the use of HVIGI in treating refractory tendinopathy [47, 48, 50], but more randomised controlled trials are needed in order to recommend its use.

References

1. Couppé C, Kongsgaard M, Aagaard P, Hansen P, Bojsen-Moller J, Kjaer M, Magnusson SP. Habitual loading results in tendon hypertrophy and increased stiffness of the human patellar tendon. J Appl Physiol (1985). 2008;105:805–10.
2. Langberg H, Ellingsgaard H, Madsen T, Jansson J, Magnusson SP, Aagaard P, Kjaer M. Eccentric rehabilitation exercise increases peritendinous type I collagen synthesis in humans with Achilles tendinosis. Scand J Med Sci Sports. 2007;17:61–6.
3. Maffulli N, Wong J, Almekinders LC. Types and epidemiology of tendinopathy. Clin Sports Med. 2003;22:675–92.
4. Andarawis-Puri N, Flatow EL, Soslowsky LJ. Tendon basic science: development, repair, regeneration, and healing. J Orthop Res. 2015;33:780–4.
5. Alfredson H, Lorentzon R. Chronic tendon pain: no signs of chemical inflammation but high concentrations of the neurotransmitter glutamate. Implications for treatment? Curr Drug Targets. 2002;3:43–54.
6. Cook JL, Khan KM, Maffulli N, Purdam C. Overuse tendinosis, not tendinitis part 2: applying the new approach to patellar tendinopathy. Phys Sports Med. 2000;28:31–46.
7. Cook JL, Purdam CR. Is tendon pathology a continuum? A pathology model to explain the clinical presentation of load-induced tendinopathy. Br J Sports Med. 2009;43:409–16.
8. Scott A, Ashe MC. Common tendinopathies in the upper and lower extremities. Curr Sports Med Rep. 2006;5:233–41.
9. Lian OB, Engebretsen L, Bahr R. Prevalence of jumper's knee among elite athletes from different sports: a cross-sectional study. Am J Sports Med. 2005;33: 561–7.
10. Fredberg U, Bolvig L, Andersen NT. Prophylactic training in asymptomatic soccer players with ultrasonographic abnormalities in achilles and patellar tendons: the Danish super league study. Am J Sports Med. 2008;36:451–60.
11. Hägglund M, Zwerver J, Ekstrand J. Epidemiology of patellar tendinopathy in elite male soccer players. Am J Sports Med. 2011;39:1906–11.

12. Sobhani S, Dekker R, Postema K, Dijkstra PU. Epidemiology of ankle and foot overuse injuries in sports: a systematic review. Scand J Med Sci Sports. 2013;23:669–86.
13. Gajhede-Knudsen M, Ekstrand J, Magnusson H, Maffulli N. Recurrence of Achilles tendon injuries in elite male football players is more common after early return to play: an 11-year follow-up of the UEFA Champions League injury study. Br J Sports Med. 2013;47:763–8.
14. Lempainen L, Sarimo J, Mattila K, Vaittinen S, Orava S. Proximal hamstring tendinopathy: results of surgical management and histopathologic findings. Am J Sports Med. 2009;37:727–34.
15. Orava S. Hamstring syndrome. Oper Tech Sports Med. 1997;5:143–9.
16. Maffulli N, Longo UG, Spiezia F, Denaro V. Aetiology and prevention of injuries in elite young athletes. Med Sport Sci. 2011;56:187–200.
17. Corte-Real NM, Moreira RM, Guerra-Pinto F. Arthroscopic treatment of tenosynovitis of the flexor hallucis longus tendon. Foot Ankle Int. 2012;33:1108–12.
18. Brulhart L. Musculoskeletal ultrasound in the management of tendinopathy. Rev Med Suisse. 2015;11:612–5.
19. Larsson ME, Käll I, Nilsson-Helander K. Treatment of patellar tendinopathy – a systematic review of randomized controlled trials. Knee Surg Sports Traumatol Arthrosc. 2012;20:1632–46.
20. Cook JL, Khan KM. What is the most appropriate treatment for patellar tendinopathy? Br J Sports Med. 2001;35:291–4.
21. Peers KH, Lysens RJ. Patellar tendinopathy in athletes: current diagnostic and therapeutic recommendations. Sports Med. 2005;35:71–87.
22. Alfredson H. Conservative management of Achilles tendinopathy: new ideas. Foot Ankle Clin. 2005;10:321–9.
23. Fournier PE, Rappoport G. Tendinopathy: physiopathology and conservative treatment. Rev Med Suisse. 2005;1:1840–2. 1845–6
24. Glaser T, Poddar S, Tweed B, Webb CW. Clinical inquiries. What's the best way to treat Achilles tendinopathy? J Fam Pract. 2008;57:261–3.
25. Christensen B, Dandanell S, Kjaer M, Langberg H. Effect of anti-inflammatory medication on the running-induced rise in patella tendon collagen synthesis in humans. J Appl Physiol (1985). 2011;110:137–41.
26. Tsai WC, Hsu CC, Chou SW, Chung CY, Chen J, Pang JH. Effects of celecoxib on migration, proliferation and collagen expression of tendon cells. Connect Tissue Res. 2007;48:46–51.
27. Coombes BK, Bisset L, Brooks P, Khan A, Vicenzino B. Effect of corticosteroid injection, physiotherapy, or both on clinical outcomes in patients with unilateral lateral epicondylalgia: a randomized controlled trial. JAMA. 2013;309:461–9.
28. Coombes BK, Bisset L, Vicenzino B. Efficacy and safety of corticosteroid injections and other injections for management of tendinopathy: a systematic review of randomised controlled trials. Lancet. 2010;376:1751–67.
29. Dean BJ, Lostis E, Oakley T, Rombach I, Morrey ME, Carr AJ. The risks and benefits of glucocorticoid treatment for tendinopathy: a systematic review of the effects of local glucocorticoid on tendon. Semin Arthritis Rheum. 2014;43:570–6.
30. Struijs PA, Smidt N, Arola H, van Dijk CN, Buchbinder R, Assendelft WJ. Orthotic devices for tennis elbow. Cochrane Database Syst Rev. 2002: CD001821.
31. Andres BM, Murrell GA. Treatment of tendinopathy: what works, what does not, and what is on the horizon. Clin Orthop Relat Res. 2008;466:1539–54.
32. Malliaras P, Barton CJ, Reeves ND, Langberg H. Achilles and patellar tendinopathy loading programmes: a systematic review comparing clinical outcomes and identifying potential mechanisms for effectiveness. Sports Med. 2013;43:267–86.
33. Magnusson SP, Langberg H, Kjaer M. The pathogenesis of tendinopathy: balancing the response to loading. Nat Rev Rheumatol. 2010;6:262–8.
34. Alfredson H, Pietilä T, Jonsson P, Lorentzon R. Heavy-load eccentric calf muscle training for the treatment of chronic Achilles tendinosis. Am J Sports Med. 1998;26:360–6.
35. Romero-Rodriguez D, Gual G, Tesch PA. Efficacy of an inertial resistance training paradigm in the treatment of patellar tendinopathy in athletes: a case-series study. Phys Ther Sport. 2011;12:43–8.
36. Wang CJ, Ko JY, Chan YS, Weng LH, Hsu SL. Extracorporeal shockwave for chronic patellar tendinopathy. Am J Sports Med. 2007;35:972–8.
37. van Leeuwen MT, Zwerver J, van den Akker-Scheek I. Extracorporeal shockwave therapy for patellar tendinopathy: a review of the literature. Br J Sports Med. 2009;43:163–8.
38. Zwerver J, Hartgens F, Verhagen E, van der Worp H, van den Akker-Scheek I, Diercks RL. No effect of extracorporeal shockwave therapy on patellar tendinopathy in jumping athletes during the competitive season: a randomized clinical trial. Am J Sports Med. 2011;39:1191–9.
39. Rompe JD, Maffulli N. Repetitive shock wave therapy for lateral elbow tendinopathy (tennis elbow): a systematic and qualitative analysis. Br Med Bull. 2007;83:355–78.
40. Mouzopoulos G, Stamatakos M, Mouzopoulos D, Tzurbakis M. Extracorporeal shock wave treatment for shoulder calcific tendonitis: a systematic review. Skelet Radiol. 2007;36:803–11.
41. van der Worp H, van den Akker-Scheek I, van Schie H, Zwerver J. ESWT for tendinopathy: technology and clinical implications. Knee Surg Sports Traumatol Arthrosc. 2013;21:1451–8.
42. Rompe JD, Furia J, Maffulli N. Eccentric loading versus eccentric loading plus shock-wave treatment for midportion achilles tendinopathy: a randomized controlled trial. Am J Sports Med. 2009;37:463–70.

43. Alfredson H, Ohberg L, Forsgren S. Is vasculo-neural ingrowth the cause of pain in chronic Achilles tendinosis? An investigation using ultrasonography and colour Doppler, immunohistochemistry, and diagnostic injections. Knee Surg Sports Traumatol Arthrosc. 2003;11:334–8.
44. Alfredson H, Ohberg L. Neovascularisation in chronic painful patellar tendinosis-promising results after sclerosing neovessels outside the tendon challenge the need for surgery. Knee Surg Sports Traumatol Arthrosc. 2005;13:74–80.
45. Hoksrud A, Ohberg L, Alfredson H, Bahr R. Ultrasound-guided sclerosis of neovessels in painful chronic patellar tendinopathy: a randomized controlled trial. Am J Sports Med. 2006;34:1738–46.
46. Zeisig E, Fahlström M, Ohberg L, Alfredson H. Pain relief after intratendinous injections in patients with tennis elbow: results of a randomised study. Br J Sports Med. 2008;42:267–71.
47. Chan O, O'Dowd D, Padhiar N, Morrissey D, King J, Jalan R, Maffulli N, Crisp T. High volume image guided injections in chronic Achilles tendinopathy. Disabil Rehabil. 2008;30:1697–708.
48. Loppini M, Maffulli N. Conservative management of tendinopathy: an evidence-based approach. Muscles Ligaments Tendons J. 2012;1:134–7.
49. Drumm O, Chan O, Malliaras P, Morrissey D, Maffulli N. High-volume image-guided injection for recalcitrant medial collateral ligament injuries of the knee. Clin Radiol. 2014;69:e211–5.
50. Maffulli N, Spiezia F, Longo UG, Denaro V, Maffulli GD. High volume image guided injections for the management of chronic tendinopathy of the main body of the Achilles tendon. Phys Ther Sport. 2013;14:163–7.
51. Abat F, Gelber PE, Polidori F, Monllau JC, Sanchez-Ibañez JM. Clinical results after ultrasound-guided intratissue percutaneous electrolysis (EPI®) and eccentric exercise in the treatment of patellar tendinopathy. Knee Surg Sports Traumatol Arthrosc. 2015;23:1046–52.
52. Abat F, Valles SL, Gelber PE, Polidori F, Stitik TP, García-Herreros S, Monllau JC, Sanchez-Ibánez JM. Molecular repair mechanisms using the Intratissue Percutaneous Electrolysis technique in patellar tendonitis. Rev Esp Cir Ortop Traumatol. 2014;58:201–5.
53. Abat F, Diesel WJ, Gelber PE, Polidori F, Monllau JC, Sanchez-Ibañez JM. Effectiveness of the Intratissue Percutaneous Electrolysis (EPI®) technique and isoinertial eccentric exercise in the treatment of patellar tendinopathy at two years follow-up. Muscles Ligaments Tendons J. 2014;4:188–93.
54. Kon E, Filardo G, Di Martino A, Marcacci M. Platelet-rich plasma (PRP) to treat sports injuries: evidence to support its use. Knee Surg Sports Traumatol Arthrosc. 2011;19:516–27.
55. Engebretsen L, Steffen K, Alsousou J, Anitua E, Bachl N, Devilee R, Everts P, Hamilton B, Huard J, Jenoure P, Kelberine F, Kon E, Maffulli N, Matheson G, Mei-Dan O, Menetrey J, Philippon M, Randelli P, Schamasch P, Schwellnus M, Vernec A, Verrall G. IOC consensus paper on the use of platelet-rich plasma in sports medicine. Br J Sports Med. 2010;44:1072–81.
56. Foster TE, Puskas BL, Mandelbaum BR, Gerhardt MB, Rodeo SA. Platelet-rich plasma: from basic science to clinical applications. Am J Sports Med. 2009;37:2259–72.
57. Kajikawa Y, Morihara T, Sakamoto H, Matsuda K, Oshima Y, Yoshida A, Nagae M, Arai Y, Kawata M, Kubo T. Platelet-rich plasma enhances the initial mobilization of circulation-derived cells for tendon healing. J Cell Physiol. 2008;215:837–45.
58. Klein MB, Yalamanchi N, Pham H, Longaker MT, Chang J. Flexor tendon healing in vitro: effects of TGF-beta on tendon cell collagen production. J Hand Surg Am. 2002;27:615–20.
59. Leitner GC, Gruber R, Neumüller J, Wagner A, Kloimstein P, Höcker P, Körmöczi GF, Buchta C. Platelet content and growth factor release in platelet-rich plasma: a comparison of four different systems. Vox Sang. 2006;91:135–9.
60. Dragoo JL, Wasterlain AS, Braun HJ, Nead KT. Platelet-rich plasma as a treatment for patellar tendinopathy: a double-blind, randomized controlled trial. Am J Sports Med. 2014;42:610–8.
61. Loew LM, Brosseau L, Tugwell P, Wells GA, Welch V, Shea B, Poitras S, De Angelis G, Rahman P. Deep transverse friction massage for treating lateral elbow or lateral knee tendinitis. Cochrane Database Syst Rev. 2014;11:CD003528.
62. Green S, Buchbinder R, Hetrick S. Acupuncture for shoulder pain. Cochrane Database Syst Rev. 2005:CD005319.
63. Chong AK, Ang AD, Goh JC, Hui JH, Lim AY, Lee EH, Lim BH. Bone marrow-derived mesenchymal stem cells influence early tendon-healing in a rabbit achilles tendon model. J Bone Joint Surg Am. 2007;89:74–81.
64. Abate M, Silbernagel KG, Siljeholm C, Di Iorio A, De Amicis D, Salini V, Werner S, Paganelli R. Pathogenesis of tendinopathies: inflammation or degeneration? Arthritis Res Ther. 2009;11:235.
65. Jonsson P, Alfredson H. Superior results with eccentric compared to concentric quadriceps training in patients with jumper's knee: a prospective randomised study. Br J Sports Med. 2005;39:847–50.
66. Visnes H, Hoksrud A, Cook J, Bahr R. No effect of eccentric training on jumper's knee in volleyball players during the competitive season: a randomized clinical trial. Clin J Sport Med. 2005;15:227–34.
67. Silbernagel KG, Thomeé R, Eriksson BI, Karlsson J. Continued sports activity, using a pain-monitoring model, during rehabilitation in patients with Achilles tendinopathy: a randomized controlled study. Am J Sports Med. 2007;35:897–06.
68. Vulpiani MC, Vetrano M, Savoia V, Di Pangrazio E, Trischitta D, Ferretti A. Jumper's knee treatment with extracorporeal shock wave therapy: a long-term

follow-up observational study. J Sports Med Phys Fitness. 2007;47:323–8.
69. Furia JP. High-energy extracorporeal shock wave therapy as a treatment for insertional Achilles tendinopathy. Am J Sports Med. 2006;34:733–40.
70. Rabago D, Best TM, Zgierska AE, Zeisig E, Ryan M, Crane D. A systematic review of four injection therapies for lateral epicondylosis: prolotherapy, polidocanol, whole blood and platelet-rich plasma. Br J Sports Med. 2009;43:471–81.
71. Creaney L, Wallace A, Curtis M, Connell D. Growth factor-based therapies provide additional benefit beyond physical therapy in resistant elbow tendinopathy: a prospective, single-blind, randomised trial of autologous blood injections versus platelet-rich plasma injections. Br J Sports Med. 2011;45:966–71.
72. de Jonge S, de Vos RJ, Weir A, van Schie HT, Bierma-Zeinstra SM, Verhaar JA, Weinans H, Tol JL. One-year follow-up of platelet-rich plasma treatment in chronic Achilles tendinopathy: a double-blind randomized placebo-controlled trial. Am J Sports Med. 2011;39:1623–9.
73. de Vos RJ, Weir A, van Schie HT, Bierma-Zeinstra SM, Verhaar JA, Weinans H, Tol JL. Platelet-rich plasma injection for chronic Achilles tendinopathy: a randomized controlled trial. JAMA. 2010;303:144–9.

Part X

Stress Injuries in the Lower Limb

Stress Fractures: Current Concepts

41

João Espregueira-Mendes, André Costa,
Pedro Pessoa, and C. Niek Van Dijk

Contents

J. Espregueira-Mendes (✉)
Clínica do Dragão, Espregueira-Mendes Sports Centre – FIFA Medical Centre of Excellence, Porto, Portugal

Dom Henrique Research Centre, Porto, Portugal

Department of Orthopaedics, Minho University, Minho, Portugal

3B's Research Group–Biomaterials, Biodegradables and Biomimetics, University of Minho, Headquarters of the European Institute of Excellence on Tissue Engineering and Regenerative Medicine, AvePark, Parque de Ciência e Tecnologia, Zona Industrial da Gandra, 4805-017 Barco, Guimarães, Portugal

ICVS/3B's–PT Government Associate Laboratory, Braga/Guimarães, Portugal

A. Costa (✉)
Centro Hospitalar Vila Nova de Gaia/ Espinho E.P.E., Gaia, Portugal

Clínica do Dragão, Espregueira-Mendes Sports Centre - FIFA Medical Centre of Excellence, Porto, Portugal
e-mail: amckosta@gmail.com

P. Pessoa
Hospital Ortopédico Sant'iago do Outao, Setúbal, Portugal

C.N. Van Dijk
Department of Orthopaedic Surgery, Academic Medical Center Amsterdam, Meibergdreef 9, 1105 AZ Amsterdam, The Netherlands

41.1 Introduction

A stress fracture is, by definition, a partial or complete solution of continuity in the bone, which results from excessive repeated loads at submaximal intensity, resulting in greater bone reabsorption without equivalent bone ingrowth.

For the correct understanding of the stress fractures, it is necessary to acknowledge the bone biology and its response to stress forces. Bone is a dynamic tissue, which reacts to shear and compression forces, leading to bone transformation according to Wolff's Law in a constant remodeling and turnover process. It is the disturbance in the equilibrium between bone resorption and regeneration that leads to injury.

A stress fracture was first described by Breithaupt [1] in 1855, as an overuse fracture seen in military recruits. Soldiers reported plantar pain and edema following long marches. In the athletic population, the first clinical description

J. Espregueira-Mendes et al. (eds.), *Injuries and Health Problems in Football*,
DOI 10.1007/978-3-662-53924-8_41

was given by Devas [2] in 1958, based on the results of plain X-rays, correlating the radiological patterns with the pain and impairment.

Stress fractures are among the most common overuse injuries in physically active individuals [3, 4]. These bone injuries can affect almost any bone, although the vast majority of these fractures (up to 95%) will occur in the lower extremity [5, 6]. The most common locations for stress fractures include the tibia, metatarsals, fibula, and navicular bones; less common locations include the femur, pelvis, and sacrum.

It is essential to perform an early and accurate diagnosis, because it will be critical to promptly assess the patient, minimize the period of recovery, optimize athlete performance, and prevent injury relapse. High-risk stress fractures are particularly important to diagnose (i.e., tension side of femoral neck, tarsal navicular, and base of the fifth metatarsal) mainly because of their long recovery period.

Football injuries are commonly divided into traumatic injuries with an acute onset and overuse injuries with a gradual onset [7, 8]. Stress fractures in football players are particularly difficult to diagnose and treat, because of the specificity of the modality and unique psycho-bio-social characteristics of the football player.

The most prevalent site of stress fractures in football remains in the lesser metatarsal [9, 10].

41.2 Pathophysiology

Stress fractures can be divided in insufficiency fractures and fatigue fractures. Insufficiency fractures occur when a normal deforming force is applied to the bone with low elastic resistance (i.e., osteoporotic fractures). In contrast, fatigue fractures occur when the bone suffers an exacerbated and repeated or cyclic deforming force, although maintaining its normal elastic resistance.

Intrinsic bone factors that affect the risk of stress fracture include porosity, mineralization, density, trabecular and cortical architecture, and fatigue microdamage, which reduces the elastic modulus.

There are various theoretical models justifying the occurrence of stress fractures. Bennell [9] proposed two different models to explain the appearance of specific fractures. The primary microdamage hypothesis: particular bone sites are maximally stressed, and injury occurs when microdamage is too extensive to be repaired by normal remodeling. Conversely, the primary remodeling hypothesis is based in an accelerated bone remodeling, secondary to genetic factors, bone strain arising from exercise, systemic or reproductive hormones influence, and poor dietary intake. Since osteoclastic resorption always precedes formation in the remodeling process, microdamage may occur at these focal areas of weakness; when the bone is stimulated to submaximal forces, the remodeling process is accelerated, exposing the athlete to temporary periods of local weakness. The fracture will occur when muscle and tendon forces exceed the level of bone resistance. Other theories are based on mechanical factors as rapid load changes or pressure/area changes [11] and negative catabolism due to insufficient dieting [12].

Knowledge of the pathophysiology of bone is essential to understand the multifactorial etiology of overuse fractures that include biomechanical, hormonal, nutritional, and genetic factors. Attention should be paid to the identification of these factors in an attempt to prevent this type of injury in athletes.

Female athletes may present higher predisposition for a stress injury because of their unique hormonal environment, and other anatomic and gender factors [10, 13, 14].

41.3 Epidemiology

Stress injuries are common among athletes and military recruits, accounting for approximately 10% of overuse injuries [3].

A number of series of stress fractures among athletes have been described in the literature, but only several reports have described in detail the distribution of stress fractures of the upper and lower extremities and trunk. These studies have generally shown that the tibia is the most common site of stress fractures, followed by the metatarsal and tarsal bones [15–18]. Running activities, especially track and distance running, have been the most common sporting activities that have resulted in stress fractures [16, 19].

These injuries are more frequent in the lower extremity and often related with intrinsic factors such as age, gender, bone alignment, hormonal and nutritional, and bone density and also with extrinsic factors (training, type of shoes, type of modality) [20].

Approximately, 69% of stress fractures occur in runners, although their incidence is not negligible in football players. Aitken et al. [21] preformed an epidemiologic study describing the characteristics of all sports-related fractures; football was the first sports activity causing traumatic bone fractures and accounted for 35.5% of sports-related fractures. In contrast, stress fractures in elite footballers show low prevalence representing only 0.5% of all injuries. Ekstrand study group [8] evaluated prospectively 2379 male football players (54 professional football teams) between 2001 and 2009 and determined an incidence of stress fractures of 0.04/1000 h of football exposure, meaning that an elite team with 25 players in their main squad can expect one stress fracture every three seasons. In the same study, the majority (78%) of stress fractures in elite football players will affect the fifth metatarsal bone. Additionally, it seems there is a higher risk of developing stress injury during preseason training period and that younger players, with juvenile bone structure, are more exposed to stress lesions.

It has been suggested that the sites of occurrence of stress fractures in athletes are activity related and that specific anatomical sites are endemic to certain sports [18, 22–27]. The repeat injury mechanism in football involves rapid changes in direction and rapid acceleration, and de-acceleration movements may be the cause of high-energy bending momentum applied to the fifth metatarsal.

41.4 Risk Factors

Armstrong [28] in 2004 was the first to compare military men and women with stress fracture to uninjured controls matched by gender, age, body mass index (BMI), and preadmission aerobic physical performance and identified sustained negative energy balance as a major risk factor for stress fracture injury, leading to increased muscular fatigue, reduced bone collagen synthesis, and reduced muscular support of the long bones of the lower extremity in recruits. The most common site of stress fracture was the tibia, and female gender experienced a higher relative incidence of stress fractures, probably to concomitant hypoestrogenic state [29, 30].

Other studies [13, 31, 32] showed that the osteoporosis seen in the female athlete triad is a consequence of endothelial dysfunction, and it is related with cardiovascular effects, stress fractures, and musculoskeletal injuries. Female athletes presenting with a stress fracture should always be evaluated for female athlete triad.

Bennell [33, 34] analyzed the ground force reaction during running and concluded that physically active males with smaller bones and less resistance to bending moments are at greater risk of stress fracture than those with larger bones and greater resistance. However, in females this correlation is not linear and may indicate that other risk factors are more important in women.

Intrinsic risk factors include mechanical factors such as bone density, skeletal alignment, and body size and composition; physiological factors such as bone turnover rate, flexibility, and muscular strength and endurance; as well as hormonal and nutritional factors [35]. Extrinsic risk factors include mechanical factors such as practice surface, footwear, external loading, and physical training parameters [36].

Fujitaka [37] conducted a longitudinal study to examine the physical characteristics and environmental factors associated with college football players who sustained a fifth metatarsal stress fracture. In the injury group, toe grip strength was significantly weaker than that in the noninjury group. In addition, the logistic regression analysis suggested that toe grip strength might be associated with fifth metatarsal stress fracture injuries. There was a significantly higher frequency of fifth metatarsal stress fracture injuries affecting the nondominant leg compared with the dominant leg.

Although stress fractures result from repeated loading, the exact contribution of training factors (volume, intensity, surface) has not been clearly established [3–6, 9, 38]. From what we do know, menstrual disturbances, caloric restriction, lower bone density, muscle weakness, and leg length

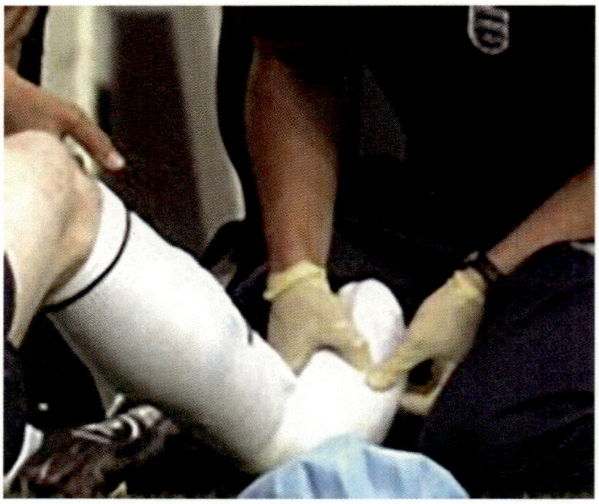

Fig. 41.1 Bone tenderness in the base of the fifth metatarsal

differences are risk factors for stress fracture (Fig. 41.1).

41.5 Clinical Presentation

The clinical onset of a stress fracture is characterized by progressive tenderness, which in an early stage may be indolent and purely neglected, only appearing after escalade in training intensity and frequency. Typically, there is an insidious onset of activity-related pain. Continuing exercise, the pain may well become more severe or occur at an earlier stage of the sports practice [1]. Often, the athlete has a history of an increase or change in the training pattern. Vague symptoms can lead to delayed diagnosis, increase of complications, impairment, and sub-achievement [39, 40]. As the stress reaction progresses to stress fracture, the symptom may turn to persistent pain even during ambulation.

History of the patient's pain and its relation to exercise is very important to determine the presence of predisposing factors. On physical examination, the most obvious feature is localized bony tenderness. Occasionally, redness, swelling, or periosteal thickening may be present at the site of the stress fracture. Special tests such as the hop test, fulcrum test, and hyperextension test should be performed as indicated by the suspected site. The diagnosis of stress fracture is primarily a clinical one; however, complementary exams will be needed to confirm the injury. Various imaging techniques can be used to confirm the diagnosis and in the majority of stress fractures, there will be no obvious abnormality on plain radiograms.

41.6 Diagnosis and Grading

Diagnosis of stress fractures is a difficult task; it takes clinical presumption, and despite positive clinical exam signs, complementary exams are mandatory. The main quest is to determine the severity and prognosis of the injury [41].

Imaging modalities, including radiography, triple-phase technetium 99 m polyphosphonate bone scanning, magnetic resonance imaging (MRI), computed tomography (CT), thermography, and tuning forks, have been used to diagnose and evaluate stress fractures. Despite the recent advances in diagnostic musculoskeletal ultrasound, its use for stress fracture diagnosis is limited. However, the relative ability of each modality to aid in the distinction of injury severity and prediction of recovery has not been comprehensively addressed. Radiography has been shown to have low sensitivity in the acute phase of bone stress injury, but it is commonly ordered to rule out other abnormalities. Technetium bone scanning historically has been considered the reference standard in the diagnosis of bone stress injury; however, specificity can be low, and positive findings in asymptomatic locations, including positive in athletes considered to be functionally healed, can be clinically misleading. MRI is increasingly recognized to have high sensitivity and specificity for bone stress injury, owing to its ability to depict subtle edema [42]. Reports of diagnosis of stress fracture with CT have also appeared in more recent literature; however, this modality is used less frequently in clinical practice. While bone stress injury grading systems have been reported for radiography, technetium bone scanning, MRI, and CT, their relative relationship to healing time has not been established (Fig. 41.2).

There is a negative relationship between clinical severity and time to healing as was the relationship between clinical severity and imaging severity.

Clinical and pain assessment is an unreliable marker of healing, and follow-up MRI and symptom resolution may be indicated to guide recommendations for the return to training.

The use of MRI evaluation allows the precise assessment of a repetitive injury to bone by allowing a more accurate diagnosis and the severity at MRI, and time to healing suggests the MRI grading system may have predictive utility (Fig. 41.3).

Arendt study group [43] showed MRI evaluation had predictive value in estimating the duration of disability, by defining a low grade of stress fracture (i.e., grade 1 and 2) and a high grade of stress fracture (i.e., grade 3 and 4). This grading system might have direct implications in the management of stress fractures, allowing more individualized treatment for the elite athletes [13].

The classification of stress fractures as high risk or low risk is important in the management of such injuries [17, 32, 44, 45]. Regarding prognosis and optimal treatment of a stress fracture cannot be answered without knowing its location, the extent of the structural damage, and the presence or absence of nonunion. High-risk fractures

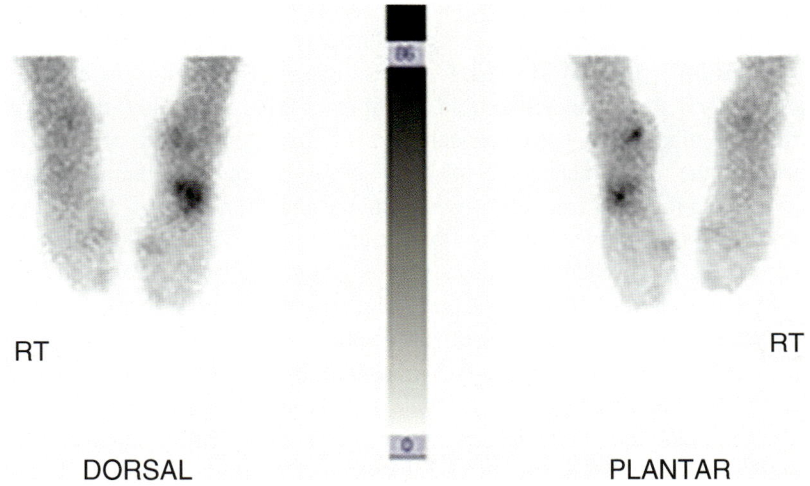

Fig. 41.2 Bone scan presenting stress fracture in the base of the fifth metatarsal bone

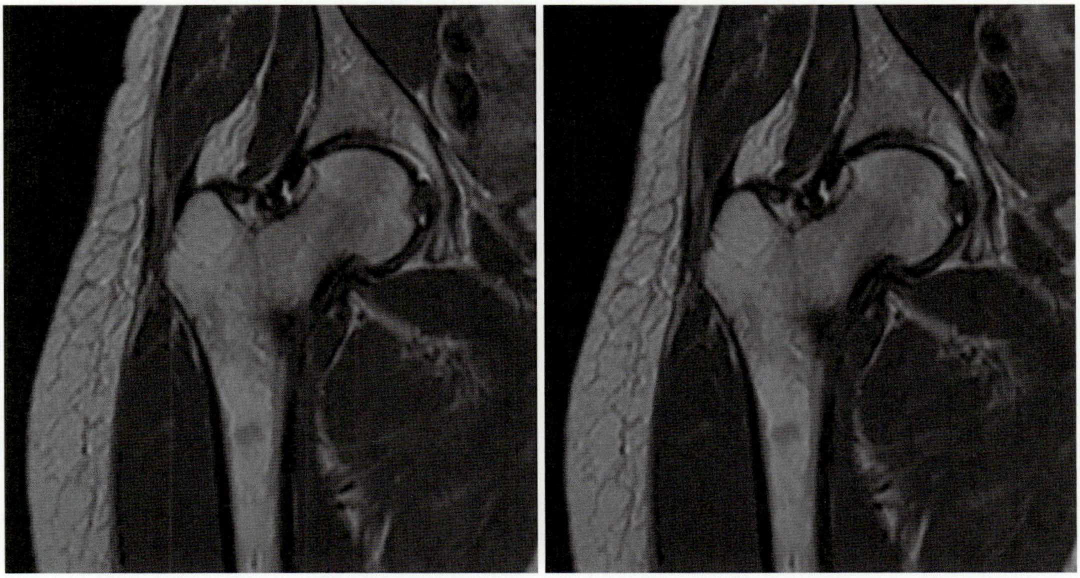

Fig. 41.3 MRI presenting proximal femur stress fracture in a male football player

include those likely to progress to complete fracture, delayed union, or nonunion, those that require surgical repair, those that require assisted weight bearing or non-weight bearing, and those occurring on the tension side of the natural biomechanical axis. The sites for high-risk fractures include the fifth metatarsal, the anterior tibia, the tarsal navicular, the femoral neck (tension side), the patella, the medial malleolus, the talar neck, and the first metatarsal sesamoids.

Fractures with a favorable natural history, those that respond well to nonsurgical management, those that allow for unassisted weight bearing, and those that occur on the compression side of the natural biomechanical axis are considered low risk [46]. Sites for low-risk fractures include the femoral shaft, the medial tibia, the fibula, the ribs, the ulnar shaft, the calcaneus, and the first through the fourth metatarsals [47].

Among the most frequently used system is the Fredericson grading system for tibial stress fractures using MRI. The Fredericson grading system [48] defines a grade 1 injury as periosteal edema only, a grade 2 injury as bone marrow edema visible on T2-weighted images only, a grade 3 injury as bone marrow edema visible on both T1-weighted and T2-weighted images, and a grade 4 injury as intracortical signal abnormalities (Table 41.1).

Table 41.1 Stress fractures MRI grading system [43]

Grade	Radiographic finding	Bone scan finding	MRI finding
1	Normal	Poorly defined area	Increased activity on STIR image
2	Normal	More intense	Poor definition on STIR and T2-weighted images
3	Discrete line	Sharp area of uptake	No focal or fusiform cortical break on T1- and T2-weighted images
4	Fracture or periosteal reaction	More intense localized transcortical uptake	Fracture line on T1- and T2-weighted images

41.7 Current Treatment Options

41.7.1 Nonoperative Treatment

Often the treatment of most stress fractures is relatively straightforward and includes decreasing activity and training intensity and sometimes weight bearing restriction or immobilization. However, patients presenting with high-risk stress fractures, such as displaced femoral neck stress fractures and fifth metatarsal base stress fractures, are more likely to have complications such as nonunion and will need surgical treatment [29, 47, 49, 50].

A two-phase protocol described by Andrish [51] can be safely implemented for the treatment of most low-risk stress fractures. Phase 1 begins with pain control provided via ice, massage, physical therapy, and oral analgesic medications. The use of nonsteroidal anti-inflammatory drug (NSAIDs) should be avoided due to its potential adverse effect and delay on bone healing. Weight bearing as tolerated is allowed for daily activities, but participation in sports should be discontinued. Walking boots can be provided for athletes who are unable to ambulate without pain.

Minimal-impact aerobic activities (using elliptical devices, cycling, pool running, and antigravity treadmill) can help maintain cardiovascular fitness. Phase 2 begins when the injured athlete has been pain-free for 10–14 days. One week after the resolution of focal bony tenderness, running may be resumed at half the usual pace and distance and should gradually be increased, allowing running to the pre-injury level over 3–6 weeks under medical supervision.

The progression and type of exercise should be individualized and dictated by the patient's pain level. To prevent progression to full fracture and associated complications, complete healing must be confirmed by complementary exams before the athlete returns to play. Antigravity treadmill is an emerging technology that may be used for the management of bone stress injuries. Antigravity treadmills provide adjustable body weight support and may promote fitness for individuals performing exercise in a hypogravity environment and have potential applications in the recovery from injury or surgery [40]. Further investigations are needed to determine the exact physiologic effect of hypogravity environment in healing stress fractures and its effect on clinical outcomes.

Pulsed ultrasound, extracorporeal shock wave therapy, and capacitive electric fields (also known as bone stimulators) [40] are noninvasive techniques applied to stress fractures to promote healing and fasten recovery. Pulsed ultrasound is thought to work by inducing aggrecan and proteoglycan synthesis in chondrocytes, thus leading to increased endochondral ossification. Extracorporeal shock wave therapy is thought to work by inducing healing via causing periosteal detachment and microfractures of the trabeculae. An electric field is known to promote bone formation in vitro and in vivo which is the working theory behind capacitative electric field devices. Additional high-quality studies are needed to clarify the clinical effects of such emerging technologies.

41.7.2 Surgical Treatment

Factors such as the site of the fracture, a higher grade of fracture, and competitive participation requirements determine whether surgery is the initial treatment of choice, although indication for operative intervention is not consensual.

Management of high-risk fractures should be more aggressive. Depending on imaging results, most of these require prompt surgery, otherwise several weeks of non-weight-bearing immobilization and rehabilitation, with high risk of disability and delayed return to sports.

A subset of stress fractures can present a high risk for progression to complete fracture, delayed union, or nonunion [44, 52]. Specific sites for this type of stress fracture are the femoral neck (tension side), the patella, the anterior cortex of the tibia, the medial malleolus, the talus, the tarsal navicular, the fifth metatarsal, and the great toe sesamoids. Tensile forces and the relative avascularity at the site of a stress-induced fracture often lead to poor healing. Therefore, high-risk stress fractures require aggressive treatment.

Begly study group [53] analyzed elite basketball professional players with stress fractures in the base of the fifth metatarsal bone and concluded that despite the success of operative management, elite athletes are at an increased risk of treatment failure likely because of the unique strenuous stresses placed on the metatarsal during sport and external demand do early return to play. Nineteen percent of the players in this study experienced a recurrence of their injury, and 12% underwent a second procedure. The use of larger 4.5 mm screws in patients with higher BMIs, screw exchange, functional bracing, shoe modifications, and the use of alternative imaging in fracture follow-up have all been proposed as methods to help prevent and manage injury recurrence. There are improved rates of union and decreased complication rates and shorter time to return to play in athletes treated operatively compared with those treated nonoperatively. Those players who did return to play did not experience a decrease in performance compared with their pre-injury statistics nor compared with matched controls.

Chuckpaiwong [34] recommends operative treatment for Types 2 to 3 fractures according to the classification of Torg [11] for fifth metatarsal fractures, in athletically active patients, and fractures that fail to unite with appropriate nonoperative treatment. This study also suggests that radiographic sclerosis of the fracture site or obliteration of the medullary canal has a negative influence on surgical outcome.

Delee [54] reports that prolonged healing time and the risk of refracture following conservative treatment demand operative treatment including bone grafting of these fractures. An axial intramedullary screw, inserted without opening the fracture site, was used in ten athletes with stress fractures of the fifth metatarsal. Union was obtained in all patients in an average of 7.5 weeks. All patients returned to their sports in an average of 8.5 weeks postoperatively (Fig. 41.4).

Granata and Roche [55, 56] suggest that intramedullary screw fixation for Jones-type fifth metatarsal fractures in high-demand athletes may be best achieved by maximizing the screw size and strength. Selecting large screws that resist

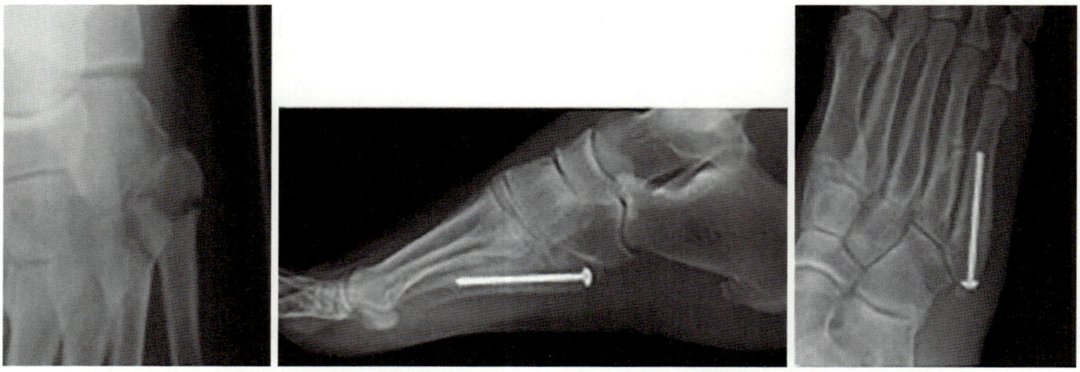

Fig. 41.4 X-ray base of fifth metatarsal fracture in a male football player (before and after surgery)

fatigue bending may be beneficial in reducing the refracture rate for this specific cohort of high-demand patients. Kerkhoffs [69] concluded that the majority of the fifth metatarsal fractures are stress fractures and mainly occur among young players. There are frequent healing problems, which might be explained by the stress nature of the injury, and with surgical treatment there are less healing problems, compared with those in conservative treatment. Mallee [18] preformed a systematic review to compare surgical and conservative treatment for high-risk stress fractures of the lower leg on return to activity, work, and sport; it remains unclear which option is most effective, but there are unsatisfying outcomes of conservative therapy in the anterior tibia. For the navicular, surgery provided an earlier return to sport [12, 18, 58–60], and when treated conservatively, weight bearing should be avoided [27]. For the fifth metatarsal, surgery provided the best results [18, 57, 61].

Surgical excision of the avulsed fragment from the proximal fifth metatarsal is a safe and effective alternative intervention when nonoperative methods fail [62].

41.8 Return to Sports

The return-to-play decision is based on the pattern, localization, and risk of the fracture [7, 57, 63]. The time to recover from a tibial stress injury has been reported to be between 4 and 20 weeks [53], suggesting that differences in injury severity can be considerable. In professional football these injuries can cause considerable problems for the individual players and the team. Because the healing time is long, these injuries normally result in 3–5 months of absence from football. It is mandatory to perform a clinical and thorough evaluation, as well as image control before the athlete restarts full activity.

Re-injury rate is not despicable, this rate is especially high for pelvic and tibia stress fractures and lower for fifth metatarsal. Re-injuries of stress fractures caused significantly longer absences than non-re-injuries [8].

41.9 Future Trends

There is limited research assessing stress fractures and other overuse injuries in football. It seems stress fractures are rare in professional men's football, but, when they occur, they cause long absences. Female players, younger age, and intensive preseason training appear to be risk factors. The change of load is the most probable explanation of stress fractures in male footballers, but insufficient caloric intake and hormonal disturbances could be a confounding factor. Further studies are needed to evaluate the possible mechanisms behind stress fractures in football.

The effectiveness of injury prevention programs in older players is promising. Therefore, targeted and effective injury prevention programs for younger players should be developed and validated [64, 65].

Regimens of bisphosphonates and vitamin D supplementation seem to have a beneficial effect for high-performance athletes. An optimal bone metabolism with sufficient daily calcium and vitamin D intake is crucial and should not only be strived for the professional but also for the recreational athlete [66, 67].

A recent prospective, randomized control trial [68] showed promising results using concentrated blood and blood marrow aspirate additionally to surgical repair with effective higher recovery rates and better functional outcomes.

References

1. Breithaupt ZR. Pathologie monschuchew fusser. Med Zeittung. 1855;24(169):170–5.
2. Devas MB. Stress fractures of the tibia in athletes or shin soreness. J Bone Joint Surg Br. 1958;40-B:227–39.
3. Bennell KL, Brukner PD. Epidemiology and site specificity of stress fractures. Clin Sports Med. 1997;16:179–96.
4. Bennell KL, Malcolm SA, Brukner PD, Green RM, Hopper JL, Wark JD, et al. A 12-month prospective study of the relationship between stress fractures and bone turnover in athletes. Calcif Tissue Int. 1998;63:80–5.
5. Bennell KL, Malcolm SA, Thomas SA, Ebeling PR, McCrory PR, Wark JD, et al. Risk factors for stress fractures in female track-and-field athletes: a retrospective analysis. Clin J Sport Med. 1995;5:229–35.
6. Bennell KL, Malcolm SA, Thomas SA, Reid SJ, Brukner PD, Ebeling PR, et al. Risk factors for stress fractures in track and field athletes. A twelve-month prospective study. Am J Sports Med. 1996;24: 810–8.
7. Dugan SA, Weber KM. Stress fractures and rehabilitation. Phys Med Rehabil Clin N Am. 2007;18:401–16.
8. Ekstrand J, Torstveit MK. Stress fractures in elite male football players. Scand J Med Sci Sports. 2012;22:341–6.
9. Bennell KL, Malcolm SA, Wark JD, Brukner PD. Models for the pathogenesis of stress fractures in athletes. Br J Sports Med. 1996;30(3):200–4.
10. Bennell KL, Malcolm SA, Wark JD, Brukner PD. Skeletal effects of menstrual disturbances in athletes. Scand J Med Sci Sports. 1997;7:261–73.
11. Torg JS, Balduini FC, Zelko RR, Pavlov H, Peff TC, Das M. Fractures of the base of the fifth metatarsal distal to the tuberosity: classification and guidelines for non-surgical and surgical management. J Bone Joint Surg Am. 1984;66:209–14.
12. Torg JS, Pavlov H, Cooley LH, Bryant MH, Arnoczky SP, Bergfeld J, et al. Stress fractures of the tarsal navicular. A retrospective review of twenty-one cases. J Bone Joint Surg Am. 1982;64:700–12.
13. Arendt EA. Stress fractures and the female athlete. Clin Orthop Relat Res. 2000;372:131–8.
14. Sundgot-Borgen J, Torstveit MK. The female football player, disordered eating, menstrual function and bone health. Br J Sports Med. 2007;41(Suppl 1):i68–72.
15. Bennell KL, Malcolm SA, Thomas SA, Wark JD, Brukner PD. The incidence and distribution of stress fractures in competitive track and field athletes. A twelve-month prospective study. Am J Sports Med. 1996;24:211–7.
16. Brukner PD, Bennell KL. Stress fractures in runners. J Back Musculoskelet Rehabil. 1995;5:341–51.
17. Kaeding CC, Miller T. The comprehensive description of stress fractures: a new classification system. J Bone Joint Surg Am. 2013;95:1214–20.
18. Mallee WH, Weel H, van Dijk CN, van Tulder MW, Kerkhoffs GM, Lin CW. Surgical versus conservative treatment for high-risk stress fractures of the lower leg (anterior tibial cortex, navicular and fifth metatarsal base): a systematic review. Br J Sports Med. 2015;49:370–6.
19. Rongstad KM, Tueting J, Rongstad M, Garrels K, Meis R. Fourth metatarsal base stress fractures in athletes: a case series. Foot Ankle Int. 2013;34:962–8.
20. Snyder RA, Koester MC, Dunn WR. Epidemiology of stress fractures. Clin Sports Med. 2006;25:37–52. viii
21. Aitken SA, Watson BS, Wood AM, Court-Brown CM. Sports-related fractures in South East Scotland: an analysis of 990 fractures. J Orthop Surg (Hong Kong). 2014;22:313–7.
22. Iwamoto J, Takeda T. Stress fractures in athletes: review of 196 cases. J Orthop Sci. 2003;8:273–8.
23. Orava S, Karpakka J, Hulkko A, Vaananen K, Takala T, Kallinen M, et al. Diagnosis and treatment of stress fractures located at the mid-tibial shaft in athletes. Int J Sports Med. 1991;12:419–22.
24. Pearce CJ, Brooks JH, Kemp SP, Calder JD. The epidemiology of foot injuries in professional rugby union players. J Foot Ankle Surg. 2011;17:113–8.
25. Pearce CJ, Zaw H, Calder JD. Stress fracture of the anterior process of the calcaneus associated with a calcaneonavicular coalition: a case report. Foot Ankle Int. 2011;32:85–8.
26. Ranawat VS, Dowell JK, Heywood-Waddington MB. Stress fractures of the lumbar pars interarticularis in athletes: a review based on long-term results of 18 professional cricketers. Injury. 2003;34:915–9.
27. Robinson M, Fulcher M. Delayed healing of a navicular stress fracture, following limited weight-bearing activity. BMJ Case Rep. 2014. Doi: 10.1136/bcr-2013-203216.
28. Armstrong 3rd DW, Rue JP, Wilckens JH, Frassica FJ. Stress fracture injury in young military men and women. Bone. 2004;35:806–16.
29. Brukner P, Bennell K. Stress fractures in female athletes. Diagnosis, management and rehabilitation. Sports Med (Auckland, NZ). 1997;24:419–29.

30. Warden SJ, Creaby MW, Bryant AL, Crossley KM. Stress fracture risk factors in female football players and their clinical implications. Br J Sports Med. 2007;41(Suppl 1):i38–43.
31. Barrack MT, Ackerman KE, Gibbs JC. Update on the female athlete triad. Curr Rev Muscoskelet Med. 2013;6:195–204.
32. Chen YT, Tenforde AS, Fredericson M. Update on stress fractures in female athletes: epidemiology, treatment, and prevention. Curr Rev Musculoskelet Med. 2013;6:173–81.
33. Bennell K, Crossley K, Jayarajan J, Walton E, Warden S, Kiss ZS, et al. Ground reaction forces and bone parameters in females with tibial stress fracture. Med Sci Sports Exerc. 2004;36:397–404.
34. Chuckpaiwong B, Queen RM, Easley ME, Nunley JA. Distinguishing Jones and proximal diaphyseal fractures of the fifth metatarsal. Clin Orthop Relat Res. 2008;466:1966–70.
35. Bennell K, Matheson G, Meeuwisse W, Brukner P. Risk factors for stress fractures. Sports Med (Auckland, NZ). 1999;28:91–122.
36. Nagel A, Fernholz F, Kibele C, Rosenbaum D. Long distance running increases plantar pressures beneath the metatarsal heads: a barefoot walking investigation of 200 marathon runners. Gait Posture. 2008;27:152–5.
37. Fujitaka K, Taniguchi A, Isomoto S, Kumai T, Otuki S, Okubo M, et al. Pathogenesis of fifth metatarsal fractures in college soccer players. Orthop J Sports Med. 2015;3:2325967115603654.
38. Crossley K, Bennell KL, Wrigley T, Oakes BW. Ground reaction forces, bone characteristics, and tibial stress fracture in male runners. Med Sci Sports Exerc. 1999;31:1088–93.
39. Carreira DS, Sandilands SM. Radiographic factors and effect of fifth metatarsal Jones and diaphyseal stress fractures on participation in the NFL. Foot Ankle Int. 2013;34:518–22.
40. Changstrom BG, Brou L, Khodaee M, Braund C, Comstock RD. Epidemiology of stress fracture injuries among US high school athletes, 2005–2006 through 2012–2013. Am J Sports Med. 2015;43:26–33.
41. Beck BR, Bergman AG, Miner M, Arendt EA, Klevansky AB, Matheson GO, et al. Tibial stress injury: relationship of radiographic, nuclear medicine bone scanning, MR imaging, and CT Severity grades to clinical severity and time to healing. Radiology. 2012;263:811–8.
42. Wright AA, Hegedus EJ, Lenchik L, Kuhn KJ, Santiago L, Smoliga JM. Diagnostic accuracy of various imaging modalities for suspected lower extremity stress fractures: a systematic review with evidence-based recommendations for clinical practice. Am J Sports Med. 2016;44:255–3.
43. Arendt EA, Griffiths HJ. The use of MR imaging in the assessment and clinical management of stress reactions of bone in high-performance athletes. Clin Sports Med. 1997;16:291–306.
44. Boden BP, Osbahr DC. High-risk stress fractures: evaluation and treatment. J Am Acad Orthop Surg. 2000;8:344–53.
45. Menge TJ, Looney CG. Medial malleolar stress fracture in an adolescent athlete. J Foot Ankle Surg. 2015;54:242–6.
46. Murray SR, Reeder MT, Udermann BE, Pettitt RW. High-risk stress fractures: pathogenesis, evaluation, and treatment. Compr Ther. 2006;32:20–5.
47. Brukner P, Bradshaw C, Bennell K. Managing common stress fractures: let risk level guide treatment. Phys Sports Med. 1998;26:39–47.
48. Fredericson M, Bergman AG, Hoffman KL, Dillingham MS. Tibial stress reaction in runners: correlation of clinical symptoms and scintigraphy with a new magnetic resonance imaging grading system. Am J Sports Med. 1995;23:472–81.
49. Patel DR. Stress fractures: diagnosis and management in the primary care setting. Pediatr Clin North Am. 2010;57:819–27.
50. Patel DS, Roth M, Kapil N. Stress fractures: diagnosis, treatment, and prevention. Am Fam Physician. 2011;83:39–46.
51. Andrish JT. The leg. In: Delee JC, Drez D, editors. Orthopaedic sports medicine: principle and practice. Philadelphia: WB Saunders; 1994.
52. Liimatainen E, Sarimo J, Hulkko A, Ranne J, Heikkila J, Orava S. Anterior mid-tibial stress fractures. Results of surgical treatment. Scand J Surg. 2009;98:244–9.
53. Begly JP, Guss M, Ramme AJ, Karia R, Meislin RJ. Return to play and performance after Jones fracture in National Basketball Association athletes. Sports Health. 2016;8:342–6.
54. DeLee JC, Evans JP, Julian J. Stress fracture of the fifth metatarsal. Am J Sports Med. 1983;11:349–53.
55. Granata JD, Berlet GC, Philbin TM, Jones G, Kaeding CC, Peterson KS. Failed surgical management of acute proximal fifth metatarsal (Jones) fractures: a retrospective case series and literature review. Foot Ankle Spec. 2015;8:454–9.
56. Roche AJ, Calder JD. Treatment and return to sport following a Jones fracture of the fifth metatarsal: a systematic review. Knee Surg Sports Traumatol Arthrosc. 2013;21:1307–15.
57. Kaeding CC, Yu JR, Wright R, Amendola A, Spindler KP. Management and return to play of stress fractures. Clin J Sport Med. 2005;15:442–7.
58. Mann JA, Pedowitz DI. Evaluation and treatment of navicular stress fractures, including nonunions, revision surgery, and persistent pain after treatment. Foot Ankle Clin. 2009;14:187–204.
59. Saxena A, Fullem B. Navicular stress fractures: a prospective study on athletes. Foot Ankle Int. 2006;27:917–21.
60. Torg JS, Moyer J, Gaughan JP, Boden BP. Management of tarsal navicular stress fractures: conservative versus surgical treatment: a meta-analysis. Am J Sports Med. 2010;38:1048–53.
61. Thevendran G, Deol RS, Calder JD. Fifth metatarsal fractures in the athlete: evidence for management. Foot Ankle Clin. 2013;18:237–54.

62. Ritchie JD, Shaver JC, Anderson RB, Lawrence SJ, Mair SD. Excision of symptomatic nonunions of proximal fifth metatarsal avulsion fractures in elite athletes. Am J Sports Med. 2011;39:2466–9.
63. Diehl JJ, Best TM, Kaeding CC. Classification and return-to-play considerations for stress fractures. Clin Sports Med. 2006;25:17–28.
64. Rossler R, Junge A, Chomiak J, Dvorak J, Faude O. Soccer injuries in players aged 7 to 12 years: a descriptive epidemiological study over 2 seasons. Am J Sports Med. 2015;44(2):309–17.
65. Tenforde AS, Sainani KL, Carter Sayres L, Milgrom C, Fredericson M. Participation in ball sports may represent a prehabilitation strategy to prevent future stress fractures and promote bone health in young athletes. PMR. 2015;7:222–5.
66. Simon MJ, Barvencik F, Luttke M, Amling M, Mueller-Wohlfahrt HW, Ueblacker P. Intravenous bisphosphonates and vitamin D in the treatment of bone marrow oedema in professional athletes. Injury. 2014;45:981–7.
67. Tenforde AS, Sayres LC, Sainani KL, Fredericson M. Evaluating the relationship of calcium and vitamin D in the prevention of stress fracture injuries in the young athlete: a review of the literature. PMR. 2010;2:945–9.
68. Weel H, Mallee WH, van Dijk CN, Blankevoort L, Goedegebuure S, Goslings JC, et al. The effect of concentrated bone marrow aspirate in operative treatment of fifth metatarsal stress fractures; a double-blind randomized controlled trial. BMC Musculoskelet Disord. 2015;16:211.
69. Kerkhoffs GM, Versteegh VE, Sierevelt IN, Kloen P, van Dijk CN. Treatment of proximal metatarsal V fractures in athletes and non-athletes. Br J Sports Med. 2012;46:644–8.

Apophysitis

42

Francesco Della Villa, Renato Andrade, Artur Pereira Castro, and Manuel Cassiano Neves

Contents

F. Della Villa (✉)
Isokinetic Medical Group, FIFA Medical Centre of Excellence, Bologna, Italy

Sport and Exercise Medicine Residency, University of Bologna, Bologna, Italy

R. Andrade
Clínica do Dragão, Espregueira-Mendes Sports Centre, FIFA Medical Centre of Excellence, Porto, Portugal

Dom Henrique Research Centre, Porto, Portugal

Faculdade de Desporto da Universidade do Porto, Porto, Portugal

A.P. Castro
Sports Traumatology of SPORTRAUMA, Lisbon, Portugal

M.C. Neves
Department Paediatric Orthopaedics, Hospital CUF Descobertas, Lisbon, Portugal

42.1 Introduction

The apophysitis is a wide and heterogeneous family of clinical conditions characterized by an often chronic and overuse mechanical stress to any apophysis of a generally immature skeletal system. These conditions, typical of a growing skeletal system, lead to a decrease of function of the affected body part due to the mechanical disruption of the over-mentioned structures. In football players the most frequent conditions of this family are those related to the lower limb. The Osgood-Schlatter (osteochondrosis of the anterior tibial tubercle (ATT)) disease is one of the most frequent apophysitis affecting the young football player. Additionally, the pubic apophysitis due to repeated stress on the proximal adductor insertion is often forgotten and can be the underlying reason (in some cases) for the chronic symptomatology of the young football player with groin pain [1].

This chapter aims to present an overview of the problem of apophysitis in football, an often overlooked problem by the scientific community.

42.2 The Aetiology of Lower Limb Apophysitis

Overuse injuries can affect multiple parts of a young athlete's body including the physis and the tendons. The bone is growing through the growth

J. Espregueira-Mendes et al. (eds.), *Injuries and Health Problems in Football*, DOI 10.1007/978-3-662-53924-8_42

plate that makes them susceptible to repetitive microinjuries in the high phases of growth but also at the extremity of the bones where the powerful muscle tendon units are attached. In the growing child/adolescent, this particular area becomes very prone to inflammation as a result of repetitive avulsion micro-traumas leading to an inflammatory stage at the tendon insertion/growth plate [2].

The musculotendinous units and their insertions into the bones are the most important factor in the development of pain in the young athlete and depend on intrinsic and extrinsic factors. Intrinsic factors include bone growth, growth of musculotendinous units, decreased bone density, skeletal maturity, muscle bulk, decreased flexibility and strength, extremity malalignment and psychological factors like high-risk behaviours. Extrinsic factors are a consequence of inappropriate changes in training, improper training surfaces, improper equipment, parental pressure, coaching pressure and peer pressure [3].

They can affect multiple parts of the body and have different clinical manifestations, and for this reason, there are multiple ways to treat and prevent the injuries in the growing child and the young adult, according to the type of presentation and the clinical manifestations.

42.3 Classification of Apophysitis

In the literature there is not a single classification for the "apophysitis" since most of the classifications are related to a specific entity/local as, for example, the Osgood-Schlatter syndrome, which is related to the tibial tuberosity. It will be helpful in terms of distinguishing the different entities to have a classification that would help directing the treatment.

42.3.1 Classification According to Type of Injury

In order to understand the different types of injuries, it is important to understand the mechanism of injury. The extremity of the bones, either at the end covered by cartilage (epiphysis) or where the tendons/muscles are attached (apophysis), can be subject to different types of trauma: avulsion lesions secondary to repetitive tractions over the site, compression lesions or shear lesions [4, 5]. The apophysitis is mostly related to an avulsion-type lesion.

42.3.2 Classification According to the Ability to Play Sports

Time can also be important to define a possible treatment approach but most important is, like the Loder's [6] classification for slipped capital femoral epiphysis, to define the ability to carry a sports activity or not. This will differentiate the acute unstable lesions from the chronic stage (stable).

For the acute lesions, we suggest to follow a modified Martin and Pipkin [7] classification applied to the treatment of avulsion of the ischial tuberosity. This basic approach updated by McKinney et al. [8] differentiated the fractures according to the degree of displacement of the fragments (Table 42.1).

In Fig. 42.1, we report a case of a 13-year-old football player that was complaining of pain over the ATT. The football player, after a kick, suddenly felt an acute local pain and the inability to bear weight. The X-ray revealed a high-riding patella with an avulsion of the ATT.

In case of a chronic lesion (type 4 of the McKinney classification), the literature is omissive, and there is a lack of consensus. Probably on this particular case, it will be crucial to combine the clinical evaluation in terms of pain with the results of imaging. This was pointed out by Kose [9] that found out that the radiologic identification of calcaneal apophysitis (Sever's disease) without the absence of clinical information was not reliable. Radiologic findings that were attributed to Sever's disease showed a wide variation between

Table 42.1 Classification of apophyseal avulsion fractures according to McKinney classification

Classification of apophyseal avulsion fractures
Type 1 nondisplaced fractures
Type 2 displacement up to 2 cm
Type 3 displacement > 2 cm
Type 4 symptomatic non-unions or painful exostosis

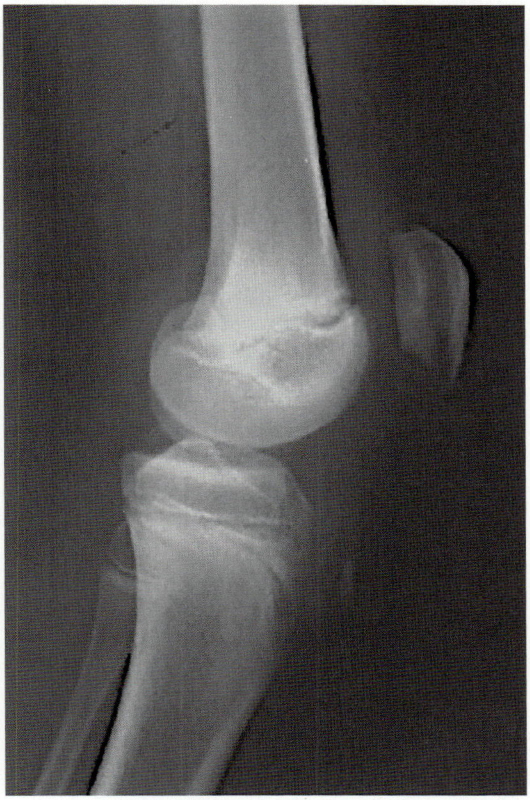

Fig. 42.1 X-ray of a 13-year-old footballer that reveals an ATT avulsion

independent observers and between separate readings by the same observer. The authors suggested that the diagnosis of calcaneal apophysitis was a clinical decision, and radiographic assessment seemed to be unnecessary. There is no specific classification regarding imaging, and several imaging tools are available for this diagnosis. For this reason it is difficult to interpret the findings.

Nakase et al. [10] in their study aimed to correlate the different findings with the degree of maturity of the bone. Tibial tuberosity development on ultrasonography was divided into three stages: sonolucent stage (stage S), individual stage (stage I) and connective stage (stage C). Age, height, quadriceps and hamstring muscle tightness and muscle strength in knee extension and flexion were determined. These findings were compared with the respective stages of development. They were able to show that thigh muscle tightness and thigh muscle performance change with the skeletal maturation of the distal attachment of the patellar tendon.

According to Arnaiz et al. [11], the MRI can be helpful in terms of differentiating the underlying pathology regarding apophysitis. They advocate that accurate identification of key MRI features of this entity may prevent misdiagnosis and inappropriate management of apophysitis.

In the early 1990s, Kujala and Orava [12] described a classification that tried to put together the clinical aspects with the observation on the different imaging modalities and relate them to the age. Although it is related to the ischial apophysitis injuries in athletes, it may be adjusted to other sites and help the clinician in terms of defining the appropriate therapy (Table 42.2).

The most important factor in the classification of the apophysitis is to differentiate the patients that are unable to play sports (acute – unstable) from the ones that still are able to play although with some restrictions (chronic – stable), since it will have a direct impact on the therapeutical indications.

Table 42.2 Classification of apophysitis and recommended imaging investigations adjusted for age according to Kujala and Orava [12]

Type of lesion	Patient's age (yrs)	Recommended imaging investigations
Tug lesions		
Apophysis (apophysitis)	13–15	X-ray, MRI (oedema)
Adult tug lesion	Adult	X-ray (sclerosis,. bone scan, CT scan
Unfused apophysis	Young adults	X-ray, bone scan, MRI
Acute avulsions		
Apophysis	13–16	X-ray, US CT scan, MRI
Muscle avulsion	Middle age	US, MRI
Small bony fragment	16–25	X-ray, US, CT scan, MRI
Large bony avulsion	16–25	X-ray
Old avulsions		
Small fragment	20–30	X-ray, US
Large fragment (pseudotumour)	18–30	X-ray

Legend: *Yrs* Years, *US* ultrasound, *CT* computed tomography, *MRI* magnetic resonance imaging

42.4 Treatment of Apophysitis

The conservative approach is often suggested as the first-line treatment in case of apophysitis. Considering the ATT apophysitis (Osgood-Schlatter disease), about 90% of patients respond well to non-operative treatment, which includes rest, icing, activity modification and rehabilitation exercises [13]. Therefore, a rehabilitation-based approach should be encouraged in most of the cases.

The surgical option should be targeted for selected cases or nonresponder chronic patients to the conservative treatment. Pihlajamäki et al. [14] reported good to excellent clinical results in almost 90% of the patients after surgical treatment of Osgood-Schlatter disease.

In this subchapter we will present a typical conservative approach to the Osgood-Schlatter patient. The crucial principles may be applied also to the other types of apophysitis.

The basis of the treatment of this common footballer apophysitis is a combination of activity modification, physical therapies and exercise programme. We adopt a rehabilitation strategy based on two main points: organizational and clinical aspects.

Regarding the organizational aspects, we really believe in the multidisciplinary approach. A sports medicine physician should guide the caregiver team consisting of a physical therapist and an athletic trainer. Appropriate facilities including a rehabilitation gym, pool and field allow a stepwise progression of the workload.

Regarding the clinical aspects, the rehabilitation protocol should always be on patient-tailored fashion and based on objective criteria progression. Our proposal consists of a three-phase protocol (Table 42.3):

1. Resolution of pain. Activity modification is crucial to change the natural progression of

Table 42.3 Conservative treatment keystones, pearls and objective criteria for moving on to the next phase

Phase	Goal	Management approach	Milestones/progression criteria	Tips and pearls
1	Resolution of pain	Tension dispersion-type knee brace Physical modalities (e.g. laser and ice)	Full ROM without pain Normal biomechanics restored	The patient should perform the exercises within a pain-free ROM Exercising in the pool will decrease the loads imposed to the lower limb and allow more active exercises Remain physically active and keep practising the sport-specific gestures
	Restore normal biomechanics	Stretching the posterior muscle chain Massage the anterior muscle chain		
	Management of the physical condition	Aerobic exercises in the gym/field		
	Enhance neuroplasticity of sport-specific movements	Neuromuscular and motor control exercises, within the football-specific gestures, in the pool		
2	Correct functional muscular imbalances	Stretching of the posterior muscle chain Eccentric exercises of the quadriceps muscles	Isokinetic bilateral asymmetry lower than 10% Isokinetic unilateral ratio within the range 50–80% Functional testing under 10% of bilateral differences	A balance between the quadriceps and hamstring muscles should be achieved A "hip strategy" instead of a "knee strategy" will decrease the tensional loads on the knee
	Decrease the load imposed to the anterior muscle chain	Neuromuscular proprioceptive exercises		
3	Reinsert the player to the field exercises and to the sport-specific gesture	On-field activities that replicate several football match situations	Re-establishment of the sport-specific gesture Recover the match fitness	A cautious progression, divided in subphases, should be follow Use different surfaces to progress in the difficulty

Legend: *ROM* Range of movement

the clinical condition. The patient should be always pain-free when performing activity. Rest is a valuable option in the first weeks of the treatment. On the other hand, we need to maintain the patient active as tolerated, once the complete rest is not recommended. Specific braces are often recommended to apply compression on the ATT and reduce the patient symptoms (Fig. 42.2a). In this first phase, it is indicated to perform exercises in the gym and in the pool. In the rehab gym, it is suggested to decrease pain using physical modalities, such as laser and ice therapy (Fig. 42.2b). Stretching of the posterior muscular chain and massage of the anterior muscle chain are indicated to restore a proper biomechanics. Aerobic activity, as tolerated, should always be maintained. In the pool, thanks to the water environment, the patient may perform more active exercises including neuroplasticity exercises for the functional sport gesture (Fig. 42.2c). The goal of this phase is the progressive control of pain without completely compromising the athlete activity.

2. Functional strengthening. In this phase the physician should think biomechanically to correct functional imbalances of the lower limb. The crucial principle is to find the balance between the quadriceps and hamstring activity and strength. The posterior chain needs to be stretched (Fig. 42.3a) properly with static and dynamic exercises, while the quadriceps muscles should be reinforced eccentrically, with a very cautious progression. Finally, in order to really reduce the amount of forces expressed by the anterior chain, a functional training (including neuromuscular

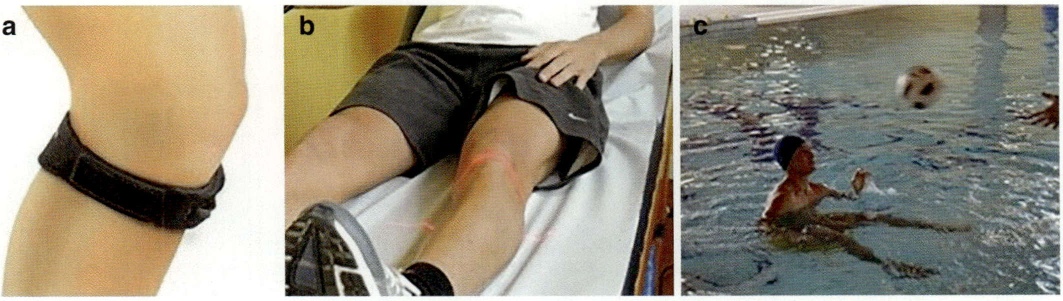

Fig. 42.2 (**a**) Compressive braces applied on the ATT. (**b**) The use of physical modalities to reduce pain and inflammation. (**c**) Football-specific exercises in the pool to maintain a proper neuromuscular control

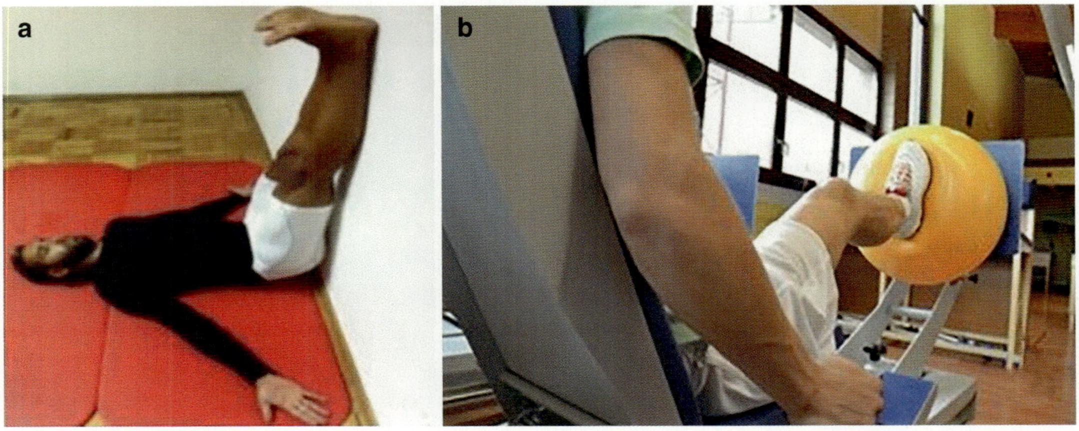

Fig. 42.3 (**a**) Stretching of the posterior muscular chain. (**b**) Eccentric strengthening of the quadriceps muscle on elastic resistance machine

and proprioceptive exercises) should be initiated. A "hip strategy" (Fig. 42.4b) instead of a "knee strategy" (Fig. 42.4a) should be enhanced in order to reduce the amount of forces applied to the knee in every single movement during the activity. The pathomechanics of the apophysitis is believed to relate with repetitive micro-traumas linked to excessive load, as explained above. Therefore, in the conservative treatment, it is suggested to think biomechanically in order to protect the lesion site. The goal of this phase is the reestablishment of muscle balance while maintaining the pain control.

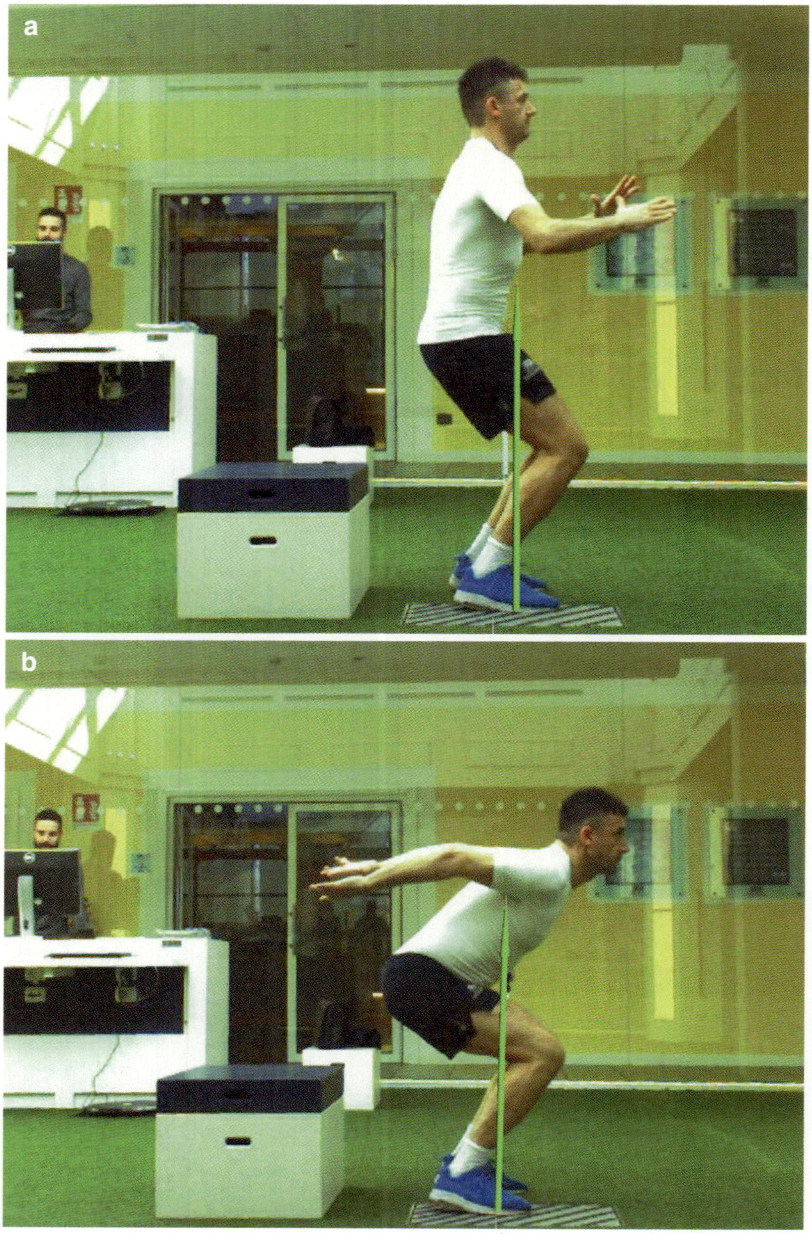

Fig. 42.4 A progression from a knee strategy (**a**) (on the *left*) (often observed in knee patient) to a more convenient movement pattern (**b**) (on the *right*) should be encouraged

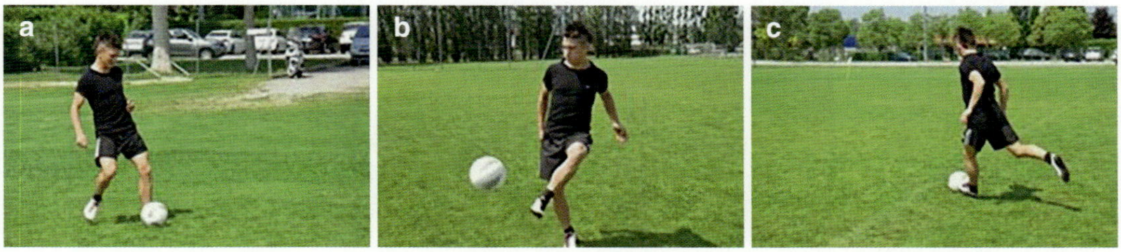

Fig. 42.5 Examples of exercises on the field. (**a**, **b**, **c**) Pain-free kicking progression is crucial for every injured footballer, and it is part of the on-field programme

3. Progressive return to activity. In this last phase, the player is ready to progress in the rehab path, and more sport-specific exercises are added to the protocol. Thus, a football-specific rehabilitation programme (Fig. 42.5) on the field is recommended in order to reinsert the sport-specific pattern in the patient's life in a controlled environment, where symptoms can be well controlled. The on-field activity should be progressive and cautious. This last phase is crucial to test patient reaction to higher loads, similar to those that will be applied on the real field and should be divided into subphases. The use of different surfaces (as sand) to progress in load modification may be indicated. The goal of this last phase is the recovery of the sport-specific gesture and a proper recovery of the match fitness.

Conclusion

Apophysitis is a frequent and often overlooked problem of the young footballer. In this chapter we tried to provide a comprehensive vision of such a big family of clinical conditions. A proper clinical and radiological diagnoses followed by an on patient-tailored treatment are key factors to reach a maximal functional recovery allowing prompt return to football.

References

1. Sailly M, Whiteley R, Read JW, Giuffre B, Johnson A, Hölmich P. Pubic apophysitis: a previously undescribed clinical entity of groin pain in athletes. Br J Sports Med. 2015;49:828–34.
2. Kerssemakers SP, Fotiadou AN, de Jonge MC, Karantanas AH, Maas M. Sport injuries in the paediatric and adolescent patient: a growing problem. Pediatr Radiol. 2009;39:471–84.
3. Cuff S, Loud K, O'Riordan M. Overuse injuries in high school athletes. Clin Pediatr. 2010;49:731–6.
4. Leahy I, Schorpion M, Ganley T. Common medial elbow injuries in the adolescent athlete. J Hand Ther. 2015;28:201–10.
5. Young SW, Safran MR. Greater trochanter apophysitis in the adolescent athlete. Clin J Sport Med. 2015;25:e57–8.
6. Loder RT, Richards BS, Shapiro PS, Reznick LR, Aronson DD. Acute slipped capital femoral epiphysis: the importance of physeal stability. J Bone Joint Surg Am. 1993;75:1134–40.
7. Martin TA, Pipkin G. Treatment of avulsion of the ischial tuberosity. Clin Orthop Relat Res. 1957;10:108–18.
8. McKinney BI, Nelson C, Carrion W. Apophyseal avulsion fractures of the hip and pelvis. Orthopedics. 2009;32:42.
9. Kose O, Celiktas M, Yigit S, Kisin B. Can we make a diagnosis with radiographic examination alone in calcaneal apophysitis (Sever's disease?). J Pediatr Orthop B. 2010;19:396–8.
10. Nakase J, Aiba T, Goshima K, Takahashi R, Toratani T, Kosaka M, Ohashi Y, Tsuchiya H. Relationship between the skeletal maturation of the distal attachment of the patellar tendon and physical features in preadolescent male football players. Knee Surg Sports Traumatol Arthrosc. 2014;22:195–9.
11. Arnaiz J, Piedra T, de Lucas EM, Arnaiz AM, Pelaz M, Gomez-Dermit V, Canga A. Imaging findings of lower limb apophysitis. AJR Am J Roentgenol. 2011;196:W316–25.
12. Kujala UM, Orava S. Ischial apophysis injuries in athletes. Sports Med. 1993;16:290–4.
13. Gholve PA, Scher DM, Khakharia S, Widmann RF, Green DW. Osgood Schlatter syndrome. Curr Opin Pediatr. 2007;19:44–50.
14. Pihlajamäki HK, Mattila VM, Parviainen M, Kiuru MJ, Visuri TI. Long-term outcome after surgical treatment of unresolved Osgood-Schlatter disease in young men. J Bone Joint Surg Am. 2009;91:2350–8.

Lower Limb Periostitis

43

João Gamelas, Luís Branco Amaral,
and Francisco Forriol

Contents

J. Gamelas (✉)
Hospital Lusíadas/Nova Medical School, Lisbon, Portugal
e-mail: jgamelas@hotmail.com

L.B. Amaral
Hospital Curry Cabral, Lisbon, Portugal

F. Forriol
School of Medicine, University CEU – San Pablo, Madrid, Spain

43.1 Introduction

Lower limb pain is fairly common, particularly among runners [1–5]. It equates to about 20% of their injuries and is naturally a big source of frustration. The most common site of shin splints is in the anterior face of the lower third of the tibia, but may extend proximally. Also they may appear in the fibula or femur or foot bones, this is more common in sprinters [6]. Periostitis in football players occurs more frequently in the pelvis and tibia. The term "shin splints" is not a specific diagnosis.

"Shin splints" is the lay term; but physicians use the term medial tibial stress syndrome (MTSS) [7] more than periostitis or exercise-related pain [8], and then "shin splints" is not a specific diagnosis (Fig. 43.1). MTSS is an overuse injury occurring among the physically active [9] and is a complex symptom seen in athletes and military personnel, which complain of exercise-induced pain along the distal posterior-medial aspect of the tibia [10]. The name given to this condition refers to pain on the posteromedial tibial border during exercise, with pain on palpation of the tibia over a length of at least 5 cm [11].

MTSS can be defined as an overuse injury that creates pain over an area covering the distal to middle third of the posteriomedial tibial border, which occurs during exercise and creates cyclic loading [12]. It is a common complaint that may stop an athlete from running [13].

J. Espregueira-Mendes et al. (eds.), *Injuries and Health Problems in Football*,
DOI 10.1007/978-3-662-53924-8_43

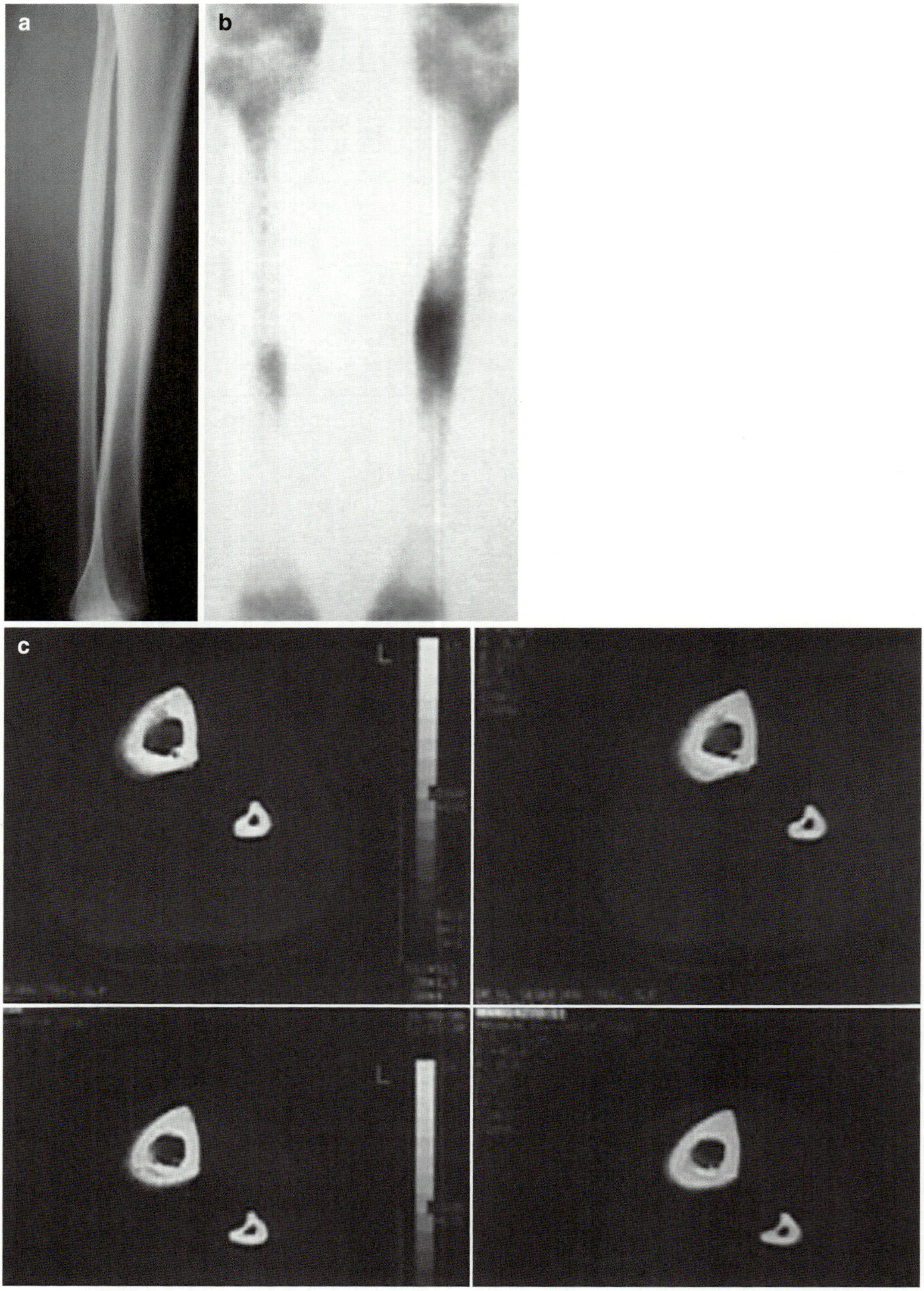

Fig. 43.1 A 21-year-old military with pain in both legs which increase with gait (**a**), left tibia periostitis with (**b**) positive scintigraphy, and (**c**) CT scan bone reaction (Courtesy of Dr. B. Vasconcelos, Lisboa, Portugal)

The evidence seems clear that shin splint pain has many different causes, and this reflects the variation in the anatomy [14]. Pain comes from a bony reaction to stress [10, 15] or from elevated pressure within muscle compartments [16, 17].

43.2 Incidence

Leg pain in athletes can be caused by many conditions, with the most frequent being MTSS. Chronic exertional compartment syndrome, stress fracture, nerve entrapment, and popliteal artery entrapment syndrome are also considerations [18]. MTSS is prevalent among military personnel, runners, and dancers, showing an incidence of 4–20% of this population [11, 12, 19, 20]. Sharma et al. [21] show that MTSS in 6608 British Army recruits had the greatest impact on training, accounting for almost 20% of all days spent in rehabilitation. Orava and Puranen [22] found that in 465 cases of exertion pain, 18% were located in the shin. MTSS was the most common overuse injury among these athletes, comprising 9.5% of all exertion injuries and 60% of leg exertion pains. Together with stress fractures of the tibia, the second most common exertion pain of the leg, it accounted for 75% of total leg pains.

43.3 Pathological and Aetiological Factors

MTSS is a common injury in active populations and has been suggested to be a result of both biomechanical and lifestyle factors [23]. Approximately 50% of all sports injuries are secondary to overuse and result from repetitive microtrauma that causes local tissue damage. Injuries are most likely with changes in mode, intensity, or duration of training and can accumulate before symptoms appear. Intrinsic factors contributing to injuries are individual biomechanical abnormalities such as malalignments, muscle imbalance, inflexibility, weakness, and instability. The most proven risk factors are overpronation of the foot and a history of previous MTSS [24]. Females are also at more risk [28].

43.3.1 General Factors

A combination of extrinsic factors, such as training errors and environmental factors, and intrinsic or anatomical factors, such as bony alignment of the extremities, flexibility deficits, and ligamentous laxity, predisposes athletes to develop overuse injuries. Hubbard et al. [25] established that the factors most influencing MTSS development were previous history of MTSS and stress fracture, years of running experience, and orthotic use (Fig. 43.2). Running injury rates increase significantly when weekly mileage extends beyond 40 miles cumulatively [26]. Common causes of running injuries include overuse, lack of rest, and activities that aggravate biomechanical predisposers of specific injuries [27]. Female gender, previous history of MTSS, fewer years of running experience, orthotic use, increased body mass index, increased navicular drop (ND), and increased external rotation hip range of motion in males are all significantly associated with an increased risk of developing MTSS [28].

A variety of physical characteristics of athletes has been proposed to be related to the risk in sustaining a sports injury [29]. Yagi et al. [30] found in females that body mass index (BMI) significantly increased the risk of MTSS and also a higher BMI was associated with a longer recovery time [11]. No significant differences were

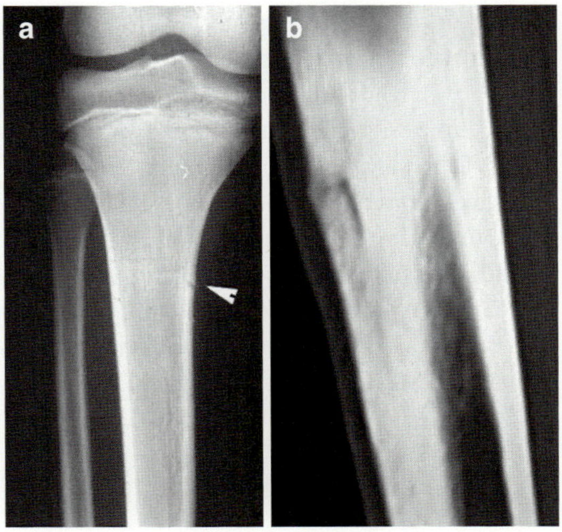

Fig. 43.2 (**a**) Proximal tibial stress fracture and (**b**) diaphyseal tibial stress fracture

found in anthropometric parameters (thigh length, leg length, foot length, and leg circumference) and body composition (the amount of minerals and body fat percentage) in a MTSS patient group [31].

43.3.2 Overstress to Bone

Overuse injuries develop when repetitive stress to bone and musculotendinous structures damage tissue at a greater rate than that at which the body can repair itself [32], and MTSS often results when bone remodelling processes adapt inadequately to repetitive stress [33]. For Devas et al. [34] and Jackson et al. [35], between pain and stress fracture, athletes may show a variety of features including periostitis, cortical demineralisation, cortical hypertrophy, or mixed patterns.

43.3.3 Compartment Syndromes

The pathogenesis is explained by increased pressure in the fascial compartment of the deep flexor muscles due to prolonged exercise. In patients susceptible to MTSS, the fascial compartments are too small to accommodate the associated 20% increase in muscle mass that typically occurs with heavy exercise [36]. The pathology of the compartment syndrome is that with exercise, a muscle retains fluid and increases bulk. Authors have demonstrated that elevated muscle compartment pressure in athletes may cause either medial-sided shin pain [16, 37] or lateral-sided shin pain [4], but this is highly contentious [10, 38]. It may be concluded that the body of evidence supports the idea that increased compartment pressure may cause shin splint pain, but not all shin splint pain is due to increased compartment pressure and that fasciotomy not only decreases the compartment pressure but decreases the muscle traction effect on the periosteum.

43.3.4 Biomechanical Factors

Biomechanical studies indicate why certain athletes are predisposed to get shin splints and may explain the pathophysiology behind elevated compartment pressure or musculotendinous tears in the aetiology of shin splints.

Malalignments of the lower extremities (average prevalence 18% and only minor deviations) did show some inconsistent relationships with the number of (specific) injuries. For pelvic obliquity, it was positive as predicted, but for malalignment of the rearfoot and a deviant footprint, it appeared to be negative. Runners with medial shin pain displayed greater frontal plane pelvic tilt excursion, peak hip internal rotation, and decreased knee flexion while running compared to a control group [13]. Leg length inequality and malalignment of the knees were not related to injuries [29]. Sommer and Vallentyne [39] found that a standing foot angle of <140° and a varus alignment of the hindfoot and/or forefoot were predictive of a previous history of MTSS.

Malalignment has also been implicated in iliotibial band syndrome, MTSS, lower extremity stress fractures, and plantar fasciitis (Fig. 43.3). Muscle inflexibility aggravates and predisposes someone to the development of a variety of overuse injuries, especially those occurring in children and adolescents, including the traction apophysitis. Flexibility deficits may be improved by an appropriate stretching protocol. Unfortunately, lower extremity malalignment is less amenable to intervention.

Foot overpronation is thus a well-documented cause of shin splints. These include tibia vara – because the foot hits the ground in an exaggerated, inverted position, therefore it must "roll over" further to make adequate ground contact and forefoot varus – because the rearfoot must "roll over" further (pronate) to compensate for the inverted forefoot and internal femoral torsion [40], because the foot may pronate to increase abduction and therefore make someone walk straighter. Increased internal rotation of the hip significantly increased the risk of MTSS [30]. Other causes of overpronation include plantarflexed fifth metatarsal, limb length inequality, various neuromuscular conditions, and tibial torsion [40]. An imbalance in foot pressure with greater pressure on the medial side than on the lateral side was the primary risk factor.

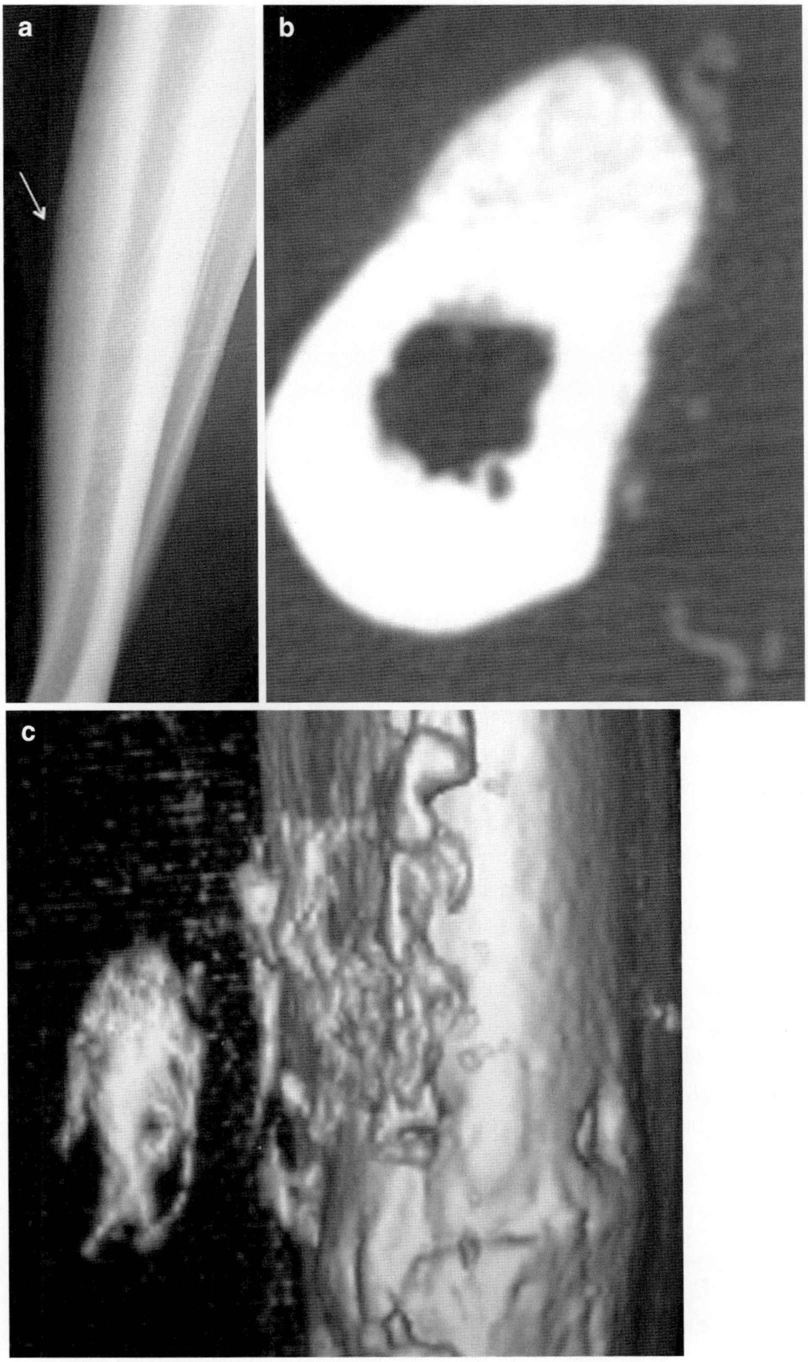

Fig. 43.3 (**a**) Recurrent tibial stress fracture in a football goalkeeper due to biomechanical alterations, meniscectomy, and foot pronation. Surgery was performed (**b** and **c**) puting BMP-7 around the fracture, both in the endomedular channel and in the tibial surface (Courtesy of Dr. A. del Corral, Madrid, Spain)

The combination of female gender and ND test measures provides an accurate prediction for the development of MTSS. Several studies [28, 41–44] have demonstrated that excessive static ND is related to the diagnosis.

Football players with MTSS have an abnormal structural deformation of their feet during the support (or stance) phase of running. This abnormal motion could be a risk factor for the development of MTSS [45].

Orthotics is often prescribed to improve lower extremity alignment. However, studies have not shown that orthotics has any effect on knee alignment, and, while they can alter subtalar joint alignment, the clinical benefit of this remains unclear. Awareness of anatomical factors that may predispose overuse injuries allows the clinician to develop individual rehabilitation programmes designed to decrease the risk of overuse injury. In addition, the clinician can advise the athlete on the importance of avoiding extrinsic factors that may also predispose overuse injury [32].

43.3.5 Muscle Fatigue in Shin Splints

It is believed that overused, fatigued muscles can cause or exacerbate the condition of shin splints. Certainly it is widely held that shin splints are most frequently seen in the underconditioned athlete trying to do too much too soon [35, 46]. Clement et al. [46] noted that earlier scientific work had suggested that muscles were able to act as "shock absorbers' and therefore absorb some of the stress of movement that would otherwise go directly to the bone. They therefore suggested that the athlete that asked his body to do too much too soon would fatigue his muscles and may decrease the shock absorption function of the muscle. Consequently, all stress would be transmitted direct to the bone, hence bone overload and periostitis. Taunton et al. [47] supported this and pointed out that biomechanical abnormality would make muscle overstress occur earlier.

43.4 Diagnostic and Physical Examination

Most importantly, the astute clinician should be persistent in observing the athlete in order to correctly diagnose and manage all the underlying problems and arrive at a satisfactory outcome [48].

Obtaining a careful history is a critical component in arriving at the correct diagnosis, and it forms the primary basis for a diagnosis of chronic compartment syndrome. A history of persistent cramping with exercise and asymptomatic rest periods with symptoms worsening over time are the major indicators of the problem. It is also important to determine whether the posterior symptoms are superficial or deep and proximal or distal, or both, and to define the exact borders of the area of pain; a common mistake is to simply pinpoint the maximal point of tenderness [1]. It is important to delineate precisely which muscles are involved. Symptoms tend to progressively worsen over time and improve with rest and reduction or cessation of exercise.

Detmer [1] proposed a clinical classification and treatment programme for MTSS. Three chronic types exist and may coexist:

Type I: tibial microfracture, bone stress reaction, or cortical fracture

Type II: periostalgia from chronic avulsion of the periosteum at the periosteal-fascial junction

Type III: chronic compartment syndrome

Bilaterality was common in type II (50%) and in type III (88%)

Chronic lower leg pain in athletes can be a frustrating problem for patients and a difficult diagnosis for clinicians [18]. In general, there are few signs associated with the condition. Most of the patients have tenderness at the site of pain. Slight oedema is sometimes noted [34] as is thickening of the subcutaneous border of the tibia.

The predominant symptom is pain felt on or around the tibia. It is felt on exertion, initially towards the end of a run; but if more severe, it can occur earlier during exercise [10]. Extremely severe cases may have pain on walking or even at rest [16]. Medial-sided tibial pain seems usually to be described as soreness or a dull aching pain [49], whereas lateral-sided pain may be more aching and cramping in quality, but this is extremely variable.

Highly developed musculature may be seen [50], and the muscle compartments may feel tense or have muscle herniae [51].

Neurological symptoms are sometimes reported, and occasionally there may be weakness and pain on passive stretching of the muscles running through the compartment [52].

Vascular disturbances are rare, even in cases when the shin splint is due to elevated compartment pressures [16, 50]. Tibial stress fractures usually exhibit well-localised tenderness and pain, often with palpable callus [15]. These are most commonly found at the lower and upper margins of the tibia. "Springing" the tibia (straining it against a fulcrum) may reproduce the pain in a stress fracture [34].

The major symptoms include paresthesia of the plantar aspect of the foot and tightness, cramping, and aching in the deep muscles posterior to the tibia.

Recurrent pain in the lower leg caused by exercise is a common problem in athletes. A recurrent tightening or tense sensation and aching in anatomically defined compartments are pathognomonic [53]. Half of the injured runners were unable to run 2×500 metres without pain after 10 weeks [54].

A comprehensive physical examination is imperative to confirm a diagnosis and should begin with an inquiry regarding the location and onset of the patient's pain and tenderness. Patient evaluation is based on meticulous history taking and physical examination. Even though the diagnosis remains clinical, imaging studies, such as plain radiographs and bone scans, are usually sufficient, although magnetic ressonance imaging (MRI) is useful in borderline cases to rule out more significant pathology [24].

43.5 Imagery

Physical examination could not differentiate between cases with medial tibial bone pain secondary to stress fractures and those with scintigraphically normal tibias [55]. Confirmation of the diagnosis requires performing the appropriate diagnostic studies, including radiographs, bone scans, magnetic ressonance angiography, compartmental pressure measurements, and arteriograms.

Diagnosis can be made by history alone in a majority of cases, but if the diagnosis is unclear, an X-ray and MRI should be considered [7]. Additional imaging such as bone and computerised tomography (CT) scans has been well studied but is of limited value. The prevalence of abnormal findings in asymptomatic subjects means that results should be interpreted with caution [11]. Clinicians should first make the clinical diagnosis of MTSS, however, because of high percentages of positive MRI scans in asymptomatic patients [12].

Aoki et al. [56] determine whether stress fractures and shin splints could be discriminated with MRI in the early phase. Stress fractures were diagnosed when consecutive radiographs showed local periosteal reaction or a fracture line, and shin splints were diagnosed in all the other cases. No MRI scans of shin splints showed an abnormally wide high signal in the bone marrow as observed on MRI scans of stress fractures.

43.6 Differential Diagnosis

The accurate diagnosis and treatment of medial tibial pain is complicated by the coexistence of periostitis and compartment syndrome. The literature [1] also suggests a third diagnostic entity, tibial stress fracture or microfracture, to be considered in medial tibial pain syndromes. The patient's history of type of exercise (running), initial symptom behaviour (quick resolution with rest), and later symptom behaviour in the presence of established painful symptoms (failure of rest, orthotics, and nonsteroidal anti-inflammatory medications) are consistent with type II disease (periostalgia with avulsion of the periosteum at the periosteal-fascial junction) [1]. Unfortunately, visits to multiple physicians without obtaining significant relief are also typical in the history of patients with periostitis [48].

The most common causes include muscle or tendon injury, MTSS, stress fracture, and exertional compartment syndrome. Less common causes of leg pain include lumbosacral radiculopathy, lumbosacral spinal stenosis, focal nerve entrapment, vascular claudication from atherosclerosis, popliteal artery entrapment syndrome, and venous insufficiency [2].

43.7 Treatment

Conservative treatment is almost always successful and includes several options, though none has proven more superior to rest. Prevention programmes do not seem to influence the rate of MTSS, though shock-absorbing insoles have reduced MTSS rates in military personnel, and shockwaves (ESWT) have shortened the duration of symptoms. Surgery is rarely indicated but has shown some promising results in patients who have not responded to all conservative options [18, 24]. Current best practice guidelines support a treatment programme of rest, cryotherapy, and a graduated walk-to-run programme [57]. The appropriate treatment depends on the aetiology of the shin splint.

43.7.1 Prevention

Training errors are commonly thought to provoke shin splints. These may include wearing inappropriate shoes, running on hard surfaces, and increasing mileage too rapidly. All these increase muscle fatigue and prevent the natural body reactions to stress from taking place. Stretching and strengthening of the leg muscles also help to prevent muscular strain. Stretching exercises, modification of training schedules, and the use of protective devices such as braces and insoles are often advocated for prevention.

Muscle strengthening is believed to help prevent the effects of fatigue on bone and muscle [46]. This usually consists of progressive exercises to the dorsi and plantar flexors of the foot. Stretching may also increase muscle shock absorption.

43.7.2 Rest

Rest is common to all treatment regimens. Rest allows time for healing and time for inflammation to settle down. It is essential though after rest gradually to reintroduce running and avoid any training errors that may have provoked the syndrome initially. It is advisable for the athlete to maintain cardiovascular fitness during rest, for example, with swimming or cycling.

43.7.3 Ice and Nonsteroidal Anti-inflammatory Drugs

These are also widely advised. They are thought to help by decreasing inflammatory reaction and also by analgesia. Ice before and after running is also recommended to control pain.

43.7.4 Correction of Biomechanical Defects

The device used will obviously depend on the biomechanical abnormality detected. The most common to be treated is overpronation. These are usually treated with an orthotic device, which is an artificial prosthesis that supports the antipronation muscles. It is usually a wedge, built up on the medial side of the heel. Other biomechanical abnormalities such as leg length discrepancy or forefoot varus can be treated by an appropriate orthotic.

43.7.5 Corticosteroid Injection

Injection of the medial tibia border with corticosteroids has been tried by some, but has very limited success.

43.7.6 Physiotherapy

Kinesio taping (KT) has gained popularity for treating musculoskeletal pathologies; however, its effect on MTSS remains uninvestigated. KT could decrease the rate of medial loading in MTSS patients. Future research might assess mechanisms by which this effect is achieved [9]. No additional large effect of the pneumatic leg brace could be found in recruits, and wearing of the brace was not feasible, since the wearing comfort was low [11].

43.7.7 Surgery

Surgery is indicated for chronic compartment syndrome. Almost 5% of the injured runners received surgical treatment [54]. Surgical management of deep compartment syndrome, consisting of fasciotomy or fasciectomy, or both, is successful for most patients [48].

Conclusion

Lower limb pain is frequent in long-distance athletes. An adequate diagnosis requires a detailed clinical history, a careful exam, the knowledge of the different types of possible pathologies, and a rational and insightful use of the possible diagnosis studies. Tibial periostitis is the most frequent cause (MTSS). Other causes are fatigue fractures and the compartmental syndromes. Especially in senior athletes, vascular and vertebral causes should also be considered.

The treatment of MTSS, like the treatment of other periostitis and fatigue fractures, requires rest, evaluation, and biomechanical corrections. The preventive measures are determinant.

References

1. Detmer D. Chronic shin splints: classification and management of medial tibial stress syndrome. Sports Med. 1986;3:436–46.
2. Fredericson M, Wun C. Differential diagnosis of leg pain in the athlete. J Am Podiatr Med Assoc. 2003;93:321–4.
3. Jones D, James S. Overuse injuries of the lower extremity: shin splints, iliotibial band friction syndrome and exertional compartment syndromes. Clin Sports Med. 1987;6:273–90.
4. Rorabeck C. Exertional tibialis posterior compartment syndrome in athletes. Clin Orthop Rel Res. 1986;208:61–4.
5. Styf J. Chronic exercise-induced pain in the anterior aspect of the lower leg: an overview of diagnosis. Sports Med. 1989;7:331–9.
6. Meyer S, Saltzman C, Albright J. Stress fractures of the foot and leg. Clin Sports Med. 1993;12:395–413.
7. Story J, Cymet TC. Shin splints: painful to have and to treat. Compr Ther. 2006;32:192–5.
8. Reinking MF. Exercise related leg pain (ERLP): a review of the literature. N Am J Sports Phys Ther. 2007:170–80.
9. Griebert MC, Needle AR, McConnell J, Kaminski TW. Lower-leg kinesio tape reduces rate of loading in participants with medial tibial stress syndrome. Phys Ther Sport. 2016;18:62–7.
10. Mubarak SJ, Gould RN, Lee YF, Schmidt DA, Hargens AR. The medial tibial stress syndrome. A cause of shin splints. Am J Sports Med. 1982;10:201–5.
11. Moen MH, Tol JL, Weir A, Steunebrink M, De Winter TC. Medial tibial stress syndrome: a critical review. Sports Med. 2009;39:523–46.
12. Craig DI. Medial tibial stress syndrome: evidence-based prevention. J Athl Train. 2008;43:316–8.
13. Loudon JK, Reiman MP. Lower extremity kinematics in running athletes with and without a history of medial shin pain. Int J Sports Phys Ther. 2012;7:356–64.
14. Bates P. Shin splints. A literature review. Brit J Sports Med. 1985;19:132–7.
15. Devas MB. Shin splints, or stress fractures of the metacarpal bone in horses, and shin soreness, or stress fractures of the tibia, in man. J Bone Joint Surg Br. 1967;49-B:310–3.
16. Puranen J, Alavaikko A. Intracompartmental pressure increase on exertion in patients with chronic compartment syndrome in the leg. J Bone Joint Surg Am. 1981;63-A:1304–9.
17. Subotnick SI. The shin splints syndrome of the lower extremity. J Am Podiatry Assoc. 1976;66:43–5.
18. Brewer RB, Gregory AJ. Chronic lower leg pain in athletes: a guide for the differential diagnosis, evaluation, and treatment. Sports Health. 2012;4:121–7.
19. Gudas CJ. Patterns of lower extremity injury in 224 runners. Compr Ther. 1980;6:50–9.
20. James SL, Bates BT, Osternis LR. Injuries to runners. Am J Sports Med. 1978;6:40–50.
21. Sharma J, Greeves JP, Byers M, Bennett AN, Spears IR. Musculoskeletal injuries in British army recruits: a prospective study of diagnosis-specific incidence and rehabilitation times. BMC Musculoskelet Disord. 2015;16:106.
22. Orava S, Puranen J. Athletes' leg pains. Br J Sports Med. 1979;13:92–7.
23. Sharma J, Weston M, Batterham AM, Spears IR. Gait retraining and incidence of medial tibial stress syndrome in army recruits. Med Sci Sports Exerc. 2014;46:1684–92.
24. Reshef N, Guelich DR. Medial tibial stress syndrome. Clin Sports Med. 2012;31:273–90.
25. Hubbard TJ, Carpenter EM, Cordova ML. Contributing factors to medial tibial stress syndrome: a prospective investigation. Med Sci Sports Exerc. 2009;41:490–6.
26. Gallo RA, Plakke M, Silvis ML. Common leg injuries of long-distance runners: anatomical and biomechanical approach. Sports Health. 2012;4:485–95.
27. Spiker AM, Dixit S, Cosgarea AJ. Triathlon: running injuries. Sports Med Arthrosc. 2012;20:206–13.
28. Newman P, Adams R, Waddington G. Two simple clinical tests for predicting onset of medial tibial stress syndrome: shin palpation test and shin oedema test. Br J Sports Med. 2012;46:861–4.
29. Twellaar M, Verstappen FT, Huson A, van Mechelen W. Physical characteristics as risk factors for sports injuries: a four year prospective study. Int J Sports Med. 1997;18:66–71.
30. Yagi S, Muneta T, Sekiya I. Incidence and risk factors for medial tibial stress syndrome and tibial stress fracture in high school runners. Knee Surg Sports Traumatol Arthrosc. 2013;21:556–63.
31. Sabeti V, Khoshraftar Yazdi N, Bizheh N. The relationship between shin splints with anthropometric characteristics and some indicators of body composition. J Sports Med Phys Fitness. 2014 Oct 6. Epub 2014 Oct 6.

32. Krivickas LS. Anatomical factors associated with overuse sports injuries. Sports Med. 1997;24:132–46.
33. Couture CJ, Karlson KA. Tibial stress injuries: decisive diagnosis and treatment of 'shin splints'. Phys Sportsmed. 2002;30:29–36.
34. Devas MB. Stress fractures of the tibia in athletes or "shin soreness". J Bone Joint Surg Br. 1958;40-B:227–39.
35. Jackson DW. Shinsplints: An Update. Phys Sports Med. 1978;6(10):50–61.
36. Schissel DJ, Godwin J. Effort-related chronic compartment syndrome of the lower extremity. Mil Med. 1999;164:830–2.
37. Wallensten R. Results of fasciotomy in patients with medial tibial syndrome or chronic anterior compartment syndrome. J Bone Joint Surg Am. 1983;65-A:1252–5.
38. D'Ambrosia RD, Zelis RF, Chuinard RG, Wilmore J. Interstitial pressure measurements in the anterior and posterior compartments in athletes with shin splints. Am J Sports Med. 1977;5:127–31.
39. Sommer HM, Vallentyne SW. Effect of foot posture on the incidence of medial tibial stress syndrome. Med Sci Sports Exerc. 1995;27:800–4.
40. Root ML, Orien WP, Weed JH. Normal and abnormal function of the foot. Los Angeles: Clinical Biomechanics Corporation; 1977.
41. Plisky MS, Rauh MJ, Heiderscheit B, Underwood FB, Tank RT. Medial tibial stress syndrome in high school cross-country runners: incidence and risk factors. J Orthop Sports Phys Ther. 2007;37:40–7.
42. Raissi GR, Cherati AD, Mansoori KD, Razi MD. The relationship between lower extremity alignment and medial tibial stress syndrome among non-professional athletes. Sports Med Arthrosc Rehabil Ther Technol. 2009;1:11.
43. Rathleff MS, Kelly LA, Christensen FB, Simonsen OH, Kaalund S, Laessoe U. Dynamic midfoot kinematics in subjects with medial tibial stress syndrome. J Am Podiatr Med Assoc. 2012;102:205–12.
44. Yüksel O, Ozgürbüz C, Ergün M, Işlegen C, Taskiran E, Denerel N, Ertat A. Inversion/eversion strength dysbalance in patients with medial tibial stress syndrome. J Sports Sci Med. 2011;10:737–42.
45. Noh B, Masunari A, Akiyama K, Fukano M, Fukubayashi T, Miyakawa S. Structural deformation of longitudinal arches during running in soccer players with medial tibial stress syndrome. Eur J Sport Sci. 2015;15:173–81.
46. Clement D, Taunton J, Smart G. A survey of overuse running injuries. Phys Sports Med. 1981;9:47–58.
47. Taunton JE, Clement DB, Webber D. Lower extremity stress fractures in athletes. Phys Sports Med. 1981;9:77–86.
48. Heinrichs K, Lachowicz WM. Concurrent periostalgia and chronic proximal deep posterior compartment syndrome in a collegiate track and field athlete: a case report. J Athl Train. 2000;35:450–2.
49. Slocum DB, James SL. Biomechanics of running. JAMA. 1968;205:97–104.
50. Mavor GE. The anterior tibial syndrome. J Bone Joint Surg Br. 1956;38-B:513–7.
51. Martens MA, Backaert M, Vermaut G, Mulier JC. Chronic leg pain in athletes due to a recurrent compartment syndrome. Am J Sports Med. 1984;12:148–51.
52. Matsen FA, Mayo KA, Sheridan GW. Monitoring of intramuscular pressure. Surgery. 1976;79:702–9.
53. Cetinus E, Uzel M, Bilgiç E, Karaoguz A, Herdem M. Exercise induced compartment syndrome in a professional footballer. Br J Sports Med. 2004;38:227–9.
54. Nielsen RO, Rønnow L, Rasmussen S, Lind M. A prospective study on time to recovery in 254 injured novice runners. PLoS One. 2014;9
55. Milgrom C, Chisin R, Gilati M, Stein M, Kachtan H, Margulies J, et al. Negative bone scans in impeding tibial stress fracture. Am J Sports Med. 1984;12:488–91.
56. Aoki Y, Yasuda K, Tohyama H, Ito H, Minami A. Magnetic resonance imaging in stress fractures and shin splints. Clin Orthop Relat Res. 2004;421:260–7.
57. Johnston E, Flynn T, Bean M, Breton M, Scherer M, Dreitzler G, et al. A randomized controlled trial of a leg orthosis versus traditional treatment for soldiers with shin splints: a pilot study. Mil Med. 2006;171:40–4.

Part XI

Toracic Concerns

Preseason Evaluation

44

Ruben Ferreira, João Pedro Araújo, Paulo Barreira, Nuno Loureiro, and Wayne Diesel

Contents

44.1 Introduction

Football demands are increasing significantly over the years. Football players are covering larger distances with higher speeds (increased covered distance with high-intensity actions), leading to an increased metabolic and physical stress during the exercise [1].

Considering this, the first step before the players start to train should be the *preseason evaluation*, in order to detect *contraindications to football practice* [2], *player's injury profile* and *player's fitness level* [3], which can be divided in three *screening levels*:

- *Life-threatening and general health conditions*
- *Injury risk factors*
- *Performance*

R. Ferreira (✉)
Football Medicine®, Abu Dhabi, UAE

Al Jazira Sports and Cultural Club – Football, Abu Dhabi, UAE

Kinesio Taping Association International, Porto, Portugal
e-mail: rubenferreira88@gmail.com

J.P. Araújo
Football Medicine®, Porto, Portugal

Al Jazira Sports and Cultural Club – Football, Abu Dhabi, UAE

Clinica do Dragão Espregueira Mendes Sports Centre – FIFA Medical Centre of Excellence, Porto, Portugal

P. Barreira
Football Medicine®, Porto, Portugal

Al Jazira Sports and Cultural Club – Football, Abu Dhabi, UAE

N. Loureiro
FC Paços de Ferreira, Paços de Ferreira, Portugal

Portuguese Cycling Federation, Lisbon, Portugal

Olympic Portuguese Committee, Lisboa, Portugal

Clinica do Dragão Espregueira Mendes Sports Centre – FIFA Medical Centre of Excellence, Porto, Portugal

W. Diesel
Miami Dolphins – American Football, Miami Gardens, FL, USA

Charlton Athletic FC and Tottenham Hotspur FC, London, UK

J. Espregueira-Mendes et al. (eds.), *Injuries and Health Problems in Football*, DOI 10.1007/978-3-662-53924-8_44

Although all being important, a hierarchy must be considered during players' assessment (see Fig. 44.1). In the preseason evaluation, priority must be given to *life-threatening and general health conditions* – addressing the person ahead of the player – and then focus on *injury risk factors*, followed by *performance* assessment.

Screening is one of the most important actions before season starts. Besides decreasing the risk of life-threatening situations [2], it will probably define a significant part of the season programme, especially individual gym routines, as it will identify the individual needs of each player (e.g. strength, flexibility, motor control imbalances) [3].

As we all know, there are an infinitive number of tests that can be performed in order to collect data [4–6]; however, due to time constraints in terms of assessment and also data analysis, any preseason screening – excluding the first level of the pyramid – should obey five rules:

- Only collect data that you know you will be able to analyse in a proper timing
- User-friendly tests
- Test reproducibility
- Only relevant tests
- Don't duplicate information

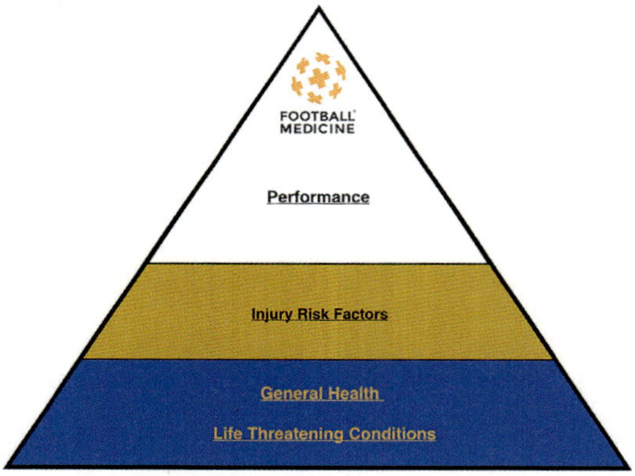

Fig. 44.1 Screening levels pyramid

44.2 FIFA and UEFA Recommendations

We recommend the reading of the documents available online on FIFA and UEFA websites – www.fifa.com and www.uefa.org.

FIFA website has a link for *medical* issues which contain many official documents including the FIFA PCMA form. This paper is a guide for a complete medical examination with cardiovascular screening (Fig. 44.2) and blood analysis. It is mandatory for clubs, involved in most of FIFA's competitions, to fill in these forms and is frequently requested by insurance companies. This document is simple, objective and easy to fill and print.

All those qualities turn the forms into an easy way to follow all the important steps of the medical screening, accomplishing, at the same time, all legal requirements for the main FIFA competitions.

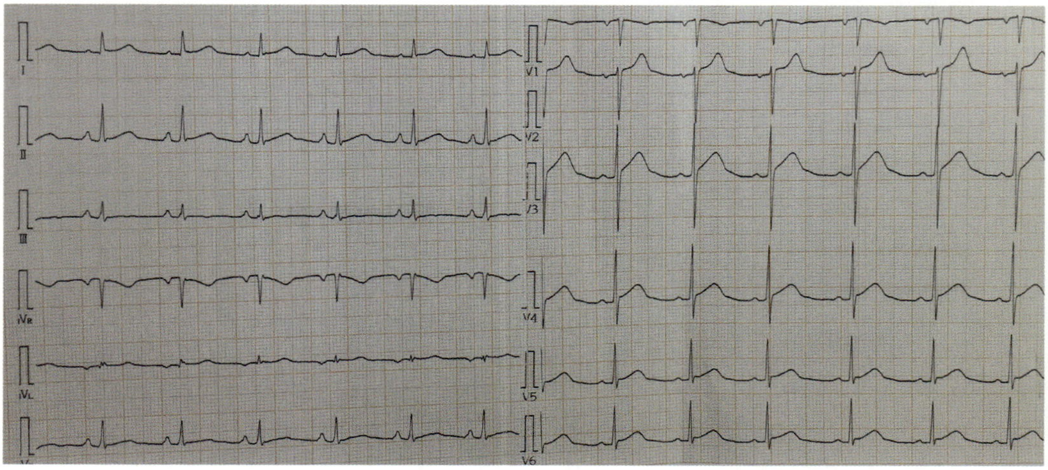

Fig. 44.2 ECG

Table 44.1 Preseason evaluation protocol

Pre-season evaluation protocol		
Life threatening conditions and general health	Injury risk factors	Performance
• Medical history	• Strength testing	• VO_2 max
• Medical physical examination	• ROM and flexibility testing	• Agility tests
• Cardiovascular screening (Fig. 44.2)	• Motor control	• Strength qualities
• Asthma and allergies screening	• Posture	• Maximum speed and sprint
• Blood and urine analysis	• Running pattern analysis	
• Musculoskeletal imaging	• Podiatrist assessment	
• Body composition and nutritional background		

44.3 Preseason Evaluation Protocol

The table below is an outline of the preseason evaluation protocol, together with the contents of each screening level (Table 44.1).

44.3.1 Life-Threatening and General Health Conditions

44.3.1.1 Medical History

Players' medical history is of major importance in the whole pre-participation examination. A careful and detailed medical interview should be conducted in a comfortable and calm setting ensuring the confidentiality of the exam. For children, the presence of an adult with knowledge about his personal and family medical history (usually the parents) is mandatory.

Many aspects should be assessed, and each clinician might have their own protocol. Nevertheless, three main domains should be accessed during this interview: family history, past medical history and present medical history. For each, we will highlight the fundamental parameters that should be assessed.

Family History

It's of paramount importance to rule out family, first or second degree, history of cardiovascular diseases that may have led to sudden death/disability or medical-advised suspension of physical activities of family (Table 44.2).

Table 44.2 Cardiovascular screening questionnaire

Cardiovascular screening questionnaire
Family history
Premature death or disability due to heart disease before 50 years of age
Personal history
Exertional chest pain or discomfort
Syncope or near-syncope
Irregular heart beat or palpitations
Shortness of breath or fatigue out of proportion to the degree of exertion

Other major and/or chronic diseases (especially with strong genetic correlations) such as asthma, type 1 diabetes and epilepsy should be part of our questionnaire.

Past Medical History

Red flag cardiovascular symptoms to be ruled out (Table 44.2)

Other chronic, major diseases or accidents (e.g. concussion)

Musculoskeletal medical history (especially long-term injuries – greater than 1 month of activity suspension – or involving hospital attendance or surgical treatment)

Present Medical History

Sports activity profile (number of games in the last 12 months, position in the field, dominant leg)

Lifestyle (harmful behaviours – smoking, alcohol consumption, drug abuse; sleep patterns; food diary)

Present medical complaints

Allergies (food, medication, physical agents, insect bites, cosmetics)

Vaccination (according to origin and residence country)
Medication and supplements (casual or chronic)

44.3.1.2 Medical Physical Examination

Normally, each doctor has his own protocol, which was built during his/her career according to guidelines and personal experience. Either you choose to follow your exam from head to toes or from system to system, the most important is to follow a sequential and systematic evaluation and to never forget the mandatory items that you can find in the UEFA and FIFA guidelines.

Next is an example of how to conduct a physical examination in a professional football player. The player should expose as much of his/her body as possible, respecting his/her personal, social and religious limitations:

- Begin the exam with a *general examination* with emphasis on the *cardiovascular system* but checking the other systems briefly. For that, you should, at least, collect the following information:
  - Height, weight
  - Skin (surgical and non-surgical wound scars, fungi, viral and bacterial infections)
  - Heart rate, blood pressure, peripheral pulses
  - Cardiac and pulmonary auscultation
  - Lymph node screening and thyroid gland palpation
  - Abdominal palpation (exclude abnormal masses, organomegaly and hernias)
  - Basic neurological examination (including reflexes, balance tests such as SOLEC, walk a straight line)
  - Exclude Marfan criteria (chest deformities, arachnodactyly of fingers and toes, long arms, scoliosis, lens dislocation, others)
- The second step will be the *musculoskeletal system* evaluation. After the cardiovascular screening, this is the major system to screen. We recommend the following sequence:
- Functional tests (important as general screening and determines the direction of the rest of the examination):
  - Walk a straight line
  - Toe walking
  - Heel walking
  - Duck walk
  - Single-leg squat
  - One-leg hop test
- Posture (sagittal, coronal and transversal planes)
- Spine examination (observe full range of motion, and perform tests including Schober's test and Gillet test)
- Lower limb length measurement
- Joint examination (special attention to shoulder and lower limbs – confirm absence of inflammatory signs, wound scars, muscle wasting or ROM restrictions, palpation of the most important ligaments and tendons such as Achilles, patellar tendons)

44.3.1.3 Blood and Urine Analysis

FIFA and UEFA recommendations are summarized in Table 44.3.

Table 44.3 FIFA and UEFA laboratorial analysis recommendations

Blood and urine analysis			
Haemoglobin	Haematocrit	Erythrocytes	Thrombocytes
Leukocytes	Sodium	Potassium	Magnesium
Cholesterol (Total)	LDL Cholesterol	HDL Cholesterol	Triglycerides
Glucose	Sedimentation Rate	Creatine	C-reactive Protein
Uric Acid	Aspartate Amino-transferase	Alanine Amino-transferase	Gamma-Glutamyl-transferase
Creatine Kinase	Iron	Ferritin	Blood Group

44.3.1.4 Musculoskeletal Imaging

Imaging technology can be used during the preseason screening according to clinical findings in the history and physical examination. However, a fast and easy systematic ultrasonography assessment of the Achilles tendon, patellar tendon and shoulder structures (in goalkeepers) can be performed if the sports medicine physician has the proper equipment and knowledge, giving us useful information regarding some of the most common pathologies in this population [7–9].

44.3.1.5 Concussion

Very recently it has been shown that college athletes were at a 2.48 times greater risk of a lower extremity injury up to 90 days post-concussion possibly due to lingering neurocognitive and motor deficits [10]. Having baseline measures on players, prior to concussion, will help return-to-play decisions and hopefully further reduce injury risk. The tests listed below are examples of what practitioners can use to establish baselines.

The United States of America Football notes that baseline screening of players using neurocognitive tools, such as ImPACT, can be used by suitably qualified staff and recommends that the Sport Concussion Assessment Tool (SCAT3), which incorporates a modified Balance Error Scoring System (BESS), should be used pitchside following suspected concussions. Players' baseline in balance and reaction time tests should also be recorded [11, 12].

44.3.1.6 Body Composition

During the pre-evaluation period, it is an ideal time to check on the player's weight, after returning from the off-season. This is also an ideal opportunity to educate players on the risks of dehydrating to make weight.

Body composition measurements, in particular percentage body fat and fat-free mass, are routinely measured in players at the start of the season and at regular intervals in-season. The widely accepted rationale behind this is that excessive adipose tissue adds 'useless' weight to the player resulting in greater energy expenditure and lower power and accelerations. What is not as widely accepted is the choice of devices to measure percentage body fat. Traditional ways include callipers and underwater weighing techniques; callipers being the simplest and cost-effective but prone to large intra-tester variances.

Dual-energy X-ray absorptiometry [DEXA] scans provide very accurate body composition measurements as well as information about bone density. Other potentially useful benefits include gaining insight in distribution of adipose in different regions of the body and even asymmetrical distribution between limbs.

44.3.1.7 Dental

Gay-Escoda et al. [13] found a significant correlation between players with poor oral health and muscle injuries. SportsInjuryLab, a company screening athletes for dental and occlusal problems (i.e. periodontitis, impacted wisdom teeth, malocclusion), has linked dental and temporomandibular joint problems to negative impacts on balance and ultimately performance or increased risk of injury [13].

Including an oral health assessment in the preseason evaluation is not common practice but may be worth considering, especially for teams that have a dentist associated with the club.

44.3.1.8 Vision

A player's ability to make the correct decision in a split second is believed to be based on three important cognitive components. These components, according to Bar-Eli [14], are perception, knowledge and decision strategies. The top decision makers use well-developed visual search strategies in both their peripheral and central vision [15] together with selective, focused and divided attention [14].

44.3.2 Injury Risk Factors

This screening level plays a significant role throughout the season because it may identify players' imbalances that should then be corrected, in order to decrease risk of injury.

Sports medicine teams should gather a *battery of tests with the best evidence available*, considering the injury risk factors, in order to apply it during the preseason evaluation. This will *identify individual players' needs/imbalances* in terms of *strength* [16], *range of motion (ROM) and flexibility* [6, 17], *motor control* [18], *posture* and *running pattern analysis* [19], [20]. Feasibility is important in a football team setup; therefore, the five rules mentioned earlier should be considered before test selection.

These battery of tests, besides identifying individual players' needs/imbalances, also have the important role of *establishing a baseline of clinical and physical features of the players*, which might be of considerable value if, in the future, they get injured and need rehabilitation. For instance, after an anterior cruciate ligament (ACL) reconstruction, and before returning to training, it is important to know if the player is able to achieve his previous knee range of motion or strength levels, and this is only possible if such data was previously collected.

After screening and analysing players' data, individual programmes should be developed in order to correct the imbalances or maintain their qualities.

44.3.2.1 Strength Testing

There is a significant amount of literature supporting the implication of strength imbalances as an injury risk factor for most of the injuries that occur in football [6, 16, 21].

It is important to assess the different types of strength, namely, *maximum strength*, *power* and *endurance*.

Maximum strength imbalances are strongly correlated with several football injuries in literature (e.g. hamstring strains, groin syndrome), making it mandatory to be assessed before season starts [16, 21, 22]. Despite the absence of evidence supporting the other strength types as injury risk factors, we still find it important to measure because it can complement player's strength profile, by providing us with a baseline of the player or leading us to a further investigation in cases where an imbalance is unveiled.

Maximum Strength

This type of strength is usually assessed using a dynamometer (Figs. 44.3 and 44.4), either isokinetic or manual. In our experience, thigh muscles acting on the knee joint (quadriceps femoris and hamstrings) are better assessed with an isokinetic dynamometer [16], whilst abductor and

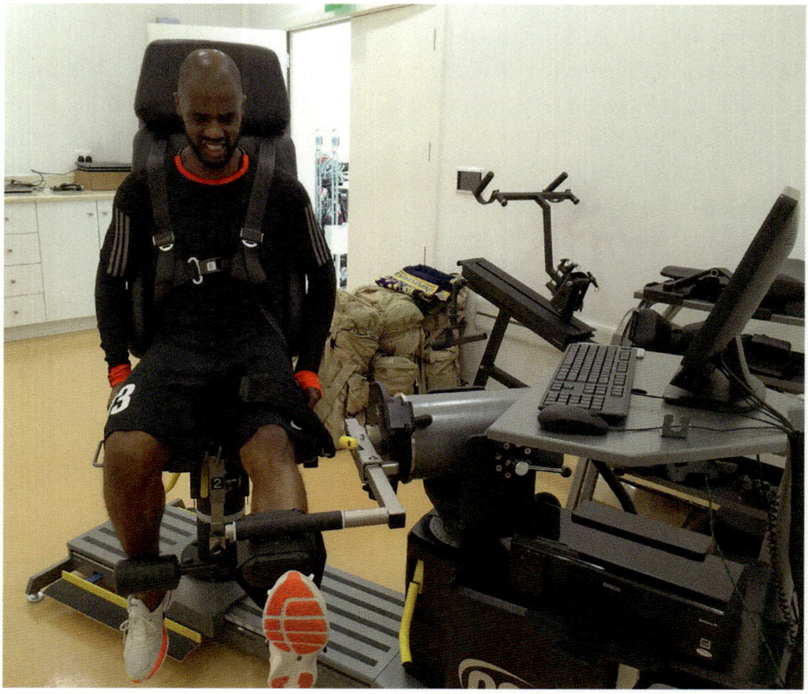

Fig. 44.3 Dynamometer isokinetic testing

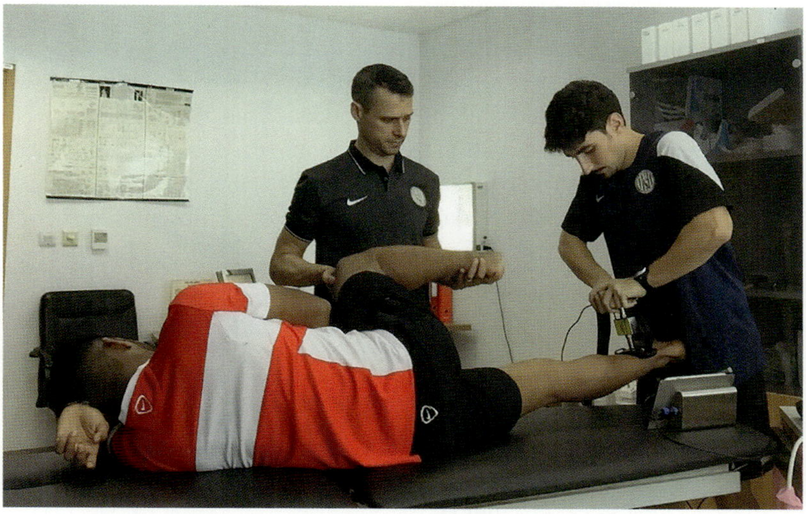

Fig. 44.4 Left hip adductor manual dynamometer testing

adductor muscles are easily assessed with manual dynamometers [22]. Ankle joint muscle maximum strength can also be assessed in an isokinetic dynamometer; however, it is not a user-friendly test to perform [5].

Clinicians should focus on agonist/antagonist strength ratios as well as contralateral imbalances [16, 22], as well as considering other specific parameters, as it will be discussed below.

Isokinetic Dynamometer [16]

As mentioned above, this device will be easily used for quadriceps (Q) and hamstring (H) strength assessment. Maximum strength will be better assessed with *low-speed testing*; however, high-speed testing will also be described in this chapter, regarding its importance to calculate *hamstring/quadriceps functional ratio* (Fig. 44.3).

Protocol

- Concentric Q and H testing – 60°/sec and 240°/sec
- Eccentric H testing – 30°/sec

Expected Outcomes

- Q and H peak torques at 60°/sec < 10% difference between sides
- H/Q conventional ratio at 60°/sec > 0, 60
- H eccentric peak torque at 30°/sec < 10% difference between sides
- H/Q functional ratio >1, 2
- H eccentric peak torque angle < 30° flexion
- Other aspects of the isokinetic outcomes can and should be assessed (e.g. curve patterns); however, it is beyond the scope of this chapter

Manual Dynamometer [22]

Groin syndrome complaints are strongly correlated with hip adductor and abductor strength imbalances, which highlight its assessment importance in football.

Abductor and adductor muscle testing can be performed using an *isometric* [make] or an *eccentric* [break] contraction, being an easy and cheap way to evaluate this muscle maximum strength. However, attention must be paid when the clinician uses the second [break] type of contraction once; an increase in the speed of the test can lead to an incorrect measure from the device and/or injury (Fig. 44.4).

Protocol

- Isometric/eccentric contraction
  - Testing position must be standardized

Expected Outcomes

- Abductor and adductor strength <10% differences between sides
- 0.90 < abductor/adductor ratio > 1.10

Sphygmomanometer Squeeze Testing [23]

Despite not being a real strength measure, this is a test found in literature to predict the risk of developing groin pain syndrome, using an adductor squeeze test measured with the sphygmomanometer between both knees that will measure pressure. It is also a useful and quick test to monitor load tolerance in season (Fig. 44.5).

Protocol

- 45° hip flexion and 90° knee flexion
- Initial sphygmomanometer pressure – 10 mm/Hg

Expected Outcome

- Squeeze pressure > 210 mm/Hg

However, this test has important limitations:

- Unable to identify the weak side
- Unable to compare between sides and calculate ratios

Power

As mentioned before in this chapter, power is another type of strength demonstration that, despite not being strongly correlated with injury risk, as previously discussed, its assessment is important to establish *players' baseline* in case of an injury occurrence or to *detect major imbalances* between sides that can prompt further investigation of the athlete.

Muscular power is a product of force and velocity; this way, its basic testing should be done with *low weights*, enabling to achieve high speed during that movement. Unlike maximal strength that is frequently assessed analytically muscle-by-muscle, power tests typically involve a *whole body functional movement* (e.g. jump), to assess the performance of all the kinetic chain [24, 25].

In football, the most frequently used power assessments are *lower limb power tests* (Fig. 44.6).

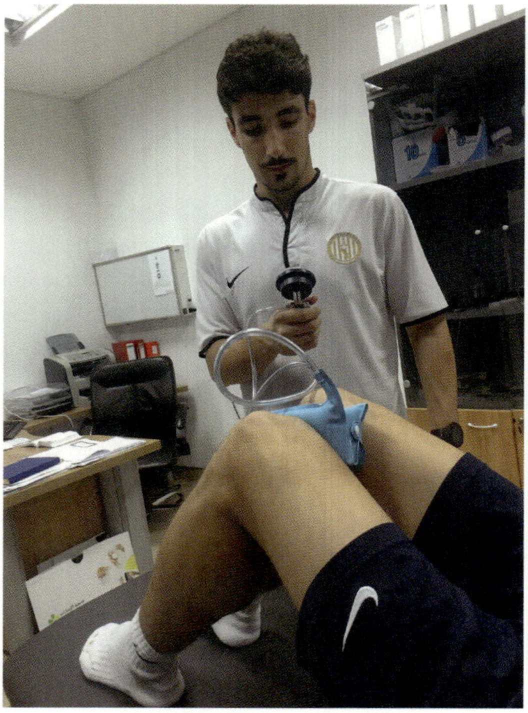

Fig. 44.5 Squeeze test with sphygmomanometer

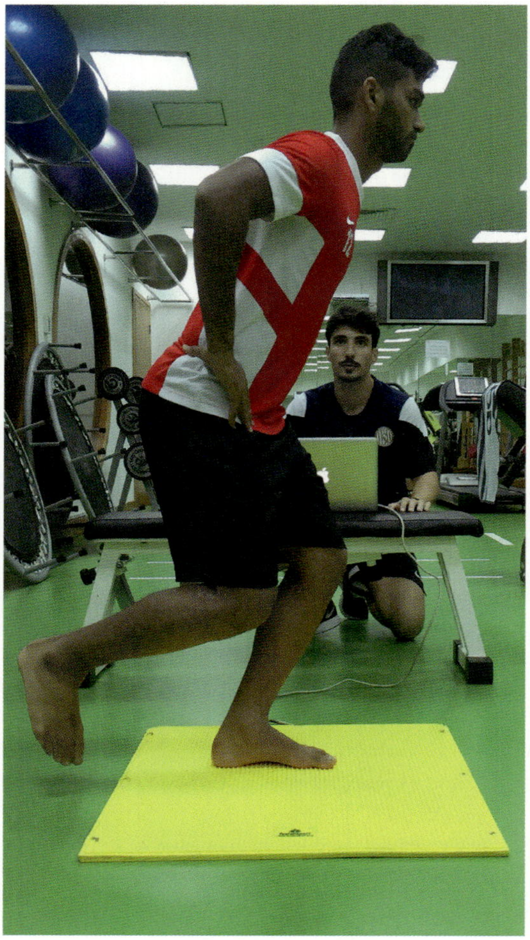

Fig. 44.6 Jump height testing with contact mat

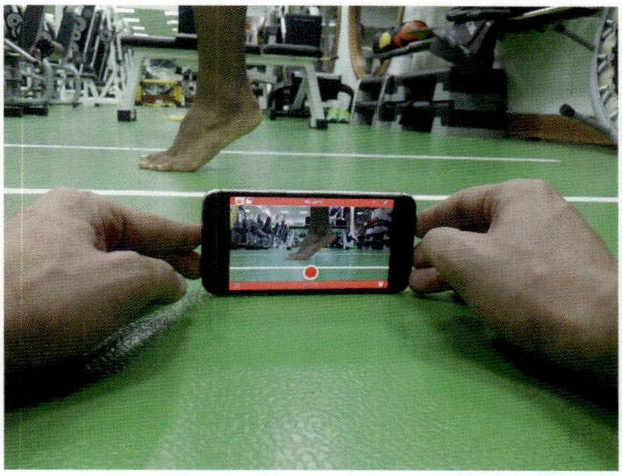

Fig. 44.7 My Jump iPhone application

Several tests are available; however, *vertical jump*, *single-leg hop* and *single-leg triple hop tests* are the most commonly used.

Vertical Jump Test [25, 26]
- Single-leg vertical jump
- Measure the height reached
- Can be assessed with photoelectric cells (e.g. Optojump), pressure-sensitive mats or video analysis (e.g. My Jump app*) [27, 28] (Fig. 44.7)

*Validated iPhone application to assess jump height

Single-Leg Hop Test [25]
- Single-leg horizontal jump
- Measure the distance between the initial contact and the landing point
- Can be assessed through video analysis or direct measure with a simple tape measure
- Careful assessment of landing mechanics [hip adduction, knee valgus, stiffness] may identify players' risk of injury such as ACL ruptures (Fig. 44.8)

Single-Leg Triple Hop Test [29]
- Three consecutive horizontal single-leg jumps
- Measure the distance between the initial contact and the finishing point
- Can be assessed through video analysis or direct measure with a simple tape measure
- As mentioned above, landing mechanics should be assessed. If any potential problems are noted, then further detailed investigation is warranted
- Limitations
  - Strongly dependent of athlete's technique and motivation
  - Performance is significantly dependent of motor control rather than strength by itself

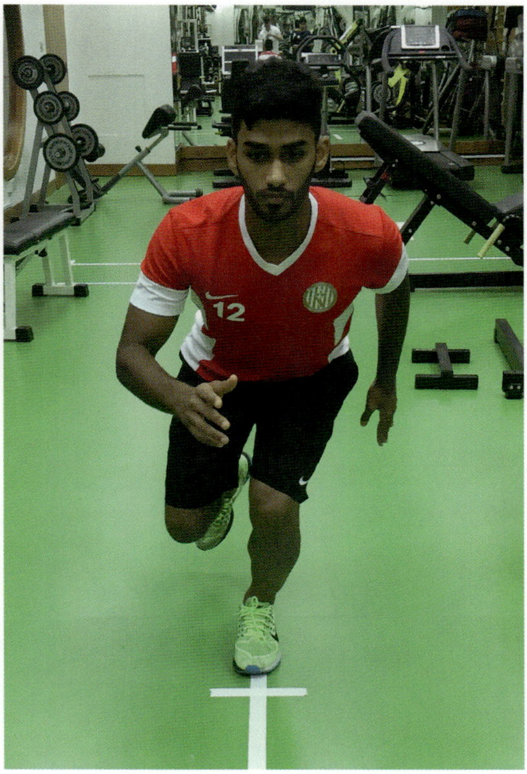

Fig. 44.8 Single-leg hop test

Endurance Strength

As discussed earlier, besides lack of evidence as an injury risk factor, endurance testing may be relevant when assessing calf muscle strength in football players, regarding its implications not only to calf injuries but also to lower limb kinematics (e.g. synergy between gastrocnemius and hamstring during landing and ACL injury risk) [30].

This way, an endurance strength test might be used for the calf muscles, focused on gastrocnemius or soleus muscle, depending on the knee flexion degree. Attention should be paid to the quality of the movement, whilst a balanced number of heel raises is expected between sides [31] (Fig. 44.9).

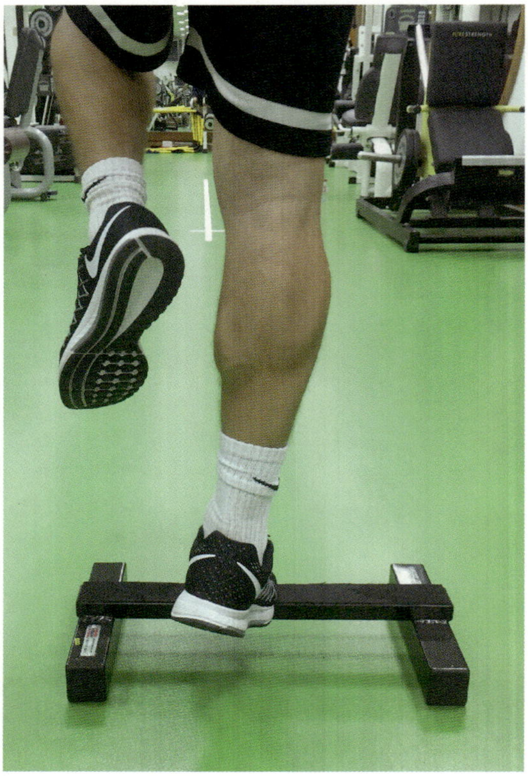

Fig. 44.9 Calf endurance test

44.3.2.2 ROM and Flexibility

This section will focus on the *most relevant tests regarding injury risk factor identification* as addressed in the *first level of the screening levels* – general health (physical examination).

In this screening, the clinician should focus on the imbalance between sides and also in significant loss of ROM/flexibility if both sides are limited (Figs. 44.10, 44.11, 44.12, 44.13, 44.14 and 44.15).

Several injuries and dysfunctional movement patterns in football are correlated with loss of mobility in the hip (e.g. groin syndrome), knee (e.g. patellofemoral syndrome) and ankle (e.g. knee dynamic valgus) joints, which is what makes this assessment mandatory in order to detect injury risk factors of the players [32–36].

44.3.2.3 Motor Control

Inadequate *movement quality* has been proposed to have a significant effect on musculoskeletal injuries. Researchers suggest that certain movement patterns might be harmful during sports' practice (e.g. excessive hip internal rotation), leading to injury [37].

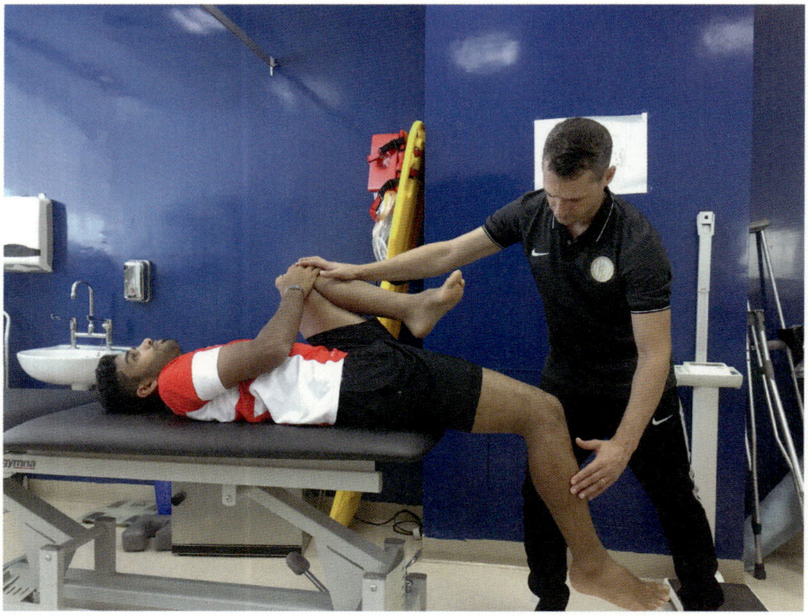

Fig. 44.10 Thomas test

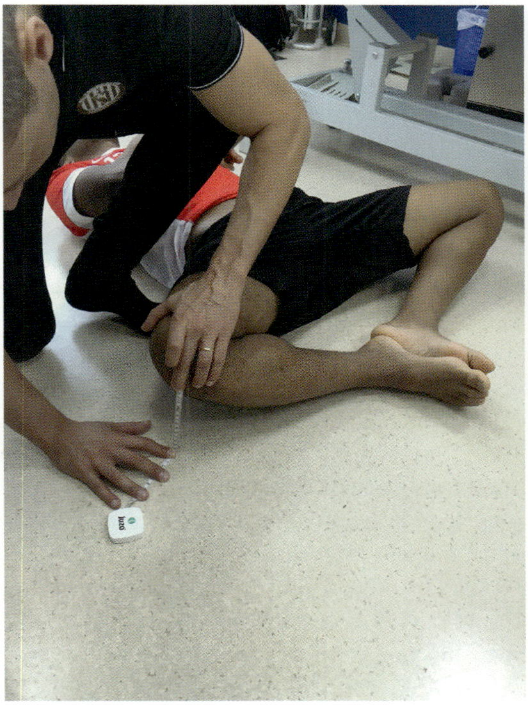

Fig. 44.11 Passive knee fallout test

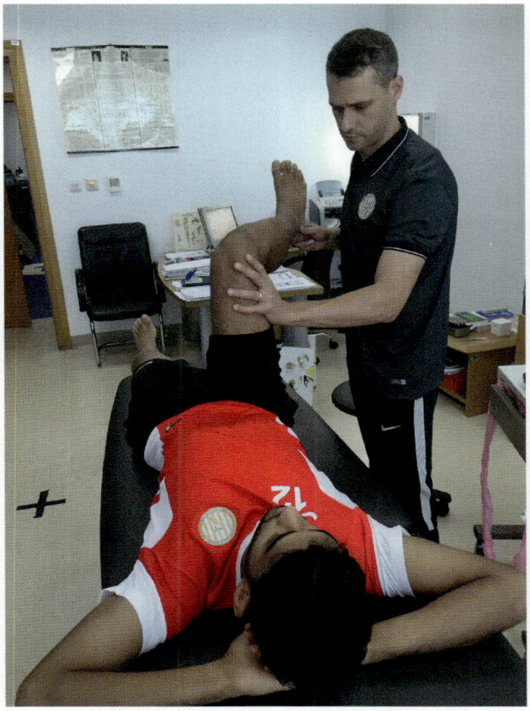

Fig. 44.12 Hip internal rotation test

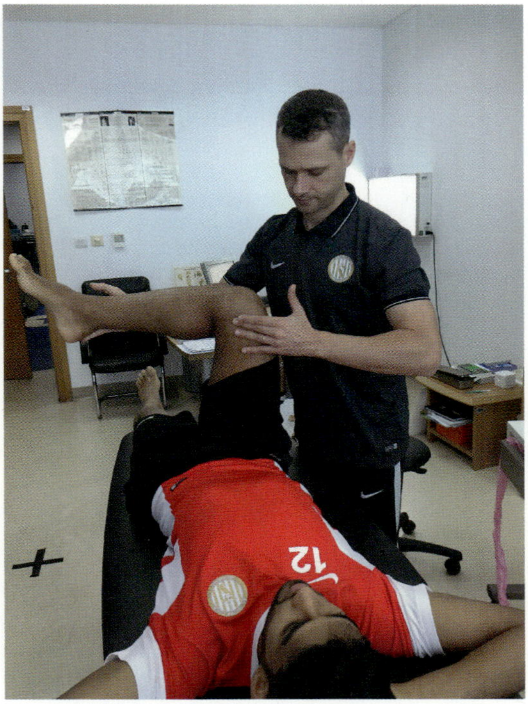

Fig. 44.13 Hip external rotation test

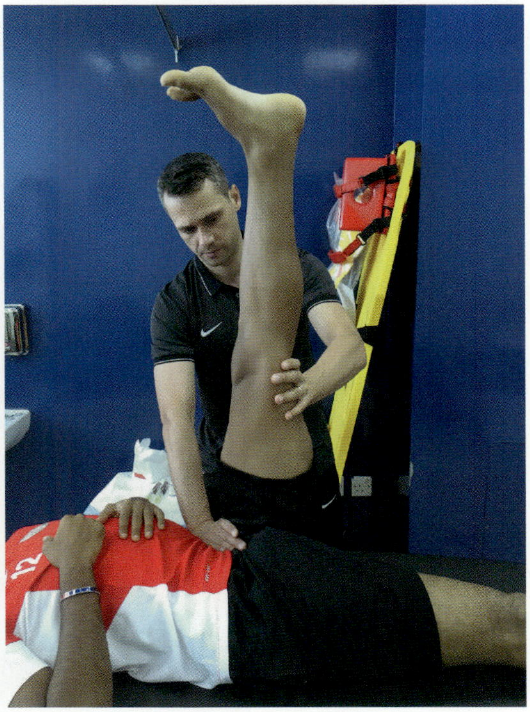

Fig. 44.14 Active-knee-extension test

Movement quality is strictly dependent of an individual's *motor control*, defined as a system responsible for the movement planning, execution and correction, whilst interpreting information gathered and processed from the afferent organs and receptors. Through this system, humans are able to select a specific motor scheme in order to perform the required task efficiently, as well as detecting movement mistakes and correcting them during the action – feedforward and feedback mechanisms [38].

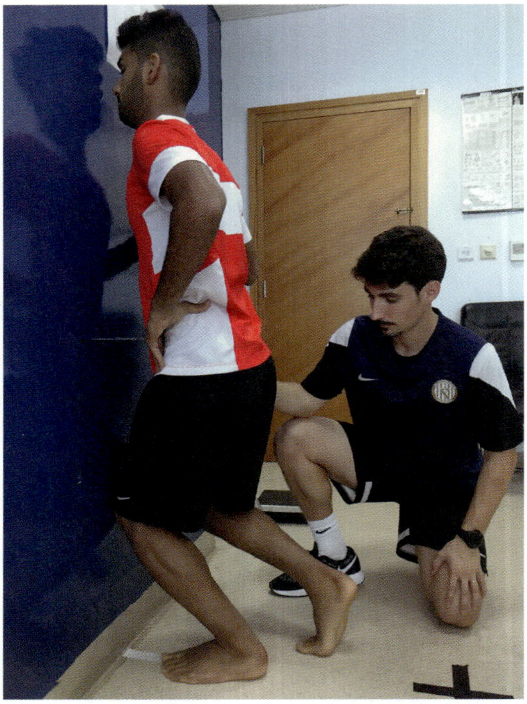

Fig. 44.15 Dorsiflexion lunge test

The aim of this screening is to detect dysfunctional movement patterns of the player during sports-specific movements (e.g. landing, decelerating, side-cutting) than can lead to increased injury risk.

Dysfunctional movement patterns have been linked to several musculoskeletal injuries in sports, both acute (e.g. ACL injury) and/or overload (e.g. patellofemoral syndrome). A significant amount of the research in this area has focused mainly on hip, knee and foot kinematics, regarding lower limb injuries due to increased dynamic valgus moments or foot overpronation [19, 20, 39].

The most frequently used movements/tests to identify motor control imbalances are the *Y-balance test* (Fig. 44.16) [40], which gives a quantitative information that correlates with lower limb injury risk, especially with ankle chronic instability, *single-leg squat* (Fig. 44.17), *landing technique* (Fig. 44.18), *side-cutting*

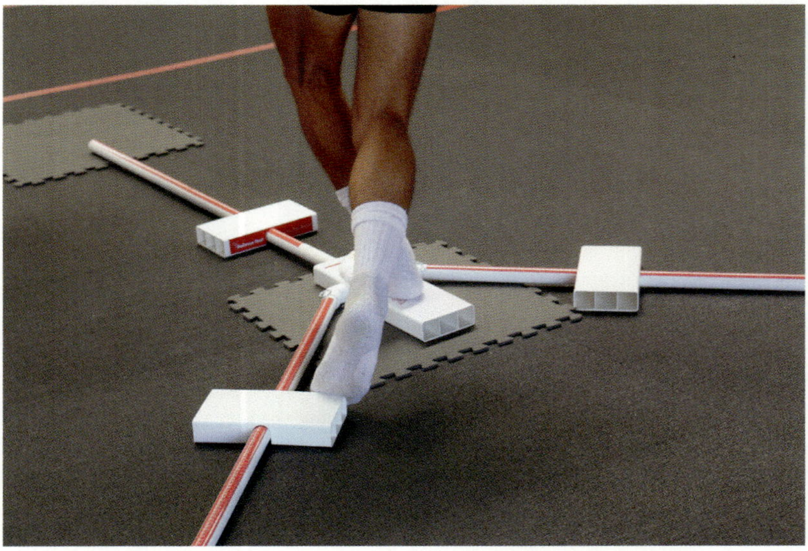

Fig. 44.16 Y-balance test

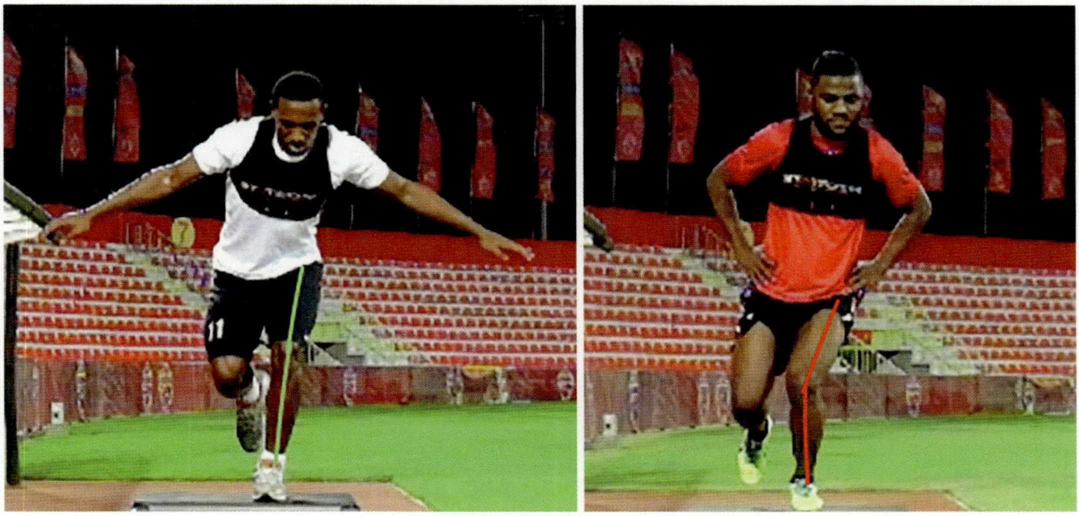

Fig. 44.17 Single-leg squat – *left*: correct pattern; *right*, dysfunctional pattern

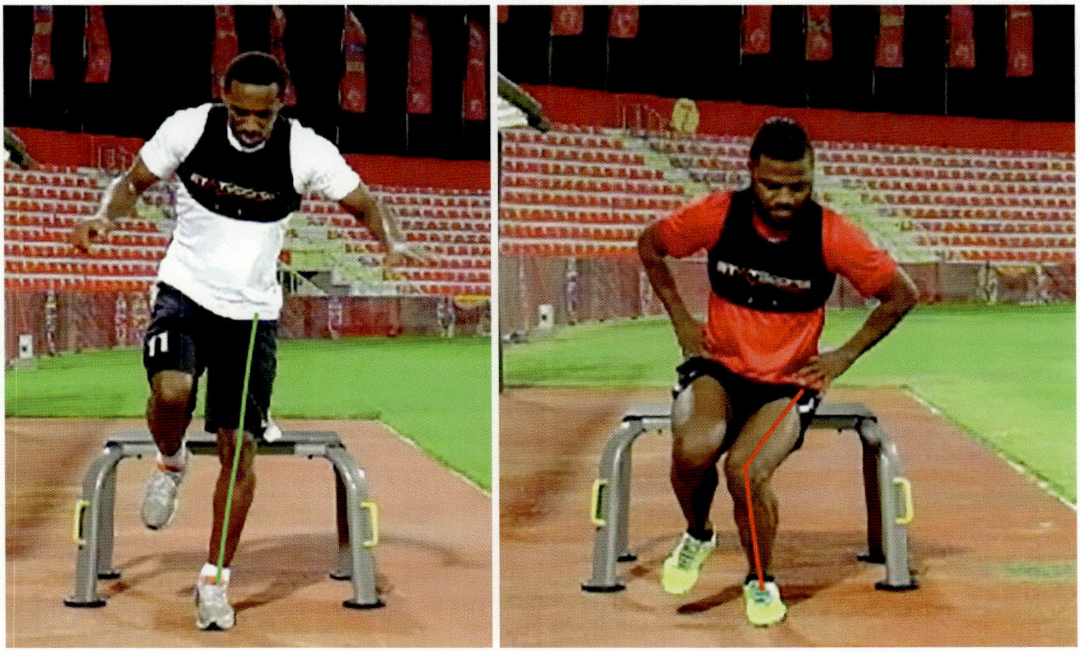

Fig. 44.18 Landing technique – *left*: correct pattern; *right*, dysfunctional pattern

(Fig. 44.19), *anterior and lateral decelerations* (Figs. 44.20 and 44.21) as well as *running technique* (the latter will be discussed further on in this chapter) [18, 19, 39, 41].

During these tests, clinicians should focus on whole body kinematics, in order to detect dysfunctional movement patterns. The most commonly identifiable ones are:

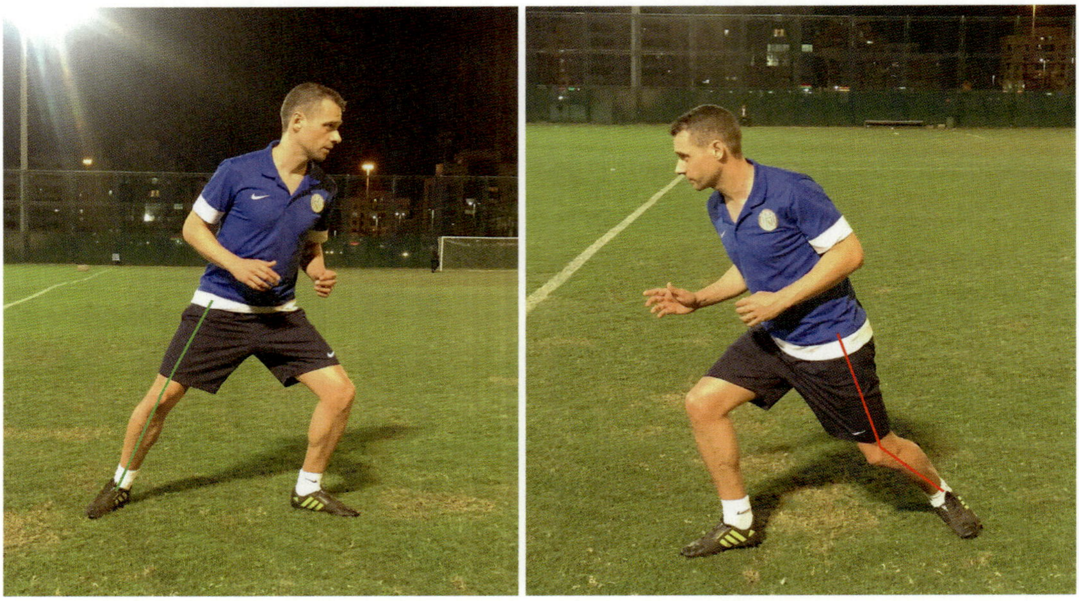

Fig. 44.19 Side-cutting – *left*: correct pattern; *right*, dysfunctional pattern

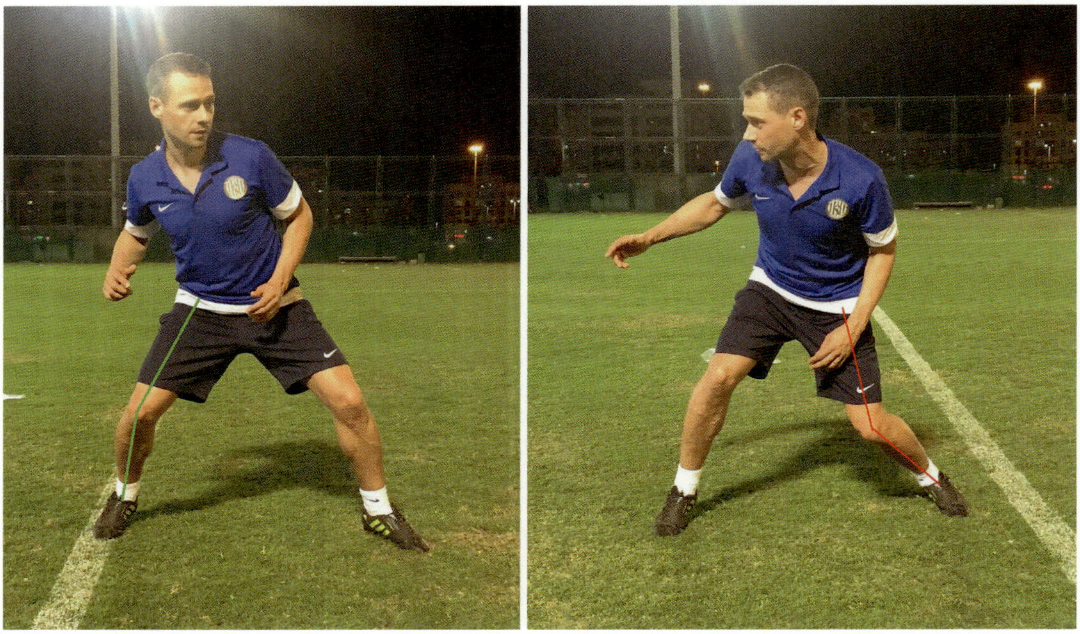

Fig. 44.20 Lateral deceleration – *left*: correct pattern; *right*, dysfunctional pattern

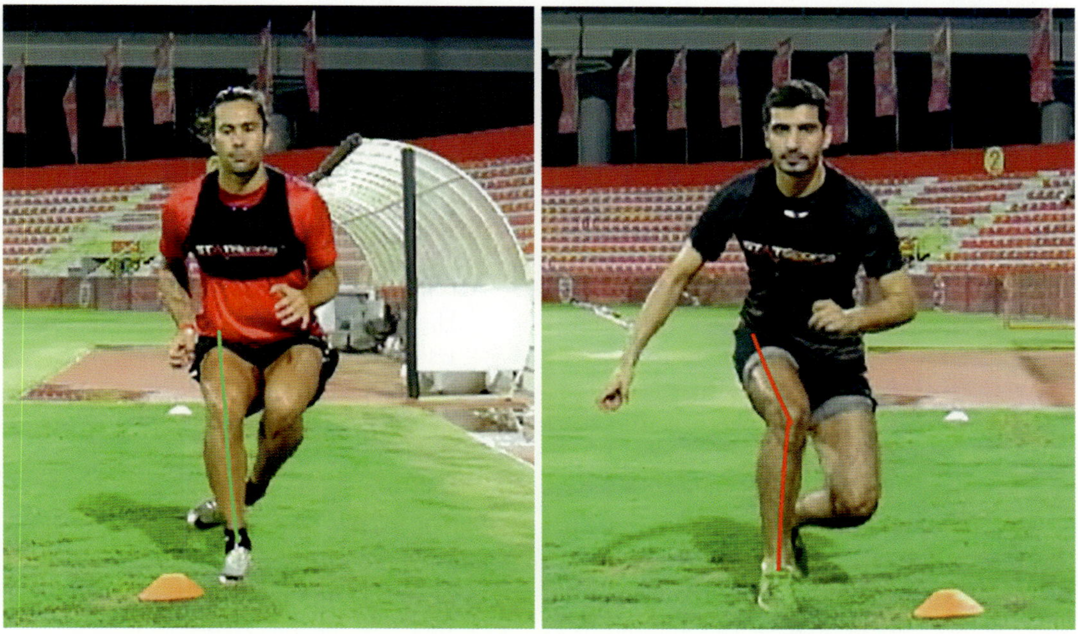

Fig. 44.21 Anterior deceleration – *left*: correct pattern; *right*, dysfunctional pattern

- Excessive foot pronation
- Decreased ankle dorsiflexion
- Knee dynamic valgus
- Excessive hip internal rotation
- Pelvic tilt

Data Collection

In order to help identify dysfunctional movement patterns during the tests, clinicians should have a *slow motion camera* in order to be able to detect not only the major but also the minor movement impairments during the tasks. A simple video analysis without any other special software is usually enough in a clinical perspective; however, for more detailed data that may be used for research purposes, *motion capture systems* (e.g. Vicon) might also be used. Apart from being considerably expensive, those systems have several limitations to use in a clinical/club setting:

- Require special infrastructures
- Specialised professional to set-up the system
- Time-consuming

Core Stability

Although controversy still exists in the literature regarding the benefits of core stabilisation training, it has been proposed by some authors that it can lead to a decrease in the injury risk in sports, due to the beneficial effects seen on whole body kinetics and kinematics (e.g. landing) [42].

Besides being a very popular concept in sports medicine, there are no widely accepted reliable tests for assessing *core stability*. However, considering its definition proposed by Kibler: "*The ability to control the position and motion of the trunk over the pelvis and to allow optimum production, transfer, and control of force and motion to the terminal segment in integrated athletic activities*", core stability is a *requirement to correct movement patterns* during sports-specific tasks, being implicated in the movements tested above [43].

Considering that there are no reliable tests to assess it, *core stability should be indirectly assessed considering the quality of the movement patterns of the previously mentioned functional tasks* [44].

44.3.2.4 Running Pattern Analysis

Running technique assessment is extremely important considering its association with several injuries in sports, especially the overuse ones. However, recent research has also correlated it with some acute injuries in sports (e.g. hamstring strain), highlighting its relevance to football practice [20].

For example, rear-foot strikers have 2.5 times greater probability of developing lower patello-femoral repetitive stress injuries than front-foot strikers, considering the decreased amount of absorbed force during the heel strike. However, front-foot strikers have an increased risk of Achilles tendon or foot and ankle injuries [45, 46].

This assessment should be aimed at detecting dysfunctional movement patterns during running that may reflect structural or functional imbalances in terms of strength, motor control or flexibility, as well as being an injury risk factor. Clinicians should pay attention to:

- Type of foot strike
- ROM balance between sides during stance phases (e.g. ankle dorsiflexion) and swing phases (e.g. knee extension)
- Foot behaviour in stance phase – especially in the frontal plane
- Shin behaviour in stance phase – especially in the frontal plane
- Knee behaviour in stance phase – especially dynamic knee valgus
- Hip behaviour in stance phase – focus on excessive internal rotation or decreased hip extension (toe off)
- Pelvic tilt in stance phase
- Increased lumbar extension during the toe off
- Asymmetrical trunk rotation

The most commonly used devices/techniques to assess athlete's running pattern are:

- Direct video analysis
  - Usually lateral and posterior assessment in treadmill – anterior view may be blocked by the treadmill itself
  - Low cost
  - User-friendly
  - Qualitative data
  - Subjective analysis
- Force platforms
  - Requires special equipment
  - Focused on foot assessment
  - Does not allow whole body analysis
  - Quantitative data
- Global Positioning Systems (GPS) – Accelerometer
  - High cost
  - User-friendly
  - Provides an easy follow-up
  - Can be used on a daily basis
  - Quantitative data showing only the imbalance between limbs
- Motion capture systems
  - Very high cost
  - Requires special infrastructures and technician to set-up the system
  - Time-consuming
  - Qualitative and quantitative data
  - Suitable for research purposes

Considering time and financial resources implicated in each device, from our perspective, direct video analysis together with the data collected from the GPS unit might be an efficient way to gather relevant information regarding athletes' running pattern.

44.3.3 Performance Testing

Football performance is not an easy subject to study because it depends not only of the *fitness* of the player but also from his *technical* and *tactical* skills. Considering this, football players' performance is often limited by their physical performance assessment.

Before assessing players' fitness level, it is extremely relevant to understand the specific *football physical demands*. Football is a hybrid sport characterised by *intermittent exercise bouts of short intense activity alternated by longer periods of low-level moderate-intensity exercise* [47].

Several tests have been proposed to assess football players' physical performance, for example, *VO_2 max, strength qualities, agility* and *maximum speed/sprint*.

44.3.3.1 VO_2 max

VO_2 max can be defined as the *upper limit on an individual's ability to take in and consume O_2* (individual versus standardized).

The importance of having a high maximal aerobic power (VO_2 max) is still being heavily debated in football, but there is some evidence suggesting that lower ranked teams have lower VO_2 max compared with teams with better performance [24, 48].

There are several validated laboratory tests that can be used to determine VO_2 max (e.g. incremental treadmill test); however, those tests lack specificity in relation to its use in a football player, because a laboratory is not able to recreate field context. Instead, there are field tests that can be performed to predict VO_2 max, of which the most commonly used are the *Cooper test* and the *Yoyo Intermittent Recovery Test*.

Although both tests can fairly accurately recreate a football context (field test), the one that best simulates football physical demands is the Yoyo Intermittent Recovery Test because, unlike Cooper Test's continuous running profile, it is composed of *bouts of high-intensity actions in between active recovery periods* [49, 50].

- *Yoyo Intermittent Recovery Test* (Fig. 44.22)
  - Focus on ability to recover after intense exercise
  - 20-m running back and forth at a controlled speed
  - 10-s active recovery between bouts
  - Incremental speed during the test
  - Stops when player is unable to maintain the speed required
  - 2–15-min duration
  - VO_2 max may be predicted with test scores using an equation
  - Test itself is a better indicator of football performance than the VO_2 max.
    - Positive correlation with player's amount of high intensity running performed during a match
    - Positive correlation with lower decrease of high intensity running towards the end of the match
    - Positive correlation with player's distance covered during a match
  - User-friendly
  - Inexpensive

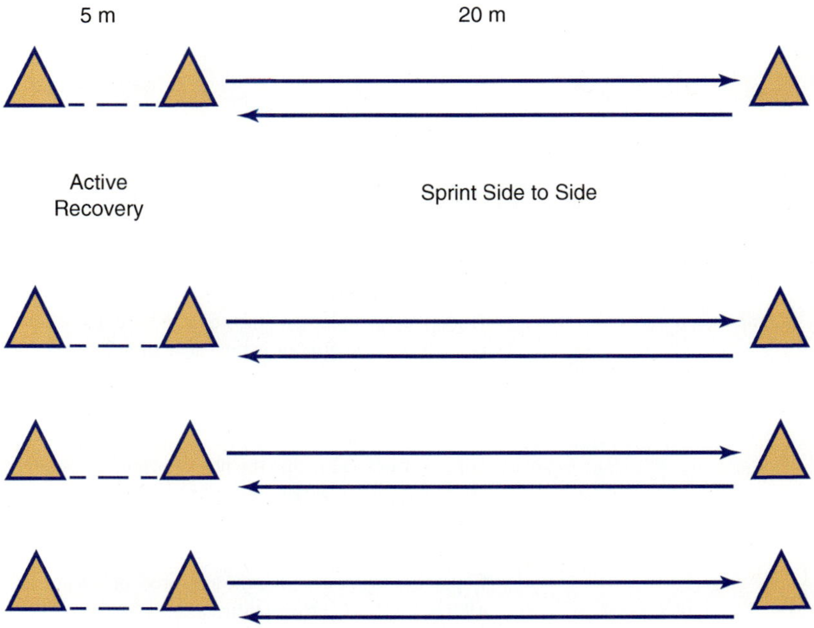

Fig. 44.22 Yoyo intermittent recovery test

After determining player's VO_2 max, sports professionals might be able to predict his aerobic and anaerobic threshold through specific equations.

44.3.3.2 Strength Qualities

In football, there are around 1000–1400 strength and power actions per match. Actions like sprinting, jumping and kicking are known to be critical in a football match; therefore, it is not surprising that maximum and power strength capabilities can distinguish competitive levels between football players [24, 48, 51].

From a mechanical perspective, *power is the product of force and velocity*, so one can expect an increase in power after an increase in force, velocity or both [52]. Considering this, it is easy to understand why maximum strength strongly correlates with performance of power tasks such as maximum speed, sprinting and jumping ability [24].

When assessing strength, sports professionals must consider that, although maximum strength positively correlates with football performance, using it in isolation to create a profile of the player may be too simplistic because *strength can be divided in different qualities* that also influence players' physical skills [52, 53], as shown in Table 44.4.

Considering the importance of closed-kinetic chain (CKC) movements to football performance (e.g. sprinting, side-cutting, decelerating), and often strength values are assessed analytically in an open-kinetic chain (OKC) pattern, sports professionals are advised to use CKC football-relevant movements to measure strength. An example of the different strength quality assessments are represented below:

Maximum Strength [55, 56]

- Concentric or isometric contraction
- Traditionally, a bilateral barbell squat may be used
  - Isometric: dynamometer or force platform – no variation on force-length and force-velocity curve and therefore are commonly used in the sports science field
  - Concentric: usually incremental load – variation on force-length and force-velocity curve
  - Squat 1-RM greater than 2x bodyweight positively correlates with better performance in sports-specific actions

Power: Low Load/High Velocity Force [52]

- To determine exact force value is expensive – force platforms – however, it can be measured indirectly using certain devices previously mentioned or through distance measurement
- Inexpensive lower body assessment
  - Vertical jump height
  - Horizontal jump distance
- Inexpensive upper body assessment
  - Medicine-ball throw distance

Table 44.4 Strength qualities and definitions (Adapted from McGuigan et al. [53]; Newton et al. [54]; Flanagan et al. [63])

FOOTBALL MEDICINE		Strength qualities
Maximum strength		Highest force value that the neuromuscular system can produce during a concentric, eccentric or isometric action, independently of time
Power P = F × V	*High load*	Highest force value that the neuromuscular system can produce during an eccentric/concentric or concentric actions, with a medium to high load (> 60% 1-RM)
	Low load	Highest force value that the neuromuscular system can produce during an eccentric/concentric or concentric actions, with a low load (0–30% 1-RM)
Rate of force development		Slope of the *force x time curve*, expressing neuromuscular system's ability to generate force rapidly
Reactive strength		Capability to produce maximum force, on a minimal timeframe, concentrically after a quick eccentric action

- Regarding football demands, this is a very important strength quality that needs to be assessed because football specific drills are performed at bodyweight and with high velocity – accelerating and jumping

Power: High-Load/Low-Velocity Force [57]
- Professionals may need a force platform or at least a contact mat in order to assess loaded (2x bodyweight) and unloaded (bodyweight) squat jump height
  - Determine *Bosco Index*, indicating player's needs in terms of force or speed – optimal score: 33%

Reactive Strength [58]
- Use of a force platform
- Perform a squat jump and a squat jump with countermovement (stretch-shortening cycle) in order to determine the *elastic index* (EI)
  - EI greater than 10–15% indicates that the player can take advantage of the elastic force and all the mechanisms of the stretch-shortening cycle
- Extremely important strength quality in running, jumping, kicking and side-cutting

Rate of Force Development [58–61]
- Slope of a time-force curve, typically measured under isometric conditions with a force platform
- Measure player's neuromuscular capability to rapidly achieve maximum strength
- Related to maximum strength and peak power output
- Important in sports performance because typically time to achieve maximum strength takes longer than the time available to do it (e.g. ground contact time of the foot on the floor is lower than the time needed to achieve maximum force)

44.3.3.3 Agility

At the moment, there is no consensus in the sports science community regarding a clear agility definition. Agility has been classically defined as the *ability to change direction rapidly and accurately*. However, some authors suggest that this definition is more prone to characterise the meaning of *changing of direction speed* rather than agility, as the latter implies a *changing of direction in response to a stimulus* – spatial and temporal agility.

Nevertheless, agility in football is usually assessed with change of direction speed tests, the *T-test* being the most commonly used (see Fig. 44.23). The player should perform the test in both directions, and then his timings should be collected [62].

44.3.3.4 Maximum Speed and Sprint Testing

Maximum speed represents one of the most valuable qualities in football, being positively correlated with players' performance. This quality may be assessed through a *sprint test*, which can be also used to determine acceleration ability.

In the past, maximum speed was calculated considering the time spent during a 30–40 m running; however, the result was significantly dependent on player's ability to accelerate. Nowadays, with the development of the GPS and its usage on the sports science field, it is possible to determine the exact maximum speed of the player, without his acceleration ability interference.

In order to achieve maximum speed, athletes usually need a sprint distance of around 60 m, however, and considering football specificity, the test may be performed instead with a 30–40 m

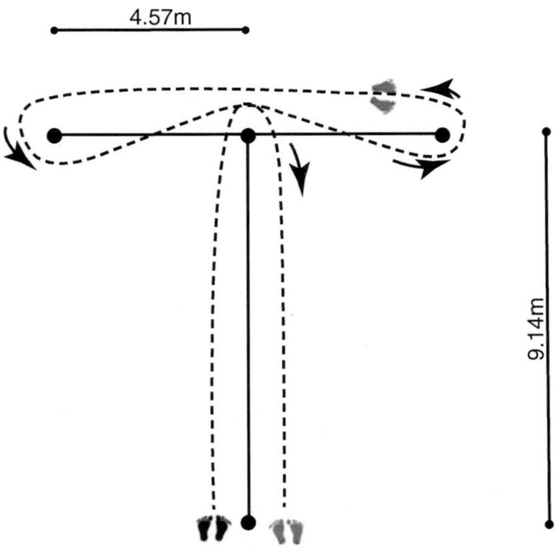

Fig. 44.23 T-test layout (Adapted from Sporis et al. [62])

sprint as players very rarely cover more than that distance whilst sprinting during games.

Conclusion

Performing a preseason evaluation of football players is an extremely important step before starting to play football because it allows sports professionals to screen for and prevent possible fatal events. In addition, this early screening will unveil players' individual needs in terms of potentially modifiable injury risk factors and fitness capabilities.

Preseason screening will further allow sports professionals to plan individual players' programmes throughout the season, decreasing injury risk and improving their performance and ultimately increasing the team's probability of success.

A conscious and meticulous choice of the tests should be taken by the sports professionals in order to respect the five rules of the preseason evaluation planning.

References

1. Barnes C, Archer DT, Hogg B, Bush M, Bradley PS. The evolution of physical and technical performance parameters in the English Premier League. Int J Sports Med. 2014;35:1–6.
2. Kramer EB, Dvorak J, Schmied C, Meyer T. F-MARC: promoting the prevention and management of sudden cardiac arrest in football. Br J Sports Med. 2015;49(9):597–8.
3. Fuller CW, Junge A, Dvorak J. Risk management: FIFA's approach for protecting the health of football players. Br J Sports Med. 2012;46(1):11–7.
4. Brukner P, Nealon A, Morgan C, Burgess D, Dunn A. Recurrent hamstring muscle injury: applying the limited evidence in the professional football setting with a seven-point programme. Br J Sports Med. 2014;48(11):929–38.
5. McCall A, Carling C, Davison M, Nedelec M, Gall FL, Berthoin S, et al. Injury risk factors, screening tests and preventative strategies: a systematic review of the evidence that underpins the perceptions and practices of 44 football (soccer) teams from various premier leagues. Br J Sports Med. 2015;49:583–9.
6. Mosler AB, Agricola R, Weir A, Hölmich P, Crossley KM. Which factors differentiate athletes with hip/groin pain from those without? A systematic review with meta-analysis. Br J Sports Med. 2015;49(12):1–12.
7. Lee JC, Mitchell AW, Healy JC. Imaging of muscle injury in the elite athlete. Br J Radiol. 2012;85:1173–85.
8. Gulati V, Jaggard M, Al-Nammari SS, Uzoigwe C, Gulati P, Ismail N, et al. Management of achilles tendon injury: A current concepts systematic review. World J Orthop. 2015;6(4):380–6.
9. Henderson RE, Walker BF, Young KJ. The accuracy of diagnostic ultrasound imaging for musculoskeletal soft tissue pathology of the extremities: a comprehensive review of the literature. Chiropr Man Therap. 2015;23:2–29.
10. Brooks MA, Peterson K, Biese K, Sanfilippo J, Heiderscheit BC, Bell DR. Concussion increases odd of sustaining a lower extremity musculoskeletal injury after return to play among collegiate athletes. Am J Sports Med. 2016;19:742–7.
11. Clark JF, Graham P, Ellis JK, Mangine RE, Rauch JT, Bixenmann B, Hasselfeld A, Divine JG, Colosimo J, Myer GD. An exploratory study of the potential effects of vision training on concussion incidence in football. Optom Vis Perform. 2015;3(2):116–25.
12. Evans KM, Ketcham CJ, Folger S, Vallabhajosula S, Hall E. Relationship between information processing and postural stability in collegiate division I NCAA athletes: does concussion history matter? Int J Phys Med Rehabil. 2015;3(2):268.
13. Gay-Escoda C, Vieira-Duarte-Pereira DM, Ardèvol J, Pruna R, Fernandez J, Valmaseda-Castellón E. Study of the effect of oral health on physical condition of professional soccer players of the Football Club Barcelona. Med Oral Patol Oral Cir Bucal. 2011;16(3):436–9.
14. Bar-Eli M, Plessner H, Raab M. Judgment, decision-making and success in sport. New Jersey: Wiley-Blackwell; 2011.
15. Vaeyens R, Lenoir M, Williams AM, Philippaerts RM. Mechanisms underpinning successful decision making in skilled youth soccer players: an analysis of visual search behaviors. J Mot Behav. 2007;39:395–408.
16. Croisier JL, Ganteaume S, Binet J, Genty M, Ferret JM. Strength imbalances and prevention of hamstring injury in professional soccer players: a prospective study. Am J Sports Med. 2008;36(8):1469–75.
17. Noronha M d, Refshauge KM, Herbert RD, Kilbreath SL. Do voluntary strength, proprioception, range of motion, or postural sway predict occurrence of lateral ankle sprain? Br J Sports Med. 2006;40(10):824–8.
18. Cortes N, Morrison S, Lunen BL, Onate JA. Landing technique affects knee loading and position during athletic tasks. J Sci Med Sport. 2012;15(2):175–81.
19. Ferber R, Kendall KD, Farr L. Changes in knee biomechanics after a hip-abductor strengthening protocol for runners with patellofemoral pain syndrome. J Athl Train. 2011;46(2):142–9.

20. Newman P, Witchalls J, Waddington G, Adams R. Risk factors associated with medial tibial stress syndrome in runners: a systematic review and meta-analysis. J Sports Med. 2013;4:229–41.
21. Bolgla LA, Malone TR, Timothy L. Comparison of hip and knee strength and neuromuscular activity in subjects with and without patellofemoral pain syndrome. Int J Sports Phys Ther. 2011;6(4):285–96.
22. Thorborg K, Branci S, Hölmich P. Eccentric and isometric hip adduction strength in male soccer players with and without adductor-related groin pain: an assessor-blinded comparison. Orthop J Sports Med. 2014;2(2):1–7.
23. Malliaras P, Hogan A, Nawrocki A, Crossley K, Schache A. Hip flexibility and strength measures: reliability and association with athletic groin pain. Br J Sports Med. 2009;43:739–44.
24. Wisløff U, Helgerud J, Hoff J. Strength and endurance of elite soccer players. Med Sci Sports Exerc. 1998;30(3):501–36.
25. Kockum B, Heijne A. Hop performance and leg muscle power in athletes: reliability of a test battery. Phys Ther Sport. 2015;16(3):222–7.
26. Mclellan CP, Lovell DI, Gass GC. The role of rate of force development on vertical jump performance. J Strength Cond Res. 2011;25(2):379–85.
27. Castagna C, Ganzetti M, Ditroilo M, Giovannelli M, Rocchetti A, Manzi V. Concurrent validity of vertical jump performance assessment systems. J Strength Cond Res. 2012;27(3):761–8.
28. Balsalobre-Fernándeza C, Glaister M, Lockey RA. The validity and reliability of an iPhone app for measuring vertical jump performance. J Sports Sci. 2015;33(15):1574–9.
29. Hamilton RT, Shultz SJ, Schmitz RJ, Perrin DH. Triple-hop distance as a valid predictor of lower limb strength and power. J Athl Train. 2008;43(2):144–51.
30. Morgan K, Donnelly C, Reinbolt J. Elevated gastrocnemius forces compensate for decreased hamstrings forces during the weight-acceptance phase of single-leg jump landing: implications for anterior cruciate ligament injury risk. J Biomech. 2014;47(13):3295–302.
31. Möller M, Lind K, Styf J, Karlsson J. The reliability of isokinetic testing of the ankle joint and a heel-raise test for endurance. Knee Surg Sports Traumatol Arthrosc. 2005;13(1):60–71.
32. Askling CM, Nilsson J, Thorstensson A. A new hamstring test to complement the common clinical examination before return to sport after injury. Knee Surg Sports Traumatol Arthrosc. 2010;18:1798–803.
33. Halabchi F, Mazaheri R, Seif-Barghi T. Patellofemoral pain syndrome and modifiable intrinsic risk factors; how to assess and address? Asian J Sports Med. 2013;4(2):85–100.
34. Reiman MP, Mather RC, Cook CE. Physical examination tests for hip dysfunction and injury. Br J Sports Med. 2013;1:1–6.
35. Nevina F, Delahunt E. Adductor squeeze test values and hip joint range of motion in Gaelic football athletes with longstanding groin pain. J Sci Med Sport. 2014;17(2):155–9.
36. Hoch MC, Farwell KE, Gaven SL, Weinhandl JT. Weight-bearing dorsiflexion range of motion and landing biomechanics in individuals with chronic ankle instability. J Athl Train. 2015;50(8):833–9.
37. Souza RB, Powers CM. Differences in hip kinematics, muscle strength, and muscle activation between subjects with and without patellofemoral pain. J Orthop Sports Phys Ther. 2009;39(1):12–9.
38. Vliet PM, Heneghan NR. Motor control and the management of musculoskeletal dysfunction. Man Ther. 2006;11:208–13.
39. Laughlin WA, Weinhandl JT, Kernozek TW, Cobb SC, Keenan KG, O'Connor KM. The effects of single-leg landing technique on ACL loading. J Biomech. 2011;44:1845–51.
40. Gonell AC, Romero JA, Soler LM. Relationship between the Y balance test scores and soft tissue injury incidence in a soccer team. Int J Sports Phys Ther. 2015;10(7):955–66.
41. Pollard C, Sigward S, Powers C. Gender differences in hip joint kinematics and kinetics during side-step cutting maneuver. Clin J Sport Med. 2007;17(1):38–42.
42. Araujo S, Cohen D, Hayes L. Six weeks of core stability training improves landing kinetics among female Capoeira athletes: a pilot study. J Hum Kinet. 2015;45:27–37.
43. Kibler W, Press J, Sciascia A. The role of core stability in athletic function. Sports Med. 2006;36(3):189–98.
44. Weir A, Darby J, Inklaar H, Koes B, Bakker E, Tol JL. Core stability: inter- and intraobserver reliability of 6 clinical tests. Clin J Sport Med. 2010;20:34–8.
45. Daoud A, Geissler G, Wang F, Saretsky J, Daoud Y, Lieberman D. Foot strike and injury rates in endurance runners: a retrospective study. Med Sci Sports Exerc. 2012;44(7):1325–34.
46. Kulmala J, Avela J, Pasanen K, Parkkari J. Forefoot strikers exhibit lower running-induced knee loading than rearfoot strikers. Med Sci Sports Exerc. 2013;45(12):2306–13.
47. Polman R, Walsh D, Bloomfield J, Nesti M. Effective conditioning of female soccer players. J Sports Sci. 2004;22:191–203.
48. Stølen T, Chamari K, Castagna C, Wisløff U. Physiology of soccer: an update. Sports Med. 2005;35(6):501–36.
49. Krustrup P, Mohr M, Amstrup T, Rysgaard T, Johansen J, Steensberg A, et al. The Yo-Yo intermittent recovery test: physiological response, reliability, and validity. Med Sci Sports Exerc. 2003;35(4):697–705.
50. Krustrup P, Mohr M, Nybo L, Jensen J, Nielsen J, Bangsbo J. The Yo-Yo IR2 test: physiological response, reliability, and application to elite soccer. Med Sci Sports Exerc. 2006;38(9):1666–73.

51. Faina M, Gallozi C, Lupo S. Definition of the physiological profile of the soccer player. London: Science and Football; 1988. p. 156–63.
52. Newton R, Kraemer W. Developing explosive muscular power: implications for a mixed methods training strategy. Strength Cond J. 1994;16(5):20–31.
53. McGuigan MR, Cormack SJ, Gill ND. Strength and power profiling of athletes: selecting tests and how to use the information for program design. Strength Cond J. 2013;35(6):7–14.
54. Newton R, Duran E. Application of Strength Diagnosis. National Strength & Conditioning Association. 2002; 24(5):50–9.
55. Young KP, Haff GG, Newton RU, Gabbett TJ, Sheppard JM. Assessment and monitoring of ballistic and maximal upper-body strength qualities in athletes. Int J Sports Physiol Perform. 2015;10(2):232–7.
56. Young KP, Haff GG, Newton RU, Sheppard JM. Reliability of a novel testing protocol to assess upper-body strength qualities in elite athletes. Int J Sports Physiol Perform. 2014;9(5):871–5.
57. Bosco C. Strength assessment with the Bosco's Test. Rome: Italian Society of Sports Science; 1999.
58. Haff GG, Stone M, O'Bryant HS, Harman E, Chris D, Johnson R, Han KH. Force-time dependent characteristics of dynamic and isometric muscle actions. J Strength Cond Res. 1997;11(4):269–72.
59. Haff GG, Carlock JM, Hartman MJ, Kilgore JL, Kawamori N, Jackson JR, Morris RT, Sands WA, Stone MH. Force- time curve characteristics of dynamic and isometric muscle actions of elite women Olympic weightlifters. J Strength Cond Res. 2005;19:741–8.
60. Stone MH, O'Bryant HS, McCoy L, Coglianese R, Lehmkuhl M, Schilling B. Power and maximum strength relationships during performance of dynamic and static weighted jumps. J Strength Cond Res. 2003;17(1):140–7.
61. Zatsiorsky VM, Kraemer W. Science and practice of strength training. 2nd ed. Champaign: Human Kinetics; 2006.
62. Sporis G, Jukic I, Milanovic L, Vucetic V. Reliability and factorial validity of agility tests for soccer players. J Strength Cond Res. 2010;24(3):679–86.
63. Flanagan EP, Comyns TM. The use of contact time and the reactive strength index to optimize fast stretch-shortening cycle training. Strength Cond J. 2008;30(5):32–8.

From Cardiac Preparticipation Evaluation to Sudden Cardiac Death

45

Pedro von Hafe, João Freitas, and Ovídio Costa

Contents

P. von Hafe (✉) • J. Freitas
Faculdade de Medicina da Universidade do Porto, Porto, Portugal

Hospital de S. João, Porto, Portugal
e-mail: mop15514@mail.telepac.pt

O. Costa
Faculdade de Medicina da Universidade do Porto, Porto, Portugal

J. Espregueira-Mendes et al. (eds.), *Injuries and Health Problems in Football*,
DOI 10.1007/978-3-662-53924-8_45

There has been growing interest in both risks and benefits of exercise, as well as the relationship between physical activity and cardiovascular health. Regular aerobic exercise improves health and may reduce the risk of fatal and nonfatal myocardial infarction. In contrast, acute vigorous physical exertion may trigger sudden death or cardiovascular events in the presence of underlying heart disease. Particularly intense exercise or sports competition may predispose athletes to an increased risk of sudden death or other major heart events.

There are several statements about the risk of sudden death associated with competitive sports participation, including in athletes with cardiovascular disease. These papers address insights and recommendations to physicians and sports institutions about secure eligibility that may contribute to the prevention of heart events during exercise including sudden cardiac death [1–5].

The incidence of sudden death in young athletes is very low (1/80,000–300,000 per year) [4]. An underlying heart disease is responsible for the majority of these deaths. A cardiac preparticipation evaluation could minimize these events by identifying subjects at risk and not permitting those at risk from taking part in competitive sports.

The general recommendations for preparticipation screening include a thorough personal and family clinical history and physical examination of the athlete. This screening should be performed by a trained physician with a long practice in the field to obtain a reliable, detailed cardiovascular history, perform a trustworthy physical exam, and recognize the possibility of heart disease.

Important clues in personal clinical history are chest pain or discomfort with exertion, unexplained syncope or near syncope concluded not to be neurocardiogenic, especially when related to exertion, and excessive dyspnea with exertion.

Most diseases responsible for sudden death in the young athlete are genetic, so the family history is of paramount importance. Family history findings that should be taken into account include antecedents in the family of premature death from heart disease before 50 years of age; major heart disease in close relative younger than 50 years old and certain cardiac conditions like hypertrophic cardiomyopathy (HCM), that is, the most common cause of sudden death in athletes; Marfan syndrome; arrhythmogenic right ventricular cardiomyopathy or dysplasia; long QT syndrome; preexcitation syndrome; Brugada syndrome or other ion channel diseases; clinically important arrhythmias; congenital coronary artery anomalies (that may contribute to almost 20% of sudden death in athletes); familial hypercholesterolemia; and premature coronary atherosclerosis.

When considering the current guidelines and recommendations, it must be noted that they are different in Europe and the USA [1–4]. Both the American College of Cardiology and the American Heart Association (AHA) agree that the obligatory screening of all athletes with an electrocardiogram (ECG) is not advised based on cost/efficacy due to the large number of tests that would be required, the low incidence of sudden death among athletes, as well as the concern for false-positive and false-negative results [3]. The AHA recommendations propose 14-point history and physical examination elements [3]. On the other hand, the European Society of Cardiology (ESC) has an opposing view and recommends resting ECG for all young athletes before they are allowed to compete [1], and the International Olympic Committee, both have endorsed such view.

Whether performed for screening or diagnostic purposes as part of the cardiac evaluation in athletes, it is critical that physicians responsible for the care of athletes be aware of ECG interpretation standards that improve disease detection and reduce false-positive results, like the so-called Seattle Criteria [6]. It is necessary to repeat annually the ECG screening given the fact that there are some cardiomyopathies that develop phenotypic evidence with time [7].

Hypertrophic cardiomyopathy is a primary and usually genetic heart disease with some known gene mutations. In this condition, there is a hypertrophied and non-dilated left ventricle. This condition is the most common structural cardiac disease responsible for sudden death in young athletes. More than 95% of cases of HCM have an ECG with clearly pathologic features [8]. The occurrence of sudden death in a family member is a marker of elevated risk for all affected members, namely, with certain genetic mutations.

Arrhythmogenic right ventricular cardiomyopathy or dysplasia (ARVC) is characterized by a myocardial atrophy and progressive replacement by fibrosis and fat that affects the right ventricle primarily and is associated with malignant ventricular arrhythmia with risk of sudden death. This condition has considerable regional variation in prevalence [9, 10]. Genetic studies have shown that it is a desmosomal cardiomyopathy that is caused by defective cell-adhesion proteins [11]. Clinical diagnosis depends on family occurrence, left bundle-branch pattern ventricular tachyarrhythmias, T-wave inversion in leads V1–V3 and epsilon waves, and signs of right ventricular dilation or segmental wall motion abnormalities, aneurysm formation, or substantial fatty deposition in the right ventricular wall demonstrated by nuclear magnetic resonance (NMR) imaging [12, 13]. Diagnostic criteria have been published and include quantitative variables [13]. Exercise might increase the arrhythmic risk in ARVC. Athletes with a definitive, borderline, or possible diagnosis of ARVC should not participate in competitive sports like football [13].

Left ventricle noncompaction (LVNC) is a recently recognized heart disease with sporadic or familial occurrence [13]. It's an uncommon entity that may result in ventricular arrhythmias, preexcitation pathways, thromboembolic events, heart failure, and sudden cardiac death [13]. Diagnosis is considered in the presence of two-layered LV chamber that involves noncompacted trabeculae with intertrabecular recesses on top of the normally compacted myocardium, limited to the distal and mid portions of the LV chamber and sparing the base [13]. Diagnosis is currently made in the presence of a ratio of noncompacted to compacted myocardium >2.3:1 in end diastole by NMR or >2.1 at end diastole by echocardiogram [14, 15]. The current recommendations of the AHA are that participation in competitive sports may be considered for asymptomatic patients with LVNC and normal systolic function, without significant ventricular tachyarrhythmias on Holter or exercise tests, and in history of unexplained syncope [13].

Brugada syndrome is a familial heart disease characterized by a particular ECG pattern associated with rapid polymorphic ventricular arrhythmia leading to sudden death.

Congenital long QT syndrome is a genetic disorder that may be associated or not with deafness and increases the risk of ventricular arrhythmia called torsade de pointes that can be precipitated by physical activity and presents with syncope or sudden death and that, in general, is associated with a history of recurrent syncope.

Genetic testing is now available for the evaluation of a patient with a suspected channelopathy like Brugada syndrome and congenital long QT syndrome.

Individuals with preexcitation syndrome including Wolff-Parkinson-White are predisposed to paroxysmal tachycardia and have an ECG with shortened PR interval with slurred upstroke of the QRS complex named delta wave. The incidence of sudden death in asymptomatic WPW is very low but may be the first clinical presentation.

Marfan syndrome is an autosomal dominant disorder that involves the connective tissue (abnormal fibrillin-1 attributable to mutations in the FBN1 gene), with physical features that include musculoskeletal, ocular, and great vessel abnormalities. It is estimated that the prevalence of this syndrome is 1 in 5000–10,000 subjects. Marfan syndrome is characterized by arachnodactyly, tall stature, kyphoscoliosis, and pectus excavatum. Death may occur from an acute aortic syndrome (aortic dissection or rupture) that may be triggered by exercise. There are other genetically triggered aortic syndromes that may increase the risk of acute aortic syndromes in athletes, including Loeys-Dietz syndrome and Ehlers-Danlos syndrome.

Mitral valve prolapse is characterized by the myxomatous degeneration of the collagen layer of the valve. It is a benign and very common condition in the general and athlete population but has been reported that could be the only heart abnormality in young athletes with sudden death. Risk factors for sudden death in patients with mitral valve prolapse includes a family history of sudden death, recurrent episodes of syncope, prolonged QT interval, moderate to severe mitral regurgitation, and complex ventricular arrhythmia.

The presence of a heart murmur must be acknowledged on physical examination. Heart auscultation must be performed in both supine and standing positions and with Valsalva maneuver to identify dynamic left ventricular outflow tract obstruction murmurs. Some findings like mid- or end-systolic clicks, single or widely split and fixed with respiration second heart sound to exclude, for example, an ostium secundum atrial septal defect, implicate more cardiovascular studies, including an echocardiogram. Femoral pulse evaluation must be made to exclude coarctation of the aorta.

After initial screening in athletes, it is consensual to obtain history and blood pressure every year in subsequent years.

Some patients must be referred for additional testing if there is any positive finding on baseline history or ECG. There are some findings in the electrocardiogram that imply other tests [5] (Table 44.1).

Table 44.1 Findings in the electrocardiogram that implies additional tests in preevaluation of athletes

P wave	
	Left atrial enlargement – negative portion of P wave on lead V1 ≥ 0.1 millivolts (mV) and ≥ 0.04 s
	Right atrial enlargement – peaked P wave in leads II and III or V1 ≥ 0.25 mV
QRS complex	
	Frontal plane axis deviation – right ≥ 120° or left −30° to −90°
	Increased voltage – amplitude of R or S wave in a standard lead ≥ 2 mV, S wave in lead V1 or V2 ≥ 3 mV, or R wave in lead V5 or V6 ≥ 3 mV
	Abnormal Q waves ≥ 0.04 s or ≥ 25% of height of ensuing R wave or QS pattern in 2 or more leads
	Right or left bundle branch block with QRS duration ≥ 0.12 s
	R or R′ wave in lead V1 ≥ 0.5 mV in amplitude and R/S ratio ≥ 1
ST segment, T waves, and QT interval	
	ST segment depression or T-wave flattening or inversion in ≥ 2 leads
	Prolongation of heart rate corrected QT interval > 0.44 s in males or > 0.46 s in females
Rhythm and conduction abnormalities	
	Premature ventricular beats or more severe ventricular arrhythmias Supraventricular tachycardia, atrial flutter, or atrial fibrillation
	Short PR interval (< 0.12 s) with or without delta wave
	Sinus bradycardia with resting heart rate ≤40 beats/min (increasing <100 beats/min during limited exercise test)

45.1 Other Testing

45.1.1 Recommendations for Patients with Congenital Heart Defects

Athletes with small interatrial or interventricular defects (open or after closure), normal right heart volume, and no pulmonary hypertension and those with a large atrial septal defect and normal pulmonary artery pressure can participate in all competitive sports. Athletes with atrial septal defect and mild pulmonary hypertension can only take part in low-intensity competitive sports, and so they must be excluded from football competitions. Pulmonary hypertension is defined here as a mean pulmonary artery pressure >25 mm Hg or a pulmonary vascular resistance index of >3 Wood units [16]. Patients with an associated pulmonary vascular obstructive disease who have cyanosis and large right-to-left shunt should not participate in competitive sports [5, 16]. Patients with hemodynamically insignificant patent ductus arteriosus (open or after closure) can take part in all competitive sports.

ECG changes occur in up to 80% of trained athletes due to an adaptation of the cardiac autonomic nervous system to exercise including sinus bradycardia or sinus arrhythmia. Profound sinus bradycardia (<30 beats/min) or marked sinus arrhythmia (pauses ≥3 s when awake) should be distinguished from sinus node dysfunction. In patients with third-degree AV block and Mobitz type II (type II second-degree), a thorough diagnostic evaluation is necessary.

There is no need to require systematic evaluation with echocardiography unless one or more of the following are present: relevant symptoms, family history of cardiovascular diseases or sudden cardiovascular death, or ECG criteria for pathologic left ventricular hypertrophy.

Further evaluation is required if suspected ostium secundum atrial septal defect, suspected arrhythmogenic right ventricular cardiomyopathy (incomplete right bundle branch block pattern associated with T-wave inversion beyond V2 to leads V3 and V4 or when accompanied by premature ventricular beats with left bundle branch block morphology), or suspected Brugada syndrome. Brugada syndrome is characterized by J wave (slow, positive deflection at R-ST junction) most perceptible in leads V1 and V2 with minimal to no changes in other leads. Diagnosis of Brugada syndrome may be confirmed by drug challenge with sodium channel blockers. In the presence of Brugada-like ECG abnormalities, analysis of ST-T segment waveform can usually differentiate between Brugada ECG and right precordial early repolarization that appears in the athlete. Brugada syndrome is characterized by downsloping ST segment with STJ/ST80 ratio > 1 [17]. Athletes show upsloping ST segment with mean STJ/ST80 ratio ≤ 1 [17]. It is obligatory to refer athletes with suspected Brugada ECG to a cardiologist with electrophysiologist knowledge for evaluation, including family history evaluation, risk stratification, and pharmacologic test with sodium channel blocking.

Usually, there is no need to further clinical evaluation if there is the presence of early repolarization, that is, a benign ECG pattern in young people and athletes. Typical characteristics of right precordial ST-T changes of early repolarization in trained athletes can easily be differentiated from arrhythmogenic right ventricular cardiomyopathy and Brugada syndrome. An ECG pattern of early repolarization in inferior/lateral leads associated with prominent terminal QRS slurring should be evaluated for idiopathic ventricular fibrillation.

If there is evidence of ST-segment depression on resting ECG (isolated or with T-wave inversion), it requires further investigation to exclude heart disease, right atrial enlargement, and right ventricular hypertrophy and implies further assessment for congenital or acquired heart disease [17]. In the case of presence of T-wave inversion with deep inverted T waves ≥ 2 mm in two or more adjacent leads, it may indicate inherited heart muscle disease requiring clinical evaluation, the study of the family, and mutation analysis when appropriate. T-wave inversion in inferior (L2, L3, aVF) or lateral leads (L1, aVL, V5, V6) is uncommon and requires further evaluation to rule out underlying heart disease. It is significant to note that minor T-wave abnormalities <2 mm in two or more leads are uncommon in athletes (occur in <0.5%) but are often seen in cardiomyopathy and may be present before evident structural changes in heart intraventricular conduction abnormalities [17]. Evidence of complete bundle branch block (QRS duration ≥ 120 ms) or hemiblock also implies cardiac assessment to evaluate for underlying pathologic causes, including exercise testing, 24-h ECG, and imaging. When bifascicular block pattern is present, it is prudent to perform ECG on athlete's family to exclude Lenègre disease, an autosomal dominant progressive cardiac conduction disease. Nonspecific intraventricular conduction abnormalities (prolonged QRS > 110 ms) may be indicative of heart muscle disease (such as ARVC) and imply further investigation [17]. Ventricular preexcitation (Wolff-Parkinson-White) assessment should include symptoms (syncope or palpitation) and family history of cardiomyopathy, preexcitation, or sudden death. To assess the risk of arrhythmia and corroborate diagnosis, it is mandatory to make 24-h ECG, exercise testing, adenosine/verapamil testing, and electrophysiological study for inducible atrioventricular reentrant tachycardia and refractory nature of the accessory pathway [17]. If there is a long QT interval, it is crucial to be aware that a corrected QT interval ≥ 500 ms is indicative of acquired or congenital long QT syndrome despite family history or symptoms including syncopal episodes. Corrected QT interval > 440 ms in male athletes and > 460 ms in female, but < 500 ms requires further assessment for diagnosis [17]. Exercise testing may assist in diagnosis confirmation [17]. In the case of short QT interval (≤ 380 ms), further evaluation is necessary to rule out metabolic causes and drugs. Of note is that short QT interval could be associated with anabolic androgenic steroid abuse in trained athletes. If there is no visible acquired source, refer the athlete for familial ECG screening and molecular genetic evaluation [17].

45.1.2 Suspicion of Hypertrophic Cardiomyopathy in an Athlete

Correct risk stratification and relevant sports ineligibility are based on the evidence that sudden death may be the first clinical manifestation of HCM, particularly in the young (<30 years). This disease is defined as unexplained left ventricular hypertrophy in the absence of other cardiac or systemic conditions that lead to ventricular wall thickness. The clinical features that support the diagnosis of HCM in the differential with hypertensive cardiomyopathy include several items. These are the familial history, the presence of right ventricular hypertrophy, late gadolinium enhancement at insertion point of the right ventricle or in localized segments of maximum thickness of the left ventricle in cardiac NMR, maximum LV wall thicknesses of 15 mm or more in whites and 20 mm in blacks, severe diastolic dysfunction, and severe disturbances of repolarization and conduction or pathological Q waves in the ECG.

In athletes under the age of 30, HCM is the first cause of sudden death (reaching more than a third of total) [18]. Preparticipation screening will increase the number of suspected cases of HCM and allow a final diagnosis in more cases. Lethal ventricular arrhythmias generally cause sudden death. High-intensity exercise may be the trigger of the arrhythmia and is considered a risk factor for sudden death. The signs and symptoms, natural history, and prognosis in HCM are variable. The estimation of risk based only on phenotypic expression is difficult. The occurrence of sudden death in a family member is a marker of high risk for all affected members. Some cases are not genotypically affected, but this is a rare finding. HCM is inherited as a Mendelian autosomal dominant trait. It should be noted that the risk associated with exercise for athletes with cardiovascular diseases is difficult to quantify, given the various situations to which individual athletes may be exposed (degree of hydration, electrolytes variations, catecholamine levels).

There can be more than 1500 mutations in any one of 11 genes which encode proteins of the sarcomere (the contractile unit of cardiac muscle), the components of which are thick or thin myosin filaments with contractile, structural, or regulatory functions, adjacent Z-disk, and calcium handling [19]. The three most common HCM-causing mutant genes are the α-myosin heavy chain, cardiac troponin T, and myosin-binding protein C. Some genetic mutations such as cardiac troponin T mutations are associated with a particular adverse prognosis. Other genes account for a minority of HCM cases, including cardiac troponin I, myosin light chains, titin, α-tropomyosin, α-actin, and α-myosin heavy chain [20]. Along the substantial number of mutant genes, there is an HCM intragenic heterogeneity: most of the mutations are missense, where a single amino acid residue is substituted with another. Myocyte disarray, fibrosis, and small vessel disease are the most common pathological features [21]. The prognostic value of mutations in asymptomatic carriers with mild or absent phenotypic expression of the disease is uncertain, but it is considered to be low. Genetic testing for the most important mutations has become available as several commercial kits. Identifying the genes responsible for HCM was thought to improve risk stratification but is now admitted that single mutations do not predict prognosis in an accurate mode. Double mutation carriers may have a higher risk of sudden cardiac death.

Diagnosis is mainly established by noninvasive cardiac imaging, namely, echocardiography and NMR. Diagnosis of HCM is based on the echocardiographic observation of the typical feature of the disease: asymmetric hypertrophy of the left ventricle (LVH), with diastolic dysfunction in association with a normal left ventricle (LV) dimension, in the absence of other cardiac or systemic diseases like hypertension or aortic stenosis associated with LVH. The presence of a systolic murmur, a systolic anterior motion of the mitral valve or a premature closure of the aortic valve is not, per se, diagnostic criteria. Most patients do not have LVOT obstruction at rest, and most of the well-documented physical findings like a systolic murmur and bifid arterial pulse are limited to patients with outflow gradients. LVH nevertheless is an independent risk factor for sudden death in young people affected by HCM and is variable in distribution and extension [18, 19]. Many patients show diffusely distributed LVH. However, almost one-third of patients have only mild wall thickening confined to a single segment. Increased left ventricle wall thicknesses range from mild (13–15 mm) to massive (30 mm [normal, ≤11 mm]) and up to 60 mm. European guidelines [1, 17] recommend a wall thickness ≥15 mm for adults to access an HCM to be diagnostic. It is relevant to note that morphological features of HCM may not be present and identified by echocardiography until adolescence, and the probability of diagnosis increases with age.

In trained athletes, modest segmental wall thickening (13–15 mm) raises the differential diagnosis between extreme physiologic LVH (i.e., athlete's heart) and mild morphologic expressions of HCM, without outflow obstruction. The differential diagnosis in this overlap gray area (about 2% of elite male athletes) in the differentiation of adaptive LVH versus HCM should be made with imaging criteria. This differentiation includes echocardiographic criteria that take in account end-diastolic diameters and a reduction of the wall thickening after 3 months of detraining that are suggestive of the athlete's heart [22, 23]. Recognition of features referring to LV dimensions, diastolic function, and brain natriuretic peptide (BNP) may be useful [24, 25]. In a pilot study, left ventricular end-diastolic diameter <45 mm, mitral deceleration time>200 ms, isovolumetric relaxation time>94 ms, tricuspid E/A<1. 63, relative wall thickness >0.445 and a BNP value at rest >9.84 pg/ml suggested an underlying cardiomyopathy [25].

NMR may be of diagnostic value when echocardiography is technically inadequate in identifying segmental LVH [26]. A model incorporating the LV end-diastolic volume and the end-diastolic mass ratio has been proposed to distinguish HCM from physiological hypertrophy in athletes [27]. This ratio has been found to be lower in patients with HCM in comparison with healthy controls and athletes. Late gadolinium enhancement in NMR may be helpful in identifying areas of intramyocardial fibrosis [26]. However, it is important to acknowledge that NMR of endurance athletes has been found to reveal abnormal findings in more than 5% of them [28].

Cardiopulmonary testing (VO2 peak value) may contribute to the differential diagnosis of HCM and the athlete's heart [26].

Genetic testing is useful in distinguishing the benign consequences of systematic athletic training from pathological LVH with the risk of sudden death. In familial assessment, it is mandatory for the proband to be informed of the familial nature and autosomal dominant transmission of HCM. Screening of first-degree relatives should be encouraged. If there is positivity for one of the most common HCM-causing genes tested, the result is definitive. Negative tests may be nondiagnostic because of false-negative results. Genetic testing has been used in the diagnosis of HCM, resulting in a group of patients with genotype positive-phenotype negative disease [29]. These cases carry the genes causing HCM but do not have evidence of disease [30]. Spontaneous transformation to LV hypertrophy in this subgroup occurs most often in adolescence [31]. The risk of sudden death in these gene-positive-phenotype-negative individuals appears, however, to be extremely low [19].

There are several other risk factors like gender (about 90% of athletic field deaths occur in men). This relative rarity in women probably could reflect lower participation rates, less intense levels of training, and the fact that women do not exercise with the same frequency than men in some of the higher-risk sports like football.

The usefulness of ECG remains crucial. The ECG have abnormalities in up to 95% of HCM patients and may present with a variety of alterations, including high QRS voltages, intra-atrial or left intraventricular conduction abnormalities, pathologic Q waves (depth >2 mm), and significant repolarization abnormalities (ST depression, negative T waves). For example, deep T-wave inversion of >2 contiguous anterior or lateral leads (but not aVR and III) are of primary concern for sports cardiologists, because they may represent the first and only sign of an inherited heart muscle disease [32].

Because of the potential and dramatic event of sudden death among young athletes, especially in the case of strong intensity sports like football players, the identification of high-risk athletes is crucial. Athletes with the definite diagnosis of HCM must be discouraged from competitive athletic participation. The distinction between physiological LV hypertrophy in trained athletes and pathological hypertrophy in HCM in affected subjects is mandatory. In the presence of HCM diagnosis, it is obligatory to perform an accurate medical qualification decision-making process. The identification of patients at low risk is easy, but individual risk stratification is difficult. This process may be very challenging, given the contending interests of the personal expectations of the athletes and the permission of the physician to protect patients from exercise situations which could provoke unacceptable risks. Of concern is the fact that an important proportion of sudden deaths in athletes may be caused by cardiovascular diseases that were not detected by screening even with ECGs [3, 33].

References

1. Corrado D, Pelliccia A, Bjornstad HH, Vanhees L, Biffi A, Borjesson M, et al. Cardiovascular preparticipation screening of young competitive athletes for prevention of sudden death: proposal for a common European protocol: Consensus Statement of the Study Group of Sport Cardiology of the Working Group of Cardiac Rehabilitation and Exercise Physiology and the Working Group of Myocardial and Pericardial Diseases of the European Society of Cardiology. Eur Heart J. 2005;26:516.
2. Maron BJ, Thompson PD, Ackerman MJ, Balady G, Berger S, Cohen D, et al., American Heart Association Council on Nutrition, Physical Activity, and Metabolism. Recommendations and considerations related to preparticipation screening for cardiovascular abnormalities in competitive athletes: 2007 update: a scientific statement from the American Heart Association Council on Nutrition, Physical Activity, and Metabolism: endorsed by the American College of Cardiology Foundation. Circulation. 2007;115:1643–55.
3. Maron BJ, Zipes DP, Kovacs RJ., American Heart Association Electrocardiography and Arrhythmias Committee of the Council on Clinical Cardiology, Council on Cardiovascular Disease in the Young, Council on Cardiovascular and Stroke Nursing, Council on Functional Genomics and Translational Biology, and the American College of Cardiology. Eligibility and disqualification recommendations for competitive athletes with cardiovascular abnormalities: preamble, principles, and general considerations: a scientific statement from the American Heart Association and American College of Cardiology. Circulation. 2015;132:e256–61.
4. Maron BJ, Friedman RA, Kligfield P, Levine BD, Viskin S, Chaitman BR, et al., American Heart Association Council on Clinical Cardiology, Advocacy Coordinating Committee, Council on Cardiovascular Disease in the Young, Council on Cardiovascular Surgery and Anesthesia, Council on Epidemiology and Prevention, Council on Functional Genomics and Translational Biology, Council on Quality of Care and Outcomes Research, and American College of Cardiology. Assessment of the 12-lead ECG as a screening test for detection of cardiovascular disease in healthy general populations of young people (12–25 years of age): a scientific statement from the American Heart Association and the American College of Cardiology. Circulation. 2014;130:1303–34.
5. Corrado D, Pelliccia A, Bjørnstad HH, Vanhees L, Biffi A, Borjesson M, et al. Cardiovascular preparticipation screening of young competitive athletes for prevention of sudden death: proposal for a common European protocol. Eur Heart J. 2005;26:516–24.
6. Drezner JA, Ackerman MJ, Anderson J, Ashley E, Asplund CA, Baggish AL, et al. Electrocardiographic interpretation in athletes: the 'Seattle Criteria'. Br J Sports Med. 2013;47:122–4.
7. Pelliccia A, Di Paolo FM, Quattrini FM, Basso C, Culasso F, Popoli G, et al. Outcomes in athletes with marked ECG repolarization abnormalities. N Engl J Med. 2008;358:152–61.
8. Calore C, Melacini P, Pelliccia A, Cianfrocca C, Schiavon M, Di Paolo FM, et al. Prevalence and clinical meaning of isolated increase of QRS voltages in hypertrophic cardiomyopathy versus athlete's heart: relevance to athletic screening. Int J Cardiol. 2013;168:4494–7.
9. Corrado D, Basso C, Pavei A, Michieli P, Schiavon M, Thiene G. Trends in sudden cardiovascular death in young competitive athletes after implementation of a preparticipation screening program. JAMA. 2006;296:1593–601.
10. Maron BJ, Doerer JJ, Haas TS, Tierney DM, Mueller FO. Sudden deaths in young competitive athletes: analysis of 1866 deaths in the United States, 1980–2006. Circulation. 2009;119:1085–92.
11. Corrado D, Thiene G. Arrhythmogenic right ventricular cardiomyopathy/dysplasia: clinical impact of molecular genetic studies. Circulation. 2006;113:1634–7.
12. Maron BJ, Towbin JA, Thiene G, Antzelevitch C, Corrado D, Arnett D, et al., American Heart Association; Council on Clinical Cardiology, Heart Failure and Transplantation Committee; Quality of Care and Outcomes Research and Functional Genomics and Translational Biology Interdisciplinary Working Groups;

Council on Epidemiology and Prevention. Contemporary definitions and classification of the cardiomyopathies: an American Heart Association Scientific Statement from the Council on Clinical Cardiology, Heart Failure and Transplantation Committee; Quality of Care and Outcomes Research and Functional Genomics and Translational Biology Interdisciplinary Working Groups; and Council on Epidemiology and Prevention. Circulation. 2006;113:1807–16.
13. Maron BJ, Udelson JE, Bonow RO, Nishimura RA, Ackerman MJ, Estes NA 3rd, et al., American Heart Association Electrocardiography and Arrhythmias Committee of the Council on Clinical Cardiology, Council on Cardiovascular Disease in the Young, Council on Cardiovascular and Stroke Nursing, Council on Functional Genomics and Translational Biology, and the American College of Cardiology. Eligibility and disqualification recommendations for competitive athletes with cardiovascular abnormalities: task force 3: hypertrophic cardiomyopathy, arrhythmogenic right ventricular cardiomyopathy and other cardiomyopathies, and myocarditis: a scientific statement from the American Heart Association and American College of Cardiology. Circulation. 2015;132:e273–80.
14. Kelley-Hedgepeth A, Towbin JA, Maron MS. Images in cardiovascular medicine. Overlapping phenotypes: left ventricular noncompaction and hypertrophic cardiomyopathy. Circulation. 2009;119:e588–9.
15. Paterick TE, Tajik AJ. Left ventricular noncompaction: a diagnostically challenging cardiomyopathy. Circ J. 2012;76:1556–62.
16. Van Hare GF, Ackerman MJ, Evangelista JA, Kovacs RJ, Myerburg RJ, Shafer KM, et al., American Heart Association Electrocardiography and Arrhythmias Committee of the Council on Clinical Cardiology, Council on Cardiovascular Disease in the Young, Council on Cardiovascular and Stroke Nursing, Council on Functional Genomics and Translational Biology, and the American College of Cardiology. Eligibility and disqualification recommendations for competitive athletes with cardiovascular abnormalities: task force 4: congenital heart disease: a scientific statement from the American Heart Association and American College of Cardiology. Circulation. 2015;132:e281–91.
17. Corrado D, Pelliccia A, Heidbuchel H, Sharma S, Link M, Basso C, et al. Recommendations for interpretation of 12-lead electrocardiogram in the athlete. Eur Heart J. 2010;31:243–59.
18. Maron BJ. Hypertrophic cardiomyopathy: a systematic review. JAMA. 2002;287:1308–20.
19. Maron BJ, Maron MS, Semsarian C. Genetics of hypertrophic cardiomyopathy after 20 years: clinical perspectives. J Am Coll Cardiol. 2012;60:705–15.
20. Gersh BJ, Maron BJ, Bonow RO, Dearani JA, Fifer MA, Link MS, et al. ACCF/AHA guidelines for the diagnosis and treatment of hypertrophic cardiomyopathy: a report of the American College of Cardiology Foundation/American Heart Association Task Force on Practice Guidelines. J Am Coll Cardiol. 2011;58:212–60.
21. Varnava AM, Elliott PM, Sharma S, McKenna WJ, Davies MJ. Hypertrophic cardiomyopathy: the interrelation of disarray, fibrosis and small vessel disease. Heart Br Card Soc. 2000;84:476–82.
22. Maron BJ. Distinguishing hypertrophic cardiomyopathy from athletes heart physiological remodelling: clinical significance, diagnostic strategies and implications for pre-participation screening. Br J Sports Med. 2009;43:649–56.
23. Pelliccia A, Maron MS, Maron BJ. Assessment of left ventricular hypertrophy in a trained athlete: differential diagnosis of physiologic athlete's heart from pathologic hypertrophy. Prog Cardiovasc Dis. 2012; 54:387–96.
24. Pagourelias ED, Efthimiadis GH, Koudi E, Zorou P, Giannoglou G, Deligiannis A, et al. Efficacy of various "classic" echocardiographic and laboratory indices in distinguishing the "gray zone" between athlete's heart and hypertrophic cardiomyopathy: a pilot study. Echocardiography. 2013;30:131–9.
25. Pagourelias ED, Giannoglou G, Kouidi E, Efthimiadis GK, Zoron P, Tziomalos K, et al. Brain natriuretic peptide and the athlete's heart: a pilot study. Int J Clin Pract. 2010;64:511–7.
26. Fioranelli M, Frajese G. Sports cardiology, from diagnosis to clinical management. 2012;ISBN 9788847027749, doi:10.1007/9788847027756. Springer.
27. Luijkx T, Cramer MJ, Buckens CF, Zaidi A, Rienks R, Mosterd A, et al. Unravelling the grey zone: cardiac MRI volume to wall mass ratio to differentiate hypertrophic cardiomyopathy and the athlete's heart. Br J Sports Med. 2015;49:1404–9.
28. Mangold S, Kramer U, Franzen E, Erz G, Bretschneider C, Seeger A, et al. Detection of cardiovascular disease in elite athletes using magnetic resonance imaging. Rofo. 2013;185:1167–74.
29. Sylvester J, Seidenburg P, Silvis M. The dilemma of genotype positive-phenotype negative hypertrophic cardiomyopathy. Curr Sports Med Rep. 2014;13: 94–9.
30. Maron BJ. Hypertrophic cardiomyopathy and other causes of sudden cardiac death in young competitive athletes, with considerations for preparticipation screening and criteria for disqualification. Cardiol Clin. 2007;25:399–414.
31. Maron BJ, Yeates L, Semsarian C. Clinical challenges of genotype positive (+)-phenotype negative (−) family members in hypertrophic cardiomyopathy. Am J Cardiol. 2011;107:604–8.
32. Wilson MG, Sharma S, Carré F, Charron P, Richard P, O'Hanlon R, et al. Significance of deep T-wave inversions in asymptomatic athletes with normal cardiovascular examinations: practical solutions for managing the diagnostic conundrum. Br J Sports Med. 2012;46:i51–8.
33. Maron BJ, Haas TS, Murphy CJ, Ahluwalia A, Rutten-Ramos S. Incidence and causes of sudden death in U.S. college athletes. J Am Coll Cardiol. 2014;63:1636–43.

Basic CPR and Cardiorespiratory Arrest: Rules and Guidelines

46

Ovídio Costa, Paulo Maia, José Ramos, and Efraim B. Kramer

Contents

O. Costa (✉)
Faculty of Medicine, University of Porto, Porto, Portugal

P. Maia
Clínica do Dragão, Espregueira-Mendes Sports Centre, FIFA Medical Centre of Excellence, Porto, Portugal

Faculty of Medicine, University of Porto, Porto, Portugal

J. Ramos
Faculty of Medicine, University of Porto, Porto, Portugal

Boavista FC, Porto, Portugal

E.B. Kramer
Department of High Performance Centre, University of Pretoria, Hatfield, Pretoria, South Africa

46.1 About Terminology

Sudden cardiac arrest (SCA) and sudden cardiac death (SCD) refer to the sudden cessation of cardiac mechanical activity with hemodynamic collapse, often due to sustained pulseless ventricular tachycardia/ventricular fibrillation. These events mostly occur in patients with evidence for ischemia due to coronary artery disease, disease of the myocardium (due to hypertrophy, fibrosis, scar replacement, or other myocardial abnormality that may or may not have been previously diagnosed), valvular abnormalities, or congenital channelopathies. The event is referred to as SCA if an intervention (e.g., defibrillation) or spontaneous reversion of the heart rhythm restores circulation. The event is called SCD if the patient dies.

46.2 Causes

Hypertrophic cardiomyopathy (HCM), arrhythmogenic right ventricular dysplasia (ARVD), and congenital channelopathies (long QT) are the most important causes of death reported in the young, and about 25% of these cases occur during sports.

Since the works of Drezner, we know that survival following out-of-hospital cardiac arrest is critically dependent on prompt recognition, early cardiopulmonary resuscitation (CPR), and access to early defibrillation. Several studies have demonstrated improved survival with the use of an

J. Espregueira-Mendes et al. (eds.), *Injuries and Health Problems in Football*, DOI 10.1007/978-3-662-53924-8_46

automated external defibrillator (AED) by trained or untrained lay responders within the first minutes following SCA [1] as well as effective hard and fast external chest compressions.

Another fact evident is the necessity to have a well-organized emergency action plan if we want to improve the ability to resuscitate cardiac arrest victims in the athlete population and public assistants. The placement of AEDs in training fields and training of persons that work with athletes have become the cornerstone of emergency response planning and the prevention of sudden cardiac death in young athletes [1–4].

46.3 Survival Rate

Drezner concluded that high school AED programs demonstrate a high survival rate (72%) either for students (85%) or adults (61%) who suffer SCA on school campuses. For those who went into SCA during physical activity, the survival rate was the same: of 18 student-athletes, 16 (89%) survived to hospital discharge, as did eight of nine (89%) adults who were arrested during physical activity. The reason seems quite obvious – the survival rate seems to be more dependent on the response time to defibrillation than the underlying pathology which is obviously very different in young athletes or in adults over 35 years of age [2].

The ability to resuscitate cardiac arrest victims is a critical component of health-related topics in the athlete population. Even with screening, there will remain people who experience sudden cardiac arrest. An effective resuscitation strategy requires multiple elements, including planning for an event, appropriate team members who can provide cardiopulmonary resuscitation (CPR), rapid availability of AEDs and other life-saving emergency medical equipment, as well as immediate telephone calls to the nearest emergency medical service (EMS).

That is the reason why any football player who collapses and is unresponsive, particularly if it occurs without contact with another player, is to be regarded as a SCA until proved otherwise.

"Any football player who collapses and displays seizure-like activity and/or agonal respirations should be regarded as a SCA" [3].

46.4 Automated External Defibrillators

AEDs are portable devices capable of detecting and successfully terminating pulseless ventricular tachycardia and ventricular fibrillation. All require human input to place the pads and turn on the device. Some are fully automated, but most are semiautomated in that they require simple continued human input, including activation of the AED to analyze the rhythm, and, then if the arrhythmia is deemed shockable, pressing a lit up button to shock. The sensitivity and specificity of AEDs to recognize ventricular tachycardia/ventricular fibrillation are excellent. AEDs may be used in children; however, the American Heart Association (AHA) recommends the use of pediatric dose attenuator systems and pediatric pads, if available, for children aged 1–8 years. AEDs require routine maintenance; battery life and system integrity require at least monthly checks, and pads have a limited shelf life-span of ≈2 years. Thus, AEDs should be part of an emergency action plan and should not be placed in isolation.

46.5 "Hands-Only CPR" and Initial Shock

More recently, evidence from randomized trials has indicated that chest compression alone – "hands-only CPR" – performed by laypersons can provide survival benefit similar to that of conventional CPR among adults who suffer witnessed arrest [4]. Given the time-sensitive nature of resuscitation, the best chances of survival occur when treatment can be delivered soon after arrest. These include immediate assessment of level of consciousness and cardiovascular status of the athlete who has collapsed unexpectedly, as well as institution of chain-of-survival actions when cardiac arrest is identified. Dispatchers [4] prioritize two questions: (1) is the patient conscious and (2) is the patient breathing normally? The term "normally" is important because it says that any breathing that does not look to be normal in an unconscious player is to be regarded as SCA. If the patient is not breathing normally, it is also important that all involuntary seizure-like movements in a collapsed player be regarded as associated with cardiac arrest, and immediate CPR and AED be initiated.

Generally, an athlete has a higher probability of being witnessed by appropriately trained bystander staff than does cardiac arrest that occurs in the general population [1, 2].

As we saw before, for any suspected SCA, the emergency medical plan (EMP) must be activated immediately followed by prompt CPR and retrieval, application, and use of an AED as soon as possible [4].

AEDs are being deployed increasingly in public venues, including schools, universities, and various sports and exercise facilities. It is recommended that the devices be deployed in a manner that results in a maximum access time of 5 min to any site on a school campus or sporting venue. While the AED is being brought to the victim's side and deployed, compression of the chest should be started by bystanders.

46.6 Rules and Guidelines on *Football Field*

According to the most recent guidelines, compression alone ("hands-only CPR") should be started at a rate of 100–120 compressions per minute without interruption for rescue breaths. As soon as the defibrillator is attached and powered up, the rhythm is analyzed. A single shock should be delivered if the device senses a shockable rhythm. If the initial rhythm is non-shockable (i.e., asystole or pulseless electrical activity), CPR should be continued. After each shock, compressions should be resumed immediately for 2 min before the next rhythm check will be undertaken by the AED. CPR may be stopped if signs of life occur in the collapsed player, e.g., player starts breathing, moves limbs, or opens eyes.

The likelihood of survival with good neurological status is directly related to the time between onset of cardiac arrest, implementation of CPR and AED use, and return of spontaneous circulation. In the adequately prepared athletic environment, including both trained staff and appropriate equipment, with the onset of the event witnessed, it is a reasonable goal to begin CPR within 60–90 s and deliver an initial shock to an athlete with a shockable rhythm in <3 min.

An emergency response plan includes preparation for cardiac arrests, including anticipation of events, placement of AEDs, and training of people to use them, access to emergency services, and simulations of real-life events.

Included in emergency response plans are monthly AED checks for integrity and battery life [1].

Conclusion

The state AED program requirements generally should include the provisions of *Good Samaritan like immunity*, medical oversight, agency notification, policies, quality assurance measures, training, AED maintenance, and post-event reporting. The AHA has developed a policy statement with the objective of guiding policymakers and other stakeholders in writing new legislation or revising existing legislation to remove potential barriers to implementation of emergency response programs that include AEDs.

Healthcare professionals should be aware of the clinical benefits of AEDs and the limited liability associated with their use. They should also consider the potential liability that could arise from failure to use AEDs as a matter of prudent public protection.

References

1. Drezner JA, Toresdahl BG, Rao AL, Huszti E, Harmon KG. Outcomes from sudden cardiac arrest in US high schools: 2-year prospective study from National Registry for AED use in sports. Br J Sports Med. 2013;47:1179–83.
2. Link MS, Myerburg RJ, Mark Estes NA. Eligibility and disqualification recommendations for competitive athletes with cardiovascular abnormalities: task force 12: emergency action plans, resuscitation, cardiopulmonary resuscitation, and automated external defibrillators. J Am Coll Cardiol. 2015;66:2434–8.
3. Dvorak J, Kramer EB, Schmied CM, Drezner JA, Zideman D, Patricios J, Correia L, Pedrinelli A, Mandelbaum B. The FIFA medical emergency bag and FIFA 11 steps to prevent sudden cardiac death: setting a global standard and promoting consistent football field emergency care. Br J Sports Med. 2013;47:1199–202.
4. Rea T. Dispatcher-directed CPR: An all-ages strategy to improve cardiac arrest survival. J Am Heart Assoc. 2014;3:e000942.

Children and Exercise

47

Rui Sales Marques, Fulgencio Molina,
and Jorge Sales Marques

Content

R.S. Marques (✉)
Physical Medicine and Rehabilitation, Centro Hospitalar do Algarve, Lagos, Portugal

Sports Medicine and Musculoskeletal Ultrasound Guide Techniques, Hospital Particular do Algarve, Alvor, Portugal

Sporting Clube Olhanense Football Team, Olhão, Algarve, Portugal

GFI Medicine, Vilamoura, Algarve, Portugal
e-mail: ruisalesmarques@gmail.com

F. Molina
Servicio de Traumatologia y Cirugia Ortopedica del Hospital Quiron Murcia, Murcia, Spain

Servicio de Traumatologia del Deporte de Sport Clinic Ripoll y de Prado, Alacant, Spain

FIFA F-Marc Sport Clinic Ripoll y de Prado- Medical Center of Excellence FIFA, Murcia, Spain

J.S. Marques
Centro Hospitalar Vila Nova de Gaia, Vila Nova de Gaia, Portugal

Pediatric and Neonatology, Centro Hospitalar Conde S. Januario, Macau, China

47.1 Introduction

Children participate in sports all over the world and should have a pre-participation physical evaluation (PPE) before the season begins.

The 2010 consensus guidelines suggest a PPE for children.

The primary goal is to maximize safe participation for all, identify medical problems with risks of life-threatening complications during participation (e.g., hypertrophic cardiomyopathy) and conditions that require a treatment plan before or during participation (e.g., hypertension), rehabilitate old musculoskeletal injuries, treat conditions that interfere with performance (e.g., exercise-induced bronchospasm), and remove unnecessary restrictions on participation.

The PPE should take place 4–6 weeks before the season starts, permitting time to evaluate and treat medical problems and/or rehabilitate musculoskeletal injuries before sports participation.

Most children with chronic medical conditions can participate in a sport at some level after appropriate evaluation and/or treatment. There are some exceptions like cervical spine stenosis and they cannot participate in contact sports.

Sudden death in the young athlete occurs with prevalence of between 1:100,000. The risk of sudden death is disproportionately higher in males. The median age was 17 years.

J. Espregueira-Mendes et al. (eds.), *Injuries and Health Problems in Football*,
DOI 10.1007/978-3-662-53924-8_47

47.2 Cardiovascular Conditions

Cardiovascular conditions causing sudden death in young athletes include:

- Hypertrophic cardiomyopathy
- Coronary artery anomalies
- Commotio cordis
- Myocarditis
- Aortic rupture (Marfan syndrome)
- Arrhythmogenic right ventricular hypertrophy
- Long QT syndrome
- Wolff-Parkinson-White syndrome
- Aortic stenosis

Most athletes who die suddenly have no symptoms of life-threatening cardiovascular disease, and the PPE is not efficient in detecting them. However, athletes suspected of having these conditions on the basis of historical or physical findings must not participate until further evaluation by a cardiologist.

Sudden cardiac death during exercise in patients with mitral valve prolapse is rare. *Athletes with mitral valve prolapse can participate in all competitive sports unless the following exist*:

- A history of syncope documented to be arrhythmogenic in origin
- A family history of sudden death associated with mitral valve prolapse
- Repetitive forms of supraventricular and ventricular arrhythmias, particularly if exaggerated by exercise
- Moderate to marked mitral regurgitation
- Prior embolic event
- Uncontrolled stage 2 hypertension – It is recommended that uncontrolled stage 2 hypertension (systolic and/or diastolic blood pressure [BP] ≥99th percentile plus 5 mmHg) or end-organ damage (e.g., retinal, renal, or cardiac changes) requires exclusion from sports participation and highly static activities until it is better controlled
- Fever – Children and adolescents with fever should be restricted from participation because fever may accompany myocarditis or other infections that can make exercise dangerous

47.3 Other Relevant Conditions

In addition to cardiovascular abnormalities, *numerous other medical conditions should be identified before clearance for sports participation because the conditions are associated with increased risk of adverse outcome or injury if left untreated. Examples of these conditions include:*

- Exercise-induced bronchoconstriction (EIB) occurs in athletes at a prevalence similar to that of the general population (9–15%), yet it may be unrecognized in the young athlete. Pulmonary disease accounts for 2% of sudden death in sports. EIB can be treated with pre-exercise medication in most patients and is not a reason to avoid exercise. The use of post-exercise spirometry in the routine PPE is not recommended
- Eating disorders (e.g., anorexia nervosa, bulimia nervosa) can manifest as excess exercise and malnutrition. Persistent exercise in the malnourished amenorrheic female athlete can cause short- and long-term consequences
- Some form of regular exercise is likely to be beneficial in most children and adolescents with diabetes mellitus. However, modifications in the pre-exercise insulin dose and additional glucose monitoring are necessary
- Athletes at risk of heat illness should follow guidelines for appropriate clothing, fluid intake, heat acclimatization, adjustment of activity level for heat and humidity levels, and timing of practices

Whether or not they are at risk of heat illness, athletes should consume fluid 2 h before prolonged exercise and every 20 min during activity. Electrolyte replacement drinks (i.e., sports drinks) are recommended after the first hour of prolonged exercise. The volume of intake varies according to the athlete's weight:

- 40 kg–500 mL, 2 h before prolonged exercise and 150 mL every 20 min during activity
- 60 kg–750 mL, 2 h before prolonged exercise and 250 mL every 20 min during activity

- Concussion – There is no evidence-based guideline regarding return to play for child athletes (i.e., 5- to 12-year-olds) following sports-related concussion. For the young athlete with repeated concussions, the decision to return to contact sports should be based on the number of concussions, the mechanism of previous concussions, the duration of recovery, and the time in between injuries
- Musculoskeletal injuries – Identifying and fully rehabilitating old musculoskeletal injuries have the greatest yield for identifying problems that will interfere with subsequent performance because injuries are common among athletes. Players with injuries to an extremity are more likely to injure that extremity during the season than an extremity that has not been injured. Proper rehabilitation can lead to lower injury rates

The athlete's history of previous injury should draw the clinician's attention to assess for residual effects. In addition to providing a plan for rehabilitating strength, endurance, and proprioceptive and flexibility deficits, the clinician should provide the athlete with a plan for returning to play. The athlete is at risk of re-injury and delayed recovery if he or she returns to competition too soon. Training errors, such as too-rapid increases in pace, distance, repetitions, or weight/resistance, are the most common factor in overuse injuries.

Another goal of the PPE is to remove unnecessary restriction on participation in sports or an exercise program because they are believed to have cardiac disease. As examples:

- One study of the morbidity of cardiac nondisease identified 93 seventh- to ninth-grade students who had "something wrong with their hearts" according to school records. After pediatric cardiology evaluation, 75 of these 93 students (81%) were found to have no cardiac disease, yet 30 of these 75 students (40%) had activity restrictions ranging from being homebound to being able to participate in physical education classes but not competitive sports
- Adolescent athletes with Osgood-Schlatter disease report stopping training and sports participation for months, and this may be with clinician advice. However, Osgood-Schlatter disease is a common problem and, although painful, should result in little if any restriction from sports activity when managed appropriately
- Obesity is a risk factor for heat injury, and exercise is an important component of obesity management, and restricting exercise is contraindicated in this setting

Incremental aerobic exercise tests are performed in children and adolescents for a variety of reasons. The primary indication is to provide the clinician with information about a young patient's physical working capacity. *The information gained from an aerobic exercise test is helpful in determining:*

- Whether a patient can perform daily activities within his or her functional capacity
- Whether he or she is responding appropriately to an exercise intervention program
- Whether chronic disease progression is affecting the patient's physical capacity

Contraindications – Exercise testing can be performed in most children. However, it is contraindicated in children with certain medical conditions. As a general rule, the exercise test should begin at a low workload so that the child becomes accustomed to the exercise and surroundings. In some cases, he or she may need to practice before beginning the test.

Exercise testing protocols may be continuous or discontinuous. When comparing results of two tests performed on an individual patient (e.g., pre- and post-exercise training), it is important to perform both tests using the same protocol and exercise modality.

- Continuous – Test protocols are usually continuous (i.e., without rest periods) and have either ramped or incremental stages
- In discontinuous exercise protocols, children are permitted to rest between stages. As an example,

each exercise stage might last 2–3 min, with 1–2 min of rest in between. Discontinuous protocols also may be more appropriate for children who are unfit and have low exercise tolerance

The average maximum heart rate in children and adolescents is considered to be 200 bpm with a wide range of individual values. It may vary by 5–10 bpm within an individual child performing different protocols. Most researchers accept an exercise test to be a maximal effort if the child's maximum heart rate is greater than 95% of predicted HRmax (i.e., HR ≥190 bpm).

- Exercise-induced bronchoconstriction (EIB) affects up to 80% of individuals who have asthma

Exercise testing is a useful tool in the diagnosis of EIB and for evaluating the exercise capacity and cardiopulmonary response to exercise in the child with asthma. Children with EIB commonly present with post-exercise coughing and chest pain; wheezing and dyspnea also may be present. The maximum heart rate criterion is not a good indicator of effort intensity in children with EIB.

- Cystic fibrosis – Compared with those with sedentary lifestyles, children, adolescents, and young adults with cystic fibrosis (CF) who exercise regularly may recover more quickly from acute illnesses. In addition, the use of exercise as an adjunct treatment to clear mucus in CF patients may result in fewer respiratory infections

In one cohort study, 109 CF patients age 7–35 years underwent pulmonary function and exercise testing and then were followed for 8 years. Survival rates were greatest among patients with the highest levels of aerobic fitness (83%, 51%, and 28% among those with VO2peak ≥82%, 59–81%, and ≤58% of predicted, respectively). Patients with higher levels of aerobic fitness were more than three times likely to survive than those with lower levels of aerobic fitness after adjustment for other risk factors.

- Idiopathic pulmonary arterial hypertension is considered by some to be a contraindication to maximal exercise testing in children, and it is not performed

Submaximal exercise testing also may be a valuable tool for assessing the prognosis and treatment of children with idiopathic pulmonary arterial hypertension. In many clinics, the 6-min walk test is given in lieu of maximal testing.

- Children and adolescents who have arthritis of any type may be less physically active than their healthy peers. Reasons for inactivity include chronic joint pain and stiffness, reduced strength, synovitis, and/or joint deformity

Children and adolescents who have arthritis appear to have decreased aerobic capacity for a variety of reasons. In one comparison study of aerobic capacity and workload completed by children with juvenile idiopathic arthritis (JIA, formerly juvenile rheumatoid arthritis, JRA) and healthy children during cycle ergometer exercise, children with JIA had a significantly lower VO2peak (33.0 mL/kg per min versus 46.9 mL/kg per min). No direct relationship was found between functional aerobic capacity and disease severity in the affected children. The authors speculated that the lower VO2peak values in children with JIA appear to be caused by either mechanical inefficiency or hypoactivity.

- In children who have neuromuscular disease, exercise performance is usually limited by decreased muscle function rather than cardiorespiratory capacity. Exercise testing of these patients can provide a quantitative assessment of the child's condition, the improvement in economy of locomotion after surgical treatment, and the potential effects of exercise stress

Contraindications for exercise testing in children and adolescents

Acute inflammatory cardiac disease (e.g., pericarditis, myocarditis, acute rheumatic heart disease)
Uncontrolled heart failure
Acute myocardial infarction
Acute pulmonary disease (e.g., acute asthma, pneumonia)
Severe systemic hypertension (e.g., blood pressure greater than 240/120 mmHg)
Acute renal disease (e.g., acute glomerulonephritis)
Acute hepatitis (within 3 months after onset)
Drug overdose affecting cardiorespiratory response to exercise (e.g., digitalis toxicity, salicylism, quinidine toxicity)
Severe aortic stenosis
Severe pulmonary stenosis

Serious ventricular dysrhythmia, especially when associated with significant cardiac disease
Coronary arterial diseases (anomalous left coronary artery, homozygous hypercholesterolemia, Kawasaki disease [acute phase])
Severe pulmonary vascular disease
Metabolic disorders (glycogenolysis types I and V)
Hemorrhagic diseases
Orthostatic hypotension

Adapted from Washington RL, Bricker JT, Alpert BS, et al. Guidelines for exercise testing in the pediatric age group. From the Committee on Atherosclerosis and Hypertension in Children, Council on Cardiovascular Disease in the Young, the American Heart Association. Circulation 1994; 90:2166 and James FW. Exercise testing in children and young adults: an overview. Cardiovasc Clin 1978; 9:187

Indications for terminating pediatric exercise testing before reaching maximal voluntary capacity level

The onset of serious cardiac arrhythmias (e.g., ventricular tachycardia, supraventricular tachycardia)
Any appearance of potential hazard to the patient
Failure of electrocardiographic monitoring system
Symptoms such as pain, headache, dizziness, or syncope, precipitated by exercise
Segmental ST depression or elevation ≥3 mm during exercise
Arrhythmia (over 25% of beats) precipitated or aggravated by exercise
Recognized types of intracardiac block precipitated by exercise

The European Society of Cardiology (ESC) has proposed guidelines for pre-participation screening for young athletes planning to begin competitive sports, which includes a standard 12-lead electrocardiogram (ECG), based upon a national screening program that has been in effect in Italy since 1982.

The following recommendations were made:

- An initial complete personal and family history and physical examination should be performed before beginning training and competition
- The evaluation should be performed by a clinician with specific training, medical skill, and cultural background to identify clinical symptoms and signs associated with cardiovascular diseases associated with sudden cardiac death (SCD). In Italy, clinicians primarily responsible for these examinations are trained in postgraduate sports medicine programs full time for 4 years and work in sports medical centers dedicated to periodic evaluation of athletes
- Screening evaluations should be repeated at least every 2 years
- A 12-lead ECG should be obtained (seeking evidence of a standardized list of abnormalities). If a specific diagnosis is considered, more detailed ECG review may be helpful
- Patients with abnormal findings on history, physical examination, family history, or ECG are referred for further testing, such as echocardiography, ambulatory monitoring, exercise treadmill testing, or cardiac magnetic ressonance imaging (MRI)

The potential advantage of the ECG is most commonly attributed to its ability to detect hypertrophic cardiomyopathy, in which the ECG is abnormal in up 95% of patients.

The routine use of ECG screening is the risk of false-positive results. The prevalence of such findings was addressed in a series of 32,652 Italian subjects who underwent routine pre-participation screening that included an ECG. The prevalence of markedly abnormal ECG patterns suggestive of significant structural heart disease was <5%. However, these results cannot be generalized to other countries. In addition to the potential impact of genetic differences, the nature of pre-participation screening is unique in Italy, where it is performed by trained and licensed sports medicine specialists who practice in dedicated sports clinics.

Over 8 years, four athletes were found to have borderline left ventricular hypertrophy (LVH) (13 mm). One was later confirmed to have hypertrophic cardiomyopathy (HCM) by genetic analysis and a second was considered to have possible HCM. In addition, 12 athletes were diagnosed with other cardiac structural abnormalities including mitral valve prolapse, myocarditis, Marfan syndrome, arrhythmogenic right ventricular cardiomyopathy, and bicuspid aortic valves. The screening ECG also can detect arrhythmogenic right ventricular cardiomyopathy, long QT syndrome, and Brugada syndrome.

Sudden cardiac death (SCD) associated with athletic activity is a rare but devastating event. Victims are usually young and apparently healthy, but many have underlying cardiovascular disease that is not diagnosed until after the event. As a result, there is great interest in detecting such abnormalities early and then defining appropriate activity restrictions for affected individuals to minimize the risk of SCD.

The majority of SCD events in athletes are due to malignant arrhythmias, usually sustained ventricular tachycardia (VT) degenerating into ventricular fibrillation (VF), or primary VF itself. Although definitions vary, "young" often refers to high school and college athletes, but applies in general to individuals under age 35 in whom SCD is usually due to congenital heart disease. Older, or "masters," athletes include individuals over age 35, in whom SCD is most commonly due to coronary heart disease (CHD).

In general, *patients with known genetic disorders that predispose to SCD* (e.g., hypertrophic cardiomyopathy, arrhythmogenic right ventricular cardiomyopathy, Marfan syndrome, long QT syndrome) should avoid recreational activities with the following characteristics:

- "Burst" exertion, involving rapid acceleration and deceleration, as is common in sprints, basketball, tennis, and football. Activities with stable energy expenditure, such as jogging, biking on level terrain, and lap swimming, are preferred
- Extreme environmental conditions (temperature, humidity, and altitude) that impact blood volume and electrolytes
- Systematic and progressive training focused on achieving higher levels of conditioning and excellence

Patients with unusual or high-risk clinical features may require greater restriction. These features include a history of syncope or pre-syncope, prior cardiac surgery, prior arrhythmic episodes, or an implantable cardioverter-defibrillator (ICD). It is widely acknowledged that SCD is the leading medical cause of death in athletes, although its exact incidence remains unclear.

An overall incidence of 1:50,000 per year in young athletes is a reasonable estimate based on existing information from retrospective cohort studies and prospective observational and cross-sectional studies. Male athletes are consistently found to be at greater risk, and there appears to be a disproportionately higher risk among male African-American athletes.

Structural heart disease can increase the risk for SCD by one or more of the following mechanisms:

- Ventricular tachyarrhythmias (most common cause)
- Bradyarrhythmia or asystole
- Syncope
- Dissection of the great vessels, as in patients with Marfan syndrome

Hypertrophic cardiomyopathy (HCM) is a relatively common disease, occurring in 0.16–0.29% of individuals in the general population (one in 350–625). *Congenital coronary artery abnormalities* were found in 12–33% of young athletes with SCD. The most common anomalies associated with SCD are the origin of the left main coronary artery from the right sinus of Valsalva and the origin of the right coronary artery from the left coronary sinus. Athletes with Marfan syndrome, familial aortic aneurysm or dissection, or congenital bicuspid aortic valve with any degree of ascending aortic enlargement should not participate in sports that involve the potential for bodily collision.

Myocarditis was present in 6–7% of cases of SCD in competitive athletes. Active myocarditis is associated with atrial and ventricular tachyarrhythmias, and bradyarrhythmias.

The incidence of SCD among competitive athletes is actually quite low, estimated to be between 1 per 50,000 athletes and 1 per 300,000 athletes.

Sudden cardiac death associated with athletic activity is a rare but devastating event. Victims are usually young and apparently healthy, but many have underlying cardiovascular disease that is not diagnosed until after the event. As a result, there is great interest in detecting such abnormalities early and then defining appropriate activity restrictions for affected individuals to minimize the risk of SCD.

Flow diagram illustrating the proposed screening protocol for young competitive athletes

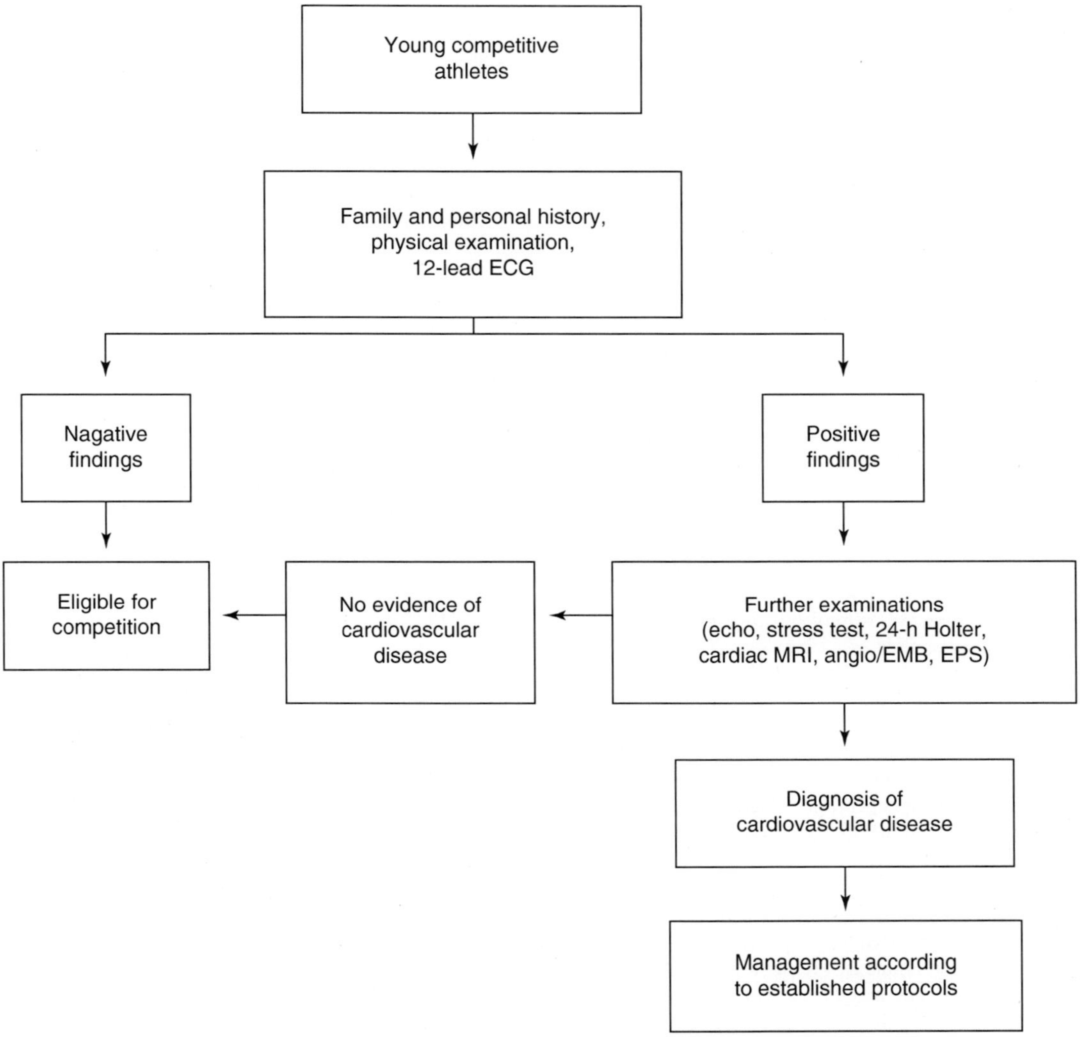

References

1. Nottin S, Vinet A, Stecken F, et al. Central and peripheral cardiovascular adaptations to exercise in endurance-trained children. Acta Physiol Scand. 2002;175:85.
2. Abu-Hasan M, Tannous B, Weinberger M. Exercise-induced dyspnea in children and adolescents: if not asthma then what? Ann Allergy Asthma Immunol. 2005;94:366.
3. Seear M, Wensley D, West N. How accurate is the diagnosis of exercise induced asthma among Vancouver schoolchildren? Arch Dis Child. 2005;90:898.
4. Javadpour SM, Selvadurai H, Wilkes DL, et al. Does carbon dioxide retention during exercise predict a more rapid decline in FEV1 in cystic fibrosis? Arch Dis Child. 2005;90:792.
5. Selvadurai HC, Blimkie CJ, Meyers N, et al. Randomized controlled study of in-hospital exercise training programs in children with cystic fibrosis. Pediatr Pulmonol. 2002;33:194.
6. Gruber W, Orenstein DM, Braumann KM, Hüls G. Health-related fitness and trainability in children with cystic fibrosis. Pediatr Pulmonol. 2008;43:953.
7. Garofano RP, Barst RJ. Exercise testing in children with primary pulmonary hypertension. Pediatr Cardiol. 1999;20:61.

8. De Caro E, Fioredda F, Calevo MG, et al. Exercise capacity in apparently healthy survivors of cancer. Arch Dis Child. 2006;91:47.
9. Pastore E, Marino B, Calzolari A, et al. Clinical and cardiorespiratory assessment in children with Down syndrome without congenital heart disease. Arch Pediatr Adolesc Med. 2000;154:408.
10. Broström E, Nordlund MM, Cresswell AG. Plantar- and dorsiflexor strength in prepubertal girls with juvenile idiopathic arthritis. Arch Phys Med Rehabil. 2004;85:1224.
11. Bar-Or O. Role of exercise in the assessment and management of neuromuscular disease in children. Med Sci Sports Exerc. 1996;28:421.
12. Takken T, Henneken T, van de Putte E, et al. Exercise testing in children and adolescents with chronic fatigue syndrome. Int J Sports Med. 2007;28:580.
13. Thompson PD, Franklin BA, Balady GJ, et al. Exercise and acute cardiovascular events placing the risks into perspective: a scientific statement from the American Heart Association Council on Nutrition, Physical Activity, and Metabolism and the Council on Clinical Cardiology. Circulation. 2007;115:2358.
14. Maron BJ, Chaitman BR, Ackerman MJ, et al. Recommendations for physical activity and recreational sports participation for young patients with genetic cardiovascular diseases. Circulation. 2004;109:2807.
15. Lampert R, Olshansky B, Heidbuchel H, et al. Safety of sports for athletes with implantable cardioverter-defibrillators: results of a prospective, multinational registry. Circulation. 2013;127:2021.
16. Maron BJ, Shirani J, Poliac LC, et al. Sudden death in young competitive athletes. Clinical, demographic, and pathological profiles. JAMA. 1996; 276:199.
17. Van Camp SP, Bloor CM, Mueller FO, et al. Nontraumatic sports death in high school and college athletes. Med Sci Sports Exerc. 1995;27:641.
18. Maron BJ, Poliac LC, Roberts WO. Risk for sudden cardiac death associated with marathon running. J Am Coll Cardiol. 1996;28:428.
19. Mitchell JH, Haskell W, Snell P, Van Camp SP. Task Force 8: classification of sports. J Am Coll Cardiol. 2005;45:1364.
20. Belonje A, Nangrahary M, de Swart H, Umans V. Major adverse cardiac events during endurance sports. Am J Cardiol. 2007;99:849.
21. Vuori I. The cardiovascular risks of physical activity. Acta Med Scand. 1986;711:205.
22. Corrado D, Basso C, Schiavon M, Thiene G. Screening for hypertrophic cardiomyopathy in young athletes. N Engl J Med. 1998;339:364.
23. Maron BJ, Thompson PD, Ackerman MJ, et al. Recommendations and considerations related to preparticipation screening for cardiovascular abnormalities in competitive athletes: 2007 update: a scientific statement from the American Heart Association Council on Nutrition, Physical Activity, and Metabolism: endorsed by the American College of Cardiology Foundation. Circulation. 2007;115:1643.
24. Roberts WO, Stovitz SD. Incidence of sudden cardiac death in Minnesota high school athletes 1993–2012 screened with a standardized pre-participation evaluation. J Am Coll Cardiol. 2013;62:1298.
25. Harmon KG, Asif IM, Klossner D, Drezner JA. Incidence of sudden cardiac death in National Collegiate Athletic Association athletes. Circulation. 2011;123:1594.
26. Eckart RE, Shry EA, Burke AP, et al. Sudden death in young adults: an autopsy-based series of a population undergoing active surveillance. J Am Coll Cardiol. 2011;58:1254.
27. Eckart RE, Scoville SL, Campbell CL, et al. Sudden death in young adults: a 25-year review of autopsies in military recruits. Ann Intern Med. 2004;141:829.
28. Virmani R, Robinowitz M, HA Jr MA. Nontraumatic death in joggers. A series of 30 patients at autopsy. Am J Med. 1982;72:874.
29. Hausmann R, Hammer S, Betz P. Performance enhancing drugs (doping agents) and sudden death – a case report and review of the literature. Int J Legal Med. 1998;111:261.
30. Maron BJ, Gardin JM, Flack JM, et al. Prevalence of hypertrophic cardiomyopathy in a general population of young adults. Echocardiographic analysis of 4111 subjects in the CARDIA study. Coronary artery risk development in (young) adults. Circulation. 1995;92:785.
31. Maron BJ, Carney KP, Lever HM, et al. Relationship of race to sudden cardiac death in competitive athletes with hypertrophic cardiomyopathy. J Am Coll Cardiol. 2003;41:974.
32. Elliott PM, Poloniecki J, Dickie S, et al. Sudden death in hypertrophic cardiomyopathy: identification of high risk patients. J Am Coll Cardiol. 2000;36:2212.
33. Gersh BJ, Maron BJ, Bonow RO, et al. 2011 ACCF/AHA guideline for the diagnosis and treatment of hypertrophic cardiomyopathy: a report of the American College of Cardiology Foundation/American Heart Association Task Force on Practice Guidelines. Circulation. 2011;124:e783.
34. Maron BJ, Ackerman MJ, Nishimura RA, et al. Task Force 4: HCM and other cardiomyopathies, mitral valve prolapse, myocarditis, and Marfan syndrome. J Am Coll Cardiol. 2005;45:1340.
35. Pelliccia A, Fagard R, Bjørnstad HH, et al. Recommendations for competitive sports participation in athletes with cardiovascular disease: a consensus document from the Study Group of Sports Cardiology of the Working Group of Cardiac Rehabilitation and Exercise Physiology and the Working Group of Myocardial and Pericardial Diseases of the European Society of Cardiology. Eur Heart J. 2005;26:1422.
36. Heidbüchel H, Corrado D, Biffi A, et al. Recommendations for participation in leisure-time physical activity and competitive sports of patients with arrhythmias and potentially arrhythmogenic conditions. Part II: ventricular arrhythmias, channelopathies

and implantable defibrillators. Eur J Cardiovasc Prev Rehabil. 2006;13:676.
37. Liberthson RR. Sudden death from cardiac causes in children and young adults. N Engl J Med. 1996;334:1039.
38. Taylor AJ, Byers JP, Cheitlin MD, Virmani R. Anomalous right or left coronary artery from the contralateral coronary sinus: "high-risk" abnormalities in the initial coronary artery course and heterogeneous clinical outcomes. Am Heart J. 1997;133:428.
39. Basso C, Maron BJ, Corrado D, Thiene G. Clinical profile of congenital coronary artery anomalies with origin from the wrong aortic sinus leading to sudden death in young competitive athletes. J Am Coll Cardiol. 2000;35:1493.
40. Graham Jr TP, Driscoll DJ, Gersony WM, et al. Task Force 2: congenital heart disease. J Am Coll Cardiol. 2005;45:1326.
41. Thompson PD, Balady GJ, Chaitman BR, et al. Task Force 6: coronary artery disease. J Am Coll Cardiol. 2005;45:1348.
42. Thiene G, Nava A, Corrado D, et al. Right ventricular cardiomyopathy and sudden death in young people. N Engl J Med. 1988;318:129.
43. Nava A, Bauce B, Basso C, et al. Clinical profile and long-term follow-up of 37 families with arrhythmogenic right ventricular cardiomyopathy. J Am Coll Cardiol. 2000;36:2226.
44. James CA, Bhonsale A, Tichnell C, et al. Exercise increases age-related penetrance and arrhythmic risk in arrhythmogenic right ventricular dysplasia/cardiomyopathy-associated desmosomal mutation carriers. J Am Coll Cardiol. 2013;62:1290.
45. Kligfield P, Devereaux RB. Is the patient with mitral valve prolapse at high risk for sudden death identifiable? In: Cheitlin MD, editor. Dilemmas in clinical cardiology. Philadelphia: FA Davis; 1990. p. 143.
46. Schwartz PJ, Priori SG, Spazzolini C, et al. Genotype-phenotype correlation in the long-QT syndrome: gene-specific triggers for life-threatening arrhythmias. Circulation. 2001;103:89.
47. Takenaka K, Ai T, Shimizu W, et al. Exercise stress test amplifies genotype-phenotype correlation in the LQT1 and LQT2 forms of the long-QT syndrome. Circulation. 2003;107:838.
48. Zipes DP, Ackerman MJ, Estes 3rd NA, et al. Task Force 7: arrhythmias. J Am Coll Cardiol. 2005;45:1354.
49. Johnson JN, Ackerman MJ. Return to play? Athletes with congenital long QT syndrome. Br J Sports Med. 2013;47:28.
50. Antzelevitch C, Brugada P, Borggrefe M, et al. Brugada syndrome: report of the second consensus conference: endorsed by the Heart Rhythm Society and the European Heart Rhythm Association. Circulation. 2005;111:659.
51. Matsuo K, Kurita T, Inagaki M, et al. The circadian pattern of the development of ventricular fibrillation in patients with Brugada syndrome. Eur Heart J. 1999;20:465.
52. Corrado D, Basso C, Buja G, et al. Right bundle branch block, right precordial st-segment elevation, and sudden death in young people. Circulation. 2001;103:710.
53. Priori SG, Napolitano C, Memmi M, et al. Clinical and molecular characterization of patients with catecholaminergic polymorphic ventricular tachycardia. Circulation. 2002;106:69.
54. Choi G, Kopplin LJ, Tester DJ, et al. Spectrum and frequency of cardiac channel defects in swimming-triggered arrhythmia syndromes. Circulation. 2004;110:2119.
55. Thompson PD, Stern MP, Williams P, et al. Death during jogging or running. A study of 18 cases. JAMA. 1979;242:1265.
56. Corrado D, Basso C, Pavei A, et al. Trends in sudden cardiovascular death in young competitive athletes after implementation of a preparticipation screening program. JAMA. 2006;296:1593.
57. Maron BJ, Thompson PD, Puffer JC, et al. Cardiovascular preparticipation screening of competitive athletes. A statement for health professionals from the Sudden Death Committee (clinical cardiology) and Congenital Cardiac Defects Committee (cardiovascular disease in the young), American Heart Association. Circulation. 1996; 94:850.
58. Maron BJ, Thompson PD, Puffer JC, et al. Cardiovascular preparticipation screening of competitive athletes: addendum: an addendum to a statement for health professionals from the Sudden Death Committee (Council on Clinical Cardiology) and the Congenital Cardiac Defects Committee (Council on Cardiovascular Disease in the Young), American Heart Association. Circulation. 1998;97:2294.
59. Maron BJ, Araújo CG, Thompson PD, et al. Recommendations for preparticipation screening and the assessment of cardiovascular disease in masters athletes: an advisory for healthcare professionals from the working groups of the World Heart Federation, the International Federation of Sports Medicine, and the American Heart Association Committee on Exercise, Cardiac Rehabilitation, and Prevention. Circulation. 2001;103:327.
60. Corrado D, Pelliccia A, Bjørnstad HH, et al. Cardiovascular pre-participation screening of young competitive athletes for prevention of sudden death: proposal for a common European protocol. Consensus Statement of the Study Group of Sport Cardiology of the Working Group of Cardiac Rehabilitation and Exercise Physiology and the Working Group of Myocardial and Pericardial Diseases of the European Society of Cardiology. Eur Heart J. 2005;26:516.
61. Corrado D, Pelliccia A, Heidbuchel H, et al. Recommendations for interpretation of 12-lead electrocardiogram in the athlete. Eur Heart J. 2010; 31:243.
62. Moyer VA, U.S. Preventive Services Task Force. Screening for coronary heart disease with electrocardi-

ography: U.S. Preventive Services Task Force recommendation statement. Ann Intern Med. 2012;157:512.
63. Pelliccia A, Maron BJ. Preparticipation cardiovascular evaluation of the competitive athlete: perspectives from the 30-year Italian experience. Am J Cardiol. 1995;75:827.
64. Maron BJ. Hypertrophic cardiomyopathy: a systematic review. JAMA. 2002;287:1308.
65. Pelliccia A, Culasso F, Di Paolo FM, et al. Prevalence of abnormal electrocardiograms in a large, unselected population undergoing pre-participation cardiovascular screening. Eur Heart J. 2007;28:2006.
66. Pelliccia A, Di Paolo FM, Corrado D, et al. Evidence for efficacy of the Italian national pre-participation screening programme for identification of hypertrophic cardiomyopathy in competitive athletes. Eur Heart J. 2006;27:2196.
67. American Academy of Family Physicians, American Academy of Pediatrics, American College of Sports Medicine. In: Bernhardt D, Roberts W, editors. Preparticipation physical evaluation. 4th ed. Elk Grove Village: American Academy of Pediatrics; 2010.
68. Roberts WO, Löllgen H, Matheson GO, et al. Advancing the preparticipation physical evaluation (PPE): an ACSM and FIMS joint consensus statement. Curr Sports Med Rep. 2014;13:395.
69. Risser WL, Hoffman HM, Bellah Jr GG, Green LW. A cost-benefit analysis of preparticipation sports examinations of adolescent athletes. J Sch Health. 1985;55:270.
70. Rice SG, American Academy of Pediatrics Council on Sports Medicine and Fitness. Medical conditions affecting sports participation. Pediatrics. 2008;121:841.
71. Maron BJ, Bodison SA, Wesley YE, et al. Results of screening a large group of intercollegiate competitive athletes for cardiovascular disease. J Am Coll Cardiol. 1987;10:1214.
72. Maron BJ, Epstein SE, Roberts WC. Causes of sudden death in competitive athletes. J Am Coll Cardiol. 1986;7:204.
73. Baggish AL, Hutter Jr AM, Wang F, et al. Cardiovascular screening in college athletes with and without electrocardiography: a cross-sectional study. Ann Intern Med. 2010;152:269.
74. Fuller CM, McNulty CM, Spring DA, et al. Prospective screening of 5,615 high school athletes for risk of sudden cardiac death. Med Sci Sports Exerc. 1997;29:1131.
75. Wilson MG, Basavarajaiah S, Whyte GP, et al. Efficacy of personal symptom and family history questionnaires when screening for inherited cardiac pathologies: the role of electrocardiography. Br J Sports Med. 2008;42:207.
76. McCambridge TM, Benjamin HJ, Brenner JS, et al. Athletic participation by children and adolescents who have systemic hypertension. Pediatrics. 2010;125:1287.
77. National High Blood Pressure Education Program Working Group on High Blood Pressure in Children and Adolescents. The fourth report on the diagnosis, evaluation, and treatment of high blood pressure in children and adolescents. Pediatrics. 2004;114:555.
78. Rupp NT, Guill MF, Brudno DS. Unrecognized exercise-induced bronchospasm in adolescent athletes. Am J Dis Child. 1992;146:941.
79. Hallstrand TS, Curtis JR, Koepsell TD, et al. Effectiveness of screening examinations to detect unrecognized exercise-induced bronchoconstriction. J Pediatr. 2002;141:343.
80. Maron BJ, Doerer JJ, Haas TS, et al. Sudden deaths in young competitive athletes: analysis of 1866 deaths in the United States, 1980–2006. Circulation. 2009;119:1085.
81. SJ Anderson, BA Griesemer, MD Johnson, TJ Martin. Climatic heat stress and the exercising child and adolescent. American Academy of Pediatrics. Committee on Sports Medicine and Fitness. Pediatrics. 2000;106:158–9.
82. Halstead ME, Walter KD, Council on Sports Medicine and Fitness. American Academy of Pediatrics. Clinical report – sport-related concussion in children and adolescents. Pediatrics. 2010;126:597.
83. Kirkwood MW, Yeates KO, Wilson PE. Pediatric sport-related concussion: a review of the clinical management of an oft-neglected population. Pediatrics. 2006;117:1359.
84. Centers for Disease Control and Prevention (CDC). Sports-related injuries among high school athletes – United States, 2005–06 school year. MMWR Morb Mortal Wkly Rep. 2006;55:1037.
85. Brooks MA, Schiff MA, Rivara FP. Identifying previous sports injury among high school athletes. Clin Pediatr (Phila). 2009;48:548.
86. Van Mechelen W, Twisk J, Molendijk A, et al. Subject-related risk factors for sports injuries: a 1-yr prospective study in young adults. Med Sci Sports Exerc. 1996;28:1171.
87. Keller CS, Noyes FR, Buncher CR. The medical aspects of soccer injury epidemiology. Am J Sports Med. 1987;15:230.
88. Schmidt-Olsen S, Jørgensen U, Kaalund S, Sørensen J. Injuries among young soccer players. Am J Sports Med. 1991;19:273.
89. Ekstrand J, Gillquist J. The avoidability of soccer injuries. Int J Sports Med. 1983;4:124.
90. Abbott HG, Kress JB. Preconditioning in the prevention of knee injuries. Arch Phys Med Rehabil. 1969;50:326.
91. Ekstrand J, Gillquist J, Liljedahl SO. Prevention of soccer. Supervision by doctor and physiotherapist injuries. Am J Sports Med. 1983;11:116.
92. Priori SG, Aliot E, Blomstrom-Lundqvist C, et al. Task Force on sudden cardiac death of the European Society of Cardiology. Eur Heart J. 2001;22:1374.
93. Rausch CM, Phillips GC. Adherence to guidelines for cardiovascular screening in current high school preparticipation evaluation forms. J Pediatr. 2009;155:584.

94. Black JL, Nader PR, Broyles SL, Nelson JA. A national survey on pediatric training and activities in school health. J Sch Health. 1991;61:245.
95. Anderson JM, Felsenthal G. Residency training in physical medicine and rehabilitation I: clinical and didactic experience. Arch Phys Med Rehabil. 1990;71:372.
96. Campbell RM, Berger S. Preventing pediatric sudden cardiac death: where do we start? Pediatrics. 2006;118:802.
97. J Goldenring. Athletic preparticipation examinations for adolescents. Report of the Board of Trustees. Group on Science and Technology, American Medical Association. Arch Pediatr Adolesc Med. 1994;148:93–8.
98. Carek PJ, Mainous 3rd AG. A thorough yet efficient exam identifies most problems in school athletes. J Fam Pract. 2003;52:127.
99. Maron BJ, Friedman RA, Kligfield P, et al. Assessment of the 12-lead ECG as a screening test for detection of cardiovascular disease in healthy general populations of young people (12–25 years of age): a scientific statement from the American Heart Association and the American College of Cardiology. Circulation. 2014;130:1303.
100. Drezner JA, Fudge J, Harmon KG, et al. Warning symptoms and family history in children and young adults with sudden cardiac arrest. J Am Board Fam Med. 2012;25:408.
101. Tretter JT, Kavey RE. Distinguishing cardiac syncope from vasovagal syncope in a referral population. J Pediatr. 2013;163:1618.
102. Maynard LM, Wisemandle W, Roche AF, et al. Childhood body composition in relation to body mass index. Pediatrics. 2001;107:344.
103. Grinsell MM, Butz K, Gurka MJ, et al. Sport-related kidney injury among high school athletes. Pediatrics. 2012;130:e40.
104. Johnson B, Christensen C, Dirusso S, et al. A need for reevaluation of sports participation recommendations for children with a solitary kidney. J Urol. 2005;174:686.
105. Viskin S. Antagonist: routine screening of all athletes prior to participation in competitive sports should be mandatory to prevent sudden cardiac death. Heart Rhythm. 2007;4:525.
106. Sharma S, Estes 3rd NA, Vetter VL, Corrado D. Clinical decisions. Cardiac screening before participation in sports. N Engl J Med. 2013;369:2049.
107. Corrado D, Basso C, Rizzoli G, et al. Does sports activity enhance the risk of sudden death in adolescents and young adults? J Am Coll Cardiol. 2003;42:1959.
108. Steinvil A, Chundadze T, Zeltser D, et al. Mandatory electrocardiographic screening of athletes to reduce their risk for sudden death proven fact or wishful thinking? J Am Coll Cardiol. 2011;57:1291.
109. Harbison AL, Hill AC, Motonaga KS, et al. Do pediatric electrophysiologists read pre-participation screening electrocardiograms more accurately than general pediatric cardiologists? J Pediatr. 2013;163:1775.
110. Maron BJ. National electrocardiography screening for competitive athletes: feasible in the United States? Ann Intern Med. 2010;152:324.
111. Hill AC, Miyake CY, Grady S, Dubin AM. Accuracy of interpretation of preparticipation screening electrocardiograms. J Pediatr. 2011;159:783.
112. Schoenbaum M, Denchev P, Vitiello B, Kaltman JR. Economic evaluation of strategies to reduce sudden cardiac death in young athletes. Pediatrics. 2012;130:e380.
113. Maron BJ, Douglas PS, Graham TP, et al. Task Force 1: preparticipation screening and diagnosis of cardiovascular disease in athletes. J Am Coll Cardiol. 2005;45:1322.
114. Maron BJ, Zipes DP. Introduction: eligibility recommendations for competitive athletes with cardiovascular abnormalities-general considerations. J Am Coll Cardiol. 2005;45:1318.

Asthma and Allergies

48

Diana Silva and André Moreira

Contents

D. Silva (✉)
Serviço de Imunologia, Faculdade de Medicina, Universidade do Porto, Porto, Portugal

Serviço de Imunoalergologia, Centro Hospitalar São João, Porto, Portugal
e-mail: disolha@gmail.com

A. Moreira
Serviço de Imunologia, Faculdade de Medicina, Universidade do Porto, Porto, Portugal

Serviço de Imunoalergologia, Centro Hospitalar São João, Porto, Portugal

Instituto de Saúde Pública da Universidade do Porto, Porto, Portugal

48.1 Asthma

A consistent body of evidence has shown that Olympic-level athletes have an increased risk for asthma and allergy, especially those who take part in endurance sports, such as swimming or running, and winter sports [1–3]. Data from the first pan-European study on allergy and asthma in Olympic athletes (the GA2 LEN Olympic study) revealed that one among four European athletes participating in the Beijing Olympic Games reported chest tightness and wheezing, whereas one out of three reported exercise-induced shortness of breath [GA2 LEN Olympic Study Coordinating Centre, Oslo, Norway, data on file]. Moreover, allergic rhinitis is a very common disease among athletes, which may negatively impact athletic performance [4]. Allergic response causes nasal and conjunctival congestion, tearing, breathing difficulties, pruritus, fatigue, and mood changes, thus affecting training and competition [5].

Asthma has a significant genetic component, but since its pathogenesis is not clear, much of its definition is descriptive: "…a chronic inflammatory disorder of the airways in which many cells

J. Espregueira-Mendes et al. (eds.), *Injuries and Health Problems in Football*,
DOI 10.1007/978-3-662-53924-8_48

and cellular elements play a role. The chronic inflammation is associated with airway hyperresponsiveness that leads to recurrent episodes of wheezing, breathlessness, chest tightness, and coughing, particularly at night or in the early morning. These episodes are usually associated with widespread, but variable, airflow obstruction within the lung that is often reversible either spontaneously or with treatment…" in the Global Initiative for Asthma (GINA) Report [6]. The pattern of inflammation in allergic asthma is characterized by T helper (Th) 2 inflammatory phenotype with a predominance of Th2 cytokines – such as interleukin-4 (IL-4), IL-5, IL-9, and IL-13. The allergic inflammation is characterized by increased IgE concentrations, mast cell degranulation, and eosinophil-mediated inflammation.

The PRACTALL initiative endorsed by the European Academy of Allergy and Clinical Immunology and the American Academy of Allergy, Asthma and Immunology defined exercise-induced asthma (EIA) as lower airway obstruction and symptoms of cough, wheezing, or dyspnea induced by exercise in patients with underlying asthma [7]. The same clinical presentation in individuals without asthma was defined as exercise-induced bronchoconstriction. These definitions are however limited by the heterogeneity in asthma expression. In fact, multiple asthma phenotypes exhibiting differences in clinical response to treatment exist, and assessment should be multidimensional, including variability in clinical, physiologic, and pathologic parameters. Two different clinical endotypes of asthma in athletes, reflecting different underlying mechanisms, have been recently suggested. The pattern of "classical asthma" is characterized by early-onset childhood asthma, methacholine responsiveness, atopy, and signs of eosinophilic airway inflammation and by another distinct phenotype with onset of symptoms during sports career, bronchial responsiveness to eucapnic hyperventilation test, and a variable association with atopic markers and eosinophilic airway inflammation [8, 9].

From the clinical point of view, the main physiological feature of asthma is intermittent and reversible airway obstruction, while the dominant pathological feature is airway inflammation sometimes associated with airway structural changes. Airway responsiveness is the tendency for airways to constrict under the influence of nonsensitizing physical stimuli such as cold air and exercise, chemical substances such as methacholine, or sensitizing agents such as allergens. Airway hyperresponsiveness can be defined as an abnormal increase in the degree to which the airways constrict upon exposure to these stimuli.

Classical postulated mechanisms behind exercise-induced asthma include the osmotic or airway-drying hypothesis [10]. As water evaporates from the airway surface liquid, it becomes hyperosmolar, thereby providing an osmotic stimulus for water to move from nearby cells. This results in shrinkage of nearby cells and the release of inflammatory mediators that causes airway smooth muscle contraction. However, this hypothesis requires that all the athletes develop bronchoconstriction at a certain point, which does not happen. This suggests that the exercise-induced bronchoconstriction explanatory model in athletes probably includes the interplay between environmental training factors, including allergens; ambient conditions such as temperature, humidity, and air quality; and athlete's personal risk factors, such as genetic and neuro-immunoendocrine determinants.

Genetic susceptibility to exercise-induced bronchospasm has been linked with the gene for the aqueous water channel aquaporin. Airway hydration during exercise is mainly dependent on the water movement, following the osmotic force generated by sodium and chloride, through aquaporin channels expressed within the apical membrane of epithelial cells. It has been suggested that functional polymorphisms of the aquaporin gene may contribute to a phenotype where hyperhidrosis, sialorrhea, and excessive tearing are traits that may predict resistance of airways to nonspecific stimulus. However, it is also possible that mechanisms affecting both water and ion movement are commonly affected by nervous system dysfunction [10].

Intensive training can have effects on autonomic regulation promoting the vagal predominance, thus regulating contractions and relaxations of the airway smooth muscle. The increased parasympathetic activity could act as a compensatory response to the sympathetic stimulation associated with frequent and intense training [11]. This could induce not only the resting bradycardia typical of athletes but also an increase in bronchomotor tone and, in turn, an increased susceptibility to the development of asthma. A dysfunctional neuroendocrine-immune interface may then play a role in the pathogenesis of exercise-induced bronchoconstriction, mainly due to release and action of neuropeptides from primary sensory nerve terminals, in a so-called neurogenic inflammation pathway. This is also clinically supported by a positive effect of inhaled anticholinergic drugs in athletes [12].

Table 48.1 Criteria set by the World Anti-Doping Agency to document asthma in athletes

A rise in FEV1 to bronchodilator ≥12 % of the baseline or predicted FEV1 and exceeds 200 ml
A fall in FEV1 ≥10 % from the baseline in response to exercise or eucapnic voluntary hyperpnea
A fall in FEV1 ≥15 % from the baseline after inhaling 22.5 ml of 4.5 g% NaCl or ≤635 mg of mannitol
A fall in FEV1 ≥20 % from the baseline in response to methacholine
PC20 ≤4 mg/ml or PD20 ≤ 400 μg (cumulative dose) or ≤200 μg (noncumulative dose) in those not taking inhaled corticosteroids (ICS) and PC20 ≤16 mg/ml or PD20 ≤1600 μg (cumulative dose) or ≤800 μg (noncumulative dose) in those taking ICS for at least 1 month

48.1.1 Diagnosing Exercise-Induced Asthma

Exercise is a powerful trigger of bronchoconstriction and symptoms in asthmatic patients and may result in avoidance of physical activity resulting in detrimental consequences to their physical and social well-being. Diagnosis demands the synthesis of medical history with respiratory symptoms, physical examination, and appropriate laboratory or field tests. Methods and thresholds to document exercise-induced bronchoconstriction may be different for recreational or competitive athletes, particularly in regulated sports. For recreational exercisers, free running for children or a simple 10 min jog for adults may be adequate to document exercise-induced bronchoconstriction (≥10% drop in lung function measured by forced expiratory volume in the first second of forced vital capacity (FEV1)). For others, the exercise challenge should elicit 90% of maximal heart rate or 40–60% of maximal ventilation during 6–8 min of exercise on a treadmill or stationary bicycle. For competitive athletes, precise criteria for diagnosing asthma have been set (Table 48.1).

48.1.2 Treatment of Exercise-Induced Asthma

Drugs effective in the treatment of asthma are likely to be effective in the treatment of EI-asthma or EI-bronchoconstriction. Inhaled β2-adrenoceptor agonists are most effective in reversing EI-asthma/bronchoconstriction and are also used for prevention [6]. The effectiveness of inhaled short-acting β-agonists such as salbutamol or terbutaline against EI-asthma/bronchoconstriction is optimal 20 min after inhalation and wanes within a few hours. Long-acting β2-agonists, such as formoterol and salmeterol, protect for up to 12 h after a single inhalation. However, only formoterol acts as fast as quick-acting beta-agonists; therefore, formoterol but not salmeterol should be chosen to reverse EI-asthma/bronchoconstriction [13]. Inhaled β2-agonists may mask worsening airway inflammation and should never be used regularly without an inhaled glucocorticoid.

Regular treatments with inhaled glucocorticoids and/or leukotriene pathway antagonists control underlying asthma and reduce EI-asthma/bronchoconstriction. Montelukast and zafirlukast are cysLT receptor-1 antagonists. H1-antihistamines have minimal effects on EI-asthma/bronchoconstriction, whereas cromones administered before exercise mildly reduce EI-bronchoconstriction. In difficult-to-control EI-asthma/bronchoconstriction, combining inhaled glucocorticoids, oral leukotriene antagonists, and/or inhaled β2-agonists may be beneficial [13].

Optimal control of underlying asthma minimizes airway narrowing during exercise. Worsening EI-asthma may be a sign of inadequate control of underlying asthma, and "step-up" therapy should be considered. On the other hand, allergic rhinitis is

Table 48.2 Drugs regulated for asthma treatment during training and competition by the World Anti-Doping Agency (WADA) in 2016

Beta-agonists		
All oral (taken by mouth and swallowed) or injected beta-2 agonists are prohibited		
Inhaled beta-2 agonists are prohibited and require a Therapeutic Use Exemption (TUE), except for albuterol (also called salbutamol) dosages under 1600 μg in any 24 h period, formoterol dosages less than 54 μg in any 24 h period, and salmeterol when taken according to manufacturer's instructions. If you use more than the amounts listed in the table below, you are required to submit a TUE for use. The presence of salbutamol in urine in excess of 1000 ng/mL is presumed not to be an intended therapeutic use of the substance and will be considered as an *adverse analytical finding* unless the *athlete* proves, through a controlled pharmacokinetic study, that the abnormal result was the consequence of the use of a therapeutic dose (maximum 1600 μg over 24 h) of inhaled salbutamol		
Inhaler brands and strengths	*Recommended dosing by manufacturer*	*WADA maximum doses per 24 h*
Advair Diskus 100/50, 250/50, or 500/50 Each has salmeterol 50mcg per puff	1 puff twice each day (100 mcg salmeterol)	Take as directed by the drug manufacturer
Advair HFA 45/21, 115/21, or 230/21Each has salmeterol 21 mcg per puff	2 puffs twice each day (84 mcg salmeterol)	Take as directed by the drug manufacturer
Albuterol 108 mcg per puffProAir, Proventil, Ventolin	1–2 puffs every 4 h as needed for wheezing	Salbutamol 108 mcg per puff: 14 puffs a day (<1600 mcg)
Dulera 100 mcg/5 mcg per puff or 200mcg/5mcg per puff	2 Puffs twice each day (20 mcg formoterol)	Formoterol 5 mcg per puff: 10 puffs a day (<54 mcg)
Foradil Aerolizer 12 mcg per puff	1 Capsule inhaled every 12 h (24 mcg formoterol)	Formoterol 12 mcg per cap: 4 puffs a day (<54 mcg)
Serevent Diskus 50 mcg per puff	1 puff twice each day (100 mcg)	Take as directed by the drug manufacturer
Symbicort 80 mcg/4.5 mcg per puff or 160 mcg/4.5 mcg per puff	2 puffs twice each day (formoterol 18 mcg)	Formoterol 4.5 mcg per puff: 12 puffs a day (<54 mcg)
Advisory		
The use of oral beta-2 agonists is prohibited even if the athlete has a TUE for the same inhaled beta-2 agonist. If the athlete's doctor prescribes an oral beta-2 agonist, the athlete should submit an application for a TUE		
Use the table above as a guide to determine the dosage of albuterol or formoterol that may be used in sport without a TUE. However, an athlete should examine his/her inhaler closely to determine the exact dose delivered		
Some dietary supplements claim to contain ingredients that have beta-2 agonist activity such as norcoclaurine. It is not known whether such products actually contain these ingredients, but USADA considers such products to be high risk		
Albuterol (urine amount over 1000 ng/mL) and formoterol (urine amount over 40 ng/mL) are "threshold substances," which means they may be used in sport without a TUE as long as they are used under a certain threshold. However, if an athlete also takes a substance that falls into the category of diuretics and masking agents, a TUE is required for albuterol or formoterol even if the athlete already has a TUE on file for the diuretic or masking agent		
The presence of albuterol in urine in excess of 1000 ng/mL is presumed *not* to be an intended therapeutic use and may be considered as an adverse analytical finding, possibly leading to a sanction		
Some inhalers have more than one active ingredient. Make sure to check all active ingredients on GlobalDRO.com		
Glucocorticosteroid		
Inhalation of glucocorticoids (e.g., for asthma) is permitted. All glucocorticosteroids are prohibited when administered by oral, intravenous, intramuscular, or rectal routes		

also a very common disease among athletes and may negatively impact athletic performance; its early recognition, diagnosis, and treatment are crucial for improving nasal function and reduce the risk of asthma during exercise and competition. Certain medications for athletes with asthma and rhinitis who participate in regulated competitions are not allowed, and physician, athletes, and coaches should be aware of the updated regulatory aspects of asthma treatment (Table 48.2).

A few notes should be taken on the effects of exercise as a non-pharmacological to asthmatic patients. At the current knowledge, evidence-based prescription of physical activity in asthma seems to be restricted to improvements in the physical fitness of the subjects. It is recommended that children and adolescents participate in at least 60 min of moderate-intensity physical activity most days of the week and preferably daily. Engagement in physical activity promotes the normal psychosocial development, neuromuscular coordination, and self-esteem. Changing from sedentary behaviors such as television viewing and computer games to moderate-intensity physical activity has been associated with enhanced overall health and prevention of chronic diseases. In asthmatics, exercise training may reduce the perception of breathlessness through strengthening of respiratory muscle and decrease the likelihood of exercise-induced symptoms by lowering the ventilation rate during exercise.

Currently, the GINA Guidelines do not include recommendations for exercise as part of the treatment for patients with asthma. Exercise is a powerful trigger for asthma symptoms. For this reason, caretakers may be reluctant to allow their asthmatic children to engage in sports practice, fearing an exacerbation of the disease. Every subject with asthma should be questioned about exercise performance, tolerance, and symptoms, but there is no reason to discourage asthmatic with a controlled disease to exercise [14].

48.2 Allergic Rhinitis

Rhinitis is defined as an inflammation of the nasal mucosa, characterized by two or more of the following symptoms: nasal congestion, anterior and posterior rhinorrhea, sneezing, and itching [15, 16]. Asthma and allergic rhinitis frequently coexist [15]. The prevalence of asthma in patients with rhinitis varies between 10 and 40%, and rhinitis seems to be an independent factor in the risk of asthma [4]. It is not still clear whether allergic rhinitis is an earlier clinical manifestation of allergic disease in atopic patients who will develop asthma or the nasal disease itself is a causative for asthma [15]. Rhinitis is classified etiologically in three main types [17]: allergic rhinitis (AR) (IgE mediated), nonallergic noninfectious rhinitis (non-IgE-mediated inflammation), and infectious rhinitis (Table 48.3) [15, 16]. Despite 30–50% of patients with rhinitis have nonallergic triggers, 44–87 % might have a mixed phenotype combining both allergic and nonallergic rhinitis mechanisms [18].

The upper airways, including the nasal cavity and its tissues, lie in a bony structure that, unlike the lower airway structure, cannot change shape [20]. Upper airways comprise an epithelium with a basement membrane and a submucosal layer, which contains venous sinusoids [20]. These vessels and mucosa glands are responsible for

Table 48.3 Rhinitis classification

I Allergic rhinitis
II Nonallergic noninfectious rhinitis A. Vasomotor rhinitis (triggered by irritant, cold air, exercise, undetermined trigger) B. Gustatory rhinitis
III Infectious rhinitis (acute infectious rhinitis, chronic rhinosinusitis)
III Occupational rhinitis A. IgE mediated (protein or chemical allergens) B. Uncertain immune mechanism (chemical respiratory sensitizers) C. Work-aggravated rhinitis
IV Rhinitis syndromes A. Hormonal induced (pregnancy or menstrual cycle induced) B. Drug induced 1. Rhinitis *medicamentosa* 2. Nonsteroidal anti-inflammatory drugs 3. Oral contraceptives 4. Antihypertensive and cardiovascular agents C. Atrophic rhinitis D. Rhinitis associated with inflammatory-immunologic disorders 1. Granulomatous infection 2. Wegener granulomatosis 3. Sarcoidosis 4. Midline granuloma 5. Churg-Strauss syndrome 6. Relapsing polychondritis 7. Amyloidosis 8. Nonallergic rhinitis with eosinophilia syndrome (NARES)
V Rhinitis by structural causes

Adapted from [19]

filtration, humidification, and warming of inhaled air, and they are regulated by autonomic nervous system reflexes [21]. Swelling of the venous sinusoids can lead to upper airway obstruction, and activation of local nerve reflexes causes sneezing, watery discharge, and vasodilation, symptoms associated with rhinitis [20].

During exercise, autonomic reflexes improve nasal efficiency [4]. In dynamic exercise training due to an increase of nasal sympathetic activity, venous sinusoids constrict. A watery discharge can also be produced, because cold air induces glandular hypersecretion [4, 20].

During training athletes are repeatedly exposed to risk factors, like allergens, but also cold air and pollutants, therefore increasing rhinitis symptoms in susceptible individuals [21]. Some experience improvement with exercise, mediated by nasal sympathetic tone, and others may have their symptoms worsen [22]. Weather conditions, like cold or dry air, and inhalation of irritants in outdoor exercise exposure can explain the worsening symptoms in some athletes [7].

Rhinitis is the most common cause of nasal symptoms in athletes [23]. Associated risk factors, such as atopy, family history of allergy, and exposure to allergens and pollution, might explain why AR prevalence has increased in all population, including athletes [15, 24]. AR is a multifactorial disease influenced by genetic and environmental interaction [25].

The World Health Organization (WHO) through the working group Allergic Rhinitis and its Impact on Asthma (ARIA) changed the classification from the time of exposure (seasonal, perennial, and occupational) to a symptomatic definition and severity characterization (Fig. 48.1). The seasonal and perennial rhinitis classification is still useful for diagnosis and immunotherapy (IT) treatment decision and can be used alongside with ARIA classification [15].

The most frequent allergic triggers are inhalant allergens, namely, mites, pollens, animals, and fungi. According to the triggers, they can cause perennial or seasonal symptoms. Preexisting rhinitis can be exacerbated by workplace irritants like smoke, cold air, and pollutants [24].

Rhinitis is largely underdiagnosed and self-managed in athletes [26]. However, it has debilitating consequences, significantly interfering with

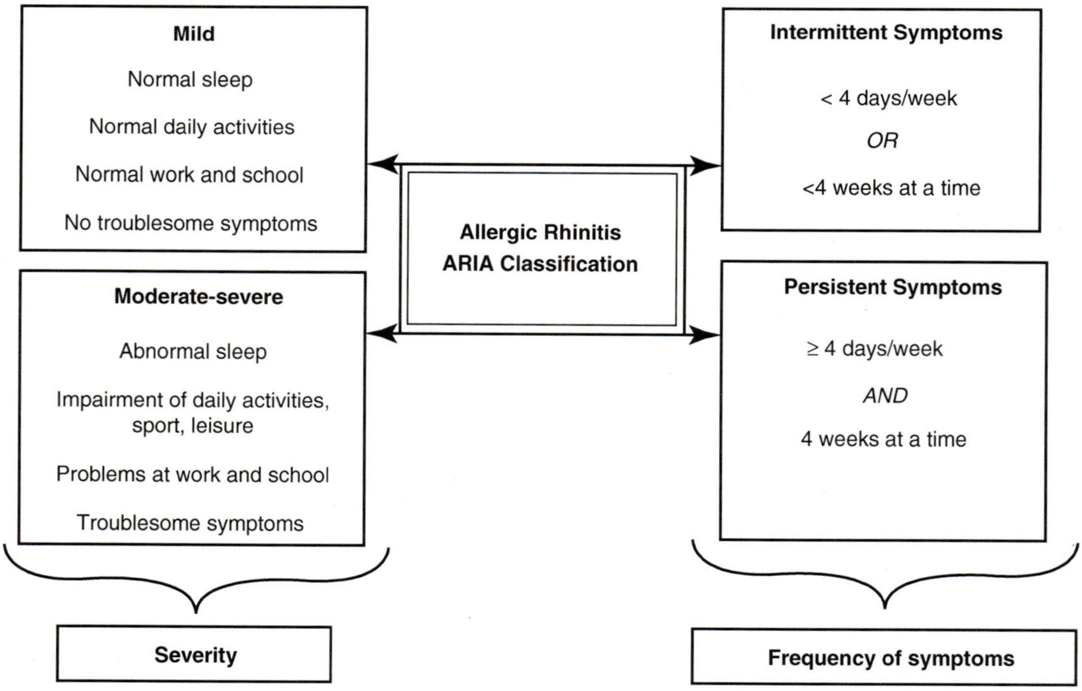

Fig. 48.1 Allergic rhinitis classification (Adapted from [15])

patient's quality of life and activity, namely, in sports practice [27]. Previous studies support its negative impact on cognitive functions, school performance, sleep, quality of life, and even behavior, which can significantly affect athletic performance [27]. This is particularly important, as a higher prevalence of rhinitis has been reported in athletes than in general population [21]. Excluding exercised-induced rhinitis, idiopathic rhinitis, and nasal symptoms related to physical, cold air, and chemical contact factors, allergic rhinitis can account for prevalence up to 30% in an athlete population.

48.2.1 Epidemiology and Risk Factors

Allergic rhinitis has a prevalence of 10–20% in the general population, which is higher in elite competitive athletes [15, 28]. In the last two decades, a prevalence range between 13.3 and 48.6% was found (Table 48.4) [21].

The allergic response causes nasal and conjunctival congestion, tearing, breathing difficulties, pruritus, fatigue, and mood changes, which might affect athletic performance [48]. Kateralis showed over spring season a negative effect of allergic rhinoconjunctivitis on performance scores (ability to train and compete). Also a resolution of those symptoms, namely, eye symptoms, and improvement on quality of life and performance scores were seen after treatment with intranasal corticosteroids [49].

During exercise, ventilation increases for a short period of time in power athletes and for longer periods in resistance athletes [4]. Most of this exercise is practiced in outdoor environments; therefore, athletes are strongly and repeatedly exposed to large amounts of aeroallergens and pollutants. This contact in training or in competition periods may increase the likelihood of exercise-induced respiratory symptoms [21]. The climate conditions, namely, the inhaled air, temperature, and humidity, also affect these patients [4, 50].

Athletes involved in outdoor sports are frequently exposed during peak allergen seasons. Indeed, major sports events frequently occur at the end of the spring and beginning of the summer [21]. Aerobiological records of pollens are used to monitor the pollen levels, and it is important for athletes to prepare themselves, particularly if they are symptomatic to some allergen. An example was the setup of an aerobiological network for the Athens Summer Olympic Games [51].

Indoor allergens, namely, mites, are not usually studied, due to the decreased frequency of contact and the specific association of more severe symptoms with endurance to outdoor exercise. However, in some more indoor sports, persistent rhinitis symptoms can occur, and it may be relevant to control this environmental exposure.

Urban-type pollution interacts with allergens and induces sensitization and triggers symptoms in allergic patients [4]. There are several studies pointing to adverse effects of outdoor air pollution, caused by carbon monoxide, nitric oxide, and ozone [21]. The two agents that most frequently affect upper respiratory airways and rhinitis are particulate matter, namely, diesel exhaust particles (DEPs) [15] and volatile organic compounds. Their peak production is from April to September in the Northern Hemisphere, and a large percentage (40%) is completely absorbed by the nasal mucosa [15]. They enhance the production of oxygen's derivatives increasing the permeability of epithelial cells [38]. Ozone increases the late-phase response to nasal allergens, increasing the eosinophilic influx after exposure, and, in the nasal mucosa, the histamine and inflammatory cells are increased in number [21].

In several studies, it has been shown that patients living in traffic-congested areas have more severe rhinitis and conjunctivitis symptoms [52]. A study in Beijing, using questionnaires in 31,829 individuals and monitoring PM10, SO2, and NO2 air levels, found a significant association between outpatient visits for allergic rhinitis and increasing air pollutant levels [53]. This finding is particularly relevant for athletes who train or compete in outdoor urban environments. So, at the Olympic Games in China, air quality was monitored in order that athletes could perform their sports safely [54]. In fact, elite athletes practice sport around the world under different

Table 48.4 Prevalence of rhinitis or seasonal allergic rhinoconjunctivitis (SARC) in athletes

Reference	Design and methods	Year of study, subjects (n)	Rhinitis/SARC* prevalence
Fitch [29]	Retrospective; medical records analysis	1976, Australian Olympics (185)	8.6
		1980, Australian Olympics (106)	7.5
Helbling [30]	Cross-sectional; questionnaire	1986, Swiss athletes (2,060)	16.8*
Kaelin [31]	Cross-sectional; questionnaire	1990, Swiss athletes (1530)	19.7%*
Potts [32]	Cross-sectional; questionnaire	1995, Canadian swimmers (738)	19.0*
Helenius [33]	Cross-sectional; skin prick tests with medical diagnosis	1996, Finnish summer athletes (162)	29.6*
Weiler [34]	Cross-sectional, questionnaire (USOC-MHQ)	1996, US Summer Olympics (699)	16.9
Weiler [35]	Cross-sectional, questionnaire (USOC-MHQ)	1998, US Winter Olympics (699)	13.3
Katelaris [36]	Cross-sectional; skin prick tests with medical diagnosis	1997/8, Australian Summer Olympics (214)	41.0/29.0*
Katelaris [28]	Cross-sectional; skin prick tests with medical diagnosis	1999, Australian Olympics/Paralympics (977)	37.0/24.0*
Lapucci [37]	Cross-sectional; skin prick tests with medical diagnosis	2000, Italian Summer Olympics (265)	25.3*
Bonadonna [38]	Cross-sectional, questionnaire on cold-induced rhinitis	2001, Italian skiers (144)	48.6
Alaranta [39]	Cross-sectional; self-reported medical diagnosis	2002, Finnish Olympic athletes (446);	26.5
		Subgroup of endurance athletes (108)	36.1
Randolph [40]	Cross-sectional; questionnaire (USOC-MHQ)	2003/4, US recreational runners (484)	34.7
Moreira [41]	Cross-sectional; self-reported medical diagnosis	2003, Finnish marathon runners (141)	17.3
Bonini [42]	Cross-sectional; medical diagnosis	2006, Italian preOlympics (98)	34.7
Macucci [43]	Cross-sectional; medical diagnosis	2006, Italian young athletes (352)	22.2
Salonen [44]	Cross-sectional; self-reported medical diagnosis	2007, Finnish young hockey players (793)	18.3
Thomas [45]	Cross-sectional; questionnaire	2008, German athletes candidates for Summer Olympic Games (291)	25*
Bonini [46]	Cross-sectional surveys from 2000 to 2012	2000–2012, Italian Olympic Delegation at Summer and Winter Olympic Games (659	26.2
Kurowski [47]	Cross-sectional; self-reported medical diagnosis	2008, Polish athletes Olympic (222)	27.0

Adapted and updated from [19]
*Seasonal Allergic Rhinoconjuntivitis

conditions and should be informed to what environment exposure they will be submitted, to adapt themselves and have appropriate preventive measures, namely, their allergic symptoms fully controlled.

Tobacco smoke is not advised in all populations, and especially in sports practice. Despite this, some athletes smoke or are exposed to passive smoke. Nasal symptoms, rhinorrhea, and nasal obstruction can occur under tobacco exposure, but these are not always consistent with increased total and specific IgEs [15].

The exposure to different environmental conditions that are specific to a particular sport also contributes to rhinitis symptoms. Rhinorrhea and nasal congestion after exposure to cold air, known as "skier's nose," can occur in normal individuals [55]. In high-performance athletes, namely, skiers, long-distance runners, and swimmers with long-term exposure to cold, the repeated cooling and drying of the mucosa results in an inflammatory infiltration of the airway mucosa, and these effects are reversed after stopping the high-performance exercise [56].

In runners, an initial decongestion of the mucosa occurs, and it is maintained nearly 30 min after stopping exercise. This reduction of nasal resistance can lead to mucosa dehydration and a rebound increase in nasal secretion to compensate it. This "runner's nose" is also integrated in differential diagnosis of allergic rhinitis [4].

Swimmers are also a specific population of athletes. Their long-term and high exposure to chlorine derivatives during regular trainings and competition at increased ventilation can induce mucosal inflammation which facilitates the responsiveness to airborne allergens and induces bronchial hyperresponsiveness. Kateralis found in a group of swimmers that they were more likely to have rhinitis symptoms and allergic sensitization than those active in other sports [36]. These results were similar when compared with healthy controls [57]. When swimmers stopped training for 2 weeks, they showed an improvement in nasal symptoms [57]. In a study comparing competitive swimmers with runners, the first experienced worsening of nasal function after training independently of being atopic [50].

48.2.2 Effects of Allergic Rhinitis on Exercise Performance

Allergic rhinitis has a negative impact on quality of life in the general population. Cognitive functions, school performance, sleep, and behavioral effects have been described, namely, in children with attention-deficit hyperactivity disorders [58]. In a questionnaire of quality of life performed during spring time, Kateralis showed poorer results in the allergic group [27]. In another study with 145 athletes with allergic rhinitis who agreed to be treated had a significant improvement of their quality of life scores under budesonide therapy [49]. In a high-level competitive swimmers population, stopping training for 2 weeks improved rhinitis-related QoL. It was not possible yet to confirm a direct association of poorly treated rhinitis and a bad exercise performance [59]; however, an indirect one can be inferred. However, it seems likely that altered airflow dynamics and ventilation and nasal obstruction can potentially have a negative effect, mainly in high-intensity activities [59]. Any factors that affect sleep, decrease ability to concentrate, or reduce physical fitness have an easy understandable impact on sports performance.

The cognitive impact (learning ability and memory) of rhinitis has been particularly studied in children [58]. Learning disability is caused as a consequence of the frequent sleep disturbances and resulting daytime sleepiness. Impaired sleep is secondary to nasal congestion which causes micro-arousal and irregular breathing, with snoring and apnea. An associated effect is school and work absenteeism and training capacity disability [58]. Correct diagnosis and management of allergic rhinitis can reduce the disease impact.

48.2.3 Diagnosis

Diagnosis of allergic rhinitis in athletes is based in the concordance of a suggestive history of allergic symptoms and physical examination and supported by diagnostic tests [15, 60].

A complete allergic history is the best diagnostic tool for rhinitis diagnosis, allowing to assess severity and guide treatment [16, 60]. The patient, namely, the athlete, may present several symptoms, namely, sneezing; anterior rhinorrhea; bilateral nasal obstruction; postnasal drip cough; itchy nose, ears, and throat; loss of smell (hyposmia or anosmia); or snoring [15, 59]. Frequently, ocular symptoms are concomitant with tearing, burning, and itching. In athletes, clinical presentation is frequently more subtle and might include poor-quality sleep, fatigue, reduced exercise performance, and difficulty to recover after more demanding exercise sessions [59]. Patient evaluation should include symptom's pattern characterization, chronicity, seasonality and triggers of nasal and related symptoms, response to treatment, presence of coexisting conditions, and the relation with training practice. It is also very important to include assessment of quality of life [16].

Physical examination of all organ systems potentially affected by allergies should be performed. Further attention should be given for the upper respiratory tract system, namely, nasal and oropharyngeal examination. In some patients, nasal examination can show bluish-gray discoloration and edema or erythema of the mucosa with clear watery rhinorrhea [60]. Infectious complications of rhinitis to which athletes seems to be more prone, like otitis and sinusitis, should be discarded during this examination [61], as well as structural causes of symptoms. It is important to explore during clinical investigations differential diagnosis for similar symptoms, like nonallergic ones.

In an athlete, when an allergic etiology is suspected, skin prick testing (SPT) with standardized allergens and/or measurement of allergen-specific IgE in serum should be used. Skin prick tests are relevant markers of the IgE-mediated allergic reaction [15, 24]. The result can depend on several variables, quality of the allergen extracts, age, and medications and is dependent on operator interpretation [15, 60]. Serum total IgE and serum-specific IgE are measured by radioimmunoassay or enzyme immunoassay and can be requested when skin tests are not possible or when SPT in association with the clinical exam is not concordant [15, 16, 24]. The sensitivity of serum-specific IgE measurements compared with SPT can vary with the immunoassay technique used [16].

Nasal and conjunctival challenge tests can be used to assess if any discrepancy occurs between history and results of skin prick test or IgE measurement and to define clinically relevant allergens in cases of multiple sensitizations [15, 24, 62].

Imaging of the nose and sino-nasal cavity is used to corroborate diagnosis and differentiate the source of sino-nasal symptoms, the relation of sino-nasal problem with surrounding structures, and the extent of the disease [60]. Plain sinus radiographs are not indicated in allergic rhinitis or rhinosinusitis diagnosis [15, 63]. Computerized tomography scanning is used to evaluate paranasal sinuses due to optimal display of air bone and soft tissue. It is indicated for differential diagnosis purposes, to exclude chronic rhinosinusitis, to eliminate rhinitis complication, and to evaluate nonresponders to treatment [15, 60]. It can be particularly useful in athletes, to exclude traumatic lesions, which occur frequently in close-contact sports, like boxing or football.

To evaluate rhinitis severity measurements of nasal obstruction and smell can be used [15]. These tests are not made in routine clinical practice but can be useful when allergen challenges are undertaken or septal surgery is contemplated [24]. Nasal patency can be monitored objectively using nasal peak inspiratory and expiratory flow, acoustic rhinometry, that measures the nasal cavity volume and rhinomanometry that measures nasal airflow and pressure [60]. In clinical practice the most frequently used is peak nasal inspiratory flow because it is simple, cheap, fast, and available and it can be used for disease home monitoring [16]. Nasal nitric oxide measurement may be a useful tool in diagnosis and management and to alert for possible mucociliary defects, but its utility in allergic rhinitis needs to be further evaluated [15, 60].

Rhinitis control is frequently monitored with control questionnaires and visual analogue scales [15]. The Rhinitis Control Assessment Test, a 6-item patient completed instrument, and Control of Allergic Rhinitis and Asthma Test (CARAT) are such examples [64, 65]. Specific questionnaires for athletes are the Allergy Questionnaire for Athletes (AQUA) that was developed by Bonini [66].

48.2.4 Management of Allergic Rhinitis in Athletes

Management of allergic rhinitis encompasses patient education, environmental control, pharmacotherapy, and allergen-specific immunotherapy. Surgical options might be used in highly selected cases [15]. Appropriate management requires an "evidence-based medicine" approach [15, 67]. For the elite athlete, it is also important to minimize the potential detrimental effects of allergic symptoms and treatment on performance [27]. Treatment requires careful planning to comply to the "anti-doping" regulations and avoid detrimental influences of treatment adverse effects [27]. Specific aims for the athlete population are the following: avoid exposure to peak levels of clinically relevant allergens and pollutants; reduce symptoms and improve nasal functions to minimize potential negative effects on sports performance; and use therapies complying with the WADA rules that do not affect performance.

Reducing allergen exposure can improve disease control and decrease the need for treatment [68]. In most cases and specifically in athletes, complete avoidance is difficult to achieve [41]. Nevertheless, measures aiming to reduce relevant allergens should be promoted. Removing carpets from the bedroom, careful and daily cleaning, and regular change of bed linen can be useful for reducing house dust mite exposure. For pollen exposure avoidance, following pollen forecasts and adapting training venues and training schedule and using appropriate face equipment may minimize exposure, at least to peak pollen levels [16, 59]. Irritants reported to cause nasal symptoms, including pollution, chlorine, and cold air, should also be minimized [16]. In order to prevent high-level exposure to these agents, training environment should be more controlled by improving ventilation systems of swimming pools and ice arenas [21] and taking measures to reduce global pollution [53].

48.2.4.1 Pharmacologic Therapy of Rhinitis in Athletes

The selection of treatment for a patient depends on multiple factors: type of rhinitis, symptom severity, age, and job [16]. In elite athletes, management of allergic rhinitis should be adapted to accommodate factors that may hazard the athletic performance, and the balance between efficacy and safety should be addressed before prescribing. In elite athletes the drug must be accepted by the most recent World Anti-Doping Agency (WADA) rules.

Antihistamines

H1-receptor antagonists block histamine at H1-receptor level (neutral antagonists or inverse agonists). They are effective in symptoms mediated by histamine, namely, rhinorrhea, sneezing, and nasal and eye itching [15]. Antihistamines can be divided accordingly into their chemical class in alkylamines, piperazine, piperidines, ethanolamines, ethylenediamines, and phenothiazines [69]. However, the most used classification is functional as first generation, which is sedating, and second generation which is relatively nonsedating [69]. Second-generation oral H1-antihistamines (e.g., rupatadine, ebastine, azelastine, levocetirizine, desloratadine, or bilastine) are recommended in the most updated guidelines as they do not have anticholinergic and sedative, cognitive, and psychomotor effects [67]. Athletes benefit the most with these recommendations, since first-generation H1-antihistamines may reduce psychomotor skills by their sedative effect and, by their anticholinergic activity, cause mucosal drying and reduce sweating and temperature regulation [21, 59]. Some authors even propose a cautious approach in the prescription of any antihistamines 24–48 h before a major competition [59].

Topical H1-antihistamine can also be used. Intranasal H1-antihistamine, like azelastine and levocabastine, is locally effective in reducing itching, sneezing, runny nose, and nasal congestion [15]. Due to their rapid effect, they can be used on demand by athletes to treat acute unexplained symptoms in the sports field [21]. Second-generation antihistamines are also used as topical treatment, like levocabastine and emedastine. They can be used in combination with mast cell stabilizers, namely, sodium cromoglycate and nedocromil, throughout allergy season [70]. Dual-action anti-allergic molecules, like olopatadine or azelastine, allow to rapidly relief symptoms, due to their antihistaminic effect, and also have a long-term effect in mast cell stabilization [68, 70].

Decongestants

Decongestants, as vasoconstrictor drugs, act on adrenergic receptor reducing nasal obstruction. Their side effects (increased blood pressure, heart rate, central nervous system stimulation) limit their use [68]. Their clinical use should be limited to a short-term (<5 days) in order to avoid rhinitis medicamentosa [67]. These drugs are frequently available alone or in combination with other anti-allergic treatments over the counter and are often used in athlete's population. There are WADA-specific anti-doping regulations of their use, for example, ephedrine and methylephedrine are prohibited when its concentration in urine is greater than 10 micrograms per milliliter and pseudoephedrine when its urine concentration is greater than 150 μg per milliliter. Athletes should be aware in order not to fall in a non-intentional doping rules violation [71].

Corticosteroids

The most efficacious and first-line treatment for allergic and nonallergic rhinitis is intranasal glucocorticosteroids [15, 24]. These medications are safe to be used in athletes and effective in all symptoms of allergic rhinitis as well as ocular symptoms [15]. It is supported by high quality of evidence [67] and meta-analysis [72] that intranasal glucocorticoids are more effective over oral and topical H1-antihistamines [67] and can be used during competition. In a cross-sectional survey in 446 athletes, treatment with corticosteroids was associated with significantly improved nasal symptoms and quality of life [39]. They have slow onset of action (12h) and maximum efficacy over weeks [68]. A recent review of Laekeman concluded that topical nasal corticosteroids require continuous therapy during at least for the symptoms duration [73].

The management of allergic rhinitis also improves asthma control and reduces asthma severity [19]. Intranasal steroids seem to prevent seasonal increase in nonspecific bronchial hyperreactivity and asthma symptoms associated with pollen exposure and seem to reduce asthma symptoms, exercise-induced bronchospasm, and bronchial responsiveness to methacholine [18]. Three post hoc studies described in the ARIA guidelines showed that allergic rhinitis treatment reduced potential utilization of healthcare for comorbid asthma [19].

Systemic corticosteroids are the last resort for allergic rhinitis treatment [68]. They are prohibited by WADA when administered orally, rectally, or by intravenous or intramuscular administration [71]. When these formulations are needed, a Therapeutic Use Exemption (TUE) should be performed for the athlete justifying its use [71].

Allergen Immunotherapy

Specific immunotherapy (IT), frequently known as allergy vaccines, is very effective in controlling symptoms of allergic rhinitis, can potentially modify the disease and their clinical benefits, and may be sustained years after discontinuing treatment [16, 67]. It is recommended in symptomatic patients, with proven allergy, whose symptoms are not controlled with pharmacological therapy, with a significant and unavoidable exposure [16, 74]. Athletes are frequently included in this group, namely, in the case of pollen-allergic athletes who train and compete in outdoor environment, with symptoms that affect their performance [21]. This treatment should be performed by trained allergist and the athlete warned not to train in a few hours after immunotherapy injection. Subcutaneous immunotherapy (SIT) is recommended in adults and children with seasonal and persistent allergic rhinitis [67]. In some cases sublingual-specific immunotherapy (SLIT) can also be used [24, 67]. Other forms of immunotherapy might be introduced, namely, intranasal allergen-specific immunotherapy in adults [67].

Other Potential Treatment Options

Antileukotrienes inhibit inflammatory mediators produced in both allergic and nonallergic rhinitis particularly after cold, allergen, and exercise challenge [21]. Recent guidelines recommend its use in seasonal allergic rhinitis in adults and children and only in children in the persistent form of rhinitis [67].

Disodium cromoglycate and sodium nedocromil are used in allergic rhinitis as intranasal preparations. They are effective in some patients and have excellent safety profile, but its use for four times a day compromises adherence [24] and is less effective than antihistamines [67]. Intranasal ipratropium bromide decreases rhinorrhea inhibiting parasympathetic stimulation, but does not act in any other rhinitis symptoms [15]. For this, it has a small role in allergic rhinitis but may be useful in winter sports ("skiers nose") increasing the ability of the nose to warm and humidify air reducing watery rhinorrhea caused by exposure to cold dry air [27].

48.3 Urticaria

Urticaria is characterized by sudden appearance of wheals, angioedema, or both that occurs secondary to the release of histamine, cytokine, and other mediators from activated mast cells [75]. Urticaria can be classified based on the duration of illness in acute (<6 weeks) or chronic (>6 weeks) [76]. Chronic urticaria can be further characterized due to their distinctly different pathological mechanisms in chronic spontaneous urticaria and inducible urticaria that include symptomatic dermographism, cold urticaria, delayed pressure, vibratory, solar, heat, contact, aquagenic and cholinergic urticaria, and vibratory angioedema [75]. It is not uncommon that both chronic spontaneous urticaria and different physical stimuli might trigger symptoms in the same patient [75]. Inducible urticaria is particularly important for athletes, as they frequently contact with physical stimuli that can trigger urticaria [77].

Cholinergic urticaria is the most common type of physical urticaria in athletes, and it is precipitated by an elevated body temperature. It occurs minutes after the onset of exercise and is characterized by the appearance, initially in the trunk and neck, of generalized flushing, combined with pruritic punctuate wheals of 2–4 mm surrounded by red flares [78]. In rare cases, systemic symptoms might occur, like hypotension, abdominal cramping, and diarrhea [77].

Another common type, particularly in winter sports, is cold-induced urticaria. It develops with changes in skin temperature after exposure to cold, but symptoms may worsen during rewarming [77]. Pruritus and hives appear mainly in cold-exposed skin areas, but extensive exposure can result in generalized urticaria and even in systemic severe reactions, like anaphylaxis [79]. Delayed pressure urticaria can occur in some athletes, particularly those with chronic localized pressure, like skaters, who have skate constantly contacting in the ankle [77]. Typically, angioedema occurs with 4–8 h delay and may persist for several hours.

Chronic urticaria has a significant impact in quality of life, and it is associated with an increased prevalence of depression, anxiety, and sleep difficulties [80]. Athletic performance might be significantly impaired if this disease is not diagnosed, and its triggers unraveled, treated, and controlled.

48.3.1 Diagnosis

The mainstay of diagnosis is a thorough clinical history, addressing the duration, frequency, triggers, and concomitant symptoms and also targeting differential diagnosis and syndromes usually related to urticarial reactions. A complete physical examination further supports diagnosis [75, 76]. The use of questionnaire, like the urticaria activity score (UAS7), might help to understand the severity of the disease and monitor its evolution through time. Diagnostic measures will depend on the patient history and urticaria subtype. In acute urticaria no routine diagnostic measures are needed. For chronic spontaneous urticaria, in the latest position paper by EAACI/GA2LEN/EDF/WAO, only very limited routine diagnostic measures are recommended including differential blood count and erythrocyte sedimentation rate or C-reactive protein. Further diagnostic procedures should be adapted accordingly to the patient clinical history and might include study of infectious diseases (e.g., *Helicobacter pylori*), type I allergy, functional autoantibodies, thyroid hormones and autoantibodies, skin tests for physical urticaria evaluation, tryptase, autologous serum skin test, and eventually a skin lesion biopsy [75].

Diagnosis of physical urticaria is particularly important in athletes, in order to avoid the trigger stimuli and also to assess response to treatment. However, for most types of physical urticaria, no validated tools exist. Cold provocation and threshold test using ice cube, cold water, and cold wind can be used to evaluate cold urticaria; nowadays, a Peltier element-based provocation device (Tempest®)[81] is used as a validated tool. For dermographism and delayed pressure urticaria, assessment tools like dermatographometer and weighted rods can be applied [75, 82]. In other physical urticaria, namely, heat, solar, and cholinergic or aquagenic urticaria, office-based methods of provocation tests have been implemented. These procedures should be performed in a standardized way to compare disease activity through time in the same patient. Contact urticaria can be demonstrated by cutaneous provocation tests, using, for example, skin prick test [75].

48.3.2 Treatment

The goal of chronic urticaria management is complete symptom control and disease remission. Therefore, the first recommendation is to avoid triggers, namely, relevant physical factors [76]. Then, pharmacological treatment using second-generation nonimpairing nonsedating H1-antihistamines is recommended as the first-line treatment. They should be used on a regular basis and not in as-needed basis [75, 76]. After 2–4 weeks of regular treatment, efficacy should be assessed, and if needed dosage should be increased up to four times the standard dose [75]. Montelukast can also be added for a 3–4 week trial. Nowadays, recommendations state that there is no additional benefit of combining different H1-antihistamines and that first-generation H1-antihistamines are no longer recommended for use in urticaria [81].

During exacerbations a short course of an oral corticosteroid can be used; however, it is mandatory for the doctor to ask for a therapeutic use exemption in athletes.

Third-line treatments include omalizumab or off-label use of cyclosporine A [81]. Omalizumab is a humanized monoclonal antibody that binds selectively to the human immunoglobulin E (IgE) in its Cε3 domain, and its efficacy and safety have been demonstrated in chronic spontaneous urticarial refractory to H1-antihistamine treatment. A previous report has been described of omalizumab use in a 14-year-old competitive athlete with recurrent exercise-induced anaphylaxis; however, despite being able to perform recreational aerobic and non-aerobic exercise, he did not resume competitive running [83]. It's use on chronic spontaneous and delayed pressure urticaria in a professional physical trainer also showed high efficacy [84]. Cyclosporine has a better risk/benefit ratio compared with long-term use of steroids, and it is recommended for patients with severe refractory disease to any dose of antihistamines [75].

48.4 Contact Dermatitis

Contact dermatitis is an inflammation that results from direct contact of a substance with the skin. It is classified in two types: contact dermatitis, a type IV delayed hypersensitivity reaction, and irritant dermatitis, which occurs due to direct contact of substances, such as solvents or chemicals, which irritate the skin after exposure [85]. Signs and symptoms mainly appear as a pruritic, eczematous eruption that has an acute phase of bright red, edematous pruritic plaques, superimposed by vesicles and excoriations. Through time, the papules and plaques turn mildly erythematous and form collarets of scale; further on, during the chronic phase, thick, lichenified plaques appear as well as hyperpigmented zones. The pattern and distribution of the lesions usually provide some guidance to the trigger of the dermatitis [86]. An athlete is particularly susceptible, as he suffers repeated exposure to trauma, heat, moisture, and contacts with several allergens and chemicals [87].

Accordingly, to the type of sports practiced, athletes contact with different synthetic and natural chemicals in their sports equipment and environment. In water sports, the use of goggles, nose plugs, and swim caps in swimmers, or the use of rubber or neoprene suits, gloves, snorkels, or mouthpieces in divers, can be associated with sensitization to benzoyl peroxide, phenol formaldehyde resin, thioureas, or antioxidants used in rubber production. Aside from equipment, water environment predisposes the appearance of irritant contact dermatitis due to the chemicals used to disinfect the pools, like chlorine [87].

In land sports, including runners and baseball, softball, and football players, they mainly react to components of rubber, leather, glues, or dyes used in tennis shoes [87]. Pedal hyperhidrosis can facilitate the leaking of thiourea compounds from a shoe and elicit acute contact dermatitis [86]. In football, the most frequently reported contact dermatitis is with football shin guards, most due to irritant contact dermatitis [88]. In sports played with a ball, one form of irritant contact dermatitis is the term "basketball pebble fingers," which is secondary to the mechanical irritation of the ball. The rubber basketball can also cause contact dermatitis, in which thiuram or mercaptobenzothiazole are the most frequent culprit agents [87]. There are only rare reports of contact dermatitis related to sports racquet use and to fiberglass in the hockey sticks [87]. Weight lifting, besides the irritant component secondary to friction due to the repeated contact, has been associated with allergic contact dermatitis to metal bars, mediated by palladium and nickel hypersensitivity [89, 90].

Besides equipment's specific topic treatments, like analgesic sprays, topical salicylates, anti-inflammatory creams or gels and massage creams, and protective adhesive taping, can be important causes of allergic contact dermatitis. Specific allergens, namely, eucalyptus oils, indomethacin and diclofenac gels, and benzocaine and lanolin, are some of the most relevant allergens.

48.4.1 Diagnosis

A comprehensive history, focusing in occupational and hobby activities, disease course, seasonal variation, and response to treatment, as well as a physical examination, including the location and morphological features of the lesions, will guide diagnosis and might provide clues regarding the source or identity of the allergen [85, 86]. Patch testing is indicated to confirm allergic contact dermatitis [91]. Usually a group of chemicals that have been proved to cause allergic contact dermatitis have been assembled into standard patch test series, namely, in the European baseline patch series, which is frequently reviewed and changed accordingly to the prevalence of clinically relevant allergens [85, 92]. The test consists of the cutaneous application of a small amount of the suspected allergen in a suitable concentration and vehicle during at least 48 h, and then the skin reaction should be read at least twice, the first time after removal of the patches (on day 2) or at day 3 and the second one 2–5 days later [91]. In some specific cases, patch testing with personal products can also be used and tested "as is" or diluted [85]. However, not all positive patch test reactions are relevant to the athlete's dermatitis. A positive patch past test that is not found to be clinically relevant is termed "contact allergy" [93].

48.4.2 Treatment

After identification of the culprit allergen, eviction recommendations should be done, with appropriate education on the recognition of the allergen in the product labels [85]. Another option is to try to create a barrier between the skin and the allergenic trigger. Treatment with topical corticosteroids improves recovery [86]. When severe and refractory cases are considered, a short course of oral corticosteroid might be needed [86].

48.5 Anaphylaxis

Anaphylaxis is defined as an acute serious life-threatening, generalized, or systematic hypersensitivity reaction that might cause death [94]. The lifetime risk is 1.6%, which is similar to what is previously reported in the literature for athletes [46, 95]. Both immunological (IgE dependent and IgE independent) and nonimmunological (direct mast cell activation) mechanisms have been related to anaphylaxis [96]. Different triggers have been described, and they usually differ between age groups and world regions. The most frequently reported are foods, venoms, drugs (including biological agents, perioperative drugs, radiocontrast media), latex, and exercise [95]. Besides potential direct triggers, an anaphylactic reaction may only occur under the presence of specific patient-related risk factors or cofactor. Patient risk factors can be age, concomitant disease (asthma, cardiovascular disease, mastocytosis), and concurrent medications like beta-blockers and ACE inhibitors. Exercise, infection, emotional stress, premenstrual status, and ethanol or nonsteroidal anti-inflammatory drugs (NSAIDs) ingestion have been described as important cofactors [94].

Five to fifteen percent of all anaphylaxis are elicited by exercise, independently of exercise intensity [97]. Food as a cofactor with exercise for anaphylaxis is described as food-dependent exercise-induced anaphylaxis (FDEIA), and it can be further classified according to the food triggers [98, 99]. If the episode occurs after ingestion of certain foods, it is described as specific food-dependent exercise-induced anaphylaxis (sFDEIA), and if it happens just after the ingestion of any food, it is designated by nonspecific food-dependent exercise-induced anaphylaxis (nsFDEIA)[100].

Exercise-induced anaphylaxis can occur both in high-level athletes and also in those that only practice exercise occasionally. It usually occurs after short-term duration and intensity physical activity and has been described both during gardening and walking activities [101]. Jogging is the most reported activity associated with exercise-induced anaphylaxis, followed by running, tennis, and football. Athletes should be informed that anaphylaxis can occur in the beginning, during, and after exercise [99, 101].

Table 48.5 Clinical criteria for diagnosing anaphylaxis

Anaphylaxis is highly likely when one of the following three criteria is fulfilled	
1.	Acute onset of an illness (minutes to several hours) with involvement of the skin, mucosal tissue, or both and at least one of the following: a. Signs or symptoms of respiratory compromise (e.g., dyspnea, wheeze-bronchospasm, stridor, hypoxemia) b. Hypotension or symptoms of end-organ dysfunction (e.g., collapse, syncope, incontinence)
2.	Two or more of the following that occur minutes to several hours after exposure to a likely allergen for that patient: a. Involvement of the skin-mucosal tissue (e.g., generalized urticaria, itch-flush, swollen lips-tongue-uvula) b. Respiratory compromise (e.g., dyspnea, wheeze-bronchospasm, stridor, hypoxemia) c. Hypotension or associated symptoms (e.g., collapse, syncope, incontinence) d. Acute onset of gastrointestinal symptoms (e.g., abdominal pain, vomiting)
3.	Hypotension after exposure to a known allergen for that patient (minutes to several hours): a. Infants and children: low systolic blood pressure (age specific) or greater than 30% decrease in systolic blood pressure[a] b. Adults: systolic blood pressure of less than 90 mmHg or greater than 30% decrease from that person's baseline %

Adapted from [96]

[a]Low systolic blood pressure for children is defined as less than 70 mmHg if less than 1 year, less than 70 mmHg (+ [2× age]) from 1 to 10 years, and less than 90 mmHg from 11 to 17 years

48.5.1 Diagnosis

Diagnosis is highly dependent on a detailed clinical history and recognition of symptoms and signs that occur minutes to hours after exposure to a known or potential trigger. A thorough description of all food, drug intake, relation to physical activity, and any potential cofactor should be studied [95]. Diagnostic criteria are described in Table 48.5. Differential diagnosis should be taken into account in order not to underdiagnose or overdiagnose anaphylaxis. Diagnosis in infants and children, elderly, and pregnant women can be more challenging; therefore, symptoms and signs are interpreted accordingly to these specific populations [95].

Serum tryptase levels in blood samples taken 15–180 min after symptom onset can be increased in about 60% of the patients and support the clinical diagnosis of anaphylaxis [94]. The gold standard for Exercise-induced anaphylaxis is an exercise challenge, preceded by food ingestion if food-dependent exercise-induced anaphylaxis is considered.

48.5.2 Treatment

Treatment for anaphylaxis and exercise-induced anaphylaxis follows consensus guidelines, which are now more strongly supported by increasingly high quality of evidence [94–96]. First, if possible, the trigger should be removed. If exercise is the considered trigger, physical activity should be ceased at the onset of symptoms [102]. Epinephrine is the medication of first choice in anaphylaxis. Early intramuscular administration in the mid-anterolateral thigh in a dose of 0.01 mg/kg of a 1:1000 (1 mg/mL) solution, to a maximum of 0.5 mg in adults (0.3 mg in children), reduces hospitalization and death [75, 94, 95]. It should be repeated at every 5–15 min, as needed [96].

It is recommended to position the patient in supine (or semi-reclining in a position of comfort if dyspneic or vomiting) with elevation of the lower extremities. H1- and H2-antihistamines and glucocorticoids are second-line medications in anaphylaxis. These medications are not lifesaving and should not be used as initial or sole treatment [96]. Glucocorticoids are used to prevent biphasic or protracted episodes of anaphylaxis [95]. At any time, if indicated, supplemental oxygen and intravenous fluid resuscitation with a crystalloid such as 0.9% (isotonic saline) can be used [94].

After an episode of anaphylaxis, all individuals should be prescribed an epinephrine auto-injector and carry an emergency action plan. Furthermore, in order to prevent recurrent anaphylaxis, they should be followed-up by a specialized physician, in order to confirm anaphylaxis triggers and educate the patient [94]. In exercise-induced anaphylaxis, it is important to understand if there is another cofactor associated. However, it is usually recommended to avoid nonsteroid anti-inflammatory medication before exercising, and, if there is an environmental trigger, like heat, cold, or humidity, exercise should be restrained in that conditions. In nsFDEIA, food ingestion should be avoided at least 2–4 h before exercise practice and at least until 1 h after [97, 99, 101, 103]. No prophylactic drugs showed any efficacy to prevent exercise-induced anaphylaxis [103]. Family members and trainer should be educated to recognize and treat an anaphylaxis, and training sessions should be supervised.

References

1. Carlsen K-H, Anderson S, Bjermer L, Bonini S, Brusasco V, Canonica W, Cummiskey J, Delgado L, Del Giacco S, Drobnic F, Haahtela T, Larsson K, Palange P, Popov T, van Cauwenberge P. Exercise-induced asthma, respiratory and allergic disorders in elite athletes: epidemiology, mechanisms and diagnosis: part I of the report from the Joint Task Force of the European Respiratory Society (ERS) and the European Academy of Allergy and Clinical Immunology (EAACI) in cooperation with GA2LEN. Allergy. 2008;63:387–403.
2. Helenius I, Tikkanen H, Haahtela T. Occurrence of exercise induced bronchospasm in elite runners: dependence on atopy and exposure to cold air and pollen. Br J Sports Med. 1998;32:125–9.
3. Bougault V, Turmel J, St-Laurent J, Bertrand M, Boulet L. Asthma, airway inflammation and epithelial damage in swimmers and cold-air athletes. Eur Respir J. 2009;33:740–6.
4. Bonini S, Bonini M, Bousquet J, Brusasco V, Canonica GW, Carlsen KH, Corbetta L, Cummiskey J, Delgado L, Del Giacco SR, Haahtela T, Jaeger S, Moretti C, Palange P, Passalacqua G, Passali D, Pedersen BK, Popov T, Rasi G, Ventura MT, Vignola AM. Rhinitis and asthma in athletes: an ARIA document in collaboration with GA2LEN. Allergy. 2006;61:681–92.
5. Dijkstra HP, Robson-Ansley P. The prevalence and current opinion of treatment of allergic rhinitis in elite athletes. Curr Opin Allergy Clin Immunol. 2011;11:103–8.
6. Bousquet J. Global initiative for asthma (GINA) and its objectives. Clin Exp Allergy. 2000;30(Suppl 1): 2–5.
7. Schwartz LB, Delgado L, Craig T, Bonini S, Carlsen KH, Casale TB, Del Giacco S, Drobnic F, van Wijk RG, Ferrer M, Haahtela T, Henderson WR, Israel E, Lotvall J, Moreira A, Papadopoulos NG, Randolph CC, Romano A, Weiler JM. Exercise-induced hypersensitivity syndromes in recreational and competitive athletes: a PRACTALL consensus report (what the general practitioner should know about sports and allergy). Allergy. 2008;63: 953–61.
8. Haahtela T, Malmberg P, Moreira A. Mechanisms of asthma in Olympic athletes – practical implications. Allergy. 2008;63:685–94.
9. Couto M, Stang J, Horta L, Stensrud T, Severo M, Mowinckel P, Silva D, Delgado L, Moreira A, Carlsen KH. Two distinct phenotypes of asthma in elite athletes identified by latent class analysis. J Asthma. 2015;52:897–904.
10. Anderson SD, Daviskas E. The mechanism of exercise-induced asthma is. J Allergy Clin Immunol. 2000;106:453–9.
11. Couto M, Silva D, Santos P, Queiros S, Delgado L, Moreira A. Exploratory study comparing dysautonomia between asthmatic and non-asthmatic elite swimmers. Rev Port Pneumol. (2006) 2015;21:22–9.

12. Stang J, Couto M, Carlsen KH, Stensrud T. Increased bronchial parasympathetic tone in elite cross-country and biathlon skiers: a randomised crossover study. Br J Sports Med. 2014;49:56–61.
13. Reddel HK, Bateman ED, Becker A, Boulet LP, Cruz AA, Drazen JM, Haahtela T, Hurd SS, Inoue H, de Jongste JC, Lemanske Jr RF, Levy ML, O'Byrne PM, Paggiaro P, Pedersen SE, Pizzichini E, Soto-Quiroz M, Szefler SJ, Wong GW, FitzGerald JM. A summary of the new GINA strategy: a roadmap to asthma control. Eur Respir J. 2015;46:622–39.
14. Moreira A, Delgado L, Haahtela T, Fonseca J, Moreira P, Lopes C, Mota J, Santos P, Rytila P, Castel-Branco MG. Physical training does not increase allergic inflammation in asthmatic children. Eur Respir J. 2008;32:1570–5.
15. Bousquet J, Khaltaev N, Cruz AA, Denburg J, Fokkens WJ, Togias A, Zuberbier T, Baena-Cagnani CE, Canonica GW, Van Weel C, Agache I, Aït-Khaled N, Bachert C, Blaiss MS, Bonini S, Boulet LP, Bousquet PJ, Camargos P, Carlsen KH, Chen Y, Custovic A, Dahl R, Demoly P, Douagui H, Durham SR, Van Wijk RG, Kalayci O, Kaliner MA, Kim YY, Kowalski ML, Kuna P, Le LTT, Lemiere C, Li J, Lockey RF, Mavale-Manuel S, Meltzer EO, Mohammad Y, Mullol J, Naclerio R, O'Hehir RE, Ohta K, Ouedraogo S, Palkonen S, Papadopoulos N, Passalacqua G, Pawankar R, Popov TA, Rabe KF, Rosado-Pinto J, Scadding GK, Simons FER, Toskala E, Valovirta E, Van Cauwenberge P, Wang DY, Wickman M, Yawn BP, Yorgancioglu A, Yusuf OM, Zar H, Annesi-Maesano I, Bateman ED, Kheder AB, Boakye DA, Bouchard J, Burney P, Busse WW, Chan-Yeung M, Chavannes NH, Chuchalin A, Dolen WK, Emuzyte R, Grouse L, Humbert M, Jackson C, Johnston SL, Keith PK, Kemp JP, Klossek JM, Larenas-Linnemann D, Lipworth B, Malo JL, Marshall GD, Naspitz C, Nekam K, Niggemann B, Nizankowska-Mogilnicka E, Okamoto Y, Orru MP, Potter P, Price D, Stoloff SW, Vandenplas O, Viegi G, Williams D. Allergic rhinitis and its impact on asthma (ARIA) 2008 update (in collaboration with the World Health Organization, GA2LEN and AllerGen). Allergy. 2008;63:8–160.
16. Wallace DV, Dykewicz MS, Bernstein DI, Blessing-Moore J, Cox L, Khan DA, Lang DM, Nicklas RA, Oppenheimer J, Portnoy JM, Randolph CC, Schuller D, Spector SL, Tilles SA. The diagnosis and management of rhinitis: an updated practice parameter. J Allergy Clin Immunol. 2008;122:S1–S84.
17. Roberts G, Xatzipsalti M, Borrego LM, Custovic A, Halken S, Hellings PW, Papadopoulos NG, Rotiroti G, Scadding G, Timmermans F, Valovirta E. Paediatric rhinitis: position paper of the European academy of allergy and clinical immunology. Allergy. 2013;68:1102–16.
18. Dykewicz MS, Hamilos DL. Rhinitis and sinusitis. J Allergy Clin Immunol. 2010;125:S103–S15.
19. Silva DM, Delgado L. Allergic rhinitis and sports. Allergic rhinitis, 1. Intech. Croatia. 2012.
20. Dahl R, Mygind N. Mechanisms of airflow limitation in the nose and lungs. Clin Exp Allergy. 1998;28(Suppl 2):17–25.
21. Delgado L, Moreira A, Capão-Filipe M. Rhinitis and its impact on sports. Allergy Clin Immunol Int. 2006;18:98–105.
22. Valero A, Serrano C, Valera JL, Barbera A, Torrego A, Mullol J, Picado C. Nasal and bronchial response to exercise in patients with asthma and rhinitis: the role of nitric oxide. Allergy. 2005;60:1126–31.
23. Navarro RR, Romero L, Williams K. Nasal issues in athletes. Curr Sports Med Rep. 2013;12:22–7.
24. Scadding GK, Durham SR, Mirakian R, Jones NS, Leech SC, Farooque S, Ryan D, Walker SM, Clark AT, Dixon TA, Jolles SR, Siddique N, Cullinan P, Howarth PH, Nasser SM. BSACI guidelines for the management of allergic and non-allergic rhinitis. Clin Exp Allergy. 2008;38:19–42.
25. Davila I, Mullol J, Ferrer M, Bartra J, del Cuvillo A, Montoro J, Jauregui I, Sastre J, Valero A. Genetic aspects of allergic rhinitis. J Investig Allergol Clin Immunol. 2009;19(Suppl 1):25–31.
26. Bonini M, Bachert C, Baena-Cagnani CE, Bedbrook A, Brozek JL, Canonica GW, Cruz AA, Fokkens WJ, Gerth van Wijk R, Grouse L, Hellings PW, Howarth P, Kalayci O, Khaltaev N, Kuna P, Larenas Linnemann D, Nekam K, Palkonen S, Papadopoulos NG, Popov TA, Price D, Rosado Pinto J, Rasi G, Ryan D, Samolinski B, Scadding GK, Schunemann HJ, Thomas DM, Triggiani M, Yorgancioglu A, Yusuf OM, Zuberbier T, Pawankar R, Bousquet J, Bonini S, Aria Initiative icwtWHOC-CfAR. What we should learn from the London Olympics. Curr Opin Allergy Clin Immunol. 2013;13:1–3.
27. Katelaris CH, Carrozzi FM, Burke TV. Allergic rhinoconjunctivitis in elite athletes: optimal management for quality of life and performance. Sports Med. 2003;33:401–6.
28. Katelaris CH, Carrozzi FM, Burke TV, Byth K. Patterns of allergic reactivity and disease in Olympic athletes. Clin J Sport Med. 2006;16:401–5.
29. Fitch KD. Management of allergic Olympic athletes. J Allergy Clin Immunol. 1984;73:722–7.
30. Helbling A, Jenoure P, Muller U. The incidence of hay fever in leading Swiss athletes. Schweiz Med Wochenschr. 1990;120:231–6.
31. Kaelin M, Brandli O. Exertional asthma in Swiss top-ranking athletes. Schweiz Med Wochenschr. 1993;123:174–82.
32. Potts J. Factors associated with respiratory problems in swimmers. Sports Med. 1996;21:256–61.
33. Helenius IJ, Tikkanen HO, Sarna S, Haahtela T. Asthma and increased bronchial responsiveness in elite athletes: atopy and sport event as risk factors. J Allergy Clin Immunol. 1998;101:646–52.
34. Weiler JM, Layton T, Hunt M. Asthma in United States Olympic athletes who participated in the 1996 summer games. J Allergy Clin Immunol. 1998;102: 722–6.
35. Weiler JM, Ryan 3rd EJ. Asthma in United States Olympic athletes who participated in the 1998

Olympic Winter Games. J Allergy Clin Immunol. 2000;106:267–71.
36. Katelaris CH, Carrozzi FM, Burke TV, Byth K. A springtime Olympics demands special consideration for allergic athletes. J Allergy Clin Immunol. 2000;106:260–6.
37. Lapucci G, Rasi G, Bonini S, Aloe L, Ambrosini B, Berlutti G, Bonini M, Caldarone G, Caselli G, Colombo G, Concu A, Del Giacco GS, Del Giacco SR, Ghiani A, Gaziani R, Lai M, Lambiase A, Manca E, Manconi PE, Matricardi PM, Pamich T, Rumi C, Todaro A, Torre A. Allergy and infectious diseases in athletes. J Allergy Clin Immunol. 2003;111:S142.
38. Bonay M, Aubier M. Pollution atmosphérique et maladies respiratoires allergiques. Med Sci (Paris). 2007;23:187–92.
39. Alaranta A, Alaranta H, Heliövaaras M, Alha P, Palmu P, Helenius I. Allergic rhinitis and pharmacological management in elite athletes. Med Sci Sports Exerc. 2005;37:707–11.
40. Randolph CC, Dreyfus D, Rundell KW, Bangladore D, Fraser B. Prevalence of allergy and asthma symptoms in recreational roadrunners. Med Sci Sports Exerc. 2006;38:2053–7.
41. Moreira A, Kekkonen R, Korpela R, Delgado L, Haahtela T. Allergy in marathon runners and effect of Lactobacillus GG supplementation on allergic inflammatory markers. Respir Med. 2007;101:1123–31.
42. Bonini M, Lapucci G, Petrelli G, Todaro A, Pamich T, Rasi G, Bonini S. Predictive value of allergy and pulmonary function tests for the diagnosis of asthma in elite athletes. Allergy. 2007;62:1166–70.
43. Macucci F, Guerrini L, Strambi M. Asthma and allergy in young athletes in Siena Province. Preliminary results. J Sports Med Phys Fitness. 2007;47:351–5.
44. Salonen RO, Pennanen AS, Vahteristo M, Korkeila P, Alm S, Randell JT. Health risk assessment of indoor air pollution in Finnish ice arenas. Environ Int. 2008;34:51–7.
45. Thomas S, Wolfarth B, Wittmer C, Nowak D, Radon K. Self-reported asthma and allergies in top athletes compared to the general population – results of the German part of the GA2LEN-Olympic study 2008. Allergy Asthma Clin Immunol. 2010;6:31.
46. Bonini M, Gramiccioni C, Fioretti D, Ruckert B, Rinaldi M, Akdis C, Todaro A, Palange P, Carlsen KH, Pelliccia A, Rasi G, Bonini S. Aida, the Italian unit of the GALENOS. Asthma, allergy and the Olympics: a 12-year survey in elite athletes. Curr Opin Allergy Clin Immunol. 2015;15:184–92.
47. Kurowski M, Jurczyk J, Krysztofiak H, Kowalski ML. Exercise-induced respiratory symptoms and allergy in elite athletes: allergy and asthma in Polish Olympic Athletes (A(2) POLO) project within GA(2) LEN initiative. Clin Respir J. 2016;10:231–8.
48. Komarow HD, Postolache TT. Seasonal allergy and seasonal decrements in athletic performance. Clin Sports Med. 2005;24:e35–50.
49. Katelaris CH, Carrozzi FM, Burke TV, Byth K. Effects of intranasal budesonide on symptoms, quality of life, and performance in elite athletes with allergic rhinoconjunctivitis. Clin J Sport Med. 2002;12:296–300.
50. Alves A, Martins C, Delgado L, Fonseca J, Moreira A. Exercise-induced rhinitis in competitive swimmers. Am J Rhinol Allergy. 2010;24:e114–7.
51. Gioulekas D, Damialis A, Papakosta D, Syrigou A, Mpaka G, Saxoni F, Patakas D. 15-year aeroallergen records. Their usefulness in Athens Olympics, 2004. Allergy. 2003;58:933–8.
52. D'Amato G, Cecchi L. Effects of climate change on environmental factors in respiratory allergic diseases. Clin Exp Allergy. 2008;38:1264–74.
53. Zhang F, Wang W, Lv J, Krafft T, Xu J. Time-series studies on air pollution and daily outpatient visits for allergic rhinitis in Beijing, China. Sci Total Environ. 2011;409:2486–92.
54. Li J, Lu Y, Huang K, Wang C, Lu J, Zhang C, Zhong N. Chinese response to allergy and asthma in Olympic athletes. Allergy. 2008;63:962–8.
55. Braat JP, Mulder PG, Fokkens WJ, van Wijk RG, Rijntjes E. Intranasal cold dry air is superior to histamine challenge in determining the presence and degree of nasal hyperreactivity in nonallergic noninfectious perennial rhinitis. Am J Respir Crit Care Med. 1998;157:1748–55.
56. Koskela HO. Cold air-provoked respiratory symptoms: the mechanisms and management. Int J Circumpolar Health. 2007;66:91–100.
57. Bougault V, Turmel J, Boulet LP. Effect of intense swimming training on rhinitis in high-level competitive swimmers. Clin Exp Allergy. 2010;40:1238–46.
58. Borres MP. Allergic rhinitis: more than just a stuffy nose. Acta Paediatr. 2009;98:1088–92.
59. Dijkstra HP, Robson-Ansley P. The prevalence and current opinion of treatment of allergic rhinitis in elite athletes. Curr Opin Allergy Clin Immunol. 2011:11(2):103–8.
60. Scadding G, Hellings P, Alobid I, Bachert C, Fokkens W, Gerth van Wijk R, Gevaert P, Guilemany J, Kalogjera L, Lund V, Mullol J, Passalacqua G, Toskala E, van Drunen C. Diagnostic tools in Rhinology EAACI position paper. Clin Transl Allergy. 2011;1:2.
61. Lim MY, Leong JL. Allergic rhinitis: evidence-based practice. Singapore Med J. 2010;51:542–50.
62. Agache I, Bilo M, Braunstahl GJ, Delgado L, Demoly P, Eigenmann P, Gevaert P, Gomes E, Hellings P, Horak F, Muraro A, Werfel T, Jutel M. In vivo diagnosis of allergic diseases – allergen provocation tests. Allergy. 2015;70:355–65.
63. Fokkens WJ, Lund VJ, Mullol J, Bachert C, Alobid I, Baroody F, Cohen N, Cervin A, Douglas R, Gevaert P, Georgalas C, Goossens H, Harvey R, Hellings P, Hopkins C, Jones N, Joos G, Kalogjera L, Kern B, Kowalski M, Price D, Riechelmann H, Schlosser R, Senior B, Thomas M, Toskala E, Voegels R, Wang de

Y, Wormald PJ. EPOS 2012: European position paper on rhinosinusitis and nasal polyps 2012. A summary for otorhinolaryngologists. Rhinology. 2012;50:1–12.
64. Fonseca JA, Nogueira-Silva L, Morais-Almeida M, Azevedo L, Sa-Sousa A, Branco-Ferreira M, Fernandes L, Bousquet J. Validation of a questionnaire (CARAT10) to assess rhinitis and asthma in patients with asthma. Allergy. 2010;65:1042–8.
65. Schatz M, Meltzer EO, Nathan R, Derebery MJ, Mintz M, Stanford RH, Dalal AA, Silvey MJ, Kosinski M. Psychometric validation of the rhinitis control assessment test: a brief patient-completed instrument for evaluating rhinitis symptom control. Ann Allergy Asthma Immunol. 2010;104:118–24.
66. Bonini M, Braido F, Baiardini I, Del Giacco S, Gramiccioni C, Manara M, Tagliapietra G, Scardigno A, Sargentini V, Brozzi M, Rasi G, Bonini S. AQUA: allergy questionnaire for athletes. Development and validation. Med Sci Sports Exerc. 2009;41:1034–41.
67. Brozek JL, Bousquet J, Baena-Cagnani CE, Bonini S, Canonica GW, Casale TB, van Wijk RG, Ohta K, Zuberbier T, Schunemann HJ. Allergic rhinitis and its impact on asthma (ARIA) guidelines: 2010 revision. J Allergy Clin Immunol. 2010;126:466–76.
68. van Cauwenberge P, Bachert C, Passalacqua G, Bousquet J, Canonica GW, Durham SR, Fokkens WJ, Howarth PH, Lund V, Malling HJ, Mygind N, Passali D, Scadding GK, Wang DY. Consensus statement on the treatment of allergic rhinitis. European Academy of Allergology and Clinical Immunology. Allergy. 2000;55:116–34.
69. Simons E. Histamine and H1-antihistamine. In: Adkinson F, editor. Middleton's allergy. 2nd ed: Mosby Elsevier, The Netherlands. 2009. p. 1517–47.
70. Leonardi A, Bogacka E, Fauquert JL, Kowalski ML, Groblewska A, Jedrzejczak-Czechowicz M, Doan S, Marmouz F, Demoly P, Delgado L. Ocular allergy: recognizing and diagnosing hypersensitivity disorders of the ocular surface. Allergy. 2012;67:1327–37.
71. WADA. World anti-doping code- The 2011 prohibited list international standard. 2011.
72. Weiner JM, Abramson MJ, Puy RM. Intranasal corticosteroids versus oral H1 receptor antagonists in allergic rhinitis: systematic review of randomised controlled trials. BMJ. 1998;317:1624–9.
73. Laekeman G, Simoens S, Buffels J, Gillard M, Robillard T, Benedetti MS, Watelet JB, Liekendael G, Ghys L, Church M. Continuous versus on-demand pharmacotherapy of allergic rhinitis: evidence and practice. Respir Med. 2010;104:615–25.
74. Jutel M, Agache I, Bonini S, Burks AW, Calderon M, Canonica W, Cox L, Demoly P, Frew AJ, O'Hehir R, Kleine-Tebbe J, Muraro A, Lack G, Larenas D, Levin M, Nelson H, Pawankar R, Pfaar O, van Ree R, Sampson H, Santos AF, Du Toit G, Werfel T, Gerth van Wijk R, Zhang L, Akdis CA. International consensus on allergy immunotherapy. J Allergy Clin Immunol. 2015;136:556–68.
75. Zuberbier T, Aberer W, Asero R, Bindslev-Jensen C, Brzoza Z, Canonica GW, Church MK, Ensina LF, Gimenez-Arnau A, Godse K, Goncalo M, Grattan C, Hebert J, Hide M, Kaplan A, Kapp A, Abdul Latiff AH, Mathelier-Fusade P, Metz M, Nast A, Saini SS, Sanchez-Borges M, Schmid-Grendelmeier P, Simons FE, Staubach P, Sussman G, Toubi E, Vena GA, Wedi B, Zhu XJ, Maurer M, European Academy of A, Clinical I, Global A, Asthma European N, European Dermatology F, World Allergy O. The EAACI/GA(2) LEN/EDF/WAO Guideline for the definition, classification, diagnosis, and management of urticaria: the 2013 revision and update. Allergy. 2014;69:868-887.
76. Bernstein JA, Lang DM, Khan DA, Craig T, Dreyfus D, Hsieh F, Sheikh J, Weldon D, Zuraw B, Bernstein DI, Blessing-Moore J, Cox L, Nicklas RA, Oppenheimer J, Portnoy JM, Randolph CR, Schuller DE, Spector SL, Tilles SA, Wallace D. The diagnosis and management of acute and chronic urticaria: 2014 update. J Allergy Clin Immunol. 2014;133:1270–7.
77. Tlougan BE, Mancini AJ, Mandell JA, Cohen DE, Sanchez MR. Skin conditions in figure skaters, ice-hockey players and speed skaters: part II – cold-induced, infectious and inflammatory dermatoses. Sports Med. 2011;41:967–84.
78. Montgomery SL. Cholinergic urticaria and exercise-induced anaphylaxis. Curr Sports Med Rep. 2015;14: 61–3.
79. Mazarakis A, Bardousis K, Almpanis G, Mazaraki I, Markou S, Kounis NG. Kounis syndrome following cold urticaria: the swimmer's death. Int J Cardiol. 2014;176:e52–3.
80. Balp MM, Vietri J, Tian H, Isherwood G. The impact of chronic urticaria from the patient's perspective: a survey in five European countries. Patient. 2015;8: 551–8.
81. Sussman G, Hebert J, Gulliver W, Lynde C, Waserman S, Kanani A, Ben-Shoshan M, Horemans S, Barron C, Betschel S, Yang WH, Dutz J, Shear N, Lacuesta G, Vadas P, Kobayashi K, Lima H, Simons FE. Insights and advances in chronic urticaria: a Canadian perspective. Allergy Asthma Clin Immunol. 2015;11:7.
82. Abajian M, Schoepke N, Altrichter S, Zuberbier T, Maurer M. Physical urticarias and cholinergic urticaria. Immunol Allergy Clin North Am. 2014;34:73–88.
83. Bray SM, Fajt ML, Petrov AA. Successful treatment of exercise-induced anaphylaxis with omalizumab. Ann Allergy Asthma Immunol. 2012;109:281–2.
84. Geller M. Successful treatment of occupational delayed pressure urticaria and angioedema with omalizumab. Ann Allergy Asthma Immunol. 2016; 116:81–2.
85. Fonacier LS, Sher JM. Allergic contact dermatitis. Ann Allergy Asthma Immunol. 2014;113:9–12.
86. Farhadian JA, Tlougan BE, Adams BB, Leventhal JS, Sanchez MR. Skin conditions of baseball, cricket, and softball players. Sports Med. 2013;43:575–89.

87. Kockentiet B, Adams BB. Contact dermatitis in athletes. J Am Acad Dermatol. 2007;56:1048–55.
88. Weston WL, Morelli JG. Dermatitis under soccer shin guards: allergy or contact irritant reaction? Pediatr Dermatol. 2006;23:19–20.
89. Gumulka M, Matura M, Liden C, Kettelarij JA, Julander A. Nickel exposure when working out in the gym. Acta Derm Venereol. 2015;95:247–9.
90. Guerra L, Misciali C, Borrello P, Melino M. Sensitization to palladium. Contact Dermatitis. 1988; 19:306–7.
91. de Waard-van der Spek FB, Darsow U, Mortz CG, Orton D, Worm M, Muraro A, Schmid-Grendelmeier P, Grimalt R, Spiewak R, Rudzeviciene O, Flohr C, Halken S, Fiocchi A, Borrego LM, Oranje AP. EAACI position paper for practical patch testing in allergic contact dermatitis in children. Pediatr Allergy Immunol. 2015;26:598–606.
92. Bruze M, Goossens A, Isaksson M. Recommendation to increase the test concentration of methylchloroisothiazolinone/methylisothiazolinone in the European baseline patch test series – on behalf of the European society of contact dermatitis and the European environmental and contact dermatitis research group. Contact Dermatitis. 2014;71:35–40.
93. Pigatto PD. Conctact dermatitis: some important topics. Eur Ann Allergy Clin Immunol. 2015;47:188–91.
94. Simons FE, Ardusso LR, Bilo MB, Cardona V, Ebisawa M, El-Gamal YM, Lieberman P, Lockey RF, Muraro A, Roberts G, Sanchez-Borges M, Sheikh A, Shek LP, Wallace DV, Worm M. International consensus on (ICON) anaphylaxis. World Allergy Organ J. 2014;7:9.
95. Simons FE, Ebisawa M, Sanchez-Borges M, Thong BY, Worm M, Tanno LK, Lockey RF, El-Gamal YM, Brown SG, Park HS, Sheikh A. 2015 update of the evidence base: World allergy organization anaphylaxis guidelines. World Allergy Organ J. 2015;8:32.
96. Simons FE, Ardusso LR, Bilo MB, El-Gamal YM, Ledford DK, Ring J, Sanchez-Borges M, Senna GE, Sheikh A, Thong BY, World Allergy O. World allergy organization guidelines for the assessment and management of anaphylaxis. World Allergy Organ J. 2011;4:13–37.
97. Barg W, Medrala W, Wolanczyk-Medrala A. Exercise-induced anaphylaxis: an update on diagnosis and treatment. Curr Allergy Asthma Rep. 2011;11:45–51.
98. Maulitz RM, Pratt DS, Schocket AL. Exercise-induced anaphylactic reaction to shellfish. J Allergy Clin Immunol. 1979;63:433–4.
99. Giacco SR-D. Exercise-induced anaphylaxis: an update. Breath. 2012;8:299–306.
100. Du Toit G. Food-dependent exercise-induced anaphylaxis in childhood. Pediatr Allergy Immunol. 2007;18:455–63.
101. Castells MC, Horan RF, Sheffer AL. Exercise-induced anaphylaxis. Curr Allergy Asthma Rep. 2003;3:15–21.
102. Bennett JR. Anaphylaxis attributed to exercise: considerations for sports medicine specialists. Phys Sportsmed. 2015;43:1–12.
103. Robson-Ansley P, Toit GD. Pathophysiology, diagnosis and management of exercise-induced anaphylaxis. Curr Opin Allergy Clin Immunol. 2010;10: 312–7.

Part XII

Prevention, Rehabilitation and Return to Sports

Injury Prevention Programs - The "FIFA 11+"

49

Nuno Pais, Paulo Beckert, Henrique Jones, and João Espregueira-Mendes

Contents

N. Pais (✉)
ULS Nordeste, Bragança, Portugal

Clínica do Dragão, Espregueira-Mendes Sports Centre - FIFA Medical Centre of Excellence, Porto, Portugal

Dom Henrique Research Centre, Porto, Portugal
e-mail: npais@espregueira.com

P. Beckert
Portuguese National Football Team, Oeiras, Portugal

Clínica CUF Alvalade, Lisbon, Portugal

H. Jones
Montijo Orthopaedic and Sports Medicine Clinic, Montijo, Portugal

J. Espregueira-Mendes
Orthopaedics Department of Minho University, Minho, Portugal

Clínica do Dragão, Espregueira-Mendes Sports Centre - FIFA Medical Centre of Excellence, Porto, Portugal

Dom Henrique Research Centre, Porto, Portugal

3B's Research Group–Biomaterials, Biodegradables and Biomimetics, University of Minho, Headquarters of the European Institute of Excellence on Tissue Engineering and Regenerative Medicine, AvePark, Parque de Ciência e Tecnologia, Zona Industrial da Gandra, 4805-017 Barco, Guimarães, Portugal

ICVS/3B's–PT Government Associate Laboratory, Braga/Guimarães, Portugal

Football is without question the world's most popular sport with an estimated 265 million registered players [1]. Much of the current growth is due to the rapid increase in the number of females playing as well as the growth in countries where football does not have a strong historical record such as the United States, China, and India [2] .

Compared with other sports, football is a vigorous sporting activity with relatively high incidence of injury [3–6]. To decrease the number of injuries, prevent early retirement, and provide a healthy and safe environment for players, preventive programs are highly recommended.

FIFA, Federation International of Football Association, comprises 206 federations, and one of its main concerns, through its Medical Commission, is to protect the players' health. Injury prevention is an important area of intervention, and therefore the foundation, in 1994, of a medical research center, FIFA Medical Assessment and Research Center (F-MARC), in order to prevent injuries and to promote safety in playing football, as well as health benefits, is a proof of this concern.

The development of injury prevention programs has been a central concern of several medical institutions involved in health care of general sportsmen and particularly with football players. The medical knowledge that the occurrence of an injury significantly increases the risk to the occurrence of a subsequent lesion (particularly if improperly rehabilitated and an unsuitable return

J. Espregueira-Mendes et al. (eds.), *Injuries and Health Problems in Football*,
DOI 10.1007/978-3-662-53924-8_49

to play and competition) is reasonable enough, in a medical perspective, for an effective investment in the development of injury prevention strategies in sports.

The types of injuries have a direct impact in preventing strategies [7]. It is possible that the noncontact injuries, which often occur in football, are likely to be prevented with the practice of regular and structured exercise programs.

Analyzing published studies about injuries prevention related to football, Bizzini and Dvorak report that 20–50 % of noncontact injuries can be avoided by prevention programs based on exercise [7, 8]. Studies such as Junge et al. [9], Soligard et al. [10], Emery et al. [11], Mandelbaum et al. [12], Steffen et al. [14], and Owoeye et al. [13] have shown evidence in the preventive effect based on exercise programs [9–14].

The "11+" is the gold standard of these programs both for amateur and competition football players, male or female, over 14 years old.

Approaching the issue of sports prevention injuries, the sequential model of actions proposed by van Mechelen has been followed by the main centers for the development and implementation of injury prevention programs.

This model outlines four essential steps for structuring and developing a prevention program.

In the first step, the problem magnitude should be established, namely, knowing the type of injury, its severity, incidence and prevalence in the sport and our target population. In this step it is crucial to resort to epidemiological studies published in the scientific literature and records.

In the second step, the mechanism of injuries and risk factors should be well known (whether of intrinsic or extrinsic nature and their possible modifications). It is essential to know that the noncontact injuries (focus of these programs) happen during the running, planting/cutting movements, and soft landings and that many of susceptible risk factors liable to be modified are related to deficiencies or imbalances involving muscle strength and neuromuscular control.

In the third step, the possible preventive measures are introduced. The "FIFA 11+" exercise program is an example of preventive measurements to be used in football in order to prevent injuries. It will be discussed below in this chapter with more detail.

Finally, the fourth step must be a repetition of the first one. The effectiveness of the recommended preventive measures should be evaluated. The "FIFA 11+" program effectiveness was demonstrated by several random studies in female and male players [10, 13–15].

49.1 The "FIFA 11+"

The "FIFA 11+" was developed in 2006 by a team of international experts from the FIFA Medical Assessment and Research Centre (F-MARC), Oslo Sports Trauma Research Center (Norway), and Santa Monica Orthopaedic and Sports Medicine Research Foundation (USA) and was based in the experience of "the 11," "PEP," and other exercise programs [12, 16–20].

The "FIFA 11+" is a complete warm-up program specially designed for football players, male or female, amateur or professional, of all levels with 14 years old or plus. This program should be performed, as a standard warm-up, at the start of each training session at least twice a week and takes around 20 min to complete. Prior to matches only the running exercises (parts one and three) should or may be performed.

This program has not only beneficial effects in preventing injuries as it contributes to the improvement of motor skills and physical performance of football players [21–23]. In Portuguese young futsal players have also been found with beneficial effects on physical parameters related to strength, balance, and motor skills [24, 25].

Scientific studies have shown that young football teams using the "FIFA 11+" as warm-up program have a significantly lower risk of injuries compared with teams that do not use it [7]. The male and female teams who perform the "FIFA 11+" regularly have 30–50 % fewer injuries in training and competition.

Its effectiveness in preventing injuries, significantly reducing the number of injuries, had been shown in a study published in 2008 by Soligard et al. (in female population 13–18 years old) and in a study by Steffen et al. [10, 14]. More recently Owoeye et al. and Silvers et al. showed, with random studies, the effectiveness of "FIFA 11+" in young male population [13, 15]. Other studies, reported by Bizzini et al. in their reviewed article published in 2015, also showed the preventive effectiveness of the "FIFA 11+" [7].

49.2 The "FIFA 11+" Structure

The "FIFA 11+" has 3 parts with a total of 15 exercises that must be performed in a specific sequence that follows a progressive and intentional warm-up. The exercises are based on good practice and scientific studies.

A key point in the program is to use the proper technique during all of the exercises. Full attention should be paid to correct posture and good body control, including straight leg alignment, knee-over-toe position, and soft landings. It is essential that the coach supervises players' performance and correct them if necessary.

The first part consists of running exercises at a slow speed combined with active stretching and controlled partner contacts.

The second part includes six sets of exercises focusing on core and leg strength, balance, and plyometrics/agility, each with three levels of increasing difficulty.

In the third part, running exercises at moderate/high speed combined with planting/cutting movements are performed.

Before the games, only the first and third parts are executed.

Each part has three levels. Players should begin at level 1, and only when the exercises are performed without any difficulty during a specific time and number of repetitions should they progress to the next level.

Regarding level upgrade, it should ideally be determined by each player. Alternatively, the group can progress in some exercises, keeping up the same level with others. To simplify, all players can progress to the next level in all exercises at the same time after 3–4 weeks of practicing.

It is estimated that the preventive effects of this program can be seen after 10–12 weeks of starting; however, it obviously depends on the frequency that players do it.

Mario Bizzini and Jiri Dvorak of FIFA Medical Assessment and Research Center (F-MARC), in the quoted article on the "FIFA 11+," highlight the fact that there are, practically, no publications on the prevention injuries of the lower limbs in professional players [7]. An exception is a study in 44 teams of several first leagues which points 5 most outstanding exercises that are part of the "FIFA 11+" exercises panel [26].

The overall structure of the "FIFA 11+" can be observed in Fig. 49.1, and all the aspects related to the program can be found at www.f-marc.com/plus.

Other age groups – children under 14 years old and veterans above 40 – as well as referees have been subjects of studies for the development of preventive programs and the evaluation of their effectiveness [27, 28].

The "FIFA 11+ Referees" is an example of one of these programs and has been worldwide distributed and included in training courses for referees.

Although "FIFA 11+" is scientifically proven to be effective in the prevention of noncontact injuries and target of numerous awareness campaigns and promotion, its dissemination and implementation on a large scale still remains a challenge for sports medicine staff in preventing injuries and promoting football practice on a safety basis and with all possible health benefits [7].

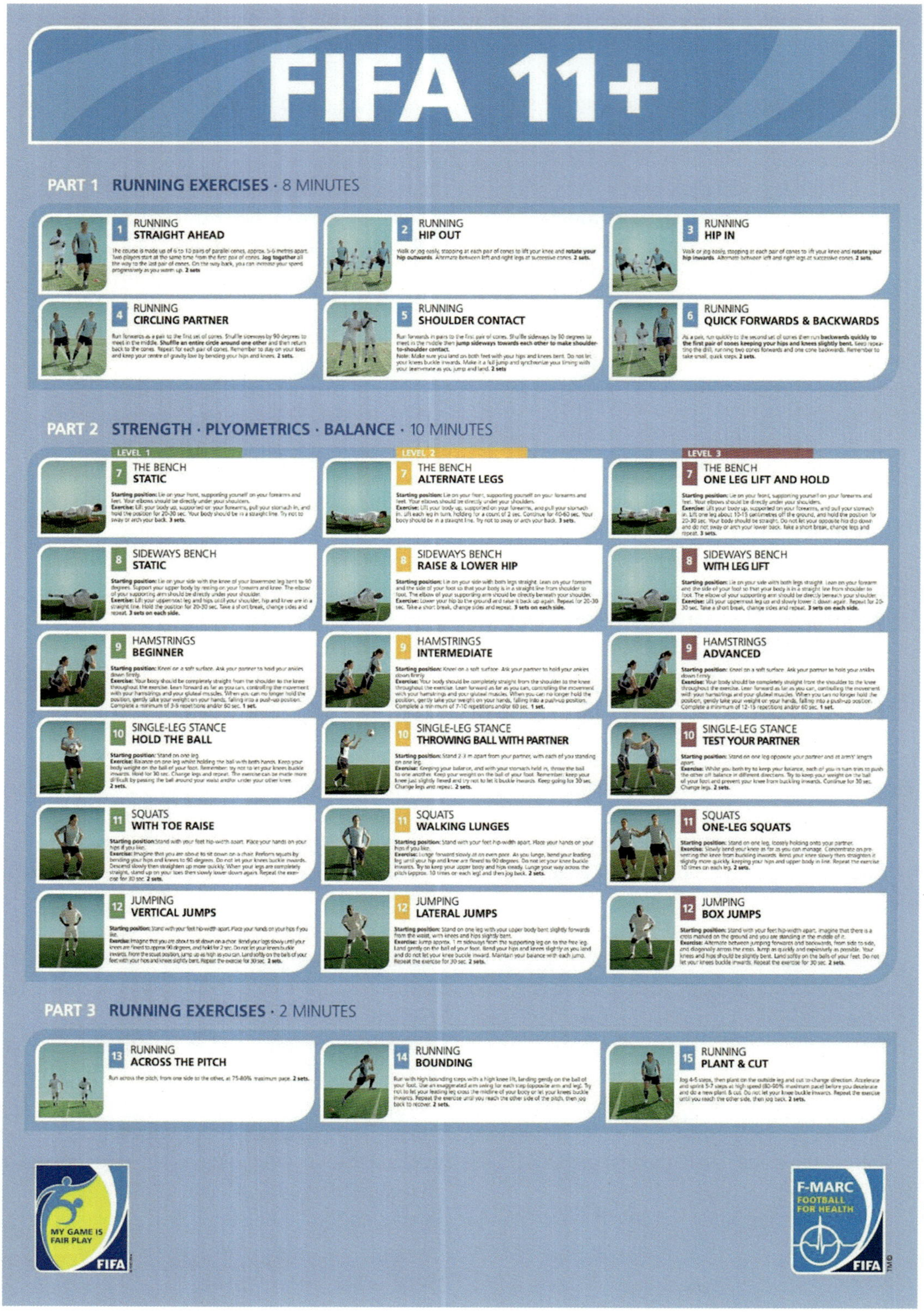

Fig. 49.1 FIFA 11+ complete warm-up program. http://www.f-marc.com/downloads/posters_generic/english.pdf

References

1. Association FIdF. FIFA Big Count 2006: 270 million people active in football. Retrieved February. 2007.
2. Engström B, Johansson C, Tornkvist H. Soccer injuries among elite female players. Am J Sports Med. 1991;19(4):372–5.
3. Hawkins RD, Fuller CW. An examination of the frequency and severity of injuries and incidents at three levels of professional football. Br J Sports Med. 1998;32(4):326–32.
4. Hawkins RD, Fuller CW. A prospective epidemiological study of injuries in four English professional football clubs. Br J Sports Med. 1999;33(3):196–203.
5. Rahnama N, Reilly T, Lees A. Injury risk associated with playing actions during competitive soccer. Br J Sports Med. 2002;36(5):354–9.
6. Kranke M. Book review: soccernomics: why England loses, why Germany and Brazil win, and why the US, Japan, Australia, Turkeyâ€" and even Iraqâ€" are destined to become the kings of the world's most popular sport. J Sports Econ. 2012;13(1):96–8.
7. Bizzini M, Dvorak J. FIFA 11+: an effective programme to prevent football injuries in various player groups worldwide – a narrative review. Br J Sports Med. 2015;49(9):577–9.
8. Bizzini M, Dvorak J. Football injury prevention. In: Volpi P, editor. Football Traumatology. New Trends. Berlin: Springer; 2015, p. 35–46.
9. Junge A, Rösch D, Peterson L, Graf-Baumann T, Dvorak J. Prevention of soccer injuries: a prospective intervention study in youth amateur players. Am J Sports Med. 2002;30(5):652–9.
10. Soligard T, Myklebust G, Steffen K, Holme I, Silvers H, Bizzini M, et al. Comprehensive warm-up programme to prevent injuries in young female footballers: cluster randomised controlled trial. BMJ Br Med J. 2009;338:95–9.
11. Emery C, Meeuwisse W. The effectiveness of a neuromuscular prevention strategy to reduce injuries in youth soccer: a cluster-randomised controlled trial. Br J Sports Med. 2010;44(8):555–62.
12. Mandelbaum BR, Silvers HJ, Watanabe DS, Knarr JF, Thomas SD, Griffin LY, et al. Effectiveness of a neuromuscular and proprioceptive training program in preventing anterior cruciate ligament injuries in female athletes 2-year follow-up. Am J Sports Med. 2005;33(7):1003–10.
13. Owoeye O, Akinbo S, Tella BA, Olawale OA. Efficacy of the FIFA 11+ warm-up programme in male youth football: a cluster randomised controlled trial. J Sports Sci Med. 2014;13(2):321–8.
14. Steffen K, Emery CA, Romiti M, Kang J, Bizzini M, Dvorak J, et al. High adherence to a neuromuscular injury prevention programme (FIFA 11+) improves functional balance and reduces injury risk in Canadian youth female football players: a cluster randomised trial. Br J Sports Med. 2013;47(12):794–802.
15. Silvers-Granelli H, Mandelbaum B, Adeniji O, Insler S, Bizzini M, Pohlig R, et al. Efficacy of the FIFA 11+ injury prevention program in the collegiate male soccer player. Am J Sports Med. 2015; 43:2628–37.
16. Junge A, Lamprecht M, Stamm H, Hasler H, Bizzini M, Tschopp M, et al. Countrywide campaign to prevent soccer injuries in Swiss amateur players. Am J Sports Med. 2011;39(1):57–63.
17. Heidt RS, Sweeterman LM, Carlonas RL, Traub JA, Tekulve FX. Avoidance of soccer injuries with preseason conditioning. Am J Sports Med. 2000;28(5):659–62.
18. Caraffa A, Cerulli G, Projetti M, Aisa G, Rizzo A. Prevention of anterior cruciate ligament injuries in soccer. Knee Surg Sports Traumatol Arthrosc. 1996; 4(1):19–21.
19. Söderman K, Werner S, Pietilä T, Engström B, Alfredson H. Balance board training: prevention of traumatic injuries of the lower extremities in female soccer players? Knee Surg Sports Traumatol Arthrosc. 2000;8(6):356–63.
20. Hewett TE, Lindenfeld TN, Riccobene JV, Noyes FR. The effect of neuromuscular training on the incidence of knee injury in female athletes a prospective study. Am J Sports Med. 1999;27(6):699–706.
21. Impellizzeri FM, Bizzini M, Dvorak J, Pellegrini B, Schena F, Junge A. Physiological and performance responses to the FIFA 11+(part 2): a randomised controlled trial on the training effects. J Sports Sci. 2013;31(13):1491–502.
22. Daneshjoo A, Rahnama N, Mokhtar AH, Yusof A. Effectiveness of injury prevention programs on developing quadriceps and hamstrings strength of young male professional soccer players. J Hum Kinet. 2013;39(1):115–25.
23. Bizzini M, Impellizzeri FM, Dvorak J, Bortolan L, Schena F, Modena R, et al. Physiological and performance responses to the "FIFA 11+"(part 1): is it an appropriate warm-up? J Sports Sci. 2013;31(13): 1481–90.
24. Brito J, Figueiredo P, Fernandes L, Seabra A, Soares JM, Krustrup P, et al. Isokinetic strength effects of FIFA's "The 11+" injury prevention training programme. Isokinet Exerc Sci. 2010;18(4):211–5.
25. Reis I, Rebelo A, Krustrup P, Brito J. Performance enhancement effects of Federation Internationale de Football Association's "The 11+" injury prevention training program in youth futsal players. Clin J Sport Med. 2013;23(4):318–20.
26. McCall A, Carling C, Nedelec M, Davison M, Le Gall F, Berthoin S, et al. Risk factors, testing and preventative strategies for non-contact injuries in professional football: current perceptions and practices of 44 teams from various premier leagues. Br J Sports Med. 2014;48:1352–57.
27. Faude O, Rößler R, Junge A. Football injuries in children and adolescent players: are there clues for prevention? Sports Med. 2013;43(9):819–37.
28. Hammes D, Aus der Fünten K, Kaiser S, Frisen E, Bizzini M, Meyer T. Injury prevention in male veteran football players – a randomised controlled trial using "FIFA 11+". J Sports Sci. 2015;33(9): 873–81.

Late Rehabilitation (On the Field) 50

Frederico Varandas, Daniel Medina, Antonio Gómez, and Stefano Della Villa

Contents

50.1 What Is It?

Late rehabilitation or *rehabilitation on field* is the last and most challenging stage in the return-to-play process of a football player. One reason for this clinical challenge is the lack of research or consensus to suggest the most effective training loads, techniques, and decision-making for improving fitness and performance during late-stage rehabilitation [1, 2].

Late rehabilitation begins when the player is clinically asymptomatic and ends when the player "returns to play." Classically, this consists of integrating the different variables worked individually until this stage (flexibility, strength, proprioception) with velocity training, power training, and football-specific skills training in the same training process. As recently proposed by Blanch et al. [3], the real challenge during this stage is to train players to meet the demands of full training and competition loads in order to ensure return to play and reduce risk of subsequent injury.

F. Varandas (✉)
Medical Department, Sporting clube Portugal, Lisbon, Portugal

Comcorpus Clinic – Sports Rehabilitation Center, Lisbon, Portugal
e-mail: ffvarandas@sporting.pt

D. Medina • A. Gómez
Sports Science and Medical Department, FC Barcelona, Catalonia, Spain

S.D. Villa
Isokinetic Medical Group, FIFA Medical Centre of Excellence, Bologna, Italy

J. Espregueira-Mendes et al. (eds.), *Injuries and Health Problems in Football*, DOI 10.1007/978-3-662-53924-8_50

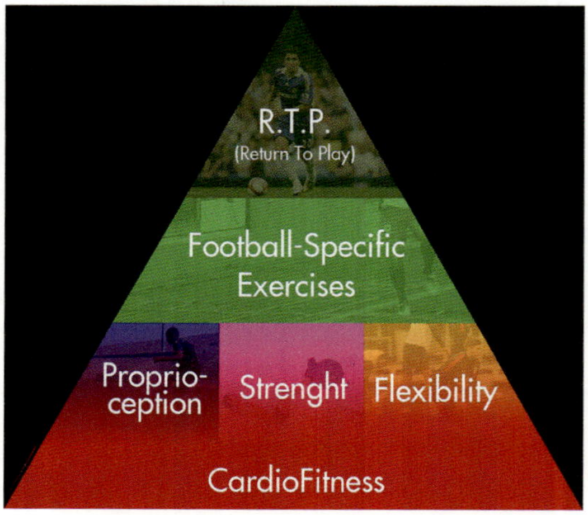

50.2 The Main Goal

The main goal is to allow a safe transition between the rehabilitation process and the training process required to accumulate load in order to provide adequate return to play and performance.

From a strictly medical point of view, we subdivide the sports rehabilitation period after injury into four stages (*1, initial stage; 2, intermediate stage; 3, advanced stage; 4, return to play*) that represent a progressive continuum of therapeutic management, according to the four typical questions the football player asks after injury: "When will I be able: **(1)** to walk normally? **(2)** to run normally? **(3)** to start training on the field? **(4)** to go back to competitions?" This strategy underlines one of the main themes of sports rehabilitation that objective criteria rather than specific timetables should guide clinical decision-making.

Late rehabilitation or *rehabilitation on field* corresponds to the third and fourth phase of the global process of sports rehabilitation.

Late rehabilitation program should be performed with on-field training, progressively exposing the player to the football-specific demands.

The phases of rehabilitation are closely related to the stages of healing:

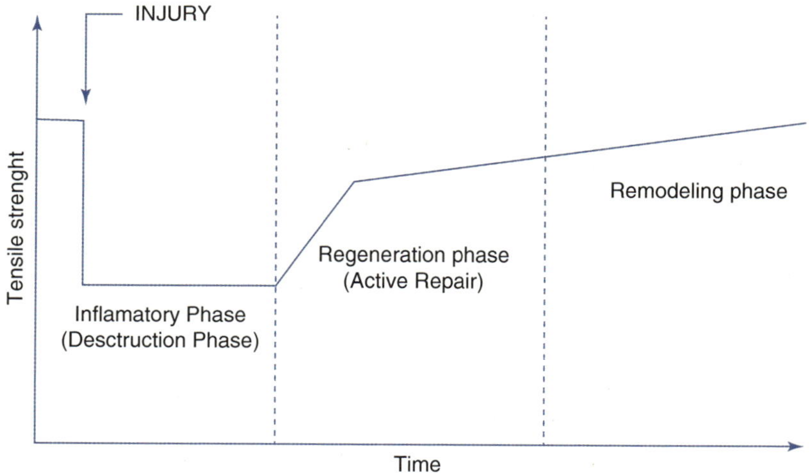

The management of injuries during the stages of healing has been established [4]; however, according to "The clinician who waits for tissue healing before clearing the athlete to return to play will probably find a short-lived career with a sporting team. So, why is there a paradox between the evidence and clinical practice regarding when the athlete should return to play? Return-to-play criteria must depend on the type of injury, demands of sports and the affected body region. Ideally, a battery of accepted clinical criteria are used to guide safe return-to-play decisions. But these are physical assessments based on clinical dogma, with little empirical evidence to support their use, and little consensus regarding what the best criteria are. This highlights the need for evidence to address this knowledge gap—ideally rigorous studies—but a good first step is to have consensus."

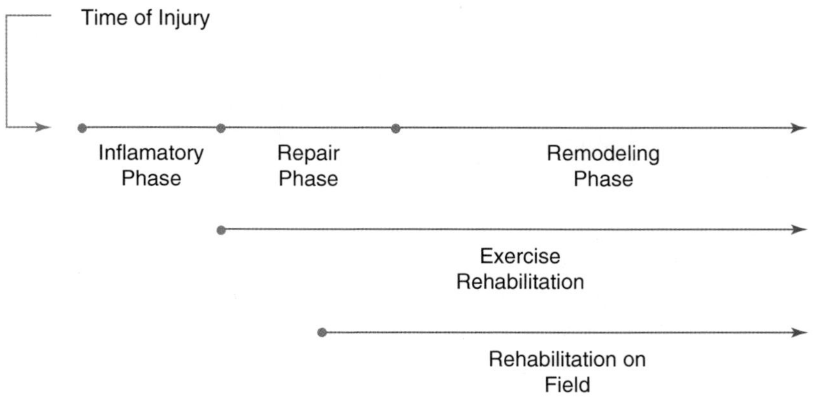

Fig. 50.1 The phases of exercise rehabilitation of the injured player

The phases of exercise rehabilitation of the injured player

	Phase 1 Cognitive Phase	Phase 2 Associative Phase	Phase 3 Autonomous Phase	Phase 4 Return to Play
AIMS	To activate and isolate the local stabilisers of the joint	To retain movement patterns and isolated muscles	Dynamic stabilisation with emphasis on skill training and functional rehabilitation	This includes the process by which the player returns to the team in a graded process until full return

Dynamic loading in the form of exercise rehabilitation can be started as soon as the repair phase has begun [6].

Exercise rehabilitation for an injury is classically described to have three phases (cognitive, associative, and autonomous) [5]. For the football player, an additional phase relevant to return to play is added. The aims of the four phases are presented in Fig. 50.1.

From the theoretical point of view, the *autonomous phase* (phase 3) and *return to play* (phase 4) form the *rehabilitation on-field* concept.

For the rehabilitation process to be successful, communication between the medical team, player, trainer, and coach is critical.

50.3 When to Start?

The criteria for starting On-Field-Rehabilitation (OFR) are a good joint stability in clinical tests, no giving-way episodes during the preceding phases, minimal or no pain (visual analogue scale [VAS] less than 3/10), minimal effusion, complete range of motion (ROM), and maximal peak torque difference less than 20% between limbs in isokinetic tests. The football player must also be able to run on the treadmill at 8 km/h for more than 10 min [7].

An extremely important criterion to reach the late stage of rehabilitation, the football player must have gained adequate strength and stability in two "key muscles": *(1) dynamic stabilizers of the hip* and *(2) core stability*. These two muscle groups are fundamental for a good rehabilitation and for the football player performance.

50.3.1 Dynamic Stabilizers of the Hip

The six short hip external rotators (superior and inferior gemellus, obturator internus and externus, quadratus femoris, and piriformis) have the capacity to provide hip joint compression and hence dynamic stability during most weight-bearing and non-weight-bearing activities.

The gluteus medius is the dominant hip abductor and is the primary lateral stabilizer of the hip during one-leg stance activities.

The gluteus maximus plays an important role in generating extension and external rotation torque and has the potential to provide hip stabilization by resisting anterior hip force. The gluteal muscles contribute at least 50% to isometric hip extension. If gluteal strength is inadequate, the hamstring muscle can be overloaded and susceptible to injury. This is especially true during sprinting activities. The gluteus maximus acts during running to control trunk flexion of the stance leg, decelerate the swing leg, and extend the hip. Any alteration in the gluteus maximus activation, strength, or endurance places greater demand on the hamstring. Overall the gluteus maximus provides powerful hip extension when sprinting, and the hamstrings help to transfer the power between the hip and the knee joints. Unlike the hamstring and quadriceps, the gluteus maximus usually is neglected in a rehabilitation program of a footballer. Definitely, the gluteus maximus is a "key muscle" for a footballer.

50.3.2 Core Stability

The musculoskeletal core of the body includes the spine, hips and pelvis, proximal lower limb, and abdominal structures. Dynamic stabilization refers to the ability to utilize strength and endurance and motor control in a functional manner through all planes of motion and action despite changes in the center of gravity.

Core exercises train the muscles in your pelvis, lower back, hips, and abdomen to work in harmony. This leads to better balance and stability on the playing field.

Strong core muscles make it easier to do everything from running technique to having a good kicking technique. The stability of the lumbopelvic region is crucial, to provide a foundation for limb movement, to support loads, and to protect the spine. Weak core muscles leave you susceptible to poor posture, lower back pain, and muscle injuries.

Each OFR session takes place outdoors on a grass or synthetic field and is integrated by gym sessions with specific strengthening, flexibility, and neuromuscular exercises. During OFR, the progression of each type of exercise is football specific and follows the principles of strength training and of increasing functional demand performed on progressively broader spaces with respect to the musculoskeletal and neuromechanical components involved in the recovery process.

50.4 Methods of Training and Rehab Interaction

The mechanistic view of human organisms inspired in analytic reductionism and classical cybernetics has deeply influenced sport theory, sport practice, and sport research in the last few decades [4].

> "Any living system, including the human body is more than the addition of its parts." Aristotle

During the last decades, influenced by the general systems theory proposed by Ludwig von Bertalanffy and the models derived from the chaos theory, a new understanding of living beings and their complexity, organization, and relationship with environment as well as their development has been stablished. From this new perspective, human beings in motion are understood as a complex and indivisible entity [5]. Football is not an exception. According to Seirul.lo [6], a new paradigm has been proposed, where the footballer is considered a hypercomplex structure configured by interactions and structures (Fig. 50.2).

According to Seirul.lo [6], these structures interact with each other and with the environment so the entire network self-structures, acquiring a different structure for each player at any given time, every time, hence the nonlinearity proposed.

This holistic paradigm shift seems ideal for team sports where continuous interaction between teammates, opponents, and objects requires a high level of self-structuring. Therefore, training becomes a unique event, where the footballer "trains and learns." Exercises should be constructed to provide this dynamic activity, i.e., practices should emphasize high variability and global approach, far from the classical analytical, repetitive, and "closed" tasks. Within that network of structures (Fig. 50.2),

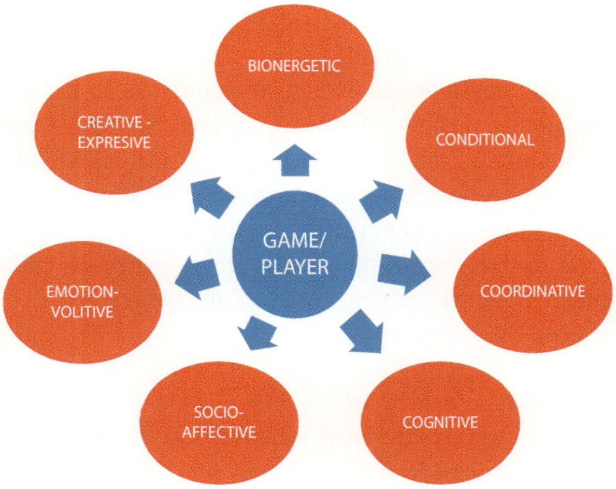

Fig. 50.2 Structures configuring the hypercomplex athlete/footballer according to Seirul.lo [6]. Each structure must be considered a manifest of underlying processes. In other words, processes, a network of dynamic relationships between systems, manifest through what we call structures. What we classically call "capacities" are nothing but a sectorial evaluation of the processes occurring in a giving system which configure a given structure

none of them is more important than the other; everything is alike. In each workout will be a distinct priority tailored to the needs of the athlete, but in the pre-match, a synthesis of all structures occurs again. In the case of injured players, once the player is ready to train on the field, as proposed by Pol [5], training should not be focused exclusively on the individual but also the collective entity (team).

> "Every engine scheme will be strengthened through the variability of practice."

The wide range of exercises (variety) of this approach has other benefits for the group work since each individual must reach a solution without requiring many individual instructions from the coach, in other words, the subject is self-organizing. Performing various exercises, and at the same time introducing variation and variability, makes the subject spontaneously discover individual movement patterns allowing to respond more effectively to the drive task proposed. We should increase the responsibility of the player in the training process, and with these actions, we'll improve motivational aspects [7].

50.4.1 Principles of Training

The so-called principles of training are defined as a set of generic rules that govern the process of developing physical fitness and are based on biological, psychological, and educational aspects. It is of paramount importance to base the planning and execution of sports programming on these principles, since proper implementation will depend largely on the success of our work [8]. These "principles" are part of the holistic approach and should not be interpreted as isolated units. We'll describe them separately in order to facilitate a better understanding.

Training loads lead to various physiological, morphological, and functional adaptations, resulting in increased physical performance. This loading must be adequate in order to avoid functional impairment and must follow these "principles."

50.4.1.1 Effective Load

Effective load intensity must exceed a "lower threshold" below which no training effect is achieved and remain under an "upper threshold" defined as the maximum tolerance level above which training effects may be harmful, leading to injury or overtraining if not identified. These thresholds are individual according to individual training levels.

50.4.1.2 Load Progression

Loading must increase gradually. Improvement in performance is a direct result of the amount and quality of work the athlete achieves in training. From the sport initiation to the top-class athlete, workload in training must increase gradually according to each individual's physiological and psychological abilities [8].

Load might be increased continuously or in a fluctuating manner. During continuous increase (monotonic), the load continuously increases without any decrease, although not necessarily always the same rate. During fluctuating increase (non-monotonic), training frequency increases first, and then training volume and workload intensity is at last increased.

50.4.1.3 Variety

The realization of the same technical and physical exercises might lead to monotony and boredom causing improvement stagnation. To overcome this problem, a wide range of training proposals should be offered. The challenge is not only changing/alternating training exercises regularly but also introducing all the structures such as conditional, cognitive, coordinative, socioaffective, etc. (Fig. 50.2) in every proposed exercise.

50.4.1.4 Optimum Balance Between Load and Recovery

Working and recovery periods are closely linked during training process in order to achieve a higher performance capacity. Classically described as the supercompensation phenomenon, recovery after each workload must be assured, either within a session or between different sessions. Recovery times are influenced by load intensity and the type of training.

50.4.1.5 Repetition and Continuity

This principle is based on the necessity for repeated actions to achieve performance improvement and ensures that repetition fixes habits, techniques, and knowledge. Without repetition and continuity in the training session's stimuli, it would be impossible to develop a good performance recovery. The body needs time to make metabolic, morphological, and structural necessary adaptations that will result in improving and maintaining fitness.

50.4.1.6 Reversibility

Training adaptations are reversible. Most of the adaptations will be reversed during inactivity periods. This rate of loss is different for each capacity, being higher for endurance and strength endurance rather than speed or the maximum force. As general rule, overall losses up to 10% of fitness in a week of total inactivity are accepted.

50.4.1.7 Periodization

The adaptation process follows different phases: growing, stabilization, and decline. It requires training to be structured in different cycles of different durations. For example, the basic training unit is a working session; a day can have one or more sessions; and a *microcycle* is a small set of workdays with a common goal: normally a week. A *mesocycle* is a set of microcycles, usually one month; and a *macrocycle* is a set of mesocycles featuring preparatory, competitive, and transition periods. For a successful recovery and performance, it is very important that each microcycle relates to the next and previous by interconnection patterns to optimize the relationship between structures.

50.4.1.8 Individuality

Each athlete is different and responds differently to training process. This is due to different intrinsic factors: genetics, age, sex, maturation, biotype, psychological factors, fitness levels, etc.; however, external factors might affect response to training process: rest, sleep, food, and environmental aspects such as temperature, altitude, etc. We should aim to design individualized training for each athlete and specific timing (especially during on-field rehabilitation). Obviously, this is not fully achievable if we establish homogeneous working groups.

50.4.1.9 Specialization and Multilateral Development

The training process during formative years requires a broad base of multilateral (or generic) training. It allows the development and settles the basis for their sporting future. As the mature athlete improves the generic work, he/she should decrease the benefit of a greater impact on specific aspects of the preparation. Since training has specific effects; it's that an energy system just improves by working that energy system. Specialization and athletic mastery are functionally based on multilateral development [8].

50.4.2 Capacities of Training

> "This is not about adding, joining, or mixing abilities; instead we should attempt to separate them as little as possible."

From the perspective of considering footballers as a hypercomplex structure (Fig. 50.2), it makes sense not to add, join, or mix abilities but more importantly to try separating them as little as possible, i.e., during the design of training situations, we should aim to be as close as possible to the structure and operation of the game of football, close to his internal logic.

Definitely, the message is to keep in mind two fundamental principles of learning for this concept: the specificity of the task and the transfer.

> "The game in football occurs globally but we can not fragment the constituent parts."

Physical capacities represent sectorial evaluations of a system from a structure [6]. All the different physical capacities are optimized to configure the physical condition of the sportsman (Fig. 50.2). Mallo [9] distinguishes endurance, strength, and speed as the three basic conditional capacities, from which strength is the most important in team sports. Each of these capacities shows a different manifestation in each playing position, and every player gives a different importance to them in his self-structuring process [6]. In addition, there are other conditional facilitating capacities as flexibility and relaxation.

As mentioned by Mallo [9], these physical capacities are worthless in themselves, as they need to be developed in interaction with coordinative and cognitive capacities (Fig. 50.2).

(a) *Coordinative capacities* support the specific skills of football players and are necessary for driving the ball, passing, shooting, etc.
(b) *Cognitive capacities* are used to integrate and to provide the best solution to each game-specific situation, in other words, optimizing the interaction between structures [9].

According to Cano [10], "the qualities and capabilities are indivisible, do not give never separated and therefore must always be united in training activities."

50.4.2.1 Strength Capacity

Exercise load is a key aspect during training programming, even more during the on-field rehab training programming. If loads are not appropriated correctly, we will not be able to achieve our goals either due to lack of stimuli or overloading.

Rehabilitation and reconditioning exercises must be functional and oriented during the whole process to the return to competition. Strengthening should follow a transition from general exercises to sport-specific exercises designed to replicate specific movement patterns of the game.

Specificity of movement speed is another key question to consider during programming. Strengthening exercises are velocity specific, which means that the speed at which an athlete trains is directly related to the speed at which strength increases.

Core stability and proprioception are strength workouts we should consider adding to any rehabilitation program, improving their demands and difficulty level under the recovery process.

50.4.2.2 Aerobic Capacity

Aerobic activities need to be worked at the submaximum and maximum capacity for the athlete including running series, running interval training, specific repeated sprints, regular weight strength routine, and specific sport-related exercises on the field.

Designing physical training programs to improve aerobic power is only limited by the coach's imagination. Various methods can be used to improve aerobic capacity; however, research [11, 12] suggests that high-intensity (running interval exercises at an intensity of

90–95% of Heart rate (HR) max for an effort/interval duration of 3–8 min are recommended) and sport-specific training (small side games between 5 and 7 four-minute efforts at approximately 90% HR max with 3 min rest between efforts) will deliver a good performance benefit.

Yo-Yo intermittent endurance test in level 2 due to his specific approach with the competition conditional data should be applied in the latest stage of the player recovery just to confirm we have the 90–95% of the aerobic capacity recovered [13].

50.4.2.3 Flexibility Capacity

Flexibility exercises should be incorporated into the overall fitness program sufficient to develop and maintain ROM. These exercises should stretch the major muscle groups and be performed a minimum of 2–3 days per week. Stretching should include appropriate static and/or dynamic techniques. According to Seirul.lo [6], flexibility will be a facilitator capacity for the recovery, inside the adjuvant training, not inside the optimizing training for the player.

50.4.2.4 Speed Capacity

Assuming accelerometer's technical limitations (included in the so-called GPS devices), we propose monitoring the athlete in terms of individualized speed peaks, symmetry of impacts (step balance), and symptom-free sport-specific patterns of movements. Ideally, the individual benchmarking will be derived from existing pre-injury match data.

For example, as proposed in the FC Barcelona (FCB) Muscle Injury Guidelines [14], running > 21 km/h free of symptoms, accelerations (most of them into 3–4 m/s^2), and total tolerance to decelerate achievement of max speed around the 90–95% of the athlete's maximum will be very useful parameters to drive our decision-making process.

Once all functional criteria described above have been achieved and strength, flexibility, and fitness have reached normal ranges, this does not mean the athlete is fully cleared to return to competition. Psychological readiness to return to play is also important in making the return-to-play transition. The current focus of rehabilitation is on restoration of physical function, and often physical and psychological readiness states do not coincide. However, no consensus is available in assessing an athlete's psychological readiness to return to play [2].

Based on FCB experience [14], a full regular week plan of training with the squad (of at least four full training sessions) without pain and free of discomfort or "fear" (adequate mindset) should be completed. During this week, performance should be monitored for individual/positional benchmarking using "GPS" and HR data as well.

This performance surveillance should be extended to competitions after the player returns to play.

References

1. Shrier I, Safai P, Charland L. Return to play following injury: whose decision should it be? Br J Sports Med 2014;48:394–401.
2. Ardern CL, Bizzini M, Bahr R. It is time for consensus on return to play after injury: five key questions. Br J Sports Med 2015; bjsports-2015-095475. Available from: http://bjsm.bmj.com/lookup/doi/10.1136/bjsports-2015-095475
3. Blanch P, Gabbett TJ. Has the athlete trained enough to return to play safely? The acute: chronic workload ratio permits clinicians to quantify a player's risk of subsequent injury. Br J sport Med. 2016;50(8):1–5.
4. Balague N, Torrents C, Hristovski R, Keith D, Araujo D. Overview of complex systems in sports. J Syst Sci Complex. 2013;26:4–13.
5. Pol R. La Preparación ¿Física? en el Fútbol. El proceso de entrenamiento desde las ciencias de la complejidad. 2ª ed. Pontevedra: MC Sports; 2013.
6. Seirul-lo F. Sistemas dinámicos y rendimiento en deportes de equipo. 1st meeting of complex systems and sport. Barcelona: INEFC; 2003.
7. Torrens C. La teoría de los sistemas dinámicos y el entrenamiento deportivo. Catalonia: University of Lleida; 2005.
8. Bompa T. Periodization: theory and methodology of training. 4th ed. Champaign: Human Kinetics; 1999.
9. Mallo J. Complex Football. From Seirul.lo´s Structured Training to Frade´s Tactical Periodisation. 1st ed. Mallo-Sainz J, editor. avier Mallo Sainz; 2015.
10. Cano O. Estudio de redes complejas. Casademont: BUTACA Fund; 2011.
11. Impellizzeri FM, Marcora SM, Castagna C, Reilly T, Sassi A, Iaia FM, et al. Physiological and performance effects of generic versus specific aerobic training in

soccer players. Int J Sports Med Germany. 2006;27:483–92.
12. Hill-Haas SV, Dawson B, Impellizzeri FM, Coutts AJ. Physiology of small-sided games training in football: a systematic review. Sports Med New Zealand. 2011;41:199–220.
13. Bradley PS, Mohr M, Bendiksen M, Randers MB, Flindt M, Barnes C, et al. Sub-maximal and maximal Yo-Yo intermittent endurance test level 2: heart rate response, reproducibility and application to elite soccer. Eur J Appl Physiol Germany. 2011;111: 969–78.
14. Pruna R, Til L, Rodas G. Muscle injuries clinical guide 3.0 January 2015 p. 1–60. [Accessed 28 Dec 2015] Available from: http://www.fcbarcelona.com/club/facilites-and-services/medical-services

ACL Risk of Reinjury: When Is It Safe to Return (Time or Criteria)

51

Stefano Della Villa, Francesco Della Villa, Margherita Ricci, Mahmut Nedim Doral, Gregory Gasbarro, and Volker Musahl

Contents

S.D. Villa • F. Della Villa • M. Ricci
Isokinetic Medical Group, FIFA Medical Centre of Excellence, Bologna, Italy

M.N. Doral
Sports Medicine Center, Hacettepe University, Ankara, Turkey

G. Gasbarro • V. Musahl (✉)
Department of Orthopaedic Surgery, University of Pittsburgh Medical Center, Pittsburgh, PA, USA
e-mail: musahlv@upmc.edu

51.1 Introduction

Anterior cruciate ligament reconstruction (ACLR) if done successfully improves stability, reduces laxity, and decreases the risk of future knee joint pathology and surgery [1, 2]. Significant advancements in surgical procedures and rehabilitation have led to improved functional outcomes and high expectations in return to sport (RTS) [3]. Despite the relatively high rate of successful outcomes following ACLR, graft failure during rehabilitation can occur [4]. In many cases, this limits an athlete's ability to return to their pre-injury level of activity with reported rates that vary from 37% to 75% [2, 4, 5]. In a recent systematic review, Ardern et al. evaluated 69 studies and 7556 participants after ACLR. On average, 81% of patients returned to some kind of sport, 65% returned to their pre-injury level of sport, and only 55% returned to competitive level sport [6]. Even though recent studies show a great difference between expectations and RTS, as RTS rates are generally reported as ranging from 60 to 80% [7–9].

One of the greatest concerns with RTS is the risk of reinjury. It is well known that the risk of sustaining a new anterior cruciate ligament (ACL) injury is 5.8% for the ipsilateral and 11.8% for the contralateral limb at a minimum of 5 years of follow-up [10]. Women have a higher incidence of ACL injury to the contralateral knee than men after reconstruction. Younger and higher-level

J. Espregueira-Mendes et al. (eds.), *Injuries and Health Problems in Football*,
DOI 10.1007/978-3-662-53924-8_51

athletes seem to be at higher risk of reinjury [11]. Graft failure may also occur as a result of errors in technique, fixation failure, or lack of biological graft incorporation into the bone tunnel [12]. Technical error has been shown to the most common etiologic factor leading to graft attrition and recurrent pathology [13]. These errors may be subdivided into the following: improper intra-articular placement of the graft, impingement of a graft in the intercondylar notch due to insufficient notchplasty or an anterior tibial tunnel, improper tensioning of the graft, or inadequate fixation [13]. A recent review found that most failures occurred 6–9 months after surgery [14].

So when is it safe to allow footballers back on the pitch? A great deal of basic science research over the last 15 years has provided insight into factors that directly influence time course and quality of graft tunnel healing [15–17]. Many of these findings however have yet to be translated to the bedside, and knowledge of the healing process in humans is limited. Strategies to enhance healing have also been explored due to great interest for earlier return to activity among competitive athletes with aggressive postoperative rehabilitation. These include the use of growth factors, periosteal augmentation, and mesenchymal stem cells [18–20].

Consistent with increasing pressures to return athletes to the field of play, methods for quantitative clinical assessment of ACL function following reconstruction have evolved. Magnetic resonance imaging (MRI) has emerged as a tool in the postoperative athlete in predicting graft health with parameters such as volume and signal intensity [21, 22]. MRI has also been used to elucidate differences in bone morphology between genders and critically evaluate postoperative patients for technical errors such as nonanatomic graft placement and graft impingement within the notch [23–25]. Similarly, electromagnetic testing and other noninvasive devices such as the KT-1000 arthrometer have recently been validated to assess ACL stability as an objective outcome measure for clinical follow-up [26–29]. Given that current parameters for return to play are largely dictated by surgeon preference and patient-reported outcomes, these quantitative measures of ACL function may help to establish a safe threshold for footballers in the immediate postoperative phase and rehabilitation process.

51.2 Clinical Strategy

51.2.1 Rehabilitation Principles

The main goal of rehabilitation following ACLR is to return the athlete to the previous level of function as quickly and as safely as possible, minimizing the risk of reinjury and degenerative changes in the joint. Recurrence after ACLR is one of the most devastating outcomes after rehabilitation and RTS. In order to reduce this phenomenon, we suggest adopting the right clinical strategy in a strong organizational context. For right clinical strategy, we mean follow a criteria-based, functional-oriented rehabilitation protocol. For strong organizational context, we mean having a proper team (including a sport medicine physician, a physical therapist, and a reconditioning specialist), a proper facility (consisting of medical offices, rehabilitation gyms, rehabilitation pool, and rehabilitation field), and a proper method (clinical strategy shared by the team).

51.2.2 Clinical Strategy

Nowadays, the most appropriate approach after ACLR is applying a criteria-based rehabilitation protocol, rather than predefined times [30–33]. Certain clinical and functional criteria must be met in order to progress throughout rehabilitation and to finally be allowed to RTS. Therefore, the time for RTS is a secondary goal, the first must be to fulfill the necessary criteria [31]. Even if criteria usually regards ROM, strength, neuromuscular control, proprioception, and endurance, validation of subjective and objective criteria for RTS is still lacking [34].

The protocol we apply in the daily clinical activity with knee patients consists of four functional steps, the so-called traffic lights, and various well-defined criteria, to be met before we proceed from one step to another:

First traffic light: walking without crutches

- Surgeon's approval
- Absence/minimal pain and swelling
- Full knee extension
- Recovery of the correct gait cycle

Second traffic light: running on a treadmill

- No pain during walking
- Knee flexion more than 120°
- Walk on a treadmill for at least 10 min without pain or swelling
- Adequate muscle tone of the trunk, thigh, and limb

Third traffic light: starting on-field rehabilitation

- Less than a 20% deficit between the two quadriceps and hamstrings at the isokinetic test
- Run on a treadmill for at least 10 min at 8 km/h without pain or swelling

Fourth traffic light: return to the team

- Surgeon's approval
- Complete ROM
- Complete recovery of muscular strength deficit at the isokinetic test
- Complete metabolic recovery (aerobic and anaerobic threshold test)
- Complete on-field rehabilitation
- Movement patterns restoration (>90 pts. at the movement analysis test)

51.2.3 Organizational Context

Regarding the organization, we suggest having a proper facility, a proper team, and a proper method in order to control the recovery process after an ACL injury. The proper facility consists of rehabilitation gyms, rehabilitation pools, and sport fields. The use of these three areas at well-defined moments is crucial for the best recovery. The rehab gym is still considered the main area with an average of 60% of the total number of sessions. During each session specific exercises are performed, together with manual and physical therapies if needed (Fig. 51.1). After the suture removal, the patient can begin rehabilitation in the pool that will cover about 20% of the total sessions. The aquatic environment offers many advantages, such as offering the opportunity of working in the absence of gravity, controlling weight-bearing progression, and introducing

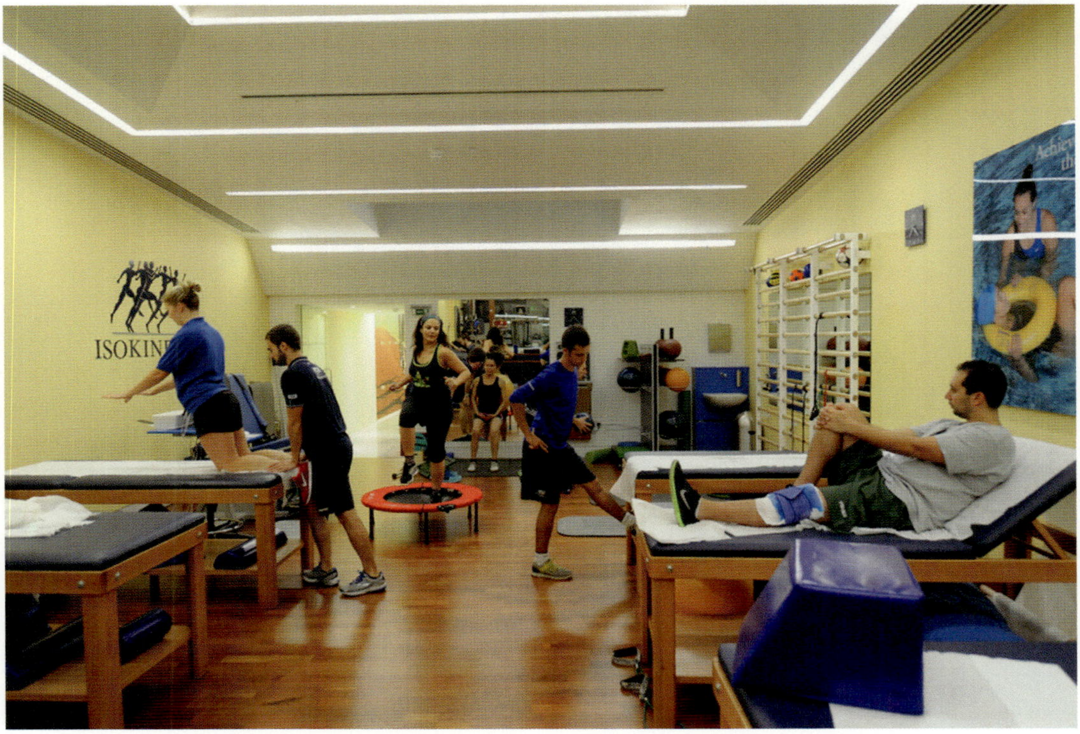

Fig. 51.1 Specific exercises performed in the gym

sport-specific movement patterns such as kicking or heading the ball. The sport field is the main facility of the last phase allowing patients to RTS.

The sport medicine team, tasked to follow the patient from the injury to RTS, consists of at least a sport medicine physician, a physiotherapist, and a reconditioning specialist. According to our method, the doctor acts as the "case manager" being in charge of the whole process. He/she plans the customized rehabilitation protocol, coordinates the team around the patient, and communicates regularly with the orthopedic surgeon. This multidisciplinary approach represents a gold standard for the recovery process. Close communication between surgical and rehabilitation team, and in the rehab team itself, is essential for successful recovery and RTS. Communication is crucial to explain the patient the goals of rehabilitation, to monitor his/her progression, and to be aware of complications.

51.2.4 Return to Sport Strategy

According to what is previously described (fourth traffic light), we allow the athlete to RTS only if certain criteria are completely satisfied. These criteria represent our RTS criteria, and we follow a potential strategy in order to accomplish each of them.

1. Recovery of muscular strength is certainly a milestone in rehabilitation, both in the literature and in our experience. Quadriceps femoris weakness is very common after ACLR and persists at long follow-up [35, 36]. We also know that strength weakness alters knee joint biomechanics and may lead to early osteoarthritis [37, 38]. It is indeed mandatory to reach the symmetry between the two limbs (100% both for extensor and flexor strength) evaluated with the isokinetic test (Fig. 51.2). In case of strength deficit, the test must be repeated until the complete recovery.

2. Metabolic recovery also plays a crucial role and has to be considered because fatigue leads to a potential risk of reinjury by altering the neuromuscular control [39]. We suggest checking aerobic and anaerobic lactate thresholds through specific tests (Fig. 51.3). Customized threshold training is subsequently proposed to guarantee a proper metabolic reconditioning. Before RTS the player has to reach the right values of aerobic and anaerobic threshold depending on the type of sport.

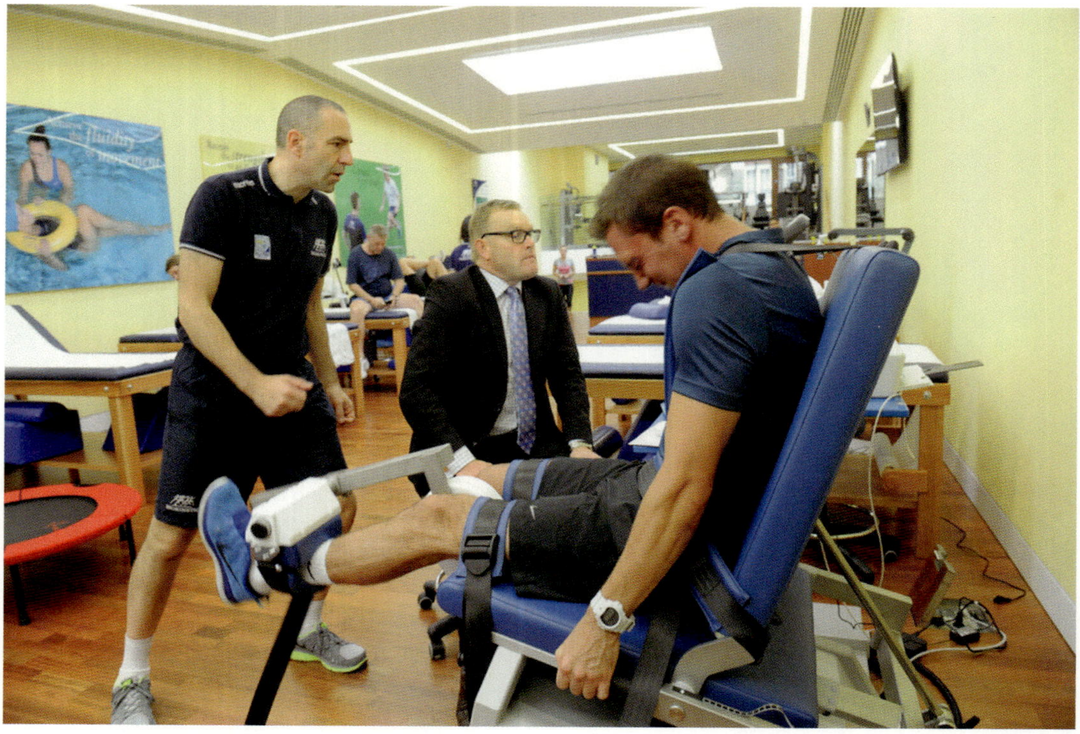

Fig. 51.2 The isokinetic test

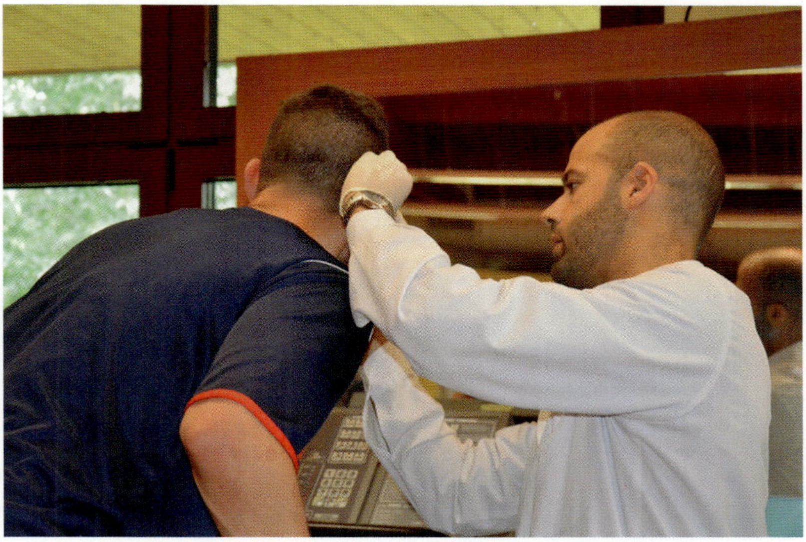

Fig. 51.3 The threshold test

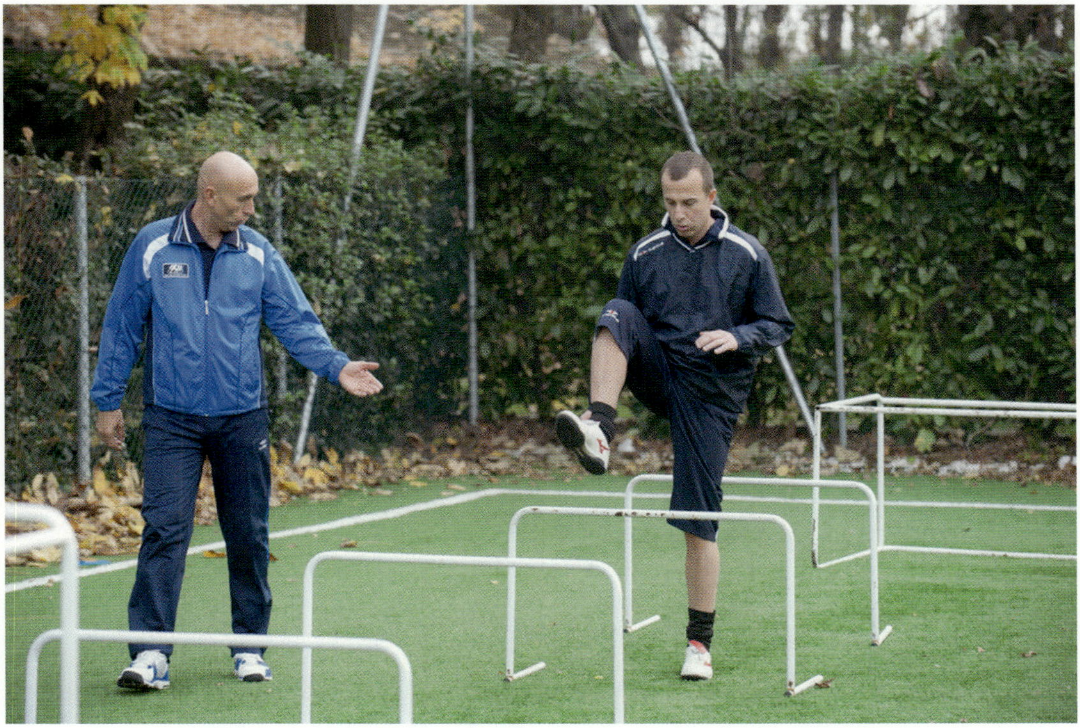

Fig. 51.4 The on-field rehabilitation

3. The on-field rehabilitation (OFR) is the most critical and important part of the recovery process. Sport-specific movements and drills are progressively reintroduced, and aerobic/anaerobic reconditioning is completed. Della Villa et al. demonstrated that a program of OFR allows earlier RTS without jeopardizing functional outcome at 5-year follow-up [40]. We also know that OFR may safely lead to complete functional recovery and return to sport [41]. The strategy we propose is to perform sport-specific supervised exercises both indoor (synthetic field) and outdoor (natural field) (Fig. 51.4). The protocol is progressive in terms of loading, complexity of

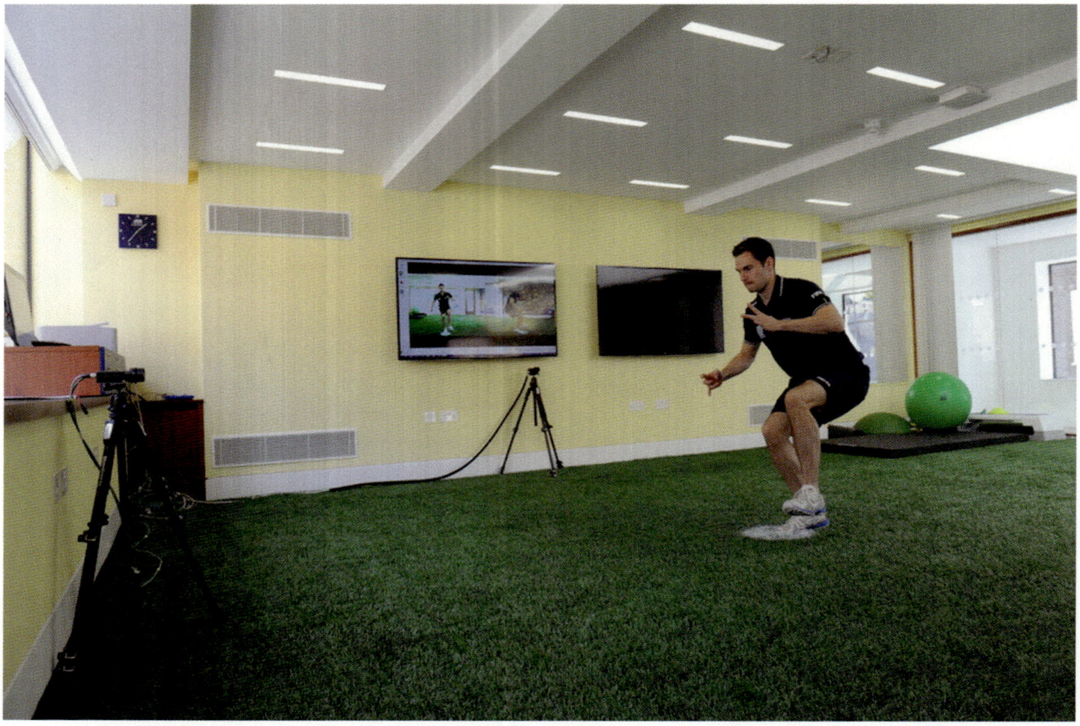

Fig. 51.5 Movement patterns evaluation

the proposed exercises, and velocity of the agility drills. Regarding the duration of the OFR, it mainly depends on the clinical issue.

4. Movement patterns restoration also needs to be pursued. We know that specific movement patterns are frequently associated with a certain type of injury. For example, a dynamic knee valgus may predict primary ACL injury, and altered neuromuscular control may predict second ACL injury after ACLR [42, 43]. These dangerous patterns have to be avoided in order to reduce the reinjury rate. Patients presenting with some kind of movement impairments need to be pro-habilitated to a more correct movement strategy. This is the main reason why we suggest performing a sport-specific movement analysis test (MAT) and correct the neuromuscular impairments (Fig. 51.5).

Apart from these well-established criteria, we know that prevention and psychological aspects are other "key points" in the modern rehabilitation landscape. The prevention concept should be early introduced in the recovery process: from the first specific intervention in the pool to the more specific neuromuscular programs to be performed on the field. The programs may be really effective in primary prevention, with a reduction up to 30% of injuries, in case of maximal compliance to the program [44]. Plus, educating the patient to a neuromuscular prevention program (to be performed at least three times a week) can be very effective in reducing the risk of reinjury. Psychological factors have been already studied; it seems that both fear (fear of reinjury and kinesiophobia) and innate personality traits play a role in the return to sport decision [45].

51.3 Quantitative Assessment

There have been numerous studies that focus more specifically on clinical measures to assess functional performance following ACL reconstruction. A recent systematic literature review found that concentric or isometric strength and the single-hop leg test for distance were most commonly used [46]. Myer et al. provided a more recent analysis on an athlete's single-limb performance using the single-limb symmetry index [47]. In their Level 3 case control study, single-limb vertical jump height and maximum vertical ground reaction force were measured on a portable force plate, but deficits were independent of time after reconstruction [47]. These measures can be difficult to extrapolate from the clinic to the playing field given the complexity of knee kinematics during athletic competition and considerations in regard to patient effort during clinical examination. Lentz et al. recently compared physical impairment and functional and psychosocial measures 6 months and 1 year following ACL reconstruction [48]. They found that elevated pain-related fear of movement and reinjury, quadriceps weakness, and reduced IKDC scores at 6 months post-op placing patients at risk for failure to return to sports at 1 year [48].

Reports in the early 1900s showed that the ACL also plays a role as a restraint to rotation of the knee [49]. Slocum and Larson first described a clinical examination that assessed rotatory knee stability [49]. Further work by Jakob and eventually Lemaire et al. on the basis of previous studies coined the term "pivot shift" to describe the anterolateral rotation laxity seen with ACL insufficiency [49]. This physical exam maneuver is characterized by abnormal anterior rotatory subluxation of the lateral tibial plateau when the medially rotated limb is under load in a few degrees of flexion. While still under load, spontaneous reduction occurs as the knee is flexed to 30° or 40°.

Despite a lack of standardization in the literature, the pivot shift is the most specific test to establish the diagnosis of ACL insufficiency before and after surgery [50–52]. On most occasions, pivot shift test grading in the clinic setting is subjective but used as an objective outcome tool to test dynamic laxity of the ACL. Standardizing the pivot shift test to improve inter-tester reliability has been the focus of recent work at our institution [53]. Several different approaches have been developed to assist in improving the pivot shift test: (1) measurement of knee laxity, (2) quantification of knee dynamics by acceleration, and (3) mechanization and instrumentation of the test [54]. A meta-analysis in 2012 found the KT-1000 arthrometer performed with maximum manual force has the highest sensitivity, specificity, accuracy, and positive predictive value for diagnosis of ACL rupture [26]. We utilize the KT-1000 arthrometer (MEDmetric Corporation) at our institution.

Improvements in measurement technology have allowed for quantification of dynamic knee motion with an electromagnetic motion tracking system. This permits characterization of the pivot shift by tibial anterior translation and/or tibial acceleration [54, 55]. The system (FASTRAK, Polhemus, Colchester, VT) at our institution uses an electromagnetic field with three receivers to measure the 6° of freedom of the knee at a high sampling rate (Fig. 51.6). To enhance repeatability, previous studies have shown that the pivot shift can be mechanized [56–58]. In the clinical setting, an examiner requires proprioceptive feedback to control the force and moment arm for each individual knee which introduces variability with regard to the examiner's unique testing maneuver. Standardized technique at our institution has been designed on the basis of the Galway and MacIntosh procedure [59]. A recent review described the most common torques used to simulate the pivot shift were 10-Nm valgus and 5-Nm internal rotation at 30 degrees of knee flexion [49]. However, great variability in technique remains, and no methodology can currently be defined as the gold standard. As such, further work is necessary before defining return to play criteria on the basis of the pivot shift maneuver.

51.3.1 Imaging Assessment

MRI has emerged as a powerful tool given its high sensitivity and specificity for diagnosis of ACL tears, graft tears, and associated injuries (Fig. 51.7). Our institutional protocol utilizes a 1.5-T magnet open-bore configuration (Magnetom Espree, Siemens Medical Solutions, Malvern, PA, USA) to image the ACL in multiple planes with different pulse sequences [60]. Clinical applications begin with preoperative

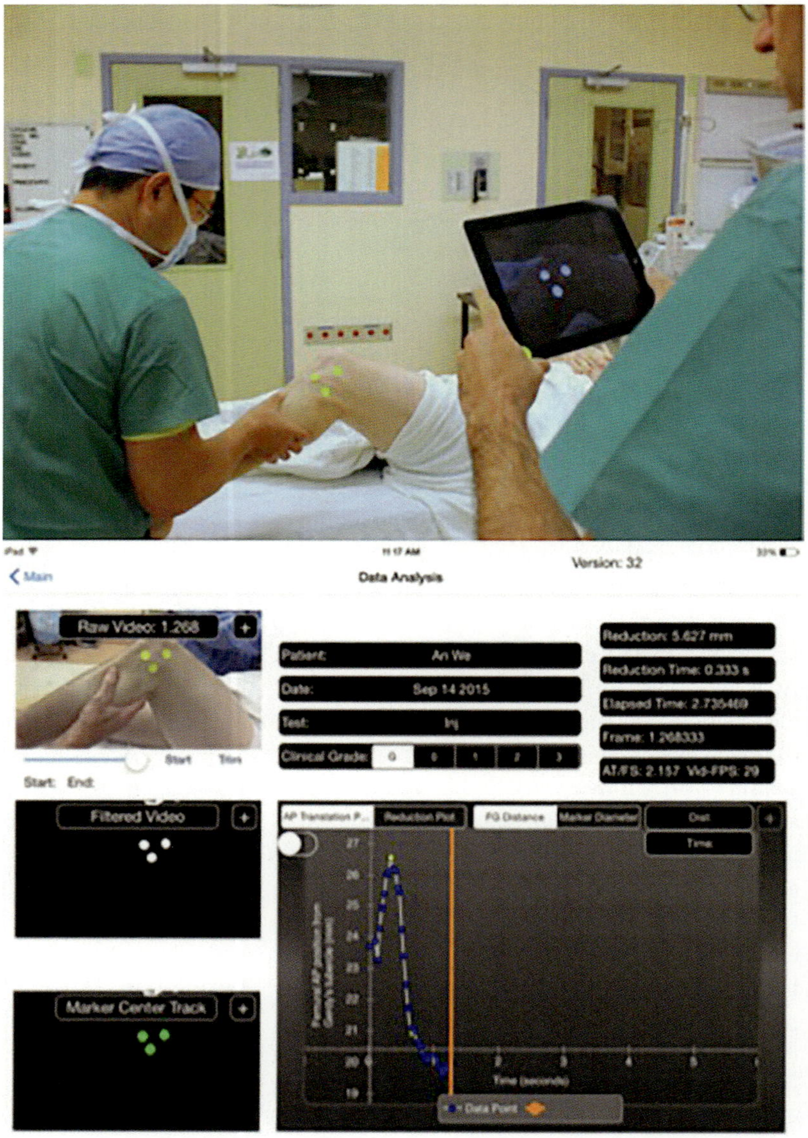

Fig. 51.6 Intraoperative pivot-shift measurements with electromagnetic motion trackers and quantification with iPad software

planning to define each athlete's unique bony morphology and ligamentous anatomy in an attempt to minimize the most common technical errors of reconstruction [60]. These errors can be critically evaluated with postoperative MRI in addition to assessment of ACL healing during the rehabilitation period [55].

Previous studies have focused on the process of graft healing and maturity or "ligamentization" and describe an early phase of increasing vascularity followed by remodeling and maturation phases [61, 62]. MRI evaluates this increase in vascularity during healing, which is represented by an increased signal in the graft and periligamentous tissues [63]. As the graft matures over time, MRI signal intensity on proton density (PD)-weighted sequences decreases [64]. Ntoulia et al. showed an increased in signal intensity at 6 months postoperative with no significant increase in signal by 12 months [64]. Contrast-enhanced studies have also been used to evaluate graft vascularity by calculating the enhancement index (ratio of signal-to-noise quotient [SNQ] before and after contrast) [65]. Autografts have been

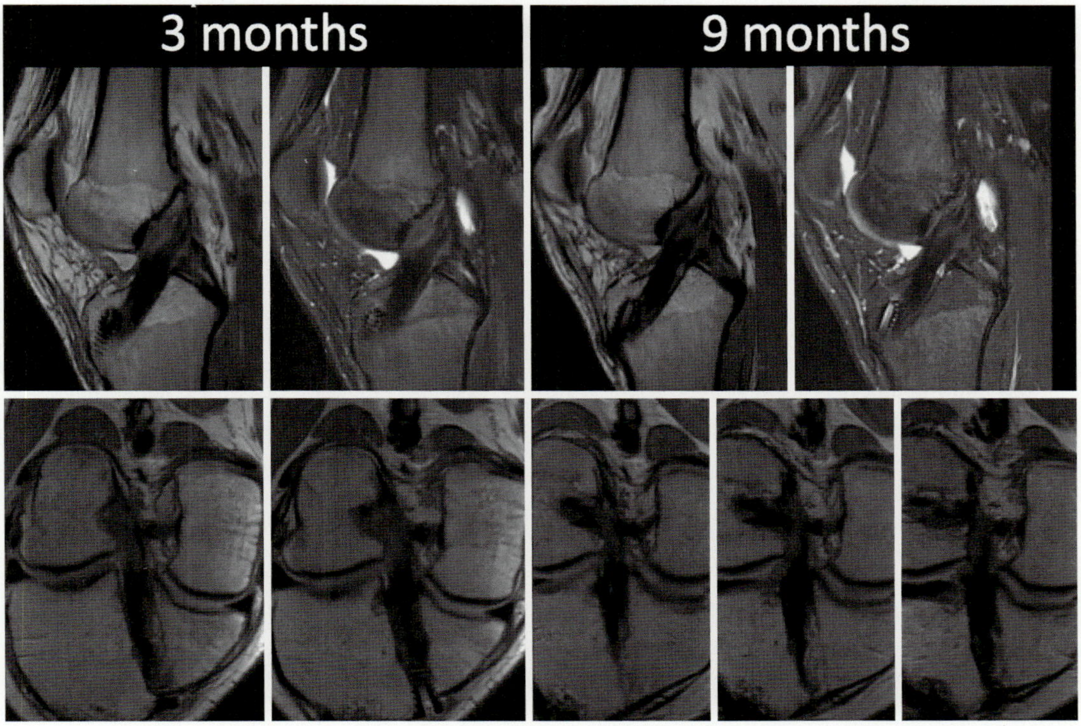

Fig. 51.7 Increased signal in ACL graft at 3 months postoperative signifies vascularity in the healing graft compared to 9 months postoperative

shown to reach peak revascularization 4–6 months after surgery, while allografts have increasing signal/noise quotient (SNQ) values 12–24 months after surgery, suggesting a slower onset and rate of revascularization [65, 66].

Variability in rates of return to play may suggest that graft healing necessary for the forces tolerated during sporting activity has not been achieved. Although signal intensity has shown promise, unrelated factors may confound interpretation such as graft impingement. One source of graft impingement is the posterior cruciate ligament, which contacts the ACL in approximately 25% of native knees [25]. Contact between the ACL graft and PCL, however, has been shown to occur in 75% of double-bundle reconstruction knees [25].

Maturation of the graft within the femoral and tibial tunnels appears to lag behind the intra-articular graft [64]. Cross-sectional imaging with MRI has been shown to be superior to plain radiographs in the assessment of tunnel healing [67]. Decreases in tunnel diameter on MRI have correlated with increased osteointegration and vascularity [67]. Sagittal oblique images, however, cannot fully visualize the boundary between the intra-femoral tunnel and intra-articular graft, and some believe coronal oblique images make evaluation of the entire course of the graft possible [68]. However, no consensus on graft visibility and prediction of graft maturation has been found, but new techniques independent of acquisition characteristics are currently being developed.

Conclusion

The current concept after ACLR is applying a criteria-based rehabilitation protocol, rather than respect prefixed times. Certain clinical and functional criteria have to be satisfied in order to progress throughout rehabilitation and to finally be allowed to RTS. The application of this kind of protocol must be emphasized to ensure optimal return to performance. Rehabilitation programs should be patient specific with respect to graft type and the biomechanical demands of an athlete's sport. In order to supplement serial examination of the postoperative athlete, new research into clinical tools and advances in imaging aim to provide objective benchmarks for safe return to play. Standardization of the pivot shift test may be a powerful tool in defining criteria for rehabilitation protocols, but further work is necessary at the current time. Correlation with serial MRI to evaluate surgical technique and graft healing may also assist with the clinical decision-making process, but no consensus in its utility has been established. The safe release of footballers to the training pitch should aim to minimize the risk of reinjury, but the scientific debate to determine the optimum time for return to sport is ongoing.

References

1. Aglietti P, Giron F, Buzzi R, Biddau F, Sasso F. Anterior cruciate ligament reconstruction: bone-patellar-bone compared with double semitendinosus and gracilis tendon graft. A prospective, randomized clinical trial. J Bone Joint Surg Am. 2004;86-A:2143–55.
2. Fithian D, Paxton E, Stone M, Luetzow WF, Csintalan RP, Phelan D, Daniel DM. Prospective trial of a treatment algorithm for the management of the anterior cruciate ligament-injured knee. Am J Sports Med. 2005;33:335–46.
3. Brukner P. Return to play – a personal perspective. Clin J Sport Med. 2005;15:459–60.
4. Yunes M, Richmond J, Engels E, Pinczewski LA. Patellar versus hamstring tendons in anterior cruciate ligament reconstruction: a meta-analysis. Arthroscopy. 2001;17:248–57.
5. Ardern C, Taylor N, Feller JA, Webster KE. Return-to-sport outcomes at 2 to 7 years after anterior cruciate ligament reconstruction surgery. Am J Sports Med. 2012;40:41–8.
6. Ardern CL, Taylor NF, Feller JA, Webster KE. Fifty-five percent return to competitive sport following anterior cruciate ligament reconstruction surgery: an updated systematic review and meta-analysis including aspects of physical functioning and contextual factors. Br J Sports Med. 2014;48:1543–52.
7. Erikson BJ, Harris JD, Cvetanovich GL, Bach BR, Bush-Joseph CA, Abrams GD, Gupta AK, McCormick FM, Cole BJ. Performance and return to sport after anterior cruciate ligament reconstruction in Male Major League Soccer players. Orthop J Sports Med. 2013;1:2325967113497189.
8. Shah VM, Andrews JR, Fleisig GS, McMichael CS, Lemak LJ. Return to play after anterior cruciate ligament reconstruction in National Football League athletes. Am J Sports Med. 2010;38:2233–9.
9. McCullough KA, Phelps KD, Spindler KP, Matava MJ, Dunn WR, Parker RD, MOON Group, Reinke EK. MOON Group: return to high school- and college-level football after anterior cruciate ligament reconstruction: a Multicenter Orthopaedic Outcomes Network (MOON) cohort study. Am J Sports Med. 2012;40:2523–9.
10. Wright RW, Magnussen RA, Dunn WR, Spindler KP. Ipsilateral graft and contralateral ACL rupture at five years or more following ACL reconstruction: a systematic review. J Bone Joint Surg Am. 2011;93(12):1159–65.
11. Shelbourne KD, Gray T, Haro HM. Incidence of subsequent injury to either knee within 5 years after anterior cruciate ligament reconstruction with patellar tendon autograft. Am J Sports Med. 2009;37:246–51.
12. Deehan D, Cawston T. The biology of integration of the anterior cruciate ligament. J Bone Joint SurgBr. 2005;87:889–95.
13. Johnson D, Swenson T, Irrgang J, Fu FH, Harner CD. Revision anterior cruciate ligament surgery: experience from Pittsburgh. Clin Orthop Relat Res. 1996;325:100–9.
14. van Eck C, Schkrohowsky J, Working Z, Irrgang JJ, Fu FH. Prospective analysis of failure rate and predictors of failure after anatomic anterior cruciate ligament reconstruction with allograft. Am J Sports Med. 2012;40:800–7.
15. Ekdahl M, Wang J, Ronga M, Fu F. Grafting healing in anterior cruciate ligament reconstruction. Knee Surg Sports Traumatol Arthrosc. 2008;16:935–47.
16. Peterson W, Laprell H. Insertion of autologous tendon grafts to the bone: a histological and immunohistochemical study of hamstring and patellar tendon grafts. Knee Surg Sports Traumatol Arthrosc. 2000;8:26–31.
17. Rodeo S, Kawamura S, Kim H, Dynybil C, Ying L. Tendon healing in a bone tunnel differs at the tunnel entrance versus the tunnel exit: an effect of graft-tunnel motion? Am J Sports Med. 2006;34:1790–800.
18. Anderson K, Seneviratne A, Izawa K, Atkinson BL, Potter HG, Rodeo SA. Augmentation of tendon healing in an intraarticular bone tunnel with use of a bone growth factor. Am J Sports Med. 2001;29:689–98.
19. Kyung H, Kim S, Oh C, Kim SJ. Tendon-to-bone tunnel healing in a rabbit model: the effect of periosteum augmentation at the tendon-to-bone interface. Knee Surg Sports Traumatol Arthrosc. 2003;11:9–15.
20. Martinek V, Latterman C, Usas A, Abramowitch S, Woo SL, Fu FH, Huard J. Enhancement of tendon-bone integration of anterior cruciate ligament graft with bone morphogenetic protein-2 gene transfer: a histological and biomechanic study. J Bone Joint Surg Am. 2002;84-A:1123–31.

21. Miyawaki M, Hensler D, Illingworth K, Irrgang JJ, Fu FH. Signal intensity on magnetic resonance imaging after allograft double-bundle anterior cruciate ligament reconstruction. Knee Surg Sports Traumatol Arthrosc. 2014;22:1002–8.
22. Biercevicz A, Akelman M, Fadale P, Hulstyn MJ, Shalvoy RM, Badger GJ, Tung GA, Oksendahl HL, Fleming BC. MRI volume and signal intensity of ACL graft predict clinical, functional, and patient-oriented outcome measures after ACL reconstruction. Am J Sports Med. 2015;43:693–9.
23. van Diek F, Wolf M, Murawski C, van Eck CF, Fu FH. Knee morphology and risk factors for developing an anterior cruciate ligament rupture: an MRI comparison between ACL-ruptured and non-injured knees. Knee Surg Sports Traumatol Arthrosc. 2014;22:987–94.
24. Vrooijjink S, Wolters F, van Eck C, et al. Measurements of knee morphometrics using MRI and arthroscopy: a comparative study between ACL-injured and non-injured subjects. Knee Surg Sports Traumatol Arthrosc. 2011;19:S12–6.
25. Kropf E, Shen W, van Eck C, et al. ACL-PCL and intercondylar notch impingement: magnetic resonance imaging of native and double-bundle ACL-reconstructed knees. Knee Surg Sports Traumatol Arthrosc. 2013;21:720–5.
26. van Eck C, Loopik M, van den Bekerom M. Methods to diagnose acute anterior cruciate ligament rupture: a meta-analysis of instrumented knee laxity tests. Knee Surg Sports Traumatol Arthrosc. 2013;21:1989–97.
27. Anderson A, Snyder R, Federspiel C, Lipscomb AB. Instrumented evaluation of knee laxity: a comparison of five arthrometers. Am J Sports Med. 1992;20:135–40.
28. Hoshino Y, Araujo P, Ahlden M, Moore CG, Kuroda R, Zaffagnini S, Karlsson J, Fu FH, Musahl V. Standardized pivot shift test improves measurement accuracy. Knee Surg Sports Traumatol Arthrosc. 2012;20:732–6.
29. Hoshino Y, Araujo P, Ahlden M, Samuelsson K, Muller B, Hofbauer M, Wolf MR, Irrgang JJ, Fu FH, Musahl V. Quantitative evaluation of the pivot shift by image analysis using the iPad. Knee Surg Sports Traumatol Arthrosc. 2013;21:975–80.
30. Adams D, Logerstedt DS, Hunter-Giordano A, Axe MJ, Snyder-Mackler L. Current concepts for anterior cruciate ligament reconstruction: a criterion-based rehabilitation progression. J Orthop Sports Phys Ther. 2012;42:601–14.
31. Kvist J. Rehabilitation following anterior cruciate ligament injury: current recommendations for sports participation. Sports Med. 2004;34:269–80.
32. Myer GD, Paterno MV, Ford KR, Quatman CE, Hewett TE. Rehabilitation after anterior cruciate ligament reconstruction: criteria-based progression through the return-to-sport phase. J Orthop Sports Phys Ther. 2006;36:385–402.
33. van Grinsven S, van Cingel RE, Holla CJ, van Loon CJ. Evidence-based rehabilitation following anterior cruciate ligament reconstruction. Knee Surg Sports Traumatol Arthrosc. 2010;18:1128–44.
34. Ellman MB, Sherman SL, Forsythe B, LaPrade RF, Cole BJ, Bach Jr BR. Return to play following anterior cruciate ligament reconstruction. J Am Acad Orthop Surg. 2015;23:283–96.
35. Palmieri-Smith RM, Thomas AC, Wojtys EM. Maximizing quadriceps strength after ACL reconstruction. Clin Sports Med. 2008;27:405–24.
36. Thomas AC, Villwock M, Wojtys EM, Palmieri-Smith RM. Lower extremity muscle strength after anterior cruciate ligament injury and reconstruction. J Athl Train. 2013;48:610–20.
37. Palmieri-Smith RM, Lepley LK. Quadriceps strength asymmetry after anterior cruciate ligament reconstruction alters knee joint biomechanics and functional performance at time of return to activity. Am J Sports Med. 2015;43:1662–9.
38. Tourville TW, Jarrell KM, Naud S. Relationship between isokinetic strength and tibiofemoral joint space width changes after anterior cruciate ligament reconstruction. Am J Sports Med. 2014;42:302–11.
39. McLean SG, Fellin RE, Suedekum N. Impact of fatigue on gender-based high-risk landing strategies. Med Sci Sports Exerc. 2007;39:502–14.
40. Della Villa S, Kon E, Filardo G, Ricci M, Vincentelli F, Delcogliano M, Marcacci M. Does intensive rehabilitation permit early return to sport without compromising the clinical outcome after arthroscopic autologous chondrocyte implantation in highly competitive athletes? Am J Sports Med. 2010;38:68–77.
41. Della Villa S, Boldrini L, Ricci M, Danelon F, Snyder-Mackler L, Nanni G, Roi GS. Clinical outcomes and return-to-sports participation of 50 soccer players after anterior cruciate ligament reconstruction through a sport-specific rehabilitation protocol. Sports Health. 2012;4:17–24.
42. Hewett TE, Myer GD, Ford KR, Heidt Jr RS, Colosimo AJ, McLean SG, et al. Biomechanical measures of neuromuscular control and valgus loading of the knee predict anterior cruciate ligament injury risk in female athletes: a prospective study. Am J Sports Med. 2005;33:492–501.
43. Paterno MV, Schmitt LC, Ford KR, Rauh MJ, Myer GD, Huang B, et al. Biomechanical measures during landing and postural stability predict second anterior cruciate ligament injury after anterior cruciate ligament reconstruction and return to sport. Am J Sports Med. 2010;38:1968–78.
44. Soligard T, Myklebust G, Steffen K, Holme I, Silvers H, Bizzini M, et al. Comprehensive warm-up program to prevent injuries in young female footballers: cluster randomized controlled trial. BMJ. 2008;337:a2469.
45. Tjong V, Murnaghan M, Nyhof-Young J, Ogilvie-Harris DJ. A qualitative investigation of the decision to return to sports after anterior cruciate ligament reconstruction: to play or not to play. Am J Sports Med. 2014;42:336–42.
46. Engelen-van Melick N, van Cingel RE, Tijssen MP. Nijhuis-van der Sanden MW. Assessment of

functional performance after anterior cruciate ligament reconstruction: a systematic review of measurement procedures. Knee Surg Sports Traumatol Arthrosc. 2012;21:869–79.
47. Myer G, Martin L, Ford K, Paterno MV, Schmitt LC, Heidt Jr RS. No association of time from surgery with functional deficits in athletes after anterior cruciate ligament reconstruction: evidence for objective return-to-sport criteria. Am J Sports Med. 2012;40:2256–63.
48. Lentz T, Zeppieri G, George S, Tillman SM, Moser MW, Farmer KW. Comparison of physical impairment, functional, and psychosocial measures based on fear of reinjury/lack of confidence and return-to-sports status after ACL reconstruction. Am J Sports Med. 2015;43:345–53.
49. Arilla F, Yeung M, Bell K, Rahnemai-Azar AA, Rothraff BB, Fu FH, et al. Experiemental execution of the simulated pivot-shift test: a systematic review of techniques. Arthroscopy. 2015;31(12):2245–54.
50. Benjaminse A, Gokeler A, van der Schans C. Clinical diagnosis of an anterior cruciate ligament rupture: a meta-analysis. J Orthop Sports Phys Ther. 2006;36:267–88.
51. Kocher M, Steadman J, Briggs K, Sterett WI, Hawkins RJ. Relationships between objective assessment of ligament stability and subjective assessment of symptoms and function after anterior cruciate ligament reconstruction. Am J Sports Med. 2004;32:629–34.
52. Leitze Z, Losee R, Jokl P, Johnson TR, Feagin JA. Implications of the pivot shift in the ACL-deficient knee. Clin Orthop Relat Res. 2005;436:229–36.
53. Musahl V, Hoshino Y, Ahlden M, Araujo P, Irrgang JJ, Zaffagnini S, et al. The pivot shift: a global user guide. Knee Surg Sports Traumatol Arthrosc. 2012;20:724–31.
54. Hoshino Y, Kuroda R, Nagamune K, Yagi M, Mizuno K, Yamaguchi M, et al. In vivo measurement of the pivot-shift test in the anterior cruciate ligament-deficient knee using an electromagnetic device. Am J Sports Med. 2007;35:1098–104.
55. Labbe D, de Guise J, Mezghani N, Godbout V, Grimard G, Baillargeon D, et al. Feature selection using a principal component analysis of the kinematics of the pivot shift phenomenon. J Biomech. 2010;43:3080–4.
56. Musahl V, Bedi A, Citak M, O'Loughlin P, Choi D, Pearle AD. Effect of single-bundle and double-bundle anterior cruciate ligament reconstructions on pivot-shift kinematics in anterior cruciate ligament- and meniscus-deficient knees. Am J Sports Med. 2011;39:289–95.
57. Musahl V, Citak M, O'Loughlin P, Choi D, Bedi A, Pearle AD. The effect of medial versus lateral meniscectomy on the stability of the anterior cruciate ligament-deficient knee. Am J Sports Med. 2010;38:1591–7.
58. Musahl V, Voos J, O'Loughlin P, Stueber V, Kendoff D, Pearle AD. Mechanized pivot shift test achieves greater accuracy than manual pivot shift test. Knee Surg Sports Traumatol Arthrosc. 2009;18:1208–13.
59. Galway H, MacIntosh D. The lateral pivot shift: a symptom and sign of anterior cruciate ligament insufficiency. Clin Orthop Relat Res. 1980;147:45–50.
60. Araujo P, van Eck C, Torabi M, Fu FH. How to optimize the use of MRI in anatomic ACL reconstruction. Knee Surg Sports Traumatol Arthrosc. 2013;21:1495–501.
61. Rabuck S, Barage M, Fu F. Anterior cruciate ligament healing and advances in imaging. Clin Sports Med. 2013;32:13–20.
62. Claes S, Verdonk P, Forsyth R, Bellemans J. The "ligamentization" process in anterior cruciate ligament reconstruction: what happens to the human graft? A systemic review of the literature. Am J Sports Med. 2011;39:2476–83.
63. Choi J, Ha J, Kim Y, Shim JC, Yang SJ, Kim JG. Relationships among tendon regeneration on MRI, flexor strength, and functional performance after anterior cruciate ligament reconstruction with hamstring autograft. Am J Sports Med. 2012;40:152–62.
64. Ntoulia A, Papadopoulou F, Ristanis S, Argyropoulou M, Georgoulis AD. Revascularization process of the bone-patellar tendon-bone autograft evaluated by contrast-enhanced magnetic resonance imaging 6 and 12 months after anterior cruciate ligament reconstruction. Am J Sports Med. 2011;39:1478–86.
65. Weiler A, Peters G, Maurer J, Unterhauser FN, Südkamp NP. Biomechanical properties and vascularity of an anterior cruciate ligament graft can be predicted by contrast-enhanced magnetic resonance imaging. A two-year study in sheep. Am J Sports Med. 2001;29:751–61.
66. Muramatsu K, Hachiya Y, Izawa H. Serial evaluation of human anterior cruciate ligament grafts by contrast-enhanced magnetic resonance imaging: comparison of allografts and autografts. Arthroscopy. 2008;24:1038–44.
67. Lajtai G, Schmiedhuber G, Unger F, Aitzetmüller G, Klein M, Noszian I, et al. Bone tunnel remodeling at the site of biodegradable interference screws used for anterior cruciate ligament reconstruction: 5-year follow-up. Arthroscopy. 2001;17:597–602.
68. Ma Y, Murawski C, Rahnemai-Azar A, Maldjian C, Lynch AD, Fu FH. Graft maturity of the reconstructed anterior cruciate ligament 6 months postoperatively: a magnetic resonance imaging evaluation of quadriceps tendon with bone block and hamstrings tendon autografts. Knee Surg Sports Traumatol Arthrosc. 2015;23:661–8.

Part XIII

Daily Medical Concerns in Football

Nutritional Guidelines for Football Players

52

António Pedro Mendes, Pedro Carvalho, and Vítor Hugo Teixeira

Contents

A.P. Mendes
Futebol Clube de Paços de Ferreira, Paços de Ferreira, Portugal

Food and Nutrition Department, Hospital Agostinho Ribeiro, Felgueiras, Portugal
e-mail: antoniopedrocm@gmail.com

P. Carvalho
Futebol Clube do Porto, Porto, Portugal

V.H. Teixeira (✉)
Futebol Clube do Porto, Porto, Portugal

Faculty of Nutrition and Food Sciences, University of Porto, Porto, Portugal

Research Centre on Physical Activity Health and Leisure, Faculty of Sport, University of Porto, Porto, Portugal
e-mail: vhugoteixeira@fcna.up.pt

52.1 Physiological Demands of Football

Football is an intermittent multiple-sprint sport characterized by repeated bouts of short duration high-intensity sprints in an endurance context that also requires the maintenance of skills throughout the match [1]. In a 90-min match, the distance covered by a football player ranges from 8 to 13 km, depending on factors like players' fitness level, field position, difficulty of the game, tactics of the team, and weather conditions [2–5]. The majority of the distance is covered by walking and low-intensity running, and it is mainly the high-intensity exercise periods that distinguish

J. Espregueira-Mendes et al. (eds.), *Injuries and Health Problems in Football*,
DOI 10.1007/978-3-662-53924-8_52

top-class players from the others. International top-class players perform 28% more high-intensity running (2.43 vs. 1.90 km) and 58% more sprinting (650 vs. 410 m) than professional players at a lower level [1]. Although players perform low-intensity activities for more than 70% of the game, heart rate and body temperature measurements suggest that average oxygen uptake for elite football players is around 70% of VO2Max with an estimated energy expenditure of 16 kcal/min [6, 7]. Since football players perform 150–250 brief, intense actions during a game [1], this indicates that the rate of anaerobic energy turnover is high during periods of a game. Even though this has not been studied directly, intense exercise during a game would lead to a high rate of creatine phosphate breakdown, which to a great extent is resynthesized in the following low-intensity exercise periods [7, 8]. The energy substrate utilized during a football match is mainly glycogen, as seen by the depletion of glycogen in some muscle fibers that could be related to fatigue toward the end of the game [9]. In high-intensity activities, such as sprints and jumps, glycogen contributes approximately 50% to ATP turnover, and the repeated sprint activity that characterizes a football match leads to a reduction in glycogen concentrations, which in turn may impair performance in the latter stages of a match [10]. In one study employing Loughborough Intermittent Shuttle Test (LIST), a protocol mimicking the demands of team sports like football, the authors found a significant reduction in muscle glycogen concentrations from before to after exercise, both in type I and type II muscle fibers [11]. A study employing the Copenhagen Soccer Test (CST) [10] found similar results: type I and type II muscle fibers exhibited significant glycogen depletion, with ~80% of fibers being completely or almost depleted (<200 mmol/kg d.w) of glycogen after 90 min of intermittent activity. These low concentrations have been shown to decrease the glycolytic rate [8]. Type II fibers seem to be the main responsible for decreases in performance when their glycogen content is low [12]. Furthermore, the depletion of muscle glycogen in the sarcoplasmic reticulum results in reductions in muscle calcium handling [13], compromising the contractile property of the muscle [14].

Fat oxidation appears to increase progressively during a game, partially compensating for the progressive lowering of muscle glycogen. Increased levels of triglycerides might occur in the second half due to elevated catecholamine concentrations. The decline in blood lactate concentration associated to an increase in plasma free fatty acids during the game confirms the change in substrate utilization during the game [8, 9].

52.2 Fatigue

Match-related fatigue is determined by a combination of central and peripheral factors. The decline in performance observed at the end of a match arises from a combination of several factors involving mechanisms from the central nervous system to the muscle cell itself and energy production [15]. Fatigue in football seems to occur at three different stages in the game: (1) after short-term intense periods in both halves, (2) in the initial phase of second half, and (3) toward the end of the game [16]. The first two stages are not directly related to nutrition issues, but fatigue at the end of the game is associated with low glycogen concentrations in a considerable number of muscle fibers.

Data from the 2014/15 Italian Serie A, English Premier League, and Spanish La Liga shows that the final 15 min of a match is the period when more goals occur and that top teams always have a better goal difference [17]. Then, it seems crucial to optimize nutritional strategies in order to reduce fatigue and maintain physical and technical performance throughout the match. In this context, it seems well established that high carbohydrate intake in order to maximize glycogen storage is a crucial strategy to enhance performance in a football match.

52.3 Carbohydrate

Carbohydrate and fat are the main fuels for training and competition, and its relative contribution to energy demands depends on several factors, such as pre-exercise carbohydrate storage, exercise frequency, intensity and duration, or even athletes' training status [18]. Since carbohydrate availability to muscle and central nervous system can be compromised when the cost of the exercise exceeds endogenous carbohydrate storage, provision of additional carbohydrate may be crucial to enhance performance in high-intensity sports [19].

Carbohydrate daily intake necessary to recover from daily training sessions depends on its intensity and duration, and it must be carefully estimated. Louise Burke and colleagues defined, in 2011, general recommendations for carbohydrate intake for daily training recovery [20]. For a highly active athlete (e.g., moderate-to-high-intensity exercise of 1–3 h/day), a 6–10 g/kg/day carbohydrate intake must be achieved. The large interval provided covers many exercise durations and intensities, and these general recommendations should be fine-tuned with individual consideration of total energy expenditure, specific training needs, and feedback from training performance [20].

52.3.1 Pre-exercise Carbohydrate Intake

For events lasting longer than 90 min of sustained/intermittent exercise, Burke et al. recommend a carbohydrate-loading strategy, consisting on a carbohydrate intake of 10–12 g/kg/day for 36–48 h [20]. It is important to choose compact carbohydrate-rich sources, low in fiber and residues, in order to meet fuel targets without compromising gut comfort. Carbohydrate loading can enhance performance of prolonged team games involving repeated high-intensity sprints, such as football [21]. Regarding the precompetitive meal, the recommendations target an intake of 1–4 g/kg of carbohydrates 1–4 h before game [22].

Consuming a carbohydrate-rich meal in the hour before a game is still a matter of debate. Most recent studies conclude that there is no effect of pre-exercise (<60 min) carbohydrate feeding on performance [23]. Furthermore, some studies claim the development of hypoglycemia in some athletes. In these individuals, it is important to plan meals in order not to develop this condition. Some options include choosing low glycaemic index (GI) carbohydrates, ingesting carbohydrate just before exercise or during a warm-up, or avoiding carbohydrate in the 90 min before exercise altogether [23].

52.3.2 Carbohydrate During a Match

The consumption of carbohydrate during a match represents an effective way of providing exogenous fuel to the muscle and central nervous system [23]. Several studies have shown a performance enhancement when carbohydrates are consumed prior and during exercise, not only in physical performance [24, 25] but also in football-related skills, such as passing, dribbling, and shooting [26–28].

Strategies providing 60 g of carbohydrate per hour seem to be effective in a football game, but it can be modified according to players' preferences. Bars, chews, gels, or drinks are effective ways for providing carbohydrate during the game [29]. Although some sports allow frequent ingestion of carbohydrate during a game, football limits the opportunity to ingest carbohydrate. Therefore, the minutes before the game and the half-time period are crucial to meet the recommendations [30].

There is accumulating evidence that the benefit from carbohydrate consumptions is due to a central effect as well. Actually, carbohydrate mouth rinse seems to improve performance during moderate- to high-intensity exercise (~60–75% VO2max), of at least 1 h duration [31]. The mechanism is probably neural, via oral receptors that activate brain regions related to the sensation of reward and pleasure. The sweetness of carbohydrate (CHO) does not influence the activation of the oral receptors [32].

52.3.3 Carbohydrate for Recovery

After exercise, timing and amount of carbohydrate consumption depend on several factors, such as the recovery period. With less than 8 h between exercise sessions, it is recommended a carbohydrate ingestion of 1.0–1.2 g/kg/h. for the first 4 h, in order to maximize glycogen synthesis [20]. The consumption of moderate to high glycemic index foods post exercise is recommended, although a recent study showed no differences in 5 km time trial performance 3 h after a low or a high glycemic index meal, consumed after a glycogen-depleting exercise [33]. When there is a large recovery period between two exercise sessions, meal frequency and carbohydrate intake are not so relevant.

Adding protein to these meals may enhance glycogen synthesis, especially when carbohydrate intake isn't high enough [20].

52.4 Hydration in Football

In a sport played outdoor like football, dehydration can have a negative impact on performance, especially when combined with heat stress. Although some individuals may be more or less sensitive to dehydration, the level generally accepted that is capable to induce performance degradations approximates >2% decrease in body mass [34]. In a football practice or match, dehydration values from 0.5% to 3.4% of body mass loss were reported [35], with higher losses being associated with temperatures from 27 °C [3] to 35 °C [36]. Data concerning dehydration and football performance is relatively scarce and inconclusive. Higher Ratings of Perceived Exertion (RPE) and slower sprint times at the end of LIST as well as a decrease of 5% on dribbling skills were observed with dehydration of 2.5% compared with 1.4% [37]. More recently after a LIST protocol, football skills and intermittent high-intensity exercise performance were similar with 2.5%, 1.1% and 0.3% of dehydration [38]. When another exercise protocol was used (Yo-Yo Intermittent Recovery Test), dehydration by 2.4% led to an increase in RPE and to a lower performance compared to 0.7% [39]. Interestingly, in this study, when players washed their mouths with plain water in a volume corresponding to 2 ml/kg body mass, without swallowing the fluid, mouth rinse resulted in 2.1% dehydration but also reduced the total distance run by the football players during the Yo-Yo Test.

Even with conflicting data, it is prudent to assess hydration status of players and try to avoid body mass losses above 2%, especially when it is known that football players start a practice or match play already in a dehydrated state, probably as a result of cumulative dehydration from previous training practices [36]. Moreover, the intake of sports beverages during a match can supply an additional source of carbohydrates, very useful in players that do not initiate the game with glycogen stores completely full.

52.5 Nutritional Interventions to Improve Skills Performance

Although the vast majority of studies regarding nutritional interventions have focused on physical performance, the possible impact of nutrition on technical performance (commonly known as skills) has become a matter of interest for the scientific community.

The results altogether are somewhat equivocal, but it seems evident that skill performance is affected by some factors which might threaten homeostasis, such as fatigue [40, 41], dehydration [42], and reductions in blood glucose concentrations [20]. The most important skills in a football match are passing and dribbling, due to its frequency, and shooting, due to its ability to decide the final result [43, 44]. The second half of a football match is usually associated with a decrease in technical skills, particularly in passing and shooting [45], with total possession and total ball distribution also suffering a reduction [41]. Proficiency in match-related skills might be even more important than high-intensity activity. A study with Premier League players found that overall technical and tactical effectiveness of the team rather than high levels of physical performance per se is a more important success determinant in football [46].

52.5.1 Carbohydrate

Although there is a lot of evidence on carbohydrate and physical performance, only a few studies evaluated its effect on football-specific technical performance. The majority of these studies used a 6–8% carbohydrate beverage before and during the exercise to investigate its effects on skills during a match simulation, and some were able to find an improved performance in dribbling [28, 47], shooting [26, 28, 48], and passing [27].

Based on the available studies, it is hard to determine an optimal dose of carbohydrate to enhance technical performance, and it remains to be determined if the current recommendations for carbohydrate intake are optimal for preservation of skills that require cognitive input. However, following the recommendations of some authors, exogenous carbohydrate intake must exceed a rate of 50 g/h [27], but the amount associated with an improvement in performance varies according to the skill observed [26].

It remains unclear whether reductions in blood glucose concentrations lead to decreased technical performance, as the influence of rebound hypoglycemia has only been studied from a physical perspective. As the glycemic response to a subsequent bout of exercise appears to be independent of carbohydrate dose [49], and high glycemic index carbohydrate intake appears to blunt rebound hypoglycemic responses [50], the provision of additional carbohydrates may enhance technical performance, particularly in the latter stages of a match.

In all studies examining carbohydrate and technical performance the mode of carbohydrate administration was a beverage, given before and during the match. Although absorption at the lower gastrointestinal tract is important to elicit carbohydrate effects on performance, carbohydrate mouth rinse without ingestion has been shown to elicit ergogenic effects [31]. In a recent review, 9 out of 11 studies regarding carbohydrate mouth rinse showed an increased performance (range from 1.50% to 11.59%) during moderate to high-intensity exercise (~75% Wmax or 65% VO2max, ~1 h duration) [31]. However, investigations on mouth rinse and football skill performance are lacking.

High carbohydrate intake several hours before a match has already been studied. In a recent study [51], football players fed with a high carbohydrate (8 g/kg body mass [BM]) diet for 3.5 days before a match had more favorable score lines than players with a low carbohydrate intake (3 g/kg BM) diet. However, a previous study [52] observed no benefit of a high carbohydrate diet (8 g/kg BM) for 48 h on shooting and dribbling performance. Further investigation is needed to understand the possible impact of high carbohydrate intake several hours before a match on technical performance, acknowledging the fact that a high carbohydrate diet 1–2 days before the match could be beneficial in muscle glycogen loading, decreasing the possibility of fatigue due to glycogen depletion toward the game.

52.5.2 Fluids

Studies regarding hydration status and technical performance are scarce and not clear. In athletes who did not ingest fluids during a 90 min match simulation, performance was deteriorated by 5% ($P < 0.05$), when compared with athletes who ingested fluids [37]. Mean heart rate, perceived exertion, serum aldosterone, osmolality, sodium, and cortisol responses during the test were also higher ($P < 0.05$) in dehydrated athletes. A study by Ali et al. [26] also showed a decrease in post-exercise shooting performance when athletes did not properly replace fuel or electrolytes during a 90 min exercise test. It is important to notice that these athletes were in a fasted and energy-depleted state.

Although the results from these studies show the importance of ingesting fluids, the conditions did not mimic real-life usual practices, and the effects of dehydration upon technical performances in football players remain unclear.

52.6 Nutritional Intake

Based on studies assessing physiological demands of football players, specific nutritional recommendations have been developed. In order to evaluate the adequacy of nutrient and energy intake in these athletes, some studies tried to analyze it using food records (weighed or estimated), food frequency questionnaires, and other less detailed methods.

52.6.1 Energy Intake and Expenditure

Most of the available investigation on energy expenditure and intake focused on adolescent and young adult football players. Overviewing available studies with accurate methodologies, we observe that energy intake is higher for male players in comparison to their female counterparts. In male adult players, two studies [53, 54] found different energy intakes: in a fourth division junior team [53], energy intake was 3030 ± 141 kcal/day, and in a first division junior team [54], it was 2796.4 ± 525 kcal/day. When assessing female players, several studies found energy intakes ranging from 1904 ± 366 kcal/day in English international players [55] to 2291 ± 310 kcal/day in American National Collegiate Athletic Association (NCAA) Division I [56].

Although higher-energy intakes are expected in men due to differences in body composition and other physiological parameters, some studies suggest that underreporting is higher in women [57, 58].

52.6.2 Carbohydrates

Most studies have reported daily CHO intakes lower than those recommended. This is somewhat surprising given the well-documented and disseminated importance of an adequate carbohydrate ingestion to maximize performance. Both fourth and first Spanish division junior teams reported mean carbohydrate intakes lower than 5 g/kg BM (4.57 ± 0.2 and 4.7 ± 1.1, respectively) [53, 54]. These intakes are lower than those recommended by Burke et al. [20].

It is necessary to understand at which extent does low to moderate carbohydrate ingestion may negatively affect performance, although it is well established the performance benefits when carbohydrate intake is high before a football match.

52.6.3 Protein

Protein needs of athletes seem to be higher than the recommended for sedentary individuals due to their potential to enhance strength, but also to provide a supply of amino acids for an increased amino acid oxidation that may occur during training and competition [59]. Many factors need to be considered when determining an optimal amount of dietary protein for exercising individuals. These factors include protein quality, energy, and carbohydrate intake, mode and intensity of exercise, and the timing of protein intake. In a review focusing on football players, the recommendation for protein intake was 1.4–1.7 g/kg [60]. Nevertheless, protein intake of adult football players typically ranges from 1.5 to 1.8 g/kg, for males, and 1.2 to 1.4 g/kg, for females [59].

These intakes are lower than the recommended in females and adequate or slightly higher in males. Timing of ingestion [61] and quality of protein intake [62] must also be considered when evaluating protein needs and outline nutritional strategies to enhance performance.

52.6.4 Fat

The dietary reference intakes set an acceptable macronutrient distribution range (AMDR) of fat as 20–35% of total calories from fat. Some authors have suggested football players to ingest <30% of total energy intake in the form of fat. In a 2009 review from the American College of Sports Medicine, athletes in general are advised to consume fats within the AMDR of 20–35% of total calories [63].

Several studies in male football players reported fat intakes over 30% [53, 54, 64], with a Spanish first division junior team reporting consumption of 37 ± 5% of energy intake from fat [54]. These values are higher than most recommendations and may limit the likelihood of achieving carbohydrate intake recommendations. Most studies regarding female athletes intake show fat intakes between 24% and 30% of total daily energy intake, although a study in Spanish teams showed a fat contribution of 37 ± 7% [65].

The proportion of dietary fatty acids and ratio n6:n3 are major factors when assessing fat intake, but only a few studies presented values for saturated, monounsaturated, and polyunsaturated fatty acids [53, 65, 66]. From the analysis of the available literature, both male and female football players consume more saturated fat than recommended (<10% of total energy intake).

The majority of studies conducted have revealed a nutritional intake pattern quite different from recommendations. There is a need to improve information availability and assure the presence of a nutritionist/dietitian in football clubs, so that nutrition intervention programs can be implemented, leading to a health and performance optimization.

52.7 Body Composition in Football

Monitoring body composition in football athletes is a very important issue and it should be performed regularly. Reported values for percent of body fat for elite football players range from 7% to 19%, estimated by skinfold equations [67]. Recently, reference values for body composition and anthropometric measures were created in Portuguese elite athletes, and the mean value for the sum of 7 skinfolds (triceps, subscapular, biceps, suprailiac, abdominal, thigh, and medial calf) was 105.5 mm in females and 58.1 mm in male footballers. Regarding body fat assessed by dual-energy X-ray absorptiometry (DXA), the mean value for male athletes was 12.1%. [68]. These values have to be framed into players' position, since goalkeepers tend to have a little more weight and body fat than other positions [69, 70]. Beyond that, the nature of effort associated to different playing positions can modify the recommended values of players' optimal body fat levels. At this regard, wide midfielders, central midfielders, fullbacks, and attackers usually cover a greater distance in high-intensity running than central defenders and could benefit from lower values of body fat [71]. It was also reported that midfielders have higher values of relative oxygen consumption, maximal heart rate, maximal running speed, and blood lactate than other positions, a physiological profile that is also associated with lower levels of body fat [70].

Although the international status of the players is not always associated with lower body fat values [69], top team players regularly have less fat and better physiological values (higher peak torque of knee extensors, running velocity at lactate threshold, and vertical jump height) in comparison to the middle and last teams of the league [72].

Ethnicity can also interfere in body composition analysis, since non-Caucasian athletes tend to have lower body fat levels [69]. Moreover, some skinfold prediction equations [73] have race as a predictor variable with total body decreasing 2–2.5% in African athletes compared to Caucasian ones.

Methods for body composition assessment will differ greatly depending on the club and the resources at its disposal. Anthropometry is a quick, relatively inexpensive, and reliable method to perform field measurements. Presenting the data as sum of skinfolds is more accurate, since it is not dependent of the equation chosen to predict body fat, but most of the times players and coaches want to know body fat percentage. At this regard, the last equation developed by Reilly et al. [67] explained 78.4% of variance in DXA. This study also showed that seven-site skinfold equation of Withers et al. [74] was the most accurate and highly correlated with DXA-derived body fat percentage. One advantage of these two equations is the incorporation of lower-body skinfold sites, since, due to loading pattern and lower-body dominance of football, it would be expected that the density of the lower limb mineral compartment increases in football players as well as muscular development, particularly the hip flexors, quadriceps, hamstrings, and ankle flexors [75]. Beyond that, a study found that anterior thigh skinfold has the highest single-skinfold correlation with DXA-determined body fat and the combination of the thigh and calf skinfolds explained more variance in body fat percentage than Durnin and Womersley's sum of 4 skinfolds equation [76]. This data reveals the importance of choosing an equation that evaluates lower-body skinfold sites, since they are more highly related to percent fat in healthy individuals than upper-body sites.

The utilization of DXA has been disseminated at elite clubs, providing an accurate assessment of fat mass, bone mineral content, and lean mass. DXA is a quick and easy to perform method and provides a precise and attractive data feedback to players [77].

52.8 Practical Nutritional Considerations in Football

Nutrition is a key factor in elite athletes' performance. Nowadays, a football season at elite level has more than 50 games, with a lot of sequences of 2 or even 3 games per week. Then, an appropriate diet is crucial to optimize match to match recovery but also to promote training adaptations. In elite football, the weekly training load is highly variable according to the number of games. In Premier League, the distance covered in training was lower in a three-game week versus one- and two-game weeks, though accumulative weekly distance was higher (35.5 ± 2.4 km), and players spent more time in speed zones >14.4 km/h [78]. So, it is certain that high carbohydrate availability is crucial to improve physical match performance, but a consistent high carbohydrate intake also attenuates molecular pathways regulating training adaptation. Thus, one of the most important practical considerations regarding nutrition in football is to periodize carbohydrate intake according to weekly training and match schedules. This could be done by offering high protein-moderate carb meals (milk, yogurts, eggs, low fat cheese, nuts, oatmeal, and whole-grains) and water as beverage option during training, in the initial days of the week, and increasing the carbohydrate availability (fruit and fruit juices, cereal bars, jam/honey sandwiches, oats) and sports drinks during training, in the day before the game. Regarding the precompetitive meal, it is not easy for most of the athletes to accomplish the recommendations (1–4 g/kg) [22], so it is very important to provide some examples of menus and adequate amount of food necessary. The club nutritionist has to be aware that in this meal the main goal is to maximize carbohydrate intake with the less possible volume of food to minimize abdominal discomfort and constraint, particularly because some athletes get nervous and anxious before the games and lose appetite.

The meal after the training session comprises an excellent opportunity to provide to athletes the nutrients needed to optimize recovery and to improve their nutritional status, since, most of the times, the other meals during the day are not supervised by the club. In this context, a recovery snack/drink is a good option following intensive, prolonged, or resistance exercise. Protein intake immediately after training guarantees a source of amino acids for muscle growth and repair. In particular, leucine appears to be an important amino acid to trigger muscle protein synthesis and adaptation [79], and current research suggests that 20–25 g protein is required in the "recovery" meal or beverage [80]. Although a lot of food combinations can be provided to accomplish these recommendations, just 1 scoop of whey protein is sufficient to provide ~2–2.5 g of leucine and 20–25 g of protein, with the advantage of players could choose the flavor and personalize their post-workout recovery drink. Beyond protein, carbohydrate needs can begin to be met simultaneously. Maltodextrins or other high glycemic index carbohydrates could be options if it is urgent to replenish liver and muscle glycogen stores, but fruit could be a very good option in this context. Particularly fruits with high amounts of phytochemicals and subsequent high antioxidant activity like cherries, pomegranate, and blueberries [81] could be a good strategy to improve players' recovery and antioxidant status. The post-workout recovery drink could also be a good way to incorporate other nutrients with a possible positive impact in players' performance like creatine, vitamin D, and n-3 fatty acids [82, 83].

52.8.1 Dietary Planning

Elite clubs are composed by players of different countries and beliefs about food. Besides food allergies/intolerances, the cultural idiosyncrasies of the players have to be taken into account when planning a menu. The provision of several options in a meal buffet is essential to guarantee that all the players are comfortable with their choice since the meals before a game should be a pleasant moment with no additional stress due to player's rejection of food options. Some specific strategies could be employed to increase the athlete's knowledge and acceptance of food:

- Soups should be served by the hotel/restaurant staff upon approval of each athlete. This procedure is much more effective in the increase of soup intake than only putting the soup pot in the buffet line
- All the foods in the buffet should be labeled with nutritional and allergens information
- The buffet layout should be managed accordingly with the nutritional priorities for the meal, since players tend to fill the plate with the first options of the buffet. In a precompetitive meal, the first options could be rich in carbohydrates (rice, pasta, potatoes, mixed carb salads), but in regular meals the buffet could start with vegetables and protein dishes, leaving the carbohydrate options for last
- Vegetable options should comprise both raw (salad) and cooked (steamed or sautéed vegetables), with different colors and textures to increase players' acceptability
- The main dish should comprise a different fish and meat option and an alternative, like spaghetti Bolognese or spaghetti with tuna, since these are regularly well accepted
- The dessert should include an easy to eat fruit option (sliced fruit, fruit salad) to increase players' acceptance and sometimes a low fat sweet alternative (baked apple, fruit crepe, etc.)

Beyond these "rules," it is also very important to hear player and staff feedback and to involve themselves in the process, asking them about their preferences and the new dishes they would like to see on the menus.

Regarding hydration issues, the use of urine color charts in bathrooms and locker rooms is an effective way to promote correct drinking habits, encouraging athletes to have a clear to light yellow (lemonade) urine. Urine specific gravity is also a good and quick method to assess hydration status, with values above 1.020 g/ml indicating dehydration. The evaluation of body mass changes during training and match play in different environmental conditions to determine individual sweating rates allows the identification of the players with poor drinking habits and consequently in a higher risk of dehydration. This method has also the advantage of individualize the hydration strategy for each player. It is also important to identify the "salty sweaters" of the team, through simple indicators like sweat that stings in the eyes or burns in an open cut, sweat that tastes salty, and gritty-feeling skin. In these players, some electrolyte powder or capsules could be incorporated in their personal sports beverage.

Conclusion

Nutrition is a strategic and crucial area in team sports and should be integrated in a multidisciplinary support team at a club. It is very important to reinforce that only with a full harmony in nutrition policy between coaches, physiologists, doctors, physiotherapists, and nutritionists, the message could be effectively transmitted to players. Food and sports nutrition is a very complex topic with a lot of (mis) information sources, and athletes are every day more interested in nutrition issues, so it is vital to have a nutritionist in the team not only to intervene directly with players in order to improve their body composition but also to define the nutrition policy of the team and the supplementation schemes and to elaborate the menus for precompetitive meals.

References

1. Mohr M, Krustrup P, Bangsbo J. Match performance of high-standard soccer players with special reference to development of fatigue. J Sports Sci. 2003;21(7):519–28.
2. Da Silva RP, Mündel T, Natali AJ, Bara Filho MG, Alfenas RC, Lima JR, Belfort FG, Lopes PR, Marins JC. Pre-game hydration status, sweat loss, and fluid intake in elite Brazilian young male soccer players during competition. J Sports Sci. 2012;30(1):37–42.

3. Duffield R, McCall A, Coutts AJ, Peiffer JJ. Hydration, sweat and thermoregulatory responses to professional football training in the heat. J Sports Sci. 2012;30(10): 957–65.
4. Maughan RJ, Watson P, Evans GH, Broad N, Shirreffs SM. Water balance and salt losses in competitive football. Int J Sport Nutr Exerc Metab. 2007; 17(6):583–94.
5. Mohr M, Nybo L, Grantham J, Racinais S. Physiological responses and physical performance during football in the heat. PLoS One. 2012;7(6): e39202.
6. Bangsbo J, Mohr M, Krustrup P. Physical and metabolic demands of training and match-play in the elite football player. J Sports Sci. 2006;24(7):665–74.
7. Bangsbo J. Physiological demands of football. Sports Sci Exch. 2014;125:1–6.
8. Bangsbo J. The physiology of soccer – with special reference to intense intermittent exercise. Acta Physiol Scand Suppl. 1994;619:1–155.
9. Krustrup P, Mohr M, Steensberg A, Bencke J, Kjaer M, Bangsbo J. Muscle and blood metabolites during a soccer game: implications for sprint performance. Med Sci Sports Exerc. 2006;38(6):1165–74.
10. Bendiksen M, Bischoff R, Randers MB, Mohr M, Rollo I, Suetta C, Bangsbo J, Krustrup P. The Copenhagen Soccer Test: physiological response and fatigue development. Med Sci Sports Exerc. 2012; 44(8):1595–603.
11. Nicholas CW, Nuttall E, Williams C. The Loughborough Intermittent Shuttle Test: a field test that simulates the activity pattern of soccer. J Sports Sci. 2000;18:97–104.
12. Greenhaff PL, Nevill ME, Soderlund K, Bodin K, Boobis LH, Williams C, Hultman E. The metabolic responses of human type I and II muscle fibres during maximal treadmill sprinting. J Physiol. 1994;478: 149–55.
13. Nielsen J, Holmberg HC, Schroder HD, Saltin B, Ortenblad N. Human skeletal muscle glycogen utilization in exhaustive exercise: role of subcellular localization and fibre type. J Physiol. 2011;589:2871–85.
14. Gejl KD, Hvid LG, Frandsen U, Jensen K, Sahlin K, Ortenblad N. Muscle glycogen content modifies SR Ca2+ release rate in elite endurance athletes. Med Sci Sports Exerc. 2014;46:496–505.
15. Nédélec M, McCall A, Carling C, Legall F, Berthoin S, Dupont G. Recovery in soccer: part I – post-match fatigue and time course of recovery. Sports Med. 2012;42(12):997–1015.
16. Mohr M, Krustrup P, Bangbo J. Fatigue in soccer: a brief review. J Sports Sci. 2005;23(6):593–9.
17. Reilly T. Motion analysis and physiological demands. In: Williams AM, Reilly T, editors. Science and soccer. London: Routledge; 2003. p. 59–72.
18. Jeukendrup AE. Modulation of carbohydrate and fat utilization by diet, exercise and environment. Biochem Soc Trans. 2003;31(6):1270–3.
19. Hargreaves M. Metabolic responses to carbohydrate ingestions: effects on exercise performance. In: Lamb DR, Murray R, editors. Perspectives in exercise science and sports medicine: the metabolic basis of performance in exercise and sport. Carmel: Cooper Publishing Group; 1999.
20. Burke LM, Hawley JA, Wong SH, Jeukendrup AE. Carbohydrates for training and competition. J Sports Sci. 2011;29(Suppl. S1):S17–27.
21. Balsom P, Wood K, Olsson P, Ekblom B. Carbohydrate intake and multiple sprint sports: with special reference to football. Int J Sports Med. 1999;20:48–52.
22. Burke LM. Fueling strategies to optimize performance: training high or training low? Scand J Med Sci Sports. 2010;20(Suppl 2):48–58.
23. Jeukendrup AE, Killer SC. The myths surrounding pre-exercise carbohydrate feeding. Ann Nutr Metab. 2010;57(Suppl 2):18–25.
24. Kirkendall D, Foster JC, Gorgan DJ, Thompson N. Effect of glucose polymer supplementation on performance of soccer players. In: Reilly T, Lees A, Davids K, Murphy W, editors. Perspectives in exercise science and sports medicine: the metabolic basis of performance in exercise and sport. London: Science and Football; 1988. p. 33–41.
25. Nicholas CW, Williams HK, Phillips G, Nowitz A. Influence of ingesting a carbohydrate-electrolyte solution on endurance capacity during intermittent, high-intensity shuttle running. J Sports Sci. 1995; 13(4):283–90.
26. Ali A, Williams C, Nicholas CW, et al. The influence of carbohydrate–electrolyte ingestion on soccer skill performance. Med Sci Sports Exerc. 2007;39: 1969–76.
27. Ali A, Williams C. Carbohydrate ingestion and soccer skill performance during prolonged intermittent exercise. J Sports Sci. 2009;27:1499–508.
28. Currell K, Conway S, Jeukendrup AE. Carbohydrate ingestion improves performance of a new reliable test of soccer performance. Int J Sport Nutr Exerc Metab. 2009;19(1):34–46.
29. Pfeiffer B, Stellingwerff T, Zaltas E, Jeukendrup AE. Oxidation of solid versus liquid CHO sources during exercise. Med Sci Sports Exerc. 2010;42(11): 2030–7.
30. Clarke ND, Drust B, MacLaren DP, Reilly T. Strategies for hydration and energy provision during soccer-specific exercise. Int J Sport Nutr Exerc Metab. 2005;15:625–40.
31. Silva T, Souza ME, Amorim JF, Stathis CG, Leandro CG, Lima-Silva AE. Can carbohydrate mouth rinse improve performance during exercise? A systematic review. Nutrients. 2014;6:1–10.
32. Chambers ES, Bridge MW, Jones DA. Carbohydrate sensing in the human mouth: effects on exercise performance and brain activity. J Physiol. 2009;587:1779–94.
33. Brown LJ, Midgley AW, Vince RV, Madden LA, McNaughton LR. High versus low glycemic index 3-h recovery diets following glycogen-depleting exercise has no effect on subsequent 5-km cycling time trial performance. J Sci Med Sport. 2013;16(5): 450–4.

34. Sawka MN, Burke LM, Eichner ER, Maughan RJ, Montain SJ, Stachenfeld NS. American College of Sports Medicine position stand. Exercise and fluid replacement. Med Sci Sports Exerc. 2007;39(2):377–90.
35. Laitano O, Runco JL, Baker L. Hydration science and strategies in football. Sports Sci Exch. 2014;27(128):1–7.
36. Aragón-Vargas LF, Moncada-Jiménez J, Hernándes-Elizondo J, Barrenechea A, Monde-Alvarado M. Evaluation of pre-game hydration status, heat stress, and fluid balance during professional soccer competition in the heat. Eur J Sport Sci. 2008;9:269–76.
37. McGregor SJ, Nicholas HK, Williams C. The influence of intermittent high-intensity shuttle running and fluid ingestion on the performance of a soccer skill. J Sports Sci. 1999;17(11):895–903.
38. Owen JA, Kehoe SJ, Oliver SJ. Influence of fluid intake on soccer performance in a temperate environment. J Sports Sci. 2013;31(1):1–10.
39. Edwards AM, Mann ME, Marfell-Jones MJ, Rankin DM, Noakes TD, Shillington DP. Influence of moderate dehydration on soccer performance: physiological responses to 45 min of outdoor match-play and the immediate subsequent performance of sport-specific and mental concentration tests. Br J Sports Med. 2007;41(6):385–91.
40. Rampinini E, Impellizzeri FM, Castagna C, Azzalin A, Ferrari Bravo D, Wisløff U. Effect of match-related fatigue on short-passing ability in young soccer players. Med Sci Sports Exerc. 2008;40(5):934–42.
41. Russell M, Rees G, Kingsley M. Technical demands of soccer match-play in the English Championship. J Strength Cond Res. 2013;27:2869–73.
42. Hillyer M, Menon K, Singh R. The effects of dehydration on skill-based performance. Int J Sports Sci. 2015;5(3):99–107.
43. Rampinini E, Impellizzeri FM, Castagna C, Coutts AJ, Wisløff U. Technical performance during soccer matches of the Italian Serie A league: effect of fatigue and competitive level. J Sci Med Sport. 2009;12(1):227–33.
44. Reilly T, Holmes M. A preliminary analysis of selected soccer skills. Phys Ed Rev. 1983;6:64–71.
45. Russell M, Benton D, Kingsley M. The effects of fatigue on soccer skills performed during a soccer match simulation. Int J Sports Physiol Perform. 2011;6:221–33.
46. Di Salvo V, Gregson W, Atkinson G, et al. Analysis of high intensity activity in Premier League soccer. Int J Sports Med. 2009;30:205–12.
47. Ostojic SM, Mazic S. Effects of a carbohydrate-electrolyte drink on specific soccer tests and performance. J Sports Sci Med. 2002;1:47–53.
48. Russell M, Kingsley M. The efficacy of acute nutritional interventions on soccer skill performance. Sports Med. 2014;44:957–70.
49. Jentjens RL, Cale C, Gutch C, et al. Effects of pre-exercise ingestion of differing amounts of carbohydrate on subsequent metabolism and cycling performance. Eur J Appl Physiol. 2003;88:444–52.
50. Moseley L, Lancaster GI, Jeukendrup AE. Effects of timing of pre-exercise ingestion of carbohydrate on subsequent metabolism and cycling performance. Eur J Appl Physiol. 2003;88:453–8.
51. Souglis AG, Chryssanthopoulos CI, Travlos AK, Zorzou AE, Gissis IT, Papadopoulos CN, Sotiropoulos AA. The effect of high vs. low carbohydrate diets on distances covered in soccer. J Strength Cond Res. 2013;27(8):2235–47.
52. Abt G, Zhou S, Weatherby R. The effect of a high-carbohydrate diet on the skill performance of midfield soccer players after intermittent treadmill exercise. J Sci Med Sport. 1998;1:203–12.
53. Ruiz F, Irazusta A, Gil S, Irazusta J, Casis L, Gil J. Nutritional intake in soccer players of different ages. J Sports Sci. 2005;23:235–42.
54. Iglesias-Gutierrez E, Garcia A, Garcia-Zapico P, Perez-Landaluce J, Patterson AM, Garcia-Roves PM. Is there a relationship between the playing position of soccer players and their food and macronutrient intake? Appl Physiol Nutr Metab. 2012;37:225–32.
55. Martin L, Lambeth A, Scott D. Nutritional practices of national female soccer players: analysis and recommendations. J Sports Sci Med. 2006;5:130–7.
56. Abood DA, Black DR, Birnbaum RD. Nutrition education intervention for college female athletes. J Nutr Educ Behav. 2004;36:135–7.
57. Macdiarmid J, Blundell J. Assessing dietary intake: who, what and why of under-reporting. Nutr Res Rev. 1998;11:231–53.
58. Novotny JA, Rumpler WV, Riddick H, Hebert JR, Rhodes D, Judd JT, Baer DJ, McDowell M, Briefel R. Personality characteristics as predictors of underreporting of energy intake on 24-h dietary recall interviews. J Am Diet Assoc. 2003;103:1146–51.
59. García-Rovés PM, García-Zapico P, Patterson ÁM, Iglesias-Gutiérrez E. Nutrient intake and food habits of soccer players: analyzing the correlates of eating practice. Nutrients. 2014;6(7):2697–717.
60. Lemon PW. Protein Requirements of Soccer. J Sports Sci. 1994;12:517–22.
61. Schoenfeld B, Aragon A, Krieger J. The effect of protein timing on muscle strength and hypertrophy: a meta-analysis. J Int Soc Sports Nutr. 2013;10:53.
62. Millward DJ, Layman DK, Tome D, Schaafsma G. Protein quality assessment: impact of expanding understanding of protein and amino acid needs for optimal health. Am J Clin Nutr. 2008;87:1576S–81S.
63. Rodriguez NR, DiMarco NM, Langley S. Position of the American Dietetic Association, Dietitians of Canada, and the American College of Sports Medicine: nutrition and athletic performance. J Am Diet Assoc. 2009;109(3):509–27.
64. Maughan RJ, Greenhaff PL, Leiper JB, Ball D, Lambert CP, Gleeson M. Diet composition and the performance of high-intensity exercise. J Sports Sci. 1997;15(3):265–75.
65. Gravina L, Ruiz F, Diaz E, Lekue JA, Badiola A, Irazusta J, Gil SM. Influence of nutrient intake on antioxidant capacity, muscle damage and white blood cell count in female soccer players. J Int Soc Sports Nutr. 2012;9:32.

66. Mullinix MC, Jonnalagadda SS, Rosenbloom CA, Thompson WR, Kicklighter JR. Dietary intake of female U.S. soccer players. Nutr Res. 2003;23: 585–93.
67. Reilly T, George K, Marfell-Jones M, Scott M, Sutton L, Wallace JA. How well do skinfold equations predict percent body fat in elite soccer players? Int J Sports Med. 2009;30(8):607–13.
68. Santos DA, Dawson JA, Matias CN, Rocha PM, Minderico CS, Allison DB, Sardinha LB, Silva AM. Reference values for body composition and anthropometric measurements in athletes. PLoS One. 2014;9(5):e97846.
69. Sutton L, Scott M, Wallace J, Reilly T. Body composition of English Premier League soccer players: influence of playing position, international status, and ethnicity. J Sports Sci. 2009;27(10):1019–26.
70. Sporis G, Jukic I, Ostojic SM, Milanovic D. Fitness profiling in soccer: physical and physiologic characteristics of elite players. J Strength Cond Res. 2009;23(7):1947–53.
71. Bradley PS, Di Mascio M, Peart D, Olsen P, Sheldon B. High-intensity activity profiles of elite soccer players at different performance levels. J Strength Cond Res. 2010;24(9):2343–51.
72. Kalapotharakos VI, Strimpakos N, Vithoulka I, Karvounidis C, Diamantopoulos K, Kapreli E. Physiological characteristics of elite professional soccer teams of different ranking. J Sports Med Phys Fitness. 2006;46(4):515–9.
73. Evans EM, Rowe DA, Misic MM, Prior BM, Arngrímsson SA. Skinfold prediction equation for athletes developed using a four-component model. Med Sci Sports Exerc. 2005;37(11):2006–11.
74. Withers RT, Craig NP, Bourdon PC, Norton KI. Relative body fat and anthropometric prediction of body density of male athletes. Eur J Appl Physiol Occup Physiol. 1987;56(2):191–200.
75. Rahnama N, Lees A, Bambaecichi E. Comparison of muscle strength and flexibility between the preferred and non-preferred leg in English soccer players. Ergonomics. 2005;48(11–14):1568–75.
76. Eston RG, Rowlands AV, Charlesworth S, Davies A, Hoppitt T. Prediction of DXA-determined whole body fat from skinfolds: importance of including skinfolds from the thigh and calf in young, healthy men and women. Eur J Clin Nutr. 2005;59(5): 695–702.
77. Collins J, Rollo I. Practical considerations in elite football. Sci Exch. 2014;27(133):1–7.
78. Anderson L, Orme P, Di Michele R, Close GL, Morgans R, Drust B, Morton JP. Quantification of training load during one-, two- and three-game week schedules in professional soccer players from the English Premier League: implications for carbohydrate periodisation. J Sports Sci. 2015;4:1–10.
79. Koopman R, Wagenmakers AJ, Manders RJ, Zorenc AH, Senden JM, Gorselink M, Keizer HA, van Loon LJ. Combined ingestion of protein and free leucine with carbohydrate increases postexercise muscle protein synthesis in vivo in male subjects. Am J Physiol Endocrinol Metab. 2005;288(4):E645–53.
80. Moore DR, Robinson MJ, Fry JL, Tang JE, Glover EI, Wilkinson SB, Prior T, Tarnopolsky MA, Phillips SM. Ingested protein dose response of muscle and albumin protein synthesis after resistance exercise in young men. Am J Clin Nutr. 2009;89(1):161–8.
81. Sousa M, Teixeira VH, Soares J. Dietary strategies to recover from exercise-induced muscle damage. Int J Food Sci Nutr. 2014;65(2):151–63.
82. Guzmán JF, Esteve H, Pablos C, Pablos A, Blasco C, Villegas JA. DHA- rich fish oil improves complex reaction time in female elite soccer players. J Sports Sci Med. 2011;10(2):301–5.
83. Morton JP. Supplements for consideration in football. Sport Sci Exc. 2014;27(130):1–8.

Supplements in Football

53

Samuel Amorim, Hernâni Gomes,
and Vítor Hugo Teixeira

Contents

53.1 Introduction

The search for dietary supplements, many times based upon superstition and ritualistic behavior, is as ancient as sport itself. Scientific understanding of the chemical and physiological nature of muscular work was followed by ergogenic aid use by athletes and rationalized as "scientific" justification. Popularity and use of ergogenic aids often have preceded scientific substantiation of claims. Whether or not these aids work, athletes will try almost anything in their search for the competitive edge, even products with demonstrated health risks [1, 2]. A 1997 poll in *Sports Illustrated* asked current and aspiring US Olympic athletes two questions. The first was whether they would take a banned performance-enhancing drug if they were guaranteed to both win their athletic event and not get suspended for drug use. The second question was whether they would take the same substance if it would enhance their ability to win every competition for the next 5 years but then result in death. Remarkably, 98% responded "yes" to the first question, and more than 50% responded "yes" to the second question [3]. The global market of

S. Amorim (✉)
Sporting Clube de Braga, Braga, Portugal
e-mail: amorimsamuel@gmail.com

H. Gomes
Rio Ave Futebol Clube, Vila do Conde, Portugal

CESPU – Institute of Research and Advanced Training in Health Sciences and Technologies, Gandra, Portugal
e-mail: hernanigomes10@gmail.com

V.H. Teixeira
Faculty of Nutrition and Food Sciences, University of Porto, Porto, Portugal

Research Centre on Physical Activity Health and Leisure, Faculty of Sport, University of Porto, Porto, Portugal

Futebol Clube do Porto, Porto, Portugal
e-mail: vhugoteixeira@fcna.up.pt

J. Espregueira-Mendes et al. (eds.), *Injuries and Health Problems in Football*,
DOI 10.1007/978-3-662-53924-8_53

supplements is a powerful one. In 2001, it was estimated at US$46 billion as reported in the *Financial Times* newspaper [4]; in 2006, the worldwide market was estimated at more than US$ 60 billion [5]; it is expected to continue to grow in the next years [6].

Dietary supplements are used by a large proportion of the general population, and the available evidence suggests that the prevalence is even higher among athletes, ranging from amateur level to elite athletes [4, 7]. The overall prevalence of the use and type of supplements used varies with the type of the sport, age, gender, and the level of competition [7, 8]. In Portugal, a study assessed the prevalence of nutritional supplements usage in national teams' athletes and found that most athletes (66%) consumed nutritional supplements, with a median consumption of four supplements per athlete [8]. In football, supplement use appears still to be increasing [9]. In 2006 World Cup, it was prescribed a mean of 1.33 supplements/player/match; 33.4% of the players that disputed the World Cups between 2002 and 2014 used supplements during the tournament [10]. A study that assessed drug use in English professional football stated that almost 58% reported using vitamin pills, 23% used mineral pills, 24% used protein powders, and 37% used creatine [11]. Footballers use rather fewer supplements than have been reported for some other athletes [12], particularly those in track and field (~85%) [13–15].

The most popular supplements in Portugal include multivitamins/minerals (67%), sports drinks (62%), and magnesium (53%) [8]. Cited reasons for supplement use are diverse, such as to aid recovery from training, for health, to improve performance, to prevent or treat an illness, to compensate for a poor diet, recommended by coach or other influential individual [7], and to have more energy/reduce fatigue [8].

Regarding football, 28% of players reported taking advice on supplement use from the club physiotherapist, 21% from a fitness trainer, and a further 21% from another sports scientist, such as a nutritionist. The club doctor was the least used source of advice, being used by just 15% of players [11]. This is in contrast with evidence published in Portugal with elite athletes (other than footballers), in which physicians were the main source of information, suggesting that Portuguese athletes perceive supplements as an issue that deserves medical attention [8]. In that work, almost one in five players (18%) reported that they used supplements without taking advice from any of the above. Some players purchase their supplies of supplements from local gyms, and, along with the purchase, they sometimes receive advice on its use. It is a matter of concern the quality of advice which players receive from this and other nonprofessional sources and the fact that some players may be given advice which encourages them to use supplements in excessively high and potentially dangerous doses [11]. Often, these supplements are used more frequently and in higher doses than recommended on the label. The reason for this behavior is the popular belief that the more supplements are taken, the better a performance will be [4].

Many athletes that take multiple supplements have nutritional habits that can be described as "unsatisfactory," implying that these athletes might benefit more from attention to the foods they ate [16]. On the other hand, a recent study stated that high-performance athletes that used nutritional supplements reported a generally higher nutritional intake from food and a lower prevalence of micronutrient inadequacy for some micronutrients [17]. The authors suggested that, perhaps, the athletes who are using or want to use nutritional supplements might be the ones who are already more concerned about nutrition-related aspects and with the least need to supplement their diet with macro- and/or micronutrients.

The decision to use a supplement should be made after careful consideration of several issues. First, it should be assessed if the supplement is safe, legal, and effective. For example, despite common perception that herbal (or natural) remedies are free of adverse effects, some supplements have been associated with severe hepatotoxicity as well an increased risk of psychiatric, autonomic, or gastrointestinal adverse events and heart palpitations [18–20]. Then, it is important to weigh the pros and the cons of using the supplement. The cons include expense, side effects, contamination causing inadvertent doping outcome, and redirection of resources from real performance-enhancing factors. The pros include assistance to meet nutritional goals (indirect performance enhancement), direct performance enhancement, and placebo effect (psychological boost) [21].

The placebo effect is a favorable outcome, arising exclusively from the belief that one received a beneficial treatment [22]. In the sport setting, athlete expectations of the likely effects on performance resulting from ingestion of substances may result in an increase or decrease of the actual performance, by mechanisms unrelated to the physiology of the substance itself [23]. Possible explanations for this event include increased motivation, higher tolerance to pain and fatigue resistance, and perhaps greater vigilance around the workout and recovery [23]. In some studies, the magnitude of the performance benefit when consuming placebo was similar to actually receiving the supplement [24]. On the other hand, it is also known that a negative belief about a particular treatment can have a negative impact on performance [25]. The negative belief about the intake of a substance with proven ergogenic value may result in a decrease of the beneficial effects of the substance's intake [26]. Given all these assumptions, it is important that, instead of simply putting the intended supplement available to the players, the sports nutritionist should briefly explain the supplement ergogenic action, dose, and timing; provide testimonials of other successful athletes; and take doubts. In this way, he would try to remove negative beliefs and foster positive beliefs (based on scientific facts, declining ethical problems). Moreover, knowing that a supplement will have little effect in a percentage of players (not susceptible individuals), they may still benefit from the placebo effect [23].

Regarding the cons of supplementation, the biggest concern for athletes who are liable to testing for the use of drugs that are prohibited in sport is the possibility that a supplement may contain something that will result in a positive doping test [27]. A failed drug test may mean temporary suspension from competition as well as damage to the athlete's reputation and perhaps permanent loss of employment and income [28]. Unlike drugs, the regulations governing the purity of dietary supplements and of the claims that can be made as to their purity and efficacy are somewhat lax. Dietary supplements are not evaluated by regulatory agencies and inaccurate labelling of ingredients is known to be a problem. Most dietary supplements will not cause problems for the athlete, and most of the companies that manufacture and supply these supplements are anxious to ensure the welfare of their customers. Nonetheless, there is compelling evidence that dietary supplements may be responsible for at least some of the positive doping results recorded by athletes [5, 29, 30]. At the request of the Medical Commission of the International Olympic Committee, the Cologne laboratory conducted a large survey [31]. Between October 2000 and November 2001, a total of 634 non-hormonal nutritional supplements were obtained in 13 countries from 215 different suppliers. Of the samples analyzed, 94 (14.8%) were found to contain hormones or prohormones that were not declared on the label. The products included amino acids and protein powders, creatine, carnitine, ribose, guarana, zinc, pyruvate, hydroxymethylbutyrate, *Tribulus terrestris*, vitamins and minerals, and herbal extracts [31]. The IOC-accredited laboratory in Vienna has analyzed a smaller number (n = 54) of supplements, all of which were purchased in Austria, and found that 12 of these (22%) contained prohibited steroids [29, 32]. In the field of practice, it is important to educate athletes in order to be cautioned against indiscriminate use of supplements. Supplements can play a role in an athlete's diet, but confirmation of their added benefit should be sought with an appropriate expert before using them. It is also essential to identify those supplements that have the slimmest chance of being contaminated with doping substances. Companies that sell products containing doping substances should definitely be avoided, and it is prudent to disregard companies with unrealistic claims in their advertisements. Contaminations can occur in many ways, which leads to possible package-to-package or even tablet-to-tablet variation. Therefore, the best available option for athletes is to only use supplements that have been analyzed in a knowledgeable laboratory on a batch-by-batch basis [33].

In addition to the contamination problem, indiscriminate supplementation may pose other problems. Nutrients ingested in excessive amounts can interact with the absorption of other nutrients, with a negative impact on its nutritional status [34]. On the other hand, supplementation with excessive amounts of a nutrient increases the risk of toxicity. Mettler et al. [35] found iron depletion and overload in 1.6% and 15% of the male recreational marathon runners, respectively, meaning that the actual risk of iron overload was higher than deficiency. Furthermore, supplementation may in some cases prevent health-promoting effects of physical exercise [36], delay muscle recovery [37, 38], and hamper training-induced adaptations [39].

53.2 Caffeine

Caffeine (1,3,7-trimethylxanthine) is a substance devoid of nutritional value, being a socially accepted drug, and probably the most widely consumed pharmacologically active substance in the world. Although it can be found in beverages such as coffee, tea, and soft drinks; cocoa- or chocolate-containing products; energy drinks; and drugs (analgesics, appetite suppressants, preparations for influenza), 75% of its consumption is carried out as coffee constituent [40, 41]. Major dietary sources of caffeine are presented in Table 53.1.

Table 53.1 Caffeine contents in foods, commonly used drinks, and non-prescription preparations

Food or drink	Serving	Caffeine (mg)
Expresso coffee	1 standard serving	107 (25–214)
Iced tea	600 mL	20–40
Chocolate milk	60 g	5–15
Dark chocolate	60 g	10–50
Coca-Cola	330 mL	43
Red Bull energy drink	250 mL	80
PowerBar sports gel	40 g	25

Adapted from Burke [78, 224]

Caffeine, as well as their metabolites (especially theophylline and paraxanthine), is structurally very similar to adenosine and can bind to their receptors on the cell membrane, thereby blocking its action [42]. Adenosine receptors are ubiquitous in the human body, which promotes the action of caffeine in various tissues simultaneously, resulting in a variety of physiological responses that interact with each other [43].

In light of current knowledge, it is not possible to explain precisely the dominant mechanism by which caffeine exerts its ergogenic action. Nevertheless, it is known that caffeine exerts broad physiological effects at central and peripheral level, in particular on the sympathetic nervous system, muscle, endocrine, cardiovascular, pulmonary, and renal levels [44, 45]. The effects of caffeine on the central nervous system possibly include changes on the level of sympathetic activity, perception of fatigue and pain, and recruitment of motor units [43]. Caffeine is known for its effects in enhancing capabilities related to alertness and ability to concentrate, including, but not limited to, sleep deprivation, possibly by stimulating the sympathetic nervous system and/or antagonism of adenosine. In this sense, there is evidence of positive effects of caffeine action in tasks such as surveillance, visual information processing, reaction time, motor learning, humor, and possibly short-term memory [46]. A meta-analysis has shown that caffeine reduces at 5.6% the degree of perceived exertion, compared to placebo, demonstrating clearly that this aspect may partially explain the ergogenic effects of caffeine in sports performance [47]. Although not consensual [48–51], especially in high- or maximum-intensity activities, some authors admit that caffeine can maintain or increase the level of firing of motor units, resulting in greater force produced by the muscle, explaining the positive effects on anaerobic performance [52]. Caffeine also exerts action at peripheral level. Caffeine can increase circulating levels of catecholamines, wherein at least this increase is not the most important parameter for ergogenic action of caffeine [43, 52]. Another mechanism proposed for the ergogenic action of caffeine is to promote the oxidation of fat and inhibiting oxidation of carbohydrates. It has been suggested that this process results in reduced dependence on muscle glycogen reserves [53]. However, although accepting the possibility that caffeine leads to the mobilization of nonesterified fatty acids from adipose tissue, there is no evidence that consequently there is an increase in fat oxidation in the muscle or an increase in muscle glycogen savings [54].

The ergogenic effect of caffeine in team sports (high intensity, intermittent) has been shown in most [55, 56] but not all studies [57]. Considering football [58], although not entirely consensual [59], it was found that caffeine intake led to improved performance through the enhancement of various parameters:

- Improvement of cognitive functioning: increased capacity of interpretation and response to visual and auditory stimuli (e.g., react more quickly and accurately to the request of a colleague-like "pass") [56]
- Reduced decline in technical capabilities during a game: increased passing accuracy; improved fine motor qualities such as ball control; improved ability to dribble [56, 60]
- Increased jumping ability, as a result of increased leg power [56, 61, 62]
- Increased countermovement jump height, average peak running speed, total running distance, number of sprint bouts, and running distance covered at a high speed [63]
- Improvement of reactive agility [64, 65]
- Higher mean sprint speed [66]
- Reduced decline in sprinting performance throughout the game [62]
- Increased number of sprints and total distance covered at high intensity [61]
- Increased peak power in sprint [67]
- Reduced decline in the ability to perform mental tasks toward the end of the game: caffeine attenuated the reduced feelings of energy and increased feelings of fatigue; resulted in more rapid responding, improved target identification, and reductions in false alarms [68]
- Altered perception of fatigue and effort that enables players to better maintain voluntary sprinting and jumping ability [62]
- Lower decline in enjoyment of physical activity toward the end of the game [62], enhanced ratings of pleasure and arousal, increased vigor, reduced fatigue, reduced rating of perceived exertion, and improved reaction time [69]

Most studies testing caffeine as ergogenic use the administration of dosages on the order of 6-mg/kg body weight [50, 55–57]. However, there is evidence demonstrating the beneficial effects of the ingestion of lower amounts of caffeine (1–3-mg/kg body weight) [46, 70, 71]. There is no dose-response relationship between caffeine intake and the benefits in endurance exercise performance, or if this relationship exists, there is a stabilization to 3-mg/kg body weight [72, 73]. On the other hand, it is known that cytochrome P450, responsible for metabolization of caffeine by the liver, becomes saturated with caffeine intake greater than 5-mg/kg body weight. Accordingly, higher doses entail the risk of producing disproportionate increases in plasma concentration of caffeine. In football, the optimal dose intake may vary according to the position on the field. The dosage required to exert an optimal effect on the visual processing is substantially lower than that required to exert an optimal effect on endurance capacity. Furthermore, although not consensual [56], it is thought that possibly a too high dose of caffeine can adversely affect processing of visual information [74]. So, considering that a goalkeeper does not need a great endurance capacity [75] and that abilities such as reaction time, alertness, and processing of visual information are crucial to his success, he should ingest a dose of 1–2-mg/kg body weight. On the other hand, a field player should ingest between 3- and 5-mg/kg body weight [74]. Doses in the range of 6–9-mg/kg of body weight can have side effects such as increased anxiety, sleep disturbances at night after an evening match [76, 77], and exaggerated increase in heart rate [78].

Caffeine is rapidly absorbed (about 20 min, in the stomach) and reaches peak concentration in blood plasma in 1 h [43]. Given that caffeine is catabolized slowly (half-life is from 4 to 6 h) and concentration in circulation is maintained near the maximum in 3–4 h following administration

[43], caffeine intake 1 h before the game (before warming up) enables an ergogenic effect during the entire game, even if there is extra time [74]. During the game, caffeine mouth rinse (alone or in combination with carbohydrates) may rapidly enhance power production, which could have benefits for specific short sprint exercise performance [67], but not maximum strength or muscular endurance performance [79].

53.3 Carnitine

Fat and carbohydrate are the primary fuel sources for skeletal muscle during a football game [80, 81]. Fat constitutes the largest energy reserve in the body, and, in terms of the amount available, it is not limiting to endurance exercise performance [82]. However, fat exhibits a relatively low maximal rate of oxidation, which begins to decline at around 65% of maximal oxygen consumption (VO_{2max}) when muscle glycogen becomes the major fuel supporting ATP homeostasis [83]. The muscle glycogen stores are limited, and it has been well established that muscle glycogen depletion, or partial depletion, in a significant number of fibers coincides with fatigue in the final phase of a football game [84–86]. As fatigue can be postponed by increasing pre-exercise muscle glycogen content [87], it is thought that augmenting the rate of fat oxidation during endurance exercise could delay glycogen depletion and improve endurance exercise performance.

Carnitine (L-3-hydroxytrimethylamminobuta noate) is a naturally occurring compound that can be synthesized from the essential amino acids lysine and methionine or ingested through diet. The rate of carnitine biosynthesis in humans has been estimated to be about 1–2-μmol/kg body wt/day [88]. Nonvegetarian humans obtain an additional ~1 mg/kg of carnitine per day from dietary sources [89]. Primary sources of carnitine are red meat and dairy products (e.g., steak, 95.7 mg/100 g) [90]. The recommended upper limit of L-carnitine supplementation is 2 g/day [91], but no adverse effects were reported following feeding up to 6 g/day for 1 year [92]. Skeletal muscle contains more than 95% of the total body carnitine (~20 g of carnitine in a 70-kg man, of which more than 19 g is in skeletal muscle), as either free or acylcarnitine [93].

Carnitine plays two essential roles in muscle energy metabolism. In the absence of carnitine, the inner mitochondrial membrane would be impermeable to long-chain fatty acids and fatty acyl-CoA esters [94]. Carnitine and carnitine palmitoyltransferase (CPT) are essential for the translocation of long-chain fatty acids into skeletal muscle mitochondria for β-oxidation. A second broad function of carnitine involves the formation of acylcarnitines from short-chain acyl-CoA. The generation of the acylcarnitine serves to buffer the small, dynamic coenzyme A pool against metabolic transients and protects against acyl-CoA accumulation, which may be deleterious to cellular function [95]. The rationale behind carnitine supplementation is that increasing muscle carnitine content could potentially increase fat oxidation during prolonged exercise, spare glycogen stores, and, thus, delay the onset of fatigue [96].

The majority of the pertinent studies in healthy humans to date have failed to increase skeletal muscle carnitine content via oral or intravenous L-carnitine administration. The bioavailability of orally administered carnitine is ~16–18% at doses of 1–2 g and may be even lower at higher doses [93]. Carnitine is transported into skeletal muscle against a considerable concentration gradient (>100-fold) which is saturated under normal conditions, and so it is unlikely that simply increasing plasma carnitine availability per se will increase muscle carnitine transport and storage [97]. A 1 g oral dose of carnitine will increment the total body carnitine pool by ~0.08 g or 0.4% [93]. However, insulin appears to stimulate skeletal muscle carnitine transport, and intravenously infusing L-carnitine in the presence of high circulating insulin (>50 mU/l) can increase muscle carnitine content by 15% [96].

A recent study [98] showed an increase in total muscle carnitine content following 2 g of carnitine plus 80 g of carbohydrate ingestion twice daily for 6 months. There was an 80% increase in free carnitine availability during

30 min of exercise at 50% VO_{2max} compared to control and a 55% reduction in muscle glycogen utilization. The study also demonstrated an improvement in exercise performance in all participants (11%, on average) during a 30-min cycle ergometer time trial in the carnitine-loaded state. Whether these improvements in endurance performance are due to glycogen sparing as a result of a carnitine-mediated increase in fat oxidation or the reported effect of carnitine on glucose disposal requires further investigation, but due to the nature of the time trial, this seems unlikely.

In which concerns to body composition, a recent study showed that a 20% increase in muscle carnitine content prevented the 1.8-kg increase in body fat mass associated with daily ingestion of a high-carbohydrate beverage [99]. Moreover, this maintenance of body mass was associated with a greater whole-body energy expenditure during low-intensity physical activity accounted for by an increase in fat oxidation. In line with the role of carnitine in the translocation of long-chain acyl groups via CPT1, these findings are most likely due to an increase in the rate of fat oxidation compared with control at rest and during low-intensity exercise [99]. Overall, however, the practical implications of this are currently unclear, and there is not enough evidence to recommend carnitine for weight loss or to increase fat oxidation [100].

Published data regarding L-carnitine supplementation on footballers is still scarce. Orer et al. [101] examined the effect of acute L-carnitine loading (3 or 4 g) on the endurance performance of footballers. The authors verified that L-carnitine supplementation taken before physical exercise prolonged time to exhaustion. Naclerio et al. [102] investigated the effects of ingesting a multi-ingredient supplement composed of carbohydrate, whey protein, glutamine, and L-carnitine on intermittent performance, perception of fatigue, immunity, and functional and metabolic markers of recovery in footballers. Although the perception of fatigue and serum myoglobin was attenuated for the multi-ingredient group, the supplement did not improve intermittent performance, inflammatory, or immune function. Finally, Guzel et al. [103] assessed the effect of acute L-carnitine supplementation on nitric oxide production and oxidative stress after exhaustive exercise in young football players. The authors found that L-carnitine supplementation (3-g dose) provides strong antioxidant action by increasing the antioxidant glutathione and nitrate-nitrite level and decreasing the thiobarbituric acid reactive substances (TBARs) level.

Research into carnitine has shown that it is a safe supplement for human consumption. Side effects have been minimal across almost all studies using the 1–3-g range of supplementation [90, 91].

53.4 Creatine

Creatine is produced from three amino acids (glycine, arginine, and methionine) endogenously by the liver (1–2 g), or it can be obtained from exogenous sources. By adequate intake, some creatine is also added to the pool, predominantly from meat and fish, with a typical diet supplying approximately 1–2 g of creatine daily [104]. Almost all the creatine in the body is stored in skeletal muscle (95%), around 60% in the phosphorylated form (phosphocreatine). It represents an average creatine pool of about 120–140 g for an average 70-kg person [105].

Phosphocreatine serves as a readily available source of phosphorus in skeletal muscle and other tissues. The fast rephosphorylation of ADP from phosphocreatine, via the creatine kinase reaction, buffers changes in ATP during transitions between rest and exercise and contributes a substantial fraction of ATP synthesis during short-duration, high-intensity exercise. Net phosphocreatine hydrolysis consumes hydrogen ions so it may also contribute to buffering of intracellular acidosis during exercise [106]. Creatine supplementation does not increase skeletal muscle protein synthesis as was thought earlier [107].

The relative importance of phosphocreatine during exercise depends on the nature of the exercise [106]. There is a consensus that exercise performance that involves short periods of extremely powerful activity (1–2 s) can be enhanced by creatine supplementation, especially if the activity is performed in repetitive bouts separated by short rest periods (30 s–1 min) [105]. On the other hand, creatine supplementation does not appear to enhance aerobic-oriented activities [106]. Highly trained athletes who participate in sports in which performance relies on repeated efforts could benefit from creatine ingestion by means of an increased ability to perform intermittent high-intensity exercise bouts [108]. This would be the case in football because high-intensity running is a crucial element of performance. Across seven seasons (2006–2007 until 2012–2013) in the English Premier League, high-intensity running distance and actions increased around 30%, and sprint distance and number of sprints increased around 35% [109]. In this context, creatine supplementation is also of particular interest for football players given that phosphocreatine stores exhibit significant declines during football match play [80].

There is compelling evidence of benefits of creatine supplementation in football. Acute creatine supplementation favorably affected repeated sprint performance and limited the decline in jumping ability [108]. On the other hand, a study with 16 male amateur football players suggests that short-term creatine supplementation does not enhances repeated high-intensity or prolonged football-specific exercise performance and body mass [110]. Creatine supplementation may also be useful during a preseason training preventing the decrement in lower-limb muscle power [111]. Additionally, creatine supplementation may also be beneficial in football players proceeding rehabilitation, with a faster recovery from muscle atrophy [112].

Most studies have employed a "loading" dose of 20 g creatine per day for 4–6 days. A more recent approach suggests that a lower dose of 3 g creatine per day will increase muscle total creatine to the same values; however it takes about 30 days [106]. To maximize creatine storage to a given dose, it is also recommended that creatine be consumed post-exercise and in conjunction with carbohydrate and/or protein feeding given that elevated insulin is known to increase muscle creatine uptake [113].

Few reports from athletes have claimed that creatine supplementation may induce muscle cramps. However, it appears that muscle cramping might be due to the intensity of exercise rather than creatine supplementation itself [104]. Despite published allegations of detrimental effects of oral creatine supplementation on liver metabolism, studies on humans have not shown any significant increase in plasma urea, nor liver enzyme activity, during 5 years of creatine supplementation. No reports have observed a modification of the glomerular filtration rate or the presence of microalbuminuria [104]. Creatine supplementation should not be used by athletes with pre-existing renal disease or those with a potential risk of renal dysfunction (diabetes, hypertension, or reduced glomerular filtration rate) [104].

Acute creatine supplementation can also induce a 1–1.5-kg gain in body mass, an effect that is greater in men compared with women [114]. Such increases in body mass are confined to fat-free mass and are likely due to an increase in intracellular water accumulation. For this reason, not all football players should be supplemented with creatine given the perception that they feel heavier and slower. It is conceivable that this increase in body mass in a weight-supported sport like football could decrease performance by increasing the energy cost of running.

53.5 Omega-3

N-3 fatty acids, a class of polyunsaturated fatty acids (PUFAs) found in various cold-water fish (salmon, mackerel, sardines, and herring), have been implicated in a number of metabolic effects with potential benefit in the sport setting [115]. N-3 fatty acids may be useful in the process of dampening inflammatory responses [116, 117], although its importance in ameliorating post-exercise inflammation is not consensual [118, 119]. The potential implications of reducing post-exercise inflammation would be reduced pain and quicker recovery time from intense exercise. Some data show beneficial effects on delayed onset of muscle soreness after only 7 days of supplementation. This suggests that chronic supplementation is not necessary for protection against muscle soreness and that supplementation could be initiated in the ~7 days prior to activity that might cause soreness, such as the preseason or intensified period of strength training [120]. It has also been suggested that n-3 PUFAs may facilitate the transport of red blood cells through the capillary bed, which could lead to enhanced oxygen delivery to skeletal muscle. There is, however, some concern that incorporating omega-3 PUFAs into cell membranes may increase the potential for lipid peroxidation, which is much more evident in athletes who undergo high oxidative stress [121]. Nevertheless, Capó et al. [122] stated that diet supplementation with a functional food rich in docosahexaenoic acid (DHA) reduced the oxidative damage in response to acute exercise in footballers. Recently, omega-3 fatty acid supplementation have been associated with beneficial effects on cardiovascular adaptation to exercise, namely, an improvement of endothelial function, possibly as a consequence of an increase in endogenous production of nitric oxide (NO) [123]. Omega-3 acids may confer a positive effect on exercise, by improving fatty acid delivery to exercising muscles via an increased blood flow. Blood flow improvements are believed to be due to an n-3 mediated suppression of n-6 eicosanoid production. A high n-6/n-3 ratio can lead to elevated levels of pro-inflammatory prostaglandins and thromboxanes. Given that these eicosanoids are pro-aggregatory vasoconstrictors, excessive amounts can lead to reductions in vascular blood flow. Supplementing with n-3 can potentially help to inhibit inflammatory eicosanoid production, as well as interacting with cyclooxygenase in a manner that reduces platelet aggregation, increases dilation of blood vessels, and improves circulatory response [124, 125]. One potential mechanism whereby n-3 supplementation may enhance benefits is via increased lipolysis and β-oxidation. Specifically, n-3 fatty acids are claimed to act as metabolic fuel partitioners, upregulating lipid oxidative enzymes and downregulating lipogenic gene expression [124]. There is evidence that n-3 PUFA supplementation results in increased protein synthesis secondary to n-3-mediated increases in cell membrane fluidity. In addition, n-3 PUFAs may enhance mTOR/p70s6k signaling, a pathway thought be involved in decreasing proteolysis by downregulating the ubiquitin-proteasome pathway [126].

Omega 3 supplementation has a markedly protective effect in suppressing exercise-induced bronchoconstriction, and this is most likely attributed to its anti-inflammatory properties [127]. It may also have an important role in recovery from injury, due to its anti-inflammatory role and its effect on muscle protein turnover. Potentially, n-3 may be helpful during immobilization to ameliorate muscle loss and boost recovery [128–131]. A key point is the question of timing of fish oil supplementation; depending on the timing of the n-3 nonesterified fatty acids (NEFA) consumption (i.e., during disuse or recovery), these compounds could either improve or worsen the muscle atrophy. Different timings targeting different biochemical events (i.e., to decrease oxidative stress/inflammation during immobilization and to increase anabolism during the recovery process) should be also tested [132]. N-3 supplementation, particularly DHA, can also be useful in the recovery process from the neurometabolic insults and structural damage to axons that occur in episodes of mild traumatic brain injury (concussion) [133, 134]. It has also been demonstrated that omega-3 PUFA can affect not only cognitive function but also mood and emotional states (e.g., depression) and may act as a mood stabilizer [135]. Guzman et al. [136] showed that supplementing female elite football players with DHA-rich fish oil for 4 weeks produced perceptual-motor benefits (i.e., improvements in complex reaction time and efficiency), which supports the view that DHA may improve performance in sports where perceptual-motor activity and decision-making are the keys to success. Although, at present, the limited human data do not support the hypothesis that omega-3 PUFA supplementation is effective in enhancing physical exercise performance, there is accumulating data that show improved athlete's health.

It has been suggested that for most athletes, ingesting approximately 1–2 g/day of EPA and DHA at a ratio of eicosapentaenoic acid (EPA) to

DHA of 2:1 would be beneficial in this context. However, it should be noted that an omega-3 PUFA (EPA+DHA) dose of ≤3.0 mg/day has been designated as safe for general consumption by the United States of America Food and Drug Administration (2004) [121]. Within the context of concussions, some current available evidence recommend intake of approximately 400 mg/day DHA [133], while other authors suggest a higher intake (10 mg/kg/day) started right after the concussion [134].

The reported health risks of fish oil supplementation include the (low) risk of contamination with toxins, such as heavy metals, dioxins, and polychlorinated biphenyl (PCBs); there is also the risk of increased bleeding or immunosuppression in case of excessive intake [121].

53.6 Buffers

Despite the fact that sprinting in a football game represents less than 10% of total distance covered, this performance is considered as one of the most critical [137]. The need of performing a sprint during a game varies, and players must be ready to perform, recover, and perform it again at the highest possible level [75].

Brief highly intense muscular effort (short sprints) depends highly on anaerobic glycolysis and leads to large accumulation of lactic acid, which can cause muscle acidification. Because of the body buffering capacity, composed by phosphates, bicarbonate, and carnosine, the H^+ concentration remains low even during the most severe exercise, allowing muscle pH to decrease from a resting value of 7.1 to no lower than 6.6–6.4 to exhaustion. Low muscle pH is believed to be the major limiter of performance and the primary cause of fatigue during maximal, all-out exercise lasting more than 20–30s [138]. Evidence shows that fatigue occurs after short-term intense periods in both halves [85].

It may be possible that in circumstances in which there is a great demand on repeated sprint ability, a player performance is limited by muscle acidosis. It appears that repeated sprint ability is related to both intracellular and extracellular buffer capacity. Increased intracellular buffer capacity should help to resist changes in muscle pH, while increases in extracellular buffer capacity may increase H^+ efflux out of the muscle cell or otherwise improve physical performance [137].

53.7 β-Alanine

β-Alanine is an amino acid that can be obtained through meat and that can be endogenously synthetized in the liver. By itself, the ergogenic properties of this amino acid are limited; however, β-alanine has been identified as the rate-limiting precursor to carnosine synthesis [139]. Carnosine (β-alanyl-L-histidine) is a cytoplasmatic intracellular dipeptide found in high concentrations in skeletal muscle (10–40-mmol/kg dry weight) [139]. It is estimated that the contribution of carnosine to the total buffering capacity in muscle may be as low as 7% [139], but it is indisputably a functional pH buffer [140]. A second mechanism that is involved in muscle fatigue is the reduction in Ca^{2+} release from the sarcoplasmic reticulum (SR). A third possible mechanism of performance improvement evoked by carnosine could be related to its antioxidative potential. However, it is clear that further research is recommended to verify the effects of ingestion of β-alanine on oxidative stress [140].

Oral carnosine supplementation is an inefficient method of augmenting muscle carnosine levels in humans, as ingested carnosine is ultimately metabolized before reaching skeletal muscle [139]. The increase of intramuscular availability of β-alanine, through a chronic loading dose, is the more effective way to increase endogenous synthesis of carnosine. Daily doses of β-alanine of 4.8–6.4 g can elevate human muscle carnosine content by 20–30% in 2 weeks [139], 60% in 4 weeks, and 80% in 10 weeks [141, 142]. Employing an incremental strategy ranging from 3.0 to 6.0 g per day may be beneficial [143].

Available literature has been somewhat conflicting regarding the effects of β-alanine on high-intensity performance. When an exercise protocol eliciting an extreme acidosis was used, a significant improvement in performance was observed

[142]. On the other hand, when exercise protocols elicit a less extreme muscular acidosis (i.e., a single bout of exercise lasting less than 60s), no effects of β-alanine have been observed [144]. Supplementation improved exercise capacity in tasks lasting 60–240 s, but not in tasks lasting under 60s in which acidosis is not likely the primary limiting factor [145]. Regarding short-duration sprint tasks, carnosine induced no significant improvements in power output in repeated 5-s bouts [146] and a 400-m race [147]. Taken together, research suggests that β-alanine supplementation is capable of improving performance in exercises resulting in an extreme intramuscular acidotic environment, such as multiple bouts of high-intensity short-term exercises, single bouts of high-intensity exercises lasting more than 60s, and single bouts undertaken when fatigue is already present. Exercises with a lower level of acidosis are unlikely to benefit from β-alanine supplementation [140, 148]. β-Alanine supplementation has a discrete ergogenic effect in exercise lasting longer than 4 min [145]. Evidence suggests that there is a small or absent ergogenic effect in endurance performance (lasting 25 min or more) [139], although anaerobic threshold can be shifted after supplementation [148].

A recent study showed that 3 weeks of β-alanine supplementation (4.5 g/d) in college football players did not result in significant improvements in fatigue rates during high-intensity anaerobic exercise, but they suggested a trend for a lower fatigue rate during prolonged (60s) high-intensity exercise. However, as supplementation continued during preseason training camp, subjective measures of fatigue were significantly lower. In addition, training volume tended to be higher in subjects supplementing with β-alanine compared with subjects consuming a placebo [149]. Another study with amateur footballers stated that 12 weeks of β-alanine supplementation improved Yo-Yo intermitent recovery (IR)2 test performance [150]. A study with female footballers showed that 30 days of β-alanine supplementation was able to improve average and peak power when performing consecutive sprints (Wingate test), although lactate did not differ from placebo [151]. Saunders et al. [152] found no effect of β-alanine supplementation (alone or in combination with sodium bicarbonate) on repeated sprints during simulated match play performed in hypoxia.

Although the scientific evidence in untrained populations is substantial, more studies need to be conducted in trained populations and in various sport disciplines in order to fully understand the value of β-alanine supplementation for performance enhancement in elite sports [140].

Daily doses should be divided in doses of 2 g or less in order to minimize side effects. Single large boluses of β-alanine have been shown to induce paresthesia and have not been effective for performance outcomes likely due to strong paresthesia, rapid changes in pH, higher excretion rates, and inability to effectively load the muscle contents. Combining β-alanine consumption with a meal has been shown to be effective for further augmenting muscle carnosine levels [139]. Washout time may vary between non-responders and responders, requiring 6–15 weeks to return to normal [139].

β-Alanine supplementation currently appears to be safe in healthy populations at recommended doses. Paresthesia is the most widely known side effect of β-alanine, being commonly experienced in individuals consuming more than 800 mg of β-alanine in a non-sustained release form. To date, there is no evidence to support that this paresthesia is harmful in any way [139]. It is possible to reach the total daily dose of 6.4 g using 1600-mg doses when using controlled-release capsules. The controlled-release capsules eliminate all symptoms of paresthesia. Four daily doses of 1600 mg may be more practical than eight daily doses of 800 mg and may also ensure greater compliance [148].

53.8 Sodium Bicarbonate

Sodium bicarbonate ($NaHCO_3$) has been investigated as a potential aid to increase the bicarbonate buffer system in blood and interstitium, enhance lactate and H^+ translocation from the myoplasm, decrease acid-base balance perturbations, prevent fatigue, and improve performance during high-intensity anaerobic exercise [153].

The exogenous intake of $NaHCO_3$ from 1 to 3 h before exercise results in an important increase in the pH and bicarbonate concentrations in blood at the beginning of an exercise session, as well as during and after it, whereas intramuscular pH and [HCO_3^-] remain apparently unchanged [154]. Muscle cell membranes are impervious to HCO_3^-, and an increase in extracellular HCO_3^- increases the pH gradient between the intracellular and extracellular environment. The effect of this increased pH gradient is to facilitate the efflux of intracellular lactate and H^+, thus reducing the fall in intracellular pH [155]. Recently, other mechanism has been proposed, stating that intracellular perturbation may be minimized by the upregulation of Na^+/H^+ or monocarboxylic transporters or a strong ion difference [156].

The optimal amount should be 0.3-g/kg body weight [157]. Timing sequences with regard to ingestion patterns vary greatly between studies. Attaining peak buffering potential while minimizing the risk of gastrointestinal distress before exercise is essential, especially if athletes are considering loading before an event [158]. For an intake of 0.3-g/kg body weight of $NaHCO_3$, 120 min are needed to reach the peak pH and an average of 100–120 min to reach maximum [HCO_3^-] [154]. The substances should be taken in or with fluid, preferably water, and in large quantities (0.5 L or greater).

The ergogenic effect of bicarbonate has been shown in 200-m freestyle swimming [159], 2 × 100-m freestyle swimming (with 10 min of passive rest between bouts) [160], repeated sprints (5 × 6s) or multiple effort bouts observed in recreational team sport [161], and high-intensity intermittent exercise performance (Yo-Yo IR2 test) [162], but not in 200–400-m run [163]. It appears that bicarbonate ingestion can enhance the performance of all-out, maximal anaerobic activities of 1–7-min duration [138].

Subjects should be familiar with possible side effects, which include gastrointestinal distress and, more rarely, gastric rupture, muscle spasms, and cardiac arrhythmias [155]. An alternative protocol can be applied, using chronic $NaHCO_3$ administration [164]. Consumption of 0.5-g/kg body weight during 5 days has ergogenic effect in anaerobic performance (Wingate test) [153]. Chronic ingestion allows subjects to perform more work during high-intensity exercise for at least 2 days after cessation of chronic $NaHCO_3$ supplementation. Moreover, athletes might use $NaHCO_3$ to improve performance without the significant side effects that are usually associated with the ingestion of $NaHCO_3$ in the doses needed. The body may be able to store the [HCO_3^-] surplus over a 5-day period and then use it to improve performance during the post-supplementation exercise [153].

53.9 Antioxidants

An antioxidant can be defined as "a compound that in a relatively low concentration, prevents or delays the oxidation of biomolecules" [165]. It is well established that physical exercise results in increased reactive oxygen species (ROS) production in active skeletal muscles. An official football match induces an increased level of oxidative stress and muscle damage throughout 48 h of the recovery period [166]. Dietary antioxidants, like vitamin C, vitamin E, carotenoids, and polyphenols, have received attention predominantly as a nutritional strategy for preventing or minimizing detrimental effects of ROS, which are generated during and after strenuous exercise [167]. Then, antioxidant supplementation has become a common practice among athletes as a mean to reduce oxidative stress, promote recovery, and enhance performance [168].

However, there is still a wide discussion whether antioxidant supplements are helpful or harmful to the athlete [169]. There is no evidence that exercise-induced radical production in skeletal muscle is detrimental to human health. Besides, regular training promotes an increase in the body's own antioxidant defense system against free radical damage [170]. Until now, requirements of antioxidant micronutrients and antioxidant compounds for athletes competing in different sport events, involving repeated sprinting, have not been determined sufficiently [171].

Actually, the evidence suggests that athletes should use caution when considering supplementation with high doses of antioxidants. A meta-analysis of 68 randomized antioxidant supplement trials (total of 232,606 human participants) concluded that dietary supplementation above the recommended dietary allowance (RDA) with beta-carotene, vitamin A, and vitamin E does not improve health outcomes and may increase mortality [172]. Furthermore, in athletes, antioxidant supplementation can prevent important exercise-induced adaptations in skeletal muscle [173]. Indeed, compelling evidence indicates that exercise-induced ROS production serves as a required signal to promote the expression of numerous skeletal muscle proteins including antioxidant enzymes, mitochondrial proteins, and heat-shock proteins [174]. Some studies in athletes [37–39, 173, 175, 176] indicate that high levels of antioxidant supplementation can blunt the training adaptation to exercise, and one study including football players [177] refers that the antioxidant supplementation group had a lower increase in Vo_{2max} compared with the placebo group.

Further research is required to establish firmly whether antioxidant supplementation is beneficial or harmful to athletes. However, at present, there is limited scientific evidence to recommend antioxidant supplements to athletes. In fact, the consumption of a diet that is nutritionally well balanced can provide a sufficient antioxidant intake, during exercise training, to maintain an appropriate physiological antioxidant status in reference to current recommendations [178].

Some athletes may not consume well-balanced diets, and therefore these individuals could be deficient in antioxidant intake. Prior to the recommendation in using antioxidant supplements, it should be enhanced the importance to nutrition education in athletes. In other situations, moderate and timely limited antioxidant supplementation may be indicated. In cases of high-altitude training periods, it would also be recommended, since radical production is intensified and endogenous defense weakened in hypoxia [179]. Nevertheless, the optimal bioavailability and combined action of multiple phytochemical and antioxidant compounds derived from fruits, vegetables, whole grains, and nuts cannot be replaced by supplementation. In any case, we have to consider the positive and negative effects of free radicals and that the right balance between these and antioxidants is necessary for health and optimal training effectiveness. Antioxidant supplementation may reduce ROS levels, but it is difficult to assume an improvement in athletic performance, only in cases of altitude training [180]. Like other nutritional supplements, it is not a case of "the more, the better."

53.10 Probiotics

Probiotics are live microorganisms which, when administered in adequate amounts, modify the bacterial population that inhabits our gut and modulate immune function by their interaction with the gut-associated lymphoid tissue, leading to positive effects on the systemic immune system [181]. However, it should be noted that such effects are dose and strain dependent [182]. Probiotics modify the intestinal microbiota such that the numbers of beneficial bacteria increase and usually the numbers of species considered harmful are decreased. Such changes are associated with a range of potential benefits to the health and functioning of the digestive system, as well as modulation of immune function [183]. A recent meta-analysis of the effect of probiotics in respiratory virus infections in the general population showed that 28 out of 33 studies reported beneficial effects [184]. Athletes engaging in prolonged intense exercise may be more susceptible to upper respiratory tract illness (URTI), than individuals participating in moderate exercise or sedentary [185]. In athletes, these symptoms are generally trivial, but no matter whether the cause is infectious or allergic inflammation, they can cause an athlete to interrupt training, underperform, or even miss an important competition [181].

Although there are few published studies of the effectiveness of probiotic use in athletes, there is growing interest in examining their potential to help maintain overall general health, enhance immune function, or reduce URTI incidence and symptom severity/duration. A randomized double-blind intervention study investigated 141 runners taking either a placebo or *L. rhamnosus* daily during 3 months of training period before a marathon race with follow-up during 2 weeks. Although there were no significant differences in the number of episodes of respiratory or gastrointestinal tract illness, the duration of gastrointestinal symptom episodes in the probiotic group was shorter than in the placebo group during the training period (2.9 vs 4.3 days) and during the 2 weeks after the marathon (1.0 vs 2.3 days) [186]. Another study in elite runners showed that supplementation in *L. fermentum* decreased the number of days of respiratory illness [187]. A substantial reduction was also observed in URTI incidence among male but not among female athletes after 77 days of *L. fermentum* supplementation. It remains unclear the differences between the sexes [188]. Probiotic supplementation ingested on a daily basis reduces the number of participants who report any incidence of an infectious symptom in 30 highly trained elite rugby players. The investigators used capsules containing three acid-resistant strains of bacteria (*Lactobacillus gasseri*, 2.6 billion colony-forming units (CFUs); *Bifidobacterium bifidum*, 0.2 billion organisms; *Bifidobacterium longum*, 0.2 billion organisms) [189]. They observed a significant reduction in the number of URTI or gastrointestinal episodes in participants on the probiotic intervention compared to the placebo and significant reduction in the number of days reporting any symptoms during the probiotic treatment compared with a placebo.

Unfortunately there are still no studies of probiotic supplementation in football players, and given the small number of studies that have examined the effects of probiotic supplementation in athletes, it is somewhat premature to issue definitive recommendations. Yet, oral probiotics in athletes, particularly those containing *Lactobacillus* strains, are a promising area of research. Probiotics may reduce the risk of respiratory and gastrointestinal illness during stressful periods of training and competition. More research is required to clarify issues of strains, dose response, mechanisms, and best practice models for probiotic implementation in the sporting community.

53.11 Vitamin D

Vitamin D is classified as a fat-soluble vitamin but acts functionally as a hormone and has a structure that is similar to steroid hormones. Humans acquire vitamin D from two different sources, endogenous production after sun exposure or via the diet (from food or supplementation). From diet, vitamin D can be found in various food products such as fatty fish, eggs, and dairy products and through various vitamin D analogues produced synthetically in a laboratory. The major source of vitamin D is provided from cutaneous synthesis via exposure to ultraviolet B (UVB) radiation in sunlight [190]. Cutaneous synthesis of vitamin D, however, is dependent on factors including time of exposure, season, latitude, cloud cover, smog, skin pigmentation, sunscreen coverage, and age [191].Vitamin D deficiency is a common but under recognized problem within the global population. The main cause of vitamin D deficiency could arise from the fact that sun exposure be connoted negatively on health. However, moderate sun exposure is the primary means of obtaining vitamin D in humans because it is unlikely to get adequate amounts through diet [192]. Dark-skinned athletes, athletes who live at more poleward latitudes, wear extensive clothing, regularly use sunblock, or consciously avoid the sun, are all at risk for vitamin D deficiency [193]. Although there is no consensus on optimal serum levels of 25(OH)D, vitamin D deficiency is defined by most experts as a total level of less than 20 ng/mL (50 nmol/L). Vitamin D insufficiency is defined as a level of 20–31 ng/mL, and a level of 32 ng/mL (80 nmol/L) or greater is indicative of sufficient levels [194]. Vitamin D inadequacy (serum 25(OH)D <32 ng/mL) was determined in a total of 2313 athletes from different modalities. Fifty six percent (44–67%) of them had vitamin D inadequacy that significantly varied by geographical location [194]. In football players the reality is not very different. A sample of 28 healthy professional football players, white Caucasians, from two First Division teams of Spain provided a blood sample in October and in early February [195]. Two thirds of players had insufficient vitamin D in early February, and almost a third of the group with 25(OH)D above 40 ng/mL in mid-October were below 30 ng/mL in early February. This study suggests that serum 25(OH) D of approximately 48.8 ng/mL is necessary in mid-October to ensure vitamin D sufficiency (30 ng/mL) at the beginning of February. In another study [196], 20 professional male Premier League football players, of varying nationalities, provided a sample in the summer and the winter. Serum 25(OH)D significantly decreased between summer (41.6 ± 8.4 ng/mL) and winter (20.4 ± 7.6 ng/mL) months. All 20 players exhibited a decrease in vitamin D concentration within this time period, where the mean decrement was 21.2 ± 6.0 ng/mL. The two players who were dark skinned exhibited the lowest serum 25(OH)D values in both summer (28 and 27.2 ng/mL, respectively) and winter (8.8 and 15.6 ng/mL, respectively). Also Polish professional football players ($n = 24$) had lower levels of 25(OH)D after the winter period compared to the summer period (24.96 ± 9.11 ng/ml vs 30.82 ± 9.04 ng/ml) [197]. Finally, in 342 professional footballers based in Qatar, 84% of them had 25(OH)D concentrations less than 30 ng/mL; 12% were severely deficient (<10 ng/mL), and there was a significant difference in 25(OH)D level depending on the country of origin of the player. Total body mass and lean mass were significantly higher in players with 25(OH)D levels greater than 20 ng/mL, when compared with the players with less than 10 ng/mL. However, there was no consistent association found between lower-limb isokinetic peak torque and 25(OH)D concentration [198].

The effects of vitamin D are not limited to bone metabolism. A recent systematic review found a moderate to strong inverse associations between 25(OH)D concentrations and cardiovascular diseases, serum lipid concentrations, inflammation, glucose metabolism disorders, weight gain, infectious diseases, multiple sclerosis, mood disorders, declining cognitive function, impaired physical functioning, and all-cause mortality [199].

The discovery of the vitamin D receptor in human skeletal muscle has led to increased research indicating a direct effect on skeletal muscle activity [200]. It has been long recognized that vitamin D deficiency is associated with muscle weakness, particularly proximal muscle weakness, and that this resolves with correction of deficiency [201]. Evidence from the Russian and German literature at the turn of the twentieth century suggests that UVB exposure makes a positive impact upon athletic performance [193]. However, these studies did not simultaneously measure markers of vitamin D status and were not made using the rigorous scientific standards employed today. Vitamin D affects skeletal muscle by indirect mechanisms, by the change of calcium and phosphate balance, and by direct mechanisms through activation of muscle cells in the vitamin D receptor triggering the transcription of genes involved in differentiation and proliferation of muscle cells [202]. There may be even an influence of vitamin D receptors polymorphisms on musculoskeletal injury. In professional football players, it was found that the *Apa*I polymorphism may be associated with the severity of musculoskeletal injury [203].

Emerging evidence also suggests that vitamin D plays important roles in immune and inflammatory modulation and therefore has the potential to impact upon the health, training, and performance of athletes. A low level of vitamin D in collegiate athletes during the spring was correlated with the frequency of the disease, including common cold, influenza, and gastroenteritis, and would benefit from supplementation during the winter to prevent seasonal decreases in 25(OH)D concentrations [204]. Recent research has provided evidence to suggest that maintaining adequate vitamin D status may reduce stress fracture risk, total body inflammation, common infectious illness [205], and enhance strength recovery after anterior cruciate ligament surgery recovery [206]. Poor vitamin D status has been linked to upper respiratory tract infection in young Finnish athletes [207] and elevated concentrations of systemic inflammatory markers in runners [208].

There is convincing evidence that the majority of football players have low levels of vitamin D, the question is how it impacts the performance. Increases in force and power production have been studied in athletes with positive results during a randomized placebo-controlled study in ten male professional football players [209] after 8 weeks of supplementation of either 5000 IU/day of vitamin D3 or a placebo; the vitamin D3 group had a significant increase in serum 25(OH) D levels and a significant improvement in both their 10-m sprint times and vertical jump when compared to the placebo group. A significant correlation between 25(OH)D levels and performance parameters was found in 67 Caucasian male professional football players [210]. This study demonstrated a linear relationship was seen between pre- and post-off-season measurements of 25(OH)D and muscle strength indicated by squat jump, countermovement jump, sprinting ability (10- and 20-m sprint), and VO_2max. However, other studies have shown no significant benefit of vitamin D supplementation in athletes with moderately deficient or adequate levels indicating that these performance benefits might be limited to individuals with significant vitamin D deficiency [211]. The largest improvements in performance will probably occur in those with the lowest levels; that is, a significant improvement in athletic performance may occur when levels increase from 15 to 30 ng/mL, but less improvement will occur when levels increase from 30 to 50 ng/ml [193]. Regular consumption of vitamin D-fortified foods is not likely to result in sufficient status in the absence of UVB exposure [212]. Habitual exposure to the arms, legs, and back several times a week for 5 min (for fair-skinned individuals) to 30 min (for darker-skinned individuals) at close to solar noon without sunscreen usually leads to sufficient vitamin D synthesis in summer months [191]. To account for the seasonal variation in ultraviolet B radiation during winter, daily supplementation with 5000 IU of vitamin D3 appears a safe and tolerable dose to restore circulating 25(OH)D concentrations to sufficient levels, thus promoting immune and bone function and potentially improving training adaptations through modulation of muscle mass [211]. Athletes, who often believe more is better, should be cautioned that daily supplementation with more than 10,000 IU could lead to toxicity [213].

53.12 Whey Protein

Although protein is not considered ergogenic to exercise performance, protein ingestion in close proximity to the exercise stimulus increases skeletal muscle protein synthesis (MPS) and thereby facilitates post-exercise skeletal muscle remodeling processes. To this end, ingestion of 20–30 g of protein is sufficient to induce maximal rates of MPS [214]. Additionally, because of its rapid rates of digestion and elevated leucine concentration, whey proteins are a better choice to both soy and casein protein sources [215]. Leucine is one of the three branched-chain amino acid that has to be provided in the diet. Besides serving as building blocks for protein synthesis, leucine can also regulate the rate of protein synthesis via a stimulatory effect on enzymes involved in the translation of specific mRNAs. From a nutrition perspective, the use of some supplements such as leucine may partially attenuate the decrease in MPS through the activation of mTOR [216]. Leucine is an essential amino acid found in greater amounts in proteins of high biological value, such as whey protein. Available data indicate that the amount of leucine required to reach an optimal effect is 1.5–2.5 g in young individuals, which is the normal content in around 20 g of high-quality protein [217]. The ingestion of 3 g of leucine, isolated or contained in protein, is capable of activating MPS [218] and would be indicated in a football player in rehabilitation process recovering from muscle atrophy [219]. Given that liquid protein induces higher plasma aminoacidemia than solid protein sources, it would be an interesting practice to provide a whey-based liquid protein immediately after games [220]. In the context of training days, 20–25 g of protein can be easily consumed through whole foods, although occasionally it may be more practical to deliver protein in the form of a protein shake or drink that delivers the exact amount of protein in a convenient form. It is also beneficial for players to consume 30–40 g of casein-based protein prior to sleep so as to stimulate MPS and promote overnight recovery [221].

The catabolite of leucine, β-hydroxy-β-methylbutyrate, ingested at 3 g per day has also been reported to be an effective supplement in the activation of MPS, although further research is needed before its use can be recommended, especially in consideration for the injured player [222]. Another product of leucine metabolism, alfa-hydroxy-isocaproic acid, may also be of interest in muscle mass increase in football players [223].

Despite lacking evidence of whey protein in performance of football players, it would be recommended to consider in moments like post-match and post-training ingestion of 20–30 g of whey protein to induce maximal rates of MPS, thereby promoting recovery and training adaptation.

References

1. Applegate EA, Grivetti LE. Search for the competitive edge: a history of dietary fads and supplements. J Nutr. 1997;127:869S–73S.
2. Morente-Sanchez J, Zabala M. Doping in sport: a review of elite athletes' attitudes, beliefs, and knowledge. Sports Med. 2013;43:395–411.
3. Silver MD. Use of ergogenic aids by athletes. J Am Acad Orthop Surg. 2001;9:61–70.
4. Van Thuyne W, Van Eenoo P, Delbeke FT. Nutritional supplements: prevalence of use and contamination with doping agents. Nutr Res Rev. 2006;19:147–58.
5. Geyer H, Parr MK, Koehler K, Mareck U, Schanzer W, Thevis M. Nutritional supplements cross-contaminated and faked with doping substances. J Mass Spectrom. 2008;43:892–902.
6. NBJ's Global Supplement & Nutrition Industry Report 2012. An analysis of markets, trends, competition and strategy in the Global Nutrition Industry. Nutr Bus J. 2012.
7. Maughan RJ, Greenhaff PL, Hespel P. Dietary supplements for athletes: emerging trends and recurring themes. J Sports Sci. 2011;29(Suppl 1):S57–66.
8. Sousa M, Fernandes MJ, Moreira P, Teixeira VH. Nutritional supplements usage by Portuguese athletes. Int J Vitam Nutr Res. 2013;83:48–58.
9. Tscholl P, Junge A, Dvorak J. The use of medication and nutritional supplements during FIFA World Cups 2002 and 2006. Br J Sports Med. 2008;42:725–30.
10. Tscholl PM, Vaso M, Weber A, Dvorak J. High prevalence of medication use in professional football tournaments including the World Cups between 2002 and 2014: a narrative review with a focus on NSAIDs. Br J Sports Med. 2015;49:580–2.
11. Waddington I, Malcolm D, Roderick M, Naik R. Drug use in English professional football. Br J Sports Med. 2005;39:e18.
12. de Silva A, Samarasinghe Y, Senanayake D, Lanerolle P. Dietary supplement intake in national-level Sri Lankan athletes. Int J Sport Nutr Exerc Metab. 2010;20:15–20.
13. Maughan RJ, Depiesse F, Geyer H, International Association of Athletics F. The use of dietary supplements by athletes. J Sports Sci. 2007;25(Suppl 1):S103–13.
14. Tscholl P, Alonso JM, Dolle G, Junge A, Dvorak J. The use of drugs and nutritional supplements in top-level track and field athletes. Am J Sports Med. 2010;38:133–40.
15. Aljaloud SO, Ibrahim SA. Use of dietary supplements among professional athletes in Saudi Arabia. J Nutr Metab. 2013;2013:245349.
16. Maughan RJ, King DS, Lea T. Dietary supplements. J Sports Sci. 2004;22:95–113.
17. Sousa M, Fernandes MJ, Carvalho P, Soares J, Moreira P, Teixeira VH. Nutritional supplements use in high-performance athletes is related with lower nutritional inadequacy from food. J Sport Health Sci. 2015;5:368–74.
18. Pittler MH, Schmidt K, Ernst E. Adverse events of herbal food supplements for body weight reduction: systematic review. Obes Rev. 2005;6:93–111.
19. Yellapu RK, Mittal V, Grewal P, Fiel M, Schiano T. Acute liver failure caused by 'fat burners' and dietary supplements: a case report and literature review. Can J Gastroenterol. 2011;25:157–60.
20. Molinari M, Watt KD, Kruszyna T, Nelson R, Walsh M, Huang WY, Nashan B, Peltekian K. Acute liver failure induced by green tea extracts: case report and review of the literature. Liver Transpl. 2006;12:1892–5.
21. Burke L, Deakin V. Clinical sports nutrition. 3rd ed. New York: McGraw-Hill; 2006.
22. Beedie CJ, Stuart EM, Coleman DA, Foad AJ. Placebo effects of caffeine on cycling performance. Med Sci Sports Exerc. 2006;38:2159–64.
23. Beedie CJ, Foad AJ. The placebo effect in sports performance: a brief review. Sports Med. 2009;39:313–29.
24. Duncan MJ, Lyons M, Hankey J. Placebo effects of caffeine on short-term resistance exercise to failure. Int J Sports Physiol Perform. 2009;4:244–53.
25. Beedie CJ, Coleman DA, Foad AJ. Positive and negative placebo effects resulting from the deceptive administration of an ergogenic aid. Int J Sport Nutr Exerc Metab. 2007;17:259–69.
26. McClung M, Collins D. "Because I know it will!": placebo effects of an ergogenic aid on athletic performance. J Sport Exerc Psychol. 2007;29:382–94.
27. van der Merwe PJ, Grobbelaar E. Unintentional doping through the use of contaminated nutritional supplements. S Afr Med J. 2005;95:510–1.
28. Striegel H, Vollkommer G, Horstmann T, Niess AM. Contaminated nutritional supplements – legal protection for elite athletes who tested positive: a case report from Germany. J Sports Sci. 2005;23:723–6.

29. Maughan RJ. Contamination of dietary supplements and positive drug tests in sport. J Sports Sci. 2005;23: 883–9.
30. Kamber M, Baume N, Saugy M, Rivier L. Nutritional supplements as a source for positive doping cases? Int J Sport Nutr Exerc Metab. 2001;11:258–63.
31. Geyer H, Parr MK, Mareck U, Reinhart U, Schrader Y, Schanzer W. Analysis of non-hormonal nutritional supplements for anabolic-androgenic steroids – results of an international study. Int J Sports Med. 2004;25:124–9.
32. Burke LM, Castell LM, Stear SJ. BJSM reviews: A-Z of supplements: dietary supplements, sports nutrition foods and ergogenic aids for health and performance part 1. Br J Sports Med. 2009;43:728–9.
33. de Hon O, Coumans B. The continuing story of nutritional supplements and doping infractions. Br J Sports Med. 2007;41:800–5.
34. de Oliveira KJ, Donangelo CM, de Oliveira Jr AV, da Silveira CL, Koury JC. Effect of zinc supplementation on the antioxidant, copper, and iron status of physically active adolescents. Cell Biochem Funct. 2009;27:162–6.
35. Mettler S, Zimmermann MB. Iron excess in recreational marathon runners. Eur J Clin Nutr. 2010;64: 490–4.
36. Ristow M, Zarse K, Oberbach A, Kloting N, Birringer M, Kiehntopf M, Stumvoll M, Kahn CR, Bluher M. Antioxidants prevent health-promoting effects of physical exercise in humans. Proc Natl Acad Sci U S A. 2009;106:8665–70.
37. Teixeira VH, Valente HF, Casal SI, Marques AF, Moreira PA. Antioxidants do not prevent postexercise peroxidation and may delay muscle recovery. Med Sci Sports Exerc. 2009;41:1752–60.
38. Close GL, Ashton T, Cable T, Doran D, Holloway C, McArdle F, MacLaren DP. Ascorbic acid supplementation does not attenuate post-exercise muscle soreness following muscle-damaging exercise but may delay the recovery process. Br J Nutr. 2006;95:976–81.
39. Gomez-Cabrera MC, Domenech E, Romagnoli M, Arduini A, Borras C, Pallardo FV, Sastre J, Vina J. Oral administration of vitamin C decreases muscle mitochondrial biogenesis and hampers training-induced adaptations in endurance performance. Am J Clin Nutr. 2008;87:142–9.
40. Nawrot P, Jordan S, Eastwood J, Rotstein J, Hugenholtz A, Feeley M. Effects of caffeine on human health. Food Addit Contam. 2003;20:1–30.
41. Keisler BD, Armsey 2nd TD. Caffeine as an ergogenic aid. Curr Sports Med Rep. 2006;5:215–9.
42. Goldstein ER, Ziegenfuss T, Kalman D, Kreider R, Campbell B, Wilborn C, Taylor L, Willoughby D, Stout J, Graves BS, Wildman R, Ivy JL, Spano M, Smith AE, Antonio J. International society of sports nutrition position stand: caffeine and performance. J Int Soc Sports Nutr. 2010;7:5.
43. Graham TE. Caffeine and exercise: metabolism, endurance and performance. Sports Med. 2001;31:785–807.
44. Burke L, Cort M, Cox G, Crawford R, Desbrow B, Farthing L, Minehan M, Shaw N, Warnes O. Supplements and sports foods. In: Burke L, Deakin V, editors. Clinical sports nutrition. 3rd ed. Sydney/London: McGraw-Hill; 2006. p. 485–579.
45. Wilmore JH, Costill DL, Kenney WL. Ergogenic aids and sport. In: Wilmore JH, Costill DL, Kenney WL, editors. Physiology of sport and exercise. 4th ed. Champaign/Leeds: Human Kinetics; 2008.
46. Lieberman HR, Tharion WJ, Shukitt-Hale B, Speckman KL, Tulley R. Effects of caffeine, sleep loss, and stress on cognitive performance and mood during U.S. Navy SEAL training. Sea-Air-Land. Psychopharmacology. 2002;164:250–61.
47. Doherty M, Smith PM. Effects of caffeine ingestion on rating of perceived exertion during and after exercise: a meta-analysis. Scand J Med Sci Sports. 2005;15:69–78.
48. Tarnopolsky MA. Effect of caffeine on the neuromuscular system – potential as an ergogenic aid. Appl Physiol Nutr Metab. 2008;33:1284–9.
49. Greer F, Morales J, Coles M. Wingate performance and surface EMG frequency variables are not affected by caffeine ingestion. Appl Physiol Nutr Metab. 2006;31:597–603.
50. Lorino AJ, Lloyd LK, Crixell SH, Walker JL. The effects of caffeine on athletic agility. J Strength Cond Res. 2006;20:851–4.
51. Astorino TA, Roberson DW. Efficacy of acute caffeine ingestion for short-term high-intensity exercise performance: a systematic review. J Strength Cond Res. 2010;24:257–65.
52. Davis JK, Green JM. Caffeine and anaerobic performance: ergogenic value and mechanisms of action. Sports Med. 2009;39:813–32.
53. Ahrendt DM. Ergogenic aids: counseling the athlete. Am Fam Physician. 2001;63:913–22.
54. Graham TE, Battram DS, Dela F, El-Sohemy A, Thong FS. Does caffeine alter muscle carbohydrate and fat metabolism during exercise? Appl Physiol Nutr Metab. 2008;33:1311–8.
55. Stuart GR, Hopkins WG, Cook C, Cairns SP. Multiple effects of caffeine on simulated high-intensity team-sport performance. Med Sci Sports Exerc. 2005;37: 1998–2005.
56. Foskett A, Ali A, Gant N. Caffeine enhances cognitive function and skill performance during simulated soccer activity. Int J Sport Nutr Exerc Metab. 2009; 19:410–23.
57. Paton CD, Hopkins WG, Vollebregt L. Little effect of caffeine ingestion on repeated sprints in team-sport athletes. Med Sci Sports Exerc. 2001;33: 822–5.
58. Morton JP. Supplements for consideration in football. Sports Sci Exch. 2014;27:1–8.
59. Pettersen SA, Krustrup P, Bendiksen M, Randers MB, Brito J, Bangsbo J, Jin Y, Mohr M. Caffeine supplementation does not affect match activities and fatigue resistance during match play in young football players. J Sports Sci. 2014;32:1958–65.

60. Russell M, Kingsley M. The efficacy of acute nutritional interventions on soccer skill performance. Sports Med. 2014;44:957–70.
61. Del Coso J, Munoz-Fernandez VE, Munoz G, Fernandez-Elias VE, Ortega JF, Hamouti N, Barbero JC, Munoz-Guerra J. Effects of a caffeine-containing energy drink on simulated soccer performance. PLoS One. 2012;7:e31380.
62. Gant N, Ali A, Foskett A. The influence of caffeine and carbohydrate coingestion on simulated soccer performance. Int J Sport Nutr Exerc Metab. 2010;20:191–7.
63. Lara B, Gonzalez-Millan C, Salinero JJ, Abian-Vicen J, Areces F, Barbero-Alvarez JC, Munoz V, Portillo LJ, Gonzalez-Rave JM, Del Coso J. Caffeine-containing energy drink improves physical performance in female soccer players. Amino Acids. 2014;46:1385–92.
64. Duvnjak-Zaknich DM, Dawson BT, Wallman KE, Henry G. Effect of caffeine on reactive agility time when fresh and fatigued. Med Sci Sports Exerc. 2011;43:1523–30.
65. Jordan JB, Korgaokar A, Farley RS, Coons JM, Caputo JL. Caffeine supplementation and reactive agility in elite youth soccer players. Pediatr Exerc Sci. 2014;26:168–76.
66. Kingsley M, Penas-Ruiz C, Terry C, Russell M. Effects of carbohydrate-hydration strategies on glucose metabolism, sprint performance and hydration during a soccer match simulation in recreational players. J Sci Med Sport. 2014;17:239–43.
67. Beaven CM, Maulder P, Pooley A, Kilduff L, Cook C. Effects of caffeine and carbohydrate mouth rinses on repeated sprint performance. Appl Physiol Nutr Metab. 2013;38:633–7.
68. Maridakis V, O'Connor PJ, Tomporowski PD. Sensitivity to change in cognitive performance and mood measures of energy and fatigue in response to morning caffeine alone or in combination with carbohydrate. Int J Neurosci. 2009;119:1239–58.
69. Ali A, O'Donnell J, Von Hurst P, Foskett A, Holland S, Starck C, Rutherfurd-Markwick K. Caffeine ingestion enhances perceptual responses during intermittent exercise in female team-game players. J Sports Sci. 2015;34:1–12.
70. Cox GR, Desbrow B, Montgomery PG, Anderson ME, Bruce CR, Macrides TA, Martin DT, Moquin A, Roberts A, Hawley JA, Burke LM. Effect of different protocols of caffeine intake on metabolism and endurance performance. J Appl Physiol. 2002;93:990–9.
71. Bridge CA, Jones MA. The effect of caffeine ingestion on 8 km run performance in a field setting. J Sports Sci. 2006;24:433–9.
72. Bruce CR, Anderson ME, Fraser SF, Stepto NK, Klein R, Hopkins WG, Hawley JA. Enhancement of 2000-m rowing performance after caffeine ingestion. Med Sci Sports Exerc. 2000;32:1958–63.
73. Anderson ME, Bruce CR, Fraser SF, Stepto NK, Klein R, Hopkins WG, Hawley JA. Improved 2000-meter rowing performance in competitive oarswomen after caffeine ingestion. Int J Sport Nutr Exerc Metab. 2000;10:464–75.
74. Hespel P, Maughan RJ, Greenhaff PL. Dietary supplements for football. J Sports Sci. 2006;24:749–61.
75. Stolen T, Chamari K, Castagna C, Wisloff U. Physiology of soccer: an update. Sports Med. 2005;35:501–36.
76. Drake C, Roehrs T, Shambroom J, Roth T. Caffeine effects on sleep taken 0, 3, or 6 hours before going to bed. J Clin Sleep Med. 2013;9:1195–200.
77. Nedelec M, Halson S, Abaidia AE, Ahmaidi S, Dupont G. Stress, sleep and recovery in elite soccer: a critical review of the literature. Sports Med. 2015;45(10):1387–400.
78. Burke LM. Caffeine and sports performance. Appl Physiol Nutr Metab. 2008;33:1319–34.
79. Clarke ND, Kornilios E, Richardson DL. Carbohydrate and caffeine mouth rinses do not affect maximum strength and muscular endurance performance. J Strength Cond Res. 2015;29(10):2926–31.
80. Krustrup P, Mohr M, Steensberg A, Bencke J, Kjaer M, Bangsbo J. Muscle and blood metabolites during a soccer game: implications for sprint performance. Med Sci Sports Exerc. 2006;38:1165–74.
81. Bangsbo J, Iaia FM, Krustrup P. Metabolic response and fatigue in soccer. Int J Sports Physiol Perform. 2007;2:111–27.
82. Miller SL, Wolfe RR. Physical exercise as a modulator of adaptation to low and high carbohydrate and low and high fat intakes. Eur J Clin Nutr. 1999;53(Suppl 1):S112–9.
83. van Loon LJ, Greenhaff PL, Constantin-Teodosiu D, Saris WH, Wagenmakers AJ. The effects of increasing exercise intensity on muscle fuel utilisation in humans. J Physiol. 2001;536:295–304.
84. Mohr M, Krustrup P, Bangsbo J. Match performance of high-standard soccer players with special reference to development of fatigue. J Sports Sci. 2003;21:519–28.
85. Mohr M, Krustrup P, Bangsbo J. Fatigue in soccer: a brief review. J Sports Sci. 2005;23:593–9.
86. Bangsbo J. Physiological demands of football. Sports Sci Exch. 2014;27:1–8.
87. Saltin B. Metabolic fundamentals in exercise. Med Sci Sports. 1973;5:137–46.
88. Rebouche CJ. Kinetics, pharmacokinetics, and regulation of L-carnitine and acetyl-L-carnitine metabolism. Ann N Y Acad Sci. 2004;1033:30–41.
89. Stephens FB, Evans CE, Constantin-Teodosiu D, Greenhaff PL. Carbohydrate ingestion augments L-carnitine retention in humans. J Appl Physiol (1985). 2007;102:1065–70.
90. Kraemer WJ, Volek JS, Dunn-Lewis C. L-carnitine supplementation: influence upon physiological function. Curr Sports Med Rep. 2008;7:218–23.
91. Hathcock JN, Shao A. Risk assessment for carnitine. Regul Toxicol Pharmacol. 2006;46:23–8.
92. Burke LM, Castell LM, Stear SJ, Rogers PJ, Blomstrand E, Gurr S, Mitchell N, Stephens FB, Greenhaff PL. BJSM reviews: A-Z of nutritional supplements: dietary supplements, sports nutrition foods and ergogenic aids for health and performance part 4. Br J Sports Med. 2009;43:1088–90.

93. Brass EP. Carnitine and sports medicine: use or abuse? Ann N Y Acad Sci. 2004;1033:67–78.
94. Karlic H, Lohninger A. Supplementation of L-carnitine in athletes: does it make sense? Nutrition. 2004;20:709–15.
95. Brass EP. Supplemental carnitine and exercise. Am J Clin Nutr. 2000;72:618S–23S.
96. Stephens FB, Constantin-Teodosiu D, Greenhaff PL. New insights concerning the role of carnitine in the regulation of fuel metabolism in skeletal muscle. J Physiol. 2007;581:431–44.
97. Stephens FB, Galloway SD. Carnitine and fat oxidation. Nestle Nutr Inst Workshop Ser. 2013;76: 13–23.
98. Wall BT, Stephens FB, Constantin-Teodosiu D, Marimuthu K, Macdonald IA, Greenhaff PL. Chronic oral ingestion of L-carnitine and carbohydrate increases muscle carnitine content and alters muscle fuel metabolism during exercise in humans. J Physiol. 2011;589:963–73.
99. Stephens FB, Wall BT, Marimuthu K, Shannon CE, Constantin-Teodosiu D, Macdonald IA, Greenhaff PL. Skeletal muscle carnitine loading increases energy expenditure, modulates fuel metabolism gene networks and prevents body fat accumulation in humans. J Physiol. 2013;591:4655–66.
100. Jeukendrup AE, Randell R. Fat burners: nutrition supplements that increase fat metabolism. Obes Rev. 2011;12:841–51.
101. Orer GE, Guzel NA. The effects of acute L-carnitine supplementation on endurance performance of athletes. J Strength Cond Res. 2014;28:514–9.
102. Naclerio F, Larumbe-Zabala E, Cooper R, Allgrove J, Earnest CP. A multi-ingredient containing carbohydrate, proteins L-glutamine and L-carnitine attenuates fatigue perception with no effect on performance, muscle damage or immunity in soccer players. PLoS One. 2015;10:e0125188.
103. Atalay Guzel N, Erikoglu Orer G, Sezen Bircan F, Coskun Cevher S. Effects of acute L-carnitine supplementation on nitric oxide production and oxidative stress after exhaustive exercise in young soccer players. J Sports Med Phys Fitness. 2015;55:9–15.
104. Poortmans JR, Rawson ES, Burke LM, Stear SJ, Castell LM. A-Z of nutritional supplements: dietary supplements, sports nutrition foods and ergogenic aids for health and performance. Part 11. Br J Sports Med. 2010;44:765–6.
105. Bemben MG, Lamont HS. Creatine supplementation and exercise performance: recent findings. Sports Med. 2005;35:107–25.
106. Terjung RL, Clarkson P, Eichner ER, Greenhaff PL, Hespel PJ, Israel RG, Kraemer WJ, Meyer RA, Spriet LL, Tarnopolsky MA, Wagenmakers AJ, Williams MH. American College of Sports Medicine roundtable. The physiological and health effects of oral creatine supplementation. Med Sci Sports Exerc. 2000;32:706–17.
107. Louis M, Poortmans JR, Francaux M, Berre J, Boisseau N, Brassine E, Cuthbertson DJ, Smith K, Babraj JA, Waddell T, Rennie MJ. No effect of creatine supplementation on human myofibrillar and sarcoplasmic protein synthesis after resistance exercise. Am J Physiol Endocrinol Metab. 2003;285:E1089–94.
108. Mujika I, Padilla S, Ibanez J, Izquierdo M, Gorostiaga E. Creatine supplementation and sprint performance in soccer players. Med Sci Sports Exerc. 2000;32:518–25.
109. Barnes C, Archer DT, Hogg B, Bush M, Bradley PS. The evolution of physical and technical performance parameters in the English Premier League. Int J Sports Med. 2014;35:1095–100.
110. Williams J, Abt G, Kilding AE. Effects of creatine monohydrate supplementation on simulated soccer performance. Int J Sports Physiol Perform. 2014;9: 503–10.
111. Claudino JG, Mezencio B, Amaral S, Zanetti V, Benatti F, Roschel H, Gualano B, Amadio AC, Serrao JC. Creatine monohydrate supplementation on lower-limb muscle power in Brazilian elite soccer players. J Int Soc Sports Nutr. 2014;11:32.
112. Hespel P, Derave W. Ergogenic effects of creatine in sports and rehabilitation. Subcell Biochem. 2007;46:245–59.
113. Robinson TM, Sewell DA, Hultman E, Greenhaff PL. Role of submaximal exercise in promoting creatine and glycogen accumulation in human skeletal muscle. J Appl Physiol (1985). 1999;87:598–604.
114. Mihic S, MacDonald JR, McKenzie S, Tarnopolsky MA. Acute creatine loading increases fat-free mass, but does not affect blood pressure, plasma creatinine, or CK activity in men and women. Med Sci Sports Exerc. 2000;32:291–6.
115. Calder PC. Dietary modification of inflammation with lipids. Proc Nutr Soc. 2002;61:345–58.
116. Nieman DC, Bishop NC. Nutritional strategies to counter stress to the immune system in athletes, with special reference to football. J Sports Sci. 2006;24: 763–72.
117. Venkatraman JT, Pendergast DR. Effect of dietary intake on immune function in athletes. Sports Med. 2002;32:323–37.
118. Toft AD, Thorn M, Ostrowski K, Asp S, Moller K, Iversen S, Hermann C, Sondergaard SR, Pedersen BK. N-3 polyunsaturated fatty acids do not affect cytokine response to strenuous exercise. J Appl Physiol (1985). 2000;89:2401–6.
119. Walsh NP, Gleeson M, Pyne DB, Nieman DC, Dhabhar FS, Shephard RJ, Oliver SJ, Bermon S, Kajeniene A. Position statement. Part two: maintaining immune health. Exerc Immunol Rev. 2011;17: 64–103.
120. Jouris KB, McDaniel JL, Weiss EP. The effect of omega-3 fatty acid supplementation on the inflammatory response to eccentric strength exercise. J Sports Sci Med. 2011;10:432–8.
121. Mickleborough TD. Omega-3 polyunsaturated fatty acids in physical performance optimization. Int J Sport Nutr Exerc Metab. 2013;23:83–96.
122. Capo X, Martorell M, Sureda A, Llompart I, Tur JA, Pons A. Diet supplementation with DHA-enriched food in football players during training season enhances the mitochondrial antioxidant capabilities in blood mononuclear cells. Eur J Nutr. 2015;54:35–49.

123. Zebrowska A, Mizia-Stec K, Mizia M, Gasior Z, Poprzecki S. Omega-3 fatty acids supplementation improves endothelial function and maximal oxygen uptake in endurance-trained athletes. Eur J Sport Sci. 2015;15:305–14.
124. Tiryaki-Sonmez G, Schoenfeld B, Vatansever-Ozen S. Omega-3 fatty acids and exercise: a review of their combined effects on body composition and physical performance. Biomed Hum Kinet. 2011;3:23–9.
125. Walser B, Giordano RM, Stebbins CL. Supplementation with omega-3 polyunsaturated fatty acids augments brachial artery dilation and blood flow during forearm contraction. Eur J Appl Physiol. 2006;97:347–54.
126. Smith GI, Atherton P, Reeds DN, Mohammed BS, Rankin D, Rennie MJ, Mittendorfer B. Omega-3 polyunsaturated fatty acids augment the muscle protein anabolic response to hyperinsulinaemia-hyperaminoacidaemia in healthy young and middle-aged men and women. Clin Sci (Lond). 2011;121:267–78.
127. Simopoulos AP. Omega-3 fatty acids and athletics. Curr Sports Med Rep. 2007;6:230–6.
128. Wall BT, van Loon LJ. Nutritional strategies to attenuate muscle disuse atrophy. Nutr Rev. 2013;71: 195–208.
129. Tipton KD. Nutrition for acute exercise-induced injuries. Ann Nutr Metab. 2010;57(Suppl 2):43–53.
130. Tipton KD. Dietary strategies to attenuate muscle loss during recovery from injury. Nestle Nutr Inst Workshop Ser. 2013;75:51–61.
131. Wall BT, Morton JP, van Loon LJ. Strategies to maintain skeletal muscle mass in the injured athlete: nutritional considerations and exercise mimetics. Eur J Sport Sci. 2015;15:53–62.
132. Magne H, Savary-Auzeloux I, Remond D, Dardevet D. Nutritional strategies to counteract muscle atrophy caused by disuse and to improve recovery. Nutr Res Rev. 2013;26:149–65.
133. Barrett EC, McBurney MI, Ciappio ED. Omega-3 fatty acid supplementation as a potential therapeutic aid for the recovery from mild traumatic brain injury/concussion. Adv Nutr. 2014;5:268–77.
134. Trojian TH, Jackson E. Omega-3 polyunsaturated fatty acids and concussions: treatment or not? Curr Sports Med Rep. 2011;10:180–5.
135. Fontani G, Corradeschi F, Felici A, Alfatti F, Migliorini S, Lodi L. Cognitive and physiological effects of Omega-3 polyunsaturated fatty acid supplementation in healthy subjects. Eur J Clin Investig. 2005;35:691–9.
136. Guzman JF, Esteve H, Pablos C, Pablos A, Blasco C, Villegas JA. DHA- rich fish oil improves complex reaction time in female elite soccer players. J Sports Sci Med. 2011;10:301–5.
137. Reilly T, Cabri J, Araújo D. Science and football V: the proceedings of the Fifth World Congress on Science and Football. London: Routledge; 2005.
138. Wilmore JH, Costill DL, Kenney WL. Physiology of sport and exercise. 4th ed. Champaign/Leeds: Human Kinetics; 2008.
139. Trexler ET, Smith-Ryan AE, Stout JR, Hoffman JR, Wilborn CD, Sale C, Kreider RB, Jager R, Earnest CP, Bannock L, Campbell B, Kalman D, Ziegenfuss TN, Antonio J. International society of sports nutrition position stand: beta-alanine. J Int Soc Sports Nutr. 2015;12:30.
140. Derave W, Everaert I, Beeckman S, Baguet A. Muscle carnosine metabolism and beta-alanine supplementation in relation to exercise and training. Sports Med. 2010;40:247–63.
141. Harris RC, Tallon MJ, Dunnett M, Boobis L, Coakley J, Kim HJ, Fallowfield JL, Hill CA, Sale C, Wise JA. The absorption of orally supplied beta-alanine and its effect on muscle carnosine synthesis in human vastus lateralis. Amino Acids. 2006;30:279–89.
142. Hill CA, Harris RC, Kim HJ, Harris BD, Sale C, Boobis LH, Kim CK, Wise JA. Influence of beta-alanine supplementation on skeletal muscle carnosine concentrations and high intensity cycling capacity. Amino Acids. 2007;32:225–33.
143. Quesnele JJ, Laframboise MA, Wong JJ, Kim P, Wells GD. The effects of beta-alanine supplementation on performance: a systematic review of the literature. Int J Sport Nutr Exerc Metab. 2014;24:14–27.
144. Hoffman J, Ratamess NA, Ross R, Kang J, Magrelli J, Neese K, Faigenbaum AD, Wise JA. Beta-alanine and the hormonal response to exercise. Int J Sports Med. 2008;29:952–8.
145. Hobson RM, Saunders B, Ball G, Harris RC, Sale C. Effects of beta-alanine supplementation on exercise performance: a meta-analysis. Amino Acids. 2012; 43:25–37.
146. Sweeney KM, Wright GA, Glenn Brice A, Doberstein ST. The effect of beta-alanine supplementation on power performance during repeated sprint activity. J Strength Cond Res. 2010;24:79–87.
147. Derave W, Ozdemir MS, Harris RC, Pottier A, Reyngoudt H, Koppo K, Wise JA, Achten E. Beta-alanine supplementation augments muscle carnosine content and attenuates fatigue during repeated isokinetic contraction bouts in trained sprinters. J Appl Physiol (1985). 2007;103:1736–43.
148. Artioli GG, Gualano B, Smith A, Stout J, Lancha Jr AH. Role of beta-alanine supplementation on muscle carnosine and exercise performance. Med Sci Sports Exerc. 2010;42:1162–73.
149. Hoffman JR, Ratamess NA, Faigenbaum AD, Ross R, Kang J, Stout JR, Wise JA. Short-duration beta-alanine supplementation increases training volume and reduces subjective feelings of fatigue in college football players. Nutr Res. 2008;28:31–5.
150. Saunders B, Sunderland C, Harris RC, Sale C. Beta-alanine supplementation improves YoYo intermittent recovery test performance. J Int Soc Sports Nutr. 2012;9:39.
151. Rodriguez Rodriguez F, Delgado Ormeno A, Rivera Lobos P, Tapia Aranda V, Cristi-Montero C. Effects of ss-alanine supplementation on wingate tests in university female footballers. Nutr Hosp. 2015;31:430–5.
152. Saunders B, Sale C, Harris RC, Sunderland C. Effect of sodium bicarbonate and beta-alanine on repeated sprints during intermittent exercise performed in hypoxia. Int J Sport Nutr Exerc Metab. 2014;24:196–205.

153. Douroudos II, Fatouros IG, Gourgoulis V, Jamurtas AZ, Tsitsios T, Hatzinikolaou A, Margonis K, Mavromatidis K, Taxildaris K. Dose-related effects of prolonged NaHCO3 ingestion during high-intensity exercise. Med Sci Sports Exerc. 2006;38:1746–53.
154. Requena B, Zabala M, Padial P, Feriche B. Sodium bicarbonate and sodium citrate: ergogenic aids? J Strength Cond Res. 2005;19:213–24.
155. Maughan RJ. Encyclopaedia of sports medicine. Vol.7, Nutrition in sport. Oxford: Blackwell Science; 2000.
156. Raymer GH, Marsh GD, Kowalchuk JM, Thompson RT. Metabolic effects of induced alkalosis during progressive forearm exercise to fatigue. J Appl Physiol (1985). 2004;96:2050–6.
157. Castell LM, Burke LM, Stear SJ, McNaughton LR, Harris RC. BJSM reviews: A-Z of nutritional supplements: dietary supplements, sports nutrition foods and ergogenic aids for health and performance part 5. Br J Sports Med. 2010;44:77–8.
158. McNaughton LR, Siegler J, Midgley A. Ergogenic effects of sodium bicarbonate. Curr Sports Med Rep. 2008;7:230–6.
159. Lindh AM, Peyrebrune MC, Ingham SA, Bailey DM, Folland JP. Sodium bicarbonate improves swimming performance. Int J Sports Med. 2008;29:519–23.
160. Mero AA, Keskinen KL, Malvela MT, Sallinen JM. Combined creatine and sodium bicarbonate supplementation enhances interval swimming. J Strength Cond Res. 2004;18:306–10.
161. Bishop D, Edge J, Davis C, Goodman C. Induced metabolic alkalosis affects muscle metabolism and repeated-sprint ability. Med Sci Sports Exerc. 2004;36:807–13.
162. Krustrup P, Ermidis G, Mohr M. Sodium bicarbonate intake improves high-intensity intermittent exercise performance in trained young men. J Int Soc Sports Nutr. 2015;12:25.
163. Brisola GM, Miyagi WE, da Silva HS, Zagatto AM. Sodium bicarbonate supplementation improved MAOD but is not correlated with 200- and 400-m running performances: a double-blind, crossover, and placebo-controlled study. Appl Physiol Nutr Metab. 2015;40:931–7.
164. Mc Naughton L, Thompson D. Acute versus chronic sodium bicarbonate ingestion and anaerobic work and power output. J Sports Med Phys Fitness. 2001;41:456–62.
165. Aalt B, RMMH G. Nutritional antioxidants: it is time to categorise. In: Lamprecht M, editor. Antioxidants in sport nutrition. Boca Raton: CRC Press; 2014. p. 17–38.
166. Silva JR, Ascensao A, Marques F, Seabra A, Rebelo A, Magalhaes J. Neuromuscular function, hormonal and redox status and muscle damage of professional soccer players after a high-level competitive match. Eur J Appl Physiol. 2013;113:2193–201.
167. Jackson MJ. Free radicals generated by contracting muscle: by-products of metabolism or key regulators of muscle function? Free Radic Biol Med. 2008; 44:132–41.
168. Peternelj TT, Coombes JS. Antioxidant supplementation during exercise training: beneficial or detrimental? Sports Med. 2011;41:1043–69.
169. Draeger CL, Naves A, Marques N, Baptistella AB, Carnauba RA, Paschoal V, Nicastro H. Controversies of antioxidant vitamins supplementation in exercise: ergogenic or ergolytic effects in humans? J Int Soc Sports Nutr. 2014;11:4.
170. Fisher-Wellman K, Bloomer RJ. Acute exercise and oxidative stress: a 30 year history. Dyn Med. 2009;8:1.
171. Margaritis I, Rousseau AS. Does physical exercise modify antioxidant requirements? Nutr Res Rev. 2008;21:3–12.
172. Bjelakovic G, Nikolova D, Gluud LL, Simonetti RG, Gluud C. Mortality in randomized trials of antioxidant supplements for primary and secondary prevention: systematic review and meta-analysis. JAMA. 2007;297:842–57.
173. Paulsen G, Cumming KT, Holden G, Hallen J, Ronnestad BR, Sveen O, Skaug A, Paur I, Bastani NE, Ostgaard HN, Buer C, Midttun M, Freuchen F, Wiig H, Ulseth ET, Garthe I, Blomhoff R, Benestad HB, Raastad T. Vitamin C and E supplementation hampers cellular adaptation to endurance training in humans: a double-blind, randomised, controlled trial. J Physiol. 2014;592:1887–901.
174. Powers SK, Jackson MJ. Exercise-induced oxidative stress: cellular mechanisms and impact on muscle force production. Physiol Rev. 2008;88:1243–76.
175. Leonardo-Mendonca RC, Concepcion-Huertas M, Guerra-Hernandez E, Zabala M, Escames G, Acuna-Castroviejo D. Redox status and antioxidant response in professional cyclists during training. Eur J Sport Sci. 2014;14:830–8.
176. Ristow M, Zarse K, Oberbach A, Klöting N, Birringer M, Kiehntopf M, Stumvoll M, Kahn CR, Blüher M. Antioxidants prevent health-promoting effects of physical exercise in humans. Proc Natl Acad Sci. 2009;106:8665–70.
177. Skaug A, Sveen O, Raastad T. An antioxidant and multivitamin supplement reduced improvements in VO(2) max. J Sports Med Phys Fitness. 2014;54:63–9.
178. Neubauer O, Reichhold S, Nics L, Hoelzl C, Valentini J, Stadlmayr B, Knasmuller S, Wagner KH. Antioxidant responses to an acute ultra-endurance exercise: impact on DNA stability and indications for an increased need for nutritive antioxidants in the early recovery phase. Br J Nutr. 2010;104:1129–38.
179. Pialoux V, Mounier R, Rock E, Mazur A, Schmitt L, Richalet JP, Robach P, Brugniaux J, Coudert J, Fellmann N. Effects of the 'live high-train low'

method on prooxidant/antioxidant balance on elite athletes. Eur J Clin Nutr. 2009;63:756–62.
180. Braakhuis AJ, Hopkins WG. Impact of dietary antioxidants on sport performance: a review. Sports Med. 2015;45:939–55.
181. Gleeson M. Nutritional support to maintain proper immune status during intense training. Nestle Nutr Inst Workshop Ser. 2013;75:85–97.
182. Borchers AT, Selmi C, Meyers FJ, Keen CL, Gershwin ME. Probiotics and immunity. J Gastroenterol. 2009;44:26–46.
183. Gleeson M, Siegler JC, Burke LM, Stear SJ, Castell LM. A to Z of nutritional supplements: dietary supplements, sports nutrition foods and ergogenic aids for health and performance – part 31. Br J Sports Med. 2012;46:377–8.
184. King S, Glanville J, Sanders ME, Fitzgerald A, Varley D. Effectiveness of probiotics on the duration of illness in healthy children and adults who develop common acute respiratory infectious conditions: a systematic review and meta-analysis. Br J Nutr. 2014;112:41–54.
185. Nieman DC. Exercise, upper respiratory tract infection, and the immune system. Med Sci Sports Exerc. 1994;26:128–39.
186. Kekkonen RA, Vasankari TJ, Vuorimaa T, Haahtela T, Julkunen I, Korpela R. The effect of probiotics on respiratory infections and gastrointestinal symptoms during training in marathon runners. Int J Sport Nutr Exerc Metab. 2007;17:352–63.
187. Cox AJ, Pyne DB, Saunders PU, Fricker PA. Oral administration of the probiotic Lactobacillus fermentum VRI-003 and mucosal immunity in endurance athletes. Br J Sports Med. 2010;44:222–6.
188. West NP, Pyne DB, Cripps AW, Hopkins WG, Eskesen DC, Jairath A, Christophersen CT, Conlon MA, Fricker PA. Lactobacillus fermentum (PCC(R)) supplementation and gastrointestinal and respiratory-tract illness symptoms: a randomised control trial in athletes. Nutr J. 2011;10:30.
189. Haywood BA, Black KE, Baker D, McGarvey J, Healey P, Brown RC. Probiotic supplementation reduces the duration and incidence of infections but not severity in elite rugby union players. J Sci Med Sport. 2014;17:356–60.
190. Macdonald HM. Contributions of sunlight and diet to vitamin D status. Calcif Tissue Int. 2013;92:163–76.
191. Holick MF. Vitamin D deficiency. N Engl J Med. 2007;357:266–81.
192. Holick MF, Chen TC. Vitamin D deficiency: a worldwide problem with health consequences. Am J Clin Nutr. 2008;87:1080S–6S.
193. Cannell JJ, Hollis BW, Sorenson MB, Taft TN, Anderson JJ. Athletic performance and vitamin D. Med Sci Sports Exerc. 2009;41:1102–10.
194. Farrokhyar F, Tabasinejad R, Dao D, Peterson D, Ayeni OR, Hadioonzadeh R, Bhandari M. Prevalence of vitamin D inadequacy in athletes: a systematic-review and meta-analysis. Sports Med. 2015;45:365–78.
195. Galan F, Ribas J, Sanchez-Martinez PM, Calero T, Sanchez AB, Munoz A. Serum 25-hydroxyvitamin D in early autumn to ensure vitamin D sufficiency in mid-winter in professional football players. Clin Nutr. 2012;31:132–6.
196. Morton JP, Iqbal Z, Drust B, Burgess D, Close GL, Brukner PD. Seasonal variation in vitamin D status in professional soccer players of the English Premier League. Appl Physiol Nutr Metab. 2012;37:798–802.
197. Kopec A, Solarz K, Majda F, Slowinska-Lisowska M, Medras M. An evaluation of the levels of vitamin D and bone turnover markers after the summer and winter periods in polish professional soccer players. J Hum Kinet. 2013;38:135–40.
198. Hamilton B, Whiteley R, Farooq A, Chalabi H. Vitamin D concentration in 342 professional football players and association with lower limb isokinetic function. J Sci Med Sport. 2014;17:139–43.
199. Autier P, Boniol M, Pizot C, Mullie P. Vitamin D status and ill health: a systematic review. Lancet Diabetes Endocrinol. 2014;2:76–89.
200. Bischoff HA, Borchers M, Gudat F, Duermueller U, Theiler R, Stahelin HB, Dick W. In situ detection of 1,25-dihydroxyvitamin D3 receptor in human skeletal muscle tissue. Histochem J. 2001;33:19–24.
201. Gunton JE, Girgis CM, Baldock PA, Lips P. Bone muscle interactions and vitamin D. Bone. 2015;80:89–94.
202. Ceglia L, Harris SS. Vitamin D and its role in skeletal muscle. Calcif Tissue Int. 2013;92:151–62.
203. Massidda M, Corrias L, Bachis V, Cugia P, Piras F, Scorcu M, Calo CM. Vitamin D receptor gene polymorphisms and musculoskeletal injuries in professional football players. Exp Ther Med. 2015;9:1974–8.
204. Halliday TM, Peterson NJ, Thomas JJ, Kleppinger K, Hollis BW, Larson-Meyer DE. Vitamin D status relative to diet, lifestyle, injury, and illness in college athletes. Med Sci Sports Exerc. 2011;43:335–43.
205. Larson-Meyer DE, Willis KS. Vitamin D and athletes. Curr Sports Med Rep. 2010;9:220–6.
206. Barker T, Martins TB, Hill HR, Kjeldsberg CR, Trawick RH, Weaver LK, Traber MG. Low vitamin D impairs strength recovery after anterior cruciate ligament surgery. J Evid Based Complement Altern Med. 2011;16:201–9.
207. Laaksi I, Ruohola JP, Tuohimaa P, Auvinen A, Haataja R, Pihlajamaki H, Ylikomi T. An association of serum vitamin D concentrations < 40 nmol/L with acute respiratory tract infection in young Finnish men. Am J Clin Nutr. 2007;86:714–7.
208. Willis KS, Smith DT, Broughton KS, Larson-Meyer DE. Vitamin D status and biomarkers of inflammation in runners. Open Access J Sports Med. 2012;3:35–42.
209. Close GL, Russell J, Cobley JN, Owens DJ, Wilson G, Gregson W, Fraser WD, Morton JP. Assessment of

vitamin D concentration in non-supplemented professional athletes and healthy adults during the winter months in the UK: implications for skeletal muscle function. J Sports Sci. 2013;31:344–53.
210. Koundourakis NE, Androulakis NE, Malliaraki N, Margioris AN. Vitamin D and exercise performance in professional soccer players. PLoS One. 2014;9: e101659.
211. Close GL, Leckey J, Patterson M, Bradley W, Owens DJ, Fraser WD, Morton JP. The effects of vitamin D(3) supplementation on serum total 25[OH]D concentration and physical performance: a randomised dose-response study. Br J Sports Med. 2013;47:692–6.
212. Cannell JJ, Hollis BW. Use of vitamin D in clinical practice. Altern Med Rev. 2008;13:6–20.
213. Larson-Meyer DE, Burke LM, Stear SJ, Castell LM. A–Z of nutritional supplements: dietary supplements, sports nutrition foods and ergogenic aids for health and performance: part 40. Br J Sports Med. 2013;47:118–20.
214. Moore DR, Robinson MJ, Fry JL, Tang JE, Glover EI, Wilkinson SB, Prior T, Tarnopolsky MA, Phillips SM. Ingested protein dose response of muscle and albumin protein synthesis after resistance exercise in young men. Am J Clin Nutr. 2009;89:161–8.
215. Tang JE, Moore DR, Kujbida GW, Tarnopolsky MA, Phillips SM. Ingestion of whey hydrolysate, casein, or soy protein isolate: effects on mixed muscle protein synthesis at rest and following resistance exercise in young men. J Appl Physiol (1985). 2009;107: 987–92.
216. van Loon LJ. Leucine as a pharmaconutrient in health and disease. Curr Opin Clin Nutr Metab Care. 2012;15:71–7.
217. Ranchordas MK, Blomstrand E, Calder PC, Burke LM, Stear SJ, Castell LM. A-z of nutritional supplements: dietary supplements, sports nutrition foods and ergogenic aids for health and performance – part 23. Br J Sports Med. 2011;45:830–1.
218. Katsanos CS, Kobayashi H, Sheffield-Moore M, Aarsland A, Wolfe RR. A high proportion of leucine is required for optimal stimulation of the rate of muscle protein synthesis by essential amino acids in the elderly. Am J Physiol Endocrinol Metab. 2006;291:E381–7.
219. Milsom J, Barreira P, Burgess DJ, Iqbal Z, Morton JP. Case study: muscle atrophy and hypertrophy in a premier league soccer player during rehabilitation from ACL injury. Int J Sport Nutr Exerc Metab. 2014;24:543–52.
220. Burke LM, Winter JA, Cameron-Smith D, Enslen M, Farnfield M, Decombaz J. Effect of intake of different dietary protein sources on plasma amino acid profiles at rest and after exercise. Int J Sport Nutr Exerc Metab. 2012;22:452–62.
221. Res PT, Groen B, Pennings B, Beelen M, Wallis GA, Gijsen AP, Senden JM, Lj VANL. Protein ingestion before sleep improves postexercise overnight recovery. Med Sci Sports Exerc. 2012;44:1560–9.
222. Molfino A, Gioia G, Rossi Fanelli F, Muscaritoli M. Beta-hydroxy-beta-methylbutyrate supplementation in health and disease: a systematic review of randomized trials. Amino Acids. 2013;45:1273–92.
223. Mero AA, Ojala T, Hulmi JJ, Puurtinen R, Karila TA, Seppala T. Effects of alfa-hydroxy-isocaproic acid on body composition, DOMS and performance in athletes. J Int Soc Sports Nutr. 2010;7:1.
224. Desbrow B, Hughes R, Leveritt M, Scheelings P. An examination of consumer exposure to caffeine from retail coffee outlets. Food Chem Toxicol. 2007;45:1588–92.

Doping Control in Football

54

Basil Ribeiro and Martin J. Vaso

Contents

B. Ribeiro (✉)
Sports Medicine, Rio Ave FC, Performance and Health Unit of the Portuguese Federation of Football, Vila Nova de Gaia, Portugal
e-mail: basil@sapo.pt

M.J. Vaso
FIFA, Zurich, Switzerland
e-mail: Martin.Vaso@fifa.org

J. Espregueira-Mendes et al. (eds.), *Injuries and Health Problems in Football*,
DOI 10.1007/978-3-662-53924-8_54

54.1 Introduction

The main aim of the doping control is not to identify athletes with an atypical finding (ATF) or with an analytical adverse finding (AAF), but just the opposite: to avoid the consumption of a prohibited substance or the use of a method of doping. The education and spread of information related to doping, together with the doping control session itself in- and out-of-competition, are an enormous force of dissuasion. Special attention should be given to young athletes, who may be vulnerable and consume banned substances with the promise of a successful career. Inappropriate advice has been countered with educational sessions and a distribution of thousands of educational leaflets on doping and banned substances, in particular during the World and European youth final rounds.

The doping control is supported on principles of moral and sports ethics and is intended to be fair, universal, and efficient. In order to be harmonized worldwide and "encourage the consistency of the anti-doping processes," the World Anti-Doping Code (the Code) was created. The intention is that any doping control undertaken anywhere in the world in- and out-of-competition on a local or international scale is performed with the same conditions, the same laboratory procedures, and with respect to the rights and duties of the athlete.

The athlete must be aware that they are responsible for the issues related to the doping control, including the presence of a prohibited substance (or its metabolites) that may be found in their biological samples. It is the athlete's duty to make sure that no prohibited substance enters their body and that no prohibited method is used. Also, they must know that the intention to use a substance or method is considered a violation of the Code and is subject to a penalty. During the doping control session, the athlete must be alert and check that no mistake has occurred. For instance, they must verify if the numbers in the bottles with the samples match those on the form. The athlete is also responsible for the "whereabouts."

54.2 Is Doping a Problem in Football?

Football is the sport with more anti-doping controls than other football types, according to the Testing Figures of the World Anti-Doping Agency (2013: American football, 721 tests; Rugby, 6126 tests; football, 28,002 tests) [2]. There are thousands of samples collected around the world, and international sporting organizations such as UEFA and FIFA are focusing a lot of effort toward this struggle.

UEFA has been very active to ensure a clean sport and for the values of fair play to be respected. The number of biological samples has been increasing over the years as can be seen in Table 54.1.

Like other organizations, UEFA is changing their strategy and is collecting a lot of samples in the out-of-competition setting (around 25% during the season 2013/2014), in particular more blood samples (250 out-of-competition versus 88 in-competition). Although a lot of samples were collected, only one tested positive (methylecgonine, a metabolite of cocaine), and the player was banned for 18 months [1].

FIFA is also very committed in the fight against doping. Before the start of the last FIFA World Cup in Brazil in 2014, players of all participating teams were subjected to out-of-competition doping controls, and samples of urine and blood were collected from all of them. During the tournament, the players were also submitted to in-competition doping controls. In order to ensure an even more reliable procedure,

Table 54.1 Number of blood and urine samples collected by UEFA [1]

Season	1998/1999	2004/2005	2013/2014
UEFA Champions League	62	212	804 urine + 318 blood
UEFA Cup/ Europa League	48	224	556 urine + 20 blood
UEFA Intertoto Cup	8	24	Not applied
Futsal competitions	0	12	104
Youth competitions	0	64	288
Women's competitions	0	28	104
UEFA Super Cup	4	4	4
Total 1	152	568	1860 urine + 338 blood
EURO	44	124	Not applied
Total 2	**196**	**692**	**1860 urine + 338 blood**

Source: UEFA – number of blood and urine samples collected by UEFA

all samples were analyzed at a laboratory in Lausanne, Switzerland, which means that FIFA had to organize a very complicated operation to obtain the samples in Brazil and have them sent securely and safely to Switzerland and analyzed. As one of the first federations worldwide, FIFA tested the players in 2015 for gene doping.

Table 54.2 includes all samples (urine and blood, in- and out-of-competition) collected by FIFA and UEFA worldwide during 2013. In total, 28,002 urine and blood samples were collected [3]. The ATF and AAF are shown. The AAF includes the presence of a prohibited substance or method, which means, for instance, that a prohibited substance was found in the urine. This occurred in 140 cases (0.5%). The atypical finding occurred 270 times (0.96%). No AAF or ATF occurred in the blood samples.

In Portugal, the Portuguese Authority for Doping control (ADoP) collected 3404 samples in all sports during 2013 [4]. These included 1086 samples collected from football players (728 in- and 358 out-of-competition samples). There were 35 analytical adverse findings

Table 54.2 Samples analyzed and reported by accredited laboratories in Anti-Doping Administration and Management System (ADAMS) [2]

	In-competition				Out-of-competition		
2013		Total samples	ATF	AAF	Total samples	ATF	AAF
UEFA	Urine	1369	15	3	473	8	0
	Blood	36	0	0	50	0	0
FIFA	Urine	920	1	5	372	4	0
	Blood	16	0	0	12	0	0
All world	Urine	21,638	159	128	5697	111	12
	Blood	494	0	0	173	0	0

Source: WADA – Samples analyzed and reported by accredited laboratories in ADAMS

(1.03%) in all sports. For football, there were five AAF (0.46%); the substances found being cannabinoids (1), diuretic (2), and cocaine (2). During 2014, ADoP collected 1120 samples in football (805 in- and 315 out-of-competition), three were AAF, and none included cannabinoid or cocaine. These kinds of substances are troublesome in other countries as well. In 2013 in Italy, amateur and professional football players presented seven AAF (0.5%), and the substances detected were tetrahydrocannabinol (1), cocaine (3), betamethasone (2), and clostebol (2). In Spain during the 2011/2012 football season, as well as in futsal and women's football, several AAF were found to have the consumption of cannabinoids and cocaine.

Is doping a problem in football? The answer is yes, because there are still players with an AAF, and quite a large and unexpected number of those are due the consumption of so-called social drugs (cannabinoids and cocaine). The number has been decreasing, however, for two reasons in particular. Firstly, in 2013, World Anti-Doping Agency (WADA) raised the threshold of disqualification for use of cannabinoids from 20 ng/ml to 150 ng/ml, which means that any low-level or long-time consumers are no longer caught [2]. But this must not tranquilize the low consumers, because it is never known how much is needed to have a positive result. The second reason and much more importantly is the education program implemented by World and National Anti-Doping Organizations. Thanks to them, athletes are learning that it is not worth consuming social drugs as they are bad for their health, social life, and sports career. Doping controls are still needed, however, to ensure athletes avoid this kind of behavior. The sanctions for cannabis are never 2 years. The vast majority of cannabis positives lead to a sanction ranging from a reprimand to a 6-month ban, but there are cases where athletes received a 2-year ban for cannabis. With the new code, it might be even more.

54.3 The Code [2]

The Code was approved in 2003 and was implemented on 2004. It was subjected to two revisions, first in 2009 and the second which entered into force on 1 January 2015. Several amendments and updates have been made since its creation. One of the revisions introduced the concept of the "nonanalytical" rule violations, in which case there may be no positive doping sample, but there is a behavior that may constitute a violation (whereabouts failure, for an example, see below). Another revision with the new Code is the sanctions for intentional doping, which have been increased from 2 to 4 years, though a more flexible regime is applicable regarding positive tests involving social drugs or contamination. Furthermore, staff surrounding the athlete (i.e., doctor, coach, nurse, etc.) can now be punished as well if there is complicity or if they assisted or promoted doping.

This is a fundamental document that harmonizes all doping procedures and specifies penalties relevant for all sports and in all countries.

The objectives are:

- To protect the fundamental right of the athletes to participate in sports competitions

without doping and to promote health, justice, and equality among all the athletes in the world
- To guarantee harmonized, coordinated, and efficient programs at national and international levels for detection, punition, and prevention of the doping

According to the Code, the following constitute anti-doping rule violations:

- Presence of a prohibited substance or its metabolites or markers in an athlete's sample
- Use or attempted use by an athlete of a prohibited substance or a prohibited method
- Evading, refusing, or failing to submit to sample collection
- Whereabouts failures
- Tampering or attempted tampering with any part of doping control
- Possession of a prohibited substance or a prohibited method
- Trafficking or attempted trafficking in any prohibited substance or prohibited method
- Administration or attempted administration to any athlete in-competition of any prohibited substance or prohibited method or administration or attempted administration to any athlete out-of-competition of any prohibited substance or any prohibited substance method that is prohibited out-of-competition
- Complicity
- Prohibited association

54.4 The International Standards [2, 3]

To achieve the goals, the Code is supported by five International Standards mandatory for all stakeholders, which are related to the following operational and technical areas:

- Prohibited list
- Testing and investigation
- Laboratories
- Therapeutic use exemption (TUE)
- Protection of privacy and personal information

54.4.1 Standard No. 1: Substances and Methods Prohibited in Sport

A list of prohibited substances and methods is published every year and is valid for the entire year starting 1 January, unless new drugs and/or methods arise in the meantime. A new list was published in September 2014 (valid 1 January 2015). It is divided by substances and methods prohibited at all times (in- and out-of-competition) and substances and methods prohibited only in-competition (stimulants, narcotics, cannabinoids, and glucocorticoids) and in several categories. The glucocorticoids are only prohibited when administered by oral, intramuscular, intravenous, or rectal routes. The methods on the list (manipulation of the blood and blood components, chemical and physical manipulation, and gene doping) are prohibited at all times. For some sports, there are special considerations, for instance, in motorized sports such as archery, in powerboating, and in air sports in-competition, the equivalent of alcohol (ethanol) in blood greater than 0.10 gr/L is forbidden. In addition, beta blockers are not allowed in-competition in some sports such as archery, billiards, and automobile, among others.

The Code considers a substance or method as doping when two of the following three criteria are met:

(a) The substance or method, alone or in combination, has the potential to enhance or enhances performance
(b) The use of the substance or method represents an actual or potential health risk to the athlete
(c) The substance or method violates the spirit of sport described in the introduction to the Code

54.4.2 Standard No. 2: Testing and Investigation

WADA states that the purpose of this standard is to plan for effective testing and to maintain the integrity and identity of samples, from notifying the athlete to transporting the samples to the lab.

The new International Standard for Testing and Investigation came into effect on 1 January 2015.

Everything related to a control, including the programming, the notification of the athlete, the collection of the samples, and their transportation to an accredited laboratory, is under this standard. The selection of the player is very well defined. Additionally, all procedures once the athlete has provided the sample including the pouring to the bottles and the check for the specific gravity are regulated. When there is not enough quantity (at least 90 ml) or it does not have the right specific gravity (over 1005 on a refractometer reading or over 1010 on a lab strip reading), the standard regulates the next procedures. In general, no alcohol is permitted in the doping control room.

It is worthwhile mentioning, since this might act as a deterrent, that some urine and blood samples are stored for reanalyzing in the future which could identify substances that are not detectable today.

54.4.3 Standard No. 3: Laboratories

This standard regulates the procedures of all accredited laboratories (by WADA). The proceedings must be equal in all laboratories in order to achieve the same result and report no matter where the sample is analyzed. It is supported by technical documents with specific criteria that must be respected by the laboratories. The accomplishment of these goals is necessary to receive accreditation from WADA.

There are 32 accredited laboratories worldwide. In Europe there are 18 in total, and countries such as Germany (Koln and Dresden) and Spain (Barcelona and Madrid) even have two. There is one in Lisbon, Portugal. In Africa, there is only one (South Africa), and in South and Central America, there are only three (in Colombia, Mexico, and Cuba).

54.4.4 Standard No. 4: Therapeutic Use Exemption (TUE)

Before becoming an athlete, a football player is just another person who can become sick and has the right to be properly treated with any kind of medication even it is included in WADA's list. Once a football player becomes an athlete, any time they need a medication that is prohibited, after considering any alternative medication or treatment, before use, they must apply for a TUE to either the National Anti-Doping Organization (NADO) or to UEFA or FIFA. The application form can be downloaded from the respective site, and all sections must be completed in block capital letters. The athlete must be aware that an incomplete or an illegible form will not be considered and will be returned for completion.

There are various criteria that must be met for a TUE to be granted according to the WADA International Standard for TUEs (citation):

- The prohibited substance or prohibited method in question is needed to treat an acute or chronic medical condition, such that the athlete would
- Experience a significant impairment to health if the prohibited substance or prohibited method was to be withheld
- The therapeutic use of the prohibited substance or prohibited method is highly unlikely to produce any additional enhancement of performance beyond what might be anticipated by a return to the athlete's normal state of health following the treatment of the acute or chronic medical condition
- There is no reasonable therapeutic alternative to the use of the prohibited substance or prohibited method
- The necessity for the use of the prohibited substance or prohibited method is not a consequence, wholly or in part, of the prior use (without a TUE) of a substance or method which was prohibited at the time of such use

The TUE application form should be signed by the player and their doctor and must include a comprehensive medical history and the results of all relevant medical investigations (blood analyses, tests, imaging studies) and then sent to a confidential fax number. In the case of UEFA, it is sent to the Medical and Anti-Doping Unit (fax: +41229903131), and for FIFA, it is sent to Medicine and Science Department, Anti-Doping

Unit. It is very important to know that before the TUE is granted, the player cannot take the prohibited substance or the prohibited method unless there is a serious medical emergency. Only in this case, it is permissible to apply for a TUE retroactively, but it should be taken into consideration that it will be only granted if there was a clear medical justification for the emergency use. Medical reports must be sent to support the application. An example is an anaphylactic crisis that can jeopardize the athlete's life and so it is permissible to administer intravenous cortisone and/or intramuscular adrenaline. In its site, WADA mentions that a TUE in an anaphylaxis case is retroactive in nature. On the same page, there is link to obtain "Medical Information to Support the Decisions" of TUEs for several diseases (arterial hypertension, diabetes mellitus, adrenal insufficiency, asthma, growth hormone insufficiency, etc.). In this section, there is a very helpful summarized description of every disease, which includes the diagnosis (medical history, diagnostic criteria, and relevant medical information), the best medical treatment (name of the prohibited substance, route of administration, dose, frequency, and recommended duration of treatment), other permitted and alternative treatments, health consequences in case of interruption of the treatment, treatment monitoring, duration of the TUE, and additional care.

According to the WADA International Standard for TUEs, the TUE should be granted as soon as possible and should not take any longer than 21 days after the submission of the TUE application [2]. However, it usually does not take so long, and in some countries, like Portugal, it can sometimes take between 3 and 4 days to receive the answer by the registered post. In the case of UEFA, a TUE is faxed, and a copy sent to the team, the National Association/Federation, NADO, FIFA, and WADA.

Special consideration must be mentioned about a player involved in an international competition, at team level and national level as well, where they must request prior authorization from UEFA or FIFA by means of a UEFA or FIFA TUE application form, and not to NADO. A UEFA TUE is valid for all UEFA, FIFA, and national-level competitions, and a FIFA TUE is valid for UEFA and for FIFA competitions and for national level. A NADO TUE is not valid for UEFA or FIFA competitions (though there are exceptions). It is necessary to send to UEFA or to FIFA the NADO TUE with the initial application form and the relevant translated medical information before the start of the competition, advisedly 21 days before the beginning.

54.4.5 Standard No. 5: Protection of Privacy and Personal Information

The aim of this standard is to guarantee that all persons involved in the doping control process respect the privacy of the athlete and all information they may aware of, namely, the "whereabouts" system, the TUE, and the doping control session itself. It includes the seal from the management of the results where a public and private divulgence cannot occur. WADA published several statements and clarifications about the protection of this sensitive information which can be consulted on their website.

54.5 Anti-Doping Administration and Management System (ADAMS) [2]

The ADAMS is a web-based database management system created by WADA to coordinate anti-doping activities and assist everybody involved in anti-doping to implement the Code. It's free, accessible in any place, and easy to use, as WADA is described as "designed to assist organizations in carrying out their anti-doping operations." It is also available in various languages (English, French, Spanish, German, Italian, Japanese, Arabic, Dutch, Chinese, Korean, Polish, Portuguese, Suomi, Bulgarian, Serbian, Czech, and Russian). Data related to laboratory results, therapeutic use exemptions, and anti-doping rule violations can be found here, and this allows a better communication among the organizations involved in this fight. It allows data sharing in a secure place with restricted access and guaranteed transparency and efficiency. It also replaces the less secure email and fax communication. Every player can have an ADAMS account. Since last year, there is a free ADAMS app for smartphones, and "using their Android or iPhone, athletes can enter, check, and change their whereabouts details at any time with just a few clicks. Using mobile notifications, the app also helps the athletes to remember their obligations to submit whereabouts, including the relevant deadlines to do so. The App can be downloaded at the Google Play Store." This is a huge investment that costs annually US$200 000 to keep all the information secure.

Core functionalities:

- Facilitate the operation of the *whereabouts system*, since any athlete anywhere in the world can enter, actualize, and change the information related to their location. The whereabouts can be modified by sending an SMS to ADAMS. It is also allowed to transfer this obligation to an authorized person, such as an agent. At the team level, usually there is a dedicated officer responsible for this issue. However, it is important to remember that all activities related to an anti-doping issue, including this one, in the first instance, are under the responsibility of the player. With this system, the athlete only needs to submit the information once, and other anti-doping organizations will have access to it. For the athletes included in a passport program, the information will be retained for 8 years and, for others, 18 months. In order to learn and facilitate the submission process, the player can watch a tutorial movie on YouTube (look for "ADAMS Whereabouts tutorial" in Google, for instance)
- Online management of the *Therapeutic Use Exemptions* (TUE), notification of those involved in the process and, after approval, the player can print their Certificate of Approval. Doctors and athletes can submit the petition online. All medical reports will be deleted from the system 18 months after the TUE expiry date and the TUE itself 8 years after the approval date
- *Test planning and results management*. With this tool, it is easier to make the schedule for the in- and out-of-competition doping control program and to avoid the duplication of tests performed by the various anti-doping organizations. In the case of a negative analytical finding, all relevant documents are deleted 18 months after the doping control mission, but when there is a positive analytical finding, the relevant documents will be deleted only 8 years after the date of the test from the system
- The *laboratory results* are stored in this system as well. WADA-accredited laboratories submit the test results to the appropriate authorities via ADAMS, who are notified of the results. A lot of information regarding analyses of thousands of urine and blood samples are annually collected and stored. Though WADA has access to all laboratory results, the testing authority only has access to their results
- The *hematological passport* is also stored in the system and can be automatically calculated. There is an automatic notification of an atypical passport finding and an automatic reporting to WADA. There is one passport for each athlete
- For further information or questions please write to adams@wada-ama.org

54.6 The Biological Passport [2, 3]

The biological passport (BP) is a registration and monitoring of various biological markers of a player. It is based on the biological stability of the human physiology. It monitors players' selected biomarkers over time, providing intelligence for target testing.

It started in 2008 when the Union Cycliste Internationale (UCI) started to collect and store this data. The registration of the results from urine and blood samples over time can define a unique biological profile of an athlete, and a "normal" value is applied to that player. Whenever they are subjected to a doping control, the results must be around that value, inside a range calculated with a mathematical formula. There is an intrapersonal comparison of the results. If the results are not in that range, then further investigation is needed, and, in the end, the athlete might have an ATF and receive a penalty as described by the Code.

This is a very simple, intelligent, and cost-effective strategy. Sometimes, a player may be using substances on an intermittent and/or low-dose basis which could go undetected, but can have an effect in the player's biological profile. The laboratory does not look for the prohibited substance in the urine or blood sample, for example, but looks for its effect. The substance itself might not be directly detected, and only the effects of doping are revealed. Instead of looking for erythropoietin (EPO), which is very expensive, it is more cost-effective and quicker to look for the hemoglobin concentration and for the hematocrit. If the hematocrit is higher than it should be, it might indicate a recent blood transfusion or the use of EPO. If it is too low, then a blood withdrawal might be considered. However, it is mandatory to test 10% of all tests in football for erythropoiesis-stimulating agent (ESA).

There are three modules, in different phases of development and implementation:

- The blood module, to detect EPO and any EPO developed in the future
- The steroid module, related to the anabolic androgenic steroids
- The endocrine module, related to the growth hormone and to the IGF-1

FIFA introduced the BP before the last World Cup (2014) and carried on during the competition. Before the beginning of the tournament, the athletes of all participating teams were subjected to an out-of-competition doping control, where blood and urine samples were collected. All data was stored to create the athletes' profile. In September 2014, the Executive Committee of UEFA approved the introduction of an athlete biological passport during the 2015/2016 season for the UEFA Champions League.

This strategy has already provided some results, not in football, but in other sports. There are at least 50 athletes banned worldwide because of irregularities in their biological passport. Athletics is the sport with the most athletes banned at the moment, a total of 36: Russia (17), Portugal (5), Turkey (3), Morocco, Saudi Arabia, and Ukraine (1). The second sport is cycling: Italy (4), Spain (4), and Portugal (3).

54.7 The Whereabouts [2, 3]

An out-of-competition doping control can only be effective if the player can be found. This tool can provide valuable information to locate the athlete to be subjected to a doping control without notice, and, in this way, a good anti-doping program is guaranteed. There is a Registered Testing Pool (RTP) where the athletes indicated by international or national sports organizations are included. The whereabouts are fulfilled four times per year, and the player must indicate a place (home, club, school, training camp, etc.) and a period of 60 min where they can be found during each of the 90 days of that period. A prevision of the completion schedules must also be provided. It is against the Code not to provide this information. It is important to clarify that a player can also be tested as an out-of-competition or in a target testing doping control outside that time period. Whenever the training schedule changes or for any other reason, the player can update the information by SMS, fax, email, or via ADAMS (except for FIFA yet in this case). This online tool allows athletes access anytime and anywhere to update their whereabouts information. It is strongly advised that the athlete knows in advance where to send any changing information, since there will be consequences if they are not found in the place and at the time previously indicated, unless there is a very good reason that can be explained later during the disciplinary process. The player can have an agent or a team representative to submit the whereabouts depending of the registered pool, but the athlete must be aware that they are the only one responsible for that and cannot blame these people if problems occur.

54.8 Selection of the Players for the Doping Control In-Competition [2, 3]

International organizations such as FIFA and UEFA select four players from each team for the doping control. They are drawn by lots at half time during a match, and only the first two players from each team (envelope 1 and 2) will actually undergo the control, unless for a very special reason that is not possible (e.g., evacuation of a player to the hospital because of injury). In this case, the player will be replaced by one of the reserves. Fifteen minutes before the end of the match, the names of the players are revealed (envelopes opened), and they are written in the summons form. Both the doping control officer (DCO) and the player representative must sign this form. A copy will be given to the representative. At a national level, usually only two players are drawn by lots 15 min before the end of the match, and their names are revealed at that moment. From the time of notification until the end of the control session, the player must always be under direct observation by the DCO or by the chaperone. As soon as the match is over, the player must go straight to the doping control room and in no circumstances is allowed to go first to the dressing room. The DCO may however grant, in circumstances as below, a delay in reporting to the doping control room, provided that the athlete can kept all times under direct observation:

- Media commitments/flash interview
- Urgent medical care
- Participation in a ceremony
- Other circumstances with a valid justification

The player is not allowed to leave the doping control room without authorization of the DCO, and they can change clothes.

In an out-of-competition testing, the player drawn by lots has 60 min to report to the DCO after notification.

54.9 The Sample Collection Session [2, 3]

The doping control officer (DCO) is responsible for the session and must pay a lot of attention at all times, but especially on the athlete identification, informing them of their rights and duties, and on the collection, identification, and sealing of the sample. All relevant information must be written down on the forms provided by the national or international authority. The DCO must record if it is an in- or an out-of-competition control. Only authorized persons are allowed to be in the doping control room, and an interpreter might be included. Only non-alcoholic beverages are allowed, and these must be served in unopened and sealed plastic bottles. It is the player's responsibility of all food consumed.

The athlete has the chance to choose the equipment to be used in the procedure. They first choose a sealed and sterilized beaker for the collection of the urine sample and then a box with two sealed and numbered bottles (sample "A" and sample "B"). The athlete must check if all the equipment is correctly intact and sealed.

The player shall urinate into the beaker under direct supervision of the DCO or an assistant (same gender as the player). At least 90 ml of urine must be collected. If it is not enough, the player will be asked to provide an additional sample (collected into a new sealed and sterilized beaker) later. The first collected sample will then be mixed with the new sample in the beaker. If the volume of urine is still below 90 ml, the entire procedure must be repeated.

It is the responsibility of the athlete to control the integrity of the sample until it is sealed in the bottles. The athlete has the possibility to pour the urine from the beaker into the bottles. If this is the case, the DCO will explain the procedure. If it is not, then the DCO will proceed and that must be indicated on the form. The first urine must go to bottle "B" (30 ml), and the rest, at least 60 ml, must go to bottle "A." A small amount of urine must be left in the beaker to be tested for the suitable specific gravity for analysis. This will validate the samples. If it is greater than 1005 (refractometer reading) or 1010 (lab strips reading) the samples will be considered good. If this is not found, then the entire process must be repeated in order to collect another urine sample. This must be indicated on the form. After the bottles have been properly sealed, the player must check all the code numbers on the bottles, caps, box, and form. At the end, the player, the accompanying person (if applicable), and the DCO must sign the form. The athlete at this moment has the opportunity to write any comment or complaints about the doping control session. They will also be asked to indicate (and sign) if the remaining urine can be used for scientific research after the laboratory work.

Conclusion

To write this chapter, the web pages of WADA, FIFA, UEFA, and ADoP were visited. This paper is not a substitution of any documents published on their websites which are the official positions of each organization. The purpose of this chapter is to provide a global overview of the anti-doping control. It is strongly recommended to read the World Anti-Doping Code (Code) and the Anti-Doping Regulations of the international organizations.

References

1. UEFA Anti-Doping Regulations. http://www.uefa.org/protecting-the-game/anti-doping/index.html. Accessed february 2017.
2. World Anti-Doping Agency. https://www.wada-ama.org/. Accessed May and June 2015.
3. FIFA Anti-Doping Regulations. http://resources.fifa.com/mm/document/footballdevelopment/medical/01/17/17/09/anti-doping2015en_neutral.pdf. Accessed May and June 2015.
4. ADoP – Autoridade de Antidopagem de Portugal. http://www.adop.pt/. Accessed May and June 2015.

Psychology Help in the Injured Player

55

Jorge Silvério and Filipa Reis

Contents

J. Silvério (✉)
Clínica do Dragão, Espregueira-Mendes Sports Centre - FIFA Medical Centre of Excellence, Porto, Portugal
e-mail: silverioj@gmail.com

F. Reis
Porto, Portugal
e-mail: filipareis.ucp@gmail.com

55.1 Introduction

Sport injuries threaten athletes' career and success [1]. Some injuries are minor and do not have any impact, instead others can end a career and have consequences on athletes' quality of life.

Getting injured is a traumatic experience for athletes: what they have devoted so much time and energy can be suddenly, without warning, taken away [2]. Additionally, participating in athletics has many benefits. Deutsch [3] recognizes that participation provides a means of developing physical mastery, positive self-concept, autonomy, and self-control. When the positive reinforcements of sport and the individual's association with the athletic role abruptly cease with the onset of injury, an athlete may question their identity and experience a sense of loss.

An injury does not affect exclusively physical capabilities but also contextual and psychological aspects. In some situations, injuries can deprive athletes of their compensation increasing life stress and determine fear of reinjury, sensation of loss, and negative emotions [4–6]. The negative impact of injury depends only in part on how much time athletes have spent in sport. For example, high performers experience major feeling of loss and mood disturbance, but they also have more psychological resources to cope with the situation because of their stronger athletic identity [7].

The injury is usually seen as a physical problem which starts from the occurrence of injury

J. Espregueira-Mendes et al. (eds.), *Injuries and Health Problems in Football*,
DOI 10.1007/978-3-662-53924-8_55

and ends when the athlete is back in "business," playing or competing. This injury influences the athlete's daily routines, emotions, behavior, social contacts, and even values in life.

According to these facts, the sport injury should be seen as much more than just a physical problem. Psychological responses to an injury must be taken in notice and integrated in the treatment plan because athletic injury, whether temporary or permanent, is and always will be a painfully disruptive and uncontrollable interruption in an athlete's life.

55.2 Causes of the Injuries: Risk Factors

Most of the lesions suffered by athletes are caused by the high demands of the competitive sport: attain great results in a short period of time, lack of psychological preparation, growing physical loads, disrespect of the adaptation time that the body needs to adapt to progressively higher demands, etc [8].

Several studies define different physiological and psychological factors affecting athletic injury risk.

During the last years, more and more researchers have claimed that two major impact factors could affect the occurrence of sport injuries [9]:

1. Internal risk factors: physical factors (problems of structural alignment, lack of flexibility, lack of muscular strength) and personal factors (demographic variables, coping and psychological skills, behavior factors, injury history, and variations associated with the maturity)
2. External risk factors: inadequate rehabilitation from a previous injury, training errors, game conditions, equipment, mixture of age groups, trainers and parents' behaviors, and the sports organization

A number of models contain proposals that specify relationships between psychological factors and an increased athletic injury risk [10]. Lavaellee and Flint [11] found that there were positive relationships between high competitive anxiety and injury. There are also studies claiming that mood states could be related to injury occurrence. Williams, Hogan, and Andersen [12] demonstrated that athletes with positive states of mind early in the season experienced fewer injuries during the season.

We cannot say there is a particular type of personality more prone to be injured [13, 14] because the research so far has failed to prove that particular personality characteristics are associated to injuries. However, a sensation-seeking person can be more willing to practice some higher-risk sports such as skiing, motorbike, and escalade, which have more probability to cause injuries than other sports [8].

55.3 Mental Constitution of Injuries: Emotional and Behavioral Experience

Injury is an inherent consequence of athletic participation that not only affects patients' physically but also their self-concept, self-esteem, belief system, values, commitments, and emotional balance. Athletic injury can be an imposing source of stress, and athletes often experience feelings of tension, confusion, hostility, loneliness, fear, irritability, and anxiety. Feelings of guilt and being ignored can also be experienced by the athlete [15].

Initially, the researchers agreed that after an injury, the athlete passes by a five-stage process:

1. Immediately after the injury, *negation phase*
2. After he gains consciousness, *rage* succeeds
3. He starts *seeking reasons* for suffering the injury
4. After having success on the other phases, *depression* begins
5. *Acceptance* of the injury

According to Hardy and Crace [16], the time an athlete spends in each of the phases depends on his personality and the support he receives from the others (family, team, coach, organization).

Actually, the common understanding is that the injury experience is not so rigid and only takes three categories of responses [17]:

1. Injury-relevant information processing: the injured athlete gathered information related to the injury and recognizes the negative consequences
2. Emotional upheaval and reactive behavior: as soon as the athlete realizes that he is injured, he experiences a set of emotions such as shock, disbelief, denial, isolation, and self-pity
3. Positive outlook and coping: the athlete accepts the injury and deals with starting coping efforts, has a good attitude, and is relieved to see the progression in his recovery

Most athletes go through these three general stages, but the time spent on each stage varies from days to months. Athletes can also experience the toughness of the same stages very differently, when one goes through it very easily, others can experience it to be very hard to go through [18].

Petitpas and Danish [19] describe other reactions and phases:

1. Identity loss: his self-concept as an athlete becomes diffusing because of the effects of injury
2. Fear and anxiety: the thoughts about reinjuring and being replaced by other teammates are overwhelming
3. Lack of confidence: as an injured player cannot practice, he can diminish confidence in his abilities
4. Performance decrements: because of the lack of confidence and less time of practice, athlete's performance can decrement when they return to practice

The athlete's response to injury can be viewed as occurring at three levels: cognitive, emotional, and behavioral.

Athletes' emotional (e.g., frustration, anger sadness, relief) and behavioral responses (e.g., isolation, tardiness, adherence) are determined by how the athlete sees and interprets one's injury and coping skills to deal with it. Additionally Bianco [20] notes that the direction of influence can also go in reverse direction, from behavioral outcomes to emotions followed by cognitions. Even though the injury is generally seen as primary stressor, the way the injury is perceived is the most important. In other words the fact that injury has occurred is less important than its meaningfulness [21].

Cognitive response is determined firstly by how the athlete sees the injury's potential seriousness and effects on the athlete and secondly by how athlete's personal and social resources are available to cope with demands of the injury [20].

The consequences of an injury are not only in terms of pain and suffering but also in self-concept, quality of life, mood alterations, sleep disturbance, depression, and anger and, directly or indirectly, through all these effects, can also affect relationships.

This inability to continue sports participation is devastating and hinders the recovery process and consequently affects the way athletes mentally deal with future injuries [22].

Fortunately, today the traditional thinking of considering an injury a mere biological problem has been surpassed, and the role of psychological factors and his treatment is widely recognized. So if we treat an injury physically, we must treat it also from the psychological point of view [23].

55.4 Psychological Intervention

Dealing with an injury from the psychological perspective is just as important to recovery as the physiological rehabilitation. As said by Crossman (pp. 335), "while many athletes spend hours and much energy each day physically preparing for competition, more often than not they are unprepared psychologically to handle the stress associated with an unforeseen or unexpected injury" [2]. Athletes have access to resources for physical rehabilitation, but often the psychological distress caused by injury goes untreated. According to Chan, Hagger, and Spray [24], emotional disturbance does occur post-injury, and injured athletes should be given the opportunity to discuss their feelings. In fact, patients express relief at being given the opportunity to confide concerns privately, away from the presence of persons who may have a vested interest in their athletic performance.

The psychological intervention can be divided in two different levels: prevention and rehabilitation.

At the preventive level, psychologists can intervene in athletes at injury risk: the ones with negative life stresses, with an increase in daily hassles, previous injuries, and poor coping resources [25]. Moreover if an athlete experiences anger and aggression during a competition or has competitive trait anxiety, the risk of injury increases.

> The combination of stress history, poor coping resources and personality factors results in what theorists call an elevated stress response. This involves increased muscle tension, increased distractibility, and a narrowing of attention so that the athlete is not as aware of or responsible to critical events or cues. Prolonged exposure to stress also changes the body's endocrine system, making a person more susceptible to illness and slowing down the healing process [25, p. 218].

Palmi [26] talks about three risk factors: the medical-physiological, psychological, and sports related and consequently suggests four intervention strategies:

1. Improving the basic information given to the athlete about the risk factors, the best preparation, and the habits to prevent injuries
2. Learning psychological resources to reduce the probability of injuries such as relaxation after finishing hard training sessions
3. Planning the training and the competition with realistic goals adapting to his own condition and in order to avoid overtraining
4. Improving technical resources because how much an athlete is ready to do a task, the less probability to get injured

On the rehabilitation side, a psychologist intervention can address these aspects:

- Establish a relationship of confidence with the athlete
- Educate the athlete about the injury and the recovery process
- The athlete must accept his responsibilities in the treatment trying to actively seek information about the lesion and what he can do in order to recover as soon as possible
- The athlete must define clear, specific, and realistic goals with a time frame in a short, medium, and long term for the rehabilitation process and for the return to practices and competition
- The athlete should know how to get support from friends, family, teammates, and trainers
- The athlete must work mentally in his recovery process taking consciousness of his attitude toward the injury, building positive self-talk about the recovery process, and if he cannot practice physically, he can mentally rehearse and practice
- The athlete cannot isolate himself from friends and family
- Teach the athlete how to cope with the possible setbacks

55.5 Psychological Models for Sport Injury Rehabilitation

Through the years, several psychological models have been proposed in order to contextualize the rehabilitation process following sport injury, such as the biopsychosocial model, the cognitive appraisal, the stage models, and finally the motivation-based models.

55.5.1 Biopsychosocial Model

Brewer [27, 28] considers seven dimensions to explain the sport injury rehabilitation process as a whole (Fig. 55.1): injury characteristics, social demographic factors, biological factors, psychological factors, social and contextual factors, intermediate biopsychological outcomes, and sport injury rehabilitation outcomes.

The process starts with an injury. Injury characteristics (type, cause and severity, history of previous injuries) and athlete characteristics (age, gender, ethnicity, socioeconomic status)

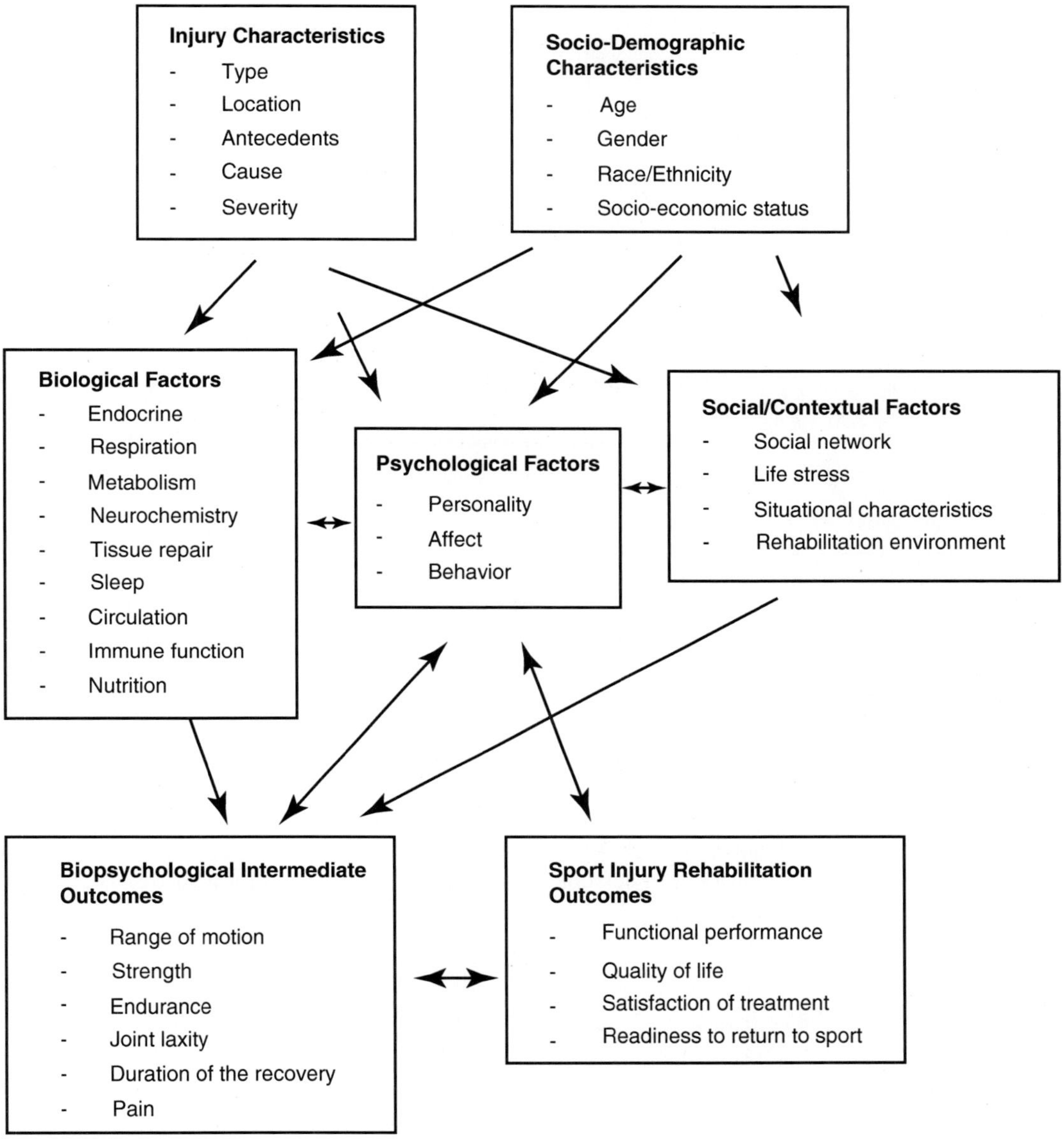

Fig. 55.1 The biopsychosocial model [27, 28]

affect athlete's biological, psychological, and social-contextual dimensions.

Subsequently, these three dimensions influence the biopsychological intermediate outcomes, such as strength and endurance of a muscle and perception of pain. Finally, these intermediate outcomes will contribute to better outcomes in rehabilitation, such as satisfaction on the treatment and functional performance after injury.

55.5.2 Cognitive Appraisal Models

The cognitive appraisal models attribute a central role to cognition in determining individual reaction to sport injury [29]. According to this model, personal and situational factors influence cognitive appraisal of the individual (coping, beliefs, and attributions), which determine their emotional response (e.g., fear of reinjury, anger, or depression). This emotional response influences

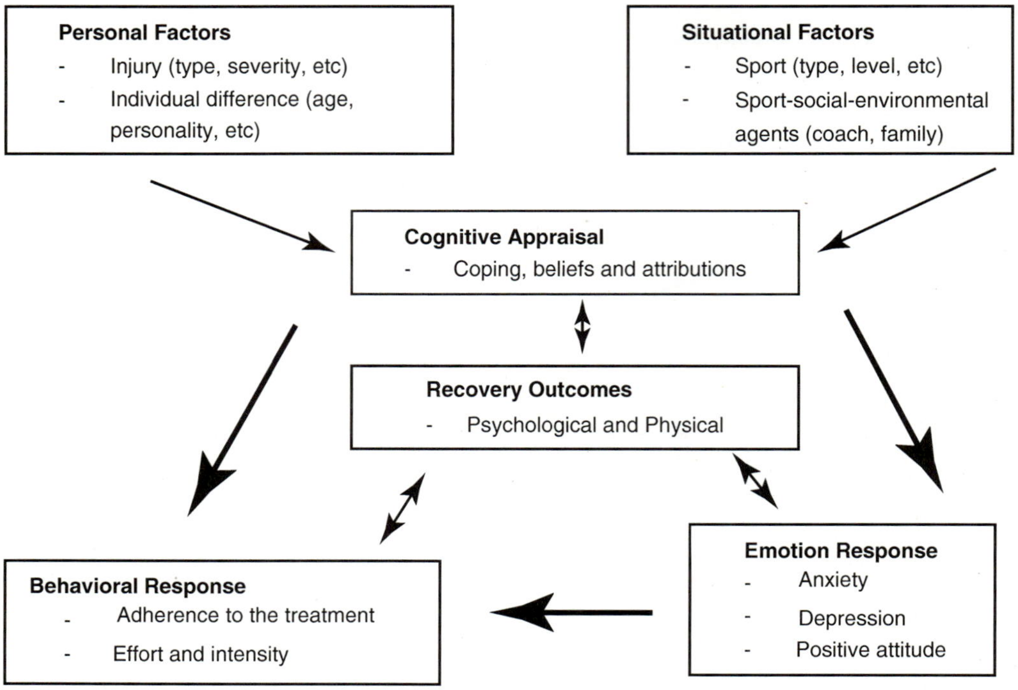

Fig. 55.2 Cognitive appraisal and psychological response to the sport injury [31]

the athlete's behavior that consequently contributes to the success of the program [30].

Weise-Bjornstal and colleagues [31] added to this model a personality dimension as a personal factor (Fig. 55.2).

55.5.3 Stage Models

Stage models provide a succession of emotions and attitudes occurring following sport injury. At the beginning, authors defend five different stages: denial, anger, bargaining, depression, and acceptance [32].

More recently, O'Connor et al. [1] have proposed the "affective cycle of injury" that includes three different responses to injury: denial, distress, and determined coping, as a more flexible and general way.

By denying, the athlete refuses and negates the consequences, the severity, and the impact of the injury on quality of life. Normally this stage occurs at the beginning of rehabilitation, and it's adaptive to the injury. If it persists during the following stages, the psychological intervention is required.

Negative emotions such as anxiety, depression, anger, fear, and feeling of loss contribute to distress stage. Despite being more common at the earlier stages of rehabilitation, distress may occur during the later stage because of the frustration of recovery against the desire to return to sport.

After a passive attitude, the athlete starts to cope with the new situation by evaluating resources, setting realistic goals, maintaining commitment, and cooperating with the staff. Determined coping occurs generally at the latter stages of the rehabilitation, when the athlete has overcome denial and has become able to manage distress.

Emotional response to injury may change during a month, a week, and also in the course of the day [30].

55.5.4 Motivation-Based Models

Motivation is an essential aspect influencing on successful recovery process [33], and it could be divided into internal and external motivation.

Agreeing to self-determination theory, there is a continuum from demotivation (lack of intention to act) to intrinsic motivation (internal satisfaction). Between this continuum, there exist external factors (team influence, punishments, and rewards) that control athlete's motivation and behaviors during the process. The highest level of self-determination is characterized by internally regulated behaviors translating intrinsic satisfaction and enjoyment in the performing action [30].

Another motivational-based model is the trans-contextual model [34], which explains how motivation is transferable from a context to another one and how sport motivation and injury rehabilitation are related. This relationship occurs in three different levels [35]: specific, contextual, and global.

The first considers that the athlete is autonomous and independent and enjoys exercising to succeed in the recovery process. At the contextual motivation, social agents (coach, psychologist, teammates) influence the behavior of athletes. If injured athletes perceived autonomy support from them, they may increase their autonomous motivation in following the treatment. At a global level, specific and contextual motivations are presented, and the causality orientation of the athlete determines their type of motivation for the rehabilitation.

According to the type of motivation, a different reaction to the treatment occurs in terms of commitment, persistence, and satisfaction [30].

55.6 Psychological Skills

A variety of psychological strategies may be useful during the rehabilitation and in the reentry period. Santi and Pietrantoni [30] describe different types of interventions: educational interventions, goal setting, imagery, self-talk, biofeedback, and social support-based interventions. Relaxation is another cognitive strategy that has been used to reduce stress, anxiety, and mental/physical strain [36].

According to the models previously presented, we can intervene on cognitive appraisal of athletes through self-talk, but also providing them biological information and feedback about their recovery. Emotions can be managed through education and imagery. Finally athletes' motivation may be enhanced by intervening directly on the athlete through goal setting or with the provision of social support [30].

These techniques can be provided and educated during rehabilitation to help the athlete cope with pain, anxiety, and negative and irrational thinking and to maintain or regain motivation and compliance [37].

The use of psychological skills training during rehabilitation from the sport injury has been found to be beneficial during the recovery.

55.6.1 Educational Intervention

Research has shown how the athletes do not have a clear vision of the rehabilitation process immediately after the injury, and this can determine negative emotion and demotivation. On the other hand, an athlete that has shown better knowledge of the rehabilitation process is more realistic toward their situation reducing depressive symptoms [38].

The injured athletes often have irrational thoughts about their injury: some injured athletes tend to either exaggerate the extent of their injury or downplay it [36]. To minimize the risk for this to happen, it is important that the medical staff educates the athlete realistically about the injury, rehabilitation process, and prognosis [18].

55.6.2 Goal Setting

Setting goals determines an enhancement in motivation and commitment and provides a direction in order to optimize the recovery. The goal setting should include short-term, medium-term, and long-term goals depending on the injury severity and the prognosis of it. The goals set should be specific, measurable, acceptable, realistic, time based, evaluated, and recorded [37]. A goal setting satisfies the need for athletes, coaches, and other sport professionals to manage the return to sport, avoiding unrealistic goals and overexpectations. An effective goal setting reduces athletes' anxiety and improves their self-confidence. As a result, the athlete adheres more to the program and perceives the treatment as more effective [39].

55.6.3 Imagery

This specific technique is used to create mental images, feelings, and sensations related to a desired outcome that is happening now or has already happened. Imagery can be an audio, kinesthetic, smell, and taste experience, divided in internal (the athlete feels inside) or external (the athlete views oneself from outside). By using all senses, mentally and physically, the athlete rehearses the desired state [18].

Research has shown how athletes adopting this technique during the rehabilitation have a better return to the competition [40].

55.6.4 Self-Talk

Athletes are used to battle with their feelings during the games and competitions and trying to set their feelings on optimal level for their best performance [18].

This kind of inner conversation is called self-talk as a psychological technique, and it is an active process, which can be affected. Self-talk influences a person's thoughts which are linked to one's emotions.

The process of changing the negative thoughts to positive is called thought stopping, and, as the name tells, it involves stopping the negative thoughts and replacing them with positive ones using a mental cue [36].

Naoi and Ostrow [6] propose a protocol for the implementation of these cognitive interventions following sport injury:

1. Expressing feelings and thoughts – in this phase the psychologist uses techniques such as active listening, reflection, and clarification
2. Identifying negative thoughts – athletes are asked to write down or talk about their thoughts and identify the negative ones
3. Looking in a positive light – athletes try to find positive aspects of the injury, and the psychologist helps them in providing examples and changing them into positive ones
4. Selecting statement – athletes identify three positive thoughts and write them on a paper
5. Reading statements – athletes read the three positive thoughts to the researcher, and after this they practice self-talk
6. Maintaining – participants keep the paper and should read and repeat to themselves at least once a day; they should also monitor their thoughts during the following sessions

55.6.5 Biofeedback

Biofeedback interventions are based on the use of computerized equipment, which provides immediate feedbacks.

In a biofeedback intervention, sensors are applied on the person and send signals to a computer. The computer receives signals and gives information to the athlete about his/her physiological functions, such as electromyography (EMG), heart rate, skin conductance, or blood pressure. The psychologist, the physiotherapist, or the coach may mediate the information and help the athlete in the interpretation [41].

Making athletes aware of their own physiological state may change their interpretation of symptoms. A similar change in cognitive appraisal affects emotional and behavioral responses and may improve athletes' health and performance [42].

In the specific context of sport injury rehabilitation, biofeedback is helpful because it provides athletes with information that can make them more self-confident and reduce their anxiety and negative thoughts about the return [28].

55.6.6 Relaxation

By increasing the athletes' awareness of their physiological and psychological arousal level, relaxation techniques can help injured athletes regulate their levels of arousal for achieving optimal outcomes [22].

The skill of relaxation gives the athlete a change control over one's own mind and thoughts

[18]. Evidence showed that relaxation can reduce the feelings of depression, frustration, and anger through lowering heart rate, breathing rate, metabolic rate, and blood pressure [36].

Other benefits for relaxation are, for example, an increased ability to focus, stress relief, and decreased sleeping problems [18].

55.6.7 Social Support

Support interventions are based on the assumption that an increased support reduces the perception of negative psychological or physical symptoms through the enhancement of coping strategies. According to the hierarchical model of motivation [34, 35], motivation derived from social context influences the motivation of injured athletes.

When it comes to training and competition, having the support of family, friends, and teammates may just be an athlete's secret weapon to improving sports success and performance.

Social support can be from a family member, a friend, a teammate, a physiotherapist, and the coach which usually are called the "significant others" [18].

According to the existent literature, we can distinguish four types of support: emotional, instrumental (tangible aid), informational (providing information), and appraisal (evaluating the situation) [43].

In Udry's research [44], the patients have indicated three types of social support to be salient: emotional support, informational support, and tangible support.

1. Emotional support includes expressions of concern, empathy, niceness, and behaviors such as listening, physical presence, etc
2. Informational support is defined as information provision in an attempt to help individuals engage in problem-solving efforts and includes the provision of sound technical information
3. Tangible support includes effective practical assistance and the provision of technically competent medical care

For the social support to be effective, the right type of support has to be provided at the right times. In the first stages of the injury, the athlete usually needs mostly emotional support, and over time informational and tangible support are more expected [18].

Emotional and instrumental support is mainly provided by family and friends, an essential part of the injured athlete's social network [43].

The role of the teammates can vary from minimal to profound, depending, for example, on the time of the injury in relation to the competitive season [44]. Teammates can be an important source of all types of social support (emotional, informational, and tangible) [18]. In order to enhance peer support, it is possible to organize meetings among athletes. During these meetings, injured athletes may discuss about their feelings, concerns, and ways to cope with the stress [30].

The physiotherapists have an essential role in sport injury rehabilitation, obviously physiologically, but also psychologically [18].

The physiotherapist should be trained on multiple areas and should have an under-standing of the principles of physical therapy, biomechanics, psychology, exercise prescription, and nutrition.

The coach's role in an athlete's life is very relevant in helping the athlete in the recovery process [18].

The other sports medicine personnel involved in the rehabilitation process can act in order to [14]:

- Educate and inform the athlete about the injury and recuperation process
- Use appropriate motivation
- Demonstrate empathy and support
- Have a supportive personality (warm and open and does not exaggerate confidence)
- Foster positive interaction and customize training
- Demonstrate competence and confidence
- Encourage the athlete's confidence

Social support-based interventions have different effects depending on the source and type of support [30]. For example, emotional support provided by family, physiotherapist, and others has an effect in reducing depression; instead informational support reduces anxiety and increases self-confidence. Finally, appraisal support provided by other injured athletes determines an enhancement in coping strategies, treatment motivation and satisfaction, and a reduced fear of reinjury [22, 43].

One of the toughest things for an injured athlete to deal with is the self-expectations and also with the expectations from others (family, trainers, managers, teammates, supporters, and friends) about his recovery and returning to practices and competitions.

Conclusion

The injury is usually seen as a physical problem which starts from the occurrence of injury and ends when the athlete is back in "business," playing and competing. Additionally the injury can affect also athlete's emotions, behavior, social contacts, and even values in life [18]. With changes in daily routine, a decrease in sources of pleasure and modifications in team participation, the athlete may question their self-identity. To help prevent loss of identity when injury occurs, the parents, coaches, and training staff should help athletes recognize other strengths in addition to their athletic skills [44].

Increasing attention has been given to the development and implementation of psychological interventions during the sport injury rehabilitation process in recent years [45].

Recent researches about the successful rehabilitation of injured athletes indicate that psychological skills are not only important but essential during the rehabilitation of injured athletes [46–48]. Moreover the athletes should be willing to listen, to maintain a positive attitude, and to be intrinsically motivated and willing to learn about the injury and rehabilitation techniques. On the other hand, the role of the psychologist is to improve athlete's communication skills, keep them involved with their team and coaches, and help them in setting realistic goals [49].

As more people involved in athletics recognize the importance of sport psychology, they could help erase the stigma surrounding psychological help. A more inclusive approach may encourage athletes to face the emotional challenges that come along with athletic injury and, consequently, rehabilitation could be expedited [50].

References

1. O'Connor E, Heil J, Harmer P, Zimmerman I. Injury. In: Taylor J, Wilson G, editors. Applying sport psychology. Champaign: Human Kinetics; 2005. p. 187–206.
2. Crossman J. Psychological rehabilitation from sport injuries. Sports Med. 1997;23:334–6.
3. Deutsch RE. The psychological implications of sports related injuries. Int J Sports Psychol. 1985;16:232–7.
4. Sparkes AC. Illness, premature career-termination, and the loss of self: a biographical study of an elite athlete. In: Jones RL, Armour KM, editors. Sociology of sport: theory and practice. Harlow: Longman; 2000. p. 14–32.
5. Vergeer I. Exploring the mental representation of athletic injury: a longitudinal case study. Psychol Sport Exerc. 2006;7:99–114.
6. Naoi A, Ostrow A. The effects of cognitive and relaxations interventions on injured athletes' mood and pain during rehabilitation. J Sport Psychol. 2008;10:1.
7. Rees T, Mitchell I, Evans L, Hardy L. Stressors, social support and psychological responses to sport injury in high- and low-performance standard participants. Psychol Sport Exerc. 2010;11:505–12.
8. Dosil J. Psicología de la actividad física y del deporte. Madrid: McGraw Hill; 2004.
9. Malina R, Bouchard C, Bar-Or O. Growth, maturation and physical activity. Champaign: Human Kinetics; 2004.
10. Ivarsson A, Johnson U. Psychological factors as predictors of injuries among senior soccer players. A prospective study. J Sports Sci Med. 2010;9:347–52.
11. Lavaellee L, Flint F. The relationship of stress, competitive anxiety, mood state, and social support to athletic injury. J Athl Train. 1996;31:296–9.
12. Williams JM, Hogan TD, Andersen MB. Positive states of mind and athletic injury risk. Psychosom Med. 1993;55:468–72.
13. Silvério J, Srebro S. Como ganhar usando a cabeça. 5th ed. Porto: Afrontamento; 2012.
14. Weinberg R, Gould D. Foundations of sport and exercise psychology. Champaign: Human Kinetics; 2014.
15. Covassin T, Beidler E, Ostrowski J, Wallace J. Psychosocial aspects of rehabilitation in sports. Sports Med. 2012;9:352–69.
16. Hardy J, Crace K. Dealing with injury. Sport Psychol Train Bull. 1980;6:1–8.
17. Udry E, Gould D, Bridges D. Down but not out: athlete responses to season ending ski injuries. Psychol Sport Exerc. 1997;3:229–48.
18. Turunen A. Injured athlete in team sports – how to help the athlete psychologically through the injury. 2012. https://www.theseus.fi/bitstream/handle/10024/54183/rurunen%20antti.pdf. Accessed 19 Sept 2015.

19. Petitpas A, Danish S. Caring for injured athletes. In: Murphy S, editor. Sport psychology interventions. Champaign: Human Kinetics; 2014. p. 255–81.
20. Bianco TM. Psychological bases of sports injuries. Morgantown: West Virginia University; 2007.
21. Henschen KP, Shelley GA. Psychological bases of sports injuries. Morgantown: West Virginia University; 2007.
22. Reese LM, Pittsinger R, Yang J. Effectiveness of psychological intervention following sport injury. J Sport Health Sci. 2012;1:71–9.
23. Silvério J. Mental constitution. In: Mayr H, Menétrev J, Zaffagnini S, editors. Prevention of injuries and overuse in sports. Berlin: Springer; 2016.
24. Chan DKC, Hagger MS, Spray CM. Treatment motivation for rehabilitation after a sport injury: application of the trans-contextual model. Psychol Sport Exerc. 2011;12:83–92.
25. Brown C. Injuries: the psychology of recovery and rehab. In: Murphy S, editor. The sport psych handbook. Champaign: Human Kinetics; 2005. p. 215–35.
26. Palmi J. Aspectos psicosociales en la prevención y recuperación de lesiones deportivas. In: Rodríguez L, Gusi N, editors. Manual de prevención e rehabilitación de lesiones deportivas. Madrid: Síntesis; 2002.
27. Brewer BW. Psychology of sport injury rehabilitation. In: Tenenbaum G, Eklund R, editors. Handbook of sport psychology. Hoboken: Wiley; 2007. p. 404–24.
28. Brewer BW. Injury prevention and rehabilitation. In: Brewer BW, editor. Sport psychology. Chichester: Wiley-Blackwell; 2009. p. 83–96.
29. Brewer BW. Review and critique of models of psychological adjustment to athletic injury. J Appl Sport Psychol. 1994;6:87–100.
30. Santi G, Pietrantoni L. Psychology of sport injury rehabilitation: a review of models and interventions. J Hum Sport Exerc. 2013;8:1029–44.
31. Weise-Bjornstal DM, Smith AM, Shaffer SM, Morrey MA. An integrated model of response to sport injury: psychological and sociological dynamics. J Appl Sport Psychol. 1998;10:46–69.
32. Kübler-Ross E. On death and dying. London: Routledge; 1969.
33. Taylor A, Marlow C. Coping with sport injuries: psychological strategies for rehabilitation. New York: Oxford University Press; 2001.
34. Hagger MS, Chatzisarantis NLD, Barkoukis V, Wang CKJ, Baranowski J. Perceived autonomy support in physical education and leisure-time physical activity: a cross-cultural evaluation of the trans-contextual model. J Educ Psychol. 2005;97:376–90.
35. Vallerand RJ. Deci and Ryan's self-determination theory: a view from the hierarchical model of intrinsic and extrinsic motivation. Psychol Inq. 2000;11:312–8.
36. Crossman J. Coping with sports injury: psychological strategies for rehabilitation. New York: Oxford University Press; 2001.
37. Gordon S, Potter M, Hamer P. Coping with sport injuries: psychological strategies for rehabilitation. New York: Oxford University Press; 2001.
38. Francis SR, Andersen MB, Maley P. Physiotherapists' and male professional athletes' views on psychological skills for rehabilitation. J Sci Med Sport. 2000; 3:17–29.
39. Evans L, Hardy L. Injury rehabilitation: a goal-setting intervention study. Res Q Exerc Sport. 2002;73:310–9.
40. Vitale F. Recupero e prevenzione dell'infortunio sportivo: una ricerca sul contributo della pratica mentale (imagery). Giorn Ital Psicol Sport. 2011;10:42–7.
41. Peper E, Harvey R, Takabayashi N. Biofeedback an evidence based approach in clinical practice. Jpn J Biofeedback Res. 2009;36:3–10.
42. Thompson M, Thompson L. The biofeedback book: an introduction to basic concepts in applied psychophysiology. Wheat Ridge: Association for Applied Psychophysiology and Biofeedback; 2003.
43. Hogan BE, Linden W, Najarian B. Social support interventions. Do they work? Clin Psychol Rev. 2002;22:381–440.
44. Udry E. Coping with sport injuries: psychological strategies for rehabilitation. New York: Oxford University Press; 2001.
45. Stiler-Ostrowski JL, Gould DR, Covassin T. An evaluation of an educational intervention in psychology of injury for athletic training students. J Athl Train. 2009;44:482–9.
46. Driediger M, Hall CR, Callow N. Imagery use by injured athletes: a qualitative analysis. J Sports Sci. 2006;24:261–71.
47. Evans L, Hare R, Mullen R. Imagery use during rehabilitation from injury. J Imagery Res Sport Phys Activ. 2006;1:1–19.
48. Sordoni CA, Hall CR, Forwell L. The use of imagery by athletes during injury rehabilitation. J Sport Rehabil. 2000;9:329–38.
49. Wiese DM, Weiss MR, Yukelson DP. Sport psychology in the training room: a survey of athletic trainers. J Sport Psychol. 1991;5:15–21.
50. Klenk C. Psychological response to injury, recovery, and social support: a survey of athletes at an NCAA Division I University. http://digitalcommons.uri.edu/srhonorsprog/. Accessed 19 Sept 2015.

Sex Before Games?

56

Pedro Vendeira

Contents

P. Vendeira, MD, PhD, FECSM
President of the Portuguese Society of Andrology, Sexual Medicine and Reproduction, Porto, Portugal

Urological/Andrological Private Practice, Porto, Portugal

Fellow of the European Committee for Sexual Medicine, Porto, Portugal

Medical Competence in Clinical Sexology by the Board of the Portuguese Medical Association, Lisbon, Portugal

Educational Committee of the European Society for Sexual Medicine (ESSM), Porto, Portugal

Educational Committee of the International Society for Sexual Medicine (ISSM), Porto, Portugal
e-mail: pvendeira@gmail.com

56.1 Sex Before Games? An Old Taboo or Maybe Not!

Since many decades, this controversy involves coaches, sport physicians, physical trainers, and players. But is this a myth or a reality? As healthcare providers, how can we advise athletes concerning sex before the big game? As we are not actually ready to answer this question on evidence-based medicine, we must ask at this point: IS IT GOOD, OR IS IT BAD? Let us take a look at some testimonies.

NO TO SEX – According to Plato, "Olympians should avoid sex before competition." This is the oldest written testimony. Antonio Miguel, former football player and Head of Medical Services of Club Universidad Nacional Plumas (Mexican football first division), says "In the '60s coaches gave us potassium nitrate because (according to them), this would inhibit the sexual desire, which made it widely used in prisons, convents, barracks and similar. However, there is no scientific evidence for such properties." Also, the all-powerful boxer Muhammad Ali (Cassius Clay) claimed that "Sex before competition zaps energy. I would not make love for six weeks before a fight."

IS IT??

YES TO SEX – According to Edson Arantes do Nascimento (Pelé), considered by many as the best football player ever lived, the testimony could not be so opposite: "I never suspended

J. Espregueira-Mendes et al. (eds.), *Injuries and Health Problems in Football*,
DOI 10.1007/978-3-662-53924-8_56

sexual encounters with my wife before a game. That thing about sex helping to relax is a verified truth." Juan Carlos Medina, general coordinator of the sports department (Tecnológico de Monterrey University), says that "Sex helps you feel relaxed. This reduces the anxiety levels before the big match." The Netherlands National Football Team (1978 World Cup in Argentina) is an example of this. "Some of those players were accompanied by their wifes, and they won the second place… I am not saying this is a determinant factor, but it brings support." George Best – the "greatest player to ever pull on the green shirt of Northern Ireland" – used to say, "Sex is good? If the scientists say so, then it must be right. Sex the night before a match is a routine for me. It certainly didn't do me any harm."

After all, WHO IS RIGHT?

Well, if it was so bad, why did the INTERNATIONAL OLYMPIC COMMITTEE distribut 150,000 condoms to athletes competing in London 2012??? AT LEAST THEY BELIEVE IN SAFE SEX – a wonderful healthcare move!!!

Anyway, the fact is that some athletes admitted that the Olympics are not only a stage for world records and medals. In the Olympic Village, sexual relationships ARE COMMON among competitors (quite a different story compared to previous decades). BUT, one-night stands could alter a player's performance because these emotional situations wear you out more than physical ones.

BUT IS IT ALL A QUESTION OF EMOTIONS?????????

Probably not, because according to Casey Stengel (legendary New York Yankees manager), "It is not the sex that wrecks this guys, it's staying up all night looking for it."

As John Bancroft (former director of the Kinsey Institute for Research in Sex, Gender, and Reproduction) said, "Having sex the night before a big match does not harm your sporting performance." "There is no physiological basis for bad news in the day after." "Well, there is always a refractory period…" Let us analyze this more carefully.

The fact is that having sex the night before competition does not alter physiological testing results: indeed measuring maximum effort grip strength test the morning after coitus and performing the same test following 6 days of abstinence show that STRENGTH and ENDURANCE of the palmar flexing muscles are not adversely affected by sex the previous night [1]. In the same way, by performing other tests in the same scenario such as balance, lateral movement, reaction time, aerobic power (stair-climbing exercise), and treadmill test, there was NO change after sexual activity. In fact, sex before the game had no effect on endurance to exhaustion on a treadmill. Considering that normal sexual intercourse between married partners expends about 25–50 calories (the energy equivalent of walking up two flights of stairs that can be restored by eating a chocolate bar), it is doubtful that sex the previous night would affect laboratory physiological performance tests [2, 3].

However, there is a need to control factors related to sexual behavior: we need to pay attention to the time of day, frequency, and duration of sexual activity, diet, fatigue, stress, and individual responses. AND NEVER FORGET that heart rate and blood pressure responses are different if sex is with a spouse of 5–10 years, compared to a new partner or in strange surroundings [4].

This leads again to:

- Casey Stengel (legendary New York Yankees manager): "These the sex that wrecks this guys, it's staying up all night looking for it."

According to Maria Cristina (Director of Sports Medicine – National Autonomous University of Mexico), "consumption of alcohol or cigarettes or lack of sleep, which sometimes accompanies sexual activity, does affect athletes' performance." MODERATION is the key: "every athlete or player, professional or amateur, can have sex as long as he or she goes to bed early, hydrates, avoids mood altering drinks and cigarettes, because all this has a negative impact on their body." WISE words.

So, it looks that a steady partner could be a better choice in the day before the game. Well, that is understandable, but even with that one, be careful with what you wish for, because as written by Ian Kerner (sexual counselor and *New York Times* best-selling author of numerous books), "one of the reasons why many athletes abstain (and they should do so…) from sex the night before the game is not because of the sex itself, but because of everything that happens around it: partying, dancing, eating, drinking, smoking,… There's nothing wrong with some good healthy comfort sex, but you have to be make sure to hit the sack and get a good night's sleep afterwards." Even with a steady partner, the day before might become quite "explosive."

Nevertheless, we should not separate physiology from psychology because they cannot live one without the other. According to Dan Trink (strength coach, personal trainer, fitness writer and nutritional consultant, and director of personal training operations at Peak Performance in NYC), "There is one factor that will trump all others when it comes to performance – his Mindset. If an athlete thinks that sex will have a negative effect on his game, it certainly will. Just as the athlete thinks that tying his shoes three times while standing on a bench wearing his favorite blue socks will improve his game, that probably will as well. Ultimately, it is the BRAIN that is the most important factor." SO, THE BRAIN…

When talking about the brain, we need to stress the calming effect of orgasm – it is unlikely to be physical exhaustion; instead PROLACTIN might be involved – it peaks a couple of hours after sex.

What about effects in alertness and aggression? These can affect the game performance, so orgasm could be harmful!!! According to McGlone and Shrier [4], "there is an optimal level of alert-ness/anxiety before a competition, and a poor performance will result from either being too anxious or not alert enough. If athletes are too anxious and restless the night before an event, then sex may be a relaxing distraction. If they are already relaxed or, like some athletes, have little interest in sex the night before the game, then a good night sleep is all they need. Individual preferences and routines should be respected. The night before is not a good time for drastic routine changes."

"Consistency is the key."

Let us go back to John Bancroft, and "Well, there is always a refractory period…."

The refractory period that follows orgasm may be as little as 20 min for a teenager, but up to 24 h for a man in late middle age. Given that professional footballers are physically fit (and presumably are not having sex 2 h before the game), any associated excessive calm is unlikely to be an issue. In fact, if male orgasm induces a state of calm and relaxation (which accounts for men's infamous tendency to smoke a cigarette, roll over, and fall asleep straight afterward), there is no evidence that this state would last until the following day [5].

What about physiology with psychology with hormones? It is classically known and accepted that testosterone is the hormone of both sexual desire and "aggression." Abstinence before the game stems from the theory that sexual "frustration" leads to increased aggression and that the act of ejaculation draws testosterone from the body, weakening the muscles. That is why abstinence could also help concentration.

So, the conclusion:

Sex will make you tired and weak the next day.

- This is a really wrong idea.

According to Emmanuele Jannini (Professor of Endocrinology, University of L'Aquila, Italy), "After 3 months without sex, which is not so uncommon for some athletes, testosterone dramatically drops" and "having sex boosts testosterone production in men, which could give guys an athletic edge." That is why "scientific studies dismiss the idea that sex before the game has a tiring effect on the athlete or that it could weaken the athlete's muscles." Moreover, in women, "orgasm blocks the release of a neuropeptide (substance P), that acts as a pain transmitter – sex might combat muscle pain in ladies." This is really good news, but as stated by Jannini (personal communication), "Some personalities need more concentration… In this case sex may be a bad idea." However, "for other athletes a bit of "extra-aggression" could be the difference between winning or losing. In this case, I would suggest a complete and satisfactory sexual intercourse the evening before the game."

The unquestionable issue is that testosterone levels are known to be higher in men who are sexually active. If you believe that testosterone is good for the game, then you need to pick your own assumptions.

Finishing with the start, we noticed different testimonies and some evidence concerning sex before the big game. No truth is certain. As a kind of take-home messages, I would stress that:

- People who have healthy sex lives end up having more confidence and self-esteem and doing better at work
- Sex must never be prohibited to athletes, because there are no evidence-based studies supporting abstinence before the game

- (IN A PROPER SETTING) Consistency and moderation are the keys
- Sex boosts testosterone production which could give guys an athletic edge
- Always respect not to have sexual intercourse 2 h before a competition event

References

1. Johnson WR. Muscular performance following coitus. J Sex Res. 1986;4:247–8.
2. Boone T, Gilmore S. Effects of sexual intercourse on maxi-mal aerobic power, oxygen pulse, and double product in male sedentary subjects. J Sports Med Phys Fitness. 1995;35:214–7.
3. Thornton J. Sexual activity and athletic performance: is there a relationship? Phys Sport Med. 1990;18:148–53.
4. McGlone S, Shrier I. Does sex the night before competition decrease performance? Clin J Sport Med. 2000;10:233–4.
5. Sztajzel J, Périat M, Marti V, Krall P, Rutishauser W. Effect of sexual activity on cycle ergometer stress test parameters, on plasmatic testosterone levels and on concentration capacity. J Sports Med Phys Fitness. 2000;40:233–9.

Part XIV

Biological Treatments and Enhancement

Hyaluronic Acid, PRP/Growth Factors, and Stem Cells in the Treatment of Osteochondral Lesions

57

Diana Ribeiro Pereira, Joana Silva-Correia, Elisaveta Kon, Hélder Pereira, Piero Volpi, João Espregueira-Mendes, Rui L. Reis, and J. Miguel Oliveira

Contents

D.R. Pereira • J. Silva-Correia • R.L. Reis
J.M. Oliveira (✉)
3B's Research Group – Biomaterials, Biodegradables and Biomimetics, University of Minho, Headquarters of the European Institute of Excellence on Tissue Engineering and Regenerative Medicine, AvePark, S. Cláudio de Barco, 4806-909 Taipas, Guimarães, Portugal

ICVS/3B's – PT Government Associated Laboratory, Porto, Portugal
e-mail: miguel.oliveira@dep.uminho.pt

E. Kon
Istituto Ortopedico Rizzoli, Bologna, Italy

H. Pereira
3B's Research Group – Biomaterials, Biodegradables and Biomimetics, University of Minho, Headquarters of the European Institute of Excellence on Tissue Engineering and Regenerative Medicine, AvePark, S. Cláudio de Barco, 4806-909 Taipas, Guimarães, Portugal

ICVS/3B's – PT Government Associated Laboratory, Porto, Portugal

Ripoll y De Prado Sports Clinic – FIFA Medical Centre of Excellence, Murcia-Madrid, Spain

Orthopedic Department Centro Hospitalar Póvoa de Varzim, Vila do Conde, Portugal

P. Volpi
Department of Orthopaedic Knee and Sports Traumatology, Humanitas Research Hospital, Rozzano, Italy

FC Internazionale Medical Staff, Milano, Italy

J. Espregueira-Mendes
Clínica do Dragão, Espregueira-Mendes Sports Centre – FIFA Medical Centre of Excellence, Porto, Portugal

Dom Henrique Research Centre, Porto, Portugal

3B's Research Group – Biomaterials, Biodegradables and Biomimetics, University of Minho, Headquarters of the European Institute of Excellence on Tissue Engineering and Regenerative Medicine, AvePark, Parque de Ciência e Tecnologia, Zona Industrial da Gandra, 4805-017 Barco, Guimarães, Portugal

ICVS/3B's – PT Government Associated Laboratory, Braga/Guimarães, Portugal

Orthopaedics Department of Minho University, Minho, Portugal

J. Espregueira-Mendes et al. (eds.), *Injuries and Health Problems in Football*,
DOI 10.1007/978-3-662-53924-8_57

57.1 Introduction

Disease of cartilage in its many presentations constitutes the condition that most often affects human joints [1]. Knee arthroscopy is still the most frequent surgical procedure in orthopedics and chondral (CD) or osteochondral (OC) defects and is observed in more than half of all knees submitted to arthroscopy [2, 3]. The high occurrence of these conditions, which many times result in functional disability, absence from work, and/or implications in other comorbidities, obviously creates a high socioeconomic impact [4]. Another aspect is that younger people increasingly adopt lifestyles which are physically demanding and these inevitably increase the risk of injury [5]. Pivoting sports are considered as a risk factor for OC defects [6, 7].

Additionally, the increasing human longevity also leads to higher frequency of cartilage degenerative conditions [5]. Degenerative changes are one of the causes of CD or OC defects and, in weight-bearing joints and limb alignment, are considered to play a role given the implication in joint biomechanics [8].

The clinical consequences resulting from articular cartilage defects are pain, swelling, mechanical symptoms, functional disability, and subsequent progression for osteoarthritis (OA) [9].

The effectiveness of "classic" therapeutic approaches for symptomatic cartilage defects is not always high or is debatable in incongruent joints (e.g., the knee) [10] or more congruent joints (e.g., the ankle) [11].

Moreover, it is recognized by the clinical community that hyaline cartilage has limited healing capacity regardless of the biomechanical or humoral environment [10].

57.2 Hyaline Cartilage Pathophysiology

The main functions of hyaline cartilage are related to facilitating joint motion by lowering either friction or shock absorption (dissipating the energy transmitted to the underlying subchondral bone) [12, 13]. The viscoelasticity of this tissue enables variable load transmission throughout the arch of movement [9].

The ultrastructure architecture of this tissue constitutes an adaptation to perform these functions. Its main constitutes are water (65–80%), extracellular matrix (ECM), and cells.

The main component of ECM is collagen fibers, mainly of type II. However, collagen types V, VI, IX, X, and XI can also be identified. A lattice-type framework combines collagen fibers with proteoglycans and hyaluronic acid. This complex framework is responsible for the unique biomechanical properties of articular (hyaline) cartilage [14]. Other proteins have been identified such as biglycan, decorin, fibromodulin, fibronectin, other link proteins, and also lipids [12]. The cellular component is the chondrocyte (2% of total volume), which is responsible for the synthesis of the ECM. These cells derive from mesenchymal stem cells. Hyaline cartilage is described as avascular and lacks innervation and thus has limited capacity to activate inflammatory response. Hyaline cartilage has been classically described in four different layers according to organization and composition: the tangential zone, intermediate zone, calcified layer, the tidemark, and the subchondral bone [15]. Together they form the cartilage unit.

Interest has been increasing about the interactions between cartilage and subchondral bone recognizing that this represents one single functional osteochondral unit [16].

Cartilage defects might originate in the superficial layer of cartilage and progress toward deeper zones. However, some conditions (e.g., osteochondritis dissecans – OCD) can originate in the subchondral bone and only secondarily affect the overlying cartilage.

In an attempt to classify and stratify the treatment options, several scores have been proposed based on the extension of the lesion. These include magnetic resonance imaging (MRI) [17], the histological International Cartilage Research Society (ICRS) grading system [18], and the most widely accepted Outerbridge articular cartilage lesion classification system based on arthroscopic findings [19–21].

The Outerbridge system characterizes changes into grades, with grade 0 as normal, grade I as softening, grade II as fibrillation, grade III as fissuring, and grade IV as reaching the depth of bone.

The key role of the subchondral bone constitutes the primary support for one important group of surgical techniques aiming to repair OC defects by bone marrow stimulation techniques. In response to an "aggression," the subchondral bone response initiates through hematoma, stem cell migration, and neovascular ingrowth. This basic mechanism is capable of producing a repair tissue, which is different from hyaline cartilage once its main constituent is collagen type I and has lower mechanical properties. So, all these techniques ultimately originate tissue that is poorer than the original.

One of the current challenges presented to surgeons and researchers is trying to influence this process to stimulate cells, fine-tune the role of growth factors (GFs), and ultimately obtain a more effective matrix with mechanical properties similar to those of hyaline cartilage.

So, historically the first attempts to treat for OC defects included joint lavage [22] and debridement [23], augmentation procedures including Pridie's perforations [24], and microfractures (Fig. 57.1) [25, 26].

Since the early 1990s, a mosaicplasty technique has been developed by Hangody et al. [27, 28] as a method to provide autologous cartilage and underlying bone to damaged areas. However, some concerns have been raised concerning donor zone complications [29–32].

More recently, several methods have been proposed and are still under investigation including advanced regenerative medicine approaches using cells [33–38], gene therapy [36, 39], and GFs [40] for treatment of the challenging OC defects (Fig. 57.2).

Conservative treatment still has a role as the initial treatment for most patients, and most often surgery is proposed only after failure of the former. Nonoperative treatment includes nonsteroidal anti-inflammatory drugs, analgesics, rest, cryotherapy, physiotherapy, and dietary supplements (glucosamine, chondroitin, omega-3, etc.), isolated or combined [9, 20].

Nowadays, we have been assisting toward the emergence of nonoperative therapies, which are

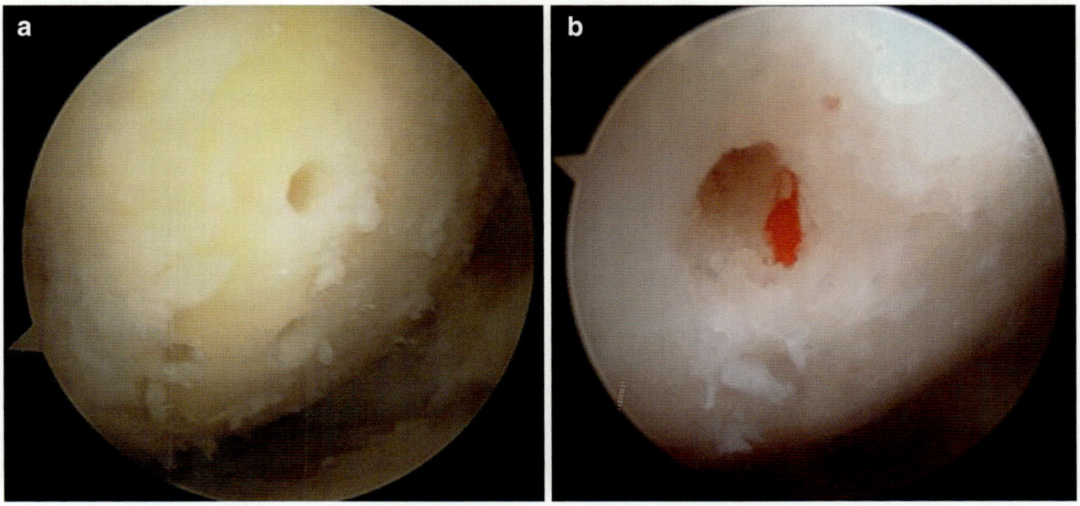

Fig. 57.1 (**a**) Arthroscopic views showing extensive OC defect on medial femoral condyle of the knee. (**b**) Blood coming out of microfracture holes bringing MSCs upon tourniquet opening

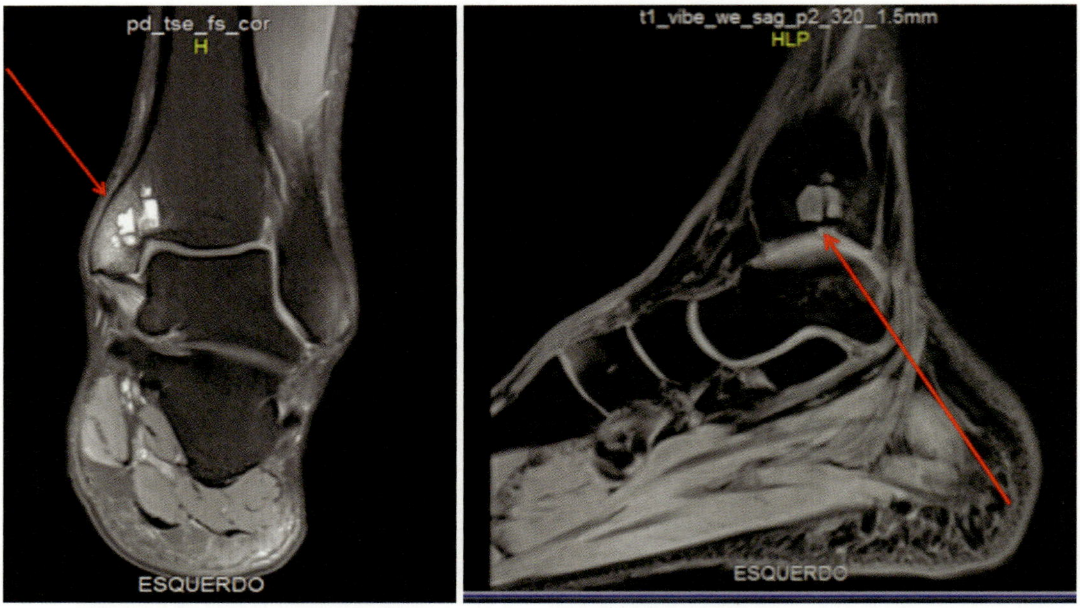

Fig. 57.2 MRI T2 images showing OC defect on the distal tibia with bone cysts formation

able to induce body self-repair and recovery from injuries. These therapies use hyaluronic acid (HA) injections, mesenchymal stem cell injection, platelet-rich plasma (PRP), serum injection, and amniotic tissue, alone or in combination. All these treatments are grouped into a new therapy named autologous regenerative therapies giving rise to a new therapeutic field named orthobiologics [17]. The fundamentals of OC tissue and the most recent developments, important basic studies, and use of orthobiologics in the clinics will be overviewed herein.

57.3 Osteochondral Tissue: Fundamentals on Anatomy and Physiology

The OC tissue has the articular cartilage layer as the foremost region of the joint, a highly flexible and supportive tissue. The unique features of cartilage tissue limit its self-renewal capabilities due to lack of vascularization and innervation [41]. Remodeling is rarely seen in cartilage due to low cell number and low metabolic activity of chondrocytes especially mature cells which produce little ECM [42, 43]. The cartilage is present in three different types in the body: hyaline cartilage, fibrocartilage, and elastic cartilage, the predominant one being hyaline cartilage which is also called articular cartilage. It is mostly composed of water, collagen, proteoglycans (PGs), proteins, and chondrocytes. Cartilaginous tissue fulfills a supportive role mainly due to its capacity to withstand high compressive loads. This behavior is intrinsically related to the ECM composition. The glycosaminoglycans (GAGs) attached to the PGs give a strongly negative charge to the ECM. In this way, osmotically active cations are attracted, leading to the entrance of water into the ECM. The intricate ECM network in articular cartilage is structured by the presence of collagen type II intertwining chondroitin, keratin sulfate (GAGs), and aggrecan (PG). The collagen type II fibrils improve the structure and the elastic strength of the cartilage. It is also believed that the existence of collagen type X is responsible for the process of mineralization happening at the interface between cartilage and bone. The overall cartilaginous tissue is formed by the same components. However, its assembly and concentrations vary in different cartilage zones. There are four different zones: superficial, middle, deep (or calcified), and subchondral bone. The presence of this calcified zone between is responsible for connecting the innermost cartilage layer and subchondral bone layer [44].

The OC tissue presents an inner region named the subchondral bone. This is the zone underlying the calcified cartilage zone and is composed of the lamella and the trabeculae [45]. The lamella can also be called the subchondral bone plate, and it is the marked zone that separates the two regions (cartilage and subchondral bone). There is a solid mass of bone underneath, defined as trabeculae. This zone is highly vascularized, and the nutrients exchanged here are utilized by both articular cartilage and subchondral bone. Apart from serving as an anchorage site to collagen fibrils, the other important roles of subchondral bone are absorption and support joint shape [46].

Damage to the articular cartilage and subsequent progression of OC defects (including OCD) and progressive OA are pathological conditions resulting in the loss of joint function. The ECM suffers a destabilization of supramolecular structures affecting collagen expression and molecular secretion [47].

57.4 Orthobiologics: Emerging Field in Sport Injury Treatments

Football is the most popular sport in the world either at amateur or professional level [48]. It is estimated that, worldwide, around 200 million individuals are active football players. But it is associated with a high risk of injury presenting 13–35 injuries per 1000 h of competition on the field [49]. Unfortunately, there is a lack of detailed information about football-related injury as to risk prevention, mechanisms, severity of injuries, and the resulting time lost to play while players recover [50, 51]. In addition, no consensus exists about study design, data collection, and pathological definitions in the epidemiological studies of football injuries to date [51]. For these reasons, epidemiological research should be carried out to devise preventive measures [52].

Over the last 20 years, a new era of medicine has been receiving a lot of attention among clinicians. Orthobiologics is an emergent field in medicine, which has a specific emphasis on tissue's healing. As previously mentioned, orthobiologics uses autologous therapies to modulate cell signaling allowing the acceleration of healing process. Sports medicine had helped to bring orthobiologics into the current medical practice. It can be attempted as cellular therapies; however, there was a paradigm shift in treatment design where no longer this treatments concern the temporary management of the pathology. Orthobiologics is somewhere in between conservative and surgical methods, and so far it has faced three evolutions over the years. Viscosupplementation, which concerns hyaluronic acid injections, was the first generation. The treatment was first applied in 1997 to relieve patients from the pain symptoms of OA. The outcome was satisfactory, and, unlike oral drug administration (NSAID), viscosupplementation was able to diminish patient's pain.

The first usage of PRP in sport medics reports to 2006. Some year after viscosupplementation usage, PRP appear as a second generation in orthobiologics. Ferrari et al. [53] was the first to use PRP in an open heart surgery. Unlike viscosupplementation, PRP is an autologous therapy and is performed to stimulate a supraphysiologic response in the body. PRP function as an enriched cocktail of bioactive proteins. The third generation in orthobiologics reports the use of mesenchymal stem cells, either from different sources such as embryonic, bone marrow, adipose, etc. Bone marrow-derived concentrate (BMDC) is often used in clinics, and it is a mixture of mesenchymal stem cell, hematopoietic cells, platelet, and cytokine involved in the regenerative potential of healing [54].

Currently, most of the orthobiologics studies carried out present considerable outcome heterogeneity, mostly being nonrandomized and nonwell classified. So, there is still the need to pursue research in a more controlled manner to achieve orthobiologics strategies that are more feasible.

57.5 Hyaluronic Acid

HA injection at the site of lesion appears as a conservative method to treat OC lesions [55]. HA is a high molecular weight and anionic biopolysaccharide [56], discovered in 1934, by Karl Meyer and his assistant John Palmerin [55]. The first medical HA application in humans was in the vitreous substitution/replacement procedure during bovine eye surgery, in the late 1950s [55]. Viscosupplementation (VS) came into clinical use in Japan and Italy in 1987 and in Canada in 1992, but in Europe and the USA, it was adopted in the second half of the 1990s. VS is the intra-articular administration of a high viscoelastic fluid into the synovial joint to reproduce and repair the rheological proprieties of the synovial fluid. VS can enhance the vital joint lubrication and shock absorption ability, essential functions for mobility improvements and pain relief. All products available on the market for VS are based on HA, a high molecular weight (105–107 Da) and unbranched glycosaminoglycan that can be found in the extracellular matrix of human tissue. While HA is used clinically, its functions are not fully known [57]. Chondroprotective effects of HA, observed in vivo, might explain the beneficial long-term effects on articular cartilage. HA also reduces pain-associated nerve impulses and sensitivity. HA is a free, non-sulfated, and negatively charged glycosaminoglycan (GAG) capable of interacting with receptors and ECM proteins [58]. HA can be derived from different sources such as rooster combs, bacterial production, and either animal or human sources [59]. Its properties (e.g., rheological properties) depend on its source. Nevertheless, HA presents high viscosity, is a water-soluble polymer, and has specific enzymatic degradation. Low and high molecular weight are the two forms of HA, differing in chain length ($\leq 2 \times 10^6$ Da and $2 \times 10^6 – \geq 4 \times 10^6$ Da, respectively). Structural and biological functions of HA are mainly chain size-related to its chains as suggested by Stern et al. [60, 61]. The interactions between tissues and HA occur through hyaladherins. Essential functions such as cell communication, motility, and morphogenesis occur due to interactions between hyaladherins and tissue receptor. These interactions occur through specific receptors, mainly CD44 and RHAMM, at the cell surface. The high molecular weight hyaluronic acid (HMWHA) molecule plays a structural role because it is able to bind 10–10,000 times its weight in water [60, 62, 63]. Thus, being osmotically active in a completely hydrated state, it is able to fill the space and act as a shock absorber as well as a lubricant. From a biological point of view, the HMW chains are anti-angiogenic and anti-inflammatory and possess immunosuppressive capacities [64, 65]. Many studies have reported a decrease in the inflammatory response and apoptosis through the downregulation of a number of factors responsible for ECM. These results suggest that HMWHA impairs the phenomena of phagocytosis, macrophage activation, and inflammatory cytokines production. However, HMWHA chains can break down into low molecular weight chains (LMWHA), which are found to have a pro-inflammatory effect. These fragments have been shown to secrete inflammatory cytokines and stimulate angiogenesis and tissue remodeling after activation of endogenous signaling pathways. They can promote the activation and maturation of dendritic cells and the release of pro-inflammatory cytokines [61, 65, 66]. Molecular changes in the ECM of damaged joints alter the composition and structure of natural HA. Along with molecule secretion and tissue remodeling, the development of pathologies also occurs [60].

HA injection, also known as viscosupplementation, appears to be a conservative method to improve the biomechanical function of the joint mainly due to HA physicochemical characteristics (i.e., hydrogel state) [67, 68]. HA is a gel-like constituent injected in the joint intra-articular cavity guided by ultrasound or X-ray fluoroscopy. It is thought that HA acts as a lubricant providing a cushion effect at the joint. However, the biological mechanism behind this role in cartilage repair remains poorly understood in medical community [69].

Positive effects of HA intra-articular injections are mainly reported in the management of osteoarthritis [70, 71]. Viscosupplementation is usually performed after surgical intervention to treat osteochondral lesions (knee and ankle) [72]. The Food and Drug Administration (FDA) regulates the use of HA for intra-articular injection. Sodium hyaluronate, hylan G-F 20, and HMWHA have received approval for clinical injections, although the biological mechanism of HA is not fully explained. Thus, some studies strongly recommend the use of HMWHA to treat OC defects. However, a strong heterogeneity in studies is

Table 57.1 Summary of studies using HA in the treatment of defects

Reference(s)	OC defect	Enrolled sample nr	Strategy applied	Outcome measure	Follow-up timing
Hakshur [74]	Knee-osteoarthritis	12	Debridement + HA injections (Euflexxa)	WOMAC VAS SF-36 KS	2, 14, 28 weeks
Kon [75]	Knee cartilage degenerative lesions and osteoarthritis	150	Platelet-rich plasma + hyaluronic acid injections	IKDC EQ VAS	2, 6 months
Doral [76]	Talar osteochondral lesions	57	Microfracture technique + hyaluronic acid injection	AOFAS Freiburg functional pain scores	1 and 2 years
Buda [77]	Talar osteochondral lesion	64	Concentrated bone marrow-derived cells + scaffold (collagen powder or Hyaluronic acid membrane)	AOFAS	53 months
Giannini [78]	Talar osteochondral lesion	49	Concentrated bone marrow-derived cells + scaffold (collagen powder or hyaluronic acid membrane)	AOFAS MRI radiography	4 years
Wong [79]	Knees with cartilage defects	56	Microfracture + Autologous bone marrow-derived mesenchymal stem cell injections + Hyaluronic acid	Tegner Lysholm IDK MRI MOCART	6 months, 1, 2 years
Mason [80]	Talar dome Full-thickness articular cartilage and subchondral bone	1	Cell-free chondroinductive implant (polyglycolic acid felt and hyaluronic acid)	–	3 years

found in clinics [73]. Nonetheless, some "off-label" (not FDA approved) HA has been used in clinical practice mainly for hip and knee OA treatments. Table 57.1 summarizes the relevant reports that make use of HA for treating OC defects. The short duration of action, due to the rapid breakdown and reabsorption of HA, is a limitation in the intra-articular injections. HA has a half-life of 17 h after intra-articular injection. Systemic HA injection at end of surgery cannot be recommended, being poorly assessed and showing benefit that are short lived accordingly to the few published studies. It has already been mentioned in clinical trials that a combination of treatments is shown to be more effective than HA alone. Additionally, there is the need to develop sustained-release approaches.

57.6 Platelet-Rich Plasma (PRP)/Growth Factors

The intrinsic physiological tissue remodeling and homeostasis is strongly influenced by GFs. GFs contribute to many processes such as chemotaxis, differentiation, proliferation, and cellular responses in OC tissues (cartilage and bone tissue). Therefore, the use of autologous and recombinant GFs is emerging in orthopedics. The main objective is to manipulate GFs and secretory proteins aiming at both cartilage and bone repair.

Bone-derived growth factors (BMPs), mainly used for bone regeneration and autologous blood-derived growth factors (used for cartilage and soft tissue regeneration), are the most widely

Table 57.2 Summary of studies using platelet-rich plasma in the treatment of OC defects

Reference(s)	OC defect	Enrolled sample nr (age/average)	Strategy applied	Outcome measure	Follow-up timing
Haleem [83]	Full-thickness cartilage defect	5	Platelet-rich fibrin glue + autologous bone marrow mesenchymal stem cells	Lysholm RHSSK X-ray MRO	1 year
Li [84]	Knee articular cartilage degeneration	30	PRP injection vs. sodium hyaluronate	IKDC WOMAC Lequese	3, 4, 6 months
Mei-Dan [85]	Talar dome osteochondra lesions	32	PRP vs. HA	AOFAS AHFS VAS stiffness/ function	28 weeks
Hart [86]	Tibio-femoral cartilage defect	50	Concentrated autologous PRPP	Lysholm Tegner IKDC Cincinnati scores	12 months
Eirale [87]	Knee-acute medial collateral ligament injury	1	PRP injections	Symptoms function	18 days
Laver [88]	High ankle sprain	16	Ultrasound-guided PRP injections	Subjective outcome	6 weeks

used GFs in clinics. The GFs can mostly be obtained from patient's own blood (autologous), and they become available after the platelet-activation procedure and are thus called PRP. The extensive clinical use of PRP (Table 57.2) for addressing OC lesions relies on its easy application and low cost [81]. PRP is part of the patient's blood plasma, composed of platelet concentrations above baseline. Normal platelet count ranges between 150,000 and 350,000 platelets/μL of human blood [82]. Clinical studies have shown efficacy of PRP using concentrated platelets (4–5 times higher than normal blood). Thus, definition of PRP concerns a concentration of 10^6 platelets/μL. To our knowledge, there are no studies showing improvements when platelet concentrations are higher than 10^6. However, biological activity of various PRP preparations may vary in efficacy. In the existing literature, the use of different terminologies for PRP is often seen as plasma rich in platelets or plasma very rich in platelets, and it also can appear as preparation rich in growth factors or platelet lysates.

The natural healing process in any tissue encompasses three major phases: (1) acute inflammatory phase (platelet clot formation is seen, degranulation of growth factors occurs, coagulation cascade is activated, and migration of granulocytes and macrophages occurs), (2) mesenchymal cell proliferation and differentiation phase, and (3) tissue regeneration by specific cells. All the three phases of the inflammatory response are regulated mainly by the platelets [89]. The most important role is at the proliferation and differentiation phase. Platelets are derived from megakaryocytes which are small blood cells with a size between 1 and 3 μm. The presence of alpha-granules in megakaryocytes produces the GFs. More than 30 bioactive proteins are found in megakaryocytes and play an important role in tissue homeostasis and healing processes. PRP, in different platelet-activation methods, are able to differentially produce growth factors [90].

Bioactive GF promotes a wide range of physiological processes such as cell proliferation, differentiation, and chemotaxis. In this way, it is understood that administration of PRP may

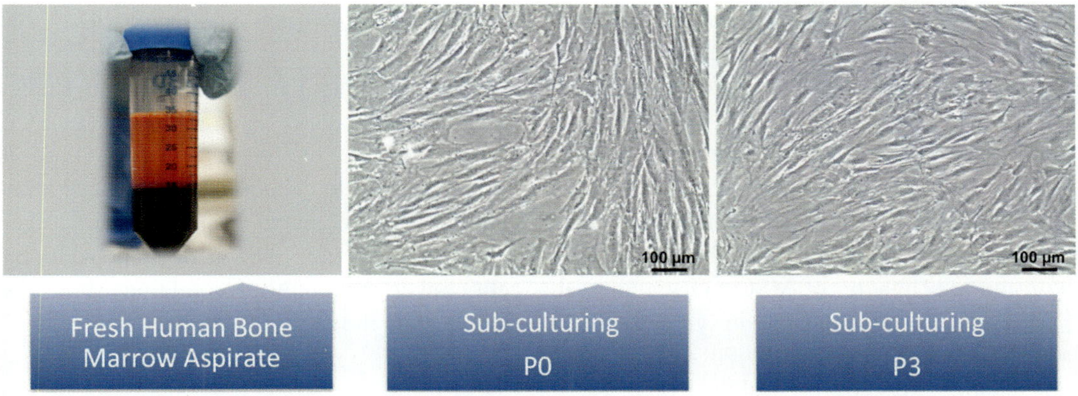

Fig. 57.3 Photomicrograph of cultured MSCs

improve healing through the action of growth factors and cytokines secreted from alpha-granules present in platelets. Tissue damage triggers a cascade of molecules to promote self-repair. Platelet-derived growth factor (PDGF), vascular endothelial growth factor (VEGF), transforming growth factor-β (TFG-β), fibroblast growth factor (FGF), and, more recently, connective tissue growth factor (CTGF) are all growth factors enriching the PRP environment to foster the regeneration of OC tissues, cartilage, and bone [91].

PRP has been employed in a wide range of clinical applications such as orthopedics including sports medicine. Many clinical questions still remain concerning the use of orthobiologics, HA, stem cells, and PRP/GF particularly regarding the therapy timing (when to start therapy and for how long), cell numbers, volume or dose, and frequency of treatment about which consensus in clinical practices has still not been reached.

57.7 Stem Cells

Large OC lesions (greater than 1 cm) cannot be addressed simply by means of using biomaterials. Stem cell-based therapies potentially allow treating these defects. Particular interest has arisen about MSCs due to their differentiation capacity toward mesodermal lineages [92]. The modulation of adult MSC pathways can lead to chondro-, osteo- and adipogenesis (chondrocytes, osteoblasts, and adipocytes, respectively) [93, 94]. MSCs are found in many different tissues in the body including the bone marrow, skin, adipose and synovial tissue, and muscles. MSCs (Fig. 57.3) are easy to prepare from aspirates such as bone marrow, adipose, or synovial tissue and are readily available from the surgery room [92, 95].

Moreover, MSCs are immunoprivileged, which can allow their transplantation without any immune response being elicited. Friedstein et al. [96] conducted the first investigation to characterize multipotent stromal precursor cells which were later on named as MSCs [97]. Depending on the harvesting site, MSCs show a better performance in certain strategies. Bone marrow stem cells are the most extensively studied. Despite the invasiveness for harvesting and isolation after collection, MSCs are ready for usage [98]. Bone marrow aspirates from the iliac crest have been used to treat focal traumatic chondral and OC defects [99–102]. Different approaches can be applied when it comes to application of MSCs. After aspiration, MSCs are capable of undergoing expansion within 2–3 weeks for further application, or the concentrated aspirate can be immediately implanted (BMDC). Usually, the use of natural matrices to embed the MSCs is employed based on platelet-rich fibrin gel [83, 101, 103–105], fibrin glue [100], collagen gel [78, 99, 100, 103, 104] or collagen scaffolds [99, 100, 105, 106], and HA [78, 101, 103, 104]. Natural matrices to embed MSCs create a cell environment that mimics the natural one, which is beneficial from a biological point of view.

In the past years, patients presenting focal chondral and OC lesions that were treated with MSCs have shown definitive clinical improvement. Knee [100, 101, 105–110] and ankle [78, 103, 104] were the two joints extensively investigated following football injuries. So far, there are no studies for periods greater than 24 months concerning treatments of focal chondral defects with the implantation of MSCs. Giannini et al. [78] reported a slight decrease in symptoms at 36 and 48 months compared to 24 months post-implantation. A study by Wakitani et al. [100] reported a long-term evidence (137 months post-surgery) of MSCs implantation taking into account only the safe use of these cells. Different studies, involving arthroscopy and MRI, assessed the efficient production of hyaline cartilage by MSCs implantation, and additionally neo-tissue formation showed good integration within 24 months postimplantation [78, 101, 103, 106, 108, 110]. Subchondral bone tissue remodeling is a longer process when compared to that of cartilage. Giannini et al. [78] have shown that, when 24 months had elapsed following MSC implantation in the talus, unhealthy subchondral tissue was formed. Two comparison studies [104, 107] of MSCs/BMDC implantation to chondrocyte implantation (ACI/MACI) found similar outcomes. However, MSCs showed better function than chondrocytes implantation did. Both strategies were able to produce neo-hyaline cartilage. Pak et al. [111] implanted autologous adipose tissue-derived stem cells in 4 patients, and all patients showed improvement after 12 weeks of treatment. The infrapatellar fat pad tissue, also known as Hoffa's body, is located under and behind the patella bone within the knee. During an arthroscopy, Hoffa's body can be removed to allow a better visualization of the knee because it is inflamed or damaged [112]. From this perspective, this tissue can be also considered a promising source of stem cells (ASCs) for use in clinics, as ASCs are already known to possess potential to differentiate into chondrocytes and osteoblasts.

Table 57.3 summarizes the relevant studies involving stem cell implantation for treating OC defects. Despite the current studies, little is known as yet as to the best dosage and cell numbers to be implanted at the defect sites. Standardization cell type and subpopulations, cell number, and culturing conditions should be performed in the clinics, in the near future.

57.8 One-Step Surgical Approaches in the Treatment of Osteochondral Defects

A major goal in orthopedics concerns the repair of OC tissues that avoids successive surgical interventions. Only a few studies have investigated the histological outcomes of one-step procedures in the treatment of articular OC lesions [99, 103, 116, 117]. Of these studies, Giannini et al. [103] combined BMC and PRP gel with HA membrane or collagen powder to treat talar OC lesions. All the patients had shown a functional improvement. Tissue remodeling was clearly observed by histological biopsies, toward hyaline-like cartilage [103]. Siclari et al. [117] harvested 5 biopsies by means of arthroscopy. Macroscopic observation revealed a whiter appearance of the repairs, some hypertrophic tissue, and irregularity at the surface. A good subchondral integration with neo-hyaline cartilage was observed in histological analysis. Enea et al. carried out an investigation that showed tissue formation and repair documented in accordance with ICRS CRA [109], even though some one-step procedures combining scaffolds have shown the presence of osteophytes formation. All the studies above mentioned are denominated in the clinics as one-step procedures. The concept of one-step implies that the patient undergoes surgery only once. In addition, the strategy itself

Table 57.3 Summary of studies using stem cells in the treatment of OC defects

Reference(s)	OC defect	Enrolled sample nr	Strategy applied	Outcome measure	Follow-up timing
Nejadnik [107]	Cartilage damage	72	First-generation autologous chondrocyte implantation vs. autologous bone marrow-derived mesenchymal stem cells	ICRS IKDC Lyshol, Tegner	3, 6, 9, 12, 18, and 24 months
Pak [111]	Hip osteonecrosis and knee OA	2	Autologous adipose-tissue-derived stem cells + hyaluronic acid + platelet rich plasma + calcium chloride + dexamethasone	MRI Pain score	Case report
Gobbi [105]	Chondral lesions	15	Bone marrow aspirate concentrate + collagen I/III matrix	X-rays MRI VAS IKDC KOOS Lysholm MARX SF-36 Tegner	1, 2 years
Teo [113]	Patellar OCD	23	Autologous chondrocyte implantation vs. cultured bone marrow stem cell	CT scans IKDC Tegner-Lysholm Lysholm-Gillquist	6, 12, and 24 months
Kasemkijwattana [106]	Large traumatic cartilage defect	2	Autologous bone marrow mesenchymal stem cells implantation	KOOS IKDC	30, 31 months
Gigante [114]	Isolated lesions at the medial femoral condyle	5	Autologous matrix (collagen) + bone marrow concentrate	ICRS CRA Histology	12 months
Koh [115]	Secondary knee OA	25	Infrapatellar fat pad mesenchymal stem cells injections	Lysholm Tegner VAS	16.4 months

satisfies all the requirements for good regeneration of the affected tissue. Commonly in these strategies, what is envisioned is an approach with more than one orthobiologic components. Others have also been mentioned in Table 57.4. The recent use of multilayered scaffolds composed of collagen type I with hydroxyapatite nanoparticles is also appealing [118]. This one-step procedure has as its final goal the treatment of chondral and osteochondral knee defects at once.

Table 57.4 Summary of studies using combinatorial substances used in the treatment of OC defects

Reference(s)	OC defect	Enrolled sample nr (age/average)	Strategy applied	Outcome measure	Follow-up timing
Kuroda [99]	Full-thickness articular cartilage defect	1	Autologous bone marrow stromal cells + collagen scaffold	ICRS IV histologic scores	1 year
Patrascu [116]	Chondral defect	1	Cell-free polyglycolic acid + HA	Histologic scores	2 years
Giannini [103]	Talar osteochondral lesion	48	Concentrate bone marrow-derived cells and collagen powder or HA membrane	AOFAS MRI histology	24 months
Kon [118]	Knee chondral or osteochondral lesions	30	Type I collagen-hydroxyapatite nanostructured scaffold	Tegner Score IKDC MRI MOCART	2 years
Crawford [119]	Distal femoral cartilage lesions	30	NeoCart, autologous cartilage tissue implant vs. microfracture	SF-36 KOOS ADL IKDC	26 ± 2 months
Vijayan [120]	Osteochondral lesions (>5 cm^2)	14	MACI membranes with impaction grafting of the subchondral bone	Cincinnati knee score Pain score	5.2 years
Saw [121]	Chondral lesions	15	Subchondral drilling injections of HA + peripheral blood stem cells	ICRD II histologic scores MRI IKDC	18 months
Turajane [122]	Early osteoarthritic knee	5	Microdrilling mesenchymal cell stimulation + autologous-activated peripheral blood stem cells + HA	WOMAC KOO scores AAPBSC/ arthroscopic	-
Siclari [117]	Knee cartilage defect		Subchondral drilling + resorbable polymer-based implants + PRP	KOOS MRI MOCART	5 years
Enea [109]	Focal condylar lesions of knee articular cartilage	9	Collagen-covered microfracture + bone marrow concentrate	MRI	12 months

57.9 Clinical Status of Orthobiologics/Tissue Engineering Osteochondral Treatments

OC tissue engineering scaffolds are already making their way through clinical trials. A review of the clinicaltrials.gov database yielded few studies in tissue engineering (Table 57.5). Bi- or multiphasic scaffolds aiming to regenerate different tissues (cartilage and subchondral bone in osteochondral tissue) are already being studied in humans at companies and at universities such as Cartiheal LTD, National Taiwan University Hospital, Kensey Nash Corporation, Fin-Ceramica Faenza Spa, and Piramal Healthcare Canada Ltd. which are in the vanguard for TE strategies commercially available. Great efforts have been made to bring tissue engineering approaches to clinical trials, but these are as yet inconclusive. So far, fresh or frozen allografts, or modified allograft products in combination with conservative or surgical methods are the approaches closest to tissue engineering. Strategies solely concerning polymers are the most widely studied in tissue engineering field. However, as shown by Stanish et al. [123], the use

Table 57.5 Current tissue engineering and regenerative medicine strategies in clinical trials

Product	Company	Design	Trial number	Status
Biphasic osteochondral composite	National Taiwan University Hospital	Biphasic construct	NCT 01409447	Clinical trials
Agili-C biphasic implant	Cartheal Lda.	Biphasic construct	NCT 01471236	Clinical trials
Cartilage repair device	Kensey Nash Corporation	Bilayered scaffold	NCT01183637	Randomized clinical trials
MaioRegen®	Fin-Ceramica Faenza Spa	Multilayered scaffold	NCT01282034	Randomized clinical trials
BST-CarGel	Piramal Healthcare Canada Ltd	Chitosan-based gel	NCT00314236	Randomized clinical Trials

of a chitosan-based gel in conjugation with autologous whole blood applied to a microfractured cartilage lesion results in better outcomes when compared to microfracture alone. BST-CarGel treatment for 12 months' time led to better site defect filling with good repair tissue quality than microfracture treatment alone. These tissue engineering polymer strategies along with orthobiologics might be the best candidates for future clinical trials.

57.10 Final Remarks and Future Directions

At present, orthobiologics can be seen as a tissue engineering strategy that is transforming the clinics, namely, the orthopedic field. The term includes the usage of a variety of autologous substances that allow regeneration and repair of tissue. Among these it is possible to include proteins, growth factors, antibodies, viscosupplements, and cell-based therapies. In the future, the treatment strategy should not rely solely on the single application of one component. More often, a combination of autologous substances is put together to restore tissue structure and function following damage. For example, in the treatment and prevention of OA progression, stem cell-based therapies are most appealing. MSCs isolated from knee infrapatellar fat pad and PRP have also been investigated as potential therapies for treatment of knee OA. Nevertheless, there are still some areas awaiting clarification such as dose, cell density, and redosage needs. And the orthobiologics field raises some controversial questions within medical community and in the industrial field. Apart from being regulated by different bodies in different countries which have dissimilar protocols, it was expected an industrial/economical growth in orthobiologics though we have not assisted to significant advances in the markets, in the last years. Some orthobiologics currently on the market such as Adequan™ and Orthokine™ were trialed in human patients even before becoming documented. This has resulted in a higher cost for the approved products.

Cell-based therapies have been strongly developed. Clinical trials had seen an increase in numbers of experiments due to the recent approval of autologous cell therapies. However, for a product to become commercially available, the vendor has to demonstrate the safe usage of cells with regard to handling the human sample, from harvesting to application in the body. Nowadays, cell-based therapies and orthobiologics are already approved in many countries. Genzyme Tissue Repair (presently Sanofi) in the USA has autologous chondrocytes cultured in defined media (Carticel™) commercially available on the market. In Europe, by means of arthroscopic biopsy, cells are collected from the patient and expanded (first surgery required) and later implanted in a debrided chondral defect underneath a periosteal or collagen membrane flap. The fibrin glue application is performed after membrane attachment (second surgery required). Also in Europe press-fit matrices impregnated with autologous cells, named matrix-induced autologous chondrocyte implantation (MACI), received approval for clinical usage. TiGenix™ was able to create screening algorithms for chondrocyte phenotype and behavior (ChrondroCelect™). The economic impact of clinical trials is enormous. Even a small clinical trial entails a cost of millions. As well as the new therapies, the traditional approaches have been improved. Arthroscopic microfracture is still under investigation due to the lower associated costs, and it requires only a single surgery. However, a better understanding of orthobiologics therapies to validate it is still needed as a clinical strategy.

Conclusion

Tissue engineering combined with orthobiologics could be the next generation of orthopedic approaches. Engineering a whole structure capable of mimicking different tissues (cartilage, subchondral bone, and interface) in an integrated manner could be a feasible approach to regenerate osteochondral defects. Biodegradable and natural polymers, such as HA or collagen, either injectable in situ or implantable, with a good choice of autologous stem cells and autologous GFs/PRP can be the future of orthopedic regenerative medicine. In other words, advanced strategies aiming to restore the lubrication properties of the injured/diseased articulation by means of different gels that mimic the native ECM for sustaining cell functions (e.g., stem cells) and PRP stabilization at the defect area will be widely used in the clinics. On the other hand, graded and hierarchic cells/scaffolds constructs are already being extensively investigated with the aim to mimic the natural tissue-to-tissue interface. However, several challenges still need to be overcome prior its application in the clinics. The perfect balance between scaffold degradation and neo-tissue formation by ECM deposition is a crucial parameter to obtain. Overall, the new tissue has to be capable of performing natural functions while maintaining the intrinsic tissue structure. The combination of all these components from the two big areas of tissue engineering and orthobiologics ends up in a complex device. Bearing in mind all the regulatory challenges and difficulties to be overcome to obtain FDA approval, these strategies are expected to reach the market within 5–10 years.

Acknowledgments The authors thank the funds provided by Portuguese Foundation for Science and Technology (FCT) through the project OsteoCart (PTDC/CTM-BPC/115977/2009), as well as the PhD scholarship provided to Diana R. Pereira (SFRH/BD/81356/2011/). The FCT distinction attributed to J. M. Oliveira under the Investigador FCT program (IF/00423/2012) is also greatly acknowledged. This work was also carried out with the support of Fundo Europeu de Desenvolvimento Regional (FEDER) through Programa Operacional do Norte through the project Articulate (Grant agreement n° 23189). We also acknowledge European Union's Seventh Framework Programme (FP7/2007-2013) under grant agreement n° REGPOT-CT2012-316331-POLARIS.

References

1. Bitton R. The economic burden of osteoarthritis. Am J Manag Care. 2009;15:S230–5.
2. Curl WW, Krome J, Gordon ES, Rushing J, Smith BP, Poehling GG. Cartilage injuries: a review of 31,516 knee arthroscopies. Arthroscopy. 1997;13:456–60.
3. Aroen A, Loken S, Heir S, Alvik E, Ekeland A, Granlund OG, Engebretsen L. Articular cartilage lesions in 993 consecutive knee arthroscopies. Am J Sports Med. 2004;32:211–5.
4. Upmeier H, Bruggenjurgen B, Weiler A, Flamme C, Laprell H, Willich SN. Follow-up costs up to 5 years after conventional treatments in patients with cartilage lesions of the knee. Knee Surg Sports Traumatol Arthrosc. 2007;15:249–57.
5. Evans CH, Ghivizzani SC, Robbins PD. Orthopedic gene therapy in 2008. Mol Ther. 2009;17:231–44.
6. Spahn G, Wolf J, Hofmann GO, Schiele R. Prevalence and distribution of knee cartilage lesions in sportspersons and non-sportspersons: results of a retrospective arthroscopic study. Sportverletz Sportschaden. 2013; 27:39–48.
7. Takeda H, Nakagawa T, Nakamura K, Engebretsen L. Prevention and management of knee osteoarthritis and knee cartilage injury in sports. Br J Sports Med. 2011;45:304–9.
8. Craig WDJ, Ming HZ. A current review on the biology and treatment of the articular cartilage defects (part I & part II). J Musculoskelet Res. 2003;7:157–81.
9. Falah M, Nierenberg G, Soudry M, Hayden M, Volpin G. Treatment of articular cartilage lesions of the knee. Int Orthop. 2010;34:621–30.
10. Perera JR, Gikas PD, Bentley G. The present state of treatments for articular cartilage defects in the knee. Ann R Coll Surg Engl. 2012;94:381–7.
11. Zengerink M, Struijs PA, Tol JL, van Dijk CN. Treatment of osteochondral lesions of the talus: a systematic review. Knee Surg Sports Traumatol Arthrosc. 2010;18:238–46.
12. Mandelbaum BR, Browne JE, Fu F, Micheli L, Mosely Jr JB, Erggelet C, Minas T, Peterson L.

Articular cartilage lesions of the knee. Am J Sports Med. 1998;26:853–61.
13. Mankin HJ. The response of articular cartilage to mechanical injury. J Bone Joint Surg Am. 1982;64: 460–6.
14. Julkunen P, Wilson W, Jurvelin JS, Rieppo J, Qu CJ, Lammi MJ, Korhonen RK. Stress-relaxation of human patellar articular cartilage in unconfined compression: prediction of mechanical response by tissue composition and structure. J Biomech. 2008;41:1978–86.
15. Minas T, Nehrer S. Current concepts in the treatment of articular cartilage defects. Orthopedics. 1997;20:525–38.
16. Gomoll AH, Madry H, Knutsen G, van Dijk N, Seil R, Brittberg M, Kon E. The subchondral bone in articular cartilage repair: current problems in the surgical management. Knee Surg Sports Traumatol Arthrosc. 2010;18:434–47.
17. Marlovits S, Striessnig G, Resinger CT, Aldrian SM, Vecsei V, Imhof H, Trattnig S. Definition of pertinent parameters for the evaluation of articular cartilage repair tissue with high-resolution magnetic resonance imaging. Eur J Radiol. 2004;52:310–9.
18. Mainil-Varlet P, Aigner T, Brittberg M, Bullough P, Hollander A, Hunziker E, Kandel R, Nehrer S, Pritzker K, Roberts S, Stauffer E, International Cartilage Repair S. Histological assessment of cartilage repair: a report by the Histology Endpoint Committee of the International Cartilage Repair Society (ICRS). J Bone Joint Surg Am. 2003;85-A(Suppl 2): 45–57.
19. Outerbridge RE. The etiology of chondromalacia patellae. J Bone Joint Surg Br. 1961;43-B:752–7.
20. Browne JE, Branch TP. Surgical alternatives for treatment of articular cartilage lesions. J Am Acad Orthop Surg. 2000;8:180–9.
21. Outerbridge RE. Further studies on the etiology of chondromalacia patellae. J Bone Joint Surg Br. 1964;46:179–90.
22. Siparsky P, Ryzewicz M, Peterson B, Bartz R. Arthroscopic treatment of osteoarthritis of the knee: are there any evidence-based indications? Clin Orthop Relat Res. 2007;455:107–12.
23. Spahn G, Kahl E, Muckley T, Hofmann GO, Klinger HM. Arthroscopic knee chondroplasty using a bipolar radiofrequency-based device compared to mechanical shaver: results of a prospective, randomized, controlled study. Knee Surg Sports Traumatol Arthrosc. 2008;16:565–73.
24. Pridie KH. A method of resurfacing osteoarthritic knee joint. J Bone Joint Surg Br. 1959;41-B:618–9.
25. Steadman JR, Rodkey WG, Rodrigo JJ. Microfracture: surgical technique and rehabilitation to treat chondral defects. Clin Orthop Relat Res. 2001:S362–9.
26. Steadman JR, Briggs KK, Rodrigo JJ, Kocher MS, Gill TJ, Rodkey WG. Outcomes of microfracture for traumatic chondral defects of the knee: average 11-year follow-up. Arthroscopy. 2003;19:477–84.
27. Hangody L, Fules P. Autologous osteochondral mosaicplasty for the treatment of full-thickness defects of weight-bearing joints: ten years of experimental and clinical experience. J Bone Joint Surg Am. 2003;85-A(Suppl 2):25–32.
28. Hangody L, Rathonyi GK, Duska Z, Vasarhelyi G, Fules P, Modis L. Autologous osteochondral mosaicplasty. Surgical technique. J Bone Joint Surg Am. 2004;86:65–72.
29. Ahmad CS, Cohen ZA, Levine WN, Ateshian GA, Mow VC. Biomechanical and topographic considerations for autologous osteochondral grafting in the knee. Am J Sports Med. 2001;29:201–6.
30. Reddy S, Pedowitz DI, Parekh SG, Sennett BJ, Okereke E. The morbidity associated with osteochondral harvest from asymptomatic knees for the treatment of osteochondral lesions of the talus. Am J Sports Med. 2007;35:80–5.
31. Valderrabano V, Leumann A, Rasch H, Egelhof T, Hintermann B, Pagenstert G. Knee-to-ankle mosaicplasty for the treatment of osteochondral lesions of the ankle joint. Am J Sports Med. 2009;37(Suppl 1): 105S–11S.
32. Espregueira-Mendes J, Pereira H, Sevivas N, Varanda P, da Silva MV, Monteiro A, Oliveira JM, Reis RL. Osteochondral transplantation using autografts from the upper tibio-fibular joint for the treatment of knee cartilage lesions. Knee Surg Sports Traumatol Arthrosc. 2012;20:1136–42.
33. Oliveira JM, Rodrigues MT, Silva SS, Malafaya PB, Gomes ME, Viegas CA, Dias IR, Azevedo JT, Mano JF, Reis RL. Novel hydroxyapatite/chitosan bilayered scaffold for osteochondral tissue-engineering applications: scaffold design and its performance when seeded with goat bone marrow stromal cells. Biomaterials. 2006;27:6123–37.
34. Lima EG, Mauck RL, Han SH, Park S, Ng KW, Ateshian GA, Hung CT. Functional tissue engineering of chondral and osteochondral constructs. Biorheology. 2004;41:577–90.
35. Brittberg M, Lindahl A, Nilsson A, Ohlsson C, Isaksson O, Peterson L. Treatment of deep cartilage defects in the knee with autologous chondrocyte transplantation. N Engl J Med. 1994;331:889–95.
36. Che JH, Zhang ZR, Li GZ, Tan WH, Bai XD, Qu FJ. Application of tissue-engineered cartilage with BMP-7 gene to repair knee joint cartilage injury in rabbits. Knee Surg Sports Traumatol Arthrosc. 2010;18:496–503.
37. Schaefer D, Martin I, Jundt G, Seidel J, Heberer M, Grodzinsky A, Bergin I, Vunjak-Novakovic G, Freed LE. Tissue-engineered composites for the repair of large osteochondral defects. Arthritis Rheum. 2002;46:2524–34.
38. Smith GD, Richardson JB, Brittberg M, Erggelet C, Verdonk R, Knutsen G, Ashton BA, Ashton IK, Harrison PE. Autologous chondrocyte implantation and osteochondral cylinder transplantation in cartilage repair of the knee joint. J Bone Joint Surg Am. 2003;85-A:2487–8.
39. Orth P, Kaul G, Cucchiarini M, Zurakowski D, Menger MD, Kohn D, Madry H. Transplanted articu-

lar chondrocytes co-overexpressing IGF-I and FGF-2 stimulate cartilage repair *in vivo*. Knee Surg Sports Traumatol Arthrosc. 2011;133:1295–301.
40. Filardo G, Kon E, Buda R, Timoncini A, Di Martino A, Cenacchi A, Fornasari PM, Giannini S, Marcacci M. Platelet-rich plasma intra-articular knee injections for the treatment of degenerative cartilage lesions and osteoarthritis. Knee Surg Sports Traumatol Arthrosc. 2011;19:528–35.
41. Temenoff JS, Mikos AG. Review: tissue engineering for regeneration of articular cartilage. Biomaterials. 2000;21:431–40.
42. Hunziker EB. Articular cartilage repair: problems and perspectives. Biorheology. 2000;37:163–4.
43. Pacifici M, Koyama E, Iwamoto M, Gentili C. Development of articular cartilage: what do we know about it and how .may it occur? Connect Tissue Res. 2000;41:175–84.
44. Radin EL, Rose RM. Role of subchondral bone in the initiation and progression of cartilage damage. Clin Orthop Relat Res. 1986;213:34–40.
45. Madry H, van Dijk CN, Mueller-Gerbl M. The basic science of the subchondral bone. Knee Surg Sports Traumatol Arthrosc. 2010;18:419–33.
46. Kawcak CE, McIlwraith CW, Norrdin RW, Park RD, James SP. The role of subchondral bone in joint disease: a review. Equine Vet J. 2001;33:120–6.
47. Aigner T, McKenna L. Molecular pathology and pathobiology of osteoarthritic cartilage. Cell Mol Life Sci. 2002;59:5–18.
48. Inklaar H. Soccer injuries II: aetiology and prevention. Sports Med. 1994;18:81–93.
49. Hoffman M, Payne VG. The effects of proprioceptive ankle disk training on healthy subjects. J Orthop Sports Phys Ther. 1995;21:90–3.
50. Barrett DS. Proprioception and function after anterior cruciate reconstruction. J Bone Joint Surg Br. 1991;73:833–7.
51. Feuerbach JW, Grabiner MD, Koh TJ, Weiker GG. Effect of an ankle orthosis and ankle ligament anesthesia on ankle joint proprioception. Am J Sports Med. 1994;22:223–9.
52. McGuine TA, Keene JS. The effect of a balance training program on the risk of ankle sprains in high school athletes. Am J Sports Med. 2006;34: 1103–11.
53. Ferrari M, Zia S, Valbonesi M, Henriquet F, Venere G, Spagnolo S, Grasso MA, Panzani I. A new technique for hemodilution, preparation of autologous platelet-rich plasma and intraoperative blood salvage in cardiac surgery. Int J Artif Organs. 1987;10:47–50.
54. Sampson S, Botto-van Bemden A, Aufiero D. Autologous bone marrow concentrate: review and application of a novel intra-articular orthobiologic for cartilage disease. Phys Sportsmed. 2013;41:7–18.
55. Myers KR. Trends in biological joint resurfacing. Bone Joint Res. 2013;2:193–9.
56. Mano JF, Silva GA, Azevedo HS, Malafaya PB, Sousa RA, Silva SS, Boesel LF, Oliveira JM, Santos TC, Marques AP, Neves NM, Reis RL. Natural origin biodegradable systems in tissue engineering and regenerative medicine: present status and some moving trends. J R Soc Interface. 2007;4:999–1030.
57. Collins MN, Birkinshaw C. Hyaluronic acid based scaffolds for tissue engineering – a review. Carbohydr Polym. 2013;92:1262–79.
58. Bonnet F, Dunham DG, Hardingham TE. Structure and interactions of cartilage proteoglycan binding region and link protein. Biochem J. 1979;228:77–85.
59. McArthur BA, Dy CJ, Fabricant PD, Valle AG. Long term safety, efficacy, and patient acceptability of hyaluronic acid injection in patients with painful osteoarthritis of the knee. Patient Prefer Adherence. 2012;6:905–10.
60. Stern R, Asari AA, Sugahara KN. Hyaluronan fragments: an information-rich system. Eur J Cell Biol. 2006;85:699–715.
61. Stern R, Kogan G, Jedrzejas MJ, Šoltés L. The many ways to cleave hyaluronan. Biotechnol Adv. 2007;25:537–57.
62. Toole BP. Hyaluronan in morphogenesis. Semin Cell Dev Biol. 2001;12:79–87.
63. Strauss EJ, Hart JA, Miller MD, Altman RD, Rosen JE. Hyaluronic acid viscosupplementation and osteoarthritis: current uses and future directions. Am J Sports Med. 2009;37:1636–44.
64. Toole BP. Hyaluronan: from extracellular glue to pericellular cue. Nat Rev Cancer. 2004;4:528–39.
65. Bollyky P, Bogdani M, Bollyky J, Hull R, Wight T. The role of hyaluronan and the extracellular matrix in islet inflammation and immune regulation. Curr Diab Rep. 2012;12:471–80.
66. Preston M, Sherman L. Neural stem cell niches: critical roles for the hyaluronan-based matrix in neural stem cell proliferation and differentiation. Front Biosci. 2011;3:1165–79.
67. Balazs EA, Denlinger JL. Viscosupplementation: a new concept in the treatment of osteoarthritis. J Rheumatol Suppl. 1993;39:3–9.
68. Moreland LW. Intra-articular hyaluronan (hyaluronic acid) and hylans for the treatment of osteoarthritis: mechanisms of action. Arthritis Res Ther. 2003;5:54–67.
69. Bannuru RR, Natov NS, Dasi UR, Schmid CH, McAlindon TE. Therapeutic trajectory following intra-articular hyaluronic acid injection in knee osteoarthritis – meta-analysis. Osteoarthr Cart. 2011;19:611–9.
70. Wang CT, Lin J, Chang CJ, Lin YT, Hou SM. Therapeutic effects of hyaluronic acid on osteoarthritis of the knee. A meta-analysis of randomized controlled trials. J Bone Joint Surg Am. 2004;86-a: 538–45.
71. Bellamy N, Campbell J, Robinson V, Gee T, Bourne R, Wells G. Viscosupplementation for the treatment of osteoarthritis of the knee. Cochrane Database Syst Rev. 2006;2:Cd005321.

72. Legre-Boyer V. Viscosupplementation: techniques, indications, results. Orthop Traumatol Surg Res. 2015;101:S101–s8.
73. Ayhan E, Kesmezacar H, Akgun I. Intraarticular injections (corticosteroid, hyaluronic acid, platelet rich plasma) for the knee osteoarthritis. World J Orthop. 2014;5:351–61.
74. Hakshur K, Benhar I, Bar-Ziv Y, Halperin N, Segal D, Eliaz N. The effect of hyaluronan injections into human knees on the number of bone and cartilage wear particles captured by bio-ferrography. Acta Biomater. 2011;7:848–57.
75. Kon E, Mandelbaum B, Buda R, Filardo G, Delcogliano M, Timoncini A, Fornasari PM, Giannini S, Marcacci M. Platelet-rich plasma intra-articular injection versus hyaluronic acid viscosupplementation as treatments for cartilage pathology: from early degeneration to osteoarthritis. Arthroscopy. 2011;27:1490–501.
76. Doral MN, Bilge O, Batmaz G, Donmez G, Turhan E, Demirel M, Atay OA, Uzumcugil A, Atesok K, Kaya D. Treatment of osteochondral lesions of the talus with microfracture technique and postoperative hyaluronan injection. Knee Surg Sports Traumatol Arthrosc. 2012;20:1398–403.
77. Buda R, Vannini F, Cavallo M, Baldassarri M, Natali S, Castagnini F, Giannini S. One-step bone marrow-derived cell transplantation in talarosteochondral lesions: mid-term results. Joints. 2013;1:102–7.
78. Giannini S, Buda R, Battaglia M, Cavallo M, Ruffilli A, Ramponi L, Pagliazzi G, Vannini F. One-step repair in talar osteochondral lesions: 4-year clinical results and T2-mapping capability in outcome prediction. Am J Sports Med. 2013;41: 511–8.
79. Wong KL, Lee KB, Tai BC, Law P, Lee EH, Hui JH. Injectable cultured bone marrow-derived mesenchymal stem cells in varus knees with cartilage defects undergoing high tibial osteotomy: a prospective, randomized controlled clinical trial with 2 years' follow-up. Arthroscopy. 2013;29:2020–8.
80. Mason LW, Wilson-Jones N, Williams P. The use of a cell-free chondroinductive implant in a child with massive cartilage loss of the talus after an open fracture dislocation of the ankle: a case report. J Pediatr Orthop. 2014;34:e58–62.
81. Civinini R, Macera A, Nistri L, Redl B, Innocenti M. The use of autologous blood-derived growth factors in bone regeneration. Clin Cases Miner Bone Metab. 2011;8:25–31.
82. Hall MP, Band PA, Meislin RJ, Jazrawi LM, Cardone DA. Platelet-rich plasma: current concepts and application in sports medicine. J Am Acad Orthop Surg. 2009;17:602–8.
83. Haleem AM, Singergy AA, Sabry D, Atta HM, Rashed LA, Chu CR, El Shewy MT, Azzam A, Abdel Aziz MT. The clinical use of human culture-expanded autologous bone marrow mesenchymal stem cells transplanted on platelet-rich fibrin glue in the treatment of articular cartilage defects: a pilot study and preliminary results. Cartilage. 2010;1: 253–61.
84. Li M, Zhang C, Ai Z, Yuan T, Feng Y, Jia W. Therapeutic effectiveness of intra-knee-articular injection of platelet-rich plasma on knee articular cartilage degeneration. Zhongguo Xiu Fu Chong Jian Wai Ke Za Zhi. 2011;25:1192–6.
85. Mei-Dan O, Carmont MR, Laver L, Mann G, Maffulli N, Nyska M. Platelet-rich plasma or hyaluronate in the management of osteochondral lesions of the talus. Am J Sports Med. 2012;40:534–41.
86. Hart R, Safi A, Komzak M, Jajtner P, Puskeiler M, Hartova P. Platelet-rich plasma in patients with tibiofemoral cartilage degeneration. Arch Orthop Trauma Surg. 2013;133:1295–301.
87. Eirale C, Mauri E, Hamilton B. Use of platelet rich plasma in an isolated complete medial collateral ligament lesion in a professional football (soccer) player: a case report. Asian J Sports Med. 2013;4: 158–62.
88. Laver L, Carmont MR, McConkey MO, Palmanovich E, Yaacobi E, Mann G, Nyska M, Kots E, Mei-Dan O. Plasma rich in growth factors (PRGF) as a treatment for high ankle sprain in elite athletes: a randomized control trial. Knee Surg Sports Traumatol Arthrosc. 2014;23:3383–92.
89. Andia I, Maffulli N. Platelet-rich plasma for managing pain and inflammation in osteoarthritis. Nat Rev Rheumatol. 2013;9:721–30.
90. Dohan Ehrenfest DM, Rasmusson L, Albrektsson T. Classification of platelet concentrates: from pure platelet-rich plasma (P-PRP) to leucocyte- and platelet-rich fibrin (L-PRF). Trends Biotechnol. 2009;27:158–67.
91. Engelhart L, Nelson L, Lewis S, Mordin M, Demuro-Mercon C, Uddin S, McLeod L, Cole B, Farr J. Validation of the knee injury and osteoarthritis outcome score subscales for patients with articular cartilage lesions of the knee. Am J Sports Med. 2012;40:2264–72.
92. Pittenger MF, Mackay AM, Beck SC, Jaiswal RK, Douglas R, Mosca JD, Moorman MA, Simonetti DW, Craig S, Marshak DR. Multilineage potential of adult human mesenchymal stem cells. Science. 1999;284:143–7.
93. da Silva ML, Caplan AI, Nardi NB. In search of the *in vivo* identity of mesenchymal stem cells. Stem Cells. 2008;26:2287–99.
94. Williams AR, Hare JM. Mesenchymal stem cells: biology, pathophysiology, translational findings, and therapeutic implications for cardiac disease. Circ Res. 2011;109:923–40.
95. Sakaguchi Y, Sekiya I, Yagishita K, Muneta T. Comparison of human stem cells derived from various mesenchymal tissues: superiority of synovium as a cell source. Arthritis Rheum. 2005;52:2521–9.
96. Friedenstein AJ, Gorskaja JF, Kulagina NN. Fibroblast precursors in normal and irradiated mouse hematopoietic organs. Exp Hematol. 1976;4:267–74.

97. Meirelles Lda S, Fontes AM, Covas DT, Caplan AI. Mechanisms involved in the therapeutic properties of mesenchymal stem cells. Cytokine Growth Factor Rev. 2009;20:419–27.
98. Bashir J, Sherman A, Lee H, Kaplan L, Hare JM. Mesenchymal stem cell therapies in the treatment of musculoskeletal diseases. PMR. 2014;6:61–9.
99. Kuroda R, Ishida K, Matsumoto T, Akisue T, Fujioka H, Mizuno K, Ohgushi H, Wakitani S, Kurosaka M. Treatment of a full-thickness articular cartilage defect in the femoral condyle of an athlete with autologous bone-marrow stromal cells. Osteoarthr Cart. 2007;15:226–31.
100. Wakitani S, Nawata M, Tensho K, Okabe T, Machida H, Ohgushi H. Repair of articular cartilage defects in the patello-femoral joint with autologous bone marrow mesenchymal cell transplantation: three case reports involving nine defects in five knees. J Tissue Eng Regen Med. 2007;1:74–9.
101. Buda R, Vannini F, Cavallo M, Grigolo B, Cenacchi A, Giannini S. Osteochondral lesions of the knee: a new one-step repair technique with bone-marrow-derived cells. J Bone Joint Surg Am. 2010;92(Suppl 2):2–11.
102. Buda R, Vannini F, Cavallo M, Baldassarri M, Luciani D, Mazzotti A, Pungetti C, Olivieri A, Giannini S. One-step arthroscopic technique for the treatment of osteochondral lesions of the knee with bone-marrow-derived cells: three years results. Musculoskelet Surg. 2013;97:145–51.
103. Giannini S, Buda R, Vannini F, Cavallo M, Grigolo B. One-step bone marrow-derived cell transplantation in talar osteochondral lesions. Clin Orthop Relat Res. 2009;467:3307–20.
104. Giannini S, Buda R, Cavallo M, Ruffilli A, Cenacchi A, Cavallo C, Vannini F. Cartilage repair evolution in post-traumatic osteochondral lesions of the talus: from open field autologous chondrocyte to bone-marrow-derived cells transplantation. Injury. 2010;41:1196–203.
105. Gobbi A, Karnatzikos G, Scotti C, Mahajan V, Mazzucco L, Grigolo B. One-step cartilage repair with bone marrow aspirate concentrated cells and collagen matrix in full-thickness knee cartilage lesions: results at 2-year follow-up. Cartilage. 2011;2:286–99.
106. Kasemkijwattana C, Hongeng S, Kesprayura S, Rungsinaporn V, Chaipinyo K, Chansiri K. Autologous bone marrow mesenchymal stem cells implantation for cartilage defects: two cases report. J Med Assoc Thai. 2011;94:395–400.
107. Nejadnik H, Hui JH, Feng Choong EP, Tai BC, Lee EH. Autologous bone marrow-derived mesenchymal stem cells versus autologous chondrocyte implantation: an observational cohort study. Am J Sports Med. 2010;38:1110–6.
108. Gigante A, Cecconi S, Calcagno S, Busilacchi A, Enea D. Arthroscopic knee cartilage repair with covered microfracture and bone marrow concentrate. Arthrosc Tech. 2012;1:e175–80.
109. Enea D, Cecconi S, Calcagno S, Busilacchi A, Manzotti S, Gigante A. One-step cartilage repair in the knee: collagen-covered microfracture and autologous bone marrow concentrate. A pilot study. Knee. 2015;22:30–5.
110. Enea D, Cecconi S, Calcagno S, Busilacchi A, Manzotti S, Kaps C, Gigante A. Single-stage cartilage repair in the knee with microfracture covered with a resorbable polymer-based matrix and autologous bone marrow concentrate. Knee. 2013;20:562–9.
111. Pak J. Regeneration of human bones in hip osteonecrosis and human cartilage in knee osteoarthritis with autologous adipose-tissue-derived stem cells: a case series. J Med Case Rep. 2011;5:296.
112. Khan WS, Tew SR, Adesida AB, Hardingham TE. Human infrapatellar fat pad-derived stem cells express the pericyte marker 3G5 and show enhanced chondrogenesis after expansion in fibroblast growth factor-2. Arthritis Res Ther. 2008;10:R74.
113. Teo BJ, Buhary K, Tai BC, Hui JH. Cell-based therapy improves function in adolescents and young adults with patellar osteochondritis dissecans. Clin Orthop Relat Res. 2013;471:1152–8.
114. Gigante A, Calcagno S, Cecconi S, Ramazzotti D, Manzotti S, Enea D. Use of collagen scaffold and autologous bone marrow concentrate as a one-step cartilage repair in the knee: histological results of second-look biopsies at 1 year follow-up. Int J Immunopathol Pharmacol. 2011;24:69–72.
115. Koh YG, Choi YJ. Infrapatellar fat pad-derived mesenchymal stem cell therapy for knee osteoarthritis. Knee. 2012;19:902–7.
116. Patrascu JM, Freymann U, Kaps C, Poenaru DV. Repair of a post-traumatic cartilage defect with a cell-free polymer-based cartilage implant: a follow-up at two years by MRI and histological review. J Bone Joint Surg Br. 2010;92:1160–3.
117. Siclari A, Mascaro G, Kaps C, Boux E. A 5-year follow-up after cartilage repair in the knee using a platelet-rich plasma-immersed polymer-based implant. Open Orthop J. 2014;8:346–54.
118. Kon E, Delcogliano M, Filardo G, Busacca M, Di Martino A, Marcacci M. Novel nano-composite multilayered biomaterial for osteochondral regeneration: a pilot clinical trial. Am J Sports Med. 2011;39:1180–90.
119. Crawford DC, DeBerardino TM, Williams 3rd RJ. NeoCart, an autologous cartilage tissue implant, compared with microfracture for treatment of distal femoral cartilage lesions: an FDA phase-II prospective, randomized clinical trial after two years. J Bone Joint Surg Am. 2012;94:979–89.
120. Vijayan S, Bartlett W, Bentley G, Carrington RW, Skinner JA, Pollock RC, Alorjani M, Briggs TW. Autologous chondrocyte implantation for osteochondral lesions in the knee using a bilayer collagen

membrane and bone graft: a two- to eight-year follow-up study. J Bone Joint Surg Br. 2012;94: 488–92.

121. Saw KY, Anz A, Siew-Yoke Jee C, Merican S, Ching-Soong Ng R, Roohi SA, Ragavanaidu K. Articular cartilage regeneration with autologous peripheral blood stem cells versus hyaluronic acid: a randomized controlled trial. Arthroscopy. 2013;29:684–94.

122. Turajane T, Chaweewannakorn U, Larbpaiboonpong V, Aojanepong J, Thitiset T, Honsawek S, Fongsarun J, Papadopoulos KI. Combination of intra-articular autologous activated peripheral blood stem cells with growth factor addition/ preservation and hyaluronic acid in conjunction with arthroscopic microdrilling mesenchymal cell stimulation Improves quality of life and regenerates articular cartilage in early osteoarthritic knee disease. J Med Assoc Thai. 2013;96:580–8.

123. Stanish WD, McCormack R, Forriol F, Mohtadi N, Pelet S, Desnoyers J, Restrepo A, Shive MS. Novel scaffold-based BST-CarGel treatment results in superior cartilage repair compared with microfracture in a randomized controlled trial. J Bone Joint Surg Am. 2013;95:1640–50.

"Biologic" Treatment for Meniscal Repair

58

Ibrahim Fatih Cengiz, J. Miguel Oliveira,
Mitsuo Ochi, Atsuo Nakamae, Nobuo Adachi,
and Rui Luís Reis

Contents

I.F. Cengiz • J.M. Oliveira (✉) • R.L. Reis
3B's Research Group – Biomaterials, Biodegradables and Biomimetics, University Minho, Headquarters of the European Institute of Excellence on Tissue Engineering and Regenerative Medicine, Avepark-Parque de Ciência e Tecnologia, Zona Industrial da Gandra, Barco, 4805-017 Guimarães, Portugal

ICVS/3B's – PT Government Associated Laboratory, Braga, Portugal
e-mail: miguel.oliveira@dep.uminho.pt

M. Ochi • A. Nakamae • N. Adachi
Department of Orthopaedic Surgery, Integrated Health Sciences, Institute of Biomedical & Health Sciences, Hiroshima University, Hiroshima, Japan

58.1 Introduction

The meniscus of the knee is involved in load distribution, joint stability, lubrication, and nutrition of the articular cartilage. A meniscus tear or meniscectomy is thought to decrease shock absorption and joint stability. It has been reported that meniscus injuries requiring resection increase the risk of cartilage loss, and about 50% of patients develop osteoarthritis 10–20 years after their meniscectomy [1]. Therefore, meniscal repair has recently strongly recommended for preventing further articular cartilage damage. Meniscal healing is greatly influenced by the peripheral vasculature of the meniscus. Meniscal tears in the avascular zone have very limited potential to heal because of a poor blood supply. Hence, despite recent progress in meniscal repair technique, indications for meniscal tear repair in the avascular area are still limited.

There have been many procedures for enhancing the meniscal healing process of the torn meniscus in the avascular area, such as synovial abrasion [2], marrow stimulation [3], synovial autograft [4, 5], and multiple trephination to induce a "vascular access channel" [6]. Biologics are biologically active natural components, which can promote tissue healing, including but not limited to fibrin clot, platelet-rich plasma (PRP), growth factors (GFs), cytokines, stem cells, and exosomes. Herein, we describe the clinical application technique of autologous bone

J. Espregueira-Mendes et al. (eds.), *Injuries and Health Problems in Football*,
DOI 10.1007/978-3-662-53924-8_58

marrow-derived fibrin clot for meniscal repair. In addition, it also addressed the progress in the tissue repair using PRP to provide further perspective for meniscal regeneration.

58.2 Autologous Bone Marrow-Derived Fibrin Clot: Application Technique

Application of an exogenous fibrin clot made from peripheral blood is one method to augment repair and promote meniscal healing [7–10]. The fibrin clot made from peripheral blood can supply GFs that promote cellular infiltration and healing and can act as a scaffold to promote healing of degenerative meniscal tears. After the defect is filled with the fibrin clot, the sutures for meniscal repair are tightened in a "sandwich fashion." We use an autologous fibrin clot derived from bone marrow instead of a fibrin clot made from peripheral blood, because the former contains more GFs than the latter.

58.2.1 Technical Note

Before preparing the autologous fibrin clot derived from bone marrow, arthroscopy was performed to observe the condition of the meniscus. The torn margin of the meniscus and adjacent synovium was abraded with a diamond rasp to improve the vascular supply to the torn meniscus. The meniscal repair was performed using the inside-out technique, outside-in technique, or all-inside technique, depending on the condition and position of the meniscal lesion. To prepare the fibrin clot, bone marrow aspirates (10–20 ml) were collected from the proximal tibia using an 18 G needle during surgery. The bone marrow aspirates were placed into a sterile glass beaker and then stirred with a sterile glass rod in a slow, repetitive fashion. The fibrin clot began to precipitate on the surface of the stick after 4–5 min. The fibrin clot was then placed onto a sterile gauze. A plastic cannula was introduced via the arthroscopic portal entry, and the prepared clot was inserted into the joint via the cannula with a grasper or a rongeur (Fig. 58.1). Finally, the fibrin clot was placed into the meniscus defect using a probe, after which it was secured by fastening the previously made sutures (Fig. 58.2).

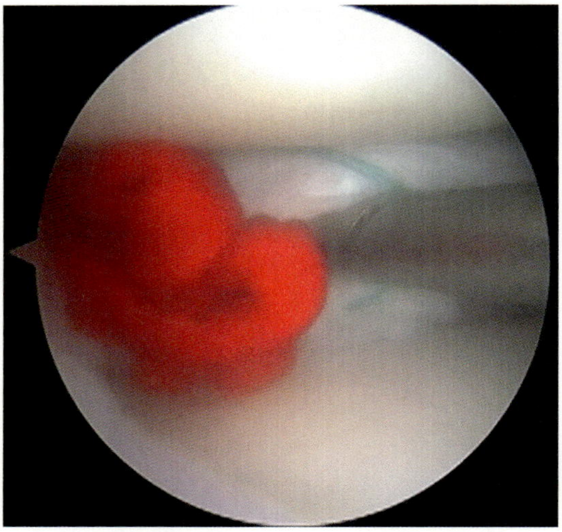

Fig. 58.1 A fibrin clot derived from bone marrow was inserted into the joint with a grasper

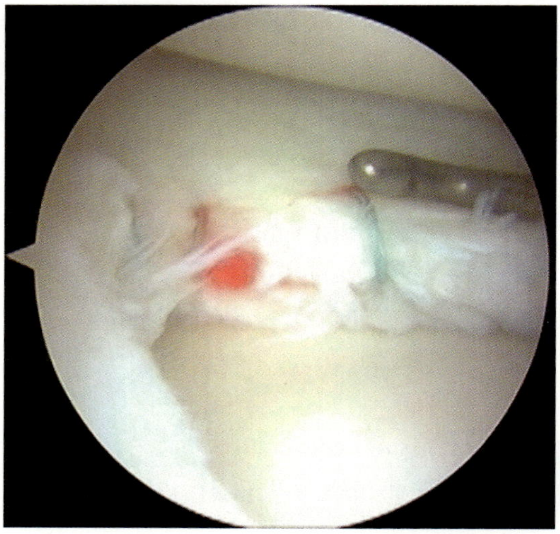

Fig. 58.2 The fibrin clot was placed into the defect in the meniscus and secured by fastening the sutures in a sandwich fashion

58.2.2 Fibrin Clot for Tissue Repair

The tissue engineering approach has been shown to have great potential for tissue regeneration and tissue repair. An autologous fibrin clot derived from peripheral blood has been used to accelerate meniscal healing for more than 20 years. In 1988, Arnoczky et al. [7] reported that a fibrin clot derived from peripheral blood improved meniscal healing in dog experiments. The fibrin clot is reported to be effective for tissue regeneration because of its biological characteristics [7–10]. It is known that the fibrin clot contains a variety of bioactive factors including several GFs and can act as a scaffold to fill the defect. In addition, the fibrin molecules of the fibrin clot serve both as storage and a release system for these bioactive factors. The major advantage of using a fibrin clot is the lack of allogenic or xenogeneic factors. Moreover, the plasticity of the prepared fibrin clot allows adaptation to various tissue topographies during implantation. The fibrin clot can be made easily in the operating theater at low cost.

For patients with meniscal tears in the avascular zone, we use an autologous fibrin clot derived from bone marrow instead of a fibrin clot made from peripheral blood. This is because we have confirmed that a bone marrow-derived fibrin clot contains more GFs such as vascular endothelial GF (VEGF), hepatocyte GF (HGF), and basic fibroblast GF (bFGF) than a peripheral blood-derived fibrin clot, and a bone marrow-derived fibrin clot has also been proven to have more potential for fibroblast proliferation than a peripheral blood-derived fibrin clot. This indicates the efficacy of a bone marrow-derived fibrin clot for tissue regeneration and clinical use (unpublished data). Our own unpublished preliminary results using a bone marrow-derived fibrin clot for meniscal repair have shown good clinical results at an average of 1 year postoperatively. Although further studies with longer-term follow-up are necessary to support a definitive conclusion, we believe that using a bone marrow-derived fibrin clot for meniscal repair is a reasonable and promising treatment option for patients with meniscal tears in the avascular zone.

58.3 Platelet-Rich Plasma (PRP)

GFs are polypeptides that have specific effects on the activity of target cell by binding to the specific receptors of the cell. The possible effects include a change in cell's gene expression, proliferation, differentiation, migration, and adhesion. These are all critical functions of cells, and employing GFs as biologics can provide positive outcomes. Platelets are small bodies, cytoplasmic fragments of megakaryocytes, without a nucleus that are found in the peripheral blood. PRP is an autologous plasma with a platelet concentration of 106 platelets per μl which is much higher than the baseline that is around 2 × 105 platelets per μl in a volume [11–13]. Platelets have vital roles in the wound healing with various proteins in the α granules [11, 14, 15]. PRP has been extensively studied for their potential therapeutic effect [16–19].

PRP is a critical source of native cytokines and GFs, as well as it contains other bioactive molecules, including but not limited to adhesive proteins (fibrin, fibronectin, and vitronectin), clotting factors, fibrinolytic factors, proteases, and antiproteases [20]. PDGF, TGF-β, FGF, IGF, VEGF, and EGF are among the GFs present in PRP [20]. Thus, use of PRP can provide increased potential to augment tissue healing [11–13]. PRP is intrinsically safe due to its autologous source, cannot cause mutation since PRP-derived GFs bind to the external surface of the cell membrane, and do not enter the cell or cell nucleus [13]. PRP is prepared from anticoagulated blood [21] and activated by clotting. Calcium chloride, thrombin, fibrin, and collagen type I are among the platelet-activating agents [22]. Platelets secrete most of the stored GFs for the first 10 min. Almost all of the stored GFs are secreted in the first hour. Then, the platelets produce more GFs for around 1 week [12, 13].

Since PRP is an autologous biologic, it is donor dependent, and there are differences due to different donors [23]. Moreover, different commercially available systems (e.g., from Biomet, Arthrex, Arteriocyte, Harvest Technologies, Medtronic, and MTF Sports Medicine) provide PRPs that are different in the number of platelet and blood cells [11, 22, 24, 25]. In a study [26], it was demonstrated that three different commercial systems provide different platelet, GF, white blood cell and red blood cell concentrations, and platelet capture efficiency. These are important source of variation in the application outcome.

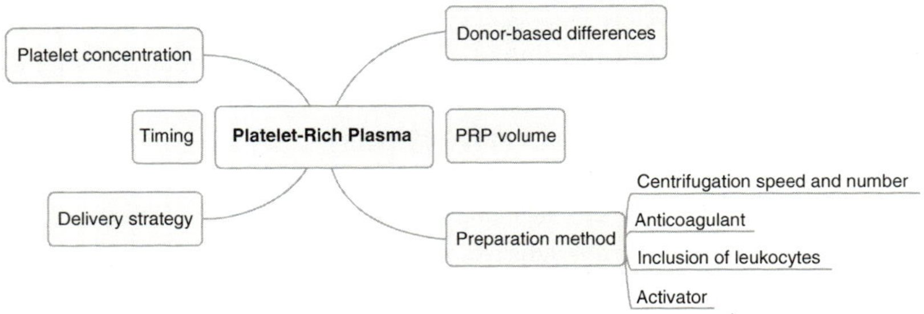

Fig. 58.3 The outcome of PRP applications is related to several factors including donor-based differences, timing and volume of PRP, platelet concentration, delivery strategy, and preparation method

Figure 58.3 illustrates the important factors affecting the outcomes of PRP application including donor-based differences, timing and volume of PRP, platelet concentration, delivery strategy, and preparation method.

The evaluation of the clinical biologic treatments can be done both with subjective outcomes and objective outcomes [27]. The clinical outcomes are the subjective including International Knee Documentation Committee (IKDC) score, Tegner Lysholm Knee Scale score, survey tools, visual analog scale, Victorian Institute of Sports Assessment, and Western Ontario and McMaster Universities osteoarthritis outcome (WOMAC) score, while the objective assessment can be done by histology, second-look arthroscopy, and medical imaging modalities, e.g., magnetic resonance imaging and ultrasound, and with the use of specific biomarkers for each GF or cytokine [27].

Effects of PRP release from collagen matrix on human meniscus cells in vitro were found to be that PRP was beneficial compared to peripheral blood to increase the growth and upregulate gene expression of collagen type I, elastin, and aggrecan [25]. The study suggested that PRP may provide a small benefit for minor meniscal defects if PRP can be accumulated. Another in vitro study showed that PRP treatment increases the 30-kDa fibronectin fragment-induced synthesis of a number of pro-inflammatory chemokines and matrix metalloproteinases by human meniscocytes and articular chondrocytes [28].

In a study with rabbit meniscocytes [29], the presence of PRP in the cell culture medium can promote cell proliferation and extracellular matrix synthesis. The mRNA expression of biglycan and decorin was upregulated while the expression of collagen type I remained the same when compared to that of with the meniscocytes cultured in medium with platelet-poor plasma or 1% fetal bovine serum. In the same study, in vivo effects of PRP were also investigated in a rabbit model. Full-thickness defects in the avascular region of meniscus showed histologically better repair at week 12 when the defects were filled with PRP incorporated in a hydrogel as compared to treatments with platelet-poor plasma incorporated in a hydrogel or hydrogel alone [29]. In a rabbit model for meniscus repair, it was reported that FGF-2 within a gelatin hydrogel significantly increased the cell proliferation and enhanced meniscal repair [30]. However, in another rabbit model study, PRP and BMP7, alone or together, did not significantly promote meniscus regeneration in avascular defects in vivo [31]. In a recent rabbit model study [32], horizontal medial meniscus tears were treated with a single injection of leukocyte-rich PRP and evaluated histologically up to 6 weeks. However, no significant differences were found between the PRP-treated group and the control group.

In a recent arthroscopic meniscus repair study [33], the differences between outcomes of the meniscus repair with and without PRP were reported to be indistinguishable in terms of functional outcome measures as well as the reoperation ratio and the proportion of patients who returned to their regular activities: sports and work. It was discussed that the study being underpowered and performed with a small sample size, a difference between groups with and without PRP augmentation, might not be detected [33].

The effects of PRP on the meniscal healing were studied in a case-control clinical study with young patients [34]. The injection of 5 ml of PRP directly into the lesion with horizontal cleavage meniscal tears following the standard open meniscal repair procedure was carried out. Clinical outcomes were reported at midterm follow-up to be only slightly improved by the in situ PRP injection [34]. In another study, one patient with a meniscal tear and knee pain was treated with percutaneous injections of a mixture of adipose tissue-derived stem cells, PRP, and hyaluronic acid (HA) and calcium chloride [35]. Even though there was no clinical improvement, the patient reported a significant decrease in pain only after injections.

PRP has been evaluated in vitro, in vivo, and clinically for other parts of the body other than meniscus, including but not limited to cartilage [36–38], rotator cuff [39–42], intervertebral disk [43–46], osteochondral tissue [36, 47, 48], muscle [49–51], ligament [52–54], and tendon [55–57]. The reported outcomes are very different and sometimes contradictory.

The effect of a combination of PRP and HA in osteoarthritis therapy was tested both in vitro and in vivo [58]. It was shown that osteoarthritis-related chemokines and cytokines can be suppressed, cartilage regeneration can be promoted, and an anti-inflammatory effect can be obtained [58]. PRP improved the patellar tendon harvest site healing in a randomized controlled trial [59]. A systematic review in 2012 [60] concluded that for the arthroscopic rotator cuff repair, PRP does not affect the retear rates or shoulder-specific outcomes. However, a systematic review in 2013 [61] analyzed the in vitro, preclinical, and clinical studies regarding the intra-articular injections of PRP. It was reported that PRP injection showed an overall benefit in preclinical studies for the healing of joint tissues, and among the high-quality clinical studies (only a few), PRP treatments showed only a benefit limited over time.

The systematic review and meta-analysis regarding the clinical benefit of PRP in orthopedics reported by Sheth et al. [62] revealed that the use of PRP is not significantly beneficial until 24 months across the randomized trials or prospective cohort studies. A small trend supporting the use of PRP exists but with wide confidence intervals. It was also reported that the literature lacks the standardization of study protocols, PRP preparations, and outcome measures [62, 63]. Nourissat et al. [64] also reported that there is no evidence-based medicine data that supports the use of PRP in arthroscopic surgery.

In an in vivo study with rabbits [65], circular defects were created with a punch in the avascular regions of menisci; the defects were treated with hyaluronic acid-collagen matrix either empty or with PRP or with mesenchymal stem cells. It was reported that cell-free treatments were not resulted with tissue healing. In a later study [66], the performance of mesenchymal stem cell-loaded scaffolds was tested in a longitudinal meniscal tear model. It was reported that for a successful avascular zone healing, stem-cell differentiation is a must; however, with the conditions in *the* study, the repair tissue was meniscus-like with a certain level of biomechanical strength. However, in the same study, treatments with PRP alone in the matrix did not provide any significant benefit [66]. It should be noted that PRP was not incorporated with cells in both studies [65, 66]. It would be interesting to see how PRP would affect the cells for the tissue healing. An in vivo study with mice [67] showed that PRP pretreatment of human articular chondrocyte-seeded scaffolds provides more cell attachment compared to ones without PRP pretreatment. It was concluded that PRP pretreatment may enhance the surface properties for cell attachment, and it can be used for meniscus tissue engineering [67].

Another use of PRP is to replace the fetal bovine serum (FBS) in cell culture [68]. It was demonstrated in an in vitro study that 10% or 20% PRP can be used instead of 10% FBS supplementation to standard cell culture medium to cultured human meniscocytes with same proliferation and gene expression level [68]. This makes it possible to avoid the clinical concerns regarding the use of FBS in cell culture medium.

58.4 Final Remarks

Fibrin clot derived from bone marrow or peripheral blood, as well as PRP can augment tissue healing. Fibrin clot and PRP contain a range of bioactive components including GFs. Fibrin clot does not have allogenic or xenogeneic factors, and its physical form fits to various tissue topographies during implantation. The clinical benefit of PRP is not yet agreed by all in the literature, and there are opposing views on the outcomes of PRP treatments; this might be due to the absence of standardization of the evaluation of the outcomes of the biological treatment studies, as well as the study designs. Due to the life-span of platelets and half-life of released GFs, the presence of GFs may not be sustained and controlled with a single PRP injection. Thus, PRP injections can be repeated on a regular basis, or their release can be controlled within a matrix/hydrogel. Besides, it is also required for a better understanding to quantify the amount of GFs released and also the duration of their biological activity. It should be also noted that GFs interact with cells and modulate cells' function. For this reason, it can be more beneficial if native and/or recruited cells need to be at the site where PRP is applied to interact with the released proteins from platelets. Additionally, for the proper evaluation of the PRP treatment, the study must be very well designed with all necessary sample groups, which was not present in some studies in the literature.

It should be also noted that the secretion of GFs is an important step. The GFs in the α granules of platelets are not complete unless they are soluble. During the GF secretion through the cell membrane, the GFs get completed by the inclusion of histone and carbohydrate side chains. Thus, no GFs will be secreted from platelets if platelets are damaged or died during the PRP preparation, and in such case, the outcome of using PRP will not be encouraging.

Acknowledgments I.F. Cengiz thanks the Portuguese Foundation for Science and Technology (FCT) for the Ph.D. scholarship (SFRH/BD/99555/2014). J. M. Oliveira also thanks the FCT for the funds provided to under the program Investigador FCT 2012 (IF/00423/2012).

References

1. Lohmander LS, Englund PM, Dahl LL, Roos EM. The long-term consequence of anterior cruciate ligament and meniscus injuries osteoarthritis. Am J Sports Med. 2007;35:1756–69.
2. Tetik O, Kocabey Y, Johnson DL. Synovial abrasion for isolated, partial thickness, undersurface, medial meniscus tears. Orthopedics. 2002;25:675.
3. Freedman KB, Nho SJ, Cole BJ. Marrow stimulating technique to augment meniscus repair. Arthroscopy. 2003;19:794–8.
4. Jitsuiki J, Ochi M, Ikuta Y. Meniscal repair enhanced by an interpositional free synovial autograft: an experimental study in rabbits. Arthroscopy. 1994;10:659–66.
5. Ochi M, Mochizuki Y, Deie M, Ikuta Y. Augmented meniscal healing with free synovial autografts: an organ culture model. Arch Orthop Trauma Surg. 1996;115:123–6.
6. Zhang Z, Arnold JA, Williams T, McCann B. Repairs by trephination and suturing of longitudinal injuries in the avascular area of the meniscus in goats. Am J Sports Med. 1995;23:35–41.
7. Arnoczky SP, Warren RF, Spivak J. Meniscal repair using an exogenous fibrin clot. An experimental study in dogs. J Bone Joint Surg Am. 1988;70:1209–17.
8. Henning CE, Lynch MA, Yearout KM, Vequist SW, Stallbaumer RJ, Decker KA. Arthroscopic meniscal repair using an exogenous fibrin clot. Clin Orthop Relat Res. 1990;252:64–72.
9. Kamimura T, Kimura M. Repair of horizontal meniscal cleavage tears with exogenous fibrin clots. Knee Surg Sports Traumatol Arthrosc. 2011;19:1154–7.
10. Ra HJ, Ha JK, Jang SH, Lee DW, Kim JG. Arthroscopic inside-out repair of complete radial tears of the meniscus with a fibrin clot. Knee Surg Sports Traumatol Arthrosc. 2013;21:2126–30.
11. Everts PA, Knape JT, Weibrich G, Schonberger J, Hoffmann J, Overdevest EP, Box HA, van Zundert A. Platelet-rich plasma and platelet gel: a review. J Extra Corpor Technol. 2006;38:174.
12. Marx RE. Platelet-rich plasma (PRP): what is PRP and what is not PRP? Implant Dent. 2001;10:225–8.
13. Marx RE. Platelet-rich plasma: evidence to support its use. J Oral Maxillofac Surg. 2004;62:489–96.
14. Pietrzak WS, Eppley BL. Platelet rich plasma: biology and new technology. J Craniofac Surg. 2005;16:1043–54.
15. Szpaderska AM, Egozi EI, Gamelli RL, DiPietro LA. The effect of thrombocytopenia on dermal wound healing. J Invest Dermatol. 2003;120:1130–7.
16. Ahmad Z, Howard D, Brooks RA, Wardale J, Henson FM, Getgood A, Rushton N. The role of platelet rich plasma in musculoskeletal science. JRSM Short Rep. 2012;3:40.
17. Braun HJ, Wasterlain AS, Dragoo JL. The use of PRP in ligament and meniscal healing. Sports Med Arthrosc. 2013;21:206–12.
18. Lopez-Vidriero E, Goulding KA, Simon DA, Sanchez M, Johnson DH. The use of platelet-rich plasma in arthroscopy and sports medicine: optimizing the healing environment. Arthroscopy. 2010;26:269–78.
19. Zhu Y, Yuan M, Meng H, Wang A, Guo Q, Wang Y, Peng J. Basic science and clinical application of platelet-rich plasma for cartilage defects and osteoarthritis: a review. Osteoarthr Cartil. 2013;21:1627–37.
20. Foster TE, Puskas BL, Mandelbaum BR, Gerhardt MB, Rodeo SA. Platelet-rich plasma from basic

science to clinical applications. Am J Sports Med. 2009;37:2259–72.
21. Araki J, Jona M, Eto H, Aoi N, Kato H, Suga H, Doi K, Yatomi Y, Yoshimura K. Optimized preparation method of platelet-concentrated plasma and noncoagulating platelet-derived factor concentrates: maximization of platelet concentration and removal of fibrinogen. Tissue Eng Part C Methods. 2011;18:176–85.
22. Taylor SA, Rodeo SA. Augmentation techniques for isolated meniscal tears. Curr Rev Muscoskelet Med. 2013;6:95–101.
23. Fréchette J-P, Martineau I, Gagnon G. Platelet-rich plasmas: growth factor content and roles in wound healing. J Dent Res. 2005;84:434–9.
24. Demange MK, de Almeida AM, Rodeo SA. Updates in biological therapies for knee injuries: tendons. Curr Rev Muscoskelet Med. 2014;7:239–46.
25. Howard D, Shepherd JH, Kew SJ, Hernandez P, Ghose S, Wardale JA, Rushton N. Release of growth factors from a reinforced collagen GAG matrix supplemented with platelet rich plasma: influence on cultured human meniscal cells. J Orthop Res. 2014;32: 273–8.
26. Castillo TN, Pouliot MA, Kim HJ, Dragoo JL. Comparison of growth factor and platelet concentration from commercial platelet-rich plasma separation systems. Am J Sports Med. 2011;39:266–71.
27. LaPrade CM, James EW, LaPrade RF, Engebretsen L. How should we evaluate outcomes for use of biologics in the knee? J Knee Surg. 2015;28:35–44.
28. Wang C-C, Lee C-H, Peng Y-J, Salter DM, Lee H-S. Platelet-rich plasma attenuates 30-kDa fibronectin fragment–induced chemokine and matrix metalloproteinase expression by meniscocytes and articular chondrocytes. Am J Sports Med. 2015;43:2481–9.
29. Ishida K, Kuroda R, Miwa M, Tabata Y, Hokugo A, Kawamoto T, Sasaki K, Doita M, Kurosaka M. The regenerative effects of platelet-rich plasma on meniscal cells in vitro and its in vivo application with biodegradable gelatin hydrogel. Tissue Eng. 2007;13:1103–12.
30. Narita A, Takahara M, Sato D, Ogino T, Fukushima S, Kimura Y, Tabata Y. Biodegradable gelatin hydrogels incorporating fibroblast growth factor 2 promote healing of horizontal tears in rabbit meniscus. Arthroscopy. 2012;28:255–63.
31. Zellner J, Taeger CD, Schaffer M, Roldan JC, Loibl M, Mueller MB, Berner A, Krutsch W, Huber MK, Kujat R. Are applied growth factors able to mimic the positive effects of mesenchymal stem cells on the regeneration of meniscus in the avascular zone? Biomed Res Int. 2014; doi: 10.1155/2014/537686.
32. Shin KH, Lee H, Kang S, Ko Y-J, Lee S-Y, Park J-H, Bae J-H. Effect of leukocyte-rich and platelet-rich plasma on healing of a horizontal medial meniscus tear in a rabbit model. Biomed Res Int. 2015; doi: 10.1155/2015/179756.
33. Griffin JW, Hadeed MM, Werner BC, Diduch DR, Carson EW, Miller MD. Platelet-rich plasma in meniscal repair: does augmentation improve surgical outcomes? Clin Orthop Relat Res. 2015;473:1665–72.
34. Pujol N, De Chou ES, Boisrenoult P, Beaufils P. Platelet-rich plasma for open meniscal repair in young patients: any benefit? Knee Surg Sports Traumatol Arthrosc. 2015;23:51–8.
35. Pak J, Lee JH, Lee SH. Regenerative repair of damaged meniscus with autologous adipose tissue-derived stem cells. Biomed Res Int. 2014; doi: 10.1155/2014/436029.
36. Milano G, Passino ES, Deriu L, Careddu G, Manunta L, Manunta A, Saccomanno MF, Fabbriciani C. The effect of platelet rich plasma combined with microfractures on the treatment of chondral defects: an experimental study in a sheep model. Osteoarthr Cartil. 2010;18:971–80.
37. Siclari A, Mascaro G, Gentili C, Cancedda R, Boux E. A cell-free scaffold-based cartilage repair provides improved function hyaline-like repair at one year. Clin Orthop Relat Res. 2012;470:910–9.
38. Spreafico A, Chellini F, Frediani B, Bernardini G, Niccolini S, Serchi T, Collodel G, Paffetti A, Fossombroni V, Galeazzi M. Biochemical investigation of the effects of human platelet releasates on human articular chondrocytes. J Cell Biochem. 2009;108:1153–65.
39. Beck J, Evans D, Tonino PM, Yong S, Callaci JJ. The biomechanical and histologic effects of platelet-rich plasma on rat rotator cuff repairs. Am J Sports Med. 2012;40:2037–44.
40. Gumina S, Campagna V, Ferrazza G, Giannicola G, Fratalocchi F, Milani A, Postacchini F. Use of platelet-leukocyte membrane in arthroscopic repair of large rotator cuff tears. J Bone Joint Surg Am. 2012;94: 1345–52.
41. Jo CH, Kim JE, Yoon KS, Shin S. Platelet-rich plasma stimulates cell proliferation and enhances matrix gene expression and synthesis in tenocytes from human rotator cuff tendons with degenerative tears. Am J Sports Med. 2012;40:1035–45.
42. Jo CH, Shin JS, Lee YG, Shin WH, Kim H, Lee SY, Yoon KS, Shin S. Platelet-rich plasma for arthroscopic repair of large to massive rotator cuff tears a randomized, single-blind, parallel-group trial. Am J Sports Med. 2013;41(10):2240–8.
43. Chen WH, Lo WC, Lee JJ, Su CH, Lin CT, Liu HY, Lin TW, Lin WC, Huang TY, Deng WP. Tissue-engineered intervertebral disc and chondrogenesis using human nucleus pulposus regulated through TGF-β1 in platelet-rich plasma. J Cell Physiol. 2006;209:744–54.
44. Chen W-H, Liu H-Y, Lo W-C, Wu S-C, Chi C-H, Chang H-Y, Hsiao S-H, Wu C-H, Chiu W-T, Chen B-J. Intervertebral disc regeneration in an ex vivo culture system using mesenchymal stem cells and platelet-rich plasma. Biomaterials. 2009;30:5523–33.
45. Gullung GB, Woodall JW, Tucci MA, James J, Black DA, McGuire RA. Platelet-rich plasma effects on degenerative disc disease: analysis of histology and imaging in an animal model. Evid Based Spine Care J. 2011;2:13.
46. Obata S, Akeda K, Imanishi T, Masuda K, Bae W, Morimoto R, Asanuma Y, Kasai Y, Uchida A, Sudo A.

Effect of autologous platelet-rich plasma-releasate on intervertebral disc degeneration in the rabbit anular puncture model: a preclinical study. Arthritis Res Ther. 2012;14:R241.
47. Mei-Dan O, Carmont MR, Laver L, Mann G, Maffulli N, Nyska M. Platelet-rich plasma or hyaluronate in the management of osteochondral lesions of the talus. Am J Sports Med. 2012;40:534–41.
48. Sun Y, Feng Y, Zhang C, Chen S, Cheng X. The regenerative effect of platelet-rich plasma on healing in large osteochondral defects. Int Orthop. 2010;34:589–97.
49. Borrione P, Grasso L, Racca S, Abbadessa G, Carriero V, Fagnani F, Quaranta F, Pigozzi F. Systemic effects of locally injected platelet rich plasma in a rat model: an analysis on muscle and bloodstream. J Biol Regul Homeost Agents. 2014;29:251–8.
50. Hammond JW, Hinton RY, Curl LA, Muriel JM, Lovering RM. Use of autologous platelet-rich plasma to treat muscle strain injuries. Am J Sports Med. 2009;37:1135–42.
51. Quarteiro ML, Tognini JRF, de Oliveira ELF, Silveira I. The effect of platelet-rich plasma on the repair of muscle injuries in rats. Rev Bras Ortop. 2015;50:586–95.
52. Murray MM, Spindler KP, Abreu E, Muller JA, Nedder A, Kelly M, Frino J, Zurakowski D, Valenza M, Snyder BD. Collagen-platelet rich plasma hydrogel enhances primary repair of the porcine anterior cruciate ligament. J Orthop Res. 2007;25:81–91.
53. Radice F, Yanez R, Gutiérrez V, Rosales J, Pinedo M, Coda S. Comparison of magnetic resonance imaging findings in anterior cruciate ligament grafts with and without autologous platelet-derived growth factors. Arthroscopy. 2010;26:50–7.
54. Silva A, Sampaio R. Anatomic ACL reconstruction: does the platelet-rich plasma accelerate tendon healing? Knee Surg Sports Traumatol Arthrosc. 2009;17:676–82.
55. Kajikawa Y, Morihara T, Sakamoto H, Matsuda K, Oshima Y, Yoshida A, Nagae M, Arai Y, Kawata M, Kubo T. Platelet-rich plasma enhances the initial mobilization of circulation-derived cells for tendon healing. J Cell Physiol. 2008;215:837–45.
56. Sampson S, Aufiero D, Meng M, Bledin A, Gillette T, Zall M. Platelet-rich plasma therapy as a first-line treatment for severe Achilles tendon tear: a case report. Int J Ther Rehabil. 2011;18:101.
57. Sánchez M, Anitua E, Azofra J, Andía I, Padilla S, Mujika I. Comparison of surgically repaired Achilles tendon tears using platelet-rich fibrin matrices. Am J Sports Med. 2007;35:245–51.
58. Chen W-H, Lo W-C, Hsu W-C, Wei H-J, Liu H-Y, Lee C-H, Chen S-YT, Shieh Y-H, Williams DF, Deng W-P. Synergistic anabolic actions of hyaluronic acid and platelet-rich plasma on cartilage regeneration in osteoarthritis therapy. Biomaterials. 2014;35:9599–607.
59. de Almeida AM, Demange MK, Sobrado MF, Rodrigues MB, Pedrinelli A, Hernandez AJ. Patellar tendon healing with platelet-rich plasma: a prospective randomized controlled trial. Am J Sports Med. 2012;40:1282–8.
60. Chahal J, Van Thiel GS, Mall N, Heard W, Bach BR, Cole BJ, Nicholson GP, Verma NN, Whelan DB, Romeo AA. The role of platelet-rich plasma in arthroscopic rotator cuff repair: a systematic review with quantitative synthesis. Arthroscopy. 2012;28:1718–27.
61. Filardo G, Kon E, Roffi A, Di Matteo B, Merli M, Marcacci M. Platelet-rich plasma: why intra-articular? A systematic review of preclinical studies and clinical evidence on PRP for joint degeneration. Knee Surg Sports Traumatol Arthrosc. 2015;23:2459–74.
62. Sheth U, Simunovic N, Klein G, Fu F, Einhorn TA, Schemitsch E, Ayeni OR, Bhandari M. Efficacy of autologous platelet-rich plasma use for orthopaedic indications: a meta-analysis. J Bone Joint Surg Am. 2012;94:298–307.
63. Metcalf KB, Mandelbaum BR, McIlwraith CW. Application of platelet-rich plasma to disorders of the knee joint. Cartilage. 2013;4:295–312.
64. Nourissat G, Mainard D, Kelberine F, SFA FAS. Current concept for the use of PRP in arthroscopic surgery. Orthop Traumatol Surg Res. 2013;99:S407–S10.
65. Zellner J, Mueller M, Berner A, Dienstknecht T, Kujat R, Nerlich M, Hennemann B, Koller M, Prantl L, Angele M. Role of mesenchymal stem cells in tissue engineering of meniscus. J Biomed Mater Res A. 2010;94:1150–61.
66. Zellner J, Hierl K, Mueller M, Pfeifer C, Berner A, Dienstknecht T, Krutsch W, Geis S, Gehmert S, Kujat R. Stem cell-based tissue-engineering for treatment of meniscal tears in the avascular zone. J Biomed Mater Res B. 2013;101:1133–42.
67. Kwak HS, Nam J, Lee J, Kim HJ, Yoo JJ. Meniscal repair in vivo using human chondrocyte-seeded PLGA mesh scaffold pretreated with platelet-rich plasma. J Tissue Eng Regen Med. 2014; doi: 10.1002/term.1938.
68. Gonzales VK, de Mulder EL, de Boer T, Hannink G, van Tienen TG, van Heerde WL, Buma P. Platelet-rich plasma can replace fetal bovine serum in human meniscus cell cultures. Tissue Eng Part C Methods. 2013;19:892–9.

Index

J. Espregueira-Mendes et al. (eds.), *Injuries and Health Problems in Football*,
DOI 10.1007/978-3-662-53924-8

T

Printed by Printforce, the Netherlands